Pediatric Nursing Procedures

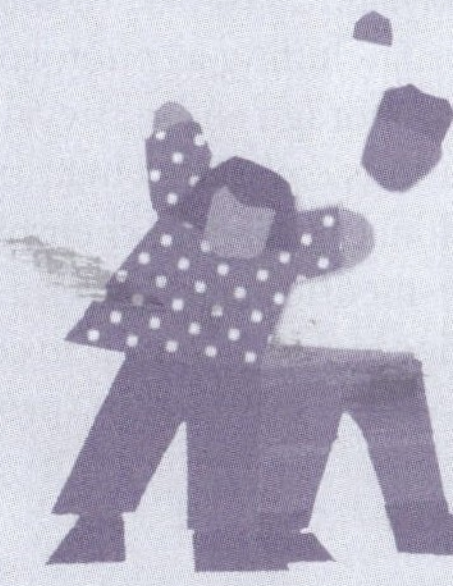

Second Edition

Vicky R. Bowden, DNSc, RN
Professor
Azusa Pacific University
Azusa, CA

Cindy Smith Greenberg, DNSc, RN, CPNP
Associate Professor
California State University, Fullerton
Fullerton, CA

Wolters Kluwer | Lippincott Williams & Wilkins
Health
Philadelphia • Baltimore • New York • London
Buenos Aires • Hong Kong • Sydney • Tokyo

Senior Acquisitions Editor: Elizabeth Nieginski
Senior Development Editor: Danielle DiPalma
Development Editor: Mackenzie Lawrence
Senior Production Editor: Debra Schiff
Director of Nursing Production: Helen Ewan
Senior Managing Editor/Production: Erika Kors
Design Coordinator: Joan Wendt
Manufacturing Manager: Karin Duffield
Indexer: Kathy Pitcoff
Compositor: Circle Graphics
Printer: Quebecor World

2nd Edition

9 8 7 6 5 4 3 2 1

ISBN: 0-7817-6682-6
ISBN: 978-0-7817-6682-1

LWW.com

To Greg, Christian and Matthew,
You make my life full and complete. Thank you for your encouragement and shared joy to see this book come to fruition.

VRB

To Jay, Erin, Jordan and Daniel,
You fill my life with laughter and remind me of what's really important. Thank you for your patience.
To my parents Barbara and William, for providing a strong foundation and always being there for me.
To Frankie and Bobbie, your memories are always in my heart.

CSG

Contributors

Diane T. Asbill, BSN, RN, IBCLC
Lactation Consultant
NC Women's and Children's Hospitals–UNC Hospitals
Chapel Hill, NC

Chapter 22: Breast Milk: Handling and Storage of Expressed Human Milk

Connie S. Austin, MSN, MAEd, CNS, RN
Dean of Health Sciences
Rio Hondo College
Whittier, CA

Chapter 52: Infection Control and Standard Precautions
Chapter 101: Range-of-Motion Exercises

Joyce S. Baker, MS, RN, PNP
Patient Service Leader
State University of New York, Upstate Medical University
Syracuse, NY

Chapter 8: Abdominal Girth
Chapter 100: Pulse Oximetry

Sharon Bauer, RN
Nurse Manager
Inpatient Pediatric Hematology Oncology (7H)
State University of New York, Upstate Medical University
Syracuse, NY

Chapter 8: Abdominal Girth
Chapter 100: Pulse Oximetry

Jan Bazner-Chandler, MSN, CNS, RN, CPNP
Assistant Professor
Azusa Pacific University
Azusa, CA

Chapter 25: Cast Care
Chapter 107: Skeletal Pin Site Care
Chapter 114: Traction Care

Nancy Blake, RN, MN, CCRN, CNAA
Director, PCS Critical Care Services
Children's Hospital of Los Angeles
Los Angeles, CA

Chapter 35: Disaster Preparedness and Response

Vicky Bowden, RN, DNSc
Professor, School of Nursing
Director of the Honors Program
Azusa Pacific University
Azusa, CA

Chapter 1: Principles of Family-Centered Care
Chapter 2: Growth and Development Milestones
Chapter 3: Teaching Children and Their Families
Chapter 4: Promoting Coping During Hospitalization
Chapter 33: Developmental Care of the Neonate
Chapter 36: Ear Irrigation
Chapter 37: Enemas
Chapter 81: Oral Care
Chapter 108: Stool Collection and Analysis
Chapter 110: Toys: Distribution, Cleaning, and Storage
Chapter 116: Urinary Catheterization: Insertion and Removal of Indwelling Catheter
Chapter 117: Urinary Catheterization: Management of Indwelling Catheter
Chapter 118: Urinary Catheterization: Self-Intermittent Catheterization
Chapter 119: Urine Collection: 24-Hour Specimen
Chapter 120: Urine Collection: Clean Catch (Midstream)
Chapter 121: Urine Collection: Indwelling Catheter
Chapter 122: Urine Collection: Routine Voided Urine Specimen
Chapter 123: Urine Collection: Straight Catheter
Chapter 124: Urine Collection: Suprapubic Aspiration

Margaret A. Brady, PhD, RN, CPNP
Director of School Nurse Credential Program and Co-director PNP Program
Azusa Pacific University
Azusa, CA

Chapter 5: Principles of Fluid and Nutritional Management
Chapter 6: Principles of Pharmacologic Management

Michelle A. Dart, RN, PNP, CDE
Summit Pediatrics
Auburn, NY

Chapter 19: Blood Glucose Monitoring

Natalie S. Deporto, CNS, PNP
Certified Asthma Educator (A-CE)
Newport Children's Medical Group
Newport Beach, CA

Chapter 9: Admission of the Child
Chapter 115: Transition Management: Discharging and Transferring the Child
Chapter 88: Pet Therapy

Trudy Dody, MS, FNP, APRN, RN, C-SPI
Upstate New York Poison Center
Syracuse, NY

Chapter 92: Poison Management

Lili Dubrow, RN
Associate Nurse
Children's Hospital of Orange County
Orange, CA

Chapter 21: Bone Marrow Aspiration

Viann Duncan, MSN, APRN, BC
Director of Admissions, Retention, and Scholarship
Lead Instructor–PsyChapter Mental Health
Azusa Pacific University
Azusa, CA

Chapter 85: Patient Identification
Chapter 102: Restraint and Seclusion
Chapter 129: Visitor Identification and Management

Dana M. Etzel-Hardman, BSN, RN, CPN
Training and Education Specialist
Children's Hospital of Pittsburgh
Pittsburgh, PA

Chapter 62: Medication Administration: Endotracheal
Chapter 63: Medication Administration: Enteral
Chapter 64: Medication Administration: Intramuscular
Chapter 65: Medication Administration: Intraosseous
Chapter 66: Medication Administration: Intravenous
Chapter 68: Medication Administration: Nasal
Chapter 69: Medication Administration: Ophthalmic
Chapter 70: Medication Administration: Oral
Chapter 71: Medication Administration: Otic
Chapter 72: Medication Administration: Rectal

Joy Ganley, RN
Clinical Systems Nurse Analyst
State University of New York, Upstate Medical University
Syracuse, NY

Chapter 12: Aerosol Treatments
Chapter 83: Oxygen Administration

Cindy Smith Greenberg, DNSc, RN, CPNP
Associate Professor
Coordinator, Undergraduate Program
California State University, Fullerton
Fullerton, CA

Chapter 7: Principles of Pain Management
Chapter 73: Medication Administration: Subcutaneous
Chapter 74: Medication Administration: Sublingual and Buccal
Chapter 75: Medication Administration: Topical
Chapter 132: Vital Signs: Pain Assessment

Carol Hafeman, MA, RN, ET
Nurse Coordinator
Children's Mercy Hospital
Kansas City, MO

Chapter 82: Ostomy Care
Chapter 136: Wound Care

Patricia Frohock Hanes, PhD(c), RN, MSN, MAEd
Assistant Professor
Azusa Pacific University
Azusa, CA

Chapter 15: Bed and Crib Choices
Chapter 98: Procedures: General Guidelines
Chapter 103: Safety Measures

Anna Marie Hefner, MSN, RN, CPNP
Associate Professor
Azusa Pacific University
Azusa, CA

Chapter 14: Bathing the Infant
Chapter 31: Circumcision Care
Chapter 34: Diapering
Chapter 40: Exchange Transfusions
Chapter 43: Feeding, Infant: Breast-Feeding and Formula-Feeding

Mary Elizabeth Hensley, MSN, RN
Clinical Nurse Specialist
St. Jude Children's Research Hospital
Stem Cell Transplant Unit
Memphis, TN
Chapter 26: Chemotherapy: Administration and Safe Handling
Chapter 27: Chemotherapy: Management of Extravasation

Ami Herberg, RN
Charge Nurse
Pediatric Intensive Care Unit
Children's Hospital of Orange County
Orange, CA
Chapter 10: Admission of the Child to the Intensive Care Unit
Chapter 20: Blood Product Administration
Chapter 55: Intravascular Therapy: Peripheral Catheters
Chapter 57: Intravascular Therapy: Totally Implantable Devices
Chapter 58: Intravascular Therapy: Tunneled Catheters
Chapter 59: Intubation
Chapter 125: Ventilators: High Frequency
Chapter 126: Ventilators: Mechanical

Diane Hudson-Barr, PhD, RN
Clinical Nurse Specialist, Newborn Critical Care Center
University of North Carolina Hospitals
Chapel Hill, NC
Chapter 90: Phototherapy
Chapter 135: Warming Devices, Use of

Dale June, BSN, RN, CPON
Staff Nurse, Chemotherapy and Biotherapy Administration
St. Jude Children's Research Hospital
Memphis, TN
Chapter 26: Chemotherapy: Administration and Safe Handling
Chapter 27: Chemotherapy: Management of Extravasation

Sara Komrowski, BSN, RN
Staff Nurse
State University of New York, Upstate Medical University
Syracuse, NY
Chapter 13: Apnea Monitors

Diane Kwaczala, RN, CNA, BC
Nurse Manager
State University of New York, Upstate Medical University
Syracuse, NY
Chapter 12: Aerosol Treatments
Chapter 83: Oxygen Administration

Michelle Santos Laabs, MSN, RN, FNP
School Nurse
Orange Unified School District
Orange, CA
Chapter 45: Hearing Screening
Chapter 95: Postural Screening
Chapter 128: Vision Screening

Debra E. Lewis, MSN, RN, CPN
Instructor
Duquesne University
Pittsburgh, PA
Education Specialist
Children's Hospital of Pittsburgh
Pittsburgh, PA
Chapter 62: Medication Administration: Endotracheal
Chapter 63: Medication Administration: Enteral
Chapter 64: Medication Administration: Intramuscular
Chapter 65: Medication Administration: Intraosseous
Chapter 66: Medication Administration: Intravenous
Chapter 68: Medication Administration: Nasal
Chapter 69: Medication Administration: Ophthalmic
Chapter 70: Medication Administration: Oral
Chapter 71: Medication Administration: Otic
Chapter 72: Medication Administration: Rectal

Mary E. MacBlane, MS, RN, PNP
Pediatric Nurse Practitioner
Neurodevelopmental Pediatrics
State University of New York, Upstate Medical University
Syracuse, NY
Chapter 28: Chest Physiotherapy
Chapter 44: Growth Parameter Assessment
Chapter 51: Incentive Spirometry

Karen A. Manning, MSN, RN, CPNP
School Nurse
Newport-Mesa Unified School District
Costa Mesa, CA
Chapter 86: Peak Flowmeters and Spacers, Use and Care of
Chapter 99: Prostheses and Orthoses

Corrine Maurins, BSN, RNC
Registered Nurse
Mary Bridge Children's Hospital and Health Center
Tacoma, WA

Chapter 38: Enteral Tubes Placement and Management: Gastrostomy, PEG, Skin-Level Devices, and Jejunostomy
Chapter 39: Enteral Tubes: Naso/Orogastric Placement and Management and Nasojejunal Management
Chapter 42: Feeding, Enteral

Catherine McCoy-Hill, MSN, RN, CCRN, CNS, ANP-C
Assistant Professor, School of Nursing
Azusa Pacific University
Azusa, CA

Chapter 46: Hemodynamic Monitoring: Central Venous Pressure
Chapter 47: Hemodynamic Monitoring: Insertion and Setup
Chapter 48: Hemodynamic Monitoring: Intraarterial Pressure
Chapter 67: Medication Administration: Intravenous Cardiovascular

Rosemary McLaughlin, MSN, RNC
Associate Professor
Union University
Jackson, TN

Chapter 16: Blood Drawing From Peripheral Sites: Heel Stick and Finger Stick
Chapter 17: Blood Drawing From Peripheral Sites: Venipuncture
Chapter 18: Blood Gas Sampling and Monitoring

Cathy McPhee, MSN, RN, NP
Instructor
Azusa Pacific University
Azusa, CA

Chapter 111: Tracheostomy: Stoma Care and Management
Chapter 112: Tracheostomy: Suctioning
Chapter 113: Tracheostomy: Tube Change

Suzan Miller-Hoover, MS, RN, CCNS
Clinical Nurse Specialist
Banner Children's Hospital at Banner Desert Medical Center
Mesa, AZ

Chapter 32: Cooling Measures, Use of
Chapter 41: Fall Prevention
Chapter 93: Postanesthesia Care
Chapter 94: Postmortem Care
Chapter 96: Potassium Infusion, Administration of
Chapter 97: Preoperative Care

Nancy P. Mitchell, MS, APRN, BC
Pediatric Nurse Practitioner
State University of New York, Upstate Medical University
Syracuse, NY

Chapter 30: Child Abuse Reporting and Documentation

Maureen T. O'Hara, MS, APRN, BC
Pediatric Nurse Practitioner
University Pediatric and Adolescent Center
State University of New York, Upstate Medical University
Syracuse, NY

Chapter 30: Child Abuse Reporting and Documentation

Nancy E. Page, MS, APRN, BC
Patient Safety Officer
Golisano Children's Hospital
State University of New York, Upstate Medical University
Syracuse, NY

Chapter 29: Chest Tubes
Chapter 76: Nasotracheal Suctioning

Lisa Philichi, MN, RN, CPNP
Pediatric Nurse Practitioner
Mary Bridge Children's Hospital Gastroenterology Clinic
Tacoma, WA

Chapter 60: Latex Precautions
Chapter 89: pH Study

Renee Pozza, PhD(c) RN, CNS, FNP
Associate Dean, Curriculum and Clinical Practice
Associate Professor
Azusa Pacific University
Azusa, CA

Chapter 49: Heparin Lock/Flush
Chapter 84: Parenteral Nutrition and Intravenous Fat Emulsion Infusion
Chapter 104: Saline Lock/Flush
Chapter 105: Sedation

Leigh D. Rabideaux, MSN, RN, CPNP
Nurse Practitioner
Children's Hospital of Orange County
Orange, CA

Chapter 24: Cardiopulmonary Resuscitation

Elaine M. Rutkowski, MSN, RN, CNS
Lecturer
California State University, Fullerton
Fullerton, CA

Chapter 130: Vital Signs: Blood Pressure

Chapter 131: Vital Signs: Heart Rate

Chapter 133: Vital Signs: Respiratory Rate

Chapter 134: Vital Signs: Temperature

Kathleen Saunders, MSN, RN, CNS
Pediatric Clinical Nurse Specialist
University of California, Irvine Medical Center
Orange, CA

Chapter 56: Intravascular Therapy: Peripherally Inserted Central Catheters

Kristin Schweizer, BSN, RN
Registered Nurse
State University of New York, Upstate Medical University
Syracuse, NY

Chapter 106: Seizure Precautions

Angela Scott, MNSc, RN, APRN, BC
Pediatric Clinical Nurse Specialist
Arkansas Children's Hospital
Little Rock, AR

Chapter 11: Advance Directives

Chapter 50: Immunizations

Chapter 53: Informed Consent

Chapter 54: Intracranial Pressure Monitoring: Assisting in Placement and Care of

Chapter 61: Lumbar Puncture

Chapter 77: Neurologic Assessment

Chapter 91: Pneumogram: Two- or Four-Channel

Chapter 127: Ventriculostomy Drain, Assisting in Placement and Care of

Pensri Smithedajkul, MSN, PNP, CNS, CCRN
Pediatric Nurse Practitioner
Pediatrics and Neonatology Medical Group of Orange County, Inc.
Santa Ana, CA

Chapter 78: Newborn Care: Immediate Needs of the Stable Newborn

Chapter 79: Newborn Care: Maintaining a Thermal Neutral Environment

Chapter 80: Newborn Care: Newborn Screening

Nicole Pando Vicioso, MSN, RN, CNS
PICU Clinical Nurse Specialist
Children's Hospital of Orange County
Orange, CA

Chapter 23: Cardiopulmonary Monitoring

Jeanne Ware, MSN, RN, FNP, WOCN
State University of New York, Upstate Medical University
Syracuse, NY

Chapter 109: Suture/Staple Removal

Rita Weinheimer, BSN
Pediatrics
State University of New York, Upstate Medical University
Syracuse, NY

Chapter 87: Pediculosis and Scabies Management

Maria-Danielle White, BSN, RN
Charge Nurse
State University of New York, Upstate Medical University
Syracuse, New York

Chapter 8: Abdominal Girth

Chapter 100: Pulse Oximetry

Reviewers

Imad Alhusami, RN
Muscat, Oman

Linda Alwine, MSN, RN
Spartanburg, South Carolina

Cheri Barber, MSN, CRNP
Coordinator, Pediatric Nurse Practitioner Program; President, NAPNAP Del/Val Chapter, Jefferson School of Nursing, Jefferson College of Health Professions, Thomas Jefferson University
Philadelphia, Pennsylvania

Anne Bisch, MSN, BSN, BS, RN
Pediatric Nurse Practitioner, Surgical Services, St. Louis Children's Hospital
St. Louis, Missouri

Mary Bjorklund, MSN, RN, CPN
Assistant Professor Nursing, Kingwood College
Kingwood, Texas

Ronald Bolan, BSN, RN, CFRN, CCRN, CEN, NREMT-P
Durham, North Carolina

Susan Bonnell, RN
Instructor, University of San Diego
San Diego, California

Anne Borgmeyer, MSN, RN, CPNP
Pediatric Nurse Practitioner, Certified Asthma Instructor, St. Louis Children's Hospital
St. Louis, Missouri

Charlotte Braaten, BSN, RN
Travel Nurse for PPR; Home Health Nurse for Oxford
Long Beach, California

Michelle Buell, MSN-CNS, RN
Instructor, Victor Valley College
Victorville, California

Virginia Carreira, MSN, RN, CCRN, CDE
Family Nurse Practitioner, Long Branch SBYSP
Long Branch, New Jersey

Rey Casas, RN
Ryerson University
Toronto, Ontario, Canada

Marcella Donkin, MSN, RN, CPNP, CCRN
Pediatric Nurse Practitioner, Pediatric Intensive Services, St. Louis Children's Hospital
St. Louis, Missouri

Debbie Donovan, MSN, BSN, CPNP
Pediatric Nurse Practitioner
Howell, New Jersey

Juanita D'Souza, BSN, RN, CCRN
Princeton, New Jersey

Susan Finn, MSN, BSN, Post-master PNP
Advanced Practice Nurse, Certified Pediatric Nurse Practitioner, Loyola University
Chicago, Illinois

Patti Gyr, MSN, RN, CPNP
Pediatric Nurse Practitioner, St. Louis Children's Hospital
St. Louis, Missouri

Cathy Haut, MS, CPNP, CCRN
Pediatric Nurse Practitioner, Acute Care; Instructor, University of Maryland School of Nursing
Baltimore, Maryland

Marie Heiligenstein, RN, CPNP
School Nurse, Madison Metropolitan School District
Madison, Wisconsin

Lisa Henry, APRN, PNP, BC
Pediatric Nurse Practitioner, Asthma Intervention Model Project, St. Louis Children's Hospital
St. Louis, Missouri

Janet Hickman, EdD, RN
Professor of Nursing and Interim Dean, Graduate Studies and Extended Education, West Chester University
West Chester, Pennsylvania

Janet Ihlenfeld, PhD, RN
Professor of Nursing, D'Youville College
Buffalo, New York

Megan Infanti, MSN, RN
Instructor, West Chester University
West Chester, Pennsylvania

Kathy Irwin, RN,C, BSN
Staff Nurse, Clinical Level III, Certified in Child and Adolescent Nursing
Springfield, Pennsylvania

Betsy Joyce, EdD, MSN, CPNP
Associate Professor Emeritus, Indiana University School of Nursing
Indianapolis, Indiana

Wren Kennedy, MSN, RN
Pediatric Nurse Practitioner in Oncology
Memphis, Tennessee

Kathleen Kreutzer, BSN, RN
Patient Care Supervisor, Pediatrics, North Suburban Medical Center
Commerce City, Colorado

Jumie Lee, RN, MSN, CPNP
Rancho Palos Verdes, California

Kristina Leppala, RN
Vantaa, Finland

Dominique Leveque, MSN, BSN, PNP
Adjunct Faculty, Indiana University School of Nursing, Indiana University and Purdue University in Indianapolis
Indianapolis, Indiana

Jamie Manley, BSN, CPN, RN
Otterbein College
Columbus, Ohio

Helen MacRonald, MS, BSN, RN
Lead Nurse for Children with Special Needs, Barts and the London NHS Trust
London, United Kingdom

Florence Miller, MSN, MPH, RN, CNS
Clinical Nurse Specialist, Pediatric Medical/Surgical Unit, Stroger Hospital
Oak Park, Illinois

Kolleen Miller-Rosser, MSN, EN, RN, Graduate Diploma (Pediatrics)
Education Coordinator, King Faisal Hospital
Riyadh, Saudi Arabia

Lynn Mohr, RN
Advocate Hope Children's Hospital
Oak Lawn, Illinois

Mary Musholt, MSN, RN, C-PNP
Nurse Consultant, UW Madison School of Nursing; Preceptor, UW Madison School of Nursing
Madison, Wisconsin

Sara Myers, BSN, RN
Western University
Mt. Albert, Ontario, Canada

Susan Parme, MSN, RN
San Diego, California

Beth Richardson, DNS, RN, CPNP
Associate Professor and Coordinator of the Pediatric Nurse Practitioner Program
Indiana University School of Nursing
Indianapolis, Indiana

Donna Ruedisueli, BSN, RN
Clinical Nurse Manager, Pediatrics/Pediatric Intensive Care, Medical University of Ohio
Toledo, Ohio

Pam Rutar, MSN, BSN, RN
CNE with the NLN; Associate Professor, Firelands Regional Medical Center School of Nursing
Sandusky, Ohio

Lori Salabad, MSN, RN, CPNP
Adjunct Faculty, Valencia Community College
Orlando, Florida

Tracy Snyder, RN
Clark State Community College
Enon, Ohio

Nancy Travis, MS, RNC, CPN, CLD, CLE, CPD
Director Women and Children's Services, The Children's Hospital of Southwest Florida
Cape Coral, Florida

Shelia Tucker, RN
Mission Hospitals
Weaverville, North Carolina

Pat Turbett, RN
Pediatric Staff Nurse, Atlantic-Cape May County Community College
Cape May Court House, New Jersey

Tracey Wagner, RN
Pediatric Nurse Educator, Fletcher Allen Healthcare, Vermont Children's Hospital
Burlington, Vermont

Julee Waldrop, MSN, BSN, BA Ed, RN
Clinical Associate Professor, School of Nursing and School of Medicine, University of North Carolina
Chapel Hill, North Carolina

Karen Wilkinson, MN, RN, ARNP
Northwest University Buntain School of Nursing
Kirkland, Washington

Preface

Our goal in compiling the second edition of the text has been to continue to provide an evidence-based text to be a clinical resource for the pediatric nurse. Since the 2003 publication of the first edition, we have been amazed and encouraged by the increased efforts of nurses and other healthcare professionals to document their standards of practice and seek national and international standardization of the practices based on best evidence.

This text is unique in that procedural skills/tasks are not adapted for children; rather, we have started with the child and his or her family as the focus of care, and demonstrate how in each contact with the child a particular procedure should be completed to ensure the intervention is developmentally appropriate for the unique needs of that child. This text is specifically designed to provide the student or the professional nurse with a quick reference of essential nursing procedures and guidelines for practice to utilize when working with the pediatric patient. The content format can be easily adapted by nurse professionals for use in organizational policy and procedure manuals.

The text is divided into two units. *Unit I, Caring for Children: Special Considerations in Healthcare*, is comprised of seven chapters that lay down foundational principles for the provision of nursing care to children and their families. Principles of family-centered care are reviewed. Growth and developmental milestones are presented and discussed as they impact teaching children and their families and providing opportunities for therapeutic play. In Unit I, considerations that are unique or important to the care of children are discussed as they impact fluid and nutritional interventions, pharmacologic interventions and pain management.

Unit II, Pediatric Guidelines and Procedures, is comprised of 129 chapters, each addressing a nursing intervention commonly performed when caring for the pediatric patient. To provide ready access to information, chapters have the following features:

- Chapters are presented in alphabetical order and given short titles that directly refer the reader to a specific procedure.
- Chapters open with **Clinical Guidelines,** bulleted points that indicate "who" can perform the procedure; "under what conditions" the procedure should be performed, and "how often." These represent the minimum safety guidelines which must be maintained to implement this procedure.
- The **Equipment** list summarizes the standard equipment needed to perform the procedure, and which should be gathered together before the procedure is performed.
- The **Child and Family Assessment and Preparation** section presents information regarding assessment of the patient prior to performance of the procedure. Developmental issues appropriate to the child's age group are included, if indicated. Concerns related to safety by developmental age, fear, mobility, comfort, and self-image are considered. Discussion includes acquiring child/family assent/consent prior to performing the procedure.
- The **Procedure** section contains the process of "how to do." It includes actions and rationale and cross-referencing to other related documents as indicated. Rationales for steps in the procedure have been thoroughly investigated, and, where possible, represent published professional standards or research presented in the literature.
- The **Child and Family Evaluation and Documentation** section notes the "how, when, and where" nursing documentation is required and describes the ongoing evaluation needed to monitor the child during and after the procedure.
- Instructions regarding how the child and caregiver would implement or modify the procedure to be completed in the home, school, or other community setting are presented in the **Community Care** section.
- **Unexpected Situations** provide a brief scenario of an unanticipated situation and the actions the nurse should implement before, during, or after the procedure.
- **References** represent the most current evidence available at publication. In a number of cases, the evidence base for a procedure has been well established in the past and no new research added to this knowledge base; thus, the literature cited reflects citations upon which the evidence for practice has been established regardless of the year in which that base was established. Some procedures do not have as strong an evidence base and would benefit from further study.

Within each chapter several pedagologic features have been included to further highlight key aspects of each procedure:

KidKare • **The KidKare icon** points out psychosocial implications for the care of the pediatric client.

caREminder • **The caREminder icon** emphasizes the main points of the procedure.

• **The Alert icon** highlight high-risk issues that may occur during a procedure.

The appendices at the end of the text provide the reader quick and easy reference to charts summarizing pediatric norms for vital signs and a list of Internet references to gain easy access to such documents as pediatric growth charts and immunization schedules.

We are certain this second edition will continue to serve as an evidence-based resource to provide consistency in the delivery of healthcare to children. We encourage you to use this resource to ensure that your clinical skills are current and based on principles that are consistent with the existing evidence, and national guidelines and standards. We also encourage you to use this text to provide family-centered care that truly focuses on the unique needs of the pediatric client.

Vicky R. Bowden
Cindy Smith Greenberg

Acknowledgments

Completing the second edition of this text has been an enjoyable journey as we once again worked with some very talented colleagues. We are thankful for the ongoing photographic contributions of Rick Williams and his willingness to show up at any time to get the right picture. We continue to be blessed with a group of clinical experts who serve as chapter contributors and resource consultants. To all of you, thanks for your work and for bringing a national perspective to the pediatric clinical practice issues presented in the text. We also had our "unofficial" advisory board. These are the colleagues that we kept coming back to over and over again to help us deliberate clinical practice issues whose evidence was unclear or conflicting in the literature. Special thanks to Margaret Brady, PhD, RN, CPNP; Linda Tirabassi, MN, RN, CPNP; Robin Koeppel, MS, RN, CPNP; Marsha Orr, MS, RN; and Kathy Saunders, MSN, RN.

Lastly, we want to thank the talented team from Lippincott Williams & Wilkins. Mackenzie Lawrence has been the most organized and efficient developmental editor we have ever had the privilege to work with on a project. Danielle DiPalma has been invaluable in guiding the direction of this book and its features, gently prodding and encouraging all of our work with Lippincott. We are grateful for her vision and commitment to our work. We appreciate the work of Debra Schiff and her production team as they brought to life our electronic documents. We owe our partnership with LWW to Elizabeth Nieginski, Senior Acquisitions Editor. She saw the potential; she had the energy, wisdom, and skills to make it happen; and she has made the completion of this text an enjoyable journey among respected friends and colleagues.

Contents

UNIT I

Caring for Children: Special Considerations in Healthcare

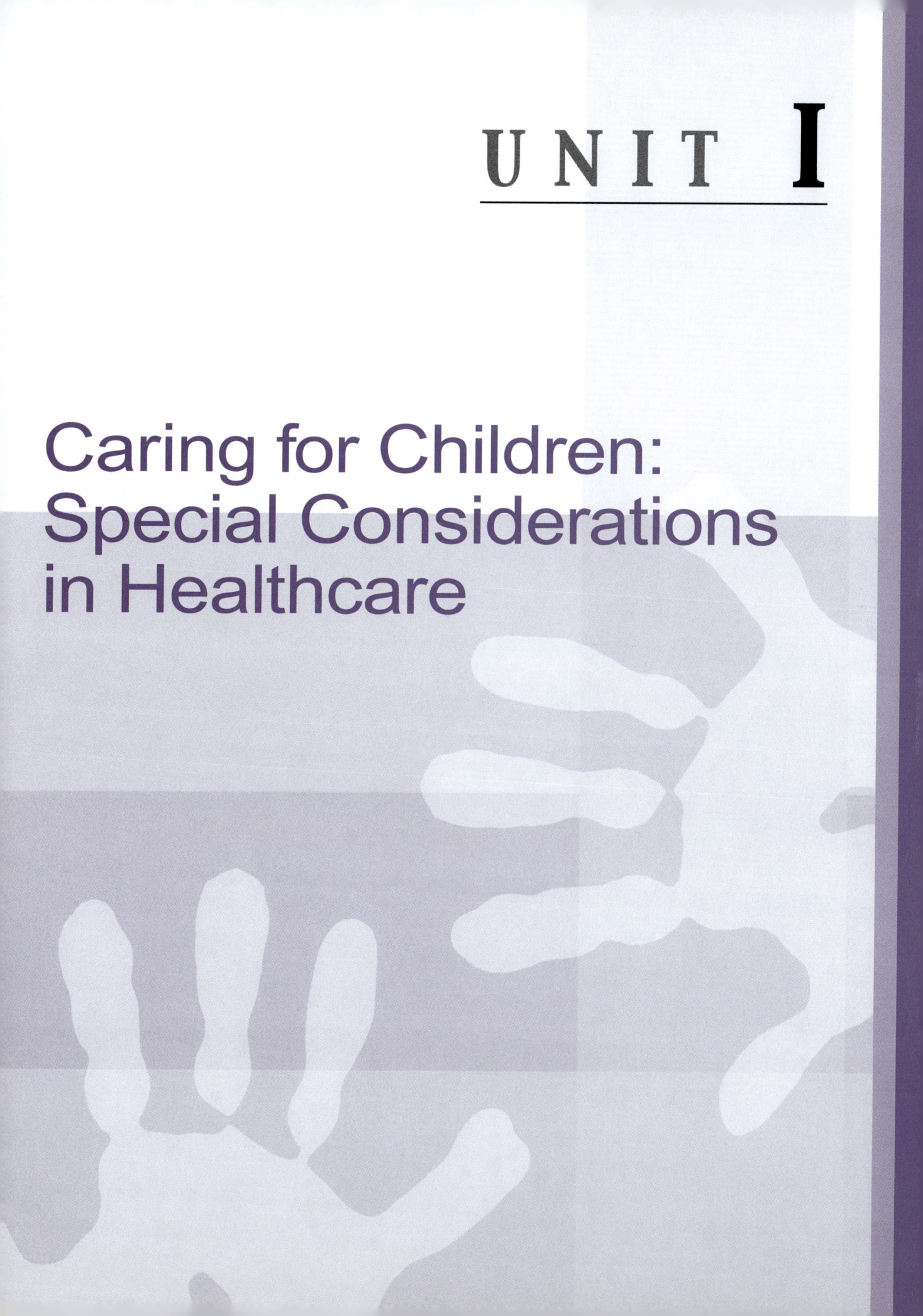

CHAPTER

1

Principles of Family-Centered Care

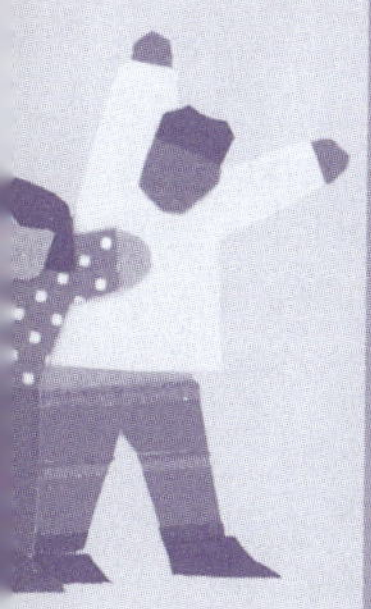

FAMILY-CENTERED CARE

Family-centered care is a philosophy of care that acknowledges the importance of the family unit as the fundamental focus of all healthcare interventions (Chart 1-1). This model of care recognizes the *collaborative* relationship between the family and the professional care provider in the pursuit of being responsive to the priorities and needs of families when they seek healthcare (Leviton, Mueller, & Kauffman, 1992; MacKean, Thurston, & Scott, 2005). This model recognizes that the family is an advocate for their child's care and that the child's voice is an essential component of the decision-making process.

ELEMENTS OF FAMILY-CENTERED CARE

Family-centered care is best understood by extracting and explaining the elements or components of this philosophy of care that work together to move an individual or an institution toward providing a family-centered approach (Chart 1-2). Each of these eight elements serves to reinforce, facilitate, and complement the implementation of the others. In pediatric healthcare, the elements of family-centered care recognize each family's uniqueness, acknowledge the influence of the family as a constant in the child's life, and emphasize the importance of providing services that demonstrate the value of collaboration between the healthcare provider, the child, and the family. Family-centered care is based on the premise that a positive adjustment to a child's level of health and well-being requires the involvement of the whole family (Shelton & Stepanek, 1994). A guide to family-centered care was published, titled *Family-Centered Care: Putting It Into Action* (Lewandowski & Tesler, 2003). This handbook provides an evidenced-based approach toward recommendations for implementing eight elements of family-centered care

FAMILY-CENTERED CARE INTERVENTIONS AND STRATEGIES

Family-centered care is a philosophy of care that must be translated into action. The relevance to the child and the family goes unnoticed unless active measures are taken to ensure that family-centered practices are integrated into every aspect of the healthcare arena. From legislation supporting family-centered practices to an interdisciplinary team focused on the needs of the entire family, the elements of family-centered care can be operationalized via a variety of unique strategies (Chart 1-3). These family-centered strategies need to continue to be

CHART 1-1 DEFINITIONS OF FAMILY-CENTERED CARE

A philosophy, a way of approaching a family rather than a set of procedures (Atkinson, 1976).

A philosophy of care based on the belief that all families are deeply caring and want to nurture their child (Edelman, 1991).

Viewing the family not as a collection of individuals but as a discrete entity, as the fundamental unit of medical care delivery (Schwenk & Hughes, 1983).

Recognizing the individual resources and needs of three partners—the child, the family, and the service providers—in an interactive system (Hanft, 1988).

The identification of problems and needs of a family and the provision of appropriate service for every family member (Yauger, 1972).

Designing services in response to needs of the total family, including the child with special needs (Friesen, Griesbach, Jacobs, Katz-Leavy, & Olson, 1988).

True partnership where family members and professionals are of mutual benefit to each other as integral members of the person's care team through the sharing of information from their unique perspectives (Shelton & Stepanek, 1994).

described in the healthcare literature, noting exactly which strategies have been truly effective in meeting family needs (Lewandowski & Tesler, 2003). In the same manner, healthcare providers need to continue to *assess* family needs, *document* how family-centered care has been implemented, *define* factors that facilitate or hinder family-centered care, and *document* the cost-effectiveness of family-centered care.

Family-centered care interventions recognize the importance of families in facilitating the growth of their children, especially children with special healthcare needs. The needs and resources of each family member and the degree to which the family wants to become involved differ with each family based on such issues as culture, spirituality, family economics, and family functioning, yet the goals remain the same: to optimize the family's ability to interact, intervene, and nurture the child during times of both physical and psychological stress. Through interdisciplinary interventions that offer education and knowledge, family, parents, and others can be empowered to make informed decisions about their child's care (Lewandowski & Tesler, 2003; Shields & Tanner, 2004).

Implementation of family-centered care interventions has elicited positive feelings from healthcare staff and

CHART 1-2 KEY ELEMENTS OF FAMILY-CENTERED CARE

The Family at the Center
Incorporating into policy and practice the recognition that the *family is the constant* in a child's life, whereas the service systems and support personnel within those systems fluctuate.

Family–Professional Collaboration
Facilitating *family–professional collaboration* at all levels of hospital, home, and community care: care of an individual child; program development, implementation, evaluation, and evolution; and policy formation.

Family–Professional Communication
Exchanging complete and unbiased information between families and professionals in a supportive manner at all times.

Cultural Diversity of Families
Incorporating into policy and practice the recognition and *honoring of cultural diversity*, strengths, and individuality within and across all families, including ethnic, racial, spiritual, social, economic, educational, and geographic diversity.

Coping Differences and Support
Recognizing and respecting *different methods of coping* and implementing comprehensive policies and programs that provide *developmental, educational, emotional, environmental, and financial supports* to meet the diverse needs of families.

Family-Centered Peer Support
Encouraging and facilitating *family-to-family support* and networking.

Specialized Service and Support Systems
Ensuring that *hospital, home, and community services and support systems* for children needing special health and developmental care and their families *are flexible, accessible, and comprehensive* in responding to diverse family-identified needs.

Holistic Perspective of Family-Centered Care
Appreciating families as families and children as children, recognizing that they possess a wide range of strengths, concerns, emotions, and aspirations beyond their need for specialized health and developmental services and support.

From Shelton, T. L., & Stepanek, J. S. (1994). *Family-centered care for children needing specialized health and developmental services.* Bethesda, MD: Association for the Care of Children's Health. Reprinted with permission.

CHART 1-3 STRATEGIES TO ENHANCE FAMILY-CENTERED CARE

Change visiting policies to promote the presence of the family at the bedside.

Establish family support groups, placing invitations to attend meetings on each child's bed.

Develop activities or programs to support the family as they make the transition from one unit (pediatric intensive care unit) to another (pediatric floor).

Be sure there are an adequate number of sleeping cots for parents.

Establish a sibling hospital visiting policy.

Encourage family visiting in the postanesthesia room.

Use parent questionnaires to better understand family needs.

Involve parents in playroom activities.

Develop mechanisms to support regular contact between the child and out-of-town parents.

Establish a parent committee or family advisory council to advise the hospital on issues of importance.

Create a parent information board containing community resources and information pamphlets.

Create a parent information and orientation program to familiarize parents with the hospital.

Provide a brief parent welcome and orientation program.

Incorporate the family in interdisciplinary conferences regarding the child's care.

Use preoperative videos and tours to ease the child's and family's fear about the pre- and postoperative process.

Establish programs to support the infant's or child's transition to home after a lengthy hospitalization.

Encourage parents to chart the child's progress.

Contract with parents to provide care for periods of time during the day.

Provide the family with a copy of the child's care path.

Coordinate and record all of the child's daily activities on a large calendar, visible to everyone.

Provide parking discount for parents.

Establish volunteer child care services for siblings while parents visit the sick child.

Call parents with reports of child's progress or send notes from the child for those hospitalized long term.

Recognize and integrate ethnic, racial, and cultural activities as appropriate into clinical setting (e.g., foods, play items, pictures on wall).

Encourage families to bring in culturally significant items such as foods and healing and religious symbols.

Aim for diversity of healthcare staff.

Encourage all family members to participate in home care activities.

In the acute care setting, provide support services such as laundry and kitchen facilities to families experiencing long hospitalizations.

Provide activities such as picnics, movies, and special events for children and their families to interact with other families who have children with the same chronic or acute condition.

reports of increased parent and child satisfaction (De Pompei, Whitford, & Beam, 1994; Gill, 1987; Heller & McKlindon, 1996; Johnson, Jeppson, & Redburn, 1992; Lewandowski & Tesler, 2003; Shields & Tanner, 2004; Stolte & Myers, 1987). Family anxiety is often reduced as the family's understanding of and involvement in the child's healthcare activities are promoted through these interventions. Family-centered care is essential to the well-being of the child and his or her family.

Bibliography

Atkinson, L. (1976). Is family-centered care a myth? *The American Journal of Maternal Child Nursing, 1*(4), 256–259.

De Pompei, P., Whitford, K., & Beam, P. (1994). One institution's effort to implement family-centered care. *Pediatric Nursing, 20*(2), 119–121, 204.

Edelman, L. (Ed.). (1991). *Getting on board: Training activities to promote the practice of family-centered care.* Bethesda, MD: Association for the Care of Children's Health.

Friesen, B., Griesbach, J., Jacobs, J., Katz-Leavy, J., & Olson, D. (1988). Caring for severely emotionally disturbed children and youth: Improving services for families. *Children Today, 17*(4), 18–22.

Gill, K. (1987). Parent participation with a family health focus: Nurses' attitudes. *Pediatric Nursing, 13*(2), 94–96.

Hanft, B. (1988). The changing environment of early intervention services: Implications for practice. *American Journal of Occupational Therapy, 42*(11), 724–731.

Heller, R., & McKlindon, D. (1996). Families as "faculty": Parents educating caregivers about family-centered care. *Pediatric Nursing, 22*(5), 428–431.

Hospital for Sick Children. (1989). *Family centered care philosophy.* Toronto, Canada: Author.

Johnson, B., Jeppson, E., & Redburn, L. (1992). *Caring for children and families: Guidelines for hospitals.* Bethesda, MD: Association for the Care of Children's Health.

Leviton, A., Mueller, M., & Kauffman, C. (1992). The family-centered consultation model: Practical applications for professionals. *Infants and Young Children, 4,* 1–8.

Lewandowski, L., & Tesler, M. (Eds.). (2003). *Family centered care: Putting it into action.* Washington, DC: American Nurses Association.

MacKean, G., Thurston, W., & Scott, C. (2005). Bridging the divide between families and health professionals' perspectives on family-centered care. *Health Expectations, 8*(1), 74–85.

Schwenk, T., & Hughes, C. (1983). The family as a patient in family medicine. *Social Science Medicine, 17,* 1–16.

Shelton, T. L., & Stepanek, J. S. (1994). *Family-centered care for children needing specialized health and developmental services.* Bethesda, MD: Association for the Care of Children's Health.

Shields, L., & Tanner, A. (2004). Pilot study of a tool to investigate perceptions of family-centered care in different care settings. *Pediatric Nursing, 30*(3), 189–197.

Stolte, K., & Myers, S. (1987). Nurses' responses to changes in maternity care. Part I. Family-centered changes and short hospitalization. *Birth, 14*(2), 82–86.

Yauger, R. (1972). Does family-centered care make a difference? *Nursing Outlook, 20*(5), 320–323.

C H A P T E R

2

Growth and Development Milestones

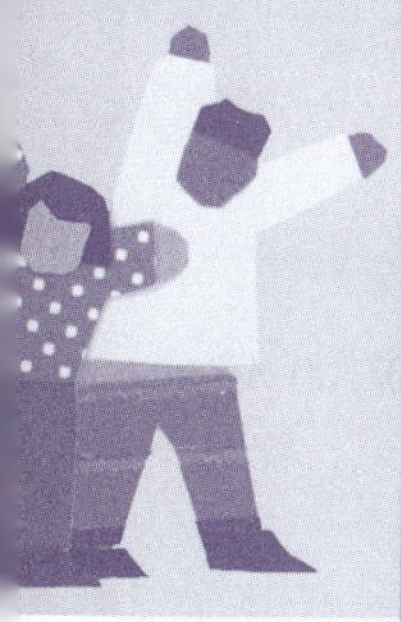

INFANTS

Newborn to 12 Months

Physical Development

NEWBORN

- Has 10% loss of birth weight in first 3 to 4 days of life
- Fluid makes up 73% of body weight
- Head circumference is 70% of adult size
- Needs to consume 120 calories per kilogram of weight per day
- Sleeps 20 to 22 hours per day, with brief waking periods of 2 to 3 hours
- Grows about 1 inch per month
- Gains 5 to 7 ounces per week
- Feeds every 2½ to 4 hours

2 TO 5 MONTHS

- Posterior fontanel closes
- Obligate (preferential) nose breathers until about 5 months
- Begins drooling

5 TO 6 MONTHS

- Doubles birth weight
- Teeth may begin to erupt
- Moves food to back of mouth and swallows during spoon feedings
- Sleeps through the night for up to 8 hours
- Goes 4 to 5 hours between feedings
- Has two to four naps per day

7 TO 9 MONTHS

- Begins teething with lower central incisors, followed by two upper incisors
- Mashes food with jaws
- Sleeps 14 to 16 hours per day, including naps

10 TO 12 MONTHS

- Sleeps 14 to 16 hours per day and still naps
- Stops drooling
- Grows about ½ inch monthly

Sexual Development

ALL INFANTS
- Oral stage: oral gratification and sucking needs (Freud)

10 MONTHS
- Begins sexual identity

Language Development

NEWBORN
- Alerting
- Social smile

2 TO 3 MONTHS
- Laughs and squeals
- Coos
- Utters single vowel sounds such as "ah" and "eh"

4 MONTHS
- Utters two-syllable vowel sounds
- Includes consonant sounds such as "m" and "b"
- Produces belly laughs
- Orients to voice of others

5 MONTHS
- Razzing
- Intersperses vowel and consonant sounds

6 MONTHS
- Babbles
- Uses about 12 speech sounds

7 MONTHS
- Makes "talking sounds" in response to parent or while others are talking
- Coos and squeals
- Vocalizes up to four different syllables

8 TO 10 MONTHS
- Uses "dada," "mama" in nonspecific way
- Responds to own name (receptive language skills develop first)
- Babbles to produce consonant sounds
- Vocalizes to toys

9 TO 12 MONTHS
- Imitates speech sounds
- Understands name and "no"
- Understands "bye" and "pat-a-cake"
- Imitates facial expressions
- Imitates definite speech sounds
- Uses jargon
- Communicates by pointing to objects and by using gestures
- Responds to simple verbal requests

12 MONTHS
- Has one word (or a few) in vocabulary
- Comprehends "give" and stops when told "no"
- Has receptive vocabulary of several dozen words
- Jabbers expressively
- Experiments with "pseudo-words"
- Deaf infants lose ability to vocalize by 1 year of age

Vision Development

NEWBORN
- Fixates on human face and demonstrates preference
- Blink reflex present

2 MONTHS
- Follows to midline
- Produces tears
- Visual acuity is hyperoptic

4 MONTHS
- Follows objects to 180 degrees

5 MONTHS
- Visual acuity 20/200
- Recognizes feeding bottle

6 MONTHS
- Inspects hands
- Fixates on object 3 feet away
- Strabismus (deviation of the eye) no longer within normal limits
- Develops hand–eye coordination

8 MONTHS
- Has permanent eye color
- Depth perception developing

10 MONTHS
- Tilts head backward to see up

12 MONTHS
- Shows smooth visual pursuit of objects with 20/100 vision
- Can follow rapidly moving objects

Hearing Development

NEWBORN
- Startles to loud noises
- Prefers high-pitched voices
- Quieted by low-pitched noises
- Responds to human voice over other noises
- Auditory behavior is reflexive; generalized body movement (blinking or crying)
- Recognizes certain sounds, ignores others; attends to quiet sounds more than loud ones—these are learned rather than reflexive behaviors
- Turns to voice (quiet listening)

5 MONTHS
- Orients to bell (looks to side)
- Stops crying in response to music

7 MONTHS
- Orients to bell (looks to side, then up)

10 MONTHS
- Localizes sound from above or below
- Orients to bell (turns directly to bell)

Gross Motor Development

NEWBORN
- Turns head when prone but cannot support head
- Adjusts posture when held at shoulder
- May squirm to corner or edge of crib when prone
- Arm and leg movements are reflexive

6 WEEKS TO 2 MONTHS
- Holds head up 45 to 90 degrees when prone
- May hold head steady when in supported sitting position

3 MONTHS
- Rolls over from back to side
- Holds head erect and steady

4 MONTHS
- When supported, sits with rounded back and flexed knees
- May bear weight on legs when assisted to stand
- Head lag disappears when pulled to sitting position

5 MONTHS
- Pulls to sitting position
- Rolls from back to stomach
- Sits alone momentarily
- Shows unilateral reaching

6 MONTHS
- Sits without support
- May creep an inch forward or backward
- Moves from place to place by rolling
- Begins drinking from a cup

7 MONTHS
- Stands while holding on
- Early stepping movements
- Begins to crawl or hitch
- Raises head spontaneously when supine

8 MONTHS
- Pulls to standing position
- Raises self to sitting position
- Palmar grasp disappears

9 MONTHS
- Walks with help
- Crawls, creeps, or hitches when permitted
- Sits down
- Holds own bottle
- Drinks from cup or glass

10 MONTHS
- Continues walking skill development with help
- Stands alone
- May climb up and down stairs
- Sits without support
- Recovers balance
- Changes from prone to sitting position

11 MONTHS
- May walk alone
- Begins to stoop and recover
- Pushes toys
- "Cruises"

12 MONTHS
- Continues walking skills
- Climbs onto sofas and chairs

Fine Motor Development

NEWBORN
- Follows to, and slightly past, midline

2 TO 3 MONTHS
- Keeps hands open predominately
- Reflex grasp replaced by voluntary grasping
- Grasps objects such as rattle in open hand
- May bring hands together at midline

3 TO 4 MONTHS
- Uses ulnar-palmar prehension with a cube
- Reaches for objects
- Hands predominately open

5 MONTHS
- Attempts to "catch" dangling objects with two hands
- Begins using of forefinger and thumb in a pincer grasp (opposable thumb—prehension)
- Retains two cubes
- Recovers rattle
- Reaches for and grasps objects

6 TO 7 MONTHS
- Can grasp at will
- Holds and manipulates objects
- Scoops pellet
- Transfers from hand to hand
- Demonstrates inferior pincer
- Bangs objects together
- Can release objects

8 TO 9 MONTHS
- Combines spoons or cubes at midline
- Retains two of three cubes offered
- Achieves neat pincer grasp of pellet
- Feeds self finger foods using only one hand
- Releases objects at will
- Rings bell
- Holds bottle and places nipple in mouth when wants it

10 TO 11 MONTHS
- Plays "pat-a-cake" (a midline skill)
- Puts several objects in a container
- Holds crayon adaptively
- Bangs two cubes together
- Looks for hidden object (object permanency) (Piaget)
- Achieves neat pincer grasp of tiny objects

Play Development

ALL INFANTS
- Engages in solitary play
- May be imitative
- Explores and manipulates

5 TO 7 MONTHS
- Resists toy pull
- Picks up tiny objects
- Plays "peek-a-boo"
- Works to get toy that is out of reach

8 TO 9 MONTHS
- Plays "pat-a-cake"
- Recognizes self in mirror

10 TO 12 MONTHS
- Plays ball with examiner
- Achieves object permanence (searches for dropped objects)

Cognitive Development

NEWBORN
Substage I (Piaget)
- Practices reflexes and reflex-like actions

1 TO 4 MONTHS
Substage II—Purposeful (Piaget)
- Reproduces reflex actions

4 TO 8 MONTHS
Substage III—Objects (Piaget)
- Oriented and imitative actions
- Accidental actions are repeated
- Develops habits
- Responds negatively to removal of a toy

8 TO 12 MONTHS
Substage IV (Piaget)
- Coordination, intentional goal direction and achievement
- Experiments with object permanence
- Imitates and models behavior
- No concept of death
- Enjoys "peek-a-boo" game
- Attempts to flee from unpleasant events
- Recognizes anticipatory signs

10 TO 12 MONTHS
- Repeats actions that elicit response from others
- Dislikes restrictions
- Shakes head for "no"
- Appears interested in picture book

Social Development

NEWBORN
- Regards face and establishes eye contact

1 TO 2 MONTHS
- Smiles responsively
- Enjoys cuddling and motion

2 TO 3 MONTHS
- Smiles spontaneously

3 TO 5 MONTHS
- Smiles at mirror image
- Shows interest in siblings
- Invites social interactions by smiling

6 MONTHS
- Exhibits stranger anxiety
- Extends arms to be held

7 TO 9 MONTHS
- Waves hands

12 MONTHS
- Demonstrates emotions of fear, anger, affection
- Can indicate desires without crying
- Offers object to a familiar adult
- Talks to mirror

Interpersonal Development

NEWBORN TO 3 MONTHS
- Self-absorbed, egocentric

4 TO 18 MONTHS
- Symbiotic phase—mother seen as an extension of child's body and needs, and vice versa

6 TO 10 MONTHS
- Exhibits stranger anxiety
- Waves arm and legs when frustrated

8 TO 24 MONTHS
- Exhibits separation anxiety
- Exhibits trust versus mistrust (Erikson)

Emotional Development

NEWBORN TO 3 MONTHS
- Feeling regulated and interested in the world
- Sensitive to parent's joyful interest in him or her

3 TO 7 MONTHS
- Forming attachments
- Highly specialized interest in the human world

8 TO 10 MONTHS
- Purposeful communication
- Can connect small units of feelings into simple patterns
- Purposeful expression of wants and needs
- Fluctuates easily between laughing and crying

10 TO 18 MONTHS
- Complex sense of self
- Communication is truly interactive, enabling toddler to tune into parents and to build appropriately on their response

Moral/Spiritual Development

ALL INFANTS
Moral—Stage I: Preconventional Level (Kohlberg)
- May be disciplined by withdrawal of stimuli (e.g., toy, food) and may experience injury related to consequences of actions. However, makes no cognitive connection between these events and distinguishing right from wrong.
- No moral concepts or rules exist

Spiritual—Stage O: Undifferentiated (Fowler)
- Not capable of formulating or communicating any conceptual ideas about self or environment
- Feelings of trust sets foundation for subsequent development of faith

TODDLERS
12 to 36 Months

Physical Development

12 MONTHS
- Head circumference equals chest circumference
- Triples birth weight to 20 pounds
- Half of adult height
- Height increases 3 inches per year for next 7 years
- Weight increases 4 to 6 pounds per year

18 TO 24 MONTHS
- Has from 10 to 14 temporary teeth
- Anterior fontanel closes
- Cuspids and first and second molars appear
- Toilet training may be accomplished
- Chest circumference exceeds head circumference
- Needs 90 to 100 calories per kilogram of weight per day

24 MONTHS
- Has 16 temporary teeth
- Average weight is 30 pounds
- Toilet training may begin; voluntary control of anal and urethral sphincters occurs
- Average 10 to 14 hours sleep, including afternoon naps

24 MONTHS TO 6 YEARS
- Needs 80 to 90 calories per kilogram of weight per day

Sexual Development

ALL TODDLERS
- Anal stage (Freud)
- Sensual pleasures shifts to anal and urethral areas
- Identification with male/female sex roles

36 MONTHS
- Knows own sex

Language Development

12 TO 18 MONTHS
- Beginning of spoken language; may occur at same time as walking, although concentration on one or the other may occur
- Recognizes nouns that stand for objects
- Uses gestures to make needs known
- Develops from 3 to 20 words
- Use of telegraphic speech, use of noun and verb to convey meaning
- Use of words may be quite inconsistent

18 TO 24 MONTHS
- Follows directions
- Points to nose, hair, eye, and so forth on demand
- Comprehends "give me that" when accompanied by a gesture

24 MONTHS
- Has 300-word vocabulary
- Gives first and last name
- Progressive comprehension of speech
- Talks without trying to convey ideas

Vision Development

18 Months
- Displays interest in pictures

24 Months
- Identifies forms
- Cooperates with Snellen testing
- Has 20/40 vision

36 Months
- Has 20/30 vision

Gross Motor Development

12 to 18 Months
- Walks well
- Throws ball
- Stoops and recovers
- Walks up stairs with help
- Begins to run
- Walks sideways and backward for 10 feet
- Stands on one foot with help
- Sits down from standing by self
- Falls frequently; often used as a way of sitting down
- Rolls large ball on floor

18 to 24 Months
- Kicks ball forward
- Throws overhand
- Walks downstairs with help—one step at a time
- Climbs
- Sits self in a small chair

24 to 36 Months
- Jumps and runs well
- Jumps from bottom step
- Jumps in place
- Balances on one foot for 1 second
- Walks on a straight line
- Tiptoes
- Broad jumps 4 to 14 inches
- Can pick up objects on floor without losing balance

36 Months
- Rides tricycle

Fine Motor Development

12 to 18 Months
- Scribbles spontaneously
- Builds tower of two blocks, then four blocks
- Dumps raisins from container after demonstration, then spontaneously
- May untie shoes
- Uses opposable thumb well (prehension)
- Shows preference for one hand or the other
- Turns pages in a book
- Uses spoon with frequent spills when getting food to mouth

18 to 24 Months
- May remove articles of clothing
- Holds pencil well enough for scribbling
- Builds tower of four cubes
- Imitates drawing a vertical line within 30 degrees
- Turns doorknobs within reach

24 to 36 Months
- Unbuttons large buttons
- Builds tower of six to eight cubes
- Can use paintbrush
- Imitates scribble
- Copies a circle
- Begins to wash and dry hands
- Drinks from cup
- Can begin brushing teeth one to two times a day
- Can take off socks and other easy-to-manipulate clothing
- Snaps large snaps
- Zips large zippers with help
- Twists caps off bottles
- Places simple shapes in correct holes
- Will disassemble objects

Play Development

12 to 18 Months
- Parallel play
- Imitates adult roles
- Imitates housework
- Will do simple household tasks

24 to 30 Months
- Uses colors
- Begins to play interactive games, such as tag
- Plays with sand, clay, Play-Doh, puzzles
- Fantasy and make-believe play
- Action games/ritualistic, such as tag or hide-and-seek

Cognitive Development

24 Months to 7 Years—Preoperational and Preconceptual; 12 to 18 Months—Substage V (Piaget)
- Production of vowel behaviors and curiosity
- Uses imitation to discover new ways of acting
- Experiments to discover how objects behave and how they can be manipulated

18 to 24 Months—Substage VI (Piaget)
- Concept of object permanency fully achieved
- Symbolic plane
- Limited concept of time (no "tomorrow")

- Very egocentric
- Animist (talks to stuffed animals)
- Imaginary playmates
- Parallel play
- Premature sense of cause and effect
- Goal-directed behavior
- Death is reversible; a temporary restriction, departure or sleep
- Bedtime very ritualistic

Social Development

12 to 18 Months
- Responds to limit setting

Interpersonal Development

0 to 18 Months
- Differentiation between "good mother/bad mother" to "good me/bad me" or "not me"
- Swings from love to hate

12 to 36 Months
- Autonomy versus shame and doubt (Erikson)

36 Months
- Self-concept begins

Emotional Development

30 to 48 Months
- Emotional ideas
- Uses symbolic communication to convey ideas in terms of complex intentions
- Explores different emotions in pretend play
- Can communicate and comprehend

Moral/Spiritual Development

All Toddlers
Moral—Stage 2: Preconventional Level (Kohlberg)
- Detects concepts of fairness and sharing
- "Instrumental–relationistic" orientation
- Satisfaction of own needs
- Conventional level; beginning
- "Good girl/nice boy"
- Approval-seeking behavior
- Above coupled with desire to please

Spiritual—Stage I: Intuitive/Projective (Fowler)
- Learns to imitate the religious affect and behavior of parents
- Mimics religious gestures but does not comprehend meaning
- Formulates own conceptions and explanations of faith and belief
- Cannot separate feelings from intellect
- Formulates imagined descriptions of God (angel, friend he or she can communicate with)

Preschool-Aged Children

3 to 6 Years

Physical Development

All Preschoolers
- Walks erect, swings arms
- Rapid skeletal development taking place
- Nutritional needs: 1,400 to 1,800 calories per kilogram of weight per day
- Loses baby fat and tummy
- Needs 12 hours of sleep a night

5 Years
- Tooth decay may be present
- Is half of adult height

6 Years
- First permanent tooth erupts, begins loss of deciduous teeth
- Weight gain average of 4 pounds per year
- Brain is 90% of adult size
- Needs 2,000 calories per day

Sexual Development

All Preschoolers: Phallic Stage (Freud)
- Much genital manipulation and exploration (particularly with other children)
- Shows intense attraction and love for parent of opposite sex (Oedipal conflict in boys, Electra conflict in girls)
- Identification with parent of same sex
- Castration anxiety; mutilation fears
- Intrusive procedures threaten body integrity
- Masturbation

Language Development

3 to 4 Years
- Uses four- to five-word sentences with adult sense of syntax
- Names body parts; recognizes colors
- Talks fluently and listens
- Comprehends "cold, tired, hungry" or at least two of these three words
- Comprehends prepositions
- Has 900-word vocabulary
- Repeats sentences of three to four words

4 to 5 Years
- Knows opposites analogies (two of three)
- Recognizes colors
- Has 1,500-word vocabulary

- Knows simple songs
- Tells exaggerated stories
- Questioning at a peak
- Asks permission
- Relates experiences and tells about activities in sequential order
- Counts to 3

5 TO 6 YEARS
- Can identify all coins
- Defines words (six of nine)
- Knows composition of objects
- Has 2,100-word vocabulary
- Can repeat sentence of 10 syllables or more
- Knows names of days, weeks, months
- Can follow commands in succession

6 YEARS
- Counts to 20
- Recognizes shapes

Vision Development

3 YEARS
- Has 20/30 vision
- Copies a circle
- Color vision fully intact

4 YEARS
- Cooperates with Snellen testing
- Copies crosses
- Maximum potential for developing amblyopia

5 YEARS
- Recognizes colors
- Copies a square

Hearing Development

ALL PRESCHOOLERS
- Cooperates on systematic audiometric tests
- Clues to hearing deficit include volume of TV, whether child responds to you, audiometric test results, intelligible speech by age 5 years

Gross Motor Development

3 YEARS
- Hops on one foot
- Rides tricycle
- Can undress self in most situations
- Catches soft object with both hands
- Jumps from low step

4 YEARS
- Skips
- Balances on one foot for 5 seconds (two out of three tries)
- Catches bounced ball (two out of three tries)
- Dresses without supervision
- Walks downstairs using alternating feet
- Twists upper body while holding feet in one place

5 YEARS
- Walks backward heel to toe (two out of three tries)
- Balances on one foot for 10 seconds (two out of three tries)
- Skips and hops on alternating feet
- Throws and catches ball well
- Jumps rope
- Jumps from height of 12 inches and lands on toes

Fine Motor Development

3 TO 4 YEARS
- Picks longer line (three out of three tries)
- Begins to use blunt scissors
- Strings large beads on shoelace

4 TO 5 YEARS
- Ties shoelaces
- Draws a man with three to six parts
- Copies a square
- Uses scissors

5 TO 6 YEARS
- Draws a man with six parts
- Copies a triangle
- Dresses without supervision
- Can print letters or numbers

Play Development

ALL PRESCHOOLERS
- Parallel/associative play
- Defines own rules
- Cooperative play
- Joins in play with others
- Plays interactive games
- Imitative play
- Dramatic play
- Solitary play
- Play with parents
- Onlooker play
- Imaginary playmates

Cognitive Development

ALL PRESCHOOLERS—PREOPERATIONAL (PIAGET)
- Egocentrism
- Omnipotence (inability to distinguish between one's own perception and that of someone else)
- Thinking is concrete and tangible; becomes more intuitive toward end of this stage

- "Transductive reasoning" from a particular event to another event
- Animism
- Magical thinking
- Artificialism (all things are "made for a purpose")
- Irreversibility (cannot backtrack steps in a thinking pattern)
- Centration (inability to consider several aspects of the situation simultaneously)
- Trial versus error
- Primitive concepts of space, time, and causality
- Uses memory
- Death is reversible, a temporary restriction, departure, or sleep
- Juxtaposition—no relationship between stated ideas

Social Development

ALL PRESCHOOLERS

- Separates easily from mother
- Magical thinking
- When permitted freedom, creativity is enhanced
- Has many fears, which are very real and logical to the child

Interpersonal Development

ALL PRESCHOOLERS

- Primitive sense of body image begins
- Initiative versus guilt (Erikson)

Emotional Development

30 TO 48 MONTHS

- Emotional thinking
- Can understand that feelings are connected ("mad because . . .")
- Added logic to expression of ideas dealing with complex intentions, wishes, and feelings

Moral/Spiritual Development

ALL PRESCHOOLERS

Moral—Stage 3: Conventional Level (Kohlberg)

- Desires to please others
- Seeks approval or attention through behaviors
- Social concern

Spiritual—Stage I: Intuitive/Projective (Fowler)

- Learns to imitate the religious affects and behavior of parents
- Mimics religious gestures but does not comprehend meaning
- Cannot separate feelings from intellect
- Formulates imagined descriptions of God (angel, friend he or she can communicate with)

SCHOOL-AGED CHILDREN

7 to 11 Years

Physical Development

ALL SCHOOL-AGED CHILDREN

- Girls by age 11 years have achieved 90% of adult height and 50% of adult weight
- Boys at age 12 years have achieved 80% of adult height and 50% of adult weight
- Striking changes in growth of long bones
- Begins Tanner stages of prepubertal development
- By 12 years of age, has all permanent teeth except second and third molars

6 TO 9 YEARS

- Sleeps 11 to 12 hours per day
- Gains 3 to 5 pounds per year
- Has 10 to 11 permanent teeth
- Arms grow longer in proportion to body

10 TO 11 YEARS

- Sleeps 10 hours per day
- Needs 2,200 to 2,500 calories a day
- Twelve-year molars erupt

Sexual Development

ALL SCHOOL-AGED CHILDREN

- Some girls have menarche as early as 10 years of age
- Normal homosexual interest
  - Latency years: sex drives repressed (Freud)

Language Development

ALL SCHOOL-AGED CHILDREN

- Augments vocabulary and cognitive skills
- Knows coin exchange

Vision Development

7 YEARS

- Has 20/20 vision

Gross Motor Development

6 YEARS

- Walks a straight line
- Has mastered all skills on Denver Developmental Screening Tests

8 YEARS

- Crouches on tiptoes
- Puts right or left foot forward on command

9 TO 11 YEARS
- Balances on one leg with eyes closed
- Catches tennis ball with one hand

Fine Motor Development

ALL SCHOOL-AGED CHILDREN
- Continually refines and improves previously learned skills
- Movements are more graceful
- Bathes unassisted
- Uses tools

Play Development

ALL SCHOOL-AGED CHILDREN
- Cooperative "team" play
- Skill play (jump rope, skating)
- Testing, model building, exploration
- Collects things and classifies them as hobbies
- Plays board games
- Reads for pleasure
- Easily engrossed in long hours of TV watching

Cognitive Development

ALL SCHOOL-AGED CHILDREN
Concrete Operations (Piaget)
- Ability to reason
- Concept of reversibility
- Classifies objects according to their characteristics
- Understands concept of conservation
- Understands concept of relativism
- Can place self in another's situation
- Serialization—masters the ordinal number line; can group and sort/place in logical order
- Fundamental skills of reading, writing, and grammar develop
- Understands concept of reciprocity
- Understands concept of identity
- Gains greater understanding of distance and directions
- Tells time
- Decentration—ability to focus on many aspects of experience

11 YEARS
- Capable of abstract and deductive reasoning
- Considers death irreversible but capricious
- Uses external/internal physiologic explanations

Social Development

ALL SCHOOL-AGED CHILDREN
- Social participation in school, neighborhood, scouting groups
- Begins to manage cooperative and competitive relationships

Interpersonal Development

ALL SCHOOL-AGED CHILDREN
- Independence within family
- Self-regulation of behavior
- Industry versus inferiority (Erikson)

Emotional Development

ALL SCHOOL-AGED CHILDREN
- Uses coping behaviors (strategies): avoidant coping, active coping, avoidant-active coping

Moral/Spiritual Development

ALL SCHOOL-AGED CHILDREN
Moral—Stage 4: Conventional (Kohlberg)
- Concern with authority figures, fixed rules in moral decisions
- Concern with obligation to duty
- Understands that a "bad" act breaks a rule or does harm
- May interpret accidents or misfortunes as punishment
- Develops a conscience and sense of values

Spiritual—Stage II: Mythical/Literal (Fowler)
- Distinguishes religious fact from fantasy
- Respects and relies on authoritative figures such as parents, priest, rabbi
- Influenced by attitude of peers toward faith
- Monomythic attitude; uses fantasies to explain events or facts he or she does not understand
- Learns to differentiate between natural and supernatural
- Perceives God in anthropomorphic imagery, has human qualities
- Description of God implies a formation of a reciprocal relationship

ADOLESCENTS

12 to 18 Years

Physical Development

- Full height not attained until ages 20 to 24 years when epiphyseal plates close
- Marked increase in muscle mass in boys related to androgen
- By age 17 years, muscle mass is two times greater in boys than girls, resulting in strength two to four times greater in boys
- Adult cardiovascular rhythms by age 16 years
- Great nutritional needs:
  Boys: 3,600 calories per day
  Girls: 2,600 calories per day
- At end of adolescence, male basal metabolic rate is about 10% greater than female rate

- Nutrition needs:
  Pregrowth spurt—1,500 to 2,400 calories per day
  Pubertal girls—2,000 to 2,500 calories per day
  Pubertal boys—2,500 to 3,000 calories per day

Sexual Development

GENITAL STAGE (FREUD)

- Learning appropriate outlets for sexual drives
- Menarche around 10 to 15 years of age in girls
- Usually cannot reproduce for 1 to 2 years after menarche because of anovulation
- Early use of oral contraceptives limits potential height
- Boy attains puberty between 12 and 16 years of age
- Tanner steps I to V usually attained between early and late adolescence

Approximate sequence of appearance of sexual characteristics in adolescence:

GIRLS

8 to 9 Years
- Hormones begin to release, sometimes causing moodiness and skin sensitivity

9 to 10 Years
- Hips start rounding out
- Breast nipples start to grow

10 to 11 Years
- Breast tissues around and under nipple begins to grow
- Downy hair near labia
- Growth spurt may begin

11 to 12 Years
- Internal and external organs continue growing (vagina, uterus, breasts, ovaries)
- Pubic hair becomes darker, coarser, and curlier

12 to 13 Years
- Underarm hair growth
- Onset of menstruation (average age, 12.8 years and about 2 years after breasts start growing)
- Pregnancy is now possible

13 to 14 Years
- There may be times when underpants are wet with a clear mucus; this is often heavier in teen years and continues naturally during adulthood, especially with ovulation and sexual arousal.

14 to 15 Years
- Earliest normal pregnancy possible
- Majority of growth spurt complete (height)

15 to 16 Years
- Deepening of voice, though not as much as in boys

BOYS

9 to 10 Years
- Hormones begin to release, sometimes causing moodiness and skin sensitivity

10 to 11 Years
- Testes become larger
- Scrotal skin becomes redder in color and coarser in texture

11 to 12 Years
- Prostate begins functioning
- Penis begins to lengthen

12 to 13 Years
- Pubic hair growth
- May experience wet dreams, spontaneous erections, ejaculations (about 1 year after testes begin to grow)
- Growth spurt may begin

13 to 14 Years
- Rapid growth of the penis occurring about 1 year after testes begin to grow
- Testes color deepens
- Two thirds of boys may experience slight growth of breast tissue, which generally subsides within 1 year but may last up to 3 years

14 to 15 Years
- Underarm hair
- Mustache begins as fine hair starting at outside lip edges about 2 years after pubic hair
- Voice change begins

15 to 16 Years
- Sperm matures and can cause pregnancy at average age of 14.6 years; 50% of boys reach this stage within the previous 2 years
- Majority of growth spurt complete (height)

16 to 17 Years
- Chest and shoulders fill out
- Facial and body hair becomes heavier
- Acne

Play Development

- Group/peer activities such as sports, academic teams
- Seeks parental-adult "limit-setting"
- Thrill-seeking behaviors

Cognitive Development

- "Pseudo-stupidity": asks "dumb" questions (Elkind)
- Difficulty reconciling concrete and formal operations
- Imaginary audience: super self-arrangement of the possible consciousness; believes everybody is watching and evaluating (Elkind)

- Personal fable: belief of being special and not subject to rational laws (Elkind)
- Apparent hypocrisy: act of expressing an idea tantamount to working for and attaining it (Elkind)

Formal Operations Development (Piaget)

- Abstraction and hypothetical/deductive reasoning
- Adaptability and flexibility
- Thinking in abstract terms
- Uses abstract symbols
- Makes conclusions drawn from set of observations
- Develops hypotheses and tests them
- Considering abstract, theoretical, and philosophical matters
- Problem solving
- Ability to comprehend purely abstract or symbolic content exists
- Ability to solve math and logic problems
- Comprehends value and belief systems in the philosophical, moral, and political realms
- Reality versus possibility—views only one
- Combinational reasoning
- Prepositional thinking
- Hypothetical-deductive reasoning
- Death is irreversible, universal, personal, but distant
- Uses natural, physiologic, and theologic explanations of death

Social Development

- Capable of sharing self with others to foster intimate relationship
- Inability to form intimate relationships may lead to sense of isolation

Interpersonal Development

- Identity versus role confusion (Erikson)

Moral/Spiritual Development

MORAL—STAGE 4: CONVENTIONAL (KOHLBERG)

12 to 16 Years

- Fixed rules in moral decisions
- Obligation to do no harm and to do duty

MORAL—STAGE 5: POSTCONVENTIONAL (KOHLBERG)

16 Years

- Social contracts understood and formulated
- Laws recognized as changeable
- Correct actions depend on standards and individual rights

MORAL—STAGE 6: ADULTHOOD (KOHLBERG)

- Abstract moral principles govern behavior
- Morality is easily separated from legality
- Orientation is based on universal ethical orientation
- Can apply situational ethics

SPIRITUAL—STAGE III: SYNTHETIC/INVENTION (FOWLER)

Preadolescent

- Reflects and questions religious beliefs from more contact with people whose values and beliefs are different
- Seeks to resolve moral conflicts by appealing to outside authority figures rather than using own inner resources
- Learns to distinguish more clearly between supernatural and natural
- Perceives God as a spirit
- Begins to understand spiritual component of individuals

SPIRITUAL—STAGE IV: INDIVIDUATING/REFLEXIVE (FOWLER)

Adolescent

- Seeks to establish and maintain balance regarding religious/spiritual questions and beliefs; may adopt "devil-may-care" attitude, go to other extreme and join zealous religious group, or suspend effort to resolve conflict

CHAPTER

3

Teaching Children and Their Families

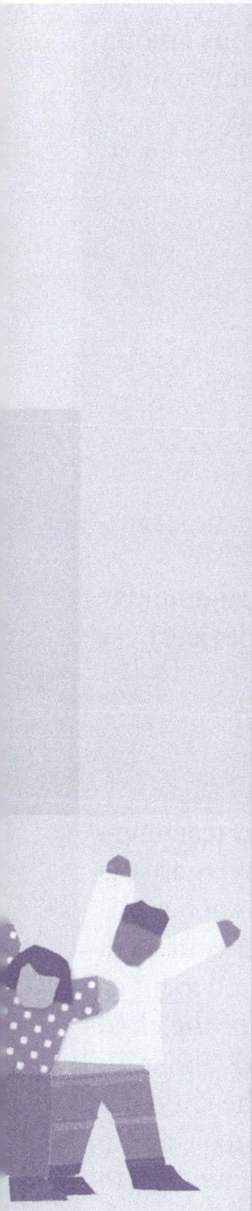

The Teaching Process

Teaching is the process by which new information is presented so that learning may occur. The method used to teach information varies depending on the needs of the learner, the time necessary for the learner to grasp the information, the methods of instruction most appropriate to the learner, and the material being taught. Individuals learn, accept, and cope with new information and situations at different rates and by different methods. Thus, the time each learner requires for each new learning experience varies. Some require more time, practice, and explanation than others. Be patient, and caution the learner to be likewise.

The learning/comprehension level varies among individuals and among children of different ages. The level of the presentation needs to adjust accordingly. Use terms and words the learner can understand. Some individuals benefit from audio and visual materials (e.g., interactive teaching on CD-ROMs, viewing videos, reading pamphlets) to help explain the content.

Three important basic learning conditions for teaching skills or procedures are as follows:

- *Contiguity:* The individual steps of the procedure must be taught in continuous order or sequence. Teaching may begin with the first step and work to the last one or may start with the last step and work backward; it does not matter as long as the steps are in sequence.
- *Practice:* This permits the individual to rehearse the sequence until each step is learned satisfactorily. Practice is most effective when the individual distributes it over a period of time rather than trying to perfect the entire sequence all at once.
- *Feedback:* This provides the learner with information about his or her progress. It is the most important variable in learning and is highly motivating to the individual. A return demonstration of learning can be critiqued and corrected.

Before providing information, the nurse must determine the learning needs of the child and family or caregivers. Throughout the initial interview, the nurse collects data about their physical and psychosocial needs. The nurse then analyzes the data to determine whether the child and family understand the situation. By identifying knowledge deficits on admission, the nurse can plan effective teaching strategies that address the family's deficits and promote coping.

Learning needs are affected by many factors, including prior experience with illness, cultural background, language skills, the patient and family's educational levels, and the child's developmental level. An educational plan must address factors to meet the child and family's information needs.

The process of patient teaching resembles the nursing process. Teaching begins with assessment of the problem and of readiness to learn and progresses to development of a plan, implementation of the plan, and evaluation of its effectiveness. During the assessment step, the nurse should determine the learner's cultural background and establish a rapport, especially when the nurse and learner come from different cultures. To promote positive patient outcomes, the nurse must adopt education strategies that enhance learning readiness and facilitate effective learning. Providing effective patient and family education has long been a professional practice standard. Because failure to teach essential information regarding healthcare and maintenance has recently become grounds for lawsuits, effective education now is also a legal requirement for nurses.

COMMUNICATING WITH THE CHILD AND FAMILY

The challenge in pediatrics is that the healthcare provider works at several different levels of communication. Among one's colleagues and peers, a specific child and his or her clinical progress may be discussed in very detailed and medically complex terms. Portions of that conversation then need to be translated into a form in which an adult (the child's parent or caregiver) can comprehend in layperson's terms the complexities of the child's condition. In addition, the child's condition, the plan of care, and the desired outcomes must be communicated to the child in a developmentally appropriate manner so that the child's input and cooperation can be incorporated into the overall plan of care. Table 3-1 and Chart 3-1 provide information regarding appropriate language considerations for pediatric patients and methods to facilitate communication with parents of acutely ill children.

APPROACHES TO TEACHING CHILDREN

Effective teaching in the pediatric population can be accomplished only when the healthcare provider approaches each child according to his or her developmental level and cognitive abilities. The 16-year-old boy with acute appendicitis, for example, will definitely have a different understanding of his condition than the 7-year-old boy in the bed next to him with the same malady. Although the 7-year-old is agonizing over the intravenous line in his hand, the 16-year-old is most likely concerned with wondering how this will impact football practice that begins in 2 weeks. Thus, each child must be approached differently in terms of how information is conveyed to him or her, the depth and breath of that information, and the means to evaluate what the child has learned.

Some general principles to remember when teaching children are as follows:

- Ask children directly how they cope with new situations.
- Ask parents what they have already told the child.
- Observe the child's behavior for clues to readiness to learn.
- Consider the child's developmental level and attention span.
- Encourage the child to ask questions.
- Use concrete terms, not technical ones.
- Use the same equipment and supplies that will be used at home.
- Present small amounts of information at a time.
- Supervise return demonstrations and several successful practice sessions for any new skills taught.
- Make expectations known clearly and simply.
- Do not offer a choice when there is none.
- Offer honest praise.

Chart 3-2 summarizes teaching considerations among the various developmental stage groups. When teaching, the variety of strategies that can be used include

- Dramatic play
- Games
- Age-appropriate books
- Coloring books
- Tours
- Audiovisuals
- CD-ROM interactive lessons
- Pictures and diagrams
- Mannequins and equipment
- Special dolls with equipment
- Poster-board displays
- Visits by other children with similar medical adjuncts (e.g., tracheotomy tubes, implanted access devices)

WORKING AS A TEAM TO MAKE TEACHING A SUCCESS

Four major parties need to be involved in the teaching–learning process with the child. The primary players are the child and the family. It is within the context of his or her primary caregivers that the child is supported, encouraged, and held responsible for the self-care needs related to his or her health. It is important to provide a means for the child to share with parents what he or she understands about his or her care and for the parents to share with the child the new skills they have also acquired to care for him or her. In addition, there must be a mechanism for family members to review what they have been taught and to share that knowledge with others at home who need to know. This means that appropriate printed literature (bilingual if necessary), illustrations, diagrams, and written instructions are provided to the family.

Another important group in the teaching–learning process is the team of healthcare providers. Communication among providers must be such that all members are aware of the family's teaching needs and there is consistency in what information is presented, how it is presented, and how outcomes are measured. The results of teaching

(text continues on page 24)

TABLE 3-1
Considerations in Choosing Language

Potentially Ambiguous	*Clearer*
The doctor will give you some "dye." *To make me die?*	The doctor will put some medicine in the tube that will help her be able to see your _____ more clearly.
Dressing, dressing change *Why are they going to undress me? Do I have to change my clothes? Will I be naked?*	Bandages; clean, new bandages
Stool collection *Why do they want to collect little chairs?*	Use child's familiar term, such as "poop," "BM," or "doody."
Urine *You're in?*	Use child's familiar term, such as "pee."
Shot *Are they mad at me? When people get shot, they're really bad hurt. Are they trying to hurt me?*	Medicine through a (small, tiny) needle
CAT scan *Will there be cats? Or something that scratches?*	Describe in simple terms and explain what the letters of the common name stand for (if child is old enough).
PICU *Pick you?*	Explain, as above.
ICU *I see you?*	Explain, as above.
IV *Ivy?*	Explain, as above.
Stretcher *Stretch her? Stretch who? Why?*	Bed on wheels
Special; funny *It doesn't look/feel special to me.*	Odd; different; unusual; strange
Gas; sleeping gas *Is someone going to pour gasoline into the mask?*	Medicine, called anesthesia. It is a kind of air you will breathe through a mask like this—to help you sleep during your operation so you won't feel anything. It is a different kind of sleep. (Explain differences.)
Put you to sleep *Like my cat was put to sleep? It never came back.*	Give you medicine that will help you go into a very deep sleep; you won't feel anything until the operation is over, then the doctor will stop giving you the medicine, so you can wake up.
Move you to the floor *Why are they going to put me on the ground?*	Unit; ward (explain why the child is being transferred, and where.)
OR (or treatment room) table *People aren't supposed to get up on tables.*	A narrow bed
Take a picture (x-rays, CT, and MRI machines are far larger than a familiar camera, move differently, and don't yield a familiar end product.)	A picture of the inside of you. (Describe appearance, sounds, and movement of the equipment.)
Flush your IV. *Flush it down the toilet?*	Explain.
Harder	***Softer***
This part will hurt.	It (you) may feel (or feel very): sore, achy, scratchy, tight, snug, full or . . . (other descriptive term).
The medicine will burn.	Some children say they feel a very warm feeling.
The room will be very cold.	Some children say they feel very cool.
The medicine will taste (or smell) bad.	The medicine may taste (or smell) different than anything you have tasted before. After you take it, will you tell me how it was for you?
Cut, open you up, slice, make a hole	The doctor will make a small opening. (Use concrete comparisons, such as "your little finger" or "a paper clip" if the opening will indeed be small.)

Continued

TABLE 3-1

Considerations in Choosing Language (continued)

Potentiation Ambiguous	*Clearer*
As big as . . . (e.g., size of an incision or of a catheter)	Smaller than
As long as . . . (e.g., for duration of a procedure)	For less time than it takes you to
As much as . . .	Less than . . .
Potentially Unfamiliar	*Concrete Explanation*
Take your vitals	Measure your temperature; see how warm your body is; see how fast and strongly your heart is working (nothing is "taken" from the child)
Electrode, leads	Sticky like a bandage, with a small wet spot in the center, and small strings that attach to the snap (monitor electrodes). Paste like wet sand, with strings with tiny metal cups that stick to the paste (EEG electrodes). The paste washes off easily afterward; the strings go into a box that will make a picture of how your heart (or brain) is working. (Show child electrodes and leads before using. Let child handle them and apply them to a doll or to self.)
Intravenous; IV	Medicine that works best when it goes right into a vein (intravenous). It's the quickest way to help you get better. (First ask the child if she knows what a vein is, and why some medicine is okay to take by mouth and others work best into a vein. Explain concept of initials if child is old enough.)
Hang your (IV) medication	Bring in new medicine in a bag, and attach it to the little tube already in your arm. The needle goes into the tube, not into your arm, so you won't feel it.
NPO	Nothing to eat. Your stomach needs to be empty. (Explain why.) You can eat and drink again as soon as . . . (Explain with concrete descriptions.)
Anesthesia	The doctor will give you medicine—you may hear it called "anesthesia." It will help you go into a very deep sleep. You will not feel anything at all. The doctors know just the right amount of medicine to give you so you will stay asleep through your whole operation. When the operation is over, the doctor stops giving you that medicine and helps you wake up.
Incision	Small opening. (Follow with discussion of how cuts and scrapes received while playing have healed in the past.)
Hard Impact	*Softer Impact*
You will have to say good-bye to your parents.	That will be the time when you say, "See you later" to your parents.
Lots of children feel sick to their stomachs and throw up when they wake up.	Your stomach has also been asleep and resting. It may need time to wake up. As your stomach wakes up, you will slowly be able to drink, and then eat food again. Some children say they feel sick while their stomachs wake up; other children say they feel fine.
You will have a sore throat when you wake up.	Your throat may feel very dry when you wake up.
You are angry/scared/sad. That was very hard for you.	How was that for you? Was it the way you thought it would be, or harder or easier? Is there something else we should tell people about this?

From Gaynard, L., Wolfer, J., Goldberger, J., Thompson, R., Redburn, L., & Laidley, L. (1990). *Psychosocial care of children in hospitals: A clinical practice manual from the ACCH Child Life Research Project* (pp. 62–65). Bethesda: ACCH. Copyright 1990. Adapted by permission.

CHART 3-1 Facilitating Communication With Parents of Acutely Ill Children

- Use active listening techniques:
  - Convey a nonhurried demeanor and minimize interruptions.
  - Position self at same level when communicating (e.g., sit down).
  - Be aware of nonverbal messages conveyed in body stance and voice inflection.
  - Consider cultural background of parents when using some techniques (e.g., maintaining eye contact is considered disrespectful in many Asian cultures).
  - Clarify what you think you heard (e.g., "You are angry because the doctors did not talk with you this morning.").
  - Encourage and accept expression of feelings (use statements such as "This is a difficult time for you.").
  - Reflect parents statements (e.g., "You feel guilty because you didn't call the doctor sooner.").
  - Ask the parents specific questions about their needs (e.g., "Do you need to go get something to eat? I will sit with Sandy while you are gone.").
  - Do not take anger personally.
- Provide information:
  - Give honest, accurate information.
  - Use short, simple explanations.
  - Be tactful in stating information, but do not try to minimize the seriousness of a situation.
  - Avoid letting long periods of time pass without giving information, especially in critical situations, even if it is only to tell the parents that the child's condition has not changed and what is being done to support the child.
  - Volunteer information freely to promote trust.
  - Teach and reinforce knowledge of disease process, treatments, and how parents can support their child.
- Be consistent:
  - Give some information over time and by different health team members.
  - Minimize the number of health team members interacting with the parents.
- Reinforce importance of the parents' role:
  - Acknowledge parents' expertise in knowing their child.
  - Encourage and provide opportunities for parents to provide physical care for the child; parents may need to be shown how they can do this (e.g., demonstrate how to bathe a child who has an intravenous line).
  - Ensure parent involvement in care conferences.

CHART 3-2 Teaching Considerations With Children

Infant

Support and educate the primary caregivers.

Calm child so that parent can focus on teaching.

Monitor infant's nonverbal cues for response to stimulation.

Rely on the parent to interpret the infant's nonverbal cues.

Allow the infant to keep the parent in view.

Use pacifiers and blankets for security devices.

Let infant play with equipment (if safe) or have diversionary toys available.

Toddler

Toddlers have a short attention span (1 to 5 minutes); thus, present information in multiple ways.

Be concrete in verbal descriptions.

Use short terms and sentences.

Toddlers can have "magical" thinking; thus, cause-and-effect processes may not be rational.

Do not talk as if child were not there.

Be attentive to their nonverbal cues (e.g., frowning, stopping activity and attending).

Explain and describe numerous times what you are doing.

Use visual aids such as puppets and dolls.

Allow the toddler to handle instruments before you use them, when possible.

Demonstrate use of instrument on parent before using on child.

Encourage the parents to be present for interactions.

Preschool-aged child

Preschool-aged children have better verbal communication (3-year-old has 900-word vocabulary, 4-year-old 1,500 words, and 6-year-old has 2,100-word vocabulary).

Their cognitive skills are improved (increased concept of time, can count, knows days of week).

Continued

CHART 3-2 TEACHING CONSIDERATIONS WITH CHILDREN (CONTINUED)

Respect the preschooler's sense of modesty.

Ease fears by allowing the child to handle equipment.

Provide opportunities to ask questions.

Use visual aids such as dolls and puppets.

Encourage dramatic play.

Listen to their "stories" of the event and clarify magical thinking.

Preschool-aged children are unable to sit still for very long.

School-aged child

Allow time for composure and privacy.

Incorporate past experiences into teaching.

Explain purpose of your activities.

Give specific information about the body part you are assessing, or they may think something is wrong.

Use teaching aids such as dolls and diagrams.

Provide explanations of function of equipment.

Integrate the child into the teaching to increase self-care and child's responsibilities (this may be difficult for the parents to do!).

Give lots of praise.

Adolescent

Provide assurance of privacy and confidentiality.

Adolescents are very concerned about loss of control.

They are preoccupied with body image.

Provide some time away from the parent.

Respect the adolescent's privacy and opinions by not prying or being judgmental.

Although the adolescent is capable of abstraction, do not overestimate this capability.

Adolescents may act as if they do not care but are really paying very close attention.

They may want detailed information.

Provide diagrams and models to ensure comprehension.

experiences with the family must be shared with other staff to ensure continuity of care. In addition, other staff may be able to contribute positive and creative interventions that further enhance the child and family's teaching experience.

Finally, the teaching–learning experience must extend to those in the community who have ongoing contact with the family. Referrals to community services with education services may be needed. Consistency between what is taught in the acute care facility and how the procedure is completed in the home or at another facility must be monitored, with corrective action taken to ensure congruence between these environments.

CHAPTER

4

Promoting Coping During Hospitalization

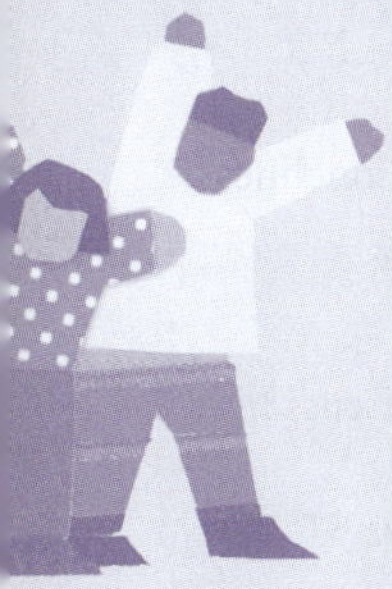

The Child's Response to Hospitalization

Children tend to respond to hospitalization with emotional upset. Seminal work by Prugh, Staub, Sands, Kirschbaum, and Lenihan (1953) revealed how children respond negatively to the stress of hospitalization, developing separation anxiety, unrealistic fears, and feelings of loss of control. These responses often manifest in withdrawal or aggressive behaviors, including crying, screaming, kicking, biting, hitting, physically resisting procedures, or ignoring requests.

Separation Anxiety

Hospitalized children between the ages of 6 months and 4 years are at the greatest risk for separation anxiety. Older children are still at risk, but increasing cognitive abilities and concept of time help them cope. Classic work by Robertson (1958) described the phases through which young children progress when separated from their parents:

- **Protest:** In this phase, the child searches for the lost parent, angrily protests, cries frequently, and rejects hospital staff. When the parent returns, the child readily goes to him or her.
- **Despair:** In this phase, the child becomes more sad and apathetic, mourning the lost parent but crying less and searching the environment less. They make few demands on their environment and those within it. When the parent returns, the child may not readily approach him or her or may cling to the parent.
- **Denial or Detachment:** In this phase, the child becomes cheerful, interested in the environment and new persons, and seemingly unaware of the lost parent (denial). The child is friendly with staff, and begins to develop superficial relationships (detachment).

caREminder

Because the child becomes increasingly "easier" to work with, it may be mistakenly interpreted that the child is coping effectively.

Children who progress to denial and detachment suffer long-term impaired parental relationships and impaired trust, which can lead to problems in establishment of close relationships, attention deficits, self-centeredness, and decreased intellectual functioning. Therefore the pediatric nurse must develop interventions that reduce separation anxiety (Table 4-1).

TABLE 4-1

Minimizing Separation Anxiety and Loss of Control

Age	Stresser	Intervention
Infant	Separation	Promote rooming-in of parents. Play peek-a-boo to promote mastery of the separation experience. Seek volunteer support for holding and stimulating the infant in the parent's absence. Provide tactile, auditory, and visual stimulation such as mobiles over the crib, cuddly toys, musical toys, or tape recordings. Minimize the number of caretakers; have consistent nurse assigned to care for the child. Provide comfort measures such as pacifier, holding, rocking, talking in a soothing voice, and cuddling.
	Loss of control	Use heparin lock intravenous device when possible. Use a crib with a canopy to allow freedom of movement in the crib. Alter the environment by using infant seat, buggy, or stroller and bringing the infant to playroom or nursing station when possible. Provide toys, such as stuffed animals, mirrors, and mobiles.
Toddler	Separation	Encourage rooming-in of parents. Teach parents to assess symptoms of stress, such as protest and withdrawal. Encourage parents to provide comfort measures. Play hide-and-seek with the child to promote mastery of the separation experience. Use doll-play to demonstrate that parents will return. Give the child time frames when parent will return: "after Sesame Street is over." Have parents bring in "transitional objects" from home to promote familiarity with the environment (e.g., favorite toys, clothes, tapes of family members' voices, photographs of family members, and pets).
	Loss of control	Promote home rituals, such as feeding and bedtime rituals. Promote dietary practices similar to those at home. Encourage autonomy by giving choices when possible, such as with toys or games. Take the child to the playroom. Provide an opportunity for medical play. Teach the parents that regression is a typical response to hospitalization and usually resolves when the child returns home.
Preschool-aged child	Separation	Use interventions for toddlers.
	Loss of control	Encourage autonomy by offering choices and participation in self-care. Take the child to the playroom. Urge the child to participate in medical and therapeutic play. Be truthful with the child.
School-aged child	Separation	Promote communication with siblings and friends. Maintain normalcy by encouraging the child to do homework from school. Be available to talk to the child. Be supportive when the child expresses feelings of loneliness. Take the child to the playroom. Explain to the parents the importance of frequent visits. Rooming-in is not necessary.
	Loss of control	Provide opportunities to discuss the medical situation. Encourage the child to discuss his or her understanding. Provide explanations of the medical situation, using diagrams, equipment, and concrete explanations. Allow opportunities for the child to achieve the developmental goal of "industry" by helping with tasks. Promote choices in care, if possible.
Adolescent	Separation	Promote peer interactions. Promote parent visitation. Teach parents the importance of the adolescent's need for control. Provide activities, such as "rap sessions," dances, and make-up sessions.
	Loss of control	Develop the plan of care with the adolescent. Respect the adolescent's need for independence. Offer choices in routines, if possible. Allow for privacy. Be open and forthright about the medical situation. Allow time to discuss this with the adolescent.

Separation anxiety is not unique to younger children. Although preschoolers exhibit fewer symptoms of restlessness, hyperactivity, and irritability, they do exhibit more somatic symptoms such as vomiting, urinary frequency, diarrhea, and dizziness.

School-aged children manifest anxiety but exhibit fewer panic reactions than younger children. Children of this age have a more developed concept of time and understand that parents need to leave and that parents will return. In addition, school-aged children are separated from their friends and school, which plays a major part in their psychosocial development. A school-aged child's anxiety is related to fear of the unknown or the unexplained, and his or her coping mechanisms usually include denial and rationalization.

Adolescents suffer separation anxiety when separated from peers rather than from parents, but it is still crucial that they are confident in their family's commitment to them. The adolescent's efforts to maintain peer contact may break hospital rules. For example, the adolescent may leave the hospital without permission, leave the unit after hours to meet peers in the lobby, use the telephone excessively (to the exclusion of participating in the hospital regimen), or refuse hospital treatments that are viewed as disfiguring or displeasing to peers.

To help prevent separation anxiety while a child is in the hospital, it is important to minimize separation of the child from his or her support systems. Allow open visitation and provide parents with the environment (e.g., sleep space, showers) and support (e.g., information, equipment) to facilitate their role as a member of the team caring for their child. Encourage friends and schoolmates to send cards, videotapes, and visit when appropriate. Bringing in transitional objects such as pictures of families and friends to put in the room can help to decrease the separation anxiety that may be felt.

Loss of Control

Hospitalized children commonly experience loss of control (Rennick, Johnston, Dougherty, Platt, & Ritchie, 2002). Unlike separation anxiety, which decreases as the child ages, control issues persist because the child is removed from the normal environment. Toddlers and preschoolers are at highest risk for loss of control. The toddler has just gained the ability to explore his or her environment. Developmental milestones such as potty training and self-feeding may be initiated or mastered. Hospitalization may interfere with the toddler's search for autonomy. A toddler who has a broken leg and is immobilized or has a peripheral IV line in her dominant hand may experience limitations if she has the ability to ambulate or feed herself. A previously potty-trained toddler who is limited to bed rest and receiving IV fluids may start having "accidents." This loss of control can be very stressful for the patient. Nurses can help alleviate this stress by allowing choices whenever possible. If the toddler is being potty trained at home, continue with the routine when hospitalized. Allow the child to feed and dress himself as much as possible. Keep the child on his home schedule and provide positive reinforcement when the child accomplishes tasks on his own.

Fears

General fears by developmental stage are important to keep in mind when children are hospitalized:

- Infants fear loud noises, sudden movements, and loss of physical and emotional support.
- Older infants fear separation, strangers, and heights.
- Toddlers fear the dark, being alone, animals, some machines, and draining tubs.
- Preschoolers fear mutilation, the unknown, the supernatural, and separation.
- School-aged children fear bodily injury, death, unsafe situations, loss of control, having a parent die, and school-related concerns.
- Adolescents fear loss of peer relationships, body disfigurement, loss of physical abilities, and death in the family.

Children who are ill or hospitalized can have more specific fears of intrusive procedures, body distortion, or mutilation. Needles and shots are often cited as what children fear most (Mahat, Scoloveno, & Cannella, 2004).

Many fears are actualized in the hospital: separation, loss of control, body mutilation, and painful events. Consider the child's fears during all interventions. Provide developmentally appropriate explanations to counter unrealistic fears and intervene to minimize trauma caused by those fears that are real (e.g., encourage parent presence during procedures or in the PACU, allow choices and have child make decisions whenever possible, use topical anesthetics and/or oral medications to reduce pain from needle sticks).

Enhancing Coping in the Hospitalized Child

The nurse must support the child in developing effective coping behaviors while in the hospital. Children use many different strategies to cope with the stress of illness, such as information seeking, social support, emotional behaviors, information limiting or avoiding, and physical exercise. This reinforces the need for individualized intervention. It is often thought that a well-prepared child copes better (Felder-Puig, Maksys, Noestlinger et al., 2003). When teaching, be alert to the child's cues indicating how much information is desired and prepare the child based on this.

To promote coping, teach the child strategies that can reduce stress, such as relaxation, imagery, distraction, and positive self-talk. Parent involvement also helps the child cope (Melnyk, Alpert-Gillis, Feinstein et al., 2004; Melnyk & Feinstein, 2001; Pelander & Leino-Kilpi, 2004).

Art

Children often reveal their fears and concerns through drawing. What children draw and how they draw it may be significant. For example, very large things may imply aggressive tendencies (often the healthcare team or equipment, such as needles, is large), whereas tiny things (the child in bed) may imply feelings of insignificance or inferiority. Based on knowledge of growth and development, the nurse can use drawings as an effective method of assessment and as a vehicle for communication with the child. In identifying the child's concerns and perceptions, the nurse can correct misconceptions and support coping skills. Use drawings for psychotherapy only if trained for such. Drawing materials are familiar to the child and nonthreatening and may support coping through distraction. Most children draw without prompting; some ask for guidance about what to draw. A broad nondirective response may help elicit issues of concern to the child (e.g., "Why don't you draw what it will be like after surgery?" or "Why don't you draw what you are thinking of right now?"). Remember, however, that not every drawing has therapeutic significance—sometimes a picture is just a picture!

Music

Music can also be used to promote coping (Chou, Wang, Chen, & Pai, 2003; Dunn, 2004; Lefevre, 2004). The child can select the music, giving him or her control over the situation and providing a familiar milieu and distraction. Honor the child's preference, although music that has a slow tempo (60 to 80 beats per minute) with low pitch at low volume is best for promoting relaxation and reducing tension (McCaffrey & Locsin, 2002). Vibroacoustic therapy, using the vibratory effects of music for relaxation, stress pain, and symptom relief, is an emerging therapy (Boyd-Brewer & McCaffrey, 2004).

Therapeutic Play

Play is one mechanism through which children cope, learn, test new ideas, and test newly acquired psychomotor skills. In other words, play is the medium through which children grow and develop. Play also provides children with a sense of control (Woon, 2004). Normative play, however, is different from therapeutic play. Normative play is activity in which children spontaneously engage and from which they derive pleasure. Therapeutic play is activity directed by the healthcare team to promote emotional and physical well-being such as playing with medical equipment during hospitalization. Therapeutic play can be used to promote coping by helping children work through hospital experiences. This may be effective for a number of reasons:

- It provides the child with information.
- The child feels a sense of control and mastery when able to manipulate the equipment and play situation.
- The nurse or child life specialist can use the session to model effective coping behaviors.

Unlike normative play, therapeutic play is goal directed. Nevertheless, both types of play should be provided in the hospital.

Although the terms often are used interchangeably, therapeutic play is different from play therapy. Play therapy is play that helps a child express and work through emotional or psychological issues. It is usually considered a form of psychotherapy that is supervised by a professional educated in play therapy methods. Play therapy may be directed by the therapist or by the child with the therapist guiding the session. Nurses and child life specialists most commonly guide children during therapeutic play sessions (Chart 4-1).

Conduct therapeutic play sessions in a protected nonthreatening environment (Chart 4-2). No treatments, doctors, or other distressing interruptions should be allowed during the play session. The healthcare professional guiding the session should be accepting of the child's play behaviors and avoid expressing approval or disapproval.

Therapeutic play includes instructional play, emotional outlet play, and physiologic-enhancing play. These types of play are always geared to the child's physical, emotional, and cognitive abilities. The nurse must incorporate play into the plan of care and value this time as essential to the child's development and emotional well-being. Do not force the child to play, however, if he or she is not emotionally or physically ready.

Child Life Programs

Child life programs became popular in the United States in the 1960s as a way to enhance family-centered care. These programs are designed to minimize stress for children and families during hospitalization and to promote the hospitalized child's continued growth and development. The American Academy of Pediatrics mandates that acute care pediatric services provide child life programs (Committee on Hospital Care, 2000).

To help the child cope successfully with hospitalization, child life programs organize interventions in the following categories:

- Preparation for hospitalization, procedures, and surgery
- Play
- Diversional activities during invasive painful procedures (e.g., lumbar punctures, IV line starts, bone marrow biopsy)
- Emotional support for parents and siblings
- Patient advocacy with hospital staff
- Promotion of family-centered environment

The child life specialist is responsible for designing and implementing interventions in each category that meet the needs of the patients and their families. To do this, child life specialists must be trained in child development and in techniques to address anxieties and fears regarding a child's condition, impending procedures, and hospitalization. Child life specialists also must be able to work in

CHART 4-1 MATERIALS/METHODS FOR USE IN THERAPEUTIC PLAY

Instructional Play

Purpose: To prepare the child for procedures or to learn about his or her disease.

- Dolls or stuffed animals dressed as doctors, nurses, children, and family members
- Hospital gowns and pajamas
- ID bracelets
- Surgical hats, masks, and booties
- Stethoscopes
- Blood pressure cuff, thermometers, and tape
- Large syringes without needles
- Bandages and dressing materials
- Equipment such as an IV pole, stretcher, and bed
- Oxygen masks
- Wash basin and towels
- Laboratory coats
- "Good Patient" stickers

Dramatic Play

Purpose: To allow the child to express anxiety or articulate fears about his or her disease or hospitalization.

- Punching bags
- Paints and crayons
- Inflatable bopper clowns
- Pegboard and hammers
- Dress-up clothes
- Puppets
- Blank books for writings stories or poetry
- Interactive video games
- Opportunities to play "doctor and nurse"
- Games such as peek-a-boo, hide-and-seek
- Sessions for telling "hospital stories"
- "Rap" groups
- Skits
- Song-writing sessions
- Water play
- Aggression play toys, such as blocks, clay, Play-Doh, punch pillows, squirt guns, and tin cans

Physiology Enhancing Play

Purpose: To allow the child to improve his or her physical health.

- Lung expansion—straw blowing, tuned bottle blowing, blowing bubbles, blowing up and popping paper bags, pinwheel spinning, kazoo or woodwind instrument playing
- Pain management—reading stories, pop-up books, telling jokes, playing musical tapes, playing video games
- Improve range of motion/muscle strength—leave toys just out of reach, take a doll on an airplane ride, arm wrestle, reach to hang up decorations, throw bean bags

an interdisciplinary setting so that therapeutic activities incorporate all aspects of care.

Because child life specialists are one of the few healthcare professionals who do not cause the child pain or discomfort, this specialist is often the one with whom the hospitalized child feels most comfortable. The child life specialist may become the primary healthcare professional to whom the child expresses feelings of anxiety, fears, and anger.

For hospitalizations that are longer than a few days, a teacher may be provided through the local school district or the child life program. Teachers provide programmed instruction and assist children in keeping current in the homework they would be completing if they were in school with other children.

Playroom

This distinctive area should be equipped to meet the unique, cultural, age-appropriate developmental needs of the population being served. Children and families should be encouraged to engage in activities there and should always feel welcome to enter.

caREminder

Any uncomfortable or painful procedures (such as an injection) should not be administered in the playroom itself. Children should feel that within the confines of this room, they are safe from intrusion and discomfort as much as possible.

To prevent the spread of infection in the playroom, follow standard precautions. Ensure that body fluids are not spread in the playroom. If a child's infectious secretions cannot be safely contained, do not permit that child in the playroom. To help minimize spread of infection, wash toys with soap and water or a 10% hypochlorite (chlorine bleach) solution after use (see Chapter 110). Also, follow the facility's guidelines for infection control in the playroom (Chart 4-3). Effective control is enhanced by consistent adherence to the policy. Toys brought from home can be contaminated with potentially dangerous bacteria and may provide unnecessary risks for nosocomial infection (Avila-Aguero, German, Paris, & Herrera, 2004). These toys must also be cleansed appropriately to prevent the spread of infections.

CHART 4-2 THERAPEUTIC PLAY

Definition: Purposeful and directive use of toys or other materials to assist children in communicating their perception and knowledge of their world and to help in gaining mastery of their environment

Activities:

Provide a quiet environment that is free from interruptions

Provide sufficient time to allow for effective play

Structure play session to facilitate desired outcome

Communicate the purpose of play session to child and parent

Discuss play activities with family

Set limits for therapeutic play session

Provide safe play equipment

Provide developmentally appropriate play equipment

Provide play equipment that stimulates creative, expressive play

Provide play equipment that stimulates role playing

Provide real or simulated hospital or medical equipment to encourage expression of knowledge and feelings about hospitalization, treatments, or illness

Supervise therapeutic play sessions

Encourage child to manipulate play equipment

Encourage child to share feelings, knowledge, and perceptions

Validate child's feelings expressed during the play session

Communicate acceptance of feelings, both positive and negative, expressed through play

Observe the child's use of play equipment

Monitor child's reactions and anxiety level throughout play session

Identify child's misconceptions or fears through comments made during (hospital role) play session

Continue play sessions on a regular basis to establish trust and reduce fear of unfamiliar equipment or treatments, as appropriate

Record observations made during play session

From McCloskey Dochterman, J., & Bulechek, G. M. (2004). *Nursing interventions classification (NIC)* (4th ed.). St. Louis: Mosby. Reprinted with permission.

Pet Therapy

Pet visitation or animal-assisted therapy involves the touching, holding, or cuddling of animals to promote therapeutic results (Hooker, Freeman, & Stewart, 2002). Pet visits distract children from the confines of their illness. Children can openly display affection and joy toward the pet. Pet visits also give children an opportunity to learn about animals. Organizations exist that provide trained animals expressly for this purpose. The animals need to be well cared for, with careful veterinary support and health screening (Chart 4-4) (Brodie, Biley, & Shewring, 2002). With the proper screening, the child's own animal may visit. If pet visitation is not possible, a videophone or use of videotapes may provide some comfort to the child while in the hospital.

PROMOTING COPING IN FAMILIES

Family coping skills are important factors to consider during a child's acute illness and hospitalization because families who face serious illness in a child (or family member) are at risk for psychosocial maladjustment (Melnyk et al., 2004). Families who use effective coping skills tend to adjust to the child's hospitalization and fare much better. Therefore, assess the family's coping skills, promote the use of effective skills, and teach additional skills if needed.

Family's Response to Hospitalization

Family members typically are affected by hospitalization based on their relationship to the child and their role in the family. Parents may exhibit responses that include fear, anxiety, helplessness, anger, and guilt. The parents' coping abilities may be reduced by financial, emotional, or work-related stressors and by the need to care for their other children as well as the hospitalized child (Board, 2004). In family-centered care, the nurse assesses the parents' response and provides intervention and support to help the family cope with the acute hospitalization of a child.

Siblings' coping skills can be affected by misperceptions about the sick child's condition and feelings of loss, parent neglect, isolation, or loneliness (Freeman, O'Dell, & Meola, 2003). The sibling may exhibit anxiety, depression, or acting-out behaviors. Difficulty in school and altered roles within the family may be apparent for the affected

CHART 4-3 INFECTION CONTROL FOR RECREATIONAL ACTIVITIES IN THE ACUTE CARE SETTING

All personnel and visitors must perform hand hygiene.
- Upon entering and leaving the unit
- When serving food to patients
- After assisting patients with toileting or diapering
- After blowing or wiping a patient's or own nose
- After removing gloves used for handling body fluids
- When leaving an isolation area or handling articles from that area
- When leaving the toilet

Prevent toys and equipment from becoming vectors for infectious agents by
- Not allowing stuffed or unwashable toys in the playroom
- Scrubbing all toys handled by infectious or drooling patients in warm soapy water and rinsing for at least 30 seconds with manual friction; spray with disinfectant, leave on surface for amount of time specified by manufacturer, rinse with water
- Wiping all nonsubmersible toys with cloth saturated with disinfectant, leave on surface for amount of time specified by manufacturer, wipe with water-moistened cloth

CHART 4-4 GUIDELINES FOR PET AND ANIMAL VISITATION

- Establish a mechanism for screening and approval of animals.
- Obtain parent's consent for the child to participate in the pet program.
- Ensure that the choice of animals complies with state and local health department regulations.
- Identify designated areas for animal visitation.
- Identify key personnel who will manage animals on location in the facility.
- Consult with the infectious disease or immunology department to determine patient restrictions regarding pet visitation.

sibling. Because pediatric care is family centered, the nurse must understand the effects of hospitalization on the patient and family and must intervene to promote effective coping by all family members.

Enhancing Coping for the Family

Parents

Parental coping is just as important as the child's coping during acute illness. Hospitalization of a seriously ill child can precipitate a crisis for the family. Parents report that the acute illness and subsequent hospitalization of a child leaves them feeling stressed, angry, uncertain, and as if they have no control (Dudley & Carr, 2004). Provide support to parents during this time. By providing appropriate information to parents about hospitalization, the nurse can reduce their anxiety during the child's hospital stay. By enhancing the parents' understanding of the child's illness, the nurse can promote their ability to cope with it. Including the parent as an active participant in developing the plan of care promotes an environment conducive to family-centered care.

Establishing rapport between parents and nurse results in more individualized care for the child. The degree of rapport is influenced by the nurse's knowledge of the child and the parent's knowledge of the nurse. The nurse's demonstration of interest in learning about the child as a person and the child's condition is important in establishing rapport (Espezel & Canam, 2003). Parents desire an interactive relationship with the healthcare providers caring for their child (Stratton, 2004). Parents need to understand and to be informed of treatments and procedures in simple terms they can understand. Having staff interact and communicate with the parent and child when providing care helps to create a sense of comfort and reassurance. Parents also have a need to "watch over" and protect their child by being with them throughout the hospitalization. In their role as "protector" of their child, having information may help them to maintain control.

Parents vary in their need for control during a child's hospitalization. One mother may regard a nurse's action (feeding the child, changing diapers) as an acceptable relinquishment of parental control. Another mother may see these actions as an indication that she is shirking her duty. Therefore, assess the parent's needs and preferences for participation in care and use this information when planning interventions to promote parent coping and satisfaction with care. Similarly, the nurse's expectations regarding parent participation in the child's care must be individualized and clearly discussed with the parent at the onset of the hospital stay.

Assisting the family in obtaining a temporary pager may enhance coping and satisfaction for children and families. Treatment of acute illness frequently involves waiting, which exacerbates anxiety and frustration. Having a pager may enable the child and family to leave the clinic or child's room to go to the cafeteria or playroom and return when paged. Having a pager also lets the parents run errands, eat, or just leave the room while the child sleeps, knowing they can be paged when the child awakens. In addition, parent coping can be enhanced by giving the unit phone number to a parent and encouraging the parent to call and speak to the nurse at any time when they are away from the hospital. These options allow the family choices that increase their control over their child's care and promote coping.

Siblings

Family-centered care also addresses the needs of siblings. Therefore, assess each sibling for risk factors that affect coping and signs of stress and ineffective coping. Children who perceive more changes in their parents' behavior and negative interpersonal effects on their lives often experience more adjustment problems (Murray, 2002). Siblings often may feel neglected or jealous of the attention that is being given to the ill sibling. The nurse can help facilitate the sibling's understanding of the illness. The sibling should be encouraged to visit and should be included in the plan of care. Social work and psychiatric consults may be necessary to help the sibling cope, especially in the case of life-threatening or terminal illnesses. Some hospitals have developed special play areas in the hospital for siblings of hospitalized children. These areas allow the sibling to visit the patient and provide a safe, nonthreatening, developmentally appropriate environment to play while the parents are with the patient. In addition, child life therapists are available to work with the siblings to help them cope with the acute hospitalization of a sibling.

KidKare Ask the siblings how they believe things are different since the child has been sick or in the hospital. Early identification of those children at high risk enables the nurse to arrange intervention and follow-up with the primary healthcare provider (Small, 2002).

Parent perceptions of effects of illness on the siblings have not been found to correlate with siblings' self-report; therefore, it is more accurate to obtain information directly from the sibling (Guite, Lobato, Kao, & Plante, 2004). On the basis of assessment findings, implement interventions to promote sibling coping. Research indicates that siblings find emotional support (e.g., empathy, encouragement, caring) and instrumental support (e.g., direct help, material aid) to be most helpful in adjusting to having a brother or sister with cancer (Murray, 2002). Encourage parents to include siblings in activities and conversations and to inform siblings of what is happening and teach them about their sibling's condition. Ideally, the routine for siblings is disturbed as little as possible, and they are able to play with their friends.

Visitation and Family Participation

Patients and families come from diverse cultural and socioeconomic backgrounds and have varying expectations of their hospital experience. Guidelines that define how the hospital can meet the family's visitation needs can serve as a useful communication tool. Guidelines can also maintain infection control and safety standards and enhance the family's satisfaction with the facility.

Parent Visitation

Separation of hospitalized children from their parents adds to the difficulty of adjusting to hospitalization. Often parental presence and participation at the bedside is a source of conflict between the family and nurse. Conflicts arise over who may visit, the number of visitors, visiting hours, and inconsistent enforcement of the policies (Griffin, 2003).

True family-centered care views parents as partners in care, not as visitors. The liberalization of visiting hours generates resistance from many healthcare team members, primarily physicians and nurses, based on several concerns, including increased physiologic stress on the child, interference with ability to provide care, and physical and emotional exhaustion of the family members. Empirical evidence through research, however, has demonstrated just the opposite.

Fortunately, the proponents of liberalized family visitation policies have had some influence (Browne, Sanchéz, Langlois, & Smith, 2004). Today, most facilities that care for children have 24-hour open visitation for parents and grandparents (Bradley, 2001). This policy encourages parents and grandparents to participate in their child's care and to room-in when possible. If parents cannot be present to support the child in person, it should not be assumed they do not care or are "bad" parents. Encourage parent participation in the child's care to the extent possible, and encourage the participation of significant others.

If parents are reluctant to visit because the child cries and protests when they leave, explain that this is a normal response to separation. If parents are absent as a result of work, sibling care, or other responsibilities, reinforce that the child will be attended to in their absence. Provide the family with the name and telephone number of a contact person knowledgeable about the child; the nurse can also initiate regular telephone contact with the family. When appropriate, assist the child in calling home. Assisting the family with logistics (e.g., handouts regarding hospital visitation policies and support services; transportation, meal, and lodging assistance) may help to increase visitation.

Sibling Visitation

Another aspect of family visitation is sibling visits. Sibling visitation is an important aspect of meeting the developmental needs of the hospitalized child and the sibling. The benefits from sibling visitation are multiple, but probably the most important is that seeing brothers and sisters helps normalize hospitalization for the patient, especially a child with a condition that requires a prolonged stay, such as cancer or certain traumatic injuries. For prolonged hospitalizations, videophones can play a key role in supplementing sibling visitation to promote increased contact between siblings on an ongoing basis. Sibling visitation also promotes adaptation of the sibling to the situation. It easily dispels misconceptions the sibling may have about the hospitalized child, such as things are "worse" than reported or the child is dead. It helps reduce separation anxiety that affects siblings when parents spend time at the hospital. Sibling visitation also promotes effective coping for the siblings at home because it provides opportunities for nurses to intervene directly, educate, allay fears, and promote a realistic understanding of the situation. Finally, it eases the strain on parents, who often face conflict between being in the hospital and supervising the children at home.

Chaos can be reduced by controlling the hours for sibling visitation and limiting the number of people who visit a child at any one time. Although sibling visitation has not been shown to be related to greater cross-infection (Roland, Russell, Richards, & Sullivan, 2001), screening siblings for infectious symptoms or exposures may protect vulnerable patients and their visitors. This type of screening can limit potential exposures to varicella (chickenpox), measles, and respiratory syncytial virus.

Support Groups

Parents usually find it helpful to discuss concerns about their ill child with other parents who have similar experiences (Mohr, 2003; Ritchie, Stewart, Ellerton et al., 2000). To facilitate this, the nurse can introduce parents to each other or refer them to a specific support group. Many types of support groups exist, ranging from disease-specific support groups to support groups for siblings, grandparents, or others. However, available groups vary from region to region. Internet support groups are rapidly evolving and have the potential to be a powerful support tool as more families become computer literate (Baum, 2004).

The unit-based support group is a particular type of support group. It is especially useful during hospitalization because it can provide a brief escape from the stress of the hospital environment. In this support group, parents can discuss their immediate concerns about hospitalization. The presence of other parents makes it easier to discuss issues that parents may have difficulty addressing individually with a staff member. These support groups usually are led by a professional, such as a pediatric nurse, child life specialist, or social worker. The group leader must have an understanding of group theory and excellent communication skills.

Having a hospital staff member lead the group helps parents solve problems that they identify in the group such as displeasure with routines or concern over a child's behavior. In a support group for an infant special care unit, for example, the support group may be led by the unit-based social worker and a translator, if needed, to provide a means for families to better understand hospitalization and vent their frustrations with it. Each week, a member of a different discipline attends the support group so parents can discuss specific questions with that representative. This type of group helps parents feel like part of the team.

EDUCATION TO SUPPORT THE CHILD AND FAMILY

Before providing information, the nurse must determine the learning needs of the child and family. Throughout the initial interview, the nurse collects data about their physical and psychosocial needs. Then the nurse analyzes the data to determine whether the child and family understand the situation. By identifying knowledge deficits on admission, the nurse can plan effective teaching strategies that address parents' and family's deficits and promote coping.

Learning needs are affected by many factors, including prior experience with illness, cultural background, language skills, the patient's and family's educational levels, and the patient's developmental level. An educational plan must address factors to meet the patient's and family's information needs.

Patient teaching may be classified in several ways. The nurse may teach individuals or groups. The acute care nurse commonly teaches about diseases, preoperative care, procedures or treatments, prescribed medications, prescribed diet, prescribed activity, and psychomotor skills. Sometimes a teaching plan incorporates several of these topics.

The process of patient teaching resembles the nursing process. Teaching begins with assessment of the problem and of readiness to learn. Then it progresses to development of a plan, implementation of the plan, and evaluation of its effectiveness. During the assessment step, the nurse should determine the learner's cultural background and establish a rapport, especially when the nurse and learner come from different cultures.

To promote positive patient outcomes, the nurse must adopt education strategies that enhance learning readiness and facilitate effective learning. Providing effective patient and family education has long been a professional practice standard. Because failure to teach essential information regarding healthcare and maintenance has recently become grounds for lawsuits, effective education now is also a legal requirement for nurses.

Hospital Tours

Whenever possible, patients and families (or prospective patients and their families) should have an opportunity to tour the acute care setting (Chart 4-5). It is especially useful before hospital admission or surgery. A successful perioperative tour can create a positive impression of the surgical experience and defuse a potentially threatening event for the child and family. It lets the child and family

CHART 4-5 GUIDELINES FOR CONDUCTING A HOSPITAL TOUR

- Keep groups small—about 10 children per group.
- Conduct the tour for 20 to 30 minutes depending on the children's attention span. The nurse or child life specialist conducting the tour should have time dedicated for the tour with no interruptions.
- Encourage parents to join the tour.
- Present the tour in a non-threatening environment, such as the hospital playroom, school classroom, or child's home.
- When unable to actually tour the site (e.g., emergency on unit, presenting at a school), use an indirect method of presenting the hospital tour, such as a puppet, film, or slide show.
- Present the tour and explanations at the child's developmental level.
- Avoid dwelling on unpleasant or threatening events or intrusive procedures.
- Give the child and parents an opportunity to ask questions.
- Give the children an opportunity for therapeutic play, using dolls and hospital equipment.
- Give the children something to take home to remind them of the hospital tour, such as a coloring book, mask, or head cover.
- Encourage parents to discuss the tour afterward with the child and clarify any concerns they may have.

meet the care providers and other staff members and to become accustomed to the environment.

If an older child is especially anxious about surgery, the facility may arrange for a tour through an operating room that is not in use, a preoperative area, and a PACU. If the child is to be admitted to the PICU after surgery, a tour of this area may be warranted. The perioperative nurse can make the tour more child friendly by using a large doll or stuffed animal to help demonstrate machinery that the child will encounter. A child may be reassured to see a teddy bear on the operating table "have a special sleep for surgery" and then "wake up" to be hugged. Explain the purposes of hospital pajamas, masks, caps, shoe covers, and gloves, and let the child try them on. Let the child hear the beeps of an electrocardiograph (ECG) machine and feel the stickiness of the ECG pads, place a pulse oximeter probe on the child's fingers or toes, put a blood pressure cuff on the child, or let the child listen to his or her own heartbeat through a stethoscope.

If the facility cannot provide tours of the operating room, substitute a photograph album, slide show, or a videotape presentation of a tour. No matter what form the tour takes, presenting a certificate to the children upon completion of the tour gives them a concrete reminder.

Some facilities have taken the hospital tour to the local community. In this outreach program, healthcare personnel use a videotape and discussion to present the hospital tour to schools and other community organizations. These presentations also act as marketing tools, enhancing the image of the hospital or surgery center to potential patients.

SUMMARY

The acute care setting is a busy and noisy environment, full of unexpected and often unpleasant events for the child and family. Anxiety, fear, pain, discomfort, surprise, separation, loss, fatigue, frustration, mistrust, and anger are common experiences for the child and family during the illness episode. It is the responsibility of all members of the healthcare team to be aware of and sensitive to these general problems. The well-trained professional can make assessments and design interventions to enhance family function and reduce the trauma associated with interactions during the acute care experience. The use of therapeutic play, playroom activities, school activities, hospital tours, and support groups can all provide creative measures to guide the child and family toward a positive beneficial experience.

Bibliography

Avila-Aguero, M. L., German, G., Paris, M. M., & Herrera, J. F. (2004). Toys in a pediatric hospital: Are they a bacterial source? *American Journal of Infection Control, 32*, 287–290.

Baum, L. S. (2004). Internet parent support groups for primary parents of a child with special healthcare needs. *Pediatric Nursing, 30*, 381–390, 401.

Board, R. (2004). Father stress during a child's critical care hospitalization. *Journal of Pediatric Healthcare, 18*, 244–249.

Boyd-Brewer, C., & McCaffrey, R. (2004). Vibroacoustic sound therapy improves pain management and more. *Holistic Nursing Practice, 18*, 111–119.

Bradley, S. (2001). Suffer the little children. The influence of nurses and parents in the evolution of open visiting in children's wards 1940–1970. *International History of Nursing Journal, 6*(2), 44–51.

Brodie, S. J., Biley, F. C., & Shewring, M. (2002). An exploration of the potential risks associated with using pet therapy in healthcare settings. *Journal of Clinical Nursing, 11*, 444–456.

Browne, J. V., Sanchéz, E., Langlois, A., & Smith, S. (2004). From visitation policies to family participation guidelines in the NICU: The experience of the Colorado Consortium of Intensive Care Nurseries. *Neonatal, Paediatric & Child Health Nursing*, 7(2), 16–23.

Chou, L. L., Wang, R. H., Chen, S. J., & Pai, L. (2003). Effects of music therapy on oxygen saturation in premature infants receiving endotracheal suctioning. *Journal of Nursing Research, 11*, 209–216.

Committee on Hospital Care, American Academy of Pediatrics. (2000). Child life services. *Pediatrics, 106*, 1156–1159.

Dudley, S. A., & Carr, J. M. (2004). Vigilance: The experience of parents staying at the bedside of hospitalized children. *Journal of Pediatric Nursing, 19,* 267–275.

Dunn, K. (2004). Music and the reduction of post-operative pain. *Nursing Standard, 18*(36), 33–39.

Espezel, H. J. E., & Canam, C. J. (2003). Parent–nurse interactions: Care of hospitalized children. *Journal of Advanced Nursing, 44,* 34–41.

Felder-Puig, R., Maksys, A., Noestlinger, C., et al. (2003). Using a children's book to prepare children and parents for elective ENT surgery: Results of a randomized clinical trial. *International Journal of Pediatric Otorhinolaryngology, 67,* 35–41.

Finkelhor, D., & Ormrod, R. (2002). *Kidnapping of juveniles: Patterns from NIBRS.* OJJDP Bulletin. Washington, DC: U.S. Department of Justice, Office of Justice Programs, Office of Juvenile Justice and Delinquency Prevention.

Freeman, K., O'Dell, C., & Meola, C. (2003). Childhood brain tumors: Children's and siblings' concerns regarding the diagnosis and phase of illness. *Journal of Pediatric Oncology Nursing, 20,* 133–140.

Griffin, T. (2003). Facing challenges of family centered care I: Conflicts over visitation. *Pediatric Nursing, 29,* 135–137.

Guite, J., Lobato, D., Kao, B., & Plante, W. (2004). Discordance between sibling and parent reports of the impact of chronic illness and disability on siblings. *Children's Healthcare, 33,* 77–92.

Hooker, S. D., Freeman, L. H., & Stewart, P. (2002). Pet therapy research: A historical review. *Holistic Nursing Practice, 16,* 17–23.

Lefevre, M. (2004). Playing with sound: The therapeutic use of music in direct work with children. *Child & Family Social Work, 9,* 333–341.

Mahat, G., Scoloveno, M. A., & Cannella, B. (2004). Comparison of children's fears of medical experiences across two cultures. *Journal of Pediatric Healthcare, 18,* 302–307.

McCaffrey, R., & Locsin, R. C. (2002). Music listening as a nursing intervention: A symphony of practice. *Holistic Nursing Practice, 16,* 70–77.

McCarthy, E. J. (2004). Malignant hyperthermia: Pathophysiology, clinical presentation, and treatment. *AACN Clinical Issues, 15,* 231–237.

Melnyk, B. M., Alpert-Gillis, L., Feinstein, N. F., et al. (2004). Creating opportunities for parent empowerment: Program effects on the mental health/coping outcomes of critically ill young children and their mothers. *Pediatrics, 113,* e597–e607.

Melnyk, B. M., & Feinstein, N. F. (2001). Mediating functions of maternal anxiety and participation in care on young children's posthospital adjustment. *Research in Nursing & Health, 24,* 18–26.

Melnyk, B. M., Small, L., & Carno, M. A. (2004). The effectiveness of parent focused interventions in improving coping/mental health outcomes of critically ill children and their parents: An evidence base to guide clinical practice. *Pediatric Nursing 30*(2), 143–149.

Mohr, W. K. (2003). The substance of a support group. *Western Journal of Nursing Research, 25,* 676–692.

Murray, J. S. (2002). A qualitative exploration of psychosocial support for siblings of children with cancer. *Journal of Pediatric Nursing, 17,* 327–337.

Pelander, T., & Leino-Kilpi, H. (2004). Quality in pediatric nursing care: Children's expectations. *Issues in Comprehensive Pediatric Nursing, 27,* 139–151.

Prugh, D., Staub, E., Sands, H., Kirschbaum, R., & Lenihan, E. (1953). A study of the emotional reactions of children and families to hospitalization and illness. *American Journal of Orthopsychiatry, 23*(1), 80–106.

Rennick, J. E., Johnston, C. C., Dougherty, G., Platt, R., & Ritchie, J. A. (2002). Children's psychological responses after critical illness and exposure to invasive technology. *Journal of Developmental and Behavioral Pediatrics, 23,* 133–144.

Ritchie, J., Stewart, M., Ellerton, M., et al. (2000). Parents' perceptions of the impact of a telephone support group intervention. *Journal of Family Nursing, 6*(1), 25–45.

Robertson, J. (1958). *Young children in hospitals.* London: Tavistock.

Roland, P., Russell, J., Richards, K. C., & Sullivan, S. C. (2001). Visitation in critical care: Processes and outcomes of a performance improvement initiative. *Journal of Nursing Care Quality, 15*(2), 26–34.

Small, L. (2002). Early predictors of poor coping outcomes in children following intensive care hospitalization and stressful medical encounters. *Pediatric Nursing, 28*(4), 339–340.

Stratton, K. M. (2004). Parents' experiences of their child's care during hospitalization. *Journal of Cultural Diversity, 11*(1), 4–11.

Woon, R. (2004). Hospital play therapy: Helping children cope with hospitalization through therapeutic play. *Singapore Nursing Journal, 31,* 16–19.

CHAPTER

5

Principles of Fluid and Nutritional Management

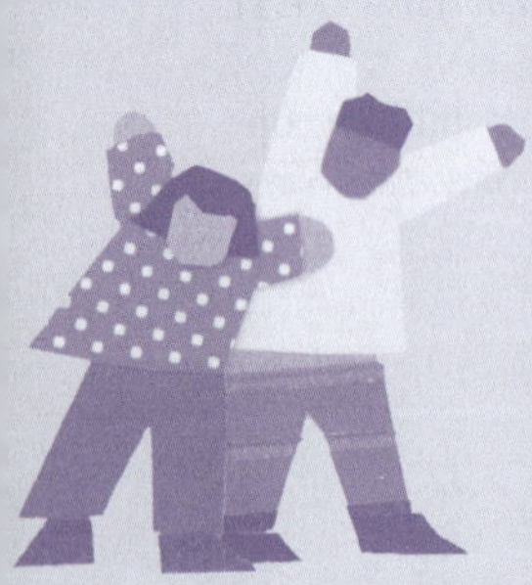

FLUIDS

Total Body Water

Water is an important solvent in the body and represents a large percentage of body weight in term infants (75%) and an even larger percentage of weight in preterm infants. In the first year of life, total body water decreases to about 60%. The percentage of total body water (TBW) to body weight remains at 60% for males but decreases to 50% for females with puberty. TBW is composed of two main components: intracellular fluid (ICF) and extracellular fluid (ECF). The fetus and newborn have a larger ECF than ICF volume. This changes with the ICF volume increasing and the ICF-to-ECF volume ratio reaching adult levels by 1 year of age (i.e., ECF is 20% to 25% of body weight compared with ICF at 30% to 40% of body weight).

The body seeks to maintain a steady state in the regulation of body water. Body water is provided through the intake of fluids and the oxidation of carbohydrates, fats, and protein. Thirst stimulates the intake of water. The kidneys, lungs, skin, and gastrointestinal tract excrete body water. Antidiuretic hormone (ADH) and renal tubular cell response to ADH are the two major mechanisms that affect renal water loss (Greenbaum, 2004).

Calculation of Fluid Requirements

The maintenance of fluid balance and correcting imbalances are important in pediatric patients. The nurse should be familiar with the formulas used to calculate fluid requirements in infants and children to verify that the correct amount is ordered and administered.

Maintenance fluids can be calculated using a formula based on body weight (in kilograms):

Weight	Fluid per Day
0–10 kg	100 mL/kg/day
11–20 kg	1,000 mL + 50 mL/kg for each kg >10 kg
>20 kg	1,500 mL + 20 mL/kg for each kg > 20 kg*

(*Maximum total fluids are normally 2,400 mL per day.)

A quick method to calculate approximate hourly rate per kilogram weight for maintenance fluid needs is as follows:

Kilogram Weight	Approximate Hourly Rate
0–10 kg	4 mL/kg/hr
10–20 kg	40 mL/hr + 2 mL/kg/hr × (wt–10 kg)
>20 kg	60 mL/hr + 1 mL/kg/hr × (wt–20 kg)*

(*Maximum rate of fluids per hour is 100 mL.)

To illustrate how this formula is used, here are two examples:

- A 13-kg child would need 1,000 mL + (50 mL × 3 = 150 mL) = 1,150 mL per day, or 47.9 or 48 mL per hour. Using the quick method for calculation of hourly rate, it is 40 mL + (2 mL × 3 = 6), or 46 mL per hour.
- A 36.5-kg child would need 1,500 mL + (20 mL × 16.5 = 330) = 1,830 mL per day, or 76.25 mL per hour. Using the quick method for calculation of hourly rate, it is 60 mL + (1 mL × 16.5), or 76.5 mL per hour.

Water is normally lost through urine, insensible loss (skin and lungs), and stool. Maintenance needs may be decreased or increased based on clinical situations. Examples of situations causing increased needs are fever, burns, tachypnea, tracheostomy, diarrhea, vomiting, nasal gastric suction, polyuria, and third space losses (shifts of fluids from intravascular space to interstitial space). Oliguria, anuria, and hypothyroidism are associated with decreased maintenance needs.

Loss of Body Weight Due to Dehydration

Clinical signs of dehydration depend on the severity of fluid loss and type of dehydration. Level of dehydration is typically classified as mild, moderate, or severe. Table 5-1 provides an outline for the clinical evaluation of dehydration. Fluid loss can be calculated based on the child's weight. Divide the weight when dehydrated by weight when healthy and calculate the percent change; then calculate the amount lost by subtracting from 100%. For example, the child's weight when healthy is 4.5 kg and current weight is 4.1 kg; divide 4.1 by 4.5 = 0.91 = 91% of healthy weight; 100 – 91 = 9% weight loss.

Quick restoration of circulatory volume is critical for infants and children who are severely dehydrated (10% to 15% dehydration estimate). In these instances, fluid imbalance must be quickly corrected. Fluid boluses of 20 mL/kg of isotonic solution (e.g., 0.9% normal saline or Ringer's lactate) over 20 minutes intravenously is used to restore circulatory volume (Greenbaum, 2004). The child with severe dehydration may need multiple fluid boluses of normal saline at a faster rate. Such boluses should be given as rapidly as possible and repeated until there are signs of improvement in circulation, such as warm skin, improved capillary refill time, and restored urine output. Reassess the child's status after each fluid bolus. Watch for signs of renal or cardiac failure while administering fluid boluses.

In selected situations, blood or colloid solutions (5% albumin, plasma, or synthetic colloids [e.g., Hetastarch, dextran]) may be used for fluid bolusing. Red blood cell

TABLE 5-1

Clinical Manifestations of Dehydration

Loss of Body Weight (%)	Clinical Manifestations	Severity
3–5	Slightly dry mucous membranes Increased thirst Decreased urine output Normal or slightly increased pulse	Mild
7–10	Tachycardia Decreased skin turgor Sunken eyes and fontanel Oliguria Poor tear production and dry mucous membranes Restless, irritable to lethargic Delayed capillary refill Cool and pale	Moderate
10–15	Rapid, weak pulse Low blood pressure Anuric Very sunken eyes and fontanel No tears, parched mucus membranes, and tenting of skin Very delayed capillary refill Lethargic to comatose	Severe

transfusions may be administered to trauma victims when signs of shock or hemodynamic instability persist despite administration of 40 to 60 mL/kg of isotonic crystalloid solution (Hazinski et al., 2002). Colloids may be used to improve fluid volume, but more research is needed to support improved outcomes. In meta-analyses that included large cross-sections of patients (children and adults), improved outcomes with colloid administration were demonstrated (Vincent, Navickis, & Wilkes, 2004), whereas others did not demonstrate improved outcomes (Roberts, Alderson, Bunn et al., 2004).

Children who are dehydrated must have their fluid and electrolyte deficits replaced and maintenance fluid needs met. The classification of dehydration based on serum sodium concentration is important in estimating water deficits. Type of dehydration and serum sodium levels is as follows:

Type	Sodium Level
Isotonic	130–150 mEq/L
Hypotonic	<130 mEq/L
Hypertonic	>150 mEq/L

Most children have isotonic dehydration. The fluid management of severe isotonic dehydration is done in a stepped approach, as outlined below.

1. Intravascular volume is restored.
   a. Receives 20 mL/kg of normal saline bolus(es) over 20 minutes or less until intravascular volume is restored.
2. Determine 24-hour water needs.
   a. Calculate maintenance water needs per kg PLUS deficit water.
3. Determine 24-hour electrolyte needs.
   a. Calculate maintenance sodium and potassium.
   b. Calculate deficit sodium and potassium.
4. Deliver appropriate fluid based on water and electrolyte needs as above.
   a. Administer ½ calculated fluid in the first 8 hours after amount delivered as bolus(es) is subtracted.
   b. Administer the remainder fluid (second ½) over the next 16 hours.

The appropriate fluid for a child with isotonic dehydration is generally D_5 ½ normal saline with 20 mEq/KCl. Children weighing 10–20 kg with only mild dehydration typically only need D_5 ¼ normal saline. The management of the child with hyponatremic dehydration is generally the same as for the child with isotonic dehydration.

Alert! *Hypernatremic dehydration is a dangerous situation and puts the child at risk for neurologic hemorrhages and thrombosis. It requires a slower correction of the fluid deficit, usually over 48 to 72 hours. Rapid correction of hypernatremic dehydration can cause rapid fluid shifts, leading to cerebral edema.*

Electrolyte replacement is calculated and determines the amount of sodium and potassium that is ordered.

caREminder

Do not add KCl until the child voids or until the serum potassium level is determined. Dehydration can be associated with acute renal failure and hyperkalemia. Carefully monitor electrolytes because children with significant dehydration are at risk for disturbances in sodium and potassium levels as well as acid–base balance.

Factors That Affect Maintenance Fluid Requirements

Factors that cause alterations in maintenance fluid requirements include the following:

Factor	Fluid Needs
Fever	Increased
Hyperventilation	Increased
Sweating	Increased
Hyperthyroidism	Variable—may be increased
Renal failure	Maintenance fluids equal to insensible losses (limit to 400 mL/m^2/24 hr) plus mL per mL of urine replacement (100% of urine replacement)

Principles of Oral Rehydration

Oral rehydration is an acceptable method to replace fluid loss and deliver maintenance fluids in selected children with vomiting and diarrhea (Burns, Dunn, Brady, Starr, & Blosser, 2004; Spandorfer, Alessandrini, Joffe, Localio, & Shaw, 2005). Diarrhea can lead to large losses of water and electrolytes and is associated with isotonic dehydration in most patients. Mild to moderate diarrheal dehydration can be treated in most children with simple oral solutions of glucose-electrolytes (e.g., World Health Organization oral rehydration salts; Rehydralyte [Ross Products, Abbott Laboratories]) and adequate supervision. For children who are vomiting, oral rehydration solutions (ORS) should begin after 1 to 2 hours of the child or infant having nothing by mouth. Key considerations in oral rehydration therapy include the following:

- Administer appropriate solution to provide replacement of needed sugars and electrolytes as ordered by the physician.
- For oral rehydration divide the total volume deficit by 4 and aim to deliver this volume of fluid during each of the 4 hours of the rehydration phase. The following amounts of ORS are generally ordered, depending on amount of fluid deficit:
  - 50 to 60 mL/kg—MILD dehydration (approximately 12 mL/kg/hr)

- 80 to 100 mL/kg—MODERATE dehydration (approximately 20 to 25 mL/kg/hr)
- PLUS (for both mild and moderate dehydrate) an additional 10 mL/kg for each diarrheal stool and 5 mL/kg for each episode of vomiting

- Begin rehydration with small amounts of the prescribed rehydration solution.
- For children younger than 2 years, give 120 mL; for children older than 2 years, give 120 mL to 240 mL slowly every hour, divided into small amounts every 15 to 20 minutes.
- If vomiting occurs, give 5 to 10 mL every few minutes until vomiting stops and then greater amounts as above; repeat unless emesis consistently occurs in amounts that exceed intake. A teaspoon or 5-mL syringe can be used for the initial administration of fluid, especially if the child is vomiting. Administer at least 5 mL of solution each minute (5mL × 60 = 300 mL). In a 10-kg infant equivalent this is equivalent to 30 mL/kg. Children larger than 15 to 20 kg can receive 10 mL per minute.

Alert! *Maintenance solutions with lower sodium concentrations (e.g., Pedialyte, Infalyte) should not be used as rehydrating solutions. Decrease ORS intake if the child appears to be well hydrated or shows signs of fluid overload.*

- Begin feeding immediately after rehydration. Give infants their regular full-strength formula. If this is not tolerated, the physician may switch the child to a lactose-free formula. Breast-fed infants should resume breastfeeding after rehydration with shorter duration and more frequent feedings. Maintenance therapy of 100 mL of ORS/kg/24 hr should be started until diarrhea stops (American Academy of Pediatrics [AAP], 2004; Greenbaum, 2004).
- Avoid solids for 4 to 6 hours and then reintroduce age-appropriate bland solids slowly and as tolerated.

NUTRITION

Energy Needs

The energy needs of children vary depending on age and other conditions. Nutrients (carbohydrates, proteins, and fats) and minerals and vitamins are needed for growth and tissue repair. The energy content of food is referred to as its kilocalorie (kcal) value. Estimated energy requirements are based on basic body metabolism, growth, and activity. The average kilocalorie requirements for children up to age 3 years are as follows (Burns et al., 2004; Butte, Cobb, Dwyer et al., 2004):

Age	Formula
0–3 months	(89 × weight {kg} – 100) + 175
4–6 months	(89 × weight {kg} – 100) + 56
7–12 months	(89 × weight {kg} – 100) + 22
13–35 months	(89 × weight {kg} – 100) + 20

An adequate nutritional intake should result in increased weight, height, and head circumference (Burns et al., 2004). (See Tables 5-2 and 5-3.)

TABLE 5-2

Normal Expected Weight Gain

Infant	Average Weekly Increase
0–3 months	210 g (8 oz)
3–6 months	140 g (5 oz)
6–12 months	85–105 g (3–4 oz)
Age Group	**Average Yearly Increase**
Toddler (1–3 years)	2–3 kg (4.4–6.6 lb)
Preschooler (3–6 years)	2 kg (4.4 lb)
School-aged (6–12 years)	3–3.5 kg (7 lb)

TABLE 5-3

Normal Expected Increase in Height

Infant	Average Monthly Increase
0–3 months	3.5 cm
3–6 months	2.0 cm
6–12 months	1.2–1.5 cm
Age Group	**Average Yearly Gain**
Toddler (1–3 years)	12 cm
Preschooler (3–6 years)	3–7 cm
School-aged (6–12 years)	6 cm
Age	**Normal Expected Increase in Head Circumference**
0–3 months	2 cm/mo
4–6 months	1 cm/mo
7–12 months	0.5 cm/mo

Plot weight, height, and head circumference as well as body mass index on Centers for Disease Control and Prevention growth grid charts to best follow the child's trajectory of growth. There are some commonly used and easy to remember general rules of weight gain. Infants generally double their birth weight by 4 to 6 months of life, triple their birth weight, and double their length by 12 months of age. The following formula can be used as a rough estimate of a child's weight based on age (Behrman, Kliegman, & Jenson, 2004):

Age	Weight in Kilograms
3–12 months	{age (months) + 9} divided by 2
1–6 years	{age (years) × 2 plus 8} divided by 2
7–12 years	{age (years) × 7 minus 5} divided by 2

A child whose body mass index is greater than the 85th percentile is considered at risk of being overweight; if the body mass index is greater than the 95th percentile, the child is considered overweight (Kavey, Daniels, Lauer et al., 2003).

Infant Feedings: Number and Volume Ingested

Chapter 43 addresses infant feeding issues such as breast-feeding and bottle-feeding techniques. Nurses frequently are asked questions about how many feedings during the day are appropriate for the normal infant and how much is typically ingested at each feeding. Infants do vary, and there is no established firm number of feedings or amount per feeding. The typical feeding pattern of breast milk or formula seen in infants is shown in Chart 5-1 (Behrman et al., 2004).

Breast-fed infants generally nurse 8 to 12 times per day in the first few weeks of life. Some infants even nurse 12 or more times. Avoid feeding intervals longer than 4 hours. After 2 weeks of age, the breast-fed infant should gain weight at a minimum rate of 20 g/day (AAP, 2004). Breast-fed infants feed more frequently than formula-fed infants, who may go 4 hours between feedings. Preterm or weak infants need more frequent feedings, often feeding every 2 to 3 hours for the first 1 or 2 months until they experience catch-up growth.

Introduction of Solid Foods

Solid foods should not be introduced sooner than 4 to 6 months of age. Earlier introduction of solids neither promotes sleeping through the night nor enhances the health of infants, and it may contribute to development of food allergies. Key points to consider when introducing solid foods are as follows:

- Use a small spoon with a long handle and rubber coating at the feeding tip that fits into the infant's mouth. It is easier for the infant to close their lips around this spoon size, and the rubber coatings helps to avoid hurting the infant with the sharp edge of a spoon.
- Food should be thin textured, not thick, to help the infant transition from a liquid diet to solids, and so it is easier for the infant to move it to the back of their throat.
- Offer rice cereal as the first solid with enough breast milk or formula to make it like thin gravy.
- Begin first feedings slowly and place a small amount of cereal in the middle portion of the infant's tongue; increase the amount and thickness of the cereal as the infant becomes used to it.
- Next, offer vegetables or fruits. Infants often prefer fruits, so it is recommended to start vegetables first so they get used to the taste before the sweeter fruits. Then, proceed to meats.
- Start with 1 to 2 teaspoons of the new food (a single-ingredient food) after the infant has mastered cereal.
- Offer new foods once a day until the infant gets accustomed to the food and wait 3 to 5 days before introducing another new food.
- Pureed vegetables should be started by at least 7 months of age.
- Pureed meats can be added by about 6 months of age.
- Avoid allergic foods for the first 12 months (e.g., wheat, nuts, egg whites, citrus, soybeans, peanuts, shellfish, strawberries, chocolate, and cow milk).

Remember to tell parents that young infants often initially push food out with their tongues until they master swallowing solids.

Establishing Healthy Nutritional Habits

Educate parents about the importance of establishing healthy nutritional habits from infancy that continue into early childhood and adolescence.

Infants and Toddlers

- Breast milk is the ideal food for infants and should be continued as long as mother and infant desire.
- Iron-fortified food cereals and formula are good sources of iron for the infant. The iron in breast milk is more bioavailable; hence, iron supplements are not needed in most breast-fed infants.
- Fat intake should not be restricted in children younger than 2 years of age; children over the age of 2 years need

CHART 5-1 TYPICAL INFANT FEEDING PATTERN FOR BREAST MILK OR FORMULA

Age	Average Number of Feedings per 24 Hours	Average Amount of Formula or Breast Milk per Feeding (mL)
By the end of the first wk	6–9	60–90
2 wk	6–8	60–90
3–4 wk	6–8	120–150
1–2 mo	5–6	120–150
2–3 mo	5–6	150–180
3–4 mo	4–5	180–210
5–7 mo	3–5	210–240
8–9 mo	3–4	210–240
10–12 mo	3	210–240

about 30% (maximum) to 20% of their calories from dietary fat for neural development (Burns et al., 2004).

- Early introduction of cow milk (before 12 months of age) and excessive cow milk intake in young children are associated with iron-deficiency anemia.
- Whole milk is recommended for children between the ages of 12 and 24 months.
- Cow milk intake should be restricted to 24 ounces per day (range, 16 to 24 ounces/day), and the intake of iron-rich foods should be encouraged.
- Start self-feeding at about 7 to 8 months of age (e.g., finger foods such as chopped pieces of ripe banana, dry unsweetened cereal, crackers); by 24 months of age, most children can feed themselves their entire meal.
- Hand-held foods need to be cut into small pieces (less than ¼ inch).
- Educate parents not to give foods that present a choking hazard (e.g., chunks of cheese, meat, peanut butter, hot dogs, whole grapes, nuts, seeds, potatoes, cherry tomatoes, raw fruits or vegetables, popcorn, hard or sticky candy, and raw carrots).
- The older infant can be given a spoon at about 10 to 12 months of age.
- Introduce a cup at 6 months of age to familiarize the child with it, not as the sole method of feeding. As the child masters cup drinking, discontinue bottle feedings by 9 to 12 months of age.
- Limit juice intake to avoid inadequate calcium intake, diarrhea, tooth decay, obesity, and failure to thrive associated with apple and pear juice consumption. If juice is given to infants younger than 1 year of age, limit to 4 to 6 ounces per day of white grape juice, which is better absorbed by infants, and offer from a cup not a bottle, which may limit the volume consumed. Do not give juice before age 6 months (AAP, 2001).

Preschool-Aged Children

- A variety of nutritious foods should be presented to the preschool-aged child.
- Appetite fluctuations are common in this age group, as are eating jags (i.e., child will only eat a few favorite foods for extended periods of time).
- The need for a children's multivitamin should be considered if the child has very limited food choices or is a picky eater.
- Most children 2 to 6 years of age need a snack or two in addition to three regular daily meals

School-Aged Children

- Variations in eating patterns that are associated with growth spurts and activity levels are common.
- Nutritious snacks need to be encouraged for children in this age group because they tend to skip meals if engrossed in favorite activities.
- Obesity is a growing problem in this age group. Be watchful for signs of obesity due to overeating, lack of exercise, and poor nutritional choices (high-fat, high-calorie, low-nutrient foods).
- Calcium supplements should be used if nutritional intake (e.g., milk and dairy products) does not meet recommended standards for calcium needs. Children ages 9 to 18 need 1,300 milligrams of calcium daily.

Adolescents

- High-energy intake is needed to support rapid growth.
- Erratic eating patterns, skipping meals, and poor nutritional choices are common problems.
- Body image distortions may lead to binge eating or anorexia nervosa.
- Poor eating habits and rapid growth place the adolescent at risk for iron, vitamin, and mineral deficiencies, and supplementation may be needed.

Food Guide Pyramid

The food guide pyramid (available at http://www.mypyramid.gov) is a useful tool to demonstrate healthy eating habits. It is designed to provide individualized guidance for intake based on age, gender, and level of physical activity. The pyramid emphasizes the five major food groups and can be used as a guide in the selection of foods so that important nutrients are part of a child's daily food intake. Fats and sweets should be used sparingly. Table 5-4 gives general recommendations for food group intake based on age and gender.

COMMON NUTRITIONAL ISSUES

Iron and Vitamin D Supplementation

Children between the ages of 6 months and 4 years and menstruating females are at greatest risk for iron-deficiency anemia, a major nutritional problem in these age groups. Supplemental iron is needed to treat iron-deficiency anemia. Therapy is directed at increasing the intake of iron-rich foods, eating a well-balanced diet, and administering supplemental iron.

> **Alert!** *Instruct parents to store iron supplements out of reach of children and to reinforce that they are medicine, not candy, because some preparations look like candy.*

Principles of iron supplementation therapy are as follows:

- Administer with water or juices high in vitamin C between meals for maximum absorption.
- Administer with food if gastrointestinal upset occurs.
- Do not administer with milk or milk products. Cereals, tea, and eggs also decrease absorption.

TABLE 5-4

Recommended Daily Intake per Food Group*

Age	Grain	Vegetable	Fruit	Milk	Meat and Beans
2–3 yr	3-ounce equivalents	1 cup	1 cup	2 cups	2-ounce equivalents
4–8 yr	4- to 5-ounce equivalents	1½ cups	1 to 1½ cups	2 cups	3- to 4-ounce equivalents
Girls 9–13 yr	5-ounce equivalents	2 cups	1½ cups	3 cups	5-ounce equivalents
Girls 14–18 yr	6-ounce equivalents	2½ cups	1½ cups	3 cups	5-ounce equivalents
Boys 9–13 yr	6-ounce equivalents	2½ cups	1½ cups	3 cups	5-ounce equivalents
Boys 14–18 yr	7-ounce equivalents	3 cups	2 cups	3 cups	6-ounce equivalents

*Information from U.S. Department of Agriculture (USDA). (2005). *Steps to a healthier you.* Retrieved September 4, 2005, from http://www.mypyramid.gov/

- Avoid contact of liquid iron preparations with the teeth because liquid iron temporarily stains enamel—use a straw or squirt medication in the back of the throat, avoiding the teeth.
- Continue treatment for 3 to 4 months after hemoglobin returns to normal levels so that iron stores can be replaced.
- Note that iron may color stools black and urine black or dark.
- Dosing is as follows:
  - For severe iron-deficiency anemia, 4 to 6 mg elemental iron/kg/day divided into three equally divided doses
  - For mild to moderate iron-deficiency anemia, 3 mg elemental iron/kg/day in one to two doses

To prevent rickets due to inadequate vitamin D intake and decreased exposure to sunlight, 200 IU of vitamin D per day is recommended for all infants, children, and adolescents. Exclusively breast-fed infants should be supplemented with a minimum intake of 200 IU of vitamin D per day beginning within the first 2 months of life (Gartner & Greer, 2003). Formula-fed infants consuming less than 500 mL per day of vitamin D–fortified formula and children and teens who do not get regular sunlight exposure or drink less than 500 mL of vitamin D–fortified milk need to take a multivitamin supplement with at least 200 IU of vitamin D (AAP, 2004).

Fat

Fats or their metabolic products are important components of cellular membranes, are needed sources of energy, insulate against changes in body temperature, and serve as the vehicle to transport fat-soluble vitamins. Because of the association with fat intake and cholesterol levels and the establishment of adult coronary artery disease in early childhood, healthy nutritional habits related to the intake of fat in childhood and adolescence are advocated. Parents and health providers should follow the American Heart Association guidelines for cardiovascular health promotion in all children and adolescents, which recommends unrestricted fat intake before 2 years of age and after age 2, limitation of foods high in saturated fats (<10% of calories/day), cholesterol (<300 mg/day), and *trans*-fatty acids. Between ages 2 and 5 years, a child should eat a fat-modified diet (less than 30% of total energy from fats). A child considered at risk for hypercholesterolemia should have a fasting lipid level measured after age 2 years. Criteria for children at risk include

- Family history of dyslipidemia;
- Incomplete or unavailable family history;
- Family (parents, grandparents, aunts and uncles) history of premature heart disease at age 55 years for men and age 65 for women (Kavey et al., 2003).

Guidelines have been established for monitoring cholesterol levels in at-risk children (Chart 5-2).

Acceptable low-density lipid cholesterol levels are less than 110 mg/dl. Levels between 110 and 130 mg/dl are borderline, and levels higher than 130 mg/dl are considered elevated. Triglyceride levels greater than the 95% for age may be a marker for some genetic forms of hyperlipidemia, even if cholesterol levels are normal. Treatment for hyperlipidemia is directed at dietary management with pharmacologic intervention in children aged 10 years or older, after a 6-month to 1-year trial of diet therapy (Burns et al., 2004).

CHART 5-2 Guidelines for Monitoring Cholesterol Levels in At-Risk Children

Fasting Cholesterol Level	Management
>170 mg/dL	Is borderline: no intervention, with follow-up in 5 years
>200 mg/dL	Is elevated: remeasure and average the two; if average is more than 170 mg/dL, a fasting lipid panel is done

CHART 5-3 RECOMMENDED DAILY ELEMENTAL CALCIUM INTAKE

Age	Recommended Daily Elemental Calcium Intake
0–6 mo	210 mg
7–12 mo	270 mg
1–3 yr	500 mg
4–8 yr	800 mg
9–18 yr	1,300 mg

Calcium

Calcium intake is important for bone mineralization, with requirements for dietary calcium intake remaining high until 25 years of age. The National Academy of Science recommends the daily amounts of elemental calcium shown in Chart 5-3 (Burns et al., 2004).

Dietary sources that are high in calcium should be part of the daily diet throughout childhood and adolescence. Children and adolescents whose diet is deficient in calcium should receive calcium supplements.

Vegetarian

Vegetarian diets are popular among teenagers. "Vegans" eat only foods of plant origins: vegetables, fruits, grains, nuts, seeds, and legumes. Lactovegetarians and ovovegetarians eat plant foods plus milk or eggs, respectively. A vegetarian diet, especially the lactovegetarian and ovovegetarian diet, can provide all necessary nutrients if vegetables are selected from different classes. However, strict vegans may have difficulty meeting protein and nutrient needs. A high incidence of vitamin B_{12} deficiency has been reported in children who are strict vegetarians. They may also become deficient in trace minerals because of the high fiber intake associated with vegan diets. To avoid such nutritional deficiencies, the child must consume plant-based proteins that complement each other and together provide a complete protein. The nutritional status of these children needs to be carefully monitored, and education about a healthy diet is essential (Dunham & Kollar, 2006).

PARENTERAL NUTRITION

Parenteral nutrition (PN) is used to deliver calories and nutrients to children who are malnourished or unable to ingest or receive enteral feeding to meet their metabolic needs for growth and repair of tissues. Chapter 84 discusses common procedures essential to the administration of PN in pediatric patients and principles of care.

PN solutions contain amino acids, glucose, electrolytes, and other additives as ordered by the prescriber and are delivered through a central or peripheral catheter. Placement of a central line is necessary to deliver solutions of greater concentrations in smaller fluid volumes than is possible using a peripheral intravenous line. Solutions that are greater than a 10% concentration of dextrose or have a protein concentration of greater than 5%, pH less than 5 or greater than 9, and an osmolality greater than 600 mOsm/L must be delivered through central infusion (Infusion Nurses Society, 2006). Infiltration of PN solution into cutaneous tissue can cause tissue sloughing and necrosis. Thus, when a peripheral line is used to deliver PN, the site must be closely and vigilantly monitored.

Careful attention to strict aseptic technique is critical when priming and maintaining intravenous lines. Prevention of microbial contamination of intravenous lines, the PN solution, and catheter access site or tubing is important because of the added risk for sepsis associated with the delivery of PN to patients. In addition, many children receiving PN also have underlying conditions that predispose them to sepsis. Likewise, monitoring electrolytes, glucose, acid–base balance, and other key indices of organ (liver and kidney) integrity is critical to determine the integrity of metabolic and organ functioning.

The prescriber ordering PN determines the child's daily nutritional requirements for calories and fluid needs. About 10% to 16% of caloric needs are provided through amino acids in either a standardized or specialized mixture (i.e., generally 1.5 to 2.5 g/kg/day of protein in an older child). Children with renal or hepatic failure are exceptions to this rule because they require lower amounts of protein. In contrast, some children have greater protein requirements, such as those with severe burns, head trauma, or sepsis (Taketomo, Hodding, & Kraus, 2004).

Most children receive a fluid maintenance level of 1,500 mL/m^2/day; requirements for preterm or very-low-birth-weight infants may vary. Caloric requirements that will be met by glucose are carefully calculated. When administering PN through a central line, glucose concentrates are begun at 10% to 12.5% and slowly advanced every day as tolerated, usually to a total of 20% to 2% dextrose solution. The rate at which the PN solution is administered must be constant; there are standards to determine the maximum amount of dextrose that should be given per kilogram of body weight per minute. Neonates are particularly sensitive to hyperglycemia and hypoglycemia if dextrose rates exceed recommended amounts per minute. When prescribing other additives, the prescriber calculates these amounts based on established guidelines for daily replacement of electrolytes, vitamins, trace elements, and minerals. Adequate amounts of calcium and phosphate are important for optimal bone mineralization especially in neonates on long-term PN.

Fatty emulsion is often ordered to provide essential fatty acids for growth and is a source of nonprotein calories. It is administered through a Y connecter in separate tubing along with the dextrose–amino acid solution over

24 hours or at a rate no greater than 0.15 to 0.2 g/kg/hr (e.g., for overnight infusions).

The nurse is closely involved in monitoring pediatric patients receiving PN. Suggested guidelines for monitoring key parameters in a hospitalized child are as follows (Taketomo et al., 2004):

Parameter	Frequency
Weight	Daily
Height and length	Weekly
Intake	Hourly (with 8- and 24-hour totals)
Output	Hourly—if catheterized and unstable—to every 8 hours or every void
Urine glucose	Twice daily
Urine specific gravity	As indicated

Blood levels are monitored for key features. Monitoring frequency depends on the condition of the patient and whether the patient is initially receiving PN or on maintenance therapy. The following is a guide to how frequently blood levels are tested for key factors:

Parameter	Initial	Maintenance
Electrolytes	Daily	1–2 weeks
Acid–base status	Until stable	As indicated
Blood urea nitrogen	Daily	Weekly
Creatinine	Daily	Weekly
Serum glucose	Daily (and as needed)	Weekly
Albumin/prealbumin	Weekly	Weekly
Triglycerides	Daily	Weekly
Liver function	Weekly	Weekly
Bilirubin (direct)	Weekly	As indicated
Complete blood count/ differential	Weekly	Weekly
Platelets, prothrombin time/partial thromboplastin time	Weekly	As indicated

ENTERAL NUTRITION

There are several key issues for the pediatric nurse to consider when administering specialized enteral feedings through access devices such as tubes, catheters, or stomas. Generally, neonates who are very low birth weight (<1,500 g) or low birth weight (<2,500 g) are considered at nutritional risk and often receive parental nutrition and progress to tube feedings before breast or nipple feeding. Similarly, children with various medical conditions may need to receive specialized nutritional support through enteral devices as part of their management plan.

The child may receive enteral feedings that are manufactured as either standard formulas or specialized formulations made up for an individualized patient. Key points to consider when administering enteral feedings through access devices are as follows:

- Identify the correct feeding for the child.
  - Label special formulations with the child's name, medical record number, product name, strength, volume, and expiration date and time.
  - Label enteral feeding "for enteral use only."
  - Check the label of the feeding formula with the patient's order for correct formula and route before administration.
  - Verify the child's identity by comparing name on the feeding with child's identification band and any other patient identifier required by the institution.
- Store feeding formulations as specified in the directions (i.e., refrigerated or at room temperature).
- Identify the length of time for administration (volume and rate) as part of the physician's order or per hospital enteral feeding protocol.
- Identify whether an enteral feeding pump is to be used for delivery.
- Maintain the cleanliness (and safety) of accessory equipment and formula and avoid contamination of materials (e.g., tubing, bag, any containers, syringes) by appropriate cleaning and regular replacement of such devices when old or contaminated. There should be a hospital protocol that addresses these issues.
- Use gloves as appropriate and follow hand hygiene considerations (Standard Precautions).
- Check for compatibility of medications with enteral feedings to avoid precipitation or tubing occlusion.
- Carefully label enteral feeding tubing and intravenous or central line tubing to avoid mixing up of lines and accidental administration of medications into the incorrect line.
- Follow timelines for removal or replacement of a new nasogastric or orogastric tubing per hospital protocol.
- Flush the tubing with the volume of water it takes to clear the tubing and the child's fluid needs or restrictions per medical order or hospital written protocol, which depends on tubing capacity.
- Monitor the child for adverse effects and clinical changes and document amount of intake, tolerance of the procedure, presence of vomiting or diarrhea, urine output, and daily weight.

The American Society for Parenteral and Enteral Nutrition has published standards of care for hospitalized pediatric patients receiving parenteral and enteral feedings (2005). Chapters 38, 39, and 42 contain additional information about the procedures to follow for inserting tubes, checking for placement, venting of tubes, and other issues related to enteral feedings.

SPECIAL DIETS

The nurse should be aware of special dietary and feeding considerations that are associated with nutritional prob-

TABLE 5-5

Feeding Considerations for Specific Medical Conditions

Medical Condition/Disease	Potential Dietary and Feeding Considerations
Cerebral palsy, neuromuscular degenerative diseases, or high spinal cord injuries	If spasticity, hypotonia, dysphagia, and/or aspiration concerns, may need enteral access devices, mechanical soft or pureed diet, adaptive spoons; careful attention to positioning to minimize chances of aspiration
Cystic fibrosis	Increased percentage of total dietary calories needed from both protein (15% to 20%) and fat (40% to 50%) categories Salt tables if excessive sweat, exercise, or fever Vitamin, mineral, and pancreatic enzyme supplements Gastrostomy feedings and/or parental nutrition may be needed
Gastroesophageal reflux	Feed infant in slightly upright position (10 to 20 degrees) Thickened formula if bottle-feeding Burp frequently
Cleft lip or palate	Semiupright (60 to 90 degrees) Adaptive nipples if bottle-feeding Burp frequently May need tube or gavage feeding if severe cleft

lems. Table 5-5 contains information about feeding and dietary considerations that need to be made for children with common diseases or conditions.

Bibliography

American Academy of Pediatrics. (2001). The use and misuse of fruit juice in pediatrics. *Pediatrics, 107,* 1210–1213.

American Academy of Pediatrics. (2004). *Pediatric nutrition handbook* (5th ed.). Elk Grove Village, IL: Author.

American Society for Parenteral and Enteral Nutrition. (2005). Standards for specialized nutrition support: Hospitalized pediatric patients. *Nutrition in Clinical Practice, 20,* 103–116.

Behrman, R. E., Kliegman, R. M., & Jenson, H. B. (Eds.). (2004). *Nelson textbook of pediatrics* (17th ed.). Philadelphia: W. B. Saunders.

Burns, C. E., Dunn, A. M., Brady, M. A., Starr, N. B., & Blosser, C. G. (Eds.). (2004). *Pediatric primary care: A handbook for nurse practitioners* (3rd ed.). Philadelphia: W. B. Saunders.

Butte, N., Cobb, K. Dwyer, J., et al. (2004). The start healthy feeding guidelines for infants and toddlers. *Journal of the American Dietetic Association, 104,* 442–454.

Dunham, L., & Kollar, L. M. (2006). Vegetarian eating for children and adolescents. *Journal of Pediatric Health Care, 20,* 27–34.

Gartner, L. M., Greer, F. R., & Section on Breastfeeding and Committee on Nutrition. (2003). Prevention of rickets and vitamin D deficiency: New guidelines for vitamin D intake. *Pediatrics, 111,* 908–910.

Greenbaum, L. (2004). Pathophysiology of body fluids and fluid therapy. In R. E. Behrman, J. M. Kliegman, & H. B. Jenson (Eds.), *Nelson textbook of pediatrics* (17th ed., pp. 190–252). Philadelphia: W. B. Saunders.

Hazinski, M. F., Zaritsky, A. L., Nadkarni, V. M., et al. (Eds.). (2002). *PALS provider manual.* Dallas, TX: American Heart Association.

Infusion Nurses Society. (2006). Infusion nursing: Standards of practice. *Journal of Infusion Nursing, 29*(1S), S1–S92.

Kavey, R. E., Daniels, S. R., Lauer, R. M., et al. (2003). American Heart Association Guidelines for primary prevention of atherosclerotic cardiovascular disease beginning in childhood. *Circulation, 107,* 1562–1566.

Roberts, I., Alderson, P., Bunn, F., et al. (2004). Colloids versus crystalloids for fluid resuscitation in critically ill patients. *The Cochrane Database of Systematic Reviews, 4,* No. CD000567.

Spandorfer, P. R., Alessandrini, E. A., Joffe, M. D., Localio, R., & Shaw, K. N. (2005). Oral versus intravenous rehydration of moderately dehydrated children: a randomized, controlled trial. *Pediatrics, 115,* 295–301.

Taketomo, C. K., Hodding, J. H., & Kraus, D. M. (2004). *Pediatric dosage handbook* (11th ed.). Hudson, OH: Lexi-Comp Inc.

Vincent, J. L., Navickis, R. J., & Wilkes, M. M. (2004). Morbidity in hospitalized patients receiving human albumin: a meta-analysis of randomized, controlled trials. *Critical Care Medicine, 32,* 2029–2038.

CHAPTER

6

Principles of Pharmacologic Management

Medication administration is one of the most challenging and critical aspects of pediatric nursing. Unlike adult medication administration, in which a "one-dose-fits-all" principle generally applies, pediatric dosing must be individualized. Pediatric medication administration must focus on age-related developmental considerations because the pharmacokinetic and pharmacodynamic drug effects are less predictable in children, especially in preterm and young infants because of their much smaller size and their organ system immaturity. Therefore, close monitoring is important. Likewise, safe administration of the right dose to the right patient at the right time through the right route is a critical issue because children are at highest risk for medication errors and are a group more vulnerable to potential side effects and overdose. Ensuring safe administration of medication is a multidisciplinary responsibility that involves the physician, pharmacist, and nurse who serve as a check and balance team. Education of nurses is a key element to ensure reliable administration of medications. This is particularly true for those nurses who administer medications that present a heightened risk of causing significant patient harm when used incorrectly.

Developmental Considerations in Pharmacokinetics and Pharmacodynamics

Children can vary greatly, from the 500-g (1.1-lb) premature newborn infant to the 100-kg (220.5-lb) overweight teenager. Thus, size and age are key factors that affect the child's ability to handle the absorption, distribution, metabolism, and elimination of drugs. For instance, although neonates are born with all the enzymes necessary for drug metabolism, only 10% to 40% of these enzymes have the ability to adequately metabolize drugs compared with that of the adult. Renal elimination of drugs in the neonate is also less efficient and takes several years to reach adult capacity, although liver function reaches adult capacity and exceeds it within the first several months of age. The age of a child is one of the most influential variables in understanding the four pharmacokinetic functions of absorption, distribution, metabolism, and elimination/excretions of drugs; this calls for differing dosages for neonates (preterm and term), infants, and young children (Mitchell, 2001; Reed & Gal, 2004). Chart 6-1 lists key developmental issues related to pharmacokinetics and the route of administration. All four pharmacokinetic functions are important considerations in the choice of medications and selecting dosages that can be safely prescribed for a child.

CHART 6-1 DEVELOPMENTAL PHARMACOKINETICS

Factors That Affect Absorption of Drugs

1. Gastrointestinal
   Gastric pH is high in neonates, with adult values by 2 years of age. Acidic drugs are more bioavailable; basic drugs have decreased bioavailability.
   Gastric and intestinal motility (transit time) is decreased in neonates and infants but increased in older infants and children.
   The bile acid pool and biliary function are diminished in the newborn and reach full capacity over the first several months of life.
2. Rectal
   Only selected drugs are suitable for rectal administration. In addition, length of exposure to the rectal mucosa affects absorption.
3. Intramuscular
   Variable in the pediatric age group secondary to (a) blood flow and vasomotor instabilities, (b) insufficient muscle tone and contraction, and (c) decreased muscle oxygenation.
4. Percutaneous
   Decreased with increased thickness of the stratum corneum and directly related to skin hydration
   Neonates and infants have increased skin permeability, allowing greater penetration of medication and a greater surface area–to–body weight ratio with potential for toxicity.
5. Intraocular
   The membranes of infants and neonates are particularly thin; ophthalmic eye medications can cause systemic effects in infants and young children.

Factors That Affect Distribution

1. Neonates have a higher proportion of total body water that rapidly reduces during the first year of life. Adult values are gradually reached by 12 years of age. This factor is an important consideration related to the water solubility of a drug.
2. Children have a lower proportion of body fat than do adults.
3. Protein binding of drugs is age dependent. Total protein concentration at birth is only 80% of adult values, which leads to more free or active drug circulation and potential for toxicity.
4. Fetal albumin in the newborn period has limited drug-binding ability.
5. An immature blood-brain barrier during the newborn period can lead to higher concentrations of drugs in the brain than at other ages.

Factors That Affect Metabolism

1. The newborn's enzymatic microsomal system is less effective.
2. Liver maturation varies among individuals; each liver enzyme becomes functional at a different rate.

Factors That Affect Elimination

1. Glomerular filtration and tubular secretion are reduced at birth.
2. There is gradual increase in renal function, with adult values reached the first 1–2 years of life.

A related concern is the mother who is breast-feeding and taking medications or herbs and whether there is the potential for harm to the infant. Certain drugs are contraindicated with breast-feeding because of their adverse effect on the developing infant. The American Academy of Pediatrics' website (www.aap.org) has information about such contraindicated drugs. Other medications may be taken by the mother with instructions about how soon before or after breast-feeding she may take the drug, taking the drug before the infant's longest sleep period, and, if necessary, the need to temporarily withhold breast-feeding. Hale's *Medications and Mother's Milk* (2004) is an excellent resource on this topic. It is also important to consider herbal supplements because they may have one or two main ingredients but may contain many other chemicals not identified on the label. Mothers often assume that herbs are natural and thus safe when breast-feeding. The Organization of Teratology Information Services (http://www.otispregnancy.org) has information on medications and herbal agents in its databases. Nurses must be aware of these issues when caring for an infant who is receiving breast milk and educate mothers about the safe use of medications and herbal teas or supplements.

THE SIX RIGHTS

The Right Medication

Selection of a medication is based on the child's need for pharmacologic therapy and the ability of the child's body to handle the drug; that is, to absorb, distribute, metabolize, and eliminate the drug. Many of the medications prescribed for pediatric patients do not have U.S. Food and Drug Administration (FDA) approval for use in pediatric patients; this practice is known as off-label use. Physicians use pediatric pharmacologic reference sources to prescribe these off-label medications and ask pediatric nurses to administer these medications. With the enactment of the

FDA's Pediatric Studies rule in 1998, new drugs that seek FDA approval and are likely to be used in children must include labeling information for pediatric use.

The nurse's responsibility in administering "the right medication" should be viewed as a multistep process. The nurse must know the indications for the medication prescribed and its potential side effects and must be knowledgeable about the child's medical illness, disease, or condition. Thus, if an unusual, unlikely, or contraindicated medication is prescribed for a pediatric patient, the nurse must clarify the order. For example, an order to give trimethoprim-sulfamethoxazole (Bactrim) to a child with a known sulfa allergy should alert the nurse to address this issue with the practitioner who prescribed the medication. Ensure that all allergies to medication are clearly visible on the patient chart, all order forms, and on the medication administration record (MAR). On a busy pediatric unit, charts of patients with the same last name can be confused, and medication orders may be written for the wrong patient. An order for furosemide (Lasix) prescribed for Mary Smith could inadvertently be written as an order in Margaret Smith's chart.

The nurse must also properly identify the medication sent from the pharmacy or taken from the patient's medication drawer with the patient's MAR. This is another step in the verification process to ensure that the correct medication is administered. Check the expiration date. Do not use expired medications; return them to the pharmacy and order a replacement medication. To reduce the chance that the wrong medication is administered, amber-coated syringes are often used as an added safeguard to help differentiate oral medications from intravenous (IV) medications that are dispensed in clear syringes from the pharmacy.

To administer the right medication, the nurse should do the following:

- Know the medication to be administered: its indication for use, action, contraindications, and side effects.
- Understand the connection between the patient's condition, illness, or disease and the use of a particular medication. If such a linkage is not present, clarify the medication order.
- Select the correct medication from the patient's medication drawer or from medications sent to the unit from the pharmacy.
- Verify the medication label with the patient's MAR. A triple verification of labels with the MAR can help to prevent medication identification errors. Check the label when first obtaining the drug, when preparing the dose, and when returning the container to the patient's medication box or discarding it.

The Right Dose

There are two "rights" in dosing. Prescribing the correct dose for the child is the first right, and dispensing the correct dose is the second.

Prescribing the Correct Dose

The nurse is responsible for knowing that the prescribed dose of medication is within safe dosage range. In pediatrics, dosages are calculated using body weight or body surface area (BSA).

To verify the right dose using body weight, look up the established standard dose from a pediatric reference and multiply the child's weight in kilograms to see whether the dose ordered is correct. For example, if the reference dose is 10 to 20 mg/kg per 24 hours divided every 6 hours and the child's weight is 10 kg, the child should receive 100 to 200 mg per 24 hours, or 25 to 50 mg every 6 hours. Compare the actual order to verify that it is within the recommended range.

A reverse calculation can also be done starting with the original order. For example, the order says to give 250 mg every 6 hours for a child weighing 10 kg. Multiply 250 mg times 4 (every 6 hours is four times a day) to find the total daily dose, which in this case is 1,000 mg per 24 hours. Divide the 1,000 mg per 24 hours by the patient's weight to obtain the milligrams per kilogram per 24 hours. Thus, 1,000 mg per 10 kg comes out 100 mg/kg per 24 hours. Look up the reference range for the drug and compare the two. In this case, the reference range is 50 to 150 mg per 24 hours; hence, the dose that was ordered (100 mg per 24 hours) is within the established reference range.

To calculate a dose using BSA, the child's height and weight are needed. Verify the correct dose from a pediatric reference source and then use a nomogram, which computes the relationship between height and weight to obtain the BSA (Figure 6-1). An alternative to using the nomogram to calculate BSA is Mosteller's formula:

$$\text{BSA}(\text{m}^2) = \sqrt{\frac{\text{weight}(\text{kg}) \times \text{height}(\text{cm})}{3{,}600}}$$

BSA is used primarily when calculating doses of cancer chemotherapeutic drugs because it is the most accurate measure for dosing medications for pediatric patients. For example, if the reference source recommends 100 mg/m^2 per 24 hours in two divided doses and the child's BSA is 0.5 m^2, then 0.5 m^2 times 100 mg equals 50 mg per 24 hours, or 25 mg every 12 hours. The actual order reads 25 mg every 12 hours (50 mg per 24 hours), so the dose ordered is within the established reference range.

Always double-check medication calculations. Misplacing a decimal point can result in the patient receiving one tenth of the required amount of medication or 10 times the ordered amount of drug. For example, if the patient is to receive 1 mg and the decimal point is misplaced while calculating, the result could be 0.1 mg or 10 mg.

When looking up reference ranges for dosing, verify the maximum amount of the medication that should be given either per dose or per 24 hours. Maximum dosage is important, especially in the overweight child. For example, if the body weight of a child weighing 100 kg was used to

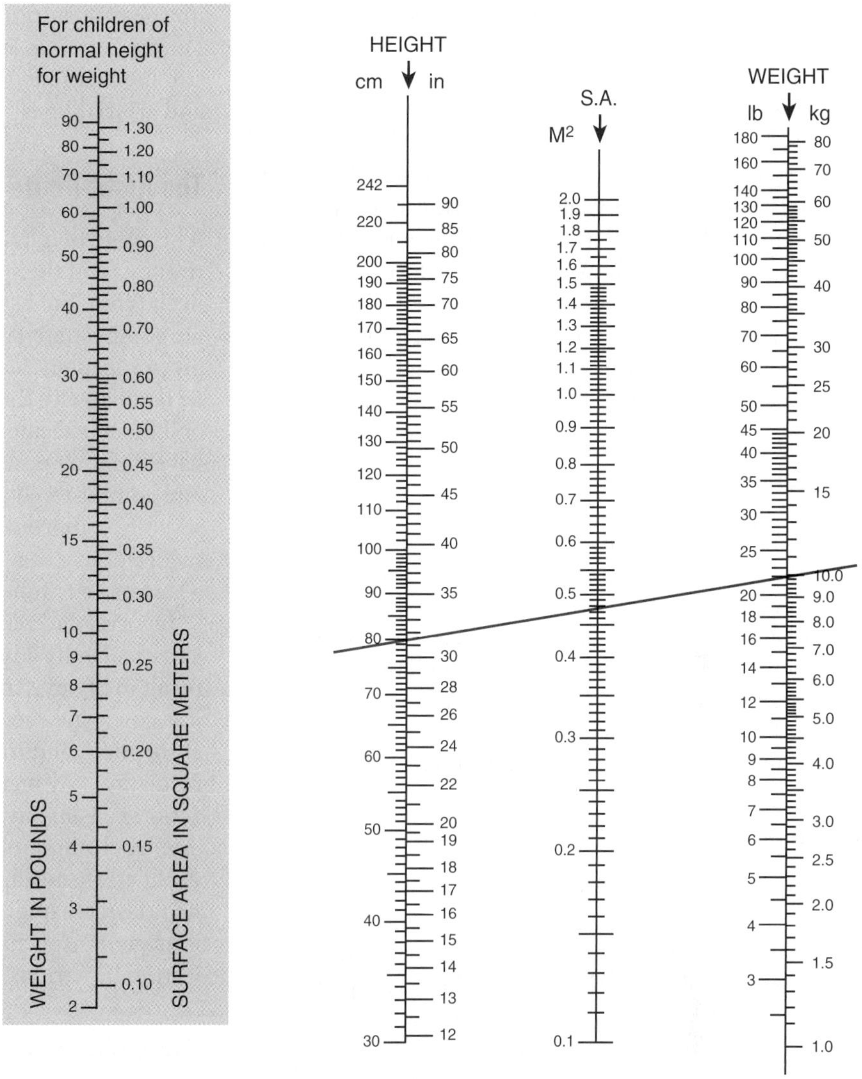

FIGURE 6-1
Nomogram for estimation of body surface area. If the child is of average size, use the shaded box on the left to find the weight (left side of box) and then the corresponding surface area (right side of box). In the nomogram on the right, the child's surface area is indicated where a straight line that intersects the height and weight levels intersects the surface area column.

determine a drug dose, the amount of drug ordered would likely exceed the capacity of the liver of the child to metabolize the drug or the renal system's ability to safely eliminate the drug. Often, adult range of dosing is used as the drug reference for children who weigh more than 50 kg (with some providers using 40 kg as the cutoff point).

Most drugs are dosed by weight; however, there are certain factors that may also influence dosing in children. Age-related metabolic changes and organ dysfunction may be factors in addition to weight that are considered in determining an appropriate dose of a medication for an individual child.

Dispensing Individual Doses

Pediatric nurses are often called on to draw up an individualized dose before administering the medication to the patient. It is important to set up equations in a consistent fashion when drawing up a medication from a multidose container or from a single-dose container that contains more medication than the ordered dose. For example, if a multidose container is labeled as cephalexin (Keflex), 250 mg per 5 mL, and the ordered amount is 200 mg of oral suspension, set up the equation as 250 mg/5 mL = 200 mg/X mL to calculate that 4 mL must be drawn up to obtain the necessary 200 mg. Similarly, an oral syringe containing ranitidine syrup, 15 mg/mL, may be sent from the pharmacy. If the order reads ranitidine, 10 mg orally, set up the equation as 15 mg/1 mL = 10 mg/X mL to calculate that the nurse would draw up 0.67 mL.

Administration of IV medication is often challenging in pediatrics, especially if the nurse must prepare a drug that comes as a powdered medication. The nurse must first dilute the powdered medication with sterile normal saline or water, determine the final concentration of medication, and then calculate how much fluid is needed to obtain the ordered amount of medication. For example, a child is to receive 225 mg of ampicillin intravenously and a 250-mg vial is sent from pharmacy. The vial says to use 1.8 mL of sterile diluent with a resulting final volume of 2 mL. The nurse sets up a math proportion and calculates that 1.8 mL of the solution is needed to obtain 225 mg of ampicillin.

Always double-check medication calculations if the drug is not sent from the pharmacy as a unit dose that contains the exact dosage of medication as ordered. Infusion times, the length of time the medication is infused over, are also important considerations for maintaining blood levels of the drug or to prevent adverse reactions. Use only recommended infusion times to deliver IV medications. Infusion times (e.g., 5, 20, 30, 60 minutes) and required fluid volume dilutions for medications are based on established concentration levels necessary to deliver IV medications; consult a reference source for dilutions and infusion times.

Key points to remember in determining the right dose include the following:

- Pediatric dosages are calculated based on weight in kilograms or BSA.
- Adult dose reference ranges, rather than kilogram dosing, may be used in children who weigh more than 50 kg (with some providers using 40 kg as the cutoff point).
- Always double-check math calculations when preparing a medication that is not supplied as an exact dose. Double-checking mathematical calculations helps to prevent mathematical errors and makes it more likely that the correct amount of medication (a portion of the amount supplied) is given to the patient.

The Right Patient

All children who are inpatients should be identified by an identification band attached to their body and not according to the bed they are in. Accurate identification serves two purposes: to reliably identify the individual as the person for whom the service or treatment is intended and to match the service or treatment to that individual. For administration of medication and other services or treatments, the Joint Commission of Accreditation of Healthcare Organizations (JCAHO) adopted a two-identifier requirement to ensure reliable identification of patients as a safety goal. Acceptable identifiers can include two of the following on a wristband: the individual's name, date of birth, assigned identification number, telephone number, or other person-specific identifier. Bar coding with two or more person-specific identifiers is also being used. Take the patient's MAR to the bedside to perform your double identifier check. Match the service about to be performed by checking the medication label with the child's identification band.

If the child does not have an identification band in place, the nurse must first identify the child before administering any medication. A parent should identify an infant or a younger child. Ask an older child his or her name and date of birth or other identifier. Be careful when there are children with the same last names on the unit or when the parents or child does not speak English. Check colored allergy bracelets to verify that the child has not had an allergic reaction to the medication about to be administered.

For IV drugs, routinely label all infusion lines to be sure that the right drug is inserted into the right infusion line. Extra caution is the rule for patients with multiple IV infusion lines and gastric infusion devices because gastric medications have been incorrectly injected into IV and arterial lines.

The Right Route

The route of administration affects the absorption, effectiveness, and the speed of action of medications, especially in children. For example, certain childhood immunizations are administrated intramuscularly (IM), whereas others are given subcutaneously (Sub-Q). Therefore, the nurse must be familiar with the various routes of administrations for all childhood vaccines. Medications given IV, IM, or Sub-Q have differing peaks and duration of action. Morphine sulfate administered IV rather than Sub-Q as ordered could severely compromise a child's respiratory status. Similarly, medications given through a jejunostomy tube rather than a gastrostomy tube have different absorption.

Incorrect administration techniques can also be problematic. Faulty administration of subcutaneous insulin can result in lipodystrophy. Application of a thick layer of topical cortisone medication can result in increased steroid absorption, and too-rapid IV infusion of vancomycin can result in "red man syndrome" (an anaphylactic-like reaction causing an erythematous maculopapular rash and intense flushing of the skin; patients may also experience dizziness, headache, chills, chest pain, and respiratory difficulties). Chapters 62 through 75 discuss techniques and important aspects to consider when administering medication by various delivery routes.

The Right Time

Medications given at the wrong interval can affect therapeutic blood levels. The use of military time helps to reduce the problem of medications being given at incorrect times. Each institution may have its own policy about scheduled times (i.e., once, twice, three, four times per day) for medication. The general rule of practice is to administer a medication within the time frame of one half hour before or after the scheduled time period. Adhering to scheduled medication times is particularly important for medications that must be given every 4, 6, or 8 hours around the clock.

There are certain situations in which the pediatric nurse must be particularly alert to timing issues. If drug blood levels are ordered at specific times to coincide with administration of certain medications at specific times, the nurse is responsible for administering the medication at the required time and notifying the laboratory of the time that the blood sample must be collected. Determining peaks and troughs of drugs is an important part of the management plan for certain medications.

Some medications should be given with meals, just before meals, on an empty stomach, or at a specified time (e.g., 2 hours after meals or at 8 a.m., 3 p.m., and 9 p.m.). Therefore, timing of those drugs is an important issue. For example, drug absorption can be altered if a certain drug is given with food, or a drug may need to be given before meals to promote effective gastrointestinal functioning. A daily dose of steroids is often given in early morning to mimic the normal physiologic response of the body. Thus, the nurse must be knowledgeable about the medications being administered and their mechanism of action.

Timing is often very important when administering oral medications to infants. Because many young infants are on demand feedings, the pediatric nurse may need to adapt the medication schedule for certain drugs based on the infant's feeding pattern.

The Right Approach

Often, individuals are less attuned to the sixth right of administering medications to children. One's approach to the child, age-appropriate explanations, and administration techniques often affect the success of administering the medication to the child in the least traumatic manner possible. Behavioral and developmental considerations of medication administration are discussed later in this chapter.

AVOIDING COMMON ERRORS IN MEDICATION ADMINISTRATION

Prescribing and Transcription Errors

Medication errors related to prescribing are generally grouped into four categories: poor handwriting, decimal errors, misused abbreviations, and incorrect calculations. Many healthcare agencies have adopted computerized medication records, which eliminate the problem of incorrect interpretation of handwriting. However, in situations when typed medication orders are not common practice, the nurse and pharmacist must carefully interpret handwritten medication orders and clarify all medication orders that are not clearly written to avoid a transcription error.

Decimal errors, the most common error in pediatric medication calculation, can be avoided by never placing a decimal and a zero after a whole number (called the trailing zero) because the decimal point might not be read correctly (e.g., 4.0 mL might be read as 40 mL; write 4 mL). A zero *should* be placed before fractions (called the leading zero) that are less than 1 (e.g., write 0.6 mL, not .6 mL, which might be confused with 6 mL if the decimal is inadvertently missed). Do not use the abbreviations q.d., q.o.d., IU, U, or u. Write out "every day" "every other day," "international unit," or "unit." It is recommended that the Latin abbreviates for the eyes and ears not be used; instead write out "right" or "left" and "ear" or "eye." Avoid other dangerous abbreviations, including μg (write mcg instead), H.S. (write out "half-strength" or "at bedtime"), S.C or S.Q. (write "Sub-Q" or "subQ"), and c.c. (write "mL"). In addition, write out "morphine sulfate" and "magnesium sulfate"; do not abbreviate because they are easily confused with one another. Prescribers are urged to write out instructions rather than using abbreviations.

Ask for clarification of medication doses that are not within the pediatric reference range. The individual who ordered the medication may have made a mathematical error or used an incorrect weight when calculating the amount of medication that was needed. Use caution when interpreting large doses above 1,000. Commas should be used for dosing units at or above 1,000 or words such as "100 thousand" or "1 million" to avoid errors.

Dispensing and Administration Errors

The pharmacist or the nurse may be involved in dispensing errors. Math errors may be made in calculating portions of medication to draw up to obtain an exact dose. If the nurse makes a math error, the amount of medication that is to be drawn up is incorrectly identified. In some situations, the amount to be drawn up is correctly calculated; however, the amount drawn up is not the amount calculated. Double-check all math calculations. Likewise, double-check to be sure that the amount needed to be drawn up (based on the nurse's calculations) is the actual amount that was drawn up.

Two registered nurses should check insulin, digoxin, and chemotherapeutic agents before they are administered. Review the original order for these medications and verify that the dose of the drug that was ordered is the amount that has been drawn up to administer to the child. For digoxin and chemotherapeutic agents, verify from the original order that, based on a reference range for the dosing and the patient's weight or BSA, the correct dose was ordered.

Smart pumps are increasingly used in hospital settings to help reduce medication administration errors. Such enhanced IV pumps contain dynamic software that is programmed to ensure that the five rights of medication administration are maintained (the sixth right, approach, cannot be ensured by technology). There are currently two types of smart pumps. The technology in type 1 pumps allows the nurse to identify the drug, its concentration, and solution providing a safety guardrail. Type 2 pumps contain the same technology found in type 1 pumps with the addition of built-in bar-code readers to identify bar-coded drug labels and to confirm unique patient identification information and record the bar-coded identification badge of the nurse (Quigley, 2004). Remember that technology is not a replacement for sound nursing judgment.

Important points for the nurse to remember to decrease medication errors include the following:

- Double-check all math calculations.
- Double-check amounts that are drawn up for dispensing.
- Clarify medication orders that are poorly handwritten.

- Use a two-nurse system to verify doses and amounts drawn up for digoxin, insulin, and chemotherapy agents.
- Verify with the pharmacist or physician unusually large volumes or dosage units for a single-patient dose.
- When a parent or patient questions whether a medication should be administered, answer questions and, if appropriate, double-check the medication order and/or call the prescriber to discuss the concern expressed by the patient or parent.

Reporting Adverse Drug Reactions and Medication Errors

Complete appropriate agency forms if an adverse drug reaction or medication error occurs. In the situation of an adverse drug reaction, identify the patient's symptoms and notify the physician and pharmacist. Hold the medication until instructed to do otherwise. Likewise, if a medication error is made, notify the physician and pharmacist immediately. Monitor the child for adverse reactions.

ADMINISTERING MEDICATION TO CHILDREN

Behavioral and Developmental Considerations

Administering medications to infants and children can be a challenge for the nurse. Explain the reason that a medication is being given and any procedure that is necessary for the administration of the medication using explanations that are simple and appropriate to the child's cognitive level. A child may cooperate more with a procedure if he or she understands why it is being done. Tips for administration of medication by pediatric age group are presented in Chart 6-2 and in the chapters that deal specifically with that method of administration (see Chapters 62 to 75).

Education About Pharmacologic Agents

Before parents and older children are discharged from a healthcare setting, they should have a basic understanding about all medications that are to be taken at home, including over-the-counter agents. Discuss the following important information (Brady, 2004):

- The reason the drug is being given, how much should be taken, and the frequency of administration. Make sure that the parent and older child know the name of the medication.
- Specific instructions about taking an "as necessary" drug or a drug that is to be taken under specific circumstances (e.g., a drug used for fever control or medications to be taken as part of a rescue plan for a child whose asthma symptoms are worsening). Cover when, how often, and how long to take "as necessary" drugs.
- Signs and symptoms that indicate the drug is effective or not effective (e.g., fever subsides or child remains febrile).
- Possible drug interactions with other medications or foods, precautions, or adverse reactions.
- Caution about the use of alternate or complementary therapies and the need to discuss these with healthcare provider before their use as they may contain dangerous elements such as iodine and heavy metals.
- Storage issues, if applicable.
- Monitoring issues (such as peak flow or blood glucose levels), if applicable.
- Pregnancy risk factors for specific drugs prescribed for female teenagers.
- Tips about administering "difficult to take" drugs.
- Written individualized medication information (essential).
- Ability to pay for prescription and over-the-counter medications, if this could be an issue.

Also assess the ability of a parent to administer a drug or for the child to self-administer a medication before discharge from a healthcare setting. Return demonstrations are an important evaluation tool to assess safe administration of medication. Indications for return demonstrations include the following:

- Administering oral medications to infants and young children
- Measuring small amounts or exact doses using a syringe
- Giving injections or delivering medications through special tubing (e.g., nasogastric, gastrostomy, or jejunostomy tubes)
- Administering ophthalmologic or nasal medications
- Using metered-dose inhalers, spacers, or inhalation equipment
- Teaching parents or patients with limited cognitive abilities or when multiple medications must be administered so that the correct dose and the correct medication are given as directed

Administration of Medication in School, Camp, or Day Care Settings

Nurses who administer medications to children in nonmedical settings, such as schools, camps, or day care, should have a written protocol that outlines the agency's regulations on administering medications. When prescription medications are administered, key elements that should be addressed in such a protocol include the need for the following:

- The child's first and last name is on the container.
- Medication is prescribed by a licensed health professional, and the name, address, and phone number of the health professional who ordered the medication appears on the container.

CHART 6-2 TIPS FOR MEDICATION ADMINISTRATION

Newborns and Young Infants

- For formula-fed babies, mix medication with a small amount of formula (3–5 mL) in a syringe. This is particularly helpful when a medication is bitter tasting. Instill the mixture into a nipple for the infant to suck.
- Unless contraindicated, hold the infant in an upright position while delivering oral medication.
- An infant who has just been fed and is sleeping deeply may not want to suck. Try to administer medications either before a feeding or when the infant is not sleeping deeply after a feeding.
- Medications that are not bitter tasting can be drawn up in a syringe (use a tuberculin syringe for volumes less than 1 mL). Slowly instill the medication in the side of the infant's mouth. Allow the infant to swallow the medication between sucking. Gently stroke the infant's cheek to elicit the suck reflex.
- For difficult-to-feed infants or those with respiratory difficulties, administer oral medication slowly. The infant may need to rest between short spurts of medication administration.

Toddlers

- Toddlers will usually take sweet-tasting oral medications in a syringe without problems. Bitter-tasting medication may need to be mixed with a small amount of juice (5 to 10 mL). Check compatibility of the medication with certain liquids. For example, Viracept (protease inhibitor) has a very bitter taste when mixed with acidic juices and should be mixed with milk. Remember that the more liquid that the medication is mixed in, the greater the volume that the child needs to take. Also, some medications are so bitter tasting that nothing will disguise their taste.
- Some pills may be crushed and mixed in applesauce, chocolate syrup, ice cream, or pudding to disguise their taste. Enteric-coated pills should not be crushed.
- If the toddler is not able to cooperate in taking medications, situate the toddler on your lap with his or her legs in between your legs. Place one of the toddler's arms behind your back and hold the other arm in one hand while administering the medication with your free hand. This is often a two-person procedure, especially if the toddler spits out the oral medication.
- In a two-person procedure, have one person hold the child in his or her lap as described above while the other person places the fingers of one hand around the child's cheek and slowly instills the oral medication from a syringe into the side of the child's mouth with the other hand. After a small amount is instilled, press the toddler's cheeks together until he or she swallows the medication; repeat this maneuver until the medication is completed.
- After the medication has been taken, praise the toddler for a job well done.

Preschool-Aged Children

- Give a simple explanation for why the medication is being given (e.g., "to help your cough go away").
- This is the time of initiative. Most preschool-aged children enjoy taking their oral medications and think it is fun to use an oral syringe. Be sure to supervise (or assist) preschool-aged children as they push the oral medication into their mouth.
- Children at this age might still refuse to take medications. In this case, the technique described for the uncooperative toddler may need to be used.
- Never lie to a child that an injection will not hurt.
- Give realistic choices that will allow the child some control over the situation (e.g., the kind of juice to take medication with, the number or type of bandages to use).
- After the medication has been taken, praise the preschooler-aged child for his or her efforts.

School-Aged and Adolescent Children

- Explain the reason that the medication is being given as appropriate to the child's cognitive level.
- Some children in these age groups may start to hide their medication and pretend they have taken the drug. Be on the alert.
- Educate children with chronic illnesses about their medications. They should know the reason that the medication is being given, side effects to watch for, and other issues related to administration and adherence. Help them develop a sense of responsibility for their own health care. Prepare them for discharge from the health setting by educating them about safe self-medication.

Additional Tips

- Never leave medications at the child's bedside unless permitted by institution policy.
- When checking medication labels, pay close attention to the spelling of the medication because many drugs have similar names.
- Prepare medications in a quiet, well-lighted area.
- Check drugs for discoloration or unusual precipitates.
- Use a calculator to check drug doses and be sure to calculate doses twice.
- Do not give a drug that another nurse has prepared.
- If medications are prepared in a syringe beforehand, label the syringe with the name of the drug, its concentration, date and time drawn, and your initials.
- Remember to remove syringes (and needle if used) from the patient's bedside and place in an appropriate sharps box.

Continued

CHART 6-2 TIPS FOR MEDICATION ADMINISTRATION (CONTINUED)

- Remember to remove caps from oral syringes before administering medications and discard in a proper receptacle. Aspiration of caps left at a child's bedside or inhaled when left in place while administering oral drugs are safety concerns.
- Be aware of drug incompatibilities with other medications or fluids. This is especially important when administering multiple intravenous (IV) medications or when the patient is receiving total parenteral nutrition or lipids.
- There should be an order by a prescriber authorized by the state in the patient chart if the nurse is to administer medication brought in from home. The pharmacist should identify the medication.
- Check the time interval between medication administrations for all PRN drugs to ensure that enough time has elapsed.
- Label external medications "for external use only" and store separately from other medications.
- Record IV fluid amounts used to deliver IV medications in the patient's intake and output record.
- Be especially careful when administering medications that are potentially toxic, such as antineoplastic drugs, digoxin, or insulin. Medications delivered by the parenteral route also demand vigilance both in preparation and while infusing.
- Use vials of sterile water or normal saline for injection as a one-time injection solution and not as multiple-dose vials.
- Be aware of potential drug–drug and drug–food interactions.
- Take a careful drug allergy history and be sure that an Allergy Alert is posted on the patient's chart and that the patient wears an Allergy Alert bracelet.
- The use of a topical anesthetic before intramuscular injections may help lessen a child's pain (see Chapter 7).

- Medication is in the original package or container.
- The date the prescription was filled and the date it expires appear on the container.
- Medication is in a childproof container.
- A statement from the healthcare provider indicates the name of the drug, the diagnosis or reason the medication is needed, and whether any serious reactions might occur or an alert for the nurse about the possibility of a serious drug reaction.
- A policy about self-administration of medication (i.e., the use of inhalers or an EpiPen) should be identified for children who are capable of self-administration, exhibit responsible behaviors, and are in need of speedy access to their medication.
- Information about security and proper storage of medications should be identified in the agency's protocol.
- Nonmedical agencies generally require a written request from the child's parent or guardian asking them to administer the medication per the healthcare provider's specific instruction.

School districts often allow non-nursing staff to administer medications to children under the training and supervision of a nurse. In such instances, the nurse is responsible for the training of those who will be administering medications and the ongoing supervision of these individuals. Documentation of such training and supervision is important.

A parent or healthcare provider may request that over-the-counter medications be administered to children in nonmedical settings. Once again, the agency should have a protocol in place to handle these requests. Often, statements from both the parent and physician are required. In such instances, each child's over the-counter medication should be labeled with the child's first and last name as well as the name and phone number of the physician who recommended the medication. Note the current date and date of expiration. Identify instructions regarding dosing and frequency as well as indications for when to notify the parent or physician that the child is not responding as anticipated.

Verbal Orders

All healthcare agencies should have a policy and protocol about nurses taking verbal orders for administration of medication. This should be a practice that is done only in emergency or unusual circumstances. The nurse who takes such orders should listen to what the physician says, write the order down, and then read the order back to the prescriber.

Resources

The Institute for Safe Medication Practices (www.ismp.org) is an excellent resource that provides education about adverse drug events and their prevention. All healthcare providers should be familiar with the National Safety Goals identified by the JCAHO (www.jcaho.org) that pertain to medication preparation and administration to pediatric patients. Pediatric nurses should be familiar with current reference handbooks that focus on pediatric and neonatal patients and have them readily available. Many hospitals subscribe to Micromedex, an online program that contains current information about pharmacologic agents. A useful source of information about complementary and alternative agents is the National Center for Complementary and Alternative Medicines (www.nccam.nih.gov).

Bibliography

Brady, M. A. (2004). Introduction to disease and pain management. In C. E. Burns, A. M. Dunn, M. A. Brady, & N. B. Starr (Eds.), *Pediatric primary care: A handbook for nurse practitioners* (3rd ed., pp. 493–515). Philadelphia: W. B. Saunders.

Hale, T. W. (2004). *Medications and mothers' milk* (11th ed.). Amarillo, TX: Pharmasoft.

Keohane, C. A., Hayes, J., Saniuk, C., Rothschild, J. M., & Bates, D. W. (2005). Intravenous medication safety and smart infusion systems: Lessons learned and future opportunities. *Journal of Intravenous Nursing, 28*, 321–328.

Mitchell, A. L. (2001). Challenges in pediatric pharmacotherapy: Minimizing medication errors. *Medscape Pharmacists* (Online). Retrieved October 30, 2004, from www.medscape.com/viewarticle/421220

Reed, M. D. & Gal, R. (2004). Principles of drug therapy. In R. E. Behrman, R. M. Kliegman, & H. B. Jenson (Eds.), *Nelson textbook of pediatrics* (17th ed., pp. 2427–2432). Philadelphia: W. B. Saunders.

Quigley, T. (2004). Smart pumps. *Advance for Nurses, 1*(7), 21–24.

CHAPTER 7

Principles of Pain Management

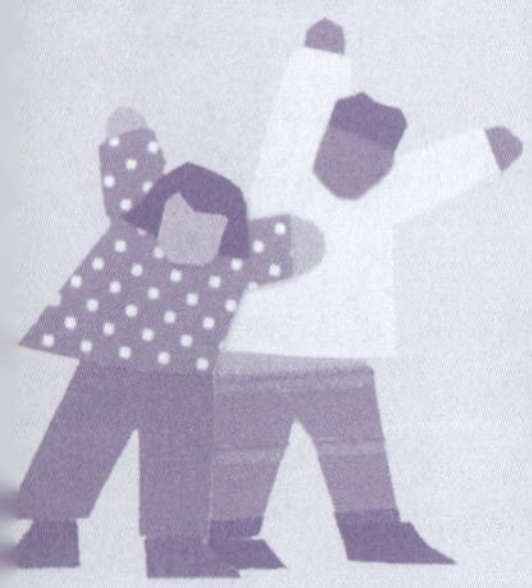

Pain has been defined by the International Association for the Study of Pain (IASP) as an unpleasant sensory and emotional experience associated with actual or potential tissue damage or described in terms of such damage (IASP, 1979). Acute (nociceptive) pain is a common adverse stimulus that occurs as the result of injury, surgery, or illness. The severity of the physical damage and physiologic response may play a role in the child's overall perception of pain. The acute pain experience generally resolves as the body heals.

Acute pain may develop into chronic pain if the pain experience extends beyond the normal trajectory of healing for the amount of tissue damage sustained. Chronic nociceptive stimulation may alter excitability in the peripheral and central nervous systems, resulting in sustained or recurrent pain with neuropathic qualities. Defining clinical characteristics of neuropathic pain are dysesthesia (impaired sensitivity to touch, such as paresthesia and cutaneous hypesthesia), hyperalgesia (excessive sensation from pain), and allodynia (nonpainful stimuli, such as light touch, is perceived as painful), motor abnormalities, and autonomic disturbances. Differing from acute pain, neuropathic pain involves the erroneous generation and transmission of information in the nervous system; it often persists and even intensifies over time.

Children experience just as much pain as adults. Although pain management has improved over the past few decades, particularly for predictable pain problems such as postoperative pain, underestimation and undertreatment of pain in children remain problems (Schechter, Berde, & Yaster, 2003; Simons et al., 2003; Stevens et al., 2003; Vincent & Denyes, 2004). Untreated pain may have significant and lifelong physiologic and psychological consequences, such as altered pain sensitivity (Grunau, 2002; Grunau et al., 2005).

The problem of untreated pain in children has been recognized by professional organizations whose members care for children. The National Association of Neonatal Nurses (NANN) has issued a position statement on pain management in infants (NANN, 1999). The American Academy of Pediatrics (AAP) and the Canadian Paediatric Society (CPS) published a joint statement underscoring the need for effective pain management in the neonate and providing recommendations for management (AAP & CPS, 2000). The AAP and the American Pain Society (APS) have issued a joint statement that reinforces the need to treat pain and suffering in all infants, children, and adolescents (AAP & APS, 2001). The APS has issued a position statement on chronic pain in children that addresses special needs in pediatric pain assessment, treatment, research, and education (APS, 2004). Effective pain management is an essential component of healthcare that encompasses initial pain assessment, therapeutic interventions, and reassessment.

INITIAL PAIN ASSESSMENT

Many factors, including emotions of anxiety, anger, depression, fear, loneliness, and fear of body intrusion, can alter perception and expression of pain. The following must be considered when assessing pain:

- Biologic factors: age (children of all ages experience pain; preterm infants likely experience even more pain than an adult when subjected to the same stimulus [Fitzgerald & Beggs, 2001; Goldschneider & Anand, 2003]); genetic characteristics (may have differing levels of neurotransmitters or response to medications); gender (biologic differences may exist [Guinsburg et al., 2000; Kim et al. 2004] coupled with societal expectations of pain response [e.g., girls may cry, boys are discouraged from crying]); and previous pain experiences (may have caused alterations in pain signal processing).
- Type of pain: acute, chronic, recurrent, extensive, minor, traumatic, surgical, or treatment.
- Psychological factors: child's coping style (e.g., information seeking versus information avoiding; if we try to teach an information avoider all about a painful event, it may increase the child's anxiety), child's perception of the pain and previous coping techniques (whether successful or not), child's perception of control (lack of control may intensify the perception of pain), and temperament (ability to adapt to situations, negative versus positive in mood and reactions).
- Cognitive factors: child's cognitive level influences his or her ability to describe pain and understanding of the pain experience.
- Cultural and societal factors: culture and society transmit accepted standards of behavior (e.g., okay to express pain, or accept it stoically because succumbing to pain is shameful).
- Parental influence: parental reaction to situation (a positive reaction may help the child cope, a negative reaction may exacerbate the child's pain); separation from parents often intensifies the child's pain experience.

An initial pain assessment includes the child's past and current pain history (see Chapter 132 for questions included in an initial history of the current pain). Ranked in hierarchical order by their importance and reliability for assessing pain are self-report, presence of pathology or a condition associated with pain, behavior, proxy ratings, and, finally, physiologic indicators of pain. Factors that influence the pain experience must also be considered. The most accurate assessment of pain uses a combination of the above. One must maintain a high index of suspicion regarding the presence of pain, particularly in nonverbal children.

Subjective Reporting

The subjective rating remains the gold standard for pain assessment: Believe that the child has pain if he or she says so. Pain in infants or other nonverbal children with cognitive impairment must be assessed using other methods. By about 18 months of age, children have words for pain; by age 3 or 4 years, children have the cognition to report degree of pain (e.g., "a lot," "a little").

Behavioral Observations

Use measures of pain-related behaviors when self-report cannot be obtained or to supplement self-report. It is important to remember that caregivers consistently underestimate a child's pain when compared with the child's self-report (Romsing, Moller-Sonnergaard, Hertel, & Rasmussen, 1996). Use of standardized rating scales and staff education produce ratings that more closely align with the patient's (Baxt et al., 2004; Colwell, Clark, & Perkins, 1996; de Rond, de Wit, van Dam, & Muller, 2000). Mothers also tend to underestimate their child's pain, but mothers' ratings are closer to the child's ratings than are nurses' (Miller, 1996).

In an infant, state (e.g., level of wakefulness or sleep) influences intensity of response to pain. Preterm infants show a less robust response to painful stimuli than term infants. Thus when an infant does not demonstrate pain behaviors, do not assume that the infant has no pain—it may be that the infant is in a sound sleep state or is too weak to respond. Behaviors that are indicators of pain in infants are

- Crying that is high-pitched, tense, and irregular and that arouses the listener.
- Facial expression with eyes tightly closed, brows lowered and drawn together, a deepened nasolabial furrow (line between outer aspect of nares and outer corner of mouth), and a square-shaped mouth with a cupped tongue.
- Simple motor responses of withdrawal from the stimulus; newborns show a generalized poorly localized response, but older infants localize more and attempt to push away or escape.

Behaviors of acute immediate pain, often associated with procedural pain experiences, change rapidly within a few minutes of the stimulus; thus reliance on these signs as indicators of acute established pain may be misleading. Behavioral responses, in addition to clinical data regarding likelihood of pain and the infant's ability to be consoled in response to comfort measures, must be considered in pain assessment.

Toddlers and preschool-aged children may lie still and rigid or be curled in a fetal position. They may clench their fists, guard or touch the painful area, and have a facial grimace of pain; they may also be irritable, sad, or depressed.

School-aged children and adolescents may try to rest quietly when in pain and may demonstrate pain behaviors similar to younger children. They typically demonstrate fewer overt pain behaviors than younger children because of increasing cognitive abilities. They understand the need for aversive procedures and can use behavioral and cognitive coping strategies to deal with pain.

Children of any age may demonstrate complex behavioral responses, which vary from child to child. Some become withdrawn and quiet, whereas others demonstrate active agitated behaviors. They may show a lack of interest in their surroundings and decreased ability to concentrate. A child may also demonstrate an alteration in sleep patterns, using activity as a coping mechanism or being unable to sleep because of the pain. Alternately, the child may sleep as a coping mechanism or from exhaustion due to pain.

Cognitive Impairment

For the child who is cognitively impaired or nonverbal, identify pain and discomfort behaviors specific to that child in conjunction with parents. Parents can reasonably estimate their child's pain using a structured pain assessment tool, although they may overestimate the child's pain in the early postoperative period (Voepel-Lewis, Malviya, & Tait, 2005). Although specific behaviors vary from child to child, classes of pain behaviors have been identified in cognitively impaired nonverbal individuals (Table 7-1). In children with cognitive impairment, pay particular attention to the cue of a twisted or distressed-looking face as an indicator of pain (Stallard et al., 2002). Fanurik, Koh, Harrison, Conrad, and Tomerlin (1998) described a useful screening method to determine whether a cognitively impaired child can accurately use a self-report pain scale.

Chronic Pain

When children experience pain of longer duration, they may forget what it feels like to be pain free and thus no longer complain of pain. The body adapts to chronic pain so that changes in vital signs are not apparent. Children with chronic pain may show disrupted sleep resulting in fatigue, irritability, and decreased ability to concentrate; developmental regression; a change in eating patterns; behavior or school problems; withdrawal from peer group activities; depression; or aggression.

Physiologic Monitoring

Pain is a stressor that activates the compensatory mechanisms of the autonomic nervous system (ANS). The ANS has two branches: the sympathetic nervous system (SNS) and the parasympathetic nervous system (PNS). SNS stimulation produces the "fight or flight" response, which results in tachycardia, peripheral vasoconstriction, diaphoresis, pupil dilation, and increased secretion of catecholamines as well as adrenocortical, thyroid, and pancreatic hormones.

Other signs of autonomic arousal are found in response to painful stimuli. Respiratory rate, systolic blood pressure, transcutaneous oxygen ($TcPo_2$) levels, heart rate, and intracranial pressure have been found to increase with painful stimuli (Johnston, Stevens, Boyer, & Porter, 2003). Conversely, decreases in respiratory rate, oxygen saturation, and $TcPo_2$ levels have also been noted in response to pain. When assessing vital sign changes, it is important to consider the influence of other factors, such as the child's position, fear, anxiety, crying, handling for procedures, medications, and clinical situation.

Research yields conflicting results, possibly because of differences in measurement, populations, and pain situations. Studies in adults and children, for example, showed a decrease in heart rate with painful stimuli (Foster, Yucha, Zuk, & Vojir, 2003; Logan, Sheffield, Lutgendorf, & Lang, 2002). Physiologic variations in response to pain warn that vital sign changes may be a general reaction to physiologic stress rather than as a specific barometer of pain. Vital sign changes may stabilize fairly quickly; thus reliance on these signs as indicators of acute established pain may be misleading. Use vital sign changes as an indicator of response considering the child's situation, behavior, and subjective reports.

Pain Assessment Tools

When selecting a method of pain assessment, consideration must be given to the developmental age of the child and the type of pain situation (e.g., procedural, postoperative, disease). Typically, assessment tools for younger children can be used with older children, but other tools require a degree of cognitive development. It is important to remember that children may regress when in pain, and a simpler tool may need to be used to ensure that the child understands proper use of the tool. Use tools that have been tested and demonstrate adequate reliability and validity. As noted previously, staff familiarity with a tool increases accuracy of the assessment; thus education regarding appropriate use of the tool is essential. For subjective ratings of pain, identify two or three tools and educate staff regarding correct usage, including developmentally appropriate selection based on the child's age and cognitive level. Use these tools to perform pain assessments. This promotes ease of comparison and tracking of adequacy of pain interventions over time. See Table 7-1 for examples of tools used to assess different types of pain, such as procedural, postoperative, and chronic or recurrent pain.

In the absence of subjective ratings, multidimensional measurement and rating tools, including behavioral observations and physiologic parameters, most accurately assess pain. Multidimensional tools may also be used to augment the subjective rating of pain.

Children older than 3 years of age can reliably report their pain. A younger child may express pain; evaluate this in the context of a multidimensional assessment. Assess ability to use pain-rating tools, such as a 0 to 10 scale, by a simple test of serialization: have the child place different-sized objects (e.g., lines, pieces of paper) in order from

TABLE 7-1

Pain Assessment Methods and Tools*

Tool Type/Population	Tool	Age/Indications for Use
Subjective Rating Scales	Direct questioning	>2 yr (with adequate cognitive abilities)
	Finger Span Scale (Merkel, 2002)	>2 yr
	Oucher (Beyer, Denyes, & Villarruel, 1992; Beyer & Knott, 1998; Yeh, 2005)	3–12 yr
	Faces Pain Scale-Revised (Hicks et al., 2001)	≥5 yr
	FACES (Wong & Baker, 1988)	3–18 yr
	Numeric 1 to 10 scale (child must understand serialization, greater than/less than)	>4 yr
	Body Outline Tool (Eland & Anderson, 1977; Savedra et al., 1989; Van Cleve & Savedra, 1993)	≥4 yr
	Colored Analog Scale (McGrath et al. 1996)	≥4 yr
	Visual Analogue Scale (Tyler, Tu, Douthit, & Chapman, 1993)	≥5 yr
	Poker Chip Tool (Hester, 1979)	4.5–13 yr
	Adolescent Pediatric Pain Tool (Savedra, Holzemer, Tesler, & Wilkie, 1993)	8–17 yr
Procedural Pain	Neonatal Facial Coding System (Grunau, Oberlander, Holsti, & Whitfield, 1998)	Preterm and term infants ≤ 4 mo
	Neonatal Infant Pain Scale (Lawrence et al., 1993)	Preterm and term infants
	Premature Infant Pain Profile (Stevens, Johnston, Petryshen, & Taddio, 1996)	Preterm and term neonates
Postoperative Pain	Premature Infant Pain Profile (McNair et al., 2004).	Preterm and term neonates
	CRIES (C, Crying; R, Requires oxygen administration; I, Increased heart rate and blood pressure; E, Expression; S, Sleeplessness) (Krechel & Bildner, 1995)	Term neonates
	Neonatal Facial Coding System (NFCS) (Peters et al., 2003)	Birth–18 mo
	FLACC (face, legs, activity, crying, consolability) (Merkel, Voepel-Lewis, Shayevitz, & Malviya, 1997; Willis, Merkel, Voepel-Lewis, & Malviya, 2003)	2 mo–7 yr
	Toddler-Preschooler Postoperative Pain Scale (Tarbell, Cohen, & Marsh, 1992)	1–5 yr
	Children's Hospital of Eastern Ontario (McGrath et al., 1985)	1–7 yr
	Parents' Postoperative Pain Measure (PPPM) (Chambers, Finley, McGrath, & Walsh, 2003)	2–12 yr
Nonverbal and Cognitive	Pain Assessment Tool (PAT) (Hodgkinson, Bear, Thorn, & Van Blaricum, 1994; Spence et al., 2005)	Preterm and term infants
	COMFORT Behavior Scale (van Dijk et al., 2000)	Birth–3 yr
	Paediatric Pain Profile (PPP) (Hunt et al., 2004)	1–18 yr
	Non-communicating Children's Pain Checklist—Revised (vocal, sleeping/eating, social, facial, activity, body/limbs, physiologic signs) (Breau, McGrath, Camfield, & Finley, 2002)	3–18 yr
	Non-communicating Children's Pain Checklist—Postoperative Version (vocal, social, facial, activity, body and limbs, physiologic signs) (Breau, Finley, McGrath, & Camfield, 2002)	3–19 yr
	Pain Indicator for Communicatively Impaired Children (PICIC) (screwed-up or distressed-looking face, screaming, tense body, difficulty in consoling, and flinching) (Stallard et al., 2002)	Tested in parents of cognitively impaired 5 to 15-yr-olds
	Individualized Numeric Rating Scale (INRS) (Solodiuk & Curley, 2003)	>3 yr
	FLACC (face, legs, activity, crying, consolability) (Malviya et al., 2006)	4–19 yr
Chronic or Recurrent Pain	Gauvain-Piquard Rating Scale (Gauvain-Piquard et al., 1987, 1991)	Long-term pain in cancer patients 2–6 yr
	Functional Disability Inventory (Claar & Walker, 2006; Walker & Greene, 1991)	8–17 yr
	Varni-Thompson Pediatric Pain Questionnaire (Varni, Thompson, & Hanson, 1987)	≥8 yr
	Pain diary	Child must be able to write and record events
	McGill Pain Questionnaire (Melzack, 1975, 1987)	≥12 yr

*Not an inclusive list; refer to other sources for in-depth discussion of different tools (e.g., Gaffney, McGrath, & Dick, 2003; Johnston, Stevens, Boyer, & Porter, 2003; Rutledge, Donaldson, & Pravikoff, 2002).

smallest to largest. If a child does not understand how to use one of the two or three tools identified for that age group, select another.

THERAPEUTIC INTERVENTIONS

Assessment of comfort level for pain is the first step in the process of pain management. Once the presence of pain is identified, interventions must be implemented to treat the pain. Pain management interventions consist of teaching the child and family about pharmacologic agents for pain relief techniques and how to use biobehavioral techniques. When selecting treatment options, one must evaluate the type and intensity of pain, the situation, and the child's characteristics (e.g., age, coping strategies, cognitive level). It is also important to discuss expectation of pain management with the child and family. Do they expect complete pain relief and absence of pain? Is this realistic in the child's situation? Build on previously successful coping and pain management techniques that the child has used. If the family believes in folk practices, incorporate these into the treatment whenever possible. Develop realistic goals for the plan of pain management in conjunction with the child and family.

Pharmacologic Management

Pain is best managed using a proactive approach. It is much more effective to anticipate pain and treat it adequately than to treat it once it is present. Medications must be administered to manage moderate to severe pain; use biobehavioral techniques to enhance the effectiveness of medications. Mild pain may be effectively managed using biobehavioral methods alone or in conjunction with nonopioid analgesics. If pain is present for most of the time, medications must be administered on an around-the-clock basis. If pain is present on an episodic basis (e.g., headaches), as-needed administration may be adequate.

Assess for pain before administering medications to obtain a baseline for determining need for medication, selecting the most effective type of medication and evaluating effectiveness of the medication after administration. Healthcare providers often assume that adolescents, because they are typically verbal and based on their increasing capacity for abstract reasoning, will tell the healthcare provider when pain medications are needed; however, this assumption may not be valid. Adolescents often assume that the healthcare provider knows when pain medication is needed and will give it; therefore assessment must be completed.

If the child can take oral medications and pain is controlled, this is optimum. Intravenous (IV) administration of medication provides a rapid onset of action and is the method of choice when treating severe pain. Avoid intramuscular injections whenever possible. This route is more painful than others, and absorption of drug is variable. Children are fearful of needles and will deny the presence of pain rather than receive an injection.

Pharmacologic medications include nonopioid analgesics, opioids, local anesthetics, and coanalgesics. Coanalgesics have a primary indication other than pain relief but also provide analgesia in certain painful conditions. These three categories of medications are typically used in combination to attack pain in a variety of ways at various points on the nociceptive pathway. By combining these analgesics, less of each individual medication is required to relieve pain, thereby reducing the potential for analgesic side effects as compared with single-agent therapy.

Nonopioid Analgesics

Nonopioids include acetaminophen and nonsteroidal anti-inflammatory drugs (NSAIDs) and salicylates. They are most effective for mild to moderate pain or can be used as a component of a multimodal approach (e.g., in conjunction with an opioid) for severe pain. Nonopioids have a ceiling effect; that is, there is a maximum dose beyond which added analgesia does not occur. The use of salicylates has decreased dramatically because of their probable association with Reye syndrome; they are now most commonly used in treating children with rheumatoid arthritis. See Maunuksela and Olkkola (2003) for a more detailed discussion of nonopioid analgesics.

Opioid Analgesics

Opioid drugs include morphine, fentanyl, hydromorphone, methadone, and meperidine. The effects of these drugs are mediated by different receptors in the central nervous system; therefore when one is not very effective, another may be. The use of meperidine is not recommended because its primary metabolite, normeperidine, is a cerebral irritant that may cause irritability, tremors, and seizures (Acute Pain Management Guideline Panel, 1992).

Concern over addiction is a common misunderstanding and may result in reluctance to administer opioids. It is important to distinguish between tolerance and physical dependence and psychological dependence. Tolerance to the drug may occur, necessitating increasing dosages to manage pain adequately. Physical dependence may occur, resulting in symptoms of withdrawal with sudden cessation of the medication after continued therapy, after as little as 7 days of continuous use (APS, 2005). To decrease the risk for withdrawal, the dose should be gradually decreased 10% to 20% per day. Psychological dependence is characterized by a compulsive craving for the drug and its use for effects other than pain relief. Addiction is extremely rare in children legitimately treated for pain, and concern over addiction should not result in inadequate pain management. Include the difference between good drugs and bad drugs and physical versus psychological dependence in child and family teaching.

Opioids may be administered by many routes, including oral, sublingual, transdermal, IV (bolus, patient-controlled analgesia [PCA], or continuous infusion), or regional analgesia (e.g., peripheral nerve blocks or epidural infusion). Injections are not recommended for the administration of analgesics and are specifically considered unacceptable for administration of pain medications to children (APS, 2003). Painful administration makes this route inconsistent with the goal of analgesic therapy.

Use of continuous infusion may decrease opioid consumption. PCA and PCA by parent (proxy) in children younger than 6 years of age experiencing both surgical and nonsurgical pain is useful (Monitto et al., 2000). However, in one study 25% of children required supplemental oxygen, 4% required naloxone for apnea and oxygen desaturation, 15% experienced vomiting, and 8% experienced pruritus (Monitto et al., 2000). Therefore the Joint Commission on Accreditation of Healthcare Organizations (2004) recommends that if PCA technology use is authorized to parents (proxies), then they should be taught the basic concept of PCA, side effects associated with opioids, and simple methods of pain assessment covering both indicators of pain and oversedation. For this to be effective, parents must be present most of the time. Although the total amount of opioid that can be administered is preset, someone else pushing the button bypasses one of the built-in safety features of the system: that an oversedated patient is not physically capable of self-administering medication.

PCA has been used in children as young as 3 years of age, but questions remain about the age at which children become cognitively capable of appropriately using this technology (Lehr & BeVier, 2003). Rather than a strict age cut-off, evaluate the child for the following criteria indicating suitability for PCA use:

- Able to activate the device
- Able to quantify pain (the child needs to activate the pump when pain is starting or increasing, not delaying treatment until pain is severe or intolerable)
- Unable to tolerate oral analgesics
- Understand the relationship between pushing the button and medication delivery
- Understand the safety mechanisms of the machine
- Report unsatisfactory pain relief

The child and family must understand that the PCA is not a panacea; it is one way to relieve pain. If the child's pain is not effectively relieved with the use of this technology, other methods of controlling pain should be considered.

Coanalgesics

Coanalgesics are drugs that play a role in pain management because of their effects of enhancing analgesia of other drugs, reducing anxiety, or exerting an analgesic effect of their own.

caREminder

Painful procedures should not be performed using only sedative medications (e.g., hypnotics, barbiturates, benzodiazepines) without the addition of analgesic drugs. Barbiturates may even cause hyperalgesia; that is, increase the child's sensitivity to pain.

Tricyclic antidepressants and selective serotonin reuptake inhibitors (SSRIs) block reuptake of neurotransmitters such as serotonin, a critical neurotransmitter in pain modulation. Tricyclic antidepressants administered for pain are given in doses that are subtherapeutic for depression. Side effects, such as somnolence and dry mouth, which are common in the first days after starting the medication, typically diminish. Encourage the child to tolerate the side effects for a few days and give the drug time to have an influence on the pain. Antihistamines are useful against histamine-induced responses and possess local anesthetic activity and central analgesia. The antiemetic effects of antihistamines also serve to address the adverse effects of opioids, nausea, vomiting, and pruritus. The potentially synergistic sedative effects of coanalgesic medications and analgesics require ongoing assessment of the child's level of sedation and analgesia. Anticonvulsants (e.g., gabapentin) are used to treat chronic and neuropathic pain and for migraine prophylaxis. Alpha agonists (e.g., clonidine) and membrane stabilizers (e.g., IV lidocaine, mexiletine) are used to treat neuropathic pain.

Dosage

Analgesic doses required to relieve pain vary by child, age, weight, route, drug, frequency, and administration techniques. Individual patient factors known to affect dose variability include type, cause, and severity of pain; ethnic and gender-related responses to analgesics; concomitant administration of other medications; past pain experiences; and previous opioid tolerance (APS, 2003). For children, initial analgesic doses are recommended as milligrams (or micrograms) per kilogram of the child's body weight. These recommendations are approximate and should be adjusted according to clinical circumstances. Refer to a reference source for dosages.

Recommended doses of analgesics and coanalgesics that have a ceiling effect generally reflect the dose required to achieve therapeutic analgesic blood levels. Recommended doses of opioids and coanalgesics that do not have an analgesic ceiling effect are considered initial recommended dosages. These dose recommendations are based on empiric evidence and clinical experience and must be titrated to achieve optimal analgesia while minimizing analgesic-related side effects.

Give special consideration to children on both ends of the age and weight spectrum. Children who exceed 50 kilograms should be started at adult dose recommendations. Calculating doses by milligrams per kilogram in larger children result in doses that exceed initial adult recommendations and therefore put these patients at an increased risk of overdose. Second, consider the smaller and younger child. The pharmacokinetics and clinical effects of opioid analgesics for infants and children older than 6 months of age are similar to adults (APS, 2003). Younger infants and neonates have slower drug clearance and longer elimination half-lives. Therefore, for preterm and term infants younger than 6 months of age, initial recommended pediatric opioid analgesic doses should be reduced to one-quarter to one-third the recommended starting dose for older children (APS, 2003).

Special dose considerations are required for children with disease processes that affect drug metabolism, elimination, and the severity of analgesic side effects. Closely monitor children with liver, renal, pulmonary, cardiac, and neuromuscular diseases when opioids are administered and as doses are titrated to achieve pain relief. Infants and children with comorbid conditions may also require reduced analgesic doses and longer intervals between doses to adjust for their altered pharmacokinetic conditions and their response to analgesics (Tobias, 2003).

Children who report decreasing pain relief from previously effective doses of opioids may be experiencing tolerance to the analgesic effects of the opioid.

caREminder

When converting the opioid-tolerant child to another opioid, equianalgesic tables provide an approximate point to dose from. The child's clinical response to analgesic dose must be evaluated and the dose titrated to provide effective pain relief.

Monitor for side effects associated with opioid administration, especially after IV or epidural administration (Chart 7-1). Opioid clearance and metabolism are immature in neonates. Therefore the dose must be titrated to effect, and infants younger than 2 months of age who are receiving opioids should initially be observed in a monitored setting until their response to the drug is determined to be safe.

CHART 7-1 Common Opioid Side Effects and Nursing Interventions

- Nausea and vomiting: Administer medications as ordered (e.g., nonsedating antiemetic, phenothiazine antiemetic, antihistamine).
- Pruritus: Apply cool compresses; administer antihistamine as ordered.
- Sedation: Assess level of consciousness; sedation may be desirable immediately after surgery but undesirable for chronic therapy, in which case, a stimulant may be ordered.
- Respiratory depression: Assess level of sedation and respiratory rate and depth; have resuscitation equipment and naloxone (antagonist) available; sedation always precedes respiratory depression; monitor sedated children closely.
- Constipation: Assess bowel sounds; administer stimulating laxative and stool softeners as ordered; encourage ambulation and increased fluid and fiber intake.
- Urinary retention: Monitor intake and output, apply a warm compress over bladder, run water, and have child ambulate if possible; may require catheterization.

Local Anesthetics

Local anesthetics should be used to alleviate pain associated with procedures (lumbar puncture, venipuncture, injection, wound repair, accessing implanted ports). Injectable anesthetics (e.g., lidocaine, procaine) are administered subcutaneously around the area to be manipulated 5 to 10 minutes before the procedure. A small needle should be used and the anesthetic buffered to reduce the stinging sensation that accompanies "caine" administration. One milliliter (mL) of bicarbonate is used to 10 mL of lidocaine, chloroprocaine, mepivacaine, or ropivacaine (Golianu, Krane, Galloway, & Yaster, 2000). After administration, the area should be tested for insensitivity before performing the procedure.

Topical (transdermal) anesthetics can be used alone or to reduce the pain of local infiltration. Lidocaine-prilocaine cream (e.g., EMLA [eutectic mixture of local anesthetics]) must be applied to intact skin at least 30 to 60 minutes before the procedure (follow manufacturer's directions), a disadvantage at times. EMLA is dosed based on child's weight and the amount of skin surface covered. Monitor the child during EMLA application to avoid accidental ingestion of the cream. Lidocaine can be dispersed in liposomes (e.g., L.M.X.4, Ferndale Labs, Maxilene, RGR Pharma) and does not require an occlusive dressing. Depth of dermal anesthesia depends on the duration of application. The analgesic effects may be equivalent to EMLA, even with the shorter application time (Eichenfield, Funk, Fallon-Friedlander, & Cunningham, 2002).

Skin refrigerants or vapocoolants, such as Frigiderm, Fluori-Methane, and ethyl chloride, are effective in reducing brief procedural pain such as injections and lumbar punctures (Abbott & Fowler-Kerry, 1995; Maikler, 1991; Reis & Holubkov, 1997). Ethyl chloride is flammable and requires adequate ventilation; thus the other vapocoolants are better choices. The refrigerant is sprayed for a few seconds (do not apply to the point of frost formation) onto the cleansed and prepared site immediately before needle insertion. Because some children experience the direct spray as noxious, a cotton ball can be saturated with the vapocoolant and then held to the site, using forceps, for 15 seconds. Anesthesia is effective immediately and lasts about 1 minute.

Iontophoresis is used over intact skin for painful procedures. Lidocaine iontophoresis has been demonstrated to reduce pain with venipuncture over placebo (Rose, Galinkin, Jantzen, & Chiavacci, 2002; Zempsky et al., 1998) and to provide similar pain relief as EMLA for insertion of IV catheters (Galinkin, Rose, Harris, & Watcha, 2002). Iontophoresis produces topical anesthesia by using a mild electrical current from a small battery-powered generator and two iontophoretic drug-delivery electrodes to push drug molecules into the skin. Numby Stuff delivers 1 mL of iontocaine (lidocaine HCl 2% with epinephrine 1:100,000) and therefore should not be used in children with a history of allergy to amide-type anesthetics, epinephrine, or sulfites (Brent, 2000). It also should not be used in children who have electrically sensitive equipment (e.g., pacemakers) or over damaged skin or new scar tissue. Place the drug-delivery electrode over the procedure site and the ground electrode over a major muscle at least 15 cm from the drug-delivery electrode. Children frequently complain of a tingling burning sensation from the electric current. To decrease this feeling, place the two electrodes far apart or place the ground electrode on a parent or nurse.

Alert! *Do not use electrode delivery on body parts supplied by end arteries. If the child complains of undue burning or pain during treatment, pause the treatment and inspect the site under the electrode. Stop the iontophoresis if excessive irritation is present or discomfort persists.*

Anesthesia occurs in 10 to 40 minutes, a major advantage over the time required for EMLA cream.

LET (lidocaine, epinephrine, tetracaine) is an anesthetic used for lacerations repair. Available as a liquid or gel, LET is applied directly on the wound and on a cotton ball or swab and held firmly for 10 to 30 minutes. Calculate the maximum lidocaine dose so as not to exceed it, especially if intradermal lidocaine is also used. LET should not be used on mucous membranes or body parts supplied by end arteries, such as the fingers or toes, or in children who are allergic to any of its components. LET should be placed on the wound for 10 to 30 minutes before suturing. Look for blanching of the wound bed to assess effectiveness.

Lidocaine jelly (2% water-soluble lubricant) should be used to minimize pain associated with urethral (Gray, 1996) and enteral tube insertion. Verify that the child has no history of allergy to amide-type anesthetics and do not use over damaged skin or mucous membranes. For urethral catheterization, insert lidocaine into the urethra 3 to 5 minutes before the procedure to allow anesthesia to occur. Use caution not to introduce lubricant into the lumen of an enteral catheter when coating the tube before insertion.

Biobehavioral Strategies (Nonpharmacologic) and Comfort Interventions

Biobehavioral techniques are used to manage mild pain and augment efficacy of medications in patients with moderate to severe pain. These biobehavioral interventions are now often termed complementary or alternative therapies.

Alert! *These interventions are not alternatives to analgesics. These techniques are adjuvants to pharmacologic management; they are never used in place of analgesic or anesthetic medications.*

Some biobehavioral methods may result in an actual reduction in pain intensity, but they are probably most effective as coping strategies. Biobehavioral techniques allow the child to play an active role, as opposed to that of a helpless victim, and give the child control or a sense of mastery over his or her response to the situation, thus often reducing distress or anxiety and ultimately resulting in decreased perception of the pain. General principles of pediatric care providing psychological support must also be followed (Chart 7-2). Examples of biobehavioral methods include cognitive-behavioral interventions such as distraction, relaxation, biofeedback, imagery, and hypnosis; biophysical management techniques include swaddling, holding, positioning, non-nutritive sucking and sweet solutions, kangaroo care, cold, heat, traditional massage, acupuncture and acupressure, and transcutaneous nerve stimulation.

Implement all interventions in a developmentally appropriate manner. Some biobehavioral interventions are not

CHART 7-2 General Principles of Psychological Support for a Child Undergoing a Painful Procedure

- Perform painful procedures in an area away from the child's bed when possible.
- Do not talk over the child—talk to the child or leave the area.
- Prepare the child for a situation; the amount and type of information is dependent on the child's cognitive level and coping style.
- Be honest regarding potential pain and sensations; for example, "Some children have told me that the stinging feeling when they put the medicine in was the worst part; you tell me what you think." Let the child know that something may hurt but that things can be done to make it not hurt as badly.
- Solicit the child's feedback and perspective: "What do you think will help you?"
- Give the child control whenever possible: "Would you like to remove the dressing?" "Do you want the IV in your right hand or left hand?"
- Recommend what the child can do ("Hold your hand very still"), not what the child should not do ("Don't move your hand").
- Provide positive reinforcement for desired actions.

appropriate for certain age groups or require a degree of cognitive development. For example:

- Cutaneous stimulation may provide too much stimuli for preterm infants; thus, when cutaneous stimulation is administered, monitor the infant for stress cues and modify the intervention based on the infant's response.
- Toddlers and preschool-aged children may not tolerate transcutaneous electrical nerve stimulation (TENS) because of the tingling sensation associated with it.
- Adolescents may be able to self-hypnotize; preschool-aged children may cooperate well with imagery.

It is beyond the scope of this text to discuss interventions in detail. For more information, the reader is referred to other sources (Chen, Joseph, & Zeltzer, 2000; Kemper & Gardiner, 2003; Kuttner & Solomon, 2003; Stevens, Gibbons, & Franck, 2000). Biobehavioral methods can broadly be categorized as cognitive-behavioral interventions and biophysical interventions (Table 7-2). Parents also play a key role in comforting and supporting their child.

Parental Involvement

Parents are an important component of pediatric pain management during both assessment and intervention. A parent who is educated about what is going to happen and what he or she can do to facilitate pain management generally feels less helpless and is better able to support the child. Parents may inadvertently encourage pain behaviors in children with chronic or recurrent pain conditions by rewarding the child with special privileges or relieving them of responsibilities due to their pain, such as school attendance and chores (Bursch, Joseph, & Zeltzer, 2003; Scharff, Leichtner, & Rappaport, 2003). Strategies to reduce parental anxiety have been associated with decreases in children's report of pain and their pain behaviors (AAP & APS, 2001). Therefore carefully prepare parents for what will happen to the child and how the parent can coach the child to cope with the procedure and pain.

During painful procedures, give parents the option to stay with their child. Reinforce that their role is to support their child, and assure them if they opt not to stay, someone

TABLE 7-2

Nonpharmacologic Pain Intervention Techniques Suggested Based on Age*

	Age				
Technique	**Infant†**	**Toddler**	**Preschool-Aged**	**School-Aged**	**Adolescent**
Cognitive-Behavioral					
Auditory stimuli	X	X	X	X	X
Biofeedback				X	X
Choices, control		X	X	X	X
Controlled breathing			X	X	X
Distraction	X	X	X	X	X
Imagery			X	X	X
Hypnosis				X	X
Modeling		X	X	X	X
Preparation	X	X	X	X	X
Relaxation			X	X	X
Biophysical					
Acupressure, acupuncture				X	X
Environmental modification	X	X	X	X	X
Holding, touch	X	X	X	X	X
Massage	X	X	X	X	X
Positioning	X	X	X	X	X
Rocking	X	X			
Sucking	X	X			
Sucrose	X				
Swaddling, containment	X				
TENS			X	X	X
Thermal application of heat or cold		X	X	X	X

*Techniques should be selected based on child's age, cognitive level, pain situation, past experience, and so forth. Several interventions may be used to augment the effectiveness of each.

†Many techniques may overstimulate an infant, particularly preterm infants who may not be able to filter out extraneous stimuli; the more immature the infant, the higher chance that overstimulation will disorient the infant. Intervene with one technique, monitor the infant for stress cues, and modify (add, decrease, or remove stimuli) based on the infant's message. Preparation of an infant includes preparing the parents.

TENS, transcutaneous electrical stimulation.

will be there to support the child. Prepare parents for how to help their child cope by giving them specific, concrete, and developmentally appropriate suggestions, such as holding the child's hand, speaking in a low and soothing voice, maintaining eye contact with the child, and distracting the child. Parents may become scared or tired when helping their child undergoing a procedure, and support from the nurse typically helps the parent recover and continue as an effective support for the child (Broome, 2000).

Cognitive-Behavioral Interventions

The goal of cognitive-behavioral interventions is to teach patients to identify, evaluate, and change sensory and thought patterns to facilitate coping behaviors (Gerik, 2005). These often work well in children who are very responsive to activities that take advantage of their natural skills of imagination. They are most effective when they draw on multiple senses: auditory, visual, tactile, and kinesthetic (e.g., encouraging the child to take an imaginary walk on a sunny beach with the waves crashing in, to feel the warm sun on his or her arms and the sand squishing between his or her toes). Behavioral techniques are designed to change either the child's own behaviors or the behaviors of the adults who interact with him or her. Encouraging active participation in mind–body strategies, also known as a coping plan, can avert attention from pain and modify behaviors that may initiate or exacerbate the pain.

Cognitive-behavioral strategies typically include combinations of the following:

- Preparation: Providing developmentally appropriate information helps the child and family develop realistic expectations of the pain and reduce the influence of fear of the unknown. Be honest if pain is anticipated. Provide concrete, objective information; model coping strategies.
- Distraction: Obtain active involvement of the child and tailor the activity to the child's developmental level and preference. Blowing bubbles or blowing on party blowers, manipulating wands or pinwheels, reading books or looking at pop-up books or books with parts that the child can manipulate, and playing virtual reality games are particularly effective activities (Wolitsky et al., 2005). The use of distraction remains a dominant strategy for reducing behavioral distress and pain despite the lack of evidence that it is effective at reducing or relieving children's pain. Therefore the use of distraction techniques should accompany pharmacologic interventions.
- Auditory stimuli: These are used both to decrease noxious noise and to increase pleasurable attention-focusing sound. Beneficial techniques include using a low-pitched and soothing voice, uterine sounds, or music (60-cycle instrumental music may be relaxing for some; older children may prefer raucous rock music; music presented through earphones also filters out environmental noise).
- Biofeedback: This gives information to the child about a physiologic function (heart rate, skin temperature, muscle tension) often through a visual display or audible tone. The child is instructed to use mental imagery to increase or decrease response in the system being monitored; reinforcement occurs when the child effects change in the system. Biofeedback requires specialized training and equipment.
- Modeling and rehearsal: These are performed to demonstrate positive coping behaviors (through an adult, a stuffed animal, another child [with permission], or videotape); provide an opportunity for the child to practice these coping techniques.
- Controlled breathing: This can focus the child's attention and help induce relaxation. Monitor for hyperventilation when using this technique. A young child can be taught to take a breath and say "ha" when exhaling; older children can take a deep breath in through the nose and exhale through pursed lips or can count to 10 while inhaling and then saying the number with each exhalation.
- Relaxation: This can help reduce anxiety and muscle tension, both of which may increase perception of pain. Controlled breathing is frequently a component of relaxation; imagery and hypnosis also induce relaxation. Practicing before the painful event increases the success of the technique. The child often requires help in implementing relaxation techniques under stressful conditions. When teaching relaxation techniques, keep the environment quiet; speak in a low, calm, measured tone; and have the child assume a comfortable position in a supportive chair or bed. There are no data to indicate that relaxation alone is effective in lessening chronic, cancer, surgical, or procedural pain, and therefore relaxation should be combined with analgesics, distraction, imagery, or hypnosis (McGrath, Dick, & Unruh, 2003).
- Imagery: The child is actively involved in visualizing a situation. Ask what the child's favorite place or activity is; also ask about fears (e.g., a fear of water), so that it is not brought into the imagery. Typically, the more senses one involves in the imagery, the more engrossing the image (imaging feeling, seeing, hearing a situation). Imagery begins with achieving a relaxed state. Guide the child to choose a favorite place. Cue the child to experience this familiar surrounding by exploring the sights, sounds, smells, and his or her feelings when in the special place.
- Hypnosis: The child enters an altered state of consciousness characterized by focused attention and profound relaxation. Hypnotic state induction should be performed under the supervision of an experienced practitioner and requires practice by the child.

Biophysical Interventions

Biophysical techniques attempt to affect physiologic responses directly during painful experiences. Biophysical strategies used to reduce pain in older children and adolescents are generally contraindicated in the high-risk neonatal population because of the physiologic response that is evoked, which may cause deleterious vital sign changes and make the infant more susceptible to intraventricular hemorrhage.

Biophysical interventions include the following:

- Environmental modification: Reduce noxious stimuli by decreasing noise (pad trash can lids, set phone ring volume to low, close doors quietly, talk at low volumes, decrease or eliminate overhead paging and radios) and light (turn lights on low, cover isolette or crib); provide periods of undisturbed rest.
- Positioning: Therapeutic positioning provides support for body alignment and reduces muscle tension over painful areas (e.g., the head of the bed is raised slightly and knees flexed to reduce pain associated with an abdominal incision). For infants, swaddling and containment provide boundaries and limit excessive motor responses due to an immature nervous system, facilitating self-regulation in preterm infants. Containment may be provided by tucking blanket rolls or prefabricated nesting around the infant and positioning the infant with extremities flexed. To provide containment during painful procedures, one caregiver should perform the procedure and another should monitor the infant for stress cues and provide support by holding the infant flexed, with the caregiver's hands supporting the child (and concurrently offering sucrose and pacifier for the infant to suck) (Stevens, Yamada, & Ohlsson, 2004; Thompson, 2005; Ward-Larson, Horn, & Gosnell, 2004). Infants older than 3 to 6 months often fight against swaddling, which may intensify anxiety and pain.
- Interpersonal contact: Holding is comforting for children of all ages and limits excessive uncontrolled movement that might exacerbate pain. The comforting benefits of holding are dependent on the child's temperament and pain situation. Use firm pressure or stroking; preterm infants respond more positively to firm pressure on their heads or heels than on the trunk. Skin-to-skin contact (kangaroo care) and holding with sucking during painful procedures reduces an infant's pain response (Johnston et al., 2003; Ludington-Hoe, Hosseini, & Torowicz, 2005; Phillips, Chantry, & Gallagher, 2005).
- Sucking: Sucking during painful stimuli such as circumcision, in addition to other analgesia such as dorsal penile nerve blocks, heel sticks, and eye examinations (Akman et al., 2002; Mitchell et al., 2004; South et al., 2005), attenuates pain distress behaviors and has a pacifying effect for preterm infants and newborns. Sucking a pacifier at a rate of at least 30 sucks per minute provides an analgesic effect (Blass & Watt, 1999). No short-term negative effects of non-nutritive sucking have been identified; data on long-term effects are not available (Pinelli, Symington, & Ciliska, 2002). Offer a pacifier or breast or encourage hand-to-mouth behaviors in infants who are undergoing painful procedures or are experiencing pain.
- Sucrose: Ingestion of sucrose decreases pain behaviors in term and preterm infants. A systematic review of the research found that a 24% solution of sucrose was effective in alleviating procedural pain in neonates (Stevens, Yamada, & Ohlsson, 2004). Other sweet-tasting solutions, such as 12.5% dextrose, 30% glucose, and 30% fructose (Akcam, 2004; Akcam & Ormeci, 2004; Akman et al., 2002), reduce pain behaviors in newborns as well but have not been studied as extensively as sucrose. Breast milk and breast-feeding are also analgesic (Aliwalas, Shah, & Shah, 2004; Phillips, Chantry, & Gallagher, 2005; Schollin, 2004; Upadhyay et al., 2004). There is no evidence that sucrose at this dose affects blood glucose; however, sucrose should be used with caution in any neonate with unstable blood glucose levels. Repeated use of sucrose for pain management is effective and safe, but more research is needed on clinical, neurobiologic, and developmental outcomes (Stevens et al., 2005).

  A pacifier can be dipped in sucrose and offered to the infant, or sucrose can be instilled by syringe followed by use of a pacifier. Use of sweet solutions and sucking may reduce pain through multisensorial pathways, thus being more effective in combination than either alone and should be offered to an infant during a painful procedure, either alone or to augment pharmacologic methods for moderate to severe pain.
- Rocking: Rocking by caregivers decreased recovery time from painful procedures in term newborns (Campos, 1994), but simulated rocking using an air mattress was not shown to be effective in decreasing pain response during painful procedures (Johnston, Stremler, Stevens, & Horton, 1997). For pain not associated with procedures, rocking may relax young children and decrease tension that might contribute to increased pain perception.
- Cutaneous stimulation: Stimulation of the skin and underlying tissues may provide benign sensory input to reduce or block transmission of painful stimuli; cutaneous stimulation also promotes blood circulation to the area. Cutaneous stimulation may be performed over painful areas, on localized areas, or by total-body massage. When direct cutaneous stimulation is not possible or tolerated, it may be applied adjacent to the painful area, between the affected area and the brain, or contralateral to the painful site. Cutaneous stimulation must be used cautiously in preterm infants because it often causes a greater intensity of response and disorganizes the infant.
  - Massage may be performed using hands or a vibrator. Use a constant rhythmic movement of moderate intensity. Light pressure is often perceived as a tickle; heavy pressure may induce more pain.

- Thermal application may involve heat, cold, or ice. For older children, cold is typically more effective in providing pain relief than heat, but heat is often better accepted. For trauma-associated pain, cold may decrease inflammation and muscle spasms. Ice massage is effective for headaches, musculoskeletal and injection pain, and brief procedures. Wrap cold and hot packs so that the pack feels cool or warm but not uncomfortable. To provide moist heat, dampen a washcloth with warm tap water and apply it directly to the area, covering it with an impermeable cover (e.g., disposable diaper or bed liner); remove as soon as the compress cools and reapply as indicated.

Alert! *Heat and cold application is not recommended for use in infants, who are more prone to thermal injury because of their skin structure. Cold may also cause hypothermia. These interventions should also be avoided in children with altered skin sensations such as spina bifida or in nonverbal children who are unable to alert care providers of temperature extremes that may cause tissue injury. Stop thermal therapies if the child complains or blanching or redness occurs; monitor skin integrity. Do not use in sleeping children or for periods longer than 30 minutes.*

- Transcutaneous electrical nerve stimulation: TENS may interfere with pain signal transmission by use of a small electrical current applied to the skin through conductive pads attached to a battery-operated generator. TENS causes a tingling sensation and may produce fear in a child.

KidKare To reduce fear, demonstrate the equipment on a parent and then apply to a nonpainful area on the child, moving to the painful area. Give the child some control over the sensation by allowing the child to adjust the TENS settings.

- Acupuncture: Acupuncture is based on the theory that energy flows along channels through the body that are connected by acupuncture points and that pain results when the energy flow is obstructed. Inserting fine needles at these acupuncture points reduces pain. Acupressure is a noninvasive derivative of acupuncture, whereby manual pressure is applied to the skin at acupuncture points. Acupressure may be more readily accepted by children than acupuncture due to children's fear of needles.

REASSESSMENT

Regular assessments of pain are necessary to evaluate adequacy of interventions and identify inadequate pain relief. Assess pain level within 1 hour after pain interventions. If the assessment identifies inadequate pain control through child report, behaviors, or physiologic parameters, best evidenced by a multidimensional pain-rating tool, then implement interventions and reassess pain at the appropriate interval.

SPECIFIC PAIN SITUATIONS

Management of pain is typically more successful using a multimodal approach. Medications are used whenever indicated, augmented by developmentally appropriate biobehavioral techniques. Specific pain situations require different methods and approaches for optimal pain management.

Procedural Pain

Often of short duration, pain associated with procedures is managed by ensuring that competent practitioners perform the procedure. Prepare the child and parents. Depending on the nature of the procedure and the child's age, cognitive level, and temperament, pain management methods include pharmacologic management of pain ranging from local anesthetics, inhaled nitrous oxide, systemic medications (anxiolytics or sedatives must not be administered without analgesia to manage the pain) to sedation following AAP guidelines (see Chapter 105); cognitive-behavioral techniques; and biophysical interventions.

Acute Pain

Acute pain is typically associated with operative procedures, trauma, and disease. Control pain as soon as possible, administering optimal doses of analgesics initially, as ordered, and titrating to the child's response (as opposed to repeated small doses). For pain that is expected to persist, around-the-clock dosing is necessary (versus on an as-needed basis). For moderate to severe pain, PCA or epidural administration of medication may provide better pain relief. Anticipate adverse effects associated with medication use (e.g., constipation with opioid use; synergistic effects of analgesics and anxiolytics and of antihistamines and antiemetics). Use biobehavioral methods to augment the pharmacologic regime. As the child's pain decreases, modify the medication regime to gradually decrease doses because analgesia medications should not be abruptly discontinued.

Chronic Pain

Management of chronic pain requires a multimodal approach that incorporates biobehavioral techniques on a routine basis, NSAIDs, opioids as necessary, local anesthetics, and coanalgesics (e.g., tricyclic antidepressants, anticonvulsants, clonidine). Biobehavioral methods are dependent on child and family preference and schedules (e.g., deep breathing and muscle relaxation or imagery every 2 hours, daily yoga, cutaneous stimulation). Teach the child to use proper body mechanics at all times. Children with persistent pain may refuse to participate in physical activities, thus losing flexibility and muscle tone. Simple stretching exercises and light weight training (as appropriate) performed for 10 to 20 minutes every day help to maintain flexibility and muscle tone.

Severe pain is a medical emergency and must be managed as such. Effective pain management in any situation requires maintaining a high index of suspicion for the presence of pain, assessment with valid and reliable multidimensional tools, use of nonpharmacologic interventions to augment pharmacologic interventions when indicated, and reassessment to evaluate adequacy of interventions. Management must be individualized for the child, family, and pain situation.

Adequate pain management is an ethical imperative. The historical undertreatment of pain in children can be ameliorated by educated practitioners. All members of the healthcare team must advocate for the patient and work as a team with the family to achieve effective pain management for children.

Bibliography

Abbott, K., & Fowler-Kerry, S. (1995). The use of a topical refrigerant anesthetic to reduce injection pain in children. *Journal of Pain and Symptom Management, 10*, 584–590.

Acute Pain Management Guideline Panel. (1992). *Acute pain management: Operative or medical procedures and trauma.* Clinical practice guideline (AHCPR Publication No. 92-0032). Rockville, MD: Agency for Health Care Policy and Research, Public Health Service, U.S. Department of Health and Human Services.

Akcam, M. (2004). Oral fructose solution as an analgesic in the newborn: A randomized, placebo-controlled and masked study. *Pediatrics International, 46*, 459–462.

Akcam, M., & Ormeci, A. R. (2004). Oral hypertonic glucose spray: A practical alternative for analgesia in the newborn. *Acta Paediatrica, 93*, 1330–1333.

Akman, I., Ozek, E., Bilgen, R., Ozdogan, T., & Cebeci, D. (2002). Sweet solutions and pacifiers for pain relief in newborn infants. *Journal of Pain, 3*, 199–202.

Aliwalas, L. L., Shah, V., & Shah, P. S. (2004). Breastfeeding or breast milk for procedural pain in neonates. *The Cochrane Database of Systematic Reviews*, (4), No. CD004950.

American Academy of Pediatrics and American Pain Society. (2001). Policy statement: The assessment and management of acute pain in infants, children, and adolescents (07). *Pediatrics, 105*, 454–461.

American Academy of Pediatrics and Canadian Paediatric Society. (2000). Policy statement: Prevention and management of pain and stress in the neonate (RE9945). *Pediatrics, 108*, 793–797.

American Pain Society (APS). (2003). *Principles of analgesic use in the treatment of acute pain and cancer pain* (5th ed.). Glenview, IL: American Pain Society.

American Pain Society (APS). (2004). *Pediatric chronic pain: A position statement.* Glenview, IL: Author. Retrieved March 21, 2006, from http://www.ampainsoc.org/advocacy/pediatric.htm

American Pain Society (APS). (2005). *Guideline for the management of cancer pain in adults and children.* Glenview, IL: Author.

Baxt, C., Kassam-Adams, N., Nance, M. L., Vivarelli-O'Neill, C., & Winston, F. K. (2004). Assessment of pain after injury in the pediatric patient: Child and parent perceptions. *Journal of Pediatric Surgery, 39*, 979–983.

Beyer, J., Denyes, M., & Villarruel, A. (1992). The creation, validation, and continuing development of the Oucher: A measure of pain intensity in children. *Journal of Pediatric Nursing, 7*, 335–346.

Beyer, J. E., & Knott, C. B. (1998). Construct validity estimation for the African-American and Hispanic versions of the Oucher scale. *Journal of Pediatric Nursing, 13*, 20–31.

Blass, E. M., & Watt, L. B. (1999). Suckling- and sucrose-induced analgesia in human newborns. *Pain, 83*, 611–623.

Breau, L. M., Finley, G. A., McGrath, P. J., & Camfield, C. S. (2002). Validation of the non-communicating children's pain checklist—postoperative version. *Anesthesiology, 96*, 528–535.

Breau, L. M., McGrath, P. J., Camfield, C. S., & Finley, G. A. (2002). Psychometric properties of the non-communicating children's pain checklist—revised. *Pain, 99*, 49–57.

Brent, A. S. G. (2000). The management of pain in the emergency department. *Pediatric Clinics of North America, 47*, 651–679.

Brinker, D. (2004). Sedation and comfort issues in the ventilated infant and child. *Critical Care Nursing Clinics of North America, 16*, 365–377.

Broome, M. E. (2000). Helping parents support their child in pain. *Pediatric Nursing, 26*, 315–317.

Bursch, B., Joseph, M. H., & Zeltzer, L. K. (2003). Pain-associated disability syndrome. In N. L. Schechter, C. B. Berde, & M. Yaster (Eds.), *Pain in infants, children, and adolescents* (2nd ed., pp. 841–848). Philadelphia: Lippincott Williams & Wilkins.

Campos, R. G. (1994). Rocking and pacifiers: Two comforting interventions for heelstick pain. *Research in Nursing and Health, 17*, 321–331.

Chambers, C. T., Finley, G. A., McGrath, P. J., & Walsh, T. M. (2003). The parents' postoperative pain measure: Replication and extension to 2- to 6-year-old children. *Pain, 105*, 437–443.

Chen, E., Joseph, M. H., & Zeltzer, L. K. (2000). Behavioral and cognitive interventions in the treatment of pain in children. *Pediatric Clinics of North America, 47*, 513–525.

Claar, R. L., & Walker, L. S. (2006). Functional assessment of pediatric pain: Psychometric properties of the Functional Disability Inventory. *Pain, 121*, 77–84.

Colwell, C., Clark, L., & Perkins, R. (1996). Postoperative use of pediatric pain scales: Children's self-report versus nurse assessment of pain intensity and affect. *Journal of Pediatric Nursing, 11*, 375–382.

Dahlquist, L. M., Busby, S. M., Slifer, K. J., et al. (2002). Distraction for children of different ages who undergo repeated needle sticks. *Journal of Pediatric Oncology Nursing, 19*, 22–34.

de Rond, M. E. J., de Wit, R., van Dam, F. S. A., & Muller, M. J. (2000). A pain monitoring program for nurses: Effects on communication, assessment and documentation of patients' pain. *Journal of Pain and Symptom Management, 20*, 424–439.

Eccleston, C., Yorke, L., Morley, S., Williams, A. C., & Mastroyannopoulou, K. (2003). Psychological therapies for the management of chronic and recurrent pain in children and adolescents. *The Cochrane Database of Systematic Reviews*, (1), No. CD003968.

Eichenfield, L. F., Funk, A., Fallon-Friedlander, S., & Cunningham, B. B. (2002). A clinical study to evaluate the efficacy of ELA-Max (4% liposomal lidocaine) as compared with eutectic mixture of local anesthetics cream for pain reduction of venipuncture in children. *Pediatrics, 109*, 1093–1099.

Eland, J. M., & Anderson, J. E. (1977). The experience of pain in children. In A. K. Jacox (Ed.), *Pain: A sourcebook for nurses and other health professionals* (pp. 453–476). Boston: Little, Brown.

Fanurik, D., Koh, J. L., Harrison, R. D., Conrad, T. M., & Tomerlin, C. (1998). Pain assessment in children with cognitive impairment: An exploration of self-report skills. *Clinical Nursing Research, 7*, 103–124.

Fitzgerald, M., & Beggs, S. (2001). The neurobiology of pain: Developmental aspects. *Neuroscientist, 7*, 246–257.

Foster, R. L., Yucha, C. B., Zuk, J., & Vojir, C. P. (2003). Physiologic correlates of comfort in healthy children. *Pain Management Nursing, 4*(1), 23–30.

Franck, L. S. (2003). Nursing management of children's pain: Current evidence and future directions for research. *NT Research, 8*, 330–353.

Franck, L. S., Greenberg, C. S., & Stevens, B. (2000). Pain assessment in infants and children. *Pediatric Clinics of North America, 47*, 487–512.

Gaffney, A., McGrath, P. J., & Dick, B. (2003). Measuring pain in children: Developmental and instrumental issues. In N. L. Schechter, C. B. Berde, & M. Yaster (Eds.), *Pain in infants, children, and adolescents* (2nd ed., pp. 241–264). Philadelphia: Lippincott Williams & Wilkins.

Galinkin, J. L., Rose, J. B., Harris, K., & Watcha, M. F. (2002). Lidocaine iontophoresis versus eutectic mixture of local anesthetics (EMLA) for IV placement in children. *Anesthesia & Analgesia, 94*, 1484–1488.

Gauvain-Piquard, A., Rodary, C., Francois, P., et al. (1991). Validity assessment of DEGR® Scale for observational rating of 2- to 6-year-old child pain. *Journal of Pain and Symptom Management, 6*, 171.

Gauvain-Piquard, A., Rodary, C., Rezvani, A., & Lemerle, J. (1987). Pain in children aged 2–6 years: A new observational rating scale elaborated in a pediatric oncology unit. Preliminary report. *Pain, 31*, 177–188.

Gerik, S. M. (2005). Pain management in children: Developmental considerations and mind-body therapies. *Southern Medical Journal, 98*, 295–302.

Goldschneider, K. R., & Anand, K. S. (2003). Long-term consequences of pain in neonates. In N. L. Schechter, C. B. Berde, & M. Yaster (Eds.), *Pain in infants, children, and adolescents* (2nd ed., pp. 58–70). Philadelphia: Lippincott Williams & Wilkins.

Golianu, B., Krane, E., Galloway, K. S., & Yaster, M. (2000). Pediatric acute pain management. *Pediatric Clinics of North America, 47*, 559–587.

Gray, M. (1996). Atraumatic urethral catheterization of children. *Pediatric Nursing, 22*, 306–310.

Grunau, R. (2002). Early pain in preterm infants: A model of long-term effects. *Clinics in Perinatology, 29*, 373–394.

Grunau, R. E., Holsti, L., Haley, D. W., et al. (2005). Neonatal procedural pain exposure predicts lower cortisol and behavioral reactivity in preterm infants in the NICU. *Pain, 113*, 293–300.

Grunau, R. E., Oberlander, T., Holsti, L., & Whitfield, M. F. (1998). Bedside application of the Neonatal Facial Coding System in pain assessment of premature infants. *Pain, 76*, 277–286.

Guinsburg, R., Peres, C. A., Almeida, M. F. B., et al. (2000). Differences in pain expression between male and female newborn infants. *Pain, 85*, 127–133.

Hadden, K. L., & von Baeyer, C. L. (2005). Global and specific behavioral measures of pain in children with cerebral palsy. *Clinical Journal of Pain, 21*, 140–146.

Hester, N. O. (1979). The preoperational child's reaction to immunization. *Nursing Research, 28*, 250–255.

Hicks, C. L., von Baeyer, C. L., Spafford, P. A., van Korlaar, I., & Goodenough, B. (2001). The Faces Pain Scale—revised: Toward a common metric in pediatric pain measurement. *Pain, 93*, 173–183.

Hodgkinson, K., Bear, M., Thorn, J., & Van Blaricum, S. (1994). Measuring pain in neonates: Evaluating an instrument and developing a common language. *Australian Journal of Advanced Nursing, 12*, 17–22.

Holsti, L., Grunau, R. E., Oberlander, T. F., Whitfield, M. F., & Weinberg, J. (2005). Body movements: An important additional factor in discriminating pain from stress in preterm infants. *Clinical Journal of Pain, 21*, 491–498.

Huang, C. M., Tung, W. S., Kuo, L. L., & Ying-Ju, C. (2004). Comparison of pain responses of premature infants to the heelstick between containment and swaddling. *Journal of Nursing Research, 12*, 31–40.

Hunt, A., Goldman, A., Seers, K., et al. (2004). Clinical validation of the Paediatric Pain Profile. *Developmental Medicine & Child Neurology, 46*, 9–18.

International Association for the Study of Pain, Subcommittee on Taxonomy. (1979). Pain terms: A list with definitions and notes on usage. *Pain, 6*, 249–252.

Joint Commission on Accreditation of Healthcare Organizations. (2005). *Comprehensive accreditation manual for hospitals: The official handbook.* Oakbrook Terrace, IL: Author.

Johnston, C. C., Stevens, B. J., Boyer, K., & Porter, F. L. (2003). Development of psychological responses to pain and assessment of pain in infants and toddlers. In N. L. Schechter, C. B. Berde, & M. Yaster (Eds.), *Pain in infants, children, and adolescents* (2nd ed., pp. 105–127). Philadelphia: Lippincott Williams & Wilkins.

Johnston, C. C., Stevens, B. J., Pinelli, J., et al. (2003). Kangaroo care is effective in diminishing pain response in preterm neonates. *Archives of Pediatrics & Adolescent Medicine, 157*, 1084–1088.

Johnston, C. C., Stremler, R. L., Stevens, B. J., & Horton, L. J. (1997). Effectiveness of oral sucrose and simulated rocking on pain response in preterm neonates. *Pain, 72*, 193–199.

Jones, M., Qazi, M., & Young, K. D. (2005). Ethnic differences in parent preference to be present for painful medical procedures. *Pediatrics, 116*, e191–197.

Kemper, K. J., & Gardiner, P. (2003). Complementary and alternative medical therapies in pediatric pain management. In N. L. Schechter, C. B. Berde, & M. Yaster (Eds.), *Pain in infants, children, and adolescents* (2nd ed., pp. 449–461). Philadelphia: Lippincott Williams & Wilkins.

Kim, H., Neubert, J. K., San Miguel, A., et al. (2004). Genetic influence on variability in human acute experimental pain sensitivity associated with gender, ethnicity and psychological temperament. *Pain, 109*, 488–496.

Kolcaba, K., & DiMarco, M. A. (2005). Comfort theory and its application to pediatric nursing. *Pediatric Nursing, 31*, 187–194.

Krause, B., & Green, S. M. (2006). Procedural sedation and analgesia in children. *Lancet, 367*, 766–780.

Krechel, S. W., & Bildner, J. (1995). CRIES: A new neonatal postoperative pain measurement score. Initial testing of validity and reliability. *Paediatric Anaesthesia, 5*, 51–63.

Kuttner, L., & Solomon, R. (2003). Hypnotherapy and imagery for managing children's pain. In N. L. Schechter, C. B. Berde, & M. Yaster (Eds.), *Pain in infants, children, and adolescents* (2nd ed., pp. 317–328). Philadelphia: Lippincott Williams & Wilkins.

LaMontagne, L., Hepworth, J. T., Cohen, F., & Salisbury, M. (2003). Cognitive-behavioral intervention affects adolescents' anxiety and pain following spinal fusion surgery. *Nursing Research, 52*, 183–190.

LaMontagne, L., Hepworth, J. T., Salisbury, M. H., & Cohen, F. (2003). Effects of coping instruction in reducing young adolescents' pain after major spinal surgery. *Orthopaedic Nursing, 22*, 398–403.

Lawrence, J., Alcock, D., McGrath, P., et al. (1993). The development of a tool to assess neonatal pain. *Neonatal Network, 12*, 59–66.

Lehr, V. T., & BeVier, P. (2003). Patient-controlled analgesia for the pediatric patient. *Orthopaedic Nursing, 22*, 298–307.

Logan, H. L., Sheffield, D., Lutgendorf, S., & Lang, E. (2002). Predictors of pain during invasive medical procedures. *The Journal of Pain, 3*, 211–217.

Ludington-Hoe, S. M., Hosseini, R., & Torowicz, D. L. (2005). Skin-to-skin contact (kangaroo care) analgesia for preterm infant heel stick. *AACN Clinical Issues, 16*, 373–387.

Maikler, V. E. (1991). Effects of a skin refrigerant/anesthetic and age on the pain responses of infants receiving immunizations. *Research in Nursing & Health, 14*, 397–403.

Malviya, S., Voepel-Lewis, T., Burke, C., Merkel, S., & Tait, A. R. (2006). The revised FLACC observational pain tool: Improved reliability and validity for pain assessment in children with cognitive impairment. *Paediatric Anaesthesia, 16*, 258–265.

Maunuksela, E. L., & Olkkola, K. T. (2003). Nonsteroidal anti-inflammatory drugs in pediatric pain management. In N. L. Schechter, C. B. Berde, & M. Yaster (Eds.), *Pain in infants, children, and adolescents* (2nd ed., pp. 171–180). Philadelphia: Lippincott Williams & Wilkins.

McGrath, P. A., Seifert, C. E., Speechley, K. N., et al. (1996). A new analogue scale for assessing children's pain: An initial validation study. *Pain, 64*, 435–443.

McGrath, P. J., Dick, B., & Unruh, A. M. (2003). Psychological and behavioral treatment of pain in children and adolescents. In N. L. Schechter, C. B. Berde, & M. Yaster (Eds.), *Pain in infants, children, and adolescents* (2nd ed., pp. 303–316). Philadelphia: Lippincott Williams & Wilkins.

McGrath, P. J., Johnson, G., Goodman, J. T., et al. (1985). CHEOPS: A behavioral scale for rating postoperative pain in children. In H. L. Fields, R. Dubner, & F. Cervero (Eds.), *Advances in pain research and therapy* (pp. 395–402). New York: Raven Press.

McNair, C., Ballantyne, M., Dionne, K., Stephens, D., & Stevens, B. (2004). Postoperative pain assessment in the neonatal intensive care unit. *Archives of Disease in Childhood. Fetal and Neonatal Edition, 89*, F537–541.

Melzack, R. (1975). The McGill Pain Questionnaire: Major properties and scoring methods. *Pain, 1*, 277–299.

Melzack, R. (1987). The short-form McGill Pain Questionnaire. *Pain, 30*, 191–197.

Merkel, S. (2002). Pain assessment in infants and young children: The finger span scale provides an estimate of pain intensity in young children. *American Journal of Nursing, 102*(11), 55–56.

Merkel, S. I., Voepel-Lewis, T., Shayevitz, J. R., & Malviya, S. (1997). The FLACC: A behavioral scale for scoring postoperative pain in young children. *Pediatric Nursing, 23*, 293–297.

Miller, D. (1996). Comparisons of pain ratings from postoperative children, their mothers, and their nurses. *Pediatric Nursing, 22*, 145–149.

Mitchell, A., Stevens, B., Mungan, N., et al. (2004). Analgesic effects of oral sucrose and pacifier during eye examinations for retinopathy of prematurity. *Pain Management Nursing, 5*, 160–168.

Monitto, C. L., Greenberg, R. S., Kost-Byerly, S., et al. (2000). The safety and efficacy of parent/nurse-controlled analgesia in patients less than six years of age. *Anesthesia & Analgesia, 91*, 573–579.

National Association of Neonatal Nurses. (1999). *Position statement on pain management in infants (#3019)*. Glenview, IL: Author.

Peters, J. W., Koot, H. M., Grunau, R. E., et al. (2003). Neonatal Facial Coding System for assessing postoperative pain in infants: Item reduction is valid and feasible. *Clinical Journal of Pain, 19*, 353–363.

Phillips, R. M., Chantry, C. J., & Gallagher, M. P. (2005). Analgesic effects of breast-feeding or pacifier use with maternal holding in term infants. *Ambulatory Pediatrics, 5*, 359–364.

Piira, T., Sugiura, T., Champion, G. D., Donnelly, N., & Cole, A. S. J. (2005). The role of parental presence in the context of children's medical procedures: A systematic review. *Child: Care, Health & Development, 31*, 233–243.

Pinelli, J., Symington, A., & Ciliska, D. (2002). Nonnutritive sucking in high-risk infants: Benign intervention or legitimate therapy? *Journal of Obstetric, Gynecologic, & Neonatal Nursing, 31*, 582–591.

Polkki, T., Vehvilainen-Julkunen, K., & Pietila, A. M. (2002). Parents' roles in using non-pharmacological methods in their child's postoperative pain alleviation. *Journal of Clinical Nursing, 11*, 526–536.

Ramelet, A. S., Abu-Saad, H. H., Bulsara, M. K., Rees, N., & McDonald, S. (2006). Capturing postoperative pain responses in critically ill infants aged 0 to 9 months. *Pediatric Critical Care Medicine, 7*, 19–26.

Reis, E. C., & Holubkov, R. (1997). Vapocoolant spray is equally effective as EMLA cream in reducing immunization pain in school-aged children. *Pediatrics, 100*, e5–e14.

Romsing, J., Moller-Sonnergaard, J., Hertel, S., & Rasmussen, M. (1996). Postoperative pain in children: Comparison between ratings of children and nurses. *Journal of Pain and Symptom Management, 11*, 42–46.

Rose, J. B., Galinkin, J. L., Jantzen, E. C., & Chiavacci, R. M. (2002). A study of lidocaine iontophoresis for pediatric venipuncture. *Anesthesia & Analgesia, 94*, 867–871.

Rutledge, D. R., Donaldson, N. E., & Pravikoff, D. S. (2002). Update 2002. Pain assessment and documentation: Pediatrics. *Online Journal of Clinical Innovations, 5*, 1–45.

Savedra, M. C., Holzemer, W. L., Tesler, M. D., & Wilkie, D. J. (1993). Assessment of postoperation pain in children and adolescents using the Adolescent Pediatric Pain Tool. *Nursing Research, 42*, 5–9.

Savedra, M. C., Tesler, M. D., Holzemer, W. L., Wilkie, D. J., & Ward, J. A. (1989). Pain location: Validity and reliability of body outline markings by hospitalized children and adolescents. *Research in Nursing & Health, 12*, 307–314.

Scharff, L., Leichtner, A. M., & Rappaport, L. A. (2003). Recurrent abdominal pain. In N. L. Schechter, C. B. Berde, & M. Yaster (Eds.). *Pain in infants, children, and adolescents* (2nd ed., pp. 719–731). Philadelphia: Lippincott Williams & Wilkins.

Schechter, N. L., Berde, C. B., & Yaster, M. (2003). Pain in infants, children and adolescents: An overview. In N. L. Schechter, C. B. Berde, & M. Yaster (Eds.), *Pain in infants, children, and adolescents* (2nd ed., pp. 3–18). Philadelphia: Lippincott Williams & Wilkins.

Schollin, J. (2004). Analgesic effect of expressed breast milk in procedural pain in neonates. *Acta Paediatrica, 93*, 453–455.

Shields, B. J., Palermo, T. M., Powers, J. D., Grewe, S. D., & Smith, G. A. (2003). Predictors of a child's ability to use a visual analogue scale. *Child Care Health Development, 29*, 281–290.

Simons, S. H., van Dijk, M., Anand, K. S., et al. (2003). Do we still hurt newborn babies? A prospective study of procedural pain and analgesia in neonates. *Archives of Pediatrics and Adolescent Medicine, 157*, 1058–1064.

Solodiuk, J., & Curley, M. A. Q. (2003). Evidence-based practice in action. Pain assessment in nonverbal children with severe cognitive impairments: The Individualized Numeric Rating Scale (INRS). *Journal of Pediatric Nursing, 18*, 295–299.

South, M. M., Strauss, R. A., South, A. P., Boggess, J. F., & Thorp, J. M. (2005). The use of non-nutritive sucking to decrease the physiologic pain response during neonatal circumcision: A randomized controlled trial. *American Journal of Obstetrics and Gynecology, 193*, 537–542.

Spence, K., Gillies, D., Johnston, L., Harrison, D., & Nagy, S. (2005). A reliable pain assessment tool for clinical assessment in the neonatal intensive care unit. *Journal of Obstetric, Gynecologic, & Neonatal Nursing, 34*, 80–86.

Stallard, P., Williams, L., Velleman, R., et al. (2002). The development and evaluation of the pain indicator of communicatively impaired children. *Pain, 98*, 145–149.

Stanford, E. A., Chambers, C. T., & Craig, K. D. (2006). The role of developmental factors in predicting young children's use of a self-report scale for pain. *Pain, 120*, 16–23.

Stevens, B., Gibbons, S., & Franck, L. S. (2000). Treatment of pain in the neonatal intensive care unit. *Pediatric Clinics of North America, 47*, 633–650.

Stevens, B., Johnston, C., Petryshen, P., & Taddio, A. (1996). The Premature Infant Pain Profile: Development and initial validation. *Clinical Journal of Pain, 12*, 13–22.

Stevens, B., McGrath, P., Gibbins, S., et al. (2003). Procedural pain in newborns at risk for neurologic impairment. *Pain, 105*, 27–35.

Stevens, B., Yamada, J., Beyene, J., et al. (2005). Consistent management of repeated procedural pain with sucrose in preterm neonates: Is it effective and safe for repeated use over time? *Clinical Journal of Pain, 21*, 543–548.

Stevens, B., Yamada, J., & Ohlsson, A. (2004). Sucrose for analgesia in newborn infants undergoing painful procedures. *The Cochrane Database of Systematic Reviews*, (3), No. CD001069.

Tarbell, S. E., Cohen, I. T., & Marsh, J. L. (1992). The toddler-preschooler postoperative pain scale: An observational scale for measuring postoperative pain in children aged 1–5: Preliminary report. *Pain, 50*, 273–280.

Thompson, D. G. (2005). Utilizing an oral sucrose solution to minimize neonatal pain. *Journal of Specialists in Pediatric Nursing, 10*, 3–10.

Tobias, J. D. (2003). Pain management for the critically ill children in the pediatric intensive care unit. In N. L. Schechter, C. B. Berde, & M. Yaster (Eds.), *Pain in infants, children, and adolescents* (2nd ed., pp. 807–840). Philadelphia: Lippincott Williams & Wilkins.

Tsao, J. C. I., & Zeltzer, L. K. (2005). Complementary and alternative medicine approaches for pediatric pain: A review of the state-of-the-science. *Evidence-Based Complementary and Alternative Medicine, 2*, 149–159.

Turner, H. N. (2005). Complex pain consultations in the pediatric intensive care unit. *AACN Clinical Issues: Advanced Practice in Acute & Critical Care, 16*, 388–395.

Tyler, D. C., Tu, A., Douthit, J., & Chapman, C. R. (1993). Toward validation of pain measurement tools for children: A pilot study. *Pain, 52*, 301–309.

Uman, L. S., Chambers, C. T., McGrath, P. J., & Kisely, S. (2005). Psychological interventions for needle-related procedural pain and distress in children and adolescents. *The Cochrane Database of Systematic Reviews*, (1), No. CD005179.

Upadhyay, A., Aggarwal, R., Narayan, S., et al. (2004). Analgesic effect of expressed breast milk in procedural pain in term neonates: A randomized, placebo-controlled, double-blind trial. *Acta Paediatrica, 93*, 518–522.

Van Cleve, L. J., & Savedra, M. C. (1993). Pain location: Validity and reliability of body outline markings by 4- to 7-year-old children who are hospitalized. *Pediatric Nursing, 19*, 217–220.

van Dijk, M., de Boer, J. B., Koot, H. M., et al. (2000). The reliability and validity of the COMFORT scale as a postoperative pain instrument in 0- to 3-year-old infants. *Pain, 84*, 367–377.

Varni, J. W., Thompson, K. L., & Hanson, V. (1987). The Varni/Thompson pediatric pain questionnaire. I. Chronic musculoskeletal pain in juvenile rheumatoid arthritis. *Pain, 28*, 27–38.

Vincent, C. V. H., & Denyes, M. J. (2004). Relieving children's pain: Nurses' abilities and analgesic administration practices. *Journal of Pediatric Nursing, 19*, 40–50.

Voepel-Lewis, T., Malviya, S., & Tait, A. R. (2005). Validity of parent ratings as proxy measures of pain in children with cognitive impairment. *Pain Management Nursing, 6*, 168–174.

Walker, L. S., & Greene, J. W. (1991). The Functional Disability Inventory: Measuring a neglected dimension of child health status. *Journal of Pediatric Psychology, 16*, 39–58.

Ward-Larson, C., Horn, R. A., & Gosnell, F. (2004). The efficacy of facilitated tucking for relieving pain of endotracheal suctioning in very low birthweight infants. *MCN: The American Journal of Maternal Child Nursing, 29*, 151–158.

Willis, M. H. W., Merkel, S. I., Voepel-Lewis, T., & Malviya, S. (2003). FLACC Behavioral Pain Assessment Scale: A comparison with the child's self-report. *Pediatric Nursing, 29*, 195–198.

Wolitsky, K., Fiyush, R., Zimand, E., Hodges, L., & Rothbaum, B. O. (2005). Effectiveness of virtual reality distraction during a painful medical procedure in pediatric oncology patients. *Psychology & Health, 20*, 817–824.

Wong, D., & Baker, C. (1988). Pain in children: Comparison of assessment scales. *Pediatric Nursing, 14*, 9–17.

Yeh, C. H. (2005). Development and validation of the Asian version of the Oucher: A pain intensity scale for children. *Journal of Pain, 6*, 526–534.

Young, K. D. (2005). Pediatric procedural pain. *Annals of Emergency Medicine, 45*, 160–171.

Zempsky, W. T., Anand, K. J. S., Sullivan, K. M., Fraser, D., & Cucina, K. (1998). Lidocaine iontophoresis for topical anesthesia before intravenous line placement in children. *Journal of Pediatrics, 132*, 1061–1063.

Zernikow, B., Meyerhoff, U., Michel, E., et al. (2005). Pain in pediatric oncology—Children's and parent's perspectives. *European Journal of Pain, 9*, 395–406.

UNIT II

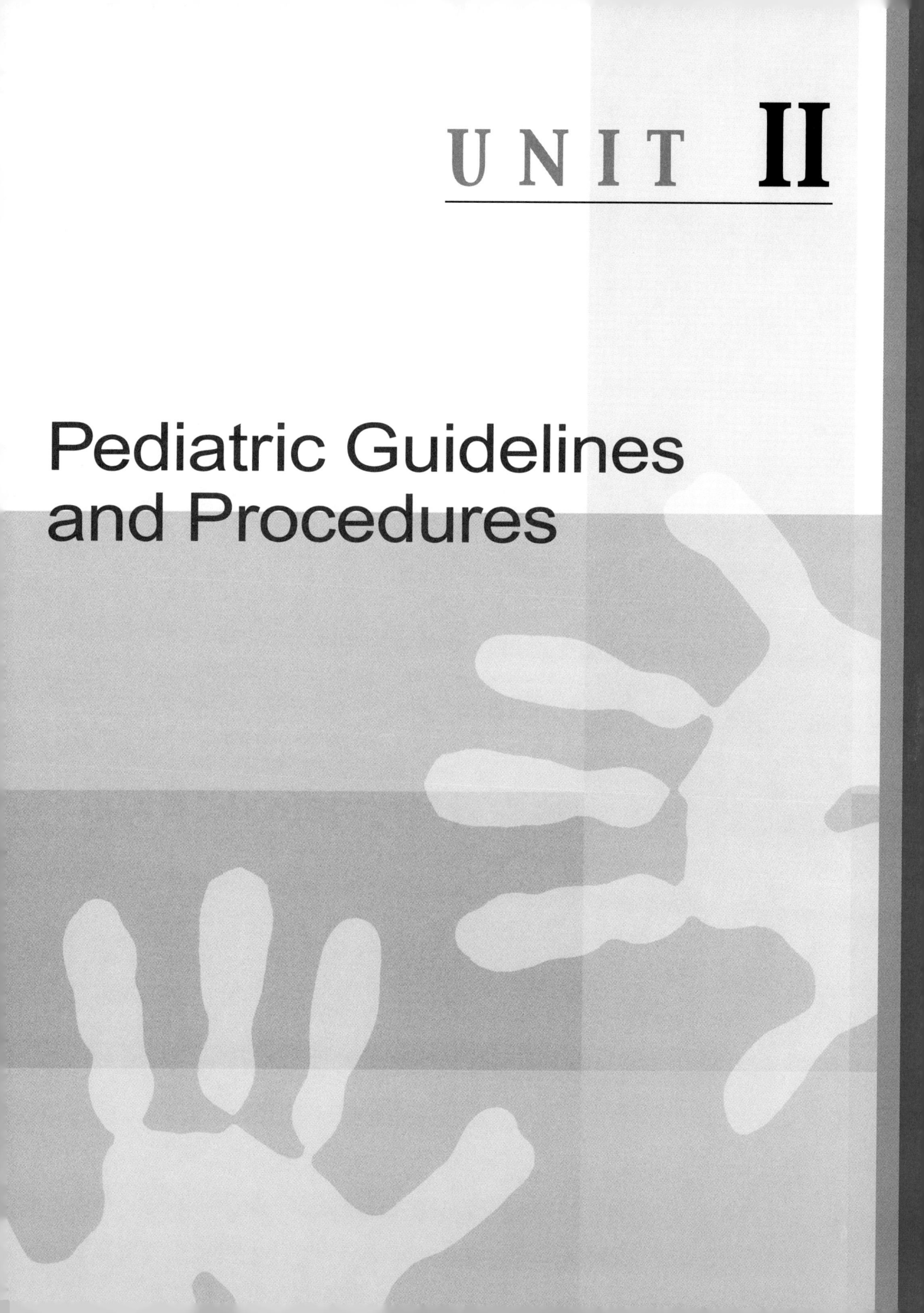

Pediatric Guidelines and Procedures

C H A P T E R
8

Abdominal Girth

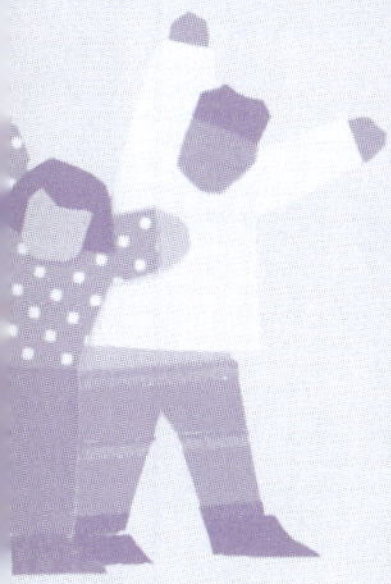

Clinical Guidelines

- Abdominal girth measurement may be performed by any healthcare provider who is educated about the technique.
- Abdominal girth is measured every 8 to 12 hours or more frequently in children who have the presence of or risk factors for abdominal distention.

Equipment

- Paper measuring tape marked in centimeters
- Ballpoint pen or marker
- Stethoscope

Child and Family Assessment and Preparation

- Determine whether the child has recently complained of abdominal pain or injury or is at risk for abdominal distention. Risk factors include gavage or enteral feeding, postoperative abdominal surgery, presence of enteral tubes for stomach or intestinal decompression, peritoneal dialysis, and prematurity (increased risk for necrotizing enterocolitis). There is little evidence to support that routine measurement of abdominal girth after suspected trauma is a reliable predictor of intraperitoneal bleeding.
- In an age-appropriate manner, explain the procedure to the child and family, including the rationale for performing the procedure and particularly the frequency with which it is done. Explain to the child that small pen marks will be made on the abdomen. Assure the child that these marks are not permanent and will wash off. Visible marks made on the child's body may be a threat to body image.

KidKare If age appropriate, allow the child to look at and touch the paper measuring tape to be used. Let the child measure the examiner's wrist or other object. Give the child time to ask questions immediately before the procedure.

caREminder

Cloth tape stretches over time, resulting in inaccurate measurements. Paper tape may be covered with clear adhesive tape to prevent paper cuts to the skin with pulling of tape. A measurement tape covered with adhesive is easy to clean with alcohol and is less likely to tear.

- Determine whether one tape will be long enough to encircle the abdomen. Two paper tapes may be taped together for added length. For accuracy, ensure that the ending mark of one tape measure lines up with the beginning mark of the other tape measure.

PROCEDURE Measuring Abdominal Girth

Steps	Rationale/Points of Emphasis
1. If available, use records and medical history information to determine previous abdominal measurements.	Provides baseline information to help evaluate findings from current assessment.
2. Perform hand hygiene.	Reduces transmission of microorganisms.
3. Auscultate bowel sounds with stethoscope before measuring abdominal girth.	Manipulating the abdomen may affect bowel sounds.
4a. The preferred position is supine with the child's knees flexed or, for an infant, hold the legs flexed at the knees and hips.	Flexing the knees helps the child's abdominal muscles to relax.
4b. If other health conditions are present, the child may need to be in a position that is therapeutic.	Some children may not tolerate a supine position for this procedure.
4c. Remove or move aside clothing that interferes with the ability to apply the measuring tape around the abdomen. Do not measure over clothing.	Any thickness of clothing affects measurement.
4d. Measure girth with the child in the same position each time.	Ensures consistency and accuracy of results.
5. Visualize the child's abdomen to evaluate for symmetry, contour, peristalsis, and abnormalities such as distention or a mass.	A protuberant abdomen may indicate fat, gaseous masses, distention, or scarring. In young children, normal protuberance of the abdomen is apparent when the child is in an upright position and disappears when the child lies down. This protuberance is due to undeveloped musculature.
6. Place your palm under child's waist and slide tape through under your own hand.	Prevents chance of paper cuts to child.
7. If serial measurements are to be made, mark exact area on either side of umbilicus at top edge and bottom edge of tape with a pen or marker.	Facilitates performing measurements at the same location for more accurate comparisons.
8. Place tape snugly across the umbilicus, but not cinching the waistline (Figure 8-1). Ensure that the tape measure is laying flat underneath the child for an accurate measurement. *Note:* Measure girth directly above the umbilicus in infants with umbilical arterial catheters or umbilical venous catheters.	Across the umbilicus is the widest part of the abdomen. Pulling the tape too tight gives an inaccurate measurement.

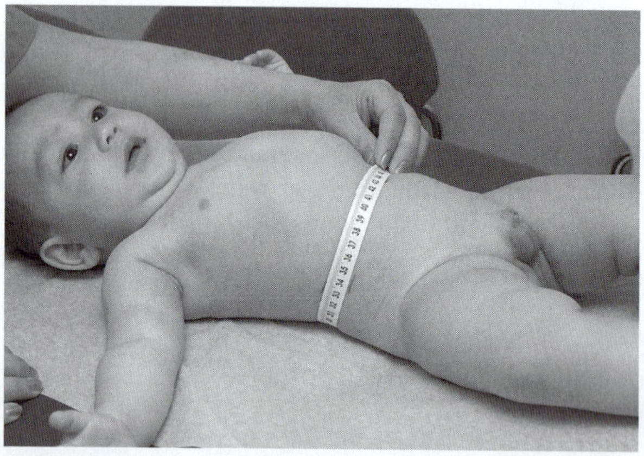

FIGURE 8-1
Measure abdominal girth over the umbilicus whenever possible. Ensure the tape measure is not taut. Marking the place of measurement ensures consistency with repeated measures.

9. Take measurements at the end of expiration.	This prevents measuring the normal abdominal distention that occurs in younger children who breathe using their abdominal muscles.

Steps	Rationale/Points of Emphasis
10a. If serial measurements are to be completed and the child is uncomfortable with movement, the tape may be left in place under the child for the next measurement.	Maintaining the tape in place prevents unnecessary movement that may cause distress to the child.
10b. Ensure that the tape is lying flat under the child. If the child wears diapers, check the tape for soiling by urine or stool at every diaper change and replace the tape as needed.	A dirty wet tape is uncomfortable and increases the risk for skin breakdown and infection.
11. Perform hand hygiene.	Reduces transmission of microorganisms.

CHILD AND FAMILY EVALUATION AND DOCUMENTATION

- Evaluate previous assessments and note any changes in abdomen, including girth, firmness, color, and bowel sounds.
- Record abdominal girth, date and time of measurement, and factors pertinent to abdominal assessment (e.g., relation to meals, bowel movements).
- Document any abdominal pain reported by child or assessed during girth measurement.
- Inform physician or nurse practitioner of any significant changes (greater than 10% of the last measurement) in abdominal girth or abdominal examination.

COMMUNITY CARE

- If parents are measuring abdominal girth at home, instruct them to
  - Mark exact area of the measurement on either side of umbilicus at top edge and bottom edge of tape with a pen or marker.
  - Complete the measurements at the same time each day and before meals.
  - Document findings on a data sheet to share information with healthcare provider.
- Instruct parents to contact the healthcare provider if
  - Abdominal girth varies significantly from the child's baseline (see following "Unexpected Situation").
  - Rapid distention of the child's abdomen is visualized and verified by measurement.
  - Child complains of ongoing abdominal pain.

Unexpected Situation

- *Child's girth measurement is significantly different from previous measurements:* Remeasure girth, ensuring that the tape measure is straight and not twisted under the child, that the measure is obtained in the same place as previous measures, and that the tape measure is placed snugly, but not cinched, around waistline. If measure is still significantly different, assess child for abdominal and respiratory distress and elevate the head of the bed to reduce pressure on the diaphragm. Notify physician.

Bibliography

Castren, M., Liukko, K., Nurmi, J., Honkanen, E., & Lindgren, L. (2004). Measurement of the abdominal circumference for the detection of intra-abdominal hemorrhage has no diagnostic value. *Acta Anaesthesiologica Scandinavica, 48*, 592–594.

Harder, H., Serra, J., Azpiroz, F., Passos, M. C., & Malagelada, J.-R. (2003). Intestinal gas distribution determines abdominal symptoms. *Gut, 52*, 1708–1713.

Langan, J. (1998). Abdominal assessment in the home: From A to Zzz. *Home Healthcare Nurse, 16*, 50–57.

Marino, B., Ogliari, C., & Basilisco, G. (2004). Effect of rectal distension on abdominal girth. *Neurogastroenterology and Motility, 16*, 497–502.

CHAPTER

9

Admission of the Child

Clinical Guidelines

- The registered nurse (RN) or licensed practical nurse (LPN) admits all children on arrival to the unit.
- Unlicensed assistive personnel (UAPs) may complete admission tasks that are consistent with their job descriptions as delegated by the registered personnel.
- The RN is accountable for the nursing assessment and must validate data obtained by the UAP.
- All assessment data gathered become a permanent part of the child's medical record.
- Children are assigned a bed, crib, isolette, warmer, or bassinet appropriate for their chronologic age, developmental age, and/or clinical condition.
- Children should be assigned to rooms based on gender, developmental age, diagnosis and seriousness of condition, communicability of illness, and projected length of stay.
- Each child must wear an identification band throughout the length of hospitalization. In the event that it is not possible to place an identification band on the child's extremity, other arrangements must be made to identify the child at all times (e.g., identification band taped to isolette).
- Principles of family-centered care should be used by all healthcare providers during the admission process and throughout the course of the child's hospitalization (see Chapter 1).

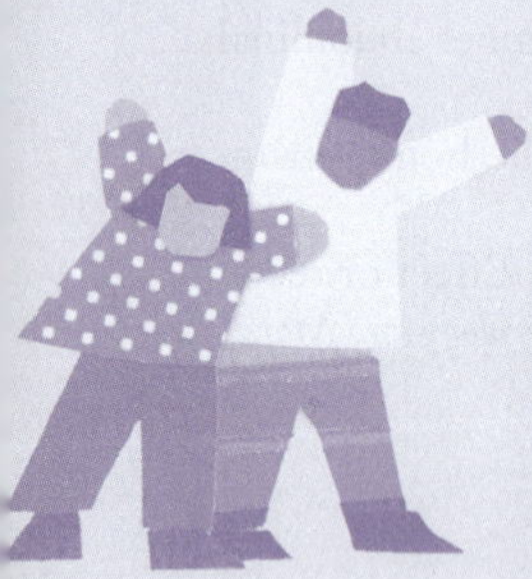

Equipment

For assigned room and personal care:

- Bed, crib, isolette, warmer, or bassinet
- Blankets, linens, bath towels, washcloths
- Washbasin
- Toiletry items (e.g., comb, soap, lotion, toothbrush, toothpaste, as applicable)
- Water pitcher and drinking glass
- Diapers and wipes (if needed)
- Diaper scale (if needed)
- Bedpan, urinal, or specimen hat (if needed)

To admit the child:

- Identification band for child (and parents, if appropriate)
- Scissors
- Measuring tape (for head circumference in patients younger than 2 years of age, recumbent length measurement, and abdominal girth measurement)

- Scale:
  - Infant scale for child 2 years of age and younger
  - Standing scale for child 3 years of age and older
  - Bed scale as indicated by the child's condition
- Thermometer
- Sphygmomanometer and blood pressure cuff (appropriate size for child)
- Stethoscope
- Pulse oximeter (as needed)
- Child and family welcome and orientation brochures
- Patient admission documentation forms
- Patient property envelope (if needed)

CHILD AND FAMILY ASSESSMENT AND PREPARATION

- Beyond infancy, children should be assigned to rooms with other children of the same gender and developmental age.
- Very sick children who may require quiet and rest should not be roomed with more active and loud children.
- Immunocompromised children should be placed in rooms with a positive airflow ventilation system and should not be placed in rooms with children who have infections.
- A child with a communicable disease should be placed in a room with a negative airflow ventilation system and should not have a roommate.
- Children with cystic fibrosis should not be cohorted in the same room unless their sputum is negative for *Burkholderia cepacia* to avoid cross-colonization of this potentially devastating organism.
- Children requiring respiratory or contact isolation should be placed in a room with a negative airflow ventilation system.

PROCEDURE **Preparing the Environment**

Steps	Rationale/Points of Emphasis
1. Perform hand hygiene.	Reduces transmission of microorganisms.
2. Obtain all necessary equipment and furniture for the room. Be sure to obtain any special equipment indicated by needs of the child.	Promotes child and family comfort by ensuring that items needed for the child's personal care are readily available. Prevents delays when immediate treatment must be initiated because of child's condition.
3. If applicable, prepare roommate and family members of roommate for arrival of new patient in the room.	Roommate may be occupying some of the space needed for the new patient, or nurse may need to take measures to help roommate secure his or her privacy in the room.
4. Check room equipment (e.g., call light, bed controls) for proper functioning.	Ensuring that all equipment is ready at bedside and in good working order prevents delays in admission and treatment process.
5. Prepare bed by adjusting to lowest horizontal position with top sheet and blanket turned down and brakes locked. Prepare bassinet or crib by ensuring that rails latch in all positions and/or brakes are locked. Prepare isolette or warmer by following manufacturers' instructions for prewarming before use.	Proper positioning of bed decreases likelihood of patient falls or back injury to staff assisting the child. Lower height of bed makes it easier and safer for child to get in and out of bed. Crib side rails must lock in place to ensure the child is not able to get out of the crib. Brakes should be in a locked position to prevent hazardous movement of the bed or crib. Isolettes and warmers must be prewarmed before patient use to ensure child is placed in environment with correct thermodynamics.
6. Arrange for a translator if necessary.	Children and family members may need the aid of a translator to communicate their concerns and understand the explanations of the healthcare providers.

PROCEDURE Assessing the Child

Steps	Rationale/Points of Emphasis
1. Greet child and family:	
• Determine whether child is addressed by a specific name or nickname.	Child will feel more comfortable and will be more likely to respond when addressed in a fashion common to him or her.
• Introduce yourself by name and title. Explain your role and responsibilities in the care of the child.	Clarifies unique roles of healthcare providers.
• Try to dispel fears and to anticipate family's questions.	Promotes friendly welcoming attitude.
2. Escort child and family to the child's room, and introduce child and family to others in room.	Acknowledges presence of others in room. **KidKare** Introduce the child to his or her roommate, and write down the children's names for each child in the room. Children are usually uncomfortable introducing themselves to other children. However, if the children know each other's names, they are more likely to talk and play together as they are recuperating.
3. Determine reliability of the person providing information about the child.	Person accompanying child may not know child's past medical history or the complete history of events that led to child's admission.
4a. Determine whether or not child has had previous hospitalizations and determine child's perception of those experiences.	Child's perceptions of and reactions to current events are likely to be strongly affected by previous experiences with hospitalization and healthcare personnel.
4b. Obtain information regarding child's temperament in relation to previous hospital or healthcare experiences.	Temperament is an important variable when considering appropriate and individualized approaches to nursing care for the hospitalized child.
5a. Assist child into bed or crib, noting his or her condition. Have child sit on parent's lap, in the bed, or in the crib during the assessment.	Child may feel less anxiety if he or she remains in the parent's arms.
5b. Make sure side rails are up if child is sitting in bed or crib.	Maintains child's safety. **KidKare** Child may wish to wear his or her own clothing.
6. Apply identification band to child and to parents (if applicable); cut off extra length if identification band is too large for child.	Identification is absolutely necessary throughout hospitalization. Child may not identify self correctly when called by name; identification bands ensure that child can be properly identified at all times. Matching identification bands for the child and parents are used as a security measure. Patient identification is a Joint Commission on Accreditation of Healthcare Organizations' (JCAHO) National Safety Goal.
7. Validate mechanism to contact family members when they are not present at the hospital.	Provides the staff with contact phone numbers, and ensures that parents can be reached at all times if needed.
8. Assess vital signs, including respirations, heart rate, temperature, blood pressure, pulse oximetry (as needed), and pain level (see Chapters 130–134).	Provides baseline parameters to compare with future findings.
9. Obtain the following information, as child's condition permits: • Height—recumbent length should be measured for all children 3 years of age and younger • Weight • Head circumference—obtain for all children 2 years of age and younger (see Chapter 44 for height, weight, and head circumference) • Abdominal girth, if warranted by child's admitting condition (see Chapter 8)	Weight is essential for calculating medication dosages for children. Measurement of height and weight allows for calculation of body surface area. Calculation of head circumference alerts healthcare workers to potential cranial problems of abnormalities. Abdominal girth is assessed if condition involves increasing abdominal girth. Weight and height information are needed as a basis for making decisions about medication administration.

Steps	Rationale/Points of Emphasis
10a. Obtain nursing history and record assessment data on admission assessment form adopted by hospital.	Provides baseline assessment data. Provides data from which to identify problems that require interdisciplinary healthcare interventions.
Alert! ***Lengthy admission procedures may be inappropriate if the child's health status appears to be deteriorating rapidly.***	
10b. Validate mechanism to contact family members when they are not present at the hospital.	Provides the staff with contact phone numbers, and ensures that parents can be reached at all times if needed.
10c. Determine and discuss health topics that are relevant to the age and development of the child (e.g., guidance and education in areas of interest or safety, diet, skin care) and that are of interest or concern to the parents.	Provides data from which to begin anticipatory guidance education in areas of interest or concern to parents.
11. Notify attending healthcare prescriber of child's arrival on unit, along with any emergent or unusual findings, and obtain admission orders. If the attending healthcare prescriber is not the primary healthcare provider, the RN or the attending physician must notify the primary healthcare provider as well.	Provides continuity of care and ensures prompt attention to the child's healthcare concerns. Establishes relationships with primary care providers, and allows for smooth transition of care.

PROCEDURE Orienting the Child and Family to the Unit

Steps	Rationale/Points of Emphasis
1. Orient and demonstrate use of: • Call light • Emergency light • Bed light • TV control • Bedside table • Bed control and side rails • Patient supplies (e.g., wash basin, toiletry items, water pitcher, drinking glass, urinal)	Child and family safety may be affected by understanding correct use of bedside equipment. Ensures that child and family know how to call for assistance.
2. Instruct child and family regarding use of bathroom facilities and monitoring intake and output. • Show location of bathroom if child is ambulating. • If output is to be monitored, show how urine is saved. If child is not toilet trained, ask parents to wrap up and save all dirty diapers until output has been measured. • If input is to be measured, instruct parents to keep track of all fluid consumed by the child. • If child is NPO, ensure that child and family members know this.	Ensures that child and family know expectations regarding urine collection and maintaining accurate intake and output records.
3a. Explain unit routine, meal schedule, visiting rules, available services and support systems, smoking policy, parking availability, cafeteria hours, and playroom hours. Provide tour of the unit. 3b. Let parents know if they may room-in with their child and/or where they can find available sleep facilities.	Having information about hospital services and support systems can help to decrease parent anxiety. It is a JCAHO standard that families be informed of the hospital's smoking policy. Allowing parents to stay at the child's bedside during the night will help to reduce the child's fears and avoid separation anxiety. Facilitates parental involvement in caregiving and decision-making practices.

Continued

Steps	Rationale/Points of Emphasis
3c. Provide family members with telephone number to unit and explain unit policies regarding who may receive information about the child's status from the healthcare providers.	The child's parents should be able to access the unit and determine the status of their child at all times. Other family members are welcome to call and make general inquiries; however, for patient confidentiality, specific health information cannot be shared due to the Health Insurance Portability and Accountability Act of 1996.
3d. Encourage parents to notify the staff when they need extra formula, snacks, diapers, or linens for the child.	Children generally eat small, frequent meals and thus may require the provision of extra snacks between the scheduled meal services.
4. Inform the child and family about other care providers who will be seeing the child during the child's hospitalization.	In some healthcare settings, especially teaching hospitals, there are a number of people who come in contact with the child and family. Reviewing this information in advance will help decrease the family's confusion.
5. Review patient's rights and advance directives as needed with parent and with child, if age appropriate (see Chapter 11).	Provides families with a summary of their rights, including the right to privacy, the right to review records, and the right to be informed about care. The Patient Self-Determination Act of 1991 requires that all healthcare agencies serving Medicaid and Medicare patients provide patients with information regarding advance directives options and the right to accept or reject medical treatment.
6a. Determine whether or not family has brought any medications, supplies, or assistive/adaptive devices from home for child's use. Discuss with physician and pharmacy which, if any, of these medications need to be identified and labeled by the pharmacy for dispensing during the hospital stay. Send all other medication home with parents or to patient property services.	Ensures medicine control during hospitalization. Prevents child from accidentally being medicated by both the family and the nursing staff. Some medications being provided at home to the child are not on the hospital formulary or are too expensive to obtain during the hospitalization, resulting in the need to have the home medications used during the hospital stay.
6b. Label all assistive/adaptive devices with the child's name and medical record number. Send any unnecessary items home with the family. Ensure items retained at the bedside are easily accessible to the child and his or her family.	Prevents child's property from getting lost. Some devices may not be needed during child's hospital stay.

PROCEDURE Securing Valuables

Steps	Rationale/Points of Emphasis
1. Place child's clothes in assigned locker or closet, and place child's toiletries in bedside stand.	Promotes cleanliness and orderliness in the room. Prevents child's clothing and supplies from getting mixed with those of a roommate.
2a. Encourage child's family to take all valuables and money home whenever possible.	Family is responsible for all items kept in child's room. **KidKare** To comfort child in the unfamiliar setting of the hospital, encourage parents to bring familiar security objects from the home for the child. Such objects may include blankets, pictures of family members, dolls, and stuffed animals. Infants may enjoy musical toys or tapes of familiar music from home.
2b. Have parents label all the child's clothing and possessions left at the bedside.	Prevents loss or having items mistakenly taken from the child's room and placed in the playroom or other area, while guaranteeing identification when found.
3a. If family is unavailable to take home valuables, use institutional records to list and place all valuables in patient property envelope while in the presence of the child or accompanying adult. Always count money in the presence of another employee.	Accounts for placement of all valuables and helps prevent loss.
3b. Describe valuable in general terms, such as "yellow metal" rather than "yellow gold" or "clear, cut stone" rather than "diamond."	Assuming an item is a diamond or piece of gold may be a false assessment of the material and subsequent value of the item. Valuables are described in terms of what is actually visualized and not presumed about the quality of the item.

Steps	Rationale/Points of Emphasis
4. In presence of witness, obtain family or guardian signature on form that documents valuables received and placed in envelope. If family or guardian is unable to sign, have another person as witness.	Verifies that witness agrees with stated list of contents and actual contents of valuables envelope.
5. Deliver envelope to patient property services or store in other secure locked location on the unit. Envelope should be labeled with child's name, room number, and patient identification number.	Valuables should be stored in a locked area to prevent loss and theft. Valuables are always labeled to ensure they can be returned to correct patient at the end of their hospital stay.
6. Return patient's copy of the signed property form to family or guardian. Place chart copy in chart. If patient is unable to keep receipt, secure receipt to inside front cover of chart until it can be given to family.	This is patient's receipt, which he or she signs when proving ownership, and clerk will also sign to release valuables.

CHILD AND FAMILY EVALUATION AND DOCUMENTATION

- Evaluate child's and family's understanding of orientation to the room and unit.
- Determine whether or not the family has other areas of concern at this time.
- Record and document nursing assessments on institutional forms.
- Initiate interdisciplinary plan of care (critical pathway) and review with child and family.

COMMUNITY CARE

- Begin discharge planning and transition management to prepare child for transition to home or to another healthcare facility.
- Notify relevant community healthcare providers of child's admission (e.g., child's general practitioner).
- Obtain referrals to additional community healthcare providers as warranted by the child's diagnosis.
- Instruct child and family to notify the healthcare provider if they have further questions or care needs.

Unexpected Situation

- *During the admission process, a toddler's mother tells you she must leave as soon as the child is admitted to the room. Upon hearing this news, the toddler starts crying loudly and clings to the mother's neck:* Crying and clinging to the parent are expected reactions of toddler when faced with separation and the realities of being left in a strange environment. Elicit more information from the parent about the length of her departure, possibilities of other family members staying with the child, and ensure that the child has favorite objects (e.g., special blanket) that can be kept with the child. Explain to the child in simple terms when the parent will return (e.g., "Mom will be back by the time the Sesame Street show is over"). Ensure the child has a consistent healthcare provider with whom he or she may develop a sense of comfort.

Bibliography

American Academy of Pediatrics. (1999). Privacy protection of health information: Patient rights and pediatrician responsibilities. *Pediatrics, 104*, 973–976.

American Academy of Pediatrics. (2003a). Facilities and equipment for the care of pediatric patients in a community hospital. *Pediatrics, 111*(5), 1120–1122.

American Academy of Pediatrics. (2003b). Physicians' role in coordinating care of hospitalized children. *Pediatrics, 111*, 707–709.

Macnab, A., Thiessen, P., McLeod, E., & Hinton, D. (2000). Parent assessment of family-centered care practices in a children's hospital. *Children's Healthcare, 29*(2), 113–128.

Pegues, D. A., Carson, L. A., Tablan, O. C., et al. (1993). Acquisition of *Pseudomonas cepacia* at summer camps for patients with cystic fibrosis. Part I. *Journal of Pediatrics, 124*, 694–792.

Schulster, L. M., Chinn, R. Y. W., Arduino, M. J., et al. (2004). *Guidelines for environmental control in health-care facilities. Recommendations of the CDC and Healthcare Infection Control Practices Advisory Committee.* Chicago, IL: American Society for Healthcare Engineering/American Hospital Association.

Wallace, M. (1995). Temperament and the hospitalized child. *Journal of Pediatric Nursing, 10*(3), 173–180.

CHAPTER

10

Admission of the Child to the Intensive Care Unit

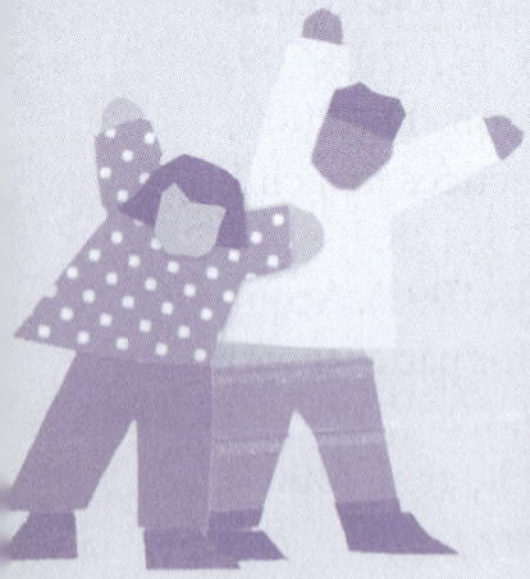

Clinical Guidelines

- A physician's order is required for admission to the intensive care unit (ICU).
- A registered nurse (RN) or licensed practical nurse (LPN) admits all children on arrival to the unit.
- Unlicensed assistive personnel (UAPs) may complete admission tasks that are consistent with their job descriptions as delegated by the registered personnel.
- The RN is accountable for the nursing assessment and must validate data obtained by the UAP.
- All assessment data gathered will become a permanent part of the child's medical record.
- Children are assigned a bed, crib, isolette, warmer, or bassinet appropriate for their developmental level and/or clinical condition.
- Each child must wear an identification band throughout the length of hospitalization. In the event that it is not possible to place an identification band on the child's extremity, other arrangements must be made to properly identify the child at all times (e.g., identification band taped to isolate).
- All children are placed on cardiorespiratory monitoring (and additional monitoring as necessary). Discontinuation of such monitoring is based on further evaluation of the child's status by the healthcare prescriber.
- Emergency medications and supplies are kept in a well-secured, easily accessible location in the ICU.
- Principles of family-centered care should be used by all healthcare providers during the admission process and throughout the course of the child's hospitalization (see Chapter 1).

Equipment

To admit the child:

- Identification band for child (and parents, if appropriate)
- Scissors
- Measuring tape (for head circumference of patients younger than 2 years of age, recumbent length measurement, and abdominal girth measurement)
- Scale:
  - Infant scale for child 2 years of age and younger
  - Standing scale for child 3 years of age and older
  - Bed scale as indicated by the child's condition

- Thermometer
- Sphygmomanometer and blood pressure cuff (appropriate size for child)
- Stethoscope
- Child and family welcome and orientation brochures
- Patient admission documentation forms
- Patient property envelope (if needed)

For assigned room and personal care:

- Bed, crib, isolette, warmer, or bassinet
- Personnel protective gear (e.g., gowns, gloves, masks, goggles/eyewear)
- Electrocardiogram lead patches
- Intravenous infusion device
- Intravenous pole
- Blankets, linens, bath towels, and washcloths
- Washbasin
- Toiletry items (e.g., comb, soap, lotion, toothbrush, toothpaste)
- Diapers and wipes (if needed)
- Diaper scale (if needed)
- Bedpan, urinal, or specimen hat (if needed)

Unit-specific supplies and equipment:

- Oxygen delivery supplies:
  - Flowmeter for O_2
  - Oxygen tubing
  - Appropriate-sized face mask and resuscitation bag
- Suction supplies:
  - Appropriate-sized sterile suction catheter (the catheter diameter should not exceed half the diameter of the airway)

Age	Catheter Size
Neonate to 18 months	5–8 French
18 to 24 months	8–10 French
2 to 7 years	8–10 French
7 to 10 years	10–14 French
11 years to adult	12–16 French

- Sterile container for sterile fluids
- Sterile gloves
- Sterile normal saline or sterile water
- Water-soluble lubricant
- Portable or wall suction machine with tubing and collection container

Intubation and ventilatory support supplies and equipment:

- Appropriate-sized laryngoscope and blades
- Appropriate-sized endotracheal tube
- Ventilator

Cardiorespiratory monitor and recorder supplies:

- Appropriate-sized electrodes
- Cardiorespiratory monitor
- Recording tape

Additional supplies:

- Defibrillator and external pacer
- Noninvasive equipment and monitoring supplies (e.g., pulse oximeter)
- Invasive equipment and monitoring (e.g., hemodynamic monitor; see Chapter 47)
- Emergency drugs and supplies
- Emergency drug calculation sheet, based on child's weight, height, and allergy status
- Length-based resuscitation tape (e.g., Braslow tape)

CHILD AND FAMILY ASSESSMENT AND PREPARATION

- Very sick children who may require quiet and rest or who may be nearing death should not be roomed near more active and loud children or children requiring extensive personnel and procedures at the bedside.
- Immunocompromised children should be placed in rooms with a positive airflow ventilation system and should not be placed near children who have infections.
- A child who has a communicable disease should be placed in a room with a negative airflow ventilation system.
- Children with cystic fibrosis should not be cohorted in the same room unless their sputum is negative for *Burkholderia cepacia* to avoid cross-colonization of this potentially devastating organism.
- Children requiring respiratory or contact isolation should be placed in a room with a negative airflow ventilation system.

PROCEDURE Preparing the Environment

Steps	Rationale/Points of Emphasis
1. Perform hand hygiene.	Reduces transmission of microorganisms.
2. Obtain all necessary equipment and furniture for the bed space or room. Be sure to obtain any special equipment indicated by needs of the child.	Promotes child and family comfort by ensuring that items needed for the child's personal care are readily available. Prevents delays when immediate treatment must be initiated because of the child's condition.
3. If applicable, prepare roommate and family members of roommate for arrival of new patient in the room.	Roommate may be occupying some of the space needed for the new patient, or nurse may need to take measures to help roommate secure his or her privacy in the room.
4. Check room equipment (e.g., suction, oxygen equipment, monitors) for proper functioning. Set age-appropriate alarm setting limits on cardiorespiratory monitor and pulse oximeter if applicable.	Ensures that all equipment is ready at bedside and in good working order prevents delays in admission and treatment process.
5. Prepare bed by adjusting to lowest horizontal position, with top sheet and blanket turned down and brakes located. (Note: If the child is arriving on a gurney, the bed should be raised to the height of the gurney to assist in transferring the child. If the bed has an in-bed scale, zero the bed according to the manufacturer's instructions.)	Proper positioning of bed decreases likelihood of patient falls or back injury to staff assisting the child. Lower height of bed makes it easier and safer for child to get in and out of bed.
Prepare bassinet or crib by ensuring that rails latch in all positions and/or brakes are locked.	Crib side rails must lock in place to ensure that the child is not able to get out of the crib. Brakes should be in a locked position to prevent hazardous movement of the bed or crib.
Prepare isolette or warmer by following manufacturer's instructions for prewarming before use.	Isolettes and warmers must be prewarmed before patient use to ensure child is placed in environment with correct thermodynamics. **caREminder** *Neonates and small infants who may have immature thermoregulatory systems may require radiant warmers or isolettes for their bed.*
6. Arrange for a translator if necessary.	Children and family members may need the aid of a translator to communicate their concerns and understand the explanations of the healthcare providers.

PROCEDURE Assessing Child

Steps	Rationale/Points of Emphasis
1. Notify healthcare prescriber of child's arrival to unit, and obtain admission orders. If the attending healthcare prescriber is not the primary healthcare provider, the registered nurse or the attending physician must notify the primary healthcare provider as well.	Provides continuity of care and ensures prompt attention to the child's healthcare concerns. In the critical care setting, the urgent healthcare needs of the child often precipitate immediate interventions by the healthcare prescriber to stabilize the child. Establishes relationships with primary care providers, and allows for smooth transition of care.
2. Greet child and family:	
• Determine whether child is addressed by a specific name or nickname.	Child will feel more comfortable and will be more likely to respond when addressed in a fashion common to him or her.
• Introduce yourself by name and title. Explain your role and responsibilities in the care of the child.	Clarifies unique roles of healthcare providers.
• Try to dispel fears and to anticipate family's questions.	Promotes friendly welcoming attitude.

Steps	Rationale/Points of Emphasis
3. If child is alert, escort child and family to the room or bed space, and introduce child and family to primary care providers (e.g., doctors, respiratory therapists).	Orients family to healthcare workers.
4. Assist child into bed, noting his or her condition. Extremely ill children may have to be moved by staff members from transferring gurney to bed.	Provides baseline parameters to compare with future findings.
5. Perform hand hygiene and don personal protective gear.	Reduces transmission of microorganisms before continuing patient assessment. Use of protective apparel is determined by child's condition (e.g., presence of blood, presence of infectious respiratory condition).
6. Determine reliability of the person providing information about the child.	Person accompanying child may not know child's past medical history or the complete history of events that led to child's admission.
7a. Determine whether or not child has had previous hospitalizations and determine child's perception of those experiences. 7b. Obtain information regarding child's temperament in relation to previous hospital or healthcare experiences.	Child's perceptions of and reactions to current events are likely to be strongly affected by previous experiences with hospitalization and healthcare personnel. Temperament is an important variable when considering appropriate and individualized approaches to nursing care for the hospitalized child.
8. Apply identification band to child and to parents (if applicable); cut off extra length if identification band is too large for child.	Identification is absolutely necessary throughout hospitalization. Child may not identify self correctly when called by name; identification bands ensure that child can be properly identified at all times. Matching identification bands for the child and parents are used as a security measure. Patient identification is a Joint Commission on Accreditation of Healthcare Organizations' (JCAHO) National Safety Goal.
9. Validate mechanism to contact family members when they are not present at the hospital.	Provides the staff with contact phone numbers, and ensures that parents can be reached at all times if needed.
10. Obtain the following information, as child's condition permits: • Height—recumbent length should be measured for all children 3 years of age and younger • Weight • Head circumference—obtain for all children 2 years of age and younger (see Chapter 44 for height, weight, and head circumference) • Abdominal girth, if warranted by child's admitting condition (see Chapter 8) **KidKare** Use of a length-based resuscitation tape may be quicker and less hazardous for the child requiring immediate medical attention.	Weight is essential for calculating medication dosages for children. Measurement of height and weight allows for calculation of body surface area. Calculation of head circumference alerts healthcare providers to potential cranial problems or abnormalities. Abdominal girth alerts healthcare providers to size of the abdominal region. **caREminder** *If the child is unconscious or clinically unstable, assessment factors such as height measures, abdominal girth measures, and evaluation of anxiety level are superseded by the need to stabilize the child's cardiac and respiratory status.*
11. Assess child's pain and anxiety level (see Chapter 132 for pain assessment).	Provides baseline parameters to compare with future measurements and pain relief.
12. Place child on cardiorespiratory monitor and pulse oximeter. Assess and obtain vital signs, including respirations, heart rate, temperature, and blood pressure (see Chapters 130–134).	Provides baseline parameters to compare with future measurements. **caREminder** *Placing the child on monitors to evaluate cardiac and respiratory status may need to be completed as soon as the child arrives in the ICU as indicated by the child's clinical condition. Children who are clinically unstable should be placed on monitors immediately and emergency measures should be used as soon as possible (e.g., initiating vascular access, administering medications).*

Continued

Steps	Rationale/Points of Emphasis
13. Obtain head-to-toe assessment, including all body systems.	Provides baseline numbers and alerts healthcare workers to potential problems or abnormalities.
14. Dispose of used equipment and waste in appropriate receptacles, and perform hand hygiene.	Standard precautions. Reduces transmission of microorganisms.
15. Complete an emergency drug calculation sheet specific for the child and post at child's bedside.	Provides information specific to the child regarding doses for emergency medications. Precalculating this information saves time if an arrest situation occurs.
16a. Obtain nursing history and record assessment data on admission assessment form adopted by hospital.	Provides baseline assessment data. Provides data from which to identify problems that require interdisciplinary healthcare interventions.
Alert! *Lengthy admission procedures may be inappropriate if the child's health status appears to be deteriorating rapidly.*	
16b. Determine and discuss health topics that are relevant to the age and development of the child (e.g., guidance and education in areas of interest or safety, diet, skin care) and that are of interest or concern to the parents.	Provides data from which to begin anticipatory guidance and education in areas of interest or concern to parents.

PROCEDURE Orienting Child and Family to the Unit

Steps	Rationale/Points of Emphasis
1. Orient and demonstrate use of: • Call light • Emergency light • Bed light • TV control • Bedside table • Bed control and side rails • Patient supplies (e.g., wash basin, toiletry items, water pitcher, drinking glass, urinal).	Child and family safety may be affected by understanding correct use of bedside equipment. Ensures that child and family know how to call for assistance.
2. Instruct child and family regarding use of bathroom facilities and monitoring intake and output. • Show location of bathroom if child is ambulating. • If output is to be monitored, show how urine is saved. If child is not toilet trained, ask parents to wrap up and save all dirty diapers until output has been measured. • If input is to be measured, instruct parents to keep track of all fluid consumed by the child. • If child is NPO, ensure that child and family members know this.	Ensures that child and family know expectations regarding urine collection and maintaining accurate intake and output records.
3a. Explain unit routine, meal schedule, visiting rules, available services and support systems, smoking policy, parking availability, and cafeteria hours. Provide tour of the unit.	Having information about hospital services and support systems can help to decrease parent anxiety. It is a JCAHO standard that families be informed of the hospital's smoking policy.
3b. Let parents know if they may room-in with their child and/or where they can find available sleep facilities.	Allowing parents to stay at the child's bedside during the night will help to minimize the child's fears and avoid separation anxiety. Facilitates parental involvement in caregiving and decision-making practices.

Steps	Rationale/Points of Emphasis
3c. Provide family members with telephone number to unit and explain unit policies regarding who may receive information about the child's status from the healthcare providers.	The child's parents should be able to access the unit and determine the status of their child at all times. Other family members are welcome to call and make general inquiries; however, for patient confidentiality, specific health information cannot be shared due to the Health Insurance Portability and Accountability Act of 1996.
3d. Encourage parents to notify the staff if they need extra formula, snacks, diapers, or linens for the child.	Children generally eat small frequent meals and thus may require the provision of extra snacks between the scheduled meal services.
3e. Introduce child and family to child life specialist and explain how age-appropriate activities can be provided at the bedside.	A child in the intensive care unit will not be visiting the playroom. Age-appropriate activities and stimulation should be provided to the child within the context of the child's condition and healthcare needs.
4. Inform the child and family about the other care providers who will be seeing the child during the child's hospitalization	In some healthcare settings, especially teaching hospitals, there are a number of people who come in contact with the child and family. Reviewing this information in advance will help decrease the child and family's confusion.
5. Review patient's rights and advance directives as needed with parent and with child if age-appropriate (see Chapter 11).	Provides families with a summary of their rights, including the right to privacy, the right to review records, and the right to be informed about care. The Patient Self-Determination Act of 1991 requires that all healthcare agencies serving Medicaid and Medicare patients provide patients with information regarding advance directives options and the right to accept or reject medical treatment.
6a. Determine whether or not family has brought medications, supplies, or assistive/adaptive devices from home for child's use. Discuss with physician and pharmacist which, if any, of these medications needs to be identified and labeled by the pharmacy for dispensing during the hospital stay. Send all other medications home with parents or to patient property services.	Ensures medicine control during hospitalization. Prevents child from accidentally being medicated by the family and the nursing staff. Some medications being provided at home to the child may not be on the hospital formulary or are too expensive to obtain during the hospitalization, resulting in the need to have the home medications used during the hospital stay.
6b. Label all assistive or adaptive devices with the child's name and medical record number. Send any unnecessary items home with the family. Ensure items retained at the bedside are easily accessible to the child and his or her family.	Prevents child's property from getting lost. Some devices may not be needed during child's hospital stay.

PROCEDURE Securing Valuables

Steps	Rationale/Points of Emphasis
1. Place child's clothes in assigned locker or closet, and place child's toiletries in bedside stand.	Promotes cleanliness and orderliness in the room. Prevents child's clothing and supplies from getting mixed with those of a roommate.
2a. Encourage child's family to take all valuables and money home whenever possible.	Family is responsible for all items kept in the child's room. **KidKare** To comfort child in the unfamiliar setting of the hospital, encourage parents to bring familiar security objects from the home for the child. Such objects may include blankets, pictures of family members, dolls, and stuffed animals. Infants may enjoy musical toys or tapes of familiar music from home.
2b. Have parents label all the child's clothing and possessions left at the bedside.	Prevents loss or having items mistakenly taken from the child's room and placed in the playroom or other area, while guaranteeing identification when found.

Continued

Steps	Rationale/Points of Emphasis
3a. If family is unavailable to take home valuables, use institutional records to list and place all valuables in patient property envelope while in the presence of the child or accompanying adult. Always count money in the presence of another employee.	Accounts for placement of all valuables and helps prevent loss.
3b. Describe valuable in general terms, such as "yellow metal" rather than "yellow gold" or "clear, cut stone" rather than "diamond."	Assuming an item is a diamond or piece of gold may be a false assessment of the material and subsequent value of the item. Valuables are described in terms of what is actually visualized and not presumed about the quality of the item.
4. In presence of witness, obtain family or guardian signature on form that documents valuables received and placed in envelope. If family or guardian is unable to sign, have another person as witness.	Verifies that witness agrees with stated list of contents and actual contents of valuables envelope.
5. Deliver envelope to patient property services or store in other secure locked location on the unit. Envelope should be labeled with child's name, room number, and patient identification number.	Valuables should be stored in a locked area to prevent loss or theft. Valuables are always labeled to ensure they can be returned to correct patient at the end of their hospital stay.
6. Return patient's copy of the signed property form to family or guardian. Place chart copy in chart. If patient is unable to keep receipt, secure receipt to inside front cover of chart until it can be given to family.	This is the patient's receipt, which he or she signs when proving ownership and clerk will also sign to release valuables.

CHILD AND FAMILY EVALUATION AND DOCUMENTATION

- Evaluate child and family understanding of orientation to the unit.
- Determine whether or not the family has other areas of concern at this time.
- Record and document nursing assessments on institutional forms.
- Initiate interdisciplinary plan of care (critical pathway) and review with child and family.

COMMUNITY CARE

- Begin discharge planning and transition management to prepare child for transition to another unit, to home, or to another healthcare facility.
- Notify relevant community healthcare providers of child's admission (e.g., child's general practitioner).
- Obtain referrals to additional community healthcare providers as warranted by the child's diagnosis.
- Instruct child and family to notify the healthcare provider if they have further questions or care needs.

Unexpected Situation

- *The child is escorted into the pediatric ICU, accompanied by his parents. During the interview process, the child's health condition changes abruptly. The child begins to vomit and has a seizure:* Immediately discontinue the interview process and attend to the immediate needs of the child. The child should be placed in a bed with cardiorespiratory equipment applied and oxygen delivered as needed. While the child's condition is being stabilized, parents may remain at the bedside per their request. A support person should be assigned to the parents to answer their questions and provide support during the stabilization process.

Bibliography

American Academy of Pediatrics. (1999). Guidelines for developing admission and discharge policies for the pediatric intensive care unit. *Pediatrics, 103*, 840–841.

American Academy of Pediatrics. (2003a). Facilities and equipment for the care of pediatric patients in a community hospital. *Pediatrics, 111*(5), 1120–1122.

American Academy of Pediatrics. (2003b). Physicians' role in coordinating care of hospitalized children. *Pediatrics, 111*, 707–709.

Heward, Y. (2003). Transfer from ward to PICU: A standard. *Paediatric Nursing, 15*(1), Critical Care: XI–XIII.

Macnab, A., Thiessen, P., McLeod, E., & Hinton, D. (2000). Parent assessment of family-centered care practices in a children's hospital. *Children's Healthcare, 29*(2), 113–128.

Maybloom, B., Chapple, J., & Davidson, L. L. (2002). Admissions for critically ill children: Where and why? *Intensive & Critical Care Nursing, 18*(3), 151–161.

Schulster, L. M., Chinn, R. Y. W., Arduino, M. J., et al. (2004). *Guidelines for environmental control in health-care facilities. Recommendations of the CDC and Healthcare Infection Control Practices Advisory Committee.* Chicago, IL: American Society for Healthcare Engineering/American Hospital Association.

C H A P T E R

11

Advance Directives

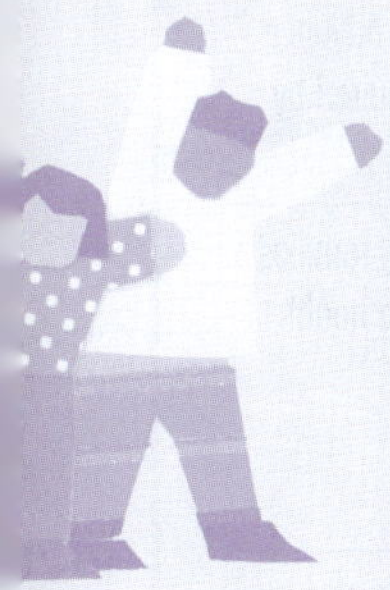

Clinical Guidelines

- On admission to the healthcare facility, all patients receive
  - A patients' rights brochure regarding patient rights, advance directives, surrogate decision making, and the forgoing of life-sustaining procedures;
  - Healthcare facility policies with respect to patients' rights, advance directives, surrogate decision making, and the forgoing of life-sustaining procedures.
- Facility protocol determines who distributes the above information (e.g., admitting personnel, nursing personnel). During the admission process, or as soon as reasonably possible thereafter, ask the family whether or not an advance directive has been completed for the child.
- If the child has an advance directive, place a copy in the medical record. If the healthcare provider believes the child's condition/circumstances have changed and that this should be reflected in the advance directive, it is the provider's responsibility to initiate the conversation with the parent or child.
- File advance directives in the medical record in a consistent section. Mark the chart on the exterior that an advance directive is present within.
- If no advance directive exists for a child, the healthcare team collaborates to discuss development of one with the family.
- Advance directives are jointly determined by the parent and child and are followed by healthcare professionals.
- An attempt should be made to resolve concerns regarding the feasibility of an advance directive order with the immediate parties involved. If unable to reach resolution, consult the institution's ethics committee or equivalent.
- Advance directives should always be developed considering the child's best interests.
- When a patient who lacks present decision-making capacity (as determined by the admitting physician in consultation with the patient's family members and close friends) is admitted to the hospital, the person responsible for documenting the admission must provide information regarding advance directives and direct questions regarding the existence of an advance directive to a relative or friend accompanying the patient, if such a person is present.
- Those who can complete the advance directive for a child include
  - Parent
  - Legal guardian
  - Emancipated minor (includes adolescent parent of child of any age)
  - A child who demonstrates the cognitive, abstract, and thinking ability to comprehend the terms of the advance directive. The advance directive requires the cosignature of a parent or legal guardian.
- When requested to do so, the healthcare team should respect the privacy and confidentiality of patients legally entitled to their own decisions (emancipated minors or those judged mature).

EQUIPMENT

- A copy of the advance directive form or a copy of previously established advance directives for that child.
- As a resource, the family should have an institutional or other guide on establishing advance directives.

CHILD AND FAMILY ASSESSMENT AND PREPARATION

- Determine the child's cognitive, developmental, and legal ability to participate in the determination of advance directives. Regardless of the legal particulars, weight should be given to the child's wishes regarding life-sustaining medical treatment.
- Determine the presence of the parent or legal guardian who is responsible for making healthcare decisions for the child. Generally, parents give permission for the treatment of children who cannot do so themselves.
- Determine the parent's ability to understand the concept and consequence of advance directive formation. Competency to make decisions at a particular time under particular circumstances must be determined. Elements of this evaluation include (1) the ability to understand and communicate information relevant to a decision, (2) the ability to reason and deliberate concerning the decision, and (3) the ability to apply a set of values to a decision that may involve conflicting elements.
- Arrange for a translator if necessary so that children and family members can better communicate their concerns and understand the explanations of the healthcare providers.
- Assess the child and family's religious and cultural beliefs that may impact life-sustaining medical treatment and end-of-life care decisions and practices. Healthcare providers must respect the family's wishes and not project their own beliefs on the family.
- Set up a multidisciplinary conference with the family as needed. Conferences prevent the family from receiving conflicting or confusing information from various healthcare providers, including consulting services.

PROCEDURE **Obtaining an Advance Directive**

Steps	Rationale/Points of Emphasis
1. Determine during the admission process whether or not the child already has an advance directive in place. If present, place a copy in the medical record. The admission note should reflect that the advance directive was obtained.	The Patient Self-Determination Act (PSDA) of 1990 requires all healthcare facilities receiving Medicare and Medicaid reimbursement to recognize the living will and durable power of attorney. In addition, it requires healthcare facilities that receive Medicare and Medicaid funds to ask patients whether they have advance directives and to provide educational materials advising patients of their rights existing under state law. Completion of an advance directive document is optional, but all healthcare facilities must provide and discuss advance directive information with each patient or parent on admission, as required by the PSDA.
2. If the child does not have an advance directive, provide the child and family with advance directive guidelines or ensure that such materials have been given to the family. These materials may include written brochures on patients' rights and establishing advance directives or a video on advance directives.	Helps child and family understand the process. According to the PSDA, families are to be provided written information regarding their rights in making healthcare decisions.
3. Discuss the prognosis for treatment, treatment options, and potential outcomes with the child and parent.	This follows the process of informed consent. The needs of the child must drive the creation of an advance directive. **caREminder** *It must be clear to the healthcare providers, the parents, and the child that the child's needs remain the primary focus. Measures necessary to ensure comfort are implemented at all times.*
4. Elicit questions from the child and parent based on the information provided.	Helps determine child's and family's understanding.

Steps	Rationale/Points of Emphasis
5. Determine the need for multidisciplinary conferences to provide the child and family with complete, comprehensive, accurate information.	Conferences prevent families from receiving conflicting or confusing information from various healthcare providers, including consulting services. **caREminder** *Children who can comprehend should hear the conclusions regarding their continued survival. Withholding this information from them can result in a breakdown in trust between themselves and those who care for them.*
6. Assist family members in coming to terms with their decision; do not take reactions personally. Support the family in efforts to communicate the decision to the child.	Individuals involved in discussing and completing an advance directive may experience emotional reactions during the process. These reactions may include anger, crying, questioning, and doubt as one considers the weight of this complex decision. Psychosocial support from trained healthcare professional resources should be readily available for the family in assisting with this potentially difficult process.
7. Have the parent or child sign the advance directive. Assure the family that the terms of the advance directive may be rescinded or altered at any time.	Provides a legal record of the decision.
8. Place a copy of the advance directive in the front of the child's medical record or in a section of the medical record especially designated for advance directives. Place a sticker signifying that advance directives are contained within on the front of the chart.	Placing the document in the same location in every medical record increases accessibility of the document. The sticker on the front of the record alerts all healthcare personnel that advance directives are present.

CHILD AND FAMILY EVALUATION AND DOCUMENTATION

- Evaluate the family's understanding of the advance directive to ensure informed decision making.
- Document the family's religious and cultural beliefs influencing end-of-life care decisions.
- Document whether or not the child has an advance directive in his or her chart. Provide the details of the advance directive in the progress notes. Documentation in the patient medical record of whether the patient has executed an advance directive is required by the PSDA.
- Clearly document in the progress notes the conversation regarding advance directives and the participation of all parents or legal guardians and the child in that conversation.
- Physician or nurse practitioner orders and the multidisciplinary plan of care must clearly reflect the extent of the advance directive and any other special requests. The orders must specify limited resuscitation, full resuscitation, or no resuscitation.

COMMUNITY CARE

- Ensure that the child's parents have a copy of the advance directive and that they have a specific place designated to maintain this information. Emphasize the importance of keeping a copy of the advance directive with whoever is caring for the child.
- The use of advance directives is increasing in pediatrics and may be encountered in the prehospital setting. It must be kept in mind that many state laws still prohibit the prehospital provider from honoring a hospital do-not-resuscitate (DNR) order. Age of the minor may also affect the provider's decision making.
- The National Education Association recommends the following be executed for a DNR in the school setting:
  - All employees who supervise the student should be briefed as to the DNR status.
  - The student should wear a medical identification bracelet indicating the DNR status.
  - The parents should speak with the emergency service that would respond to the school and have a written contract to adhere to the DNR status. A copy should remain with the parents, the school, and the emergency service.
  - The DNR plan should be reviewed annually before the child enters the next grade level.
- Instruct the child and family to notify the healthcare provider if there is a change in the status of the child and family's decisions regarding the advance directive.

Unexpected Situation

- *The child, parent, or legal guardian makes a request to withdraw the advance directive:* Immediately notify the primary physician and consult institutional policy regarding necessary steps to address in processing the request.

Bibliography

American Academy of Pediatrics, Committee on Bioethics. (1994; reaffirmed January, 2004). Guidelines on forgoing life-sustaining medical treatment. *Pediatrics, 93*, 532–536.

American Academy of Pediatrics, Committee on School Health and Committee on Bioethics. (2000). Do not resuscitate orders in schools. *Pediatrics, 105*, 878–879.

American Nurses Association (ANA) Board of Directors. (1991). *Ethics and human rights position statements: Nursing and the patient self-determination acts.* Retrieved July 10, 2006, from http://www.nursingworld.org/readroom/position/ethics/prtetsdet.htm

Badzek, L., & Kanowky, S. (2002). Mature minors and end-of-life decision making: A new development in their legal right to participation. *Journal of Nursing Law, 8*, 23–29.

Committee on Child Abuse and Neglect and Committee on Bioethics. (2000). Forgoing life-sustaining medical treatment in abused children. *Pediatrics, 106*, 1151–1153.

Fallat, M. E., Deshpande, J. K., & ACP Section on Surgery. (2004). Do-not-resuscitate orders for pediatric patients who require anesthesia and surgery. *Pediatrics, 114*, 1686–1692.

Freyer, D. R. (2004). Care of the dying adolescent: Special considerations. *Pediatrics, 113*, 381–388.

Gaunthier, D. M., & Froman, R. D. (2001). Preferences for care near the end of life: Scale development and validation. *Research in Nursing & Health, 24*, 298–306.

Hardin, S. B., & Yusufaly, Y. A. (2004). Difficult end-of-life treatment decisions: Do other factors trump advance directives? *Archives of Internal Medicine, 164*, 1531–1533.

McAdam, J. L., Stotts, N. A., Padilla, G., & Puntillo, K. (2005). Attitudes of critically ill Filipino patients and their families toward advance directives. *American Journal of Critical Care, 14*, 17–25.

McAliley, L. G., Gunning, R. S., Hudson-Barr, D. C., & Rowbottom, L. A. (2000). The use of advance directives with adolescents. *Pediatric Nursing, 26*, 471–480.

Rushton, C. (2000). Pediatric palliative care: Coming of age. In A. Romer, K. Heller, D. Weissman, & M. Solomon (Eds.), *Innovations in end-of-life care* (Vol. 2). New Rochelle, NY: Mary Ann Leibert, Inc.

Savage, T., & Michalak, D. R. (2001). Finding agreement to limit life-sustaining treatment for children who are in state custody. *Pediatric Nursing, 27*, 594–597.

Tournay, A. E. (2000). Withdrawal of medical treatment in children. *Western Journal of Medicine, 173*, 407–411.

U.S. General Accounting Office. Omnibus Budget Reconciliation Act. (1990). *Patient Self-Determination Act.*

Westley, C., & Briggs, L. A. (2004). Using the stages of change model to improve communication about advance care planning. *Nursing Forum, 39*(3), 5–12.

CHAPTER 12

Aerosol Treatments

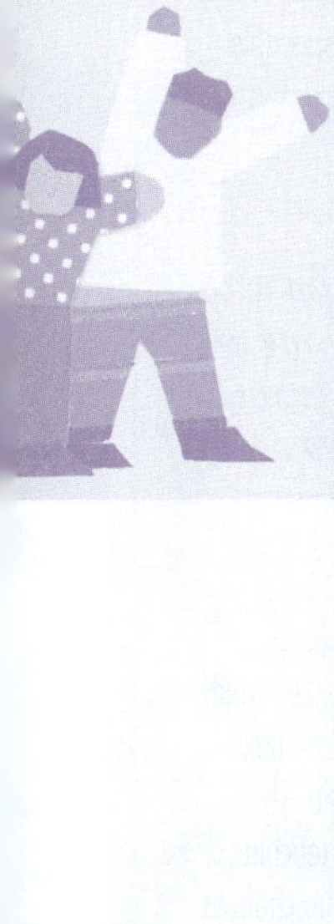

Clinical Guidelines

- The healthcare prescriber orders aerosol treatments.
- An aerosol treatment may be administered by the child, if age appropriate, or by a respiratory therapist, registered nurse (RN), licensed practical nurse (LPN), or parent or caregiver.
- Healthcare personnel responsible for delivery of aerosol treatments should have demonstrated and documented knowledge and skills related to
  - Aerosol delivery devices and their limitations
  - Assembly, care, and use of aerosol delivery devices
  - Medications being delivered, including contraindications, potential side effects, and desired outcomes
  - Recognition and response to adverse reactions during medication administration and modification of treatment accordingly
  - Performance of subjective and objective assessments to determine medication efficacy and patient's ability to use aerosol delivery devices properly
  - Provision of comprehensive patient and lay caregiver instructions
- The child, family member, or lay caregiver responsible for delivery of aerosol treatments should demonstrate
  - Proper use and understanding of aerosol delivery device and delivery technique
  - Proper assembly, cleaning, and care of aerosol delivery device and medication preparation
  - An understanding of medication purpose, dosage, indications, and side effects
  - Ability to alter medication as needed
  - Knowledge of when to report to healthcare prescriber
- Indications for aerosol treatment include the need to deliver aerosolized medications to patients in acute distress or with reduced respiratory flow, the need to modify drug concentration, and the need to deliver a topical medication in aerosol form to the lung parenchyma.
- Aerosol delivery devices are used according to the frequency of the prescribed medication.
- Aerosol treatments can be administered in a number of settings, including hospital, clinic, extended care facility, school, home, and during medical transportation.
- Continuous monitoring of the electrocardiogram is recommended when delivering a bronchodilator by a large-volume nebulizer.
- Resuscitation apparatus with airway manometer and masks of appropriate size should be available when aerosol treatments are being provided to the child.
- Standard precautions and measures to limit the transmission of microorganisms, including tuberculosis, must be adhered to at all times
  - Low oxygen systems do not require routine replacement.
  - Nasopharyngeal catheters should be changed every 24 hours.
  - Transtracheal catheters should be changed every 3 months.
  - Reservoir systems do not require routine replacement on the same child.

- Large-volume nebulizers should be changed every 24 hours.
- Oxy-Hood and reservoirs do not require routine replacement on the same child.

EQUIPMENT

- Age-appropriate aerosol delivery device that includes
  - Generator (small-volume nebulizer, large-volume nebulizer, metered-dose inhaler, or dry-powder inhaler)
  - Power source (mechanism by which the generator operates or is actuated)
  - Interface (mouthpiece, face mask) (Table 12-1)
- Ordered medication and prescribed isotonic diluent
- Disposable gloves and protective mask
- Stethoscope
- Flowmeter, if oxygen is ordered

CHILD AND FAMILY ASSESSMENT AND PREPARATION

- Determine which type of equipment would be most appropriate for use according to age and ability of child to manage mouthpiece versus face mask.
- Determine the child and family's knowledge regarding medical reason for the treatment, proper use of aerosol delivery device, ability to perform treatment, medication administration, and care of aerosol delivery equipment.
- Assess heart rate, respiratory rate, work of breathing, and breath sounds before starting treatments.

PROCEDURE Administering Aerosol Treatments

Steps	Rationale/Points of Emphasis
1. Perform hand hygiene.	Reduces transmission of microorganisms.
2a. Gather the necessary supplies.	Promotes efficient time management and provides an organized approach to the procedure.
2b. Select appropriate aerosol device (see Table 12-1).	The effectiveness of medication that is delivered in an aerosolized form depends on • Position of patient to the equipment • Particle size, ventilatory pattern, and airway architecture • Dose of medication used
3. Don gloves and a protective mask.	Protects the administrator from exposure to aerosols, medications, and patient-generated droplets. There is an increased awareness of possible health effects of aerosols, such as ribavirin and pentamidine. Recent research also warns of potential exposure effects of aerosolized antibiotics, steroids, and bronchodilators.
4. Following the specific manufacturer's directions for the equipment that is being used, assemble the aerosol delivery device, power source, and the interface (mouthpiece, face mask).	Each manufacturer has unique directions for connecting the various disposable parts of the aerosol equipment. **caREminder** *A face mask, rather than a mouthpiece, should be used with infants and children younger than 3 years of age. Using a mask attached to the nebulizer cup, which is held over the nose and mouth, enables the treatment to be dispersed as a mist, thus eliminating the need to keep a mouthpiece in place.*
5. Fill the nebulizer chamber, using a syringe to measure the precise amount of isotonic diluent or medication ordered. Close the chamber.	Diluents that are not isotonic may increase reactivity. Delivering aerosolized medications or mist is an inexact science because the actual amount of aerosolized material delivered into the lungs varies with the tidal volume of the child. The smaller the tidal volume, the smaller the actual amount of medication reaching the lungs. Precision in measuring what is being aerosolized increases the chances that the ordered amount of medication actually reaches the lungs.

Steps	Rationale/Points of Emphasis
	caREminder *Use only sterile fluids for aerosol solutions and dispense them aseptically. Medications ordered from multidose vials are handled, dispensed, and stored following the manufacturer's instructions.*
6a. Position the child and place the interface (mouthpiece, face mask) in position for delivery. When using a mouthpiece, it is important that the child seals the lips around the mouthpiece and breathes only through the mouth (Figure 12-1).	Children younger than 3 years of age are usually not able to cooperate well enough to use a mouthpiece and achieve the desired seal around the device. Use of face mask is recommended for children younger than 3 years of age.
6b. If the patient is an infant, hold him or her upright in a comforting position, supporting the head and the neck, and place the face mask over the mouth and nose.	Increasing the comfort level of the infant will increase your ability to finish the treatment without the infant crying. Crying reduces particle deposition in the lungs.
6c. For the older child, elevate the head of the bed or place him or her in a sitting position, and place the mask over his or her mouth, forming a tight seal (see Figure 83-2 in Chapter 83).	Prevents treatment from escaping without being delivered to the lungs.

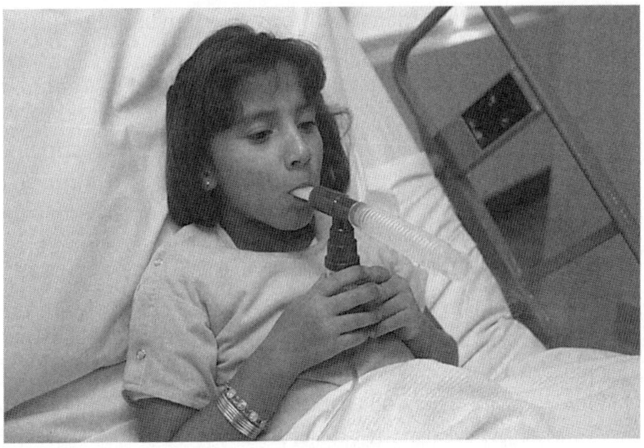

FIGURE 12-1
Remind the child to form a tight seal with his or her lips around the mouthpiece during the aerosol treatment.

7. Turn on the compressor and use for the prescribed amount of time.	With aerosol treatments, the duration may vary slightly, but an extended treatment may lead to an increase in noncompliance.
8. Carefully monitor the child's vital signs for signs and symptoms of adverse reactions to the treatment. Continue to assess child for improvement in respiratory status.	Aerosol treatment may result in adverse reactions, including tachycardia, cardiac arrhythmias, and palpitations. Delivering aerosol treatment directly to the lungs should result in stabilization of respiratory status.
9a. When finished with the treatment, remove mask from the child's face and turn off the compressor.	Equipment left operating can constitute a safety hazard.
9b. Assist the child to rinse the mouth with water after each administration of inhaled steroids.	Prevents oral irritation or overgrowth of opportunistic organisms from medication.
10. Return the child to a safe position in bed, with side rails up.	Protects child from falling out of bed.
11. Remove equipment from child's room and arrange for cleaning according to institution protocol. Dispose of waste in appropriate receptacle.	Clean equipment decreases the risk that pathogens will grow between uses. Inadequate cleaning can decrease nebulizer output by 50%. Standard precautions.
12. Perform hand hygiene.	Reduces transmission of microorganisms.

TABLE 12-1
Aerosol Devices

Type	Function	Administration Considerations
Small-volume nebulizer (SVN)	A jet nebulizer powered by compressed air	• For children older than 3 years of age who do not have an artificial airway and who are able to cooperate, a mouthpiece with an extension reservoir should be used. For children younger than 3 years of age, a facemask should be used. • An SVN with a T connector is used for children with a mechanical ventilator circuit or manual resuscitation bag. • Children with smaller tidal volumes (particularly neonates) or dyspneic children with shallow breathing may inhale less of the aerosolized agent and receive less of the dose when nebulization is continuous. • Cold, wet mist may be irritating to children and may limit the time the treatment is tolerated. • Nasal breathing will result in reduction in particle deposition. • A slow, deep inhalation with an inspiratory pause or hold is performed during SVN treatments. • A flow of 6–8 L/min and fill volume of 4 mL (depending on brand of equipment used) provides a maximum volume of delivered drug. • The sides of the SVN are periodically tapped to minimize the dead volume. • SVNs are for single-patient use only. Between treatments on the same patient, the equipment is disinfected, rinsed with sterile water, and air-dried. In the home, cleaning and rinsing with a solution of vinegar and water and air-drying is adequate.
Large-volume nebulizer (LVN)	Compressed air is used to deliver medication continuously over a period of time.	• There has been limited research into the use of this in the neonate and pediatric population. When it is used with children, however, it should be used with a facemask. • Cold, wet mist may be irritating to children and may limit the time the treatment is tolerated. • LVNs are for single-patient use only; nondisposable parts must be subject to high-level disinfection or sterilization between patients.
Metered-dose inhaler (MDI)	Pressurized canister that contains medication and propellant. A spacer device enhances delivery by decreasing the velocity of the particles and by reducing the number of large particles. A spacer device with a one-way valve (i.e., holding chamber) eliminates the need for the child to coordinate activation and inhalation, thus optimizing drug delivery.	• Children older than 3 years of age can use this with a valved-spacer device. • Children younger than 3 years of age should use a facemask. • The valved-spacer device eliminates the need for the child to coordinate inspiration and actuation. • MDI actuation occurs at the end exhalation, followed by a slow inspiration and breath hold for 10 seconds. • MDIs are for single-patient use only. Clean or replace when they appear dirty.
Dry powder inhaler (DPI)	This breath-activated device uses a gelatin capsule containing a single dose of medication and a carrier substance. The capsule is inserted into the device and then is punctured. The child's inspiratory flow disperses the dry particles and draws them into the lower airway.	• The device is appropriate for children who are able to achieve an inspiratory flow greater than or equal to 50 L/min. This usually corresponds to children older than 6 years of age. • Child must be instructed to produce a rapid inhalation in order to activate and discharge DPI fully. • DPIs are for single-patient use only. Clean or replace when they appear dirty.

Data from American Association of Respiratory Care. (1995). AARC clinical practice guideline: Selection of an aerosol device for neonatal and pediatric patients. *Respiratory Care, 40*(12), 1325–1335.

CHILD AND FAMILY EVALUATION AND DOCUMENTATION

- Evaluate child's response to the treatment, comparing findings with pretreatment assessment of work of breathing and breath sounds.
- Evaluate child, family, and caregiver's ability to perform all aspects of the procedure (e.g., delivery technique, proper administration of the medication, cleaning of the equipment).
- Document the following:
  - Respiratory status of child before and after treatment
  - Type of aerosol delivery device used
  - Name and amount of medications and diluents given
  - Frequency of treatments
  - Adverse reaction to the treatment
- Document successful training of child, family, and caregivers who will be performing this procedure.

COMMUNITY CARE

- If the family is to continue the treatments for the patient at home, arrangements should be made be to ensure that the child and family are able to complete all aspects of treatment safely and appropriately.
- Personnel performing this procedure in the home or school should be provided instruction on
  - Proper use and understanding of aerosol delivery device and delivery technique
  - Proper assembly, cleaning, and care of aerosol delivery device and medication preparation
  - An understanding of medication purpose, dosage, indications, and side effects
  - When to report child's condition and responses to treatment to healthcare prescriber
- Arrange for the necessary equipment to be provided in the home.
- Teach the family safety precautions to be used when oxygen is used in the home (see Chapter 83).
- Instruct the family to contact the healthcare provider if
  - Child's respiratory status does not improve after a treatment
  - Child exhibits side effects of medication administration

Unexpected Situation

- *Child was doing well on oxygen delivered by face mask for past hour but now is having an increased respiratory rate, and the pulse oximetry reading is 87%:* Verify that the oxygen delivery system is intact with the tubing still connected to the flowmeter and that the flowmeter is still on and at the previous setting. Assess respiratory sounds and respiratory effort, noting changes in child's status. If pulse oximetry readings remain below acceptable parameters, contact the healthcare prescriber and consider changing oxygen delivery to a nasal cannula and increasing oxygen flow rate.

Bibliography

American Association of Respiratory Care. (1995). Selection of an aerosol device for neonatal and pediatric patients. *Respiratory Care, 40*(12), 1325–1335.

American Association of Respiratory Care. (2002). Selection of an aerosol device for neonatal and pediatric patients—2002 Revision and update. *Respiratory Care, 47*(6), 707–716.

American Association of Respiratory Care. (2004). Application of continuous positive airway pressure to neonates via nasal prongs, nasopharyngeal tube or nasal mask—2004 Revision and update. *Respiratory Care, 49*(9), 1100–1108.

Cole, C. (2000). Special problems in aerosol delivery: Neonatal and pediatric considerations. *Respiratory Care, 45*(6), 646–651.

Kofman, C., Berlinski, A., Zaragoza, S., & Teper, A. (2004). Aerosol therapy for pediatric outpatients. *The Journal for Respiratory Care Practitioners, 17*(3), 26–28.

Mason, J. W., Miller, W. C., & Small, S. (1994). Comparison of aerosol delivery via circular system vs. conventional small volume nebulizer. *Respiratory Care, 39*(12), 1157–1161.

Newman, S. (1991). Aerosol generators and delivery systems. *Respiratory Care, 36*(9), 939–951.

Ranade, V. (2001). Inhalation therapy: New delivery systems. *American Journal of Therapeutics, 8*(5), 367–381.

Rubin, B. (2002). Nebulizer therapy for children: The device-patient interface. *Respiratory Care, 47*(11), 1314–1320.

CHAPTER

13

Apnea Monitors

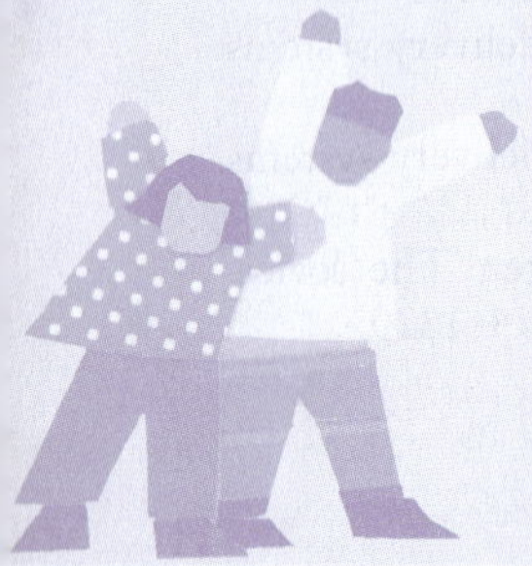

Clinical Guidelines

- In the healthcare setting, the registered nurse (RN), licensed practical nurse (LPN), or respiratory therapist is responsible for ensuring that the apnea monitor is used in accordance with the manufacturer's guidelines.
- Apnea monitoring is medically indicated for infants and children with a wide variety of acute and chronic conditions, including infants with:
  - One or more severe episodes of an apparent life-threatening event
  - Respiratory conditions requiring ongoing mechanical ventilation (continuous positive airway pressure and/or supplemental oxygen)
  - Gastroesophageal reflux with apneic episodes
  - Tracheostomies or anatomic abnormalities that make them vulnerable to airway compromise
  - Intrauterine exposure to cocaine or opiates before birth
  - Metabolic or neurologic disorders affecting respiratory control
  - Ongoing pain management using a patient-controlled analgesia device
- Unless otherwise ordered, the apnea monitor should be used continuously, except during bathing or at times when the infant is involved in interactive activities with the parent.
- Apnea monitor alarms should be on at all times during which the leads are placed on the infant.
- Use of home cardiopulmonary monitoring should be limited to specific clinical indications and implemented for a predetermined period of time. Such conditions include those listed above and premature infants at high risk for recurrent episodes of apnea, bradycardia, and/or hypoxemia after hospital discharge and those who remain technology dependent, have unstable airways, or have conditions affecting breathing regulation (American Academy of Pediatrics, Committee on Fetus and Newborn, 2003).
- The decision to discontinue home apnea monitoring should be made jointly between the family and the healthcare professionals. The use of home monitoring for the at-risk preterm infant should be discontinued approximately 43 weeks postmenstrual age or after the cessation of extreme episodes, whichever comes last (American Academy of Pediatrics, 2003).
- Home cardiopulmonary monitors should have the following features:
  - Ability to detect both a physiologic problem that results from apnea (e.g., slow heart rate) and the absence of breathing
  - Battery backup that can supply power for at least 8 hours
  - Both audio and visual alarms
  - Sensors to detect improper equipment performance
  - Safeguards to prevent inadvertent or unauthorized disabling of alarms
  - A remote alarm unit
  - An event monitor

EQUIPMENT

- Apnea monitor
- Apnea monitor belt or two electrode patches
- Apnea monitor electrode leads (two to four based on specific apnea device, usually one each of different colors)
- Apnea monitor log (optional)

CHILD AND FAMILY ASSESSMENT AND PREPARATION

- Review child's chart to determine the reason for apnea monitoring.
- Reinforce to parents reason for apnea monitoring. Explain how the equipment works, including where leads will be placed and what circumstances can cause the alarms to sound. If apneic episodes are being continuously documented, teach family members how to complete the apnea monitor log.
- Educate the parent to
  - Place the infant "Back to Sleep"
  - Provide a safe sleeping environment
  - Eliminate prenatal and postnatal tobacco smoke to prevent the risk of sudden infant death syndrome (SIDS)
- Assess the child's breath sounds and respirations to obtain baseline data before initiating monitoring.

PROCEDURE Preparing an Apnea Monitor

Steps	Rationale/Points of Emphasis
1a. Perform hand hygiene. 1b. Gather monitor, leads, and monitor belt or patches.	Reduces transmission of microorganisms. Promotes efficient time management.
2. Inspect the electrodes and lead wires for breaks or cracks.	Faulty electrodes and wires will not transmit the information needed to monitor the cardiorespiratory status of the infant.
3. Place the monitor on a sturdy level surface at least 6 inches away from walls or curtains.	The monitor operates most effectively from a firm surface. Placing the monitor against walls or curtains or on a crib mattress will muffle the sound of the alarm.
4. If an apnea monitor belt is used, inspect it for cleanliness and integrity.	Pathogens may grow in an unclean environment. Broken wires will not work effectively. **caREminder** *The electrode belt can be kept clean by handwashing it in warm soapy water and then laying it out to dry naturally. The belt should not be placed in an automatic washer or dryer because it is generally made of backed foam rubber and will come apart if exposed to harsh mechanical treatment.*
5. Position the infant on his or her back.	Several studies support the finding that healthy term infants and high-risk infants are at risk for increased episodes of apnea when placed in the side or prone position. The "Back to Sleep" campaign promoted by the American Academy of Pediatrics recommends that all infants be placed to sleep in the supine position.

PROCEDURE Using an Apnea Monitor Belt

Steps	Rationale/Points of Emphasis
1. With the child lying on his or her back, place the electrode belt under the child's back, halfway between the armpits and the bottom of the rib cage. Cut belt material to size (Figure 13-1A).	Electrodes should be placed where the greatest amount of chest excursion or respiratory movement occurs and where the heart rate can be clearly noted to monitor for either bradycardia or tachycardia. The belt covers most of the rib cage in infants and very small children because of the relatively small chest area.

Continued

Steps	Rationale/Points of Emphasis

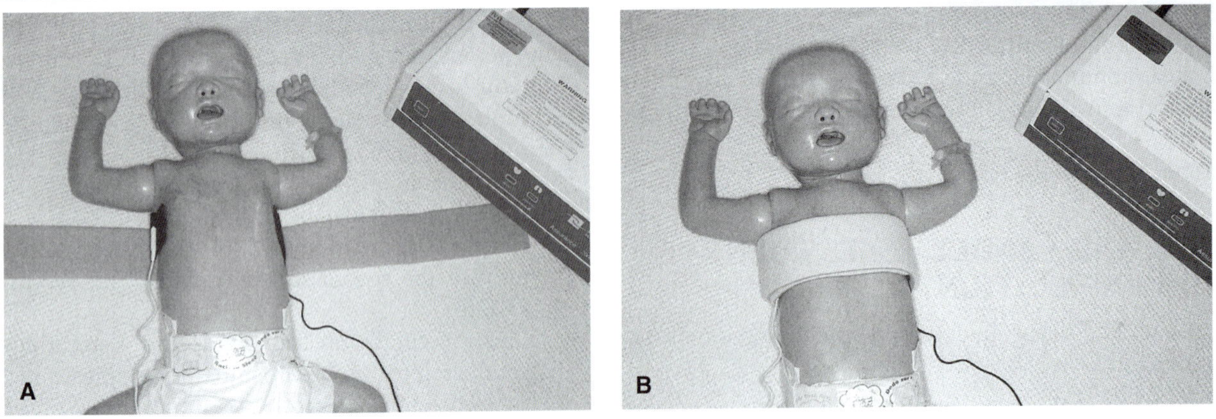

FIGURE 13-1
(**A**) With the child lying on his or her back, place the electrode belt under the child's back halfway between the armpits and the bottom of the rib cage. Cut belt material to size. (**B**) Place electrodes with lead wires attached directly below the armpits and close the Velcro fastener on the outer surface of the belt so that it fits snugly but not tightly.

Steps	Rationale/Points of Emphasis
2. Connect lead wires to each electrode. The white-tipped lead wire should be connected to the electrode that is located on the infant's *right side*. The black-tipped wire should be connected to the electrode that is located on the infant's *left side*.	Wires and electrodes conduct the chest movement and heartbeat information to the monitor. **caREminder** *Hold the lead wires only by the reinforced plastic grips at each end and insert them as far as possible into the electrodes to minimize wire damage and increase the conductivity of the electrodes.*
3. Place electrodes, with lead wires attached, directly below armpits, one on each side of the chest (Figure 13-1B). The lead wires should point toward the bottom of the belt.	Wires should be as far away from the infant's head and hands as possible. Being placed under the armpit makes them proximal to the apnea monitor and distal from the hands and mouth of the infant. **KidKare** As the infant grows, the best electrode placement to pick up respirations and heartbeat may change slightly. The apex of the heart is located at the fourth intercostal space in children younger than 7 years of age and the fifth intercostal space in children older than 7 years of age.
4. With the electrodes in their proper position, the Velcro fastener on the outer surface of the belt is closed so that the belt fits snugly but not tightly.	Ensures constant contact between the infant's skin and the electrodes. Electrodes are encased in plastic with Velcro on one side. This arrangement makes it easy to adjust their placement. The belt must not hamper the breathing movements of the chest or upper abdomen. **caREminder** *After securing the belt around the infant, an adult should be able to fit two fingers easily between the belt and the chest of the infant. Unlike adults, infants rely on the diaphragm for breathing. Anything that fits too snugly can impede respiration.*
5. Plug the distal ends of the lead wires into the apnea monitor according to the specific directions for the apnea monitor used.	Connections may be slightly different according to the specific apnea monitor that is in use.

Steps	Rationale/Points of Emphasis
6. Turn on the apnea monitor. The apnea/alarm time lapse should be preset by the respiratory therapist or by the vendor for the monitor.	Generally, when the order is given for an infant to undergo apnea monitoring, the ordering physician determines what is to be considered apnea, bradycardia, or tachycardia. The monitor alarms are then set accordingly. The U.S. Food and Drug Administration established that 20 seconds of apnea or a heart rate drop below 80 beats/min is cause for alarm.
7. Discontinue monitor when ordered by healthcare prescriber.	Continued use of the monitor when no longer needed may cause breakdown of skin under electrodes and unnecessarily limits the child's movement and activities.

PROCEDURE Using Electrode Patches

Steps	Rationale/Points of Emphasis
1. Remove electrode patches from packaging and examine them for moistness and stickiness.	Electrodes that have dried out will not adhere to the infant's skin. Electrode patches are made of plastic with one adhesive side.
2. Examine the skin of the infant to ensure there is no powder, oil, perspiration, or tissue breakdown.	Powders, oil, and perspiration interfere with adhesion and conduction. Placing an electrode over tissue that is compromised will lead to further breakdown or infection.
3a. Place the white lead to the patient's right chest above the nipple. Place the black lead to the patient's left chest above the nipple. Place the green/red lead to the patient's abdomen where respirations can be visualized (Figure 13-2).	Correct lead placement is essential for accurate monitoring of the patient's cardiorespiratory status.

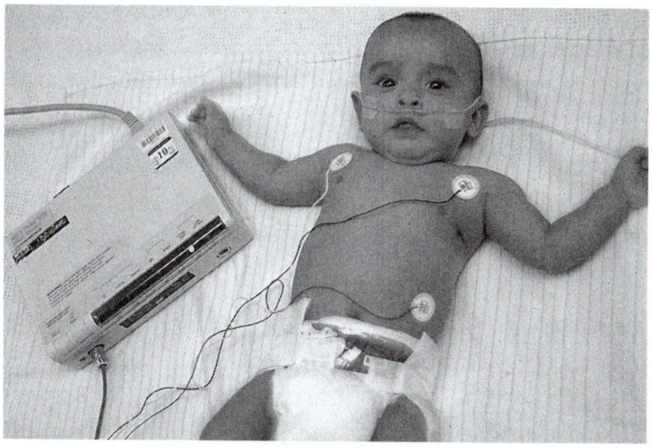

FIGURE 13-2
Place the adhesive gel side of the electrode patch above the nipple on the right and left quadrants of the chest and on either lower quadrant of the abdomen for the three lead monitors.

caREminder

A helpful pneumonic device to remember the correct placement of the leads is "white, right; smoke, above fire" (white is on the right, black above the heart).

Steps	Rationale/Points of Emphasis
3b. The inserts for the lead wires should point away from the head and hands of the infant.	Placing the wires away from the mouth and hands of the infant decreases the chance that infant will disconnect or become entangled in them.

caREminder

The exact site of electrode placement should be rotated slightly each time that the electrodes are replaced to decrease the chance

Continued

Steps	Rationale/Points of Emphasis
	that the skin will become compromised. Care should be taken that the electrodes are NEVER placed over the infant's nipple area, which is extremely sensitive and prone to breakdown. **KidKare** With a diapered patient, release one side of the folded over diaper flap, place all three wires such that they lie between the two folds of the diaper and are not touching the infant's skin, and then re-adhere the diaper flap. This secures the cords and limits the patient ability or temptation to pull on them.
4. Connect the lead wires into the apnea monitor and turn it on per the manufacturer's instructions.	Although the guiding principles are basically the same for all apnea monitors, each monitor has unique features according to its manufacturer.
5. Remove all apnea monitoring equipment from contact with the child's skin for at least 10 to 15 minutes per day. During this time, the infant should receive a daily bath or sponge bath, and the skin should be examined for redness and other signs of breakdown.	Skin needs to be exposed to remain intact. Adhesive gel that allows electrodes to adhere to the skin of the infant will break down when exposed to the corrosive effect of perspiration. If good contact is not maintained with the skin, there will be an increased number of false alarms due to poor information conduction.
6. Discontinue monitor when ordered by physician.	Continued use of the monitor when no longer needed may cause breakdown of skin under electrodes and unnecessarily limits the child's movement and activities.

PROCEDURE **Troubleshooting and Problem Solving**

Steps	Rationale/Points of Emphasis
1. Response to an apnea monitor must be immediate and thorough. If alarm sounds, assess the child for • Chest movement • Activity • Color • Respiratory and cardiac rate	Statistically, less than 20% of infants who progress from apnea to full arrest survive the crisis. Each alarm must be treated seriously until proven false. **KidKare** If the infant's color is normal and the infant is breathing, observe without stimulation. DO NOT shake the infant. Caretakers should turn on the light and look for signs of breathing. Picking up the infant without pausing to see whether the infant has truly stopped breathing makes it difficult to determine whether an apneic episode truly occurred.
2. After verifying that the infant is not in distress, check the leads for appropriate contact with either the skin or the electrode.	The most common cause of a false alarm is a loose lead or one that fails to make contact with either the skin or the electrode. Lead wires are made of multiple strands of fine fragile wire wound together to form one larger wire, which is then covered with plastic. A break in one of these small wires will trigger an alarm.
3. Check infant's skin to determine whether powder, oil, or perspiration is present. If necessary, cleanse the skin with soap and water. Rinse and dry thoroughly and then reapply the electrodes.	The points on the infant's skin where electrodes are placed must be clean and dry to maintain good contact with the electrodes.
4. If the child is in respiratory or cardiac distress, begin cardiopulmonary resuscitation procedures (see Chapter 24).	Rapid response increases the infant's chance of survival.

CHILD AND FAMILY EVALUATION AND DOCUMENTATION

- Evaluate the family's understanding of why the apnea monitor is being used.
- Determine the appropriateness of the response to the monitor alarms by the family.
- Document the following:
  - Use of apnea monitor, noting that the alarms are turned on
  - Setting and triggering alarm limits every time the monitor is turned on or the beginning of each shift.
  - Child's condition at the time of the assessment
  - Each alarm event, noting the time, date, condition, and response of the infant and the type of alarm (e.g., heart rate, loose lead)
- Document family teaching related to use of apnea monitor and response to alarms.
- When an apneic episode occurs, document the following:
  - Time of apneic episode
  - Length of episode
  - Color of child's skin
  - Activity of the child
  - If chest movement ceased
  - Respiratory or cardiac rate at time alarm sounded
  - Whether child's recovery response was spontaneous or child needed stimulation to breathe
- Document the person (company) responsible for the maintenance of the apnea monitor. Post the person's name and number where he or she can be reached if the apnea monitor malfunctions.

COMMUNITY CARE

- If the infant is to be discharged to home while still using an apnea monitor, discharge coordination with the home care company should begin as soon as possible.
- The home caregiver should be involved in all aspects of the teaching regarding the apnea monitor and response to the alarms. Family education/training should include
  - Monitoring techniques
  - Operation of the monitor, including response to alarms
  - Cardiopulmonary resuscitation
  - Minimum environmental requirements for home use, including electricity and a telephone in the home
  - Managing the monitor during transportation of child in a car/car seat
- Instruct the family about potential sources of monitor interference, including
  - Radio signals from police stations, fire stations, or airports
  - Electrical appliances such as electric blankets, electric waterbed heaters, television sets, air conditioners, and cordless telephones. Such equipment should be kept at least 1 foot away from the monitor.
- Provide references to support groups for families of infants using an apnea monitor.

Alert! ***Parents must be advised that home cardiopulmonary monitoring is not prescribed to prevent SIDS and has not been proven to prevent sudden and unexpected deaths in infants.***

- Instruct the family to contact the equipment vendor if equipment malfunctions or more supplies are needed.
- Instruct the family to contact the healthcare provider if
  - Child experiences an increasing number of apneic spells
  - Child requires an increase in stimulation efforts to return to baseline respiratory parameters

Unexpected Situations

- *A young mother is lying on a cot in the room with the infant asleep in the crib. The apnea monitor on her baby begins to alarm:* Look at the infant, noting his or her color. Look at what the monitor screens are indicating. Check the leads on the child to determine whether they are in the correct positions and are fully attached to the chest wall. Note the infant's respirations (normal, ceased, or increased from his/her baseline). Stimulate infant if needed. Document findings on the log at the bedside.
- *The infant has to be transported off the unit for a procedure:* Either obtain a physician's order to discontinue the monitor for this procedure or take the monitor with you if the child's condition is unstable. Generally, stable patients can be disconnected for a short amount of time during the day (use your nursing and assessment and judgment). Ensure you have the necessary equipment to provide ventilation and oxygenation if needed for the unstable child during transport.

Bibliography

American Academy of Pediatrics. (2003). Apnea, sudden infant death syndrome, and home monitoring. *American Academy of Pediatrics, 111*(4), 914–917.

Baker, L., & Thyer, B. (2000). Promoting parental compliance with infant home apnea monitor use. *Behavior Research & Therapy, 39*(3), 285–297.

Bennett, A. (2002). Home apnea monitoring for infants. *Advance for Nurse Practitioners, 10*(3), 48–53.

Hershberger, M., Peeke, K., Levett, J., & Spear, M. (2001). Effect of sleep position on apnea and bradycardia in high-risk infants. *Journal of Perinatology, 21*(2), 85–89.

Sychowski, S., Dodd, E., Thomas, P., Peabody, J., & Clark, R. (2001). Home apnea monitoring use in preterm infants discharged from newborn intensive care units. *Journal of Pediatrics, 139*(2), 245–248.

CHAPTER 14

Bathing the Infant

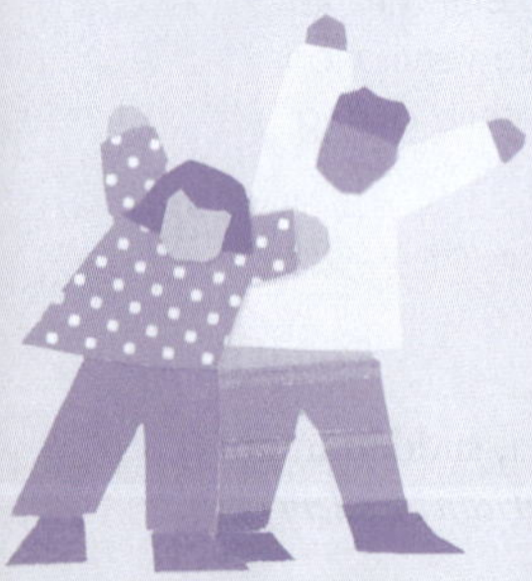

Clinical Guidelines

- Bathing is completed by a parent, registered nurse (RN), licensed practical nurse (LPN), or nursing assistant.
- The healthy newborn's first bath is given after the infant's temperature has stabilized in the normal range (98.2–99°F or 36.8–37.2°C axillary) and when appropriate care is taken to support thermal stability.
- The older infant should have a temperature between 97.5° and 98.6°F or 36.4° and 37°C axillary or orally before initiation of the bath.
- The infant is given a complete bath two to three times a week or more often, if necessary.
- Hair washing is completed with the first newborn bath and as needed thereafter.
- Between complete baths, the infant's face, neck, hands, and genital areas are washed as needed.
- The infant's age, medical condition, and neurodevelopmental stability determines the type of bath given.
  - A tub bath may be give once the umbilical cord has fallen off. Or a tub bath may be given if the infant is placed in a tub containing a shallow amount of water that does not immerse the umbilical cord.
  - The circumcised male should not be bathed in a tub until the penis is healed.

Equipment

- Warming lamp
- Dry blanket or waterproof pad
- Basin with warm water: 100°F (37.8°C)
- Nonsterile gloves
- Mild soap or cleansing agent
- Towels (at least two)
- Washcloth
- Cotton swabs or gauze wipes
- Perfume-free lotion of ointment
- Petroleum jelly
- Emollient
- Soft-bristle brush or comb
- Clean clothing and diaper
- Bedding
- Bulb syringe (if needed)

CHILD AND FAMILY ASSESSMENT AND PREPARATION

- Assess the special needs of the child before starting the bath. Some restrictions may apply to children with surgical incisions, traction, intravenous catheters, casts, urinary catheters, and artificial airways.
- Review the chart to determine the type of bath ordered (if specified), when the last bath was given, and child's last recorded temperature.
- Assess the premature infant's physiologic state (vagal tone, heart rate, oxygen saturation) to determine the appropriate timing for a sponge bath.
- Ensure that the room is warm and free of drafts. If needed, use a heat lamp to provide direct warmth to the area where the bath will be given.
- Allow the parent to participate in bathing the child, instructing her or him as necessary about any special precautions or equipment. Use bath time as an opportunity to teach about tub and water safety.
- With the older infant, the bath can be incorporated into a playful game.

PROCEDURE Giving a Sponge Bath

Steps	Rationale/Points of Emphasis
1. Gather the necessary supplies.	Promotes efficient time management and provides an organized approach to the procedure.
2. Ensure that the opposite side rail of a crib is raised. Keep isolette doors closed until equipment is ready for the bath.	Depending on the developmental level of the child, he or she could roll off the bed if side rails are left down.
3. Turn on warming lamp and ensure it is appropriate distance from infant (see Chapter 135).	Prepares environment to be thermally stable. Heat loss can occur by convection. An infant's temperature-regulating mechanisms are immature, and the infant is at high risk for heat loss, especially premature infants or very—low-birth-weight infants. Hypothermia can result in increased oxygen consumption and respiratory distress.
4. Place a dry bath blanket or waterproof pad on the bed surface of the crib or isolette.	A dry surface will reduce heat loss by conduction.
5. Fill basin or small tub with warm water. Water temperature should be about 100°F (37.8°C).	Prevents scalding of infant skin. If a thermometer is not available, test the temperature of the water with the sensitive skin on the inside of your wrist or elbow.
6. Perform hand hygiene and don gloves.	Standard precaution to reduce transmission of microorganisms.
7. Position the infant in a supine position. Loosely cover the infant at all times with a dry towel or blanket.	Keeping the total body area from being exposed to the air helps reduce heat loss.
8. Begin bath by bathing the face using cotton balls or a soft washcloth and water.	Using plain water will prevent soap from irritating the eyes.
9. When cleansing orbital area, wash from inner canthus to outer canthus, using a fresh cotton ball or clean corner of washcloth for each eye.	Following the natural tear flow will prevent the spread of microorganisms.
10. Pat bathed area dry with a clean, dry towel.	Rubbing can irritate the skin.
11a. Cleanse nose with corner of cloth or cotton ball. Remove any incrustations from the nares by using a twisted moist cotton ball or washcloth.	Moisture loosens the incrustations in the nares for easy removal.
11b. Gentle suctioning of the nares with a bulb syringe may help clear the nares of nasal secretions.	Infants and small children cannot expel the secretions in the nose by blowing through the nasal passages.
12. Wash the external ears and behind the ear by winding a damp washcloth around the index finger.	Prevents possible packing of the discharge farther down the ear canal. Prevents damage to the eardrum. **caREminder** *Never place cotton swabs or other small objects in the infant's ear canal.*

Continued

Steps	Rationale/Points of Emphasis
13a. Using a mild soap or cleansing agent, work from the shoulders to the feet in a systematic manner to wash one section of the body at a time. Pay special attention to the folds of the neck, thighs, and underarms.	Ensures that all areas of the body are bathed as efficiently as possible. The younger the infant, the more sensitive the skin is to abrasive soaps. Cleansing agents that have a neutral pH and minimal dyes and perfumes will reduce risk of future allergy sensitization to topical agents. There are no studies to support the use of antimicrobial solutions or cleansers for the purpose of bathing the infant or premature child. Using mild soap as opposed to water alone for the first newborn bath has demonstrated minimal effect on skin bacterial colonization. **caREminder** *For extremely premature infants (less than 26 weeks' gestational age), sterile water alone should be used for bathing.*
13b. Excess vernix can be removed from the newborn's skin; however, removal of all vernix is not necessary.	Studies indicate that vernix may provide antibacterial protection and promote wound healing. It may also contribute to the development of the epidermal barrier function, regulating postnatal and surface adhesion properties, heat flux, and surface electrical activities.
14. Rinse and dry each area after washing. Do not rub the skin surfaces.	Soap residue can be irritating to the infant's skin. Rubbing skin surfaces can cause chafing and irritation. ***Alert!*** ***If the infant is being monitored, observe the heart rate and oxygen saturation level. Discontinue the bath procedures if the infant's condition deteriorates.***
15. Clean the umbilical area with soap and water. Observe umbilicus for redness or drainage. Lift cord and clean base; do not wet the umbilical cord. Rinse and dry the area. Leave site open to air; do not apply alcohol, antiseptics, or antibiotics to umbilical cord stump.	Promotes drying of the stump. Prevents infection (omphalitis) that can be life threatening. Studies have shown that natural drying of the umbilical cord does not result in increased incidence of infection and that treatment with antiseptics prolongs time to cord separation.
16. Place the infant on his or her stomach. Wash, rinse, and dry the infant's back. Cover the infant with a dry towel.	Prevents loss of body heat.
17. Apply a small amount of perfume-free lotion or ointment (petroleum jelly or hydrophilic ointment) to any dry area. Vitamin C cream may also be used. Avoid the use of baby oil or baby powder.	Baby oil clogs the skin pores, and baby powder may irritate dry skin.
18. Cleanse the genital area:	
a. For females, gently wash the area from front to back, from vagina to rectum. Use a portion of the washcloth or a moistened cotton ball to cleanse the area. Use cotton ball only once to wipe area. Discard after one use and change to new cotton ball for each subsequent wipe.	Cleaning from front to back reduces risk for contamination of the urethra or vagina from the anus. Reduces transmission of microorganisms.
b. If a white substance is noted in the labial fold, do not attempt to wipe clean. Females may have blood present during diaper change.	Some mucus may be noted in the vaginal area of the neonate. Blood may be present because of maternal hormones.
c. For males, squeeze clean water over head of the penis. In the uncircumcised male, gently move the foreskin back as far as it will go, cleanse the head of the penis, and return the foreskin to the normal position. Do not force the foreskin back.	At birth, only 4% of boys have a retractile prepuce; by age 3 years, the foreskin is retractable in 90% of boys. Leaving the prepuce in a retracted position constricts the blood vessels supplying the glans penis, causing edema. Retracting the foreskin when bathing decreases the chances of having smegma accumulation, inflammation, phimosis, or adhesions.
d. In the circumcised infant, a petroleum-coated gauze bandage or petroleum jelly should be applied to the tip of the penis if the circumcision was the Gomco type. May apply an antibiotic ointment on Plastibell-type circumcision if ordered by physician.	The dressing helps prevent the circumcised area from rubbing against the diaper or sticking to the diaper as the healing process progresses.

Steps	Rationale/Points of Emphasis
19. Raise the infant's lower body by the ankles to expose the buttocks. Wash, rinse, and dry the infant's buttocks.	Wash from front to back to reduce the transmission of microorganisms from the anus.
20. Apply petroleum jelly or A&D ointment to buttock area and crease areas if indicated by redness and or breakdown of skin in the area (see Chapter 34).	Cream barrier keeps ammonia away from the infant's skin and prevents diaper rash.

Alert! *Powders should not be used on the infant. Baby powders may be accidentally aspirated by the infant. Aspiration of the particles can lead to pneumonia and even death.*

Steps	Rationale/Points of Emphasis
21. Apply a clean diaper. If the umbilical cord is still in place, adjust the top of the diaper so that it is below the umbilical area.	The umbilical area should be uncovered to prevent irritation and infection.
22. Apply emollient (e.g., Aquaphor) to the infant's skin as needed.	Emollients can prevent excessive drying, skin cracking, and fissures. Avoid products with perfumes or dyes because these substances can be absorbed and are potential contact irritants. Emollients are safe to use with premature infants.
23. If washing hair, wrap the infant in a warm blanket, securing the arms close to the body. Place the infant in a football hold position (Figure 14-1).	A warm blanket will help stabilize body temperature during hair washing. With the football hold, the infant will be securely held in place, allowing the parent a free hand to wash the infant's hair.

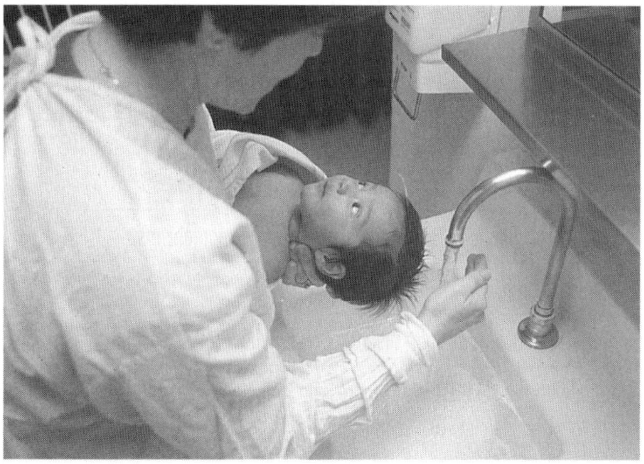

FIGURE 14-1
Hold the child securely in the "football hold" position, supporting the neck, when washing the infant's hair.

Steps	Rationale/Points of Emphasis
24. Position the infant's head over the wash basin. Lather the infant's scalp with a mild soap or shampoo.	Gentle washing helps reduce seborrhea, a scaly scalp condition commonly called "cradle cap."
25. Using a damp, soapy cloth, wash the infant's hair and rinse thoroughly. Dry with a towel.	Soap or shampoo residue may irritate the scalp if either is left at the site.
26. Comb the infant's hair with a fine-toothed comb or a soft-bristle brush.	Aids in removing crusts from the infant's scalp if cradle cap is present.
27. Remove blankets from infant after hair washing. Proceed to dress the infant in dry clothing and wrap him or her in a dry blanket. Cover his or her head with a cap or bonnet. Position for comfort and safety. Ensure the bedside rails are up or isolette doors closed.	Prevents loss of body heat. Promotes safe environment.
28. Cleanse and rinse the basin or tub. Return all equipment to its proper storage area. Dispose of waste in appropriate receptacle.	Reduces the transmission of microorganisms. Standard precautions.
29. Remove gloves and perform hand hygiene.	Reduces transmission of microorganisms.

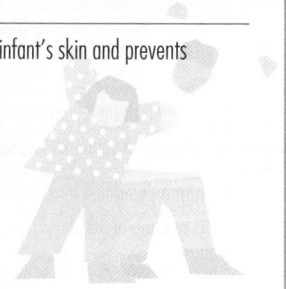

PROCEDURE Giving a Tub Bath

Steps	Rationale/Points of Emphasis
1. Gather the necessary supplies.	Promotes efficient time management and provides an organized approach to the procedure.
2. Ensure that the opposite side rail of a crib is raised. Keep isolette doors closed until equipment is ready for the bath.	Depending on the developmental level of the child, he or she could roll off the bed if side rails are left down.
3. Turn on warming lamp and ensure it is appropriate distance from infant (see Chapter 135).	Prepares environment to be thermally stable. Heat loss can occur by convection. An infant's temperature-regulating mechanisms are immature, and the infant is at high risk for heat loss, especially premature infants or very—low-birth-weight infants. Hypothermia can result in increased oxygen consumption and respiratory distress.
4. Fill basin or tub with two or three inches of warm water. Water temperature should be about 100°F (37.8°C).	An infant can drown in a few inches of water. Prevents scalding of infant skin. If a thermometer is not available, test the temperature of the water using the inside of your wrist or elbow. **caREminder** *An infant should never be left alone when bathing, whether in a tub of water or on a counter. Instruct parents to prepare for interruptions by taking the telephone off the hook or engaging the answering machine. If the doorbell rings or a sibling screams, the infant should be wrapped up in a blanket and taken with the parent no matter what phase the bathing process is at.*
5. Perform hand hygiene and don gloves.	Standard precautions to reduce transmission of microorganisms.
6. Undress the infant.	Prepares for bath.
7. Gradually slip the infant into the tub while supporting the neck and head.	An infant is unable to support his or her own head.
8. Wash the infant with the soapy cloth beginning at the shoulders and arms, continuing to the lower extremities. Cleanse the skin folds thoroughly.	Starting with the cleanest area progressing to the area that is most soiled keeps the bath water cleaner. Use soap sparingly.
9. Rinse the infant thoroughly with a clean, damp washcloth.	Rinse well so soap residue will not irritate the infant's skin.
10. Wash the infant's hair, following steps 23–26 in Sponge Bath. To position the infant for hair washing in the tub, support the infant's back and neck while allowing the head to drop backward at an angle that prevents water and soap from running into the infant's eyes.	Prevents drying of scalp and development of cradle cap. Soap and water in the eyes will cause irritation.
11. Dry the infant and dress him or her in dry clothing. Place infant in crib. Position for comfort and safety. Ensure the bedside rails are up.	Prevents loss of body heat. Promotes safe environment.
12. Cleanse and rinse the basin or tub. Return all equipment to its proper storage area. Dispose of waste in appropriate receptacle.	Reduces the transmission of microorganisms. Standard precautions.
13. Remove gloves and perform hand hygiene.	Reduces transmission of microorganisms.

CHILD AND FAMILY EVALUATION AND DOCUMENTATION

- Monitor child's response to bathing and hygiene procedures; discontinue if the child demonstrates signs of stress or hypothermia.
- Evaluate abnormal findings noted during the bath, such as umbilical redness or drainage, which may indicate infection, and report to the physician or advanced nurse practitioner.
- Document the following:
  - Completion of bath

- Assessments made of skin and general appearance of infant
- Infant's response to the bath
- Parent–child interaction during the bath
- Parental teaching completed during the bath demonstration and competencies noted upon return demonstration

COMMUNITY CARE

- Refer parents as indicated to community classes for basic infant care.
- Teach parents that an infant or young child should never be left unattended in a tub or basin.
- Instruct parents to verify that the water heater in the home is set between 120°F and 125°F, or 49°C and 52°C.
- Instruct parents to contact the healthcare provider if
  - Abnormal skin lesions are noted during the child's bath
  - Child's skin becomes scalded due to exposure to water that was too hot

Unexpected Situation

- *During the bath the infant's extremities become cold, with accompanying increases in heart rate and respiratory rate:* The infant is hypothermic. Immediately stop the bath and initiate measures to warm the infant, including quickly drying the infant, using a heat lamp, and/or placing the infant in a warm isolette or a warming bed.

Bibliography

Behring, A., Vezaeu, T., & Fink, R. (2003). Timing of the newborn first bath: A replication. *The Journal of Neonatal Nursing, 22*(1), 39–46.

Bryanton, J., Walsh, D., Barrett, M., & Gaudet, D. (2004). Tub bathing versus traditional sponge bathing for the newborn. *Journal of Obstetric, Gynecologic, and Neonatal Nursing, 33*(6), 704–712.

Karl, D. J. (1999). The interactive newborn bath: Using infant neurobehavior to connect parents and newborns. *MCN; American Journal of Maternal Child Nursing, 24*, 280–286.

Lee, H. (2002). Effects of sponge bathing on vagal tone and behavioural responses in premature infants. *Journal of Clinical Nursing, 11*(4), 510–519.

Lund, C., Kuller, J., Lane, A., Lott, J., & Raines, D. (1999). Neonatal skin care: The scientific basis for practice. *Journal of Obstetric, Gynecologic, and Neonatal Nursing, 28*(3), 241–254.

Medves, J., & O'Brien, B. (2001). Does bathing newborns remove potentially harmful pathogens from the skin? *Birth, 28*(3), 161–165.

Medves, J., & O'Brien, B. (2004). The effect of the bather and location of first bath on maintaining thermal stability in newborns. *Journal of Obstetric, Gynecologic, and Neonatal Nursing, 33*(2), 175–182.

Peters, K. L. (1998). Bathing premature infants: Physiological and behavioral consequences. *American Journal of Critical Care*, 7, 90–100.

Trotter, S. (2002). Skincare for the newborn: Exploring the potential harm of manufactured products. *RCM Midwives Journal, 5*(11), 376–378.

Varda, K., & Behnke, R. (2000). The effect of timing of initial bath on newborn's temperature. *Journal of Obstetric, Gynecologic, and Neonatal Nursing, 29*(1), 27–32.

Zupan, J., Garner, P., & Omari, A. (2004). Topical umbilical cord care at birth. *The Cochrane Database of Systematic Reviews*, (3). No. CD001057.

CHAPTER

15

Bed and Crib Choices

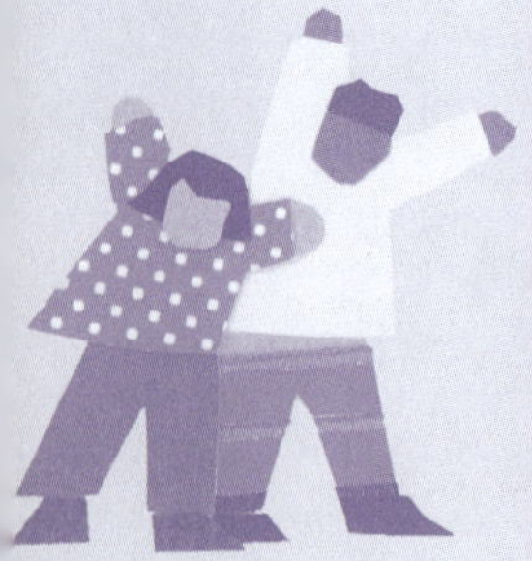

Clinical Guidelines

- Children are assigned an isolette, crib, or bed appropriate for their chronologic age, developmental age, and/or clinical condition.
- Children who exhibit growth and development parameters considered normative for their age and who show no alterations in mental status or level of consciousness may be placed in the following types of beds:
  - Premature infants and newborns: isolette or bed with radiant warmer
  - Infants and toddlers: open crib
  - Toddlers and young preschoolers: crib with enclosed bubble top
  - Older preschoolers, school-aged children, and adolescents: hospital bed
- Wheels are placed in a locked position when any isolette, crib, or bed is occupied.
- Side rails are kept in the highest position possible when the child is occupying the isolette, crib, or bed. The lower two side rails of a hospital bed may be left down for the older ambulatory child to make it easier for the child to get in and out of bed and to prevent the child from having to climb over the side rails.
- Use of specialty beds is not addressed in this procedure even though certain children may require the use of specialty beds. To identify those children who would benefit from the use of these beds, see manufacturer's guidelines and refer to institutional policies.
- The supine sleeping position ("Back to Sleep") is recommended for all preterm and term infants.

Equipment

- Isolette, crib, or bed
- Age-appropriate toys or objects that are developmentally stimulating

Child and Family Assessment and Preparation

- Determine child's age, developmental abilities, and level of consciousness.
- Determine whether or not the child has healthcare needs that warrant selection of a specialty bed.
- Explain to the child and family the importance of maintaining side rails in full upright position when the child is in the isolette, crib, or bed.

Alert! *The infant or toddler in an isolette or crib should never be left unattended with the side rails down. The parent or healthcare provider should always keep one hand on the infant or toddler when the side rails are down.*

- Discuss with parents the American Academy of Pediatrics (AAP) recommendations that premature and full-term infants should be placed for sleep in a supine (back-lying) position. A supine position confers the lowest risk for aspiration and sudden infant death syndrome (SIDS) and is the current standard of care. AAP has adopted the slogan "back to sleep and tummy to play" as part of its "Healthy Child America Back to Sleep Campaign" to decrease the occurrence of SIDS.

caREminder

Certain groups, such as African Americans, low-birth-weight infants, and infants from families with more than three children have demonstrated a higher incidence of children dying from SIDS. Effective parental education regarding infant sleeping positions can decrease risk of SIDS.

PROCEDURE General Preparations

Steps	Rationale/Points of Emphasis
1. Select and obtain an isolette, crib, or bed based the child's age, developmental abilities, level of consciousness, and medical condition (see Clinical Guidelines above).	Children placed in inappropriately selected beds are at risk for falls, strangulation, and other bodily injuries due to the incompatibility between the physical structure of the bed and the size and motor capabilities of the child. Critically ill children may require a specialty bed that includes devices to turn the child and prevent skin breakdown.
2a. Position the isolette, crib, or bed away from electrical appliances, electrical outlets, oxygen and suction outlets, equipment cords, window cords, and shelves that may be easily within reach of the child.	The young child is likely to be attracted to objects within reach and may attempt to play with them or place them in his or her mouth, which can lead to accidental injury.
2b. Explain these safety precautions to the child and family.	Child safety may be impacted by the family's correct use and positioning of isolette, crib, or bed.
3. Ensure that the isolette, crib, or bed wheels are locked.	Prevents rolling of the isolette, crib, or bed.
4. Ensure that side rails on the isolette, crib, or bed are operating correctly (Figure 15-1).	Side rails that are not operating correctly may be difficult to raise or may not latch properly once in a raised position. Side rails that do not latch properly may drop down, leaving the child vulnerable to falling out of the isolette, crib, or bed.

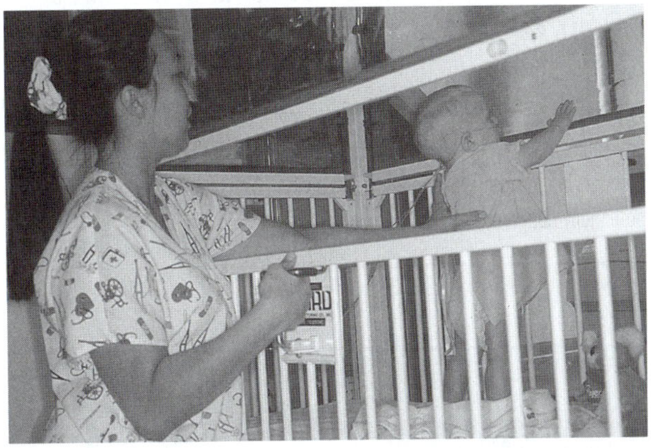

FIGURE 15-1
Latch and secure both top and side rails when the child is in the crib.

Steps	Rationale/Points of Emphasis
5. Demonstrate to family members how to operate the side rails. Reinforce importance of keeping the side rails fully raised at all times when the child is in the isolette, crib, or bed.	Family members must share equal responsibility in ensuring that side rails are up at all times.

PROCEDURE Preparing an Isolette

Steps	Rationale/Points of Emphasis
1a. Prewarm double-walled isolette before placing infant in the isolette. Time to prewarm may vary.	Isolettes circulate warm air around the infant. Prewarming decreases the heat loss from conduction from the mattress.
1b. Follow manufacturer's directions for setting the temperature of the isolette.	Ensures safe use of equipment.
1c. Set air temperature based on the neutral thermal environment table (see Chapter 79, Table 79-1) and the infant's age and weight.	Ensures environmental temperature is individualized as appropriate for the infant.
2. Place infant in the double-walled isolette with porthole covers.	Preterm infants require placement in these environments because they are unable to initiate thermogenesis due to their limited stores of fat and insufficient amounts of other chemicals, such as glucose, liver enzymes, and hormones.
3. If using a temperature probe, place the servo temperature probe on the infant over a solid meaty area (i.e., not over a hollow organ such as lungs or stomach), and ensure that the infant is not lying on the probe wires.	Servo temperature probes allow monitoring temperature without disturbing the infant and also allow monitoring temperature trends. A probe placed over a hollow organ does not provide a consistent reading of body temperature. For instance, a probe placed over the stomach fluctuates temperature readings based on the temperature of the feeding.
4a. Monitor infant's temperature every 30 minutes for 2 hours when first placed in isolette and then as indicated by infant's acuity level.	Ensures that deviations from normal temperature are detected promptly.
4b. If using a temperature probe, verify probe temperatures with electronic thermometer every 4 hours and as needed.	Correlates temperatures to ensure accuracy because probe temperatures also control the environmental temperatures.
4c. Change temperature probe site every 12–24 hours.	Probe electrodes can dry out and thus not adhere to the skin well. Poor skin adherence may alter probe readings. Accidental dislodgment can lead to overheating. **caREminder** *Minimize the number of entries into the isolette, because entering the isolette changes the ambient temperature of the environment.*
5a. Provide infant with age-appropriate visual stimulation such as black-and-white printed patterns.	Provides visual stimulation to the infant to enhance neurobehavioral development.
5b. Review with family importance of keeping objects out of isolette that would be hazardous to the infant (e.g., lotion bottles, medications, extra diapers).	Prevents infant from chewing and subsequently aspirating or suffocating on potentially dangerous objects or substances.

PROCEDURE Preparing a Crib

Steps	Rationale/Points of Emphasis
1. For the child in a covered crib, lower top rails and secure upper and lower latches of side rails in place.	The covered crib is used for older infants and toddlers who are able to stand. When latched into place, the upper structure of the crib prevents the child from falling or climbing out of the crib.
2. Place bumper pads around the inner sides of the crib if indicated.	Bumper pads are placed in cribs of small infants who may easily roll and lodge themselves against the side rails. Bumper pads are not used for children who are able to stand because they may step on them in an effort to get out of the crib.
3a. Place child in crib. Infants should be placed for sleep in a supine position. Review with the family the importance of maintaining the infant in the supine position while sleeping (Figure 5-2).	The prone sleeping position is associated with a higher incidence of SIDS. Infants who usually sleep supine are 18–20 times more likely to die of SIDS when placed in the prone position. Placing infants on their backs has been shown to reduce the

Steps	Rationale/Points of Emphasis
	risk of fever, stuffy nose, and ear infections. Childcare providers may not be aware of the latest mandates for child safety. Healthcare providers must be responsible for communicating changes to parents and referring them to resources such as AAP and the National Institute of Child Health and Human Development "Back to Sleep" Campaign. This includes visitors who might be handling the child.
3b. Provide child with age-appropriate toys or comfort items (e.g., favorite blanket, small stuffed animal).	Provides developmental stimulation to child. Familiar comfort items aid the child to feel more secure in the unfamiliar environment of the hospital.
3c. Review with family the importance of keeping objects out of the crib that would be hazardous to the child (e.g., lotion bottles, medications, extra diapers).	Prevents child from chewing and subsequently aspirating or suffocating on potentially dangerous objects or substances.
4. Place side rails in a fully upright position.	Prevents child from falling or climbing out of crib.

PROCEDURE Preparing a Hospital Bed

Steps	Rationale/Points of Emphasis
1a. Adjust bed to the lowest possible height, and place child in bed. Raise side rails. (Note: The lower two side rails may be left down for the older ambulatory child.)	The bed is positioned low to reduce injury if the child falls out of bed, and this position promotes easy exiting and entering of the bed by the child. Elevated side rails help prevent the child from falling out of bed. Placing the lower two side rails down makes it easier for the ambulatory child to get out and prevents the child from having to climb over the side rails.
1b. Demonstrate to the child and family how to operate the bed controls. Explain importance of keeping side rails up and maintaining bed at the lowest possible height at all times.	Family members must share equal responsibility in ensuring that side rails are up, the bed is positioned low, and the bed is operating properly to ensure child's safety. **KidKare** Young children should not be encouraged to play with the mechanisms to raise and lower the position of the bed, because some children have been injured or killed when a body part was stuck between the bed frame and the mattress-lowering mechanism. Some hospital beds have a lockout feature that allows staff to disable the raise/lower feature on the bed, preventing the child from using this feature independently. The lockout feature should be used if available.
2. Place call light within easy reach of the child.	Call light should be easily accessible to promote comfort and to ensure that the child is able to easily contact a healthcare provider, if needed.

CHILD AND FAMILY EVALUATION AND DOCUMENTATION

- Document the child's level of consciousness and ability to follow directions.
- Determine that the child or family members know how to use isolette, crib, or bed properly and are able to manage the side rails.
- During ongoing daily assessments, assess and document position of side rails. Reinforce parent teaching about safe use of isolette, crib, or bedside rails as needed.

COMMUNITY CARE

- Instruct parents that cribs at home should meet the following standards:

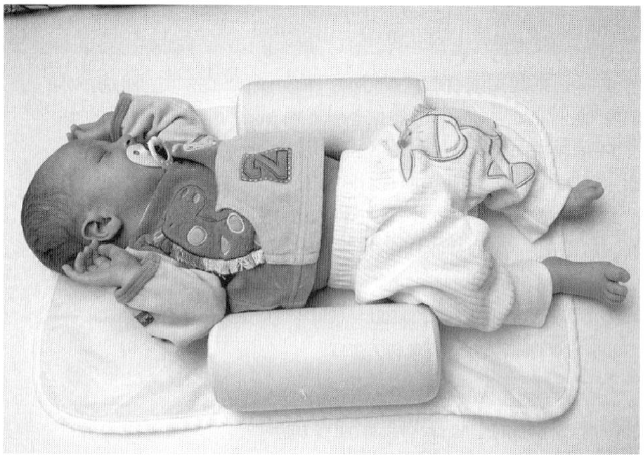

FIGURE 15-2
Commercial position devices can be purchased to assist in maintaining the infant in a supine position.

- Slats should be no wider than 2⅜ inches (6 cm) apart to ensure that the child's body cannot slip through the slats.
- Corner posts should protrude no further than 1/16 inch above end panels, because decorative knobs and posts can present a hazard by entangling the child's clothing.
- Cribs with decorative cutouts on the end boards should be avoided because these can trap a child's head or limbs. All open holes should be too small for a child's finger to get caught.
- The mattress should fit snugly with no more than two finger widths between the edge of the mattress and the crib side. A square-cornered mattress provides the best fit.
- The mattress should be no thicker than 6 inches (15 cm) and not have a soft surface.
- Bumper pads should be placed around the crib rails for newborns and very small infants. Once the child becomes more active and is able to freely move around the crib, the bumper pads should be removed. The child who is able to stand may use the bumper pad to step on to get out of the crib. Plush toys should also be removed from the crib at this time for the same reason.
- When buying a secondhand crib, it should be completely stripped and refinished before use. Cribs manufactured before 1976 were painted with lead-based paint, which is highly toxic. A child may chew on side rails and ingest old paint chips.

• To assemble and maintain the crib, instruct the parent to
  - Follow assembly directions carefully.
  - Periodically check and tighten all nuts, bolts, and screws. All small parts should be firmly attached to withstand 20 pounds of force, pull or push.
  - Check teething rails for cracks and replace when sharp edges appear.
  - Assess all support hangers and ensure that they are secure if the crib is moved or the mattress lowered.
  - Lower the mattress on a periodic basis to ensure that the height of the rail is above the child's nipple line when the child is in a standing position inside the crib. This protects the child from being able to lean out and fall out of the crib.
  - Ensure that when the mattress is in the lowest position there is a minimum of 26 inches (66 cm) between the mattress and the top of the rail.
  - Check mattress hooks regularly. A bent or broken hook can allow the mattress to fall and trap the child.
  - Never place casters (rollers) on the crib. Children can rock back and forth inside the crib and move it within reach of harmful objects.
  - Secure side rails all the way up every time the child is placed in the crib.

• To best position the crib or bed in a room, instruct the parent to
  - Place the bed or crib away from electrical outlets so that they are inaccessible to the child.
  - Place the crib or bed so that it is not directly under a window. The child may be able to push on the screen and crawl out the window. Also, should the window break, the child would be endangered.
  - Avoid placing cribs or beds against an outside wall or near a radiator to avoid extremes of temperature.
  - Place the crib so that shelves are far from the child's reach. Do not hang pictures above or within reach of the crib.
  - Keep mobiles above cribs out of the child's reach. Mobiles should be removed from the crib when the child is able to sit up.

• For ongoing safety, the parents are instructed as follows:
  - The child should be moved from a crib to a bed if the child is able to climb out unaided or is taller than 35 inches (90 cm).
  - Infants should not be allowed to sleep on a waterbed.
  - Infants should never be placed sleeping on a couch with anyone or in a bed with other children.
  - The child should not be given a pillow until he or she is sleeping in a bed.
  - Pillows and mattresses should never be covered with plastic. Such products can smother the child.

caREminder

Specially made allergy covers are available to reduce exposure to allergens that thrive in bedding (mattresses, pillows, comforters). Synthetic quilts have been associated with increased childhood wheeze.

  - Infant sleepers or sacks are preferred. Blankets, if used, must be tucked in along the sides and end of the

mattress. Infants are to be placed near the bottom of the crib. Keep the infant's feet at the foot of the bed; practice the "feet-to-foot" rule (see Figure 15-2).
  - Never cover the infant's head with the blanket.
  - Keep the room temperature between 68° and 72°F (20° and 22°C) and avoid overdressing the infant.
  - Safety rails can be placed on the side of the bed to prevent the small child from falling out of bed.
  - The child should not be placed in the upper bunk of a bunk bed until 6 years of age. Safety rails on the upper bunk are still warranted at this time.
- When using cribs provided outside the home, parents should
  - Evaluate the safety of the crib provided by a hotel, friend, or day care provider before use.
  - Ensure that any portable crib they may use is in safe working condition and has not been recalled by the manufacturer.

Unexpected Situation

- *While making patient rounds you notice that the mother of a 1-year-old has left her child in the crib with the side rails half way down on one side. The child is standing at the side rail crying:* This child is at high risk for falling from the crib. Place the side rail in its highest locked position. When the mother returns, discuss with her side rail safety concerns. Document teaching on the child's chart. If the incident continues to reoccur, further measures may need to be taken to ensure the child's safety, including placing the child on a more visible unit where healthcare providers can continually monitor parent activities and child safety.

Bibliography

American Academy of Pediatrics. (1992). Positioning and SIDS. *Pediatrics, 89*(6), 1120–1126.

American Academy of Pediatrics. (1996). Positioning and sudden infant death syndrome (SIDS): Update. *Pediatrics, 98*(6), 1216–1218.

American Academy of Pediatrics. (2000). Changing concepts of sudden infant death syndrome: Implications for infant sleeping environment and sleep position (RE 9946). *Pediatrics, 105*, 650–656.

American Academy of Pediatrics. (2004). *Healthy child care America back to sleep campaign speaker materials: Reducing the risk of SIDS in child care.* Retrieved September 4, 2004, from http://healthychildcare.org/section_SIDS.cfm

Ariagno, R., Mirmiran, M., Adams, M., et al. (2003). Effect of position on sleep, heart rate variability, and QT interval in preterm infants at 1 and 3 months' corrected age. *Pediatrics, 111*, 622–625.

Corwin, M., Lesko, S., Heeren, T., et al. (2003). Secular changes in sleep position during infancy: 1995–1999. *Pediatrics, 111*, 52–60.

Hauck, F., Moore, C., Herman, S., et al. (2002). The contribution of prone sleeping position to the racial disparity in sudden infant death syndrome: The Chicago infant mortality study. *Pediatrics, 110*, 772–780.

Hein, H., & Pettit, S. (2001). Back to sleep: Good advice for parents but not for hospitals? *Pediatrics, 107*, 537–539.

Hunt, C., Lesko, S., Vezina, R., et al. (2003). Infant sleep position and associated health outcomes. *Archives of Pediatric and Adolescent Medicine, 157*, 469–474.

Krum, A. (1999). New laws about unsafe cribs. *Parenting, 13*(2), 28.

Lyons, T., & Oates, R. (1993). Falling out of bed: A relatively benign occurrence. *Pediatrics, 92*(1), 125–127.

National Institutes of Health, National Institute of Child Heath & Human Development. (2003). *SIDS: Back to sleep campaign.* Retrieved September 4, 2004, from http://www.nichd.nih.gov/sids/sids.cfm

Pollack, H. A., & Frohna, J. G. (2002). Infant sleep placement after the back to sleep campaign. *Pediatrics, 109*(4), 608–614.

Ponsonby, A., Dwyer, T., Trevillian, L., et al. (2004). The bedding environment, sleep position, and frequent wheeze in childhood. *Pediatrics, 113*(5), 1216–1222.

Porter, R. (2000). Hotels and motels offer unsafe cribs and play areas. *Trial, 36*(6), 110–111.

Ridenour, M. (1997). Age, side height, and spindle shape of the crib in climbing over the side. *Perceptual & Motor Skills, 85*(2), 667–674.

Scherreik, S. (1998). A new parent's buying guide. *Money, 27*(4), 186–188.

CHAPTER

16

Blood Drawing From Peripheral Sites: Heel Stick and Finger Stick

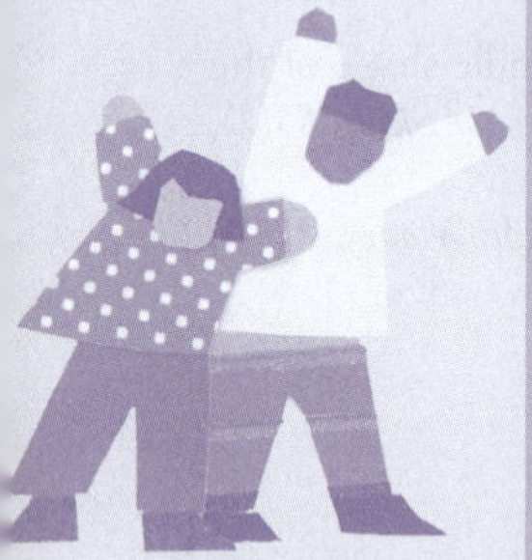

Clinical Guidelines

- Blood sampling is obtained upon a healthcare prescriber's order using aseptic technique and standard precautions.
- Blood sampling is completed by a registered nurse (RN), licensed practical nurse (LPN), healthcare prescriber, or appropriately certified technician.
- Unlicensed assistive personnel (UAPs) may perform blood drawing as delegated by the RN, upon completion of a competency program and consistent with their job description.
- Consider venipuncture for blood specimen collection because it is less painful; otherwise, use the following:
  - Heel stick in infants up to 18 months of age
  - Finger stick in children over 18 months of age who require a specimen of less than 2.5 mL

Equipment

- Mechanical (automated) lancing device or lancet
- Antiseptic wipes (75% isopropanol)
- 2 × 2 sterile wipes
- Gloves
- Specimen container or capillary tube
- Warming supplies (i.e., chemical warmer, cloth)

Child and Family Assessment and Preparation

- Assess child for signs of poor perfusion, local edema, infection at the site, and impaired blood coagulation. The presence of these findings can lead to inadequate sampling, blood specimen contamination, increased pain, and infection. Avoid edematous areas because the presence of the fluids can contaminate the blood specimen. The presence of ecchymosis or hemolyzed samples can give false results (e.g., elevated bilirubin or potassium levels). Rotate the sites of puncture to decrease these complications.
- Apply topical anesthetic (e.g., lidocaine, prilocaine) for finger stick before procedure, as time allows, and based on child's preference. The research is conflicting, but most studies indicate that topical anesthetics are not effective for the pain of heel stick. Because a risk

for methemoglobinemia exists, do not use lidocaine and prilocaine if the child is receiving methemoglobin-inducing agents (e.g., sulfonamides, acetaminophen).

- Question parents about the existence of coagulation disorders in their family history and previous signs of a blood dyscrasia (e.g., the presence of unexpected ecchymotic spots or prolonged bleeding after blood testing or injury).
- Administer vitamin K per newborn routine before heel stick to increase clotting and prevent prolonged bleeding.
- Verify physician's order for laboratory tests.
- Explain procedure to child, as appropriate, and parents.
- Prepare the child, as appropriate, to cognitive and developmental level (see Chapters 3 and 4). Provide therapeutic play as indicated, or involve a child life specialist, to allow the child to work through fears, help with the procedure (e.g., hold Band-Aid), and master control of the situation.
- Encourage parents to remain with the child during the procedure. Discuss with parents comfort measures (e.g., swaddling, use of sucrose pacifiers) and distraction techniques that they can use with their child.

PROCEDURE Performing Heel and Finger Sticks

Steps	Rationale/Points of Emphasis
1. Gather the necessary supplies, including puncture device. An automated device is recommended; refer to manufacturer's recommendations for use.	Promotes efficient time management and provides an organized approach to the procedure. Mechanical devices either puncture or incise the skin and may be less painful than lancets. A shallow incision may facilitate bleeding, healing, and reduce pain. There is an increased chance of bone penetration resulting in injury and infection (e.g., perichondritis, osteomyelitis) with puncture devices of longer length. Research on preterm infants indicates that the use of an automatic incision device for collecting repeated skin puncture samples is less traumatic than the use of a conventional manual lancet, causing less bruising and inflammation of the heel. **caREminder** *Manual lancets for pediatric patients should be no longer than 1.55 mm.*
2. Apply warming device to area for 5 to 10 minutes before puncture. The following methods are acceptable: • Commercially prepared chemical warmer • Warm cloth (<109°F or 42.8°C)	Increases blood flow and reduces hemolysis and bruising. Hematocrit and capillary blood gas samples collected from nonwarmed heels are inaccurate. Do not use microwave-warmed products because uneven heating occurs and presents a burn risk. Research on heel warming before capillary blood sampling on preterm and term infants indicates that this may be an unnecessary technique. Volume of blood, collection time, crying time, and repeat procedures have not indicated they were enhanced by prewarming the site. More research is needed.
3. Perform hand hygiene and don gloves.	Standard precaution to reduce transmission of microorganisms.
4. Remove warming device.	Leaving a warming device in contact with the skin cools by conduction.
5. Select and identify puncture site: • Heel, outer aspects (infants younger than 18 months) ▪ Lateral to an imaginary line drawn from between the fourth and fifth toes and running parallel to the lateral aspect of heel (Figure 16-1). ▪ Medial to an imaginary line drawn from the middle of the great toe and running parallel to the medial aspect of the heel. Never puncture the back of an infant's heel because the calcaneus is closest to the surface in that location. **Alert!** *Heel sticks should be 2 mm apart. Avoids puncturing through a previous puncture site that might be infected; reduces chance of cellulites.*	Using appropriate site minimizes the risk for injury (e.g., striking artery, bone, or nerve). **caREminder** *Avoid calluses, scars, and lesions. These areas will be difficult to penetrate with the lancet.*

Continued

Steps	Rationale/Points of Emphasis
• Finger (older than 18 months of age) ■ The side of the third or fourth finger, near the tip (see Figure 16-1)	
6a. Cleanse puncture site with antiseptic (75% isopropanol) and allow to dry for 30 seconds. Then dry with sterile gauze	Provides disinfection. Wiping prevents alcohol contamination of blood sample, which may cause hemolysis and errors in glucose values.
6b. If topical anesthetic cream has been used, remove before cleansing.	Residual alcohol may cause hemolysis and errors in glucose values.
7. Place extremity in a dependent position. Grasp extremity firmly; dorsiflex infant's foot for heel stick.	Facilitates blood flow to area. Prevents inadvertent movement by child; controls position of site for puncture.
8. Briskly puncture skin with selected lancing device and wipe off first drop of blood with sterile gauze.	Eliminates tissue fluids or residual alcohol potentially present in initial drop of blood, which can alter test values.

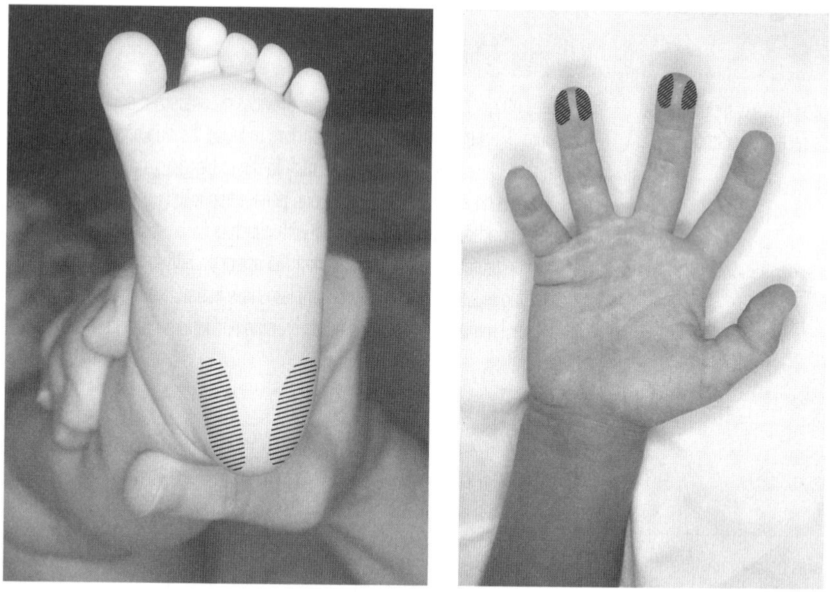

FIGURE 16-1
Sites for capillary blood specimens.

Steps	Rationale/Points of Emphasis
9a. Continue to hold puncture site in dependent position while gently applying intermittent pressure to surrounding area; collect blood in appropriate container.	Harshly squeezing the area may produce hemolyzed samples and bruising and may contaminate sample with tissue fluid.
9b. When using capillary tubes or micropipettes, hold horizontally to fill them by capillary action and fill two thirds to three fourths full. Cover the end with your finger when transferring the specimen to bedside test strip, sealing clay, or other material.	Holding tube horizontal and applying intermittent pressure facilitates blood flow. Covering the tube prevents blood loss. **caREminder** *Do not pipette orally or scrape blood into tubing. Oral pipetting greatly increases the chance of contact with potentially contaminated body fluids and scraping causes hemolysis.*
10a. Elevate extremity above level of heart. Gently press dry sterile gauze to puncture site until bleeding stops.	Facilitates hemostasis.
10b. Do not use bandages.	Bandages can lead to skin maceration and pose an aspiration hazard.
11. Properly dispose of contaminated equipment. Place lancing device in sharps container and blood-soaked gauze in a biohazard bag.	Prevents needle-stick injury and transmission of blood-borne pathogens.
12. Remove gloves and perform hand hygiene.	Reduces transmission of microorganisms. Standard precautions.

Steps	Rationale/Points of Emphasis
13. Perform bedside laboratory testing or label specimen with child's name, medical record number and unit, date and time of collection, and collector's initials.	Ensures that correct specimen is tested for the right patient.
14a. Place specimen in biohazard bag and transport specimen to laboratory, if necessary.	Standard precautions.
14b. Provide appropriate environment for transport (e.g., ice, refrigeration).	Reduces degradation of specimen before analysis.

CHILD AND FAMILY EVALUATION AND DOCUMENTATION

- Evaluate puncture site for evidence of continued bleeding; keep wound clean and dry.

Alert! ***Children with hematologic disorders and those receiving certain medications (e.g., warfarin sodium, heparin, aspirin) may have prolonged clotting times.***

- Monitor child for signs of pain and involve parents in providing comfort measures (e.g., rocking, cuddling, swaddling, talking in a quiet and soothing voice, providing pacifier, praise, presenting a small reward).
- Assess puncture wound daily for signs of infection, scarring, calcified nodules, or bruising.
- Document the following:
  - Date and time
  - Site of puncture
  - Specimens obtained
  - Amount of blood loss
  - Child's response to procedure
- Maintain running total of blood loss in neonates or when multiple samples are being obtained.

COMMUNITY CARE

- Educate parents, and child if appropriate, on proper technique for home blood sampling (i.e., device use, site selection, sharps disposal, when to obtain samples, and complication recognition); give written instructions and observe return demonstration.
- A single-use mechanical device is the option of choice for home sampling. Coordinate to ensure that proper equipment is available for home use.
- Instruct the family to contact healthcare provider if
  - The child has signs of infection
  - The child has excessive bleeding or pain
  - Laboratory values are outside of normal parameters

Unexpected Situation

- *While performing a heel puncture on a newborn, you are unable to obtain an adequate blood sample:* Assess temperature of the extremities; if cool to touch, provide warming measures before attempting redraw. Place foot in dependent position. Attempt heel stick in new location. If still unable to collect specimen, perform venipuncture.

Bibliography

American Association of Respiratory Care. (1994). Capillary blood gas sampling for neonatal and pediatric patients. *Respiratory Care, 39*, 1180–1183.

Becht, D. K., & Anderson, M. A. (1996). Using heat to reduce blood collection time in pediatric clients. *Clinical Nursing Research, 5*(4), 441–452.

Corbo, M. G., Mansi, G., Staging, A., et al. (2000). Non-nutritive sucking during heel stick procedures decreases behavioral distress in the newborn infant. *Biology of the Neonate, 77*, 162–167.

Fitzgerald, M., Millard, C., & McIntosh, N. (1989). Cutaneous hypersensitivity following peripheral tissue damage in newborn infants and its reversal with topical anaesthesia. *Pain, 39*, 31–36.

Gradin, M., & Schollin, J. (2005). The role of endogenous opioids in mediating pain reduction by orally administered glucose among newborns. *Pediatrics, 115*(4), 1004–1007.

Greenberg, C. S. (2002). A sugar-coated pacifier reduces procedural pain in newborns. *Pediatric Nursing, 28*, 271–277.

Huang, C. M., Tung, W. S., Kuo, L. L., & Ying-Ju, C. (2004). Comparison of pain responses of premature infants to the heelstick between containment and swaddling. *Journal of Nursing Research, 12*, 31–40.

Jain, A., Rutter, N., & Ratnayaka, M. (2001). Topical amethocaine gel for pain relief of heel prick blood sampling: A randomized double-blind controlled trial. *Archives of Disease in Childhood: Fetal and Neonatal Edition, 84*(1), F56–F59.

Janes, M., Pinelli, J., Landry, S., Downey, S., & Paes, B. (2002). Comparison of capillary blood sampling using an automated incision device with and without warming the heel. *Journal of Perinatology, 22*(2), 154–158.

Johnson, K., Cress, G., Connolly, N., et al. (2000). Neonatal laboratory blood sampling: Comparison of results from arterial catheters with those from an automated capillary device. *Neonatal Network, 19*, 27–34.

Larsson, B. A., Norman, M., Bjerring, P., et al. (1996). Regional variations in skin perfusion and skin thickness may contribute to varying efficacy of topical, local anaesthetics in neonates. *Paediatric Anaesthesia*, *6*(2), 107–110.

Ogawa, S., Ogihara, T., Fujiwara, E., et al. (2005). Venipuncture is preferable to heel lance for blood sampling in term neonates. *Archives of Disease in Childhood: Fetal and Neonatal Edition*, *90*(5), F432–F436.

Rho, N., Youn, S., Park, H., Kim, W., & Lee, E. (2003). Calcified nodule on the heel of a child following a single heelstick in the neonatal period. *Clinical & Experimental Dermatology*, *28*, 502–503.

Shah, V., & Ohlsson, A. (2004). Venipuncture versus heel lance for blood sampling in term neonates. *The Cochrane Database of Systematic Reviews* (4), No. CD001452.

Vertanen, H., Fellman, V., Brommels, M., & Vinikka, L. (2002). An automatic incision device for obtaining blood samples from the heels of preterm infants causes less damage than a conventional manual lancet. *Archives of Disease in Childhood: Fetal and Neonatal Edition*, *84*(1), F53–F55.

C H A P T E R

17

Blood Drawing From Peripheral Sites: Venipuncture

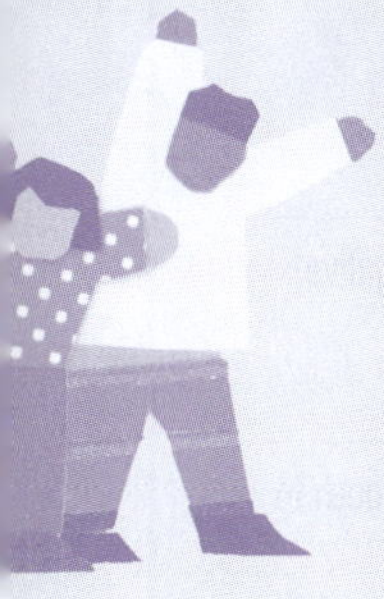

Clinical Guidelines

- Blood sampling is obtained upon a healthcare prescriber's order using aseptic technique and standard precautions.
- Venipuncture is completed by a registered nurse (RN), licensed practical nurse (LPN), healthcare prescriber, or appropriately certified technician.
- Unlicensed assistive personnel (UAPs) may perform blood drawing as delegated by the RN, upon completion of a competency program and consistent with their job description.

Equipment

- 70% alcohol pads or chlorhexidine 2 mg/mL solution or swabs
- Dry sterile gauze pads
- Tourniquet
- Small adhesive bandage
- Appropriate specimen tubes for tests ordered
- Venous access device:
  - Vacuum container needle and vacuum holder with needle protection system, or
  - A 1-inch butterfly needle with attached tubing and Luer adapter for children younger than 12 years of age, 23 gauge for children younger than 12 years of age, and 21 gauge for children older than 12 years of age
- Patient labels for specimen tubes
- Appropriate laboratory requisitions
- Gloves
- Cold pack for specimens that need to be transported cold (i.e., coagulation studies)
- Biohazard bag

Child and Family Assessment and Preparation

- Assess severity of child's illness and determine whether there is time for use of topical pain relief and amount of time that can be devoted to explanation of procedure.
- Determine whether fasting or timing of medication administration is a consideration for the test being performed.

- Assess child for previous puncture experiences and reactions to latex. Use this information in preparing child.

Alert! *If latex allergy or risk is present, institute latex allergy or latex precautions (see Chapter 60).*

- Assess child's total blood volume and associated pathology that affects oxygen-carrying capacity of blood (e.g., anemia, ongoing blood loss, shock) to determine necessity of limiting amount of blood taken. Consider amount of blood previously taken for specimen analysis and degree of total blood deficit in child. Calculate minimal amount of blood necessary to perform microanalysis of specimens; compare necessity of test versus amount of blood needed. Check with laboratory to determine the minimum amount of blood needed, particularly for a preterm infant; many tests can be run on 0.5 mL or less of blood.
- Prepare child and family for procedure as developmentally appropriate. In emergent situations, explain actions as they are implemented. Use simple clear explanations. Explain that the child needs to stay still but can yell or cry if so desired. Teach the child simple distraction techniques to assist in pain management.

KidKare Tell the child, "I need to check your blood." Be careful of statements such as, "I need to take some blood." Children may interpret this as literally all of their blood will be taken and they won't have any left.

- Encourage parents to remain with the child during the procedure. Discuss with parents distraction techniques and other pain management techniques they can use with their child.
- When not emergent, apply a topical anesthetic to two sites (see Chapter 7). Therefore if the initial puncture is unsuccessful, a second site is already prepared. When using an eutectic mixture (e.g., EMLA), it should remain on the skin for at least 60 minutes before puncture. When using a stimulated iontophoresis method, it should remain on the skin for 5 to 15 minutes before puncture.

PROCEDURE Performing Venipuncture

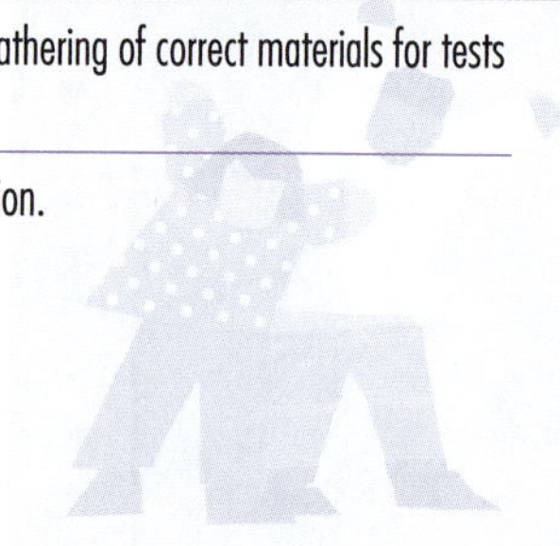

Steps	Rationale/Points of Emphasis
1. Verify orders, laboratory requisitions, and patient labels.	Prevents unneeded punctures. Allows the gathering of correct materials for tests ordered.
2. Identify the child using two different patient identifiers (see Chapter 85).	Ensures correct patient for specimen collection.

Alert! *Identify patients at risk for latex allergy and use latex precautions. Avoids latex exposure and adverse patient reactions.*

Steps	Rationale/Points of Emphasis
3. Perform hand hygiene.	Reduces transmission of microorganisms. Antibiotic-resistant gram-negative organisms frequently contaminate the hands of healthcare personnel, in addition to the usual skin flora.
4. Gather the necessary supplies based on size of child, method of collection, and tests required.	Promotes efficient time management and provides an organized approach to the procedure. Too large a needle may damage valves in the vein. Butterfly wings provide more control and thus less trauma to vessels. Use of a syringe and straight needle to draw blood is not recommended because the amount of pressure exerted cannot be controlled, the vein collapses, and damage may occur.

caREminder

Do not puncture the stopper on the specimen tubes. If the stopper is punctured, the tube will lose its vacuum, and blood will not enter the tube.

Steps	Rationale/Points of Emphasis
5. Select puncture site, using the distal veins first. Veins most commonly used are the antecubital fossa (Figure 17-1).	The median antecubital vein may not always be visible, but it is usually large and palpable. It is well supported by subcutaneous tissue and least likely to roll.

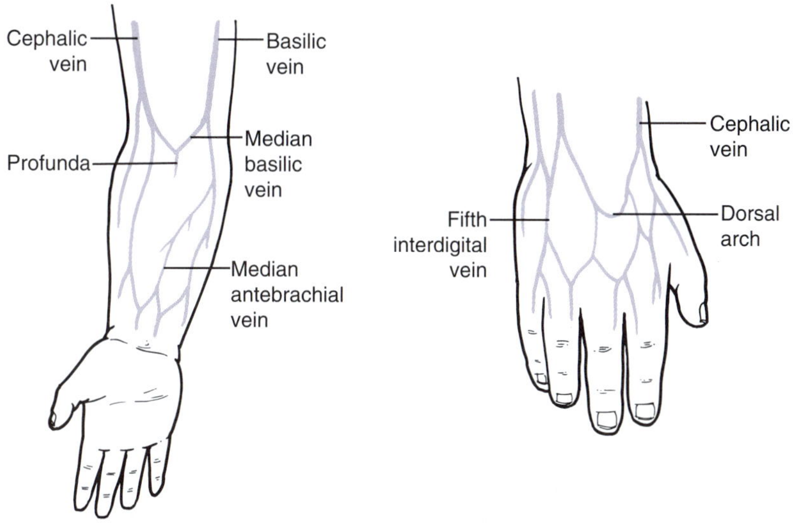

FIGURE 17-1
Veins in the upper extremities most commonly used for venipuncture sites.

> ***Alert!*** *Avoid scars, lesions, and veins above where an intravenous line is in place. Scars make entry into the vein more difficult; lesions are avoided to prevent the transfer of microorganisms. Intravenous fluids alter test results.*

Steps	Rationale/Points of Emphasis
6. Place the site in dependent position.	Facilitates blood flow to the area. **KidKare** Older children may cooperate better if they can sit up with the arm well supported on a pillow, if they are given detailed explanations, and if they are involved in decisions as appropriate (e.g., site selection). If child is younger than school age, have child lie down. A second person to assist in stabilizing the site may be helpful.
7. Don gloves.	Standard precaution to reduce transmission of microorganisms.
8. If child is able to follow commands, ask the child to make a fist.	Assists in vein distention for older children.
9. Apply tourniquet around child's extremity above the site.	Obstructs venous blood flow and causes vein distention so that the vein is easier to see and palpate.
10. Cleanse the site with alcohol or chlorhexidine using a circular motion from site outward. When using alcohol, scrub the site for 20 seconds. If using chlorhexidine, allow to dry for at least 30 seconds. Always use chlorhexidine when obtaining blood cultures. Do not touch the cleansed area again with your finger or any other unsterile object.	Moves microorganisms away from the proposed puncture site, thus decreasing the transfer of microorganisms. Alcohol is less effective than chlorhexidine in decreasing bacterial colonization and causes the greatest amount of permanent tissue damage in animal studies.

> ***Alert!*** *In infants younger than 2 months of age, remove cleansing solution, after it dries, with sterile water. Use of chlorhexidine may be associated with contact dermatitis in low-birth-weight infants.*

Continued

Steps	Rationale/Points of Emphasis
11. Remove needle shield. Anchor the child's vein with thumb of your non-dominant hand.	Prevents rolling of vein.
12. Hold the needle bevel up, positioned at a 45-degree angle over the vein. Puncture the site. If unsuccessful after two attempts, have another practitioner perform procedure.	Allows placement of needle parallel to the vein.
13a. Obtain blood using a vacuum container: Stabilize the vacuum holder and push in on the specimen tube to puncture the stopper; when first specimen tube is full, remove it from the vacuum holder while stabilizing the holder, being careful not to jar the needle; stabilizing the holder, insert succeeding tubes in holder, making sure that the stoppers are punctured on each tube to initiate blood flow; gently invert tubes containing additives 8 to 10 times.	If the needle is in the vein, the tube will begin to fill with blood.
13b. Obtain blood using butterfly: When a blood backflow is seen, insert Luer adapter into the microtainer or Vacutainer, or gently withdraw blood with a 1- or 3-mL syringe if blood for several tests is needed.	Once the specimen tube is full, vacuum stops the flow of blood. Inserting succeeding tubes quickly and evenly allows obtaining several specimens from one puncture site. Inverting tubes ensures mixture of additives. **caREminder** *If no blood flows into specimen tube or ceases to flow before an adequate sample is collected, the following steps should be taken:* • *Confirm correct needle position, change the angle of needle insertion by a few degrees.* • *Remove specimen tube and replace with a new specimen tube.* • *If the new tube does not fill with blood, remove needle as described below.* • *Evaluate need for repeat puncture.*
14. Release the tourniquet.	Prevents blood from entering surrounding tissue.
15. Note the total amount of blood withdrawn.	Provides a gauge of how much blood has been taken and when replacement may be needed.
16. Remove tourniquet.	Allows venous blood flow to resume.
17. Apply dry sterile gauze and withdraw needle. Apply pressure to puncture site until bleeding stops. Keeping the arm straight, elevate the extremity above the level of the heart.	Stops the bleeding. Elevation promotes negative pressure in vein and promotes clotting. **Alert!** *Do not bend the arm after drawing blood because it promotes hematoma formation. Children with cardiac disease should not raise their extremities because this action creates negative pressure in veins.*
18a. Place specimen in appropriate tube. 18b. Invert all tubes containing additives 8 to 10 times before specimen collection in next tube.	Ensures adequate preparation and stabilization of specimen for accurate analysis. Ensures mixture of additives. **Alert!** *Do not shake tubes. Rough specimen handling, such as forceful injection or shaking, may damage erythrocytes and alter laboratory results.*

Steps	Rationale/Points of Emphasis
19. Dispose of sharps immediately: • If using a needle-protection device, withdraw the needle back into the container until a click is heard. • When not using a needle-protection device, place the needle in the needle-protection box immediately without reshielding it.	Prevents accidental needle-stick injuries with contaminated sharps.
20. Apply small bandage, as appropriate. **Alert!** ***Bandages may present a choking hazard in infants and toddlers.***	Prevents further bleeding. Reassures children, particularly preschool-aged children, that all their blood will not leak out.
21. Label all specimen tubes with the following: • Child's name • Time and date of collection • Initials of person collecting • Medical record number	Ensures that correct specimens are tested for correct child.
22. Place in biohazard bag and transport to the laboratory.	Protects against blood contact.
23. Dispose of equipment and waste in appropriate receptacle. Remove gloves and perform hand hygiene.	Standard precautions. Reduces transmission of microorganisms.
24. Recheck puncture site.	Detects further bleeding.

CHILD AND FAMILY EVALUATION AND DOCUMENTATION

- Evaluate child and family understanding of procedure.
- Evaluate effectiveness of child and family coping during procedure. Determine whether a better coping mechanism could be used during future blood sampling. If so, teach to child and family.
- Document the following:
  - Date and time
  - Site of puncture
  - Specimens obtained
  - Amount of blood loss
  - Child's response to procedure
- Maintain running total of blood loss in neonates or when multiple samples are being obtained.

COMMUNITY CARE

- Assure parents that although the equipment used in the home may differ from that used in the hospital, it works with the same effectiveness.
- Ensure that there is a sealed needle container in the child's home. Upon completion of the procedure, dispose of the used needle in the container and make sure that it is out of reach of children in the home.
- Teach parents to monitor for signs of bleeding or infection at puncture site.
- Transport blood specimens in a cool dark container as quickly as possible to the laboratory.
- Instruct the family to contact the healthcare provider if
  - The child has signs of infection
  - The child has excessive bleeding or pain
  - Laboratory values are outside of normal parameters

Unexpected Situations

- *Unable to access vein, despite several attempts:* The extremity may be cold with subsequent vasoconstriction or the child may be dehydrated. Warming the extremity and/or hydrating the child may assist in venipuncture access. It is also helpful for a new person to be used to complete the venipuncture at a different location on the child. Transillumination (using a high-powered cold source of light) to view the deep tissue has also been shown effective to aid in establishing venous access on an infant when there has been a failed venipuncture attempt.
- *Hematoma develops at venipuncture site:* Apply pressure with gauze or cotton ball for 3 to 5 minutes or until bleeding stops.

Bibliography

Centers for Disease Control and Prevention. (2002). *Guidelines for prevention of intravascular catheter-related infections.* Retrieved July 11, 2006, from www.cdc.gov/mmwr/preview/mmwrhtml/rr5110al.htm

Dugan, L., Leech, L., Speroni, K. G., & Corriher, J. (2005). Factors affecting hemolysis rates in blood samples drawn from newly placed IV sites in the emergency department. *Journal of Emergency Nursing, 31*(4), 338–345.

Fetzer, S. (2002). Reducing venipuncture and intravenous insertion pain with eutectic mixture of local anesthetic: A meta-analysis. *Nursing Research, 51*(2), 119–124.

Goren, A., Laufer, J., Yatio, N., et al. (2001). Transillumination of the palm for venipuncture in infants. *Pediatric Emergency Care, 17*(2), 130–131.

Intravenous Nurses Society. (2006). Infusion nursing: Standards of practice. *Journal of Intravenous Nursing, 29*(1S), S1–S92.

Lund, C., Kuller, J., Lane, A., Lott, J. W., & Raines, D. A. (1999). Neonatal skin care: The scientific basis for practice. *Journal of Obstetric, Gynecologic, and Neonatal Nursing, 28*, 241–254.

MacLaren, J., & Cohne, L. (2005). Comparison of distraction strategies for venipuncture distress in children. *Journal of Pediatric Psychology, 30*(5), 387–396.

Ogawa, S., Ogihara, T., Fujiwara, E., et al. (2005). Venipuncture is preferable to heel lance for blood sampling in term neonates. *Archives of Disease in Childhood: Fetal and Neonatal Edition, 90*(5), F432–F436.

Rogers, T., & Ostrow, L. (2004). The use of EMLA cream to decrease venipuncture pain in children. *Journal of Pediatric Nursing, 19*(1), 33–39.

Shah, V., & Ohlsson, A. (2004). Venipuncture versus heel lance for blood sampling in term neonates. *The Cochrane Database of Systematic Reviews* (4), No. CD001452.

Squire, S. J., Kirchhoff, K. T., & Hissong, K. (2000). Comparing two methods of topical anesthesia used before intravenous cannulation in pediatric patients. *Journal of Pediatric Healthcare, 14*(2), 68–72.

Strand, C. L., Wajsbort, R. R., & Sturmann, K. (1993). Effect of iodophor vs. iodine tincture skin preparation on blood culture contamination rate. *Journal of the American Medical Association, 269*, 1004–1007.

Wolfram, R. (1997). Effects of parental presence during young children's venipuncture. *Pediatric Emergency Care, 13*(5), 325–328.

CHAPTER

18

Blood Gas Sampling and Monitoring

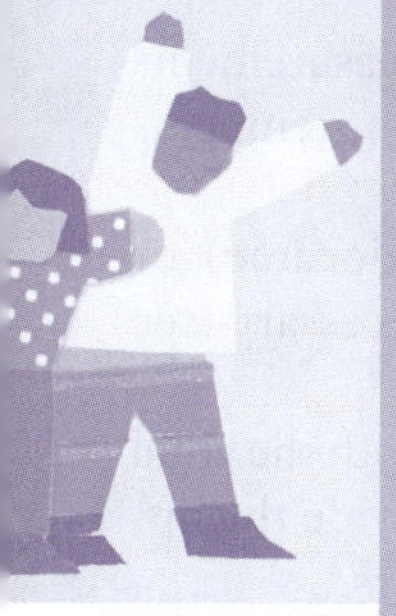

CLINICAL GUIDELINES

- Children who are physiologically compromised and/or those who need adjunctive oxygen therapy may require blood gas analysis and/or monitoring.
- Blood gas analysis provides a direct method to assess oxygenation, acid–base balance, adequacy of ventilation, hypoxic states, and evaluation of the child's response to therapy via blood sample collection.
  - Blood gas samples are obtained upon a healthcare prescriber order using aseptic technique and standard precautions.
  - Healthcare prescribers, respiratory care practitioners, and registered nurses (RNs) may collect blood gas samples after demonstrating competency by the selected route.
  - If a child is to receive frequent blood gas sampling, consider arterial line cannulation to reduce the child's discomfort, vasospasm, hematoma, or neurovascular compromise.
- Blood gas samples may be obtained from arterial lines or puncture (arterial blood gas [ABG]), capillary puncture (CBG), or, if necessary, venous blood draw (VBG). Capillary sampling is a useful alternative to arterial sampling even in presence of hypothermia and hypoperfusion, provided that hypertension is not present. CBG and VBG are not recommended for determining Po_2 of arterial blood.
- Local anesthesia is used for arterial blood gas sampling by arterial puncture in nonemergent situations (see Chapter 7).
- Continuous hemodynamic monitoring of arterial pressures by arterial cannulation also provides for direct blood gas collection. Clearly label and monitor these lines to avoid inadvertent intravenous (IV) use and possible exsanguination from dislodgment (see Chapter 48).
- Transcutaneous monitoring (Tco_2M) measures skin surface Po_2 and Pco_2, providing estimates of arterial partial pressure (Pao_2) and carbon dioxide ($Paco_2$). This estimation allows for the monitoring of arterial oxygenation and/or ventilation and for evaluation of therapeutic interventions.
  - Transcutaneous blood gas monitoring can be performed by trained healthcare prescribers, respiratory care practitioners, and RNs.
  - Those patients with poor skin integrity or adhesive allergy may not tolerate this type of monitoring.
  - If the child is hemodynamically compromised, the Tco_2M may not be an accurate measure.
  - Arterial blood gas values should be compared with transcutaneous readings taken at the time of arterial sampling to validate the transcutaneous values. Factors that may increase

the discrepancy between arterial and transcutaneous values include hyperoxemia, a hyperperfused state (e.g., shock, acidosis), improper electrode placement, use of vasoactive drugs, increase skinfold thickness, or tissue edema.
  - Manufacturer's recommendations for maintenance, operation, and safety of transcutaneous monitoring equipment should be followed.
- A basic understanding of normal arterial blood gas values is essential for accurate interpretation of blood gas results.
  pH = 7.35 to 7.45
  Pa_{CO_2} = 5 to 45 mm Hg
  Pa_{O_2} = 80 to 100 mm Hg
  Sa_{O_2} = 94% to 98%
  Base excess = 12 to 22
  H_{CO_3} = 22 to 26 mEq/L

EQUIPMENT

For Capillary Blood Gas Sampling

- Warm, moist cloth or commercially prepared warming pad
- Nonsterile gloves
- Skin antiseptic
- Preheparinized glass capillary tube
- Clay or wax sealant or cap
- Sterile lancet (1.5 mm in depth)
- Adhesive bandage
- Patient specimen label
- Ice (sample must be on ice if analysis delayed >10 minutes)
- Gauze or cotton balls
- Sharps and biohazard disposal container
- Biohazard bag for transporting the specimen to the laboratory

For Arterial Blood Gas Sampling by Arterial Puncture

- Preheparinized 1-mL syringe with cap
- 25-g needle or 25-g butterfly needle
- Nonsterile gloves
- Skin antiseptic
- Gauze or cotton balls
- Patient specimen label
- Ice (sample must be on ice if analysis delayed >10 minutes)
- Adhesive bandage
- Patient specimen label
- Biohazard bag for transporting the specimen
- Sharps and biohazard disposal container
- Anesthetic for nonemergent sampling:
  - Topical agents (see Chapter 7)
  - Local anesthetic (injectable buffered lidocaine, 1% without epinephrine)
- Ice pack for puncture site (if needed)

For Blood Gas Sampling by Indwelling Heparinized Arterial or Deep Venous Catheter

- 3-mL syringe (heparinized if discard blood will be reinfused)
- 1-mL syringe heparinized
- 3-mL heparinized normal saline flush syringe
- Nonsterile gloves
- Alcohol wipes
- Patient specimen label
- Ice (sample must be on ice if analysis delayed >10 minutes)
- Biohazard bag for transporting the specimen
- Sharps and biohazard disposal container

For Transcutaneous Blood Gas Monitoring

- Transcutaneous monitor
- Adhesive electrode rings
- Transcutaneous sensor contact gel
- Calibration gases and calibrator

CHILD AND FAMILY ASSESSMENT AND PREPARATION

- Assess child and child's medical record for:
  - History of circulatory impairment (i.e., presence of cardiac or vascular grafts). Puncture of vessels or grafts may cause hematoma and decreased circulation.
  - Prolonged clotting times or bleeding disorders that may affect clotting times
  - Impaired gas exchange related to underlying disease processes or for impaired breathing and note oxygen therapy and whether child requires continuous ventilatory assistance
  - Factors that may influence blood gas measurements (i.e., anxiety, suctioning, child's position, temperature, oxygen therapy, metabolic rate)
  - Allergies to local anesthetics (e.g., lidocaine) or latex; implement latex precautions if necessary (see Chapter 60)
- Explain the procedure, as appropriate, to both the child and the family (see Chapters 3 and 4). Provide the opportunity to ask questions and alleviate fears.
- Explain to the child and family that a lancet or needle will be used to puncture the child's skin and gain access to the blood that is needed for this procedure. A topical anesthetic may be administered with arterial punctures before the procedure to minimize the pain of this needle stick. Explain that the blood withdrawn will be used to look at the amount of oxygen in the child's blood. After the procedure, a Band-Aid or small dressing will be placed on the site.
- Reinforce the need for blood gas collection, as appropriate, to both the child and the family.

PROCEDURE Capillary Blood Gas Sampling

Steps	Rationale/Points of Emphasis
1. Gather the necessary supplies.	Promotes efficient time management and provides an organized approach to the procedure.
2. Perform hand hygiene.	Reduces transmission of microorganisms.
3. Raise the bed to a comfortable working height, or stand on a step stool at crib side.	Promotes good body mechanics and reduces back strain.
4. Select capillary puncture site (see Chapter 16).	Facilitates visualization and ease of access. **KidKare** Use the posterior curvature of the heel in children who have not begun walking and are without callus development (the great toe may be also used as an alternative in neonates). Use the finger or great toe in walking children and adults.
5. Wrap the selected foot or hand with a warmed moist cloth or commercially prepared warming pad; leave on for 5 to 10 minutes.	Warming the site arterializes the patient sample and allows for vasodilation. Inadequate warming of the site before puncture may result in capillary values that poorly correlate with arterial pH and Pco_2 values.
6. Don gloves.	Standard precaution to reduce transmission of microorganisms.
7. Remove the warming cloth or pad. Scrub the selected site with antiseptic wipe and allow to dry.	Reduces the transmission of microorganisms.
8. Ensure that end caps, lancet, capillary tube, cotton or gauze, and adhesive bandage are within easy reach.	Allows for procedure to continue quickly and efficiently. Facilitates ease of access to the equipment.
9. Puncture capillary site with sterile lancet; advance lancet at an angle so as to cut more capillary beds and generate greater blood flow.	Provides for specimen sample.
10. As indicated with nondominant hand: Grasp the foot firmly with the thumb and index finger wrapped around heel, or grasp the finger or great toe firmly with thumb and index finger wrapped around the finger or toe.	Allows for control of blood flow.
11. Gently apply pressure to heel, finger, or toe in an upward direction to drive maximum blood to the puncture site.	Provides for adequate specimen sample. Undue squeezing of the puncture site may result in venous and lymphatic contamination of the sample.
12. Release pressure periodically to allow blood to continue to build and flow.	Controls blood flow, so as not to stave off blood flow.
13. Remove the first drop of blood from puncture site with gauze or cotton using dominant hand.	Usually, the first drop of blood contains tissue fluid and thereby contaminates the blood gas sample.
14. Holding the capillary tube horizontally with the dominant hand, introduce blood into the tube.	Holding the tube horizontally prevents air entrapment.
15. Fill the entire tube with blood and cap the ends.	Maintains blood within the tube.
16. Cleanse the puncture site with gauze or cotton and apply adhesive bandage over area; do not use alcohol.	Reduces transmission of microorganisms. Alcohol stings and prolongs bleeding.
17. Place the sample in a laboratory specimen bag, label properly, and transport for analysis as soon as possible.	Allows for blood gas analysis and ensures that results are reported on correct patient. **caREminder** *Place the sample on ice if analysis will be delayed longer than 10 minutes. Ice slows oxygen metabolism.*

Continued

Steps	Rationale/Points of Emphasis
18. Return the child's bed to the lowest position or to a level that is age appropriate.	Reduces potential injury from falls.
19. Dispose of used equipment and waste in appropriate receptacle. Remove gloves and perform hand hygiene.	Standard precautions. Reduces transmission of microorganisms.

PROCEDURE Arterial Blood Gas Sampling Using Arterial Puncture

Steps	Rationale/Points of Emphasis
1. Gather the necessary supplies.	Promotes efficient time management and provides an organized approach to the procedure.
2. Perform hand hygiene.	Reduces transmission of microorganisms.
3. Raise the bed to a comfortable working height, or stand on a step stool at crib side.	Promotes good body mechanics and reduces back strain.
4. Select arterial puncture site. Perform a collateral circulation test for occlusion of the radial or ulnar (modified Allen test) by elevating the hand and compressing the ulnar and radial arteries until blanching of the hand is seen. Upon removal of pressure from one of the arteries, the redness of the hand is observed.	Facilitates visualization and ease of access. Ensures adequate blood supply to the extremity. If the test is negative (no collateral circulation), then select another site.
a. Use the radial artery as first choice.	The radial artery is small and easily stabilized as it passes over a bony groove located at the wrist.
b. Use the brachial artery as the second choice except in case of poor pulsation due to shock, obesity, or sclerotic vessel.	Studies have shown the brachial artery to be technically easier to access and more comfortable for the child.
c. Use the femoral artery in the case of altered perfusion to the upper extremity arteries or cardiopulmonary arrest.	The femoral artery is easily palpated and punctured; however, complications surrounding femoral artery puncture limit its usefulness. Also, there is greater risk for contamination from venous blood in the nearby femoral vein as well as infection because of the close proximity of the pubic area.
5. Don gloves.	Standard precaution to reduce transmission of microorganisms.
6. Position the child; have another staff member assist in holding the child.	Facilitates visualization and ease of access. Limits child's movements and promotes safer performance of procedure. **KidKare** Parents should not be responsible for securing the child but may remain to give support such as holding the child's hand.
7. Scrub the selected site with antiseptic; wipe in a circular motion, moving outward. Allow to dry.	Reduces the transmission of microorganisms.
8. In nonemergent situation, use topical anesthesia (e.g., cream or vapocoolant) and locally anesthetize the site with lidocaine.	Minimizes discomfort. **caREminder** *Verify that the child is not allergic or sensitive to topical or local anesthetics; if so, perform the procedure without them.*
9. Ensure that preheparinized 1-mL syringe with cap, 25-g needle or 25-g butterfly needle, gauze or cotton balls, patient specimen label, adhesive bandage, and biohazard bag for transporting the specimen are within reach.	Allows for procedure to continue quickly and efficiently. Facilitates ease of access to the equipment.

Steps	Rationale/Points of Emphasis
10a. Perform percutaneous puncture of the selected artery by pulling the skin taut around the pulsation with the nondominant hand and puncturing the skin slowly with the dominant hand using the 25-g needle and heparinized 1-mL syringe, bevel up, in a 45- to 60-degree angle to the artery. Keep index finger on the artery to determine which direction to advance the needle.	Provides for specimen sample.
10b. Advance the needle until the artery is punctured. Do not move the needle around as if "hunting" for the vessel.	Blood will appear in the needle hub when the artery is punctured. Excessive movement of the needle and reinsertion may cause nerve and/or artery damage and is very painful to the child.
11. Slowly and evenly withdraw required amount of blood for sample.	Prevents inadvertent aspiration of air during withdrawal. **KidKare** Accurate tests can be done with as little as 0.2 mL of sample. Use the least amount of blood needed to ensure accurate sample, particularly in neonates and children at risk for anemia.
12. Remove needle while stabilizing the barrel of the syringe and have assistant quickly apply firm continuous pressure to the puncture site with cotton or gauze for 5 minutes or until bleeding stops.	Hematomas and hemorrhage can occur if pressure is not applied quickly and correctly. If bleeding persists, place an ice pack over site and continue with firm pressure.
13. Once bleeding stops, apply adhesive bandage firmly and stretched tautly over puncture site.	Prevents further bleeding and reduces transmission of microorganisms.
14. Hold blood sample syringe upright and express any air bubbles rapidly.	Air bubbles may alter test results.
15. Seal tip of syringe immediately with cap or stopper. Roll syringe gently to mix blood with heparin to prevent clot formation.	Keep airtight to prevent alterations in results.
16. Place the sample in a laboratory specimen bag, label properly, and transport for analysis as soon as possible. Place the sample on ice if analysis will be delayed longer than 10 minutes.	Allows for blood gas analysis and results reported on correct patient. Ice slows oxygen metabolism.
17. Return the child's bed to the lowest position or to a level that is age appropriate.	Reduces potential injury from falls.
18. Dispose of used equipment and waste in appropriate receptacle. Remove gloves and perform hand hygiene.	Standard precautions. Reduces transmission of microorganisms.

PROCEDURE Blood Gas Sampling Using an Indwelling Heparinized Arterial or Deep Venous Catheter

Steps	Rationale/Points of Emphasis
1. Gather the necessary supplies.	Promotes efficient time management and provides an organized approach to the procedure.
2. Perform hand hygiene.	Reduces transmission of microorganisms.
3. Raise the bed to a comfortable working height, or stand on a step stool at crib side.	Promotes good body mechanics and reduces back strain.
4. Vigorously cleanse the aspiration stopcock or port of the indwelling catheter with an alcohol wipe.	Reduces the transmission of microorganisms.
5. Apply 3-mL syringe to aspiration port and stopcock of indwelling catheter and turn the stopcock off to the infusing fluid (or as appropriate to line setup).	Opens the system from the child to the syringe.

Continued

Steps	Rationale/Points of Emphasis
6. Withdraw twice the dead space of the syringe (approximately 1.5–2.0 mL) of discard blood.	Removes any clot material and intravenous fluid from within the catheter; accesses blood. **caREminder** *If blood discard is to be reinfused into the child, syringe must be heparinized. Heparinization of syringe reduces clotting of blood.*
7a. Turn the stopcock to a position midway between the infusing fluid and syringe connection and replace the 3-mL discard syringe with a heparinized 1-mL syringe.	Facilitates removal of blood gas sample.
7b. If blood discard is to be reinfused into the child (follow institutional guidelines), maintain sterility.	Blood discard may be reinfused in neonates and children at risk for anemia to minimize blood volume depletion.
8. Turn the stopcock off to the infusing fluid and slowly and evenly withdraw required amount of blood for sample into 1-mL syringe.	Prevents inadvertent aspiration of air during withdrawal. Decreases arterial spasm if done slowly. Accurate tests can be done with as little as 0.2 mL of sample.
9. Turn the stopcock off to the syringe; remove and cap the 1-mL syringe and momentarily set aside.	This will be used for the blood gas sample.
10. If blood is to be reinfused, visually examine discard syringe for clots; if none, apply syringe with discard fluid to stopcock, turn stopcock off to infusing fluid, and infuse contents slowly. Turn the stopcock off to the syringe. If discard will not be infused, omit this step.	Reinfusion of discard reduces blood loss with sampling and helps maintain child's blood volume. Examination of discard avoids infusing clotted blood. Rapid infusion may precipitate arteriospasm.
11. Apply 3-mL heparinized NS flush syringe to stopcock, turn off to infusing fluid, and flush catheter through of blood until line is again clear (or flush as appropriate for line setup).	Maintains patency of indwelling catheter.
12. Hold blood sample syringe upright and express any air bubbles rapidly.	Air bubbles may alter test results.
13. Place the sample in a laboratory specimen bag, label properly, and transport for analysis as soon as possible.	Allows for blood gas analysis and results reported on correct patient. Place the sample on ice if analysis will be delayed longer than 10 minutes. Ice slows oxygen metabolism.
14. Return the child's bed to the lowest position or to a level that is age appropriate.	Reduces potential injury from falls.
15. Dispose of used equipment and waste in appropriate receptacle. Remove gloves and perform hand hygiene.	Standard precautions. Reduces transmission of microorganisms.

PROCEDURE Transcutaneous Blood Gas Monitoring

Steps	Rationale/Points of Emphasis
1. Gather the necessary supplies.	Promotes efficient time management and provides an organized approach to the procedure.
2. Perform hand hygiene.	Reduces transmission of microorganisms.
3. Raise the bed to a comfortable working height, or stand on a step stool at crib side.	Promotes good body mechanics and reduces back strain.
4. Attach the appropriate sensor to the front of the machine following manufacturer's instructions.	Allows for correct monitoring of patient.

Steps	Rationale/Points of Emphasis
5. Turn the machine on and double-check for battery operation.	Ensures power to the machine.
6. Calibrate the machine according to manufacturer's instructions.	Ensures correct calibration.
7. Set alert limits.	Ensures safety of the device, especially from overheating and the possibility of a skin burn.
8. Attach the ring to the sensor face and, with a drop of sensor gel, apply to the patient.	A clean sealed application allows for accurate monitoring. Avoid bubbles, and check for a damaged membrane, which could limit the precision of the device.
9. Dispose of equipment and waste in appropriate receptacle. Perform hand hygiene.	Standard precautions. Reduces transmission of microorganisms.

Child and Family Evaluation and Documentation

- Evaluate the neurovascular status of the extremity used. Check the site for delayed hematoma formation and for impaired circulation to the distal extremity. Children with frequent blood gas draws from arterial puncture can be at increased risk for thrombosis (especially in the femoral artery).
- Monitor for large or small arterial occlusions, which can present as cold extremities, absent pulses, or petechiae.
- Evaluate for local edema, which can be caused by internal hemorrhage.
- Assess the child's tolerance and response to the procedure, the ease or difficulty of obtaining sample, and the presence of complications or adverse reactions.
- Determine whether the child and family have other areas of concern to discuss.
- Continue to assess and document the condition of the site, per institutional policy (at least once per shift or more often, as indicated by child's condition), until wound is healed; if child is discharged before healing, give discharge instructions for monitoring site. Evaluate child for signs and symptoms of infection, including fever, tachycardia, redness, swelling, or inflammation at the puncture site.
- For indwelling arterial lines, check and document circulation of extremity and integrity of line at minimum with vital sign checks or per institutional policy.
- Document the following in child's medical record for blood gas sampling:
  - Date and time procedure performed
  - Topical or local anesthetic used
  - Catheter size used or removed
  - Ease or difficulty of obtaining sample
  - Amount of blood aspirated and reinfused
  - Appearance of the puncture site
  - Presence of complications or adverse reactions
  - Child's response to and tolerance of the procedure
  - Child's temperature at the time the blood gas was obtained, position or level of activity, clinical appearance, and any adjunctive therapies such as chest tubes
  - Blood gas results. Note the amount of oxygen the child is receiving, the oxygen administration device or ventilator settings, and any noninvasive respiratory monitoring values (e.g., respiratory rate, pulse oximetry, transcutaneous values, end-tidal CO_2 values).

caREminder

Maintain running total of blood loss in neonates from sample withdrawals. Ensures circulating blood volume is not negatively impacted by ongoing blood loss.

- Document the following in child's medical record for transcutaneous monitoring:
  - Date and time of measurement
  - Transcutaneous reading
  - Child's position
  - Respiratory rate
  - Child's activity level
  - Inspired oxygen concentration or supplemental oxygen flow (specify type of oxygen delivery device)
  - Mode of ventilatory support, ventilator, or continuous positive airway pressure settings
  - Electrode placement site, electrode temperature, and time of placement
  - Clinical appearance of the child including perfusion, pallor, and skin temperature
  - Results of simultaneously obtained PaO_2, $PaCO_2$, and pH when available

Community Care

- Instruct family on the care and dressing of the wound puncture site at home and how to monitor for signs of respiratory distress and local and systemic infection.
- If the procedure will be completed in a physician's office or clinic, encourage family to discuss the procedure with the child on the trip to the office or clinic.
- Instruct the family to notify the healthcare provider if
  - Child demonstrates signs of respiratory distress
  - Infection at puncture site or systemically

Unexpected Situation

- *The capillary blood gas has been drawn and is ready for delivery to the laboratory. One hour later you return to the nurse's station and realize that the blood gas sample has not been sent for analysis:* This sample needs to be discarded and another sample drawn. Samples must be anticoagulated and obtained anaerobically with the capillary tube filled completely and air bubbles expelled. The sample should be immediately chilled or analyzed within 10–15 minutes if left at room temperature.

Bibliography

American Academy of Pediatrics, Task Force on Transcutaneous Oxygen Monitors. (1986). Report of consensus meeting. *Pediatrics, 83*, 122–126.

American Association of Respiratory Care. (1994). Capillary blood gas sampling for neonatal and pediatric patients. *Respiratory Care, 39*, 1180–1183.

American Association of Respiratory Care. (2004). Transcutaneous blood gas monitoring for neonatal and pediatric patients—2004 revision & update. *Respiratory Care, 49*(9), 1069–1972.

Berkenbosch, J. W., & Obias, J. D. (2002). Transcutaneous carbon dioxide monitoring during high-frequency oscillatory ventilation in infants and children. *Critical Care Medicine, 30*, 1024–1027.

Escalante-Kanashiro, R., & Tantalean-Da-Fieno, J. (2000). Capillary blood gases in a pediatric intensive care unit. *Critical Care Medicine, 28*, 224–226.

Matsagas, M. I., Miitsis, M., Rigopoulous, C., et al. (2004). A large radial artery false aneurysm after repeated arterial punctures, causing compartment syndrome of the forearm. *Intensive Care Medicine, 29*, 1032.

Perinatal–Pediatrics Guidelines Committee, AARC. (1994). American Association for Respiratory Care clinical practice guidelines: Capillary blood gas sampling for neonatal and pediatric patients. *Respiratory Care, 39*, 1180–1183.

Perinatal–Pediatrics Guidelines Committee, AARC. (2004). American Association for Respiratory Care clinical practice guidelines: Transcutaneous blood gas monitoring for neonatal and pediatric patients. *Respiratory Care, 49*, 1069–1072.

Rickard, C. M., Conchman, B. A., Schmidt, S. J., Dank, A., & Purdie, D. M. (2003). A discard volume twice the deadspace ensures clinically accurate arterial blood gases and electrolytes and prevents unnecessary blood loss. *Critical Care Medicine, 31*, 1654–1658.

Rüdiger, M., Töpfer, K., Hammer, H., Schmalisch, G., & Wauer, R. (2005). Survey of transcutaneous blood gas monitoring among european neonatal intensive care units. *BMC Pediatrics, 5* (30). Retrieved July 11, 2006, from http://www.biomedcentral.com/1471-2431/5/30

Tran, N. Q., Pretto, J. J., & Worsnop, C. J. (2002). A randomized controlled trial of the effectiveness of topical amethocaine in reducing pain during arterial puncture. *Chest, 122*, 1357–1360.

Yildizdas, D., Yapicioglu, H., Yilmaz, H. L., & Sertdemir, Y. (2004). Correlation of simultaneously obtained capillary, venous, and arterial blood gases of patients in a paediatric intensive care unit. *Archives of the Diseases of Childhood, 89*, 176–180.

CHAPTER

19

Blood Glucose Monitoring

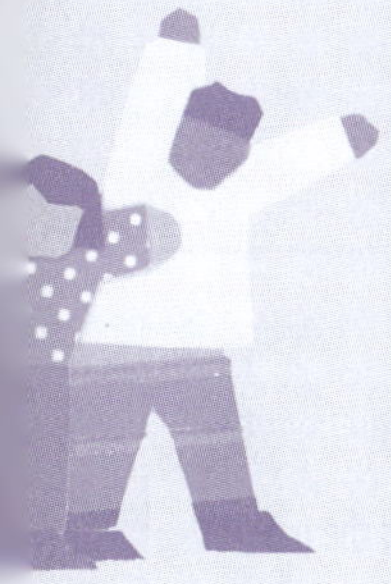

Clinical Guidelines

- Trained healthcare personnel, according to the guidelines of the institution, may perform capillary blood glucose monitoring using regularly maintained equipment and supplies.
- A trained staff member will perform the technique in resuscitation/emergency situations or when working with neonates. Children with established diabetes and other children requiring continued blood glucose monitoring may perform the procedure while supervised by a trained staff member or other adult (e.g., parent who has been trained on the procedure).
- Capillary whole blood level is measured with a blood glucose meter to gain a rapid assessment of a child's metabolic state. Blood glucose monitoring helps detect hypoglycemia and hyperglycemia (Chart 19-1). Blood glucose monitoring helps the child with diabetes reach a desired level of glycemic control.
- The blood glucose meter is tested daily for quality control or per institutional protocol.

Equipment

- Blood glucose meter
- Reagent strips
- Alcohol or alcohol wipe
- Lancet device
- Lancets
- Cotton balls or gauze pads
- Gloves
- Washcloth (if needed)
- Bandages (if needed)
- Heel-warming device (optional for use in neonates)

Child and Family Assessment and Preparation

- Assess the child and family's readiness to learn how to monitor blood glucose levels (see Chapter 3).
- Determine whether the child and family understand the procedure and its significance. Blood glucose monitoring is part of the daily routine of a child with diabetes and is a skill necessary for the child and family to learn before discharge from the hospital. Review explanation of procedure as needed.

CHART 19-1 HYPOGLYCEMIA AND HYPERGLYCEMIA

Hypoglycemia

Definition: The blood glucose level at which hypoglycemia is defined varies. A blood glucose of less than 45 mg/dL is abnormal at any age. Check with the physician caring for the child to define hypoglycemia for a specific patient.

Signs and symptoms: Feeling shaky, weak, sweaty, hungry, dizzy, light-headed, palpitations, or "butterflies" in the stomach. Signs of central nervous system hypoglycemia include visual changes, gait disturbance, change in affect or behavior, confusion, paresthesia, slurred speech, and sleepiness progressing to unconsciousness or seizure.

Causes:

A. If child has diabetes:
- Too much insulin
- Delayed food, not enough food, missed meal or snack
- Exercise without adequate adjustment in food or insulin

B. If child does not have diabetes:
- Hyperinsulinism
- Tumors
- Glycogen storage disease
- Malnutrition
- Liver disease
- Renal failure
- Cardiac failure
- Sepsis
- Ketotic hypoglycemia of childhood
- Medications: insulin, sulfonylureas, salicylates, acetaminophen, alcohol, colchicine, monoamine oxidase inhibitors, propoxyphene, haloperidol, pentamidine, perhexiline, disopyramide, propranolol

Hyperglycemia

Definition: The diagnosis of diabetes is made by the clinical symptoms and a fasting blood glucose >126 mg/dL or random blood glucose >200 mg/dL. The reading would be repeated on a different day.

Signs and symptoms of persistent elevation in blood glucose: Increased thirst, increased urination, weight loss, increased appetite, and decreased energy level.

Causes other than diabetes: Any condition of stress may cause a temporary rise in blood glucose. In children, the most common causes of stress would be from an infection or postoperative stress. All cases of hyperglycemia warrant further investigation.

- Older children or teenagers usually assist or perform their own blood glucose monitoring. Younger children have the procedure performed on them and should be given developmentally appropriate information.

KidKare A fearful young child may prefer to be held during the procedure. Holding the child provides comfort and assists in the procedure. Therapeutic play with dolls or stuffed animals performing blood glucose monitoring may also help child cope with, and learn about, the procedure.

PROCEDURE Monitoring Blood Glucose

Steps	Rationale/Points of Emphasis
1. Review the child's chart to determine the rationale and the timing for the procedure.	For the child with diabetes, it is important to perform the technique at the prescribed time for the assessment of insulin requirements and treatment of hypoglycemia. Strict glycemic control is important to prevent diabetes-related complications. For other children in whom hypoglycemia or hyperglycemia is a concern, the procedure is performed based on clinical signs and symptoms (see Chart 19-1).
2. Gather the necessary supplies.	Promotes efficient time management and provides an organized approach to the procedure.
3a. Check expiration date on strips. Perform necessary quality control on equipment per manufacturer's instructions, or verify that quality control has been done, and ensure that all equipment is functioning correctly.	Properly functioning equipment and supplies are needed for accurate results.

Steps	Rationale/Points of Emphasis
3b. When appropriate, make sure the cap is always kept on the vial of strips. Observe the strip for discoloration.	Strips are sensitive to light and humidity and may become inactivated. **caREminder** *Reagent containers that have been left open or strips that are discolored should be discarded.*
4. Load lancet in lancet device according to manufacturer's instructions.	Lancet device will be more comfortable for the child because it may not penetrate the skin as deeply as using the lancet alone. **KidKare** For the child's comfort, use a lancet device and lancet designed for pediatric blood glucose monitoring. Lancet sizes vary for use with neonates, children, and adults. Many lancet devices can be adjusted for depth of penetration. **caREminder** *Use a new lancet for each procedure.*
5. Perform hand hygiene, and don gloves. Use standard precautions throughout the procedure.	Reduces transmission of microorganisms. Protects against exposure to blood or body fluids.
6a. Select a puncture site (Figure 19-1); refer to Chapter 16. • In neonates, infants, and children who are not walking, the outer aspect of the heel is commonly used. • In infants and toddlers with diabetes, the toe pads can be used. • In a child or adult, the end or lateral aspect of the fingertip is the most common site. Check specific meter for approved alternate sites for testing (e.g., finger pads, heel of hand on thumb side and finger side, forearm, upper arm, thigh, calf, or abdomen).	Toes are acceptable because decreased sensation to this area has not occurred yet because these children do not have long-standing disease.

Alert! ***Do not use the very center of the finger pad. Fingertips have an abundance of cutaneous blood vessels; however, they are densely innervated and consequently painful. Because the center of the finger pad is very sensitive, using a site just lateral to this can help reduce the child's discomfort.***

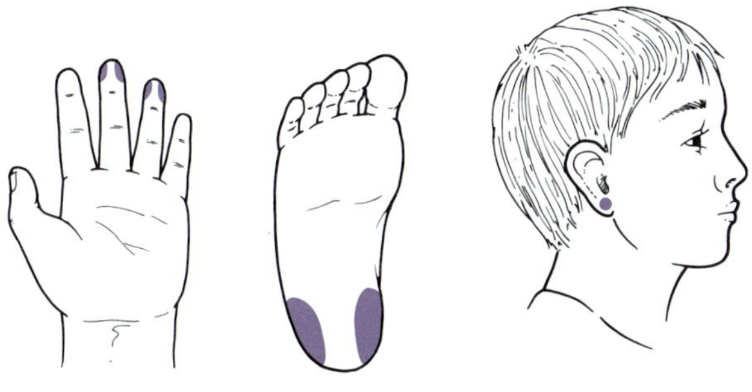

FIGURE 19-1
Puncture sites for capillary blood specimen collection for glucose monitoring.

Continued

Steps	Rationale/Points of Emphasis
6b. "Alternate site testing" (e.g., testing on heel of hand on thumb side and finger side, forearms, upper arms, thighs, calf, abdomen) is another option; refer to meter's manufacturer's instructions. When alternate sites are used, the area must be rubbed vigorously.	Alternate sites have fewer nerve endings than fingers and thus are an option for children who complain of a lot of pain with finger sticks. Alternate sites are often desirable for adolescents, who can be very sensitive about the visibility of multiple finger punctures (Figure 19-2). Vigorous rubbing helps increase circulation.

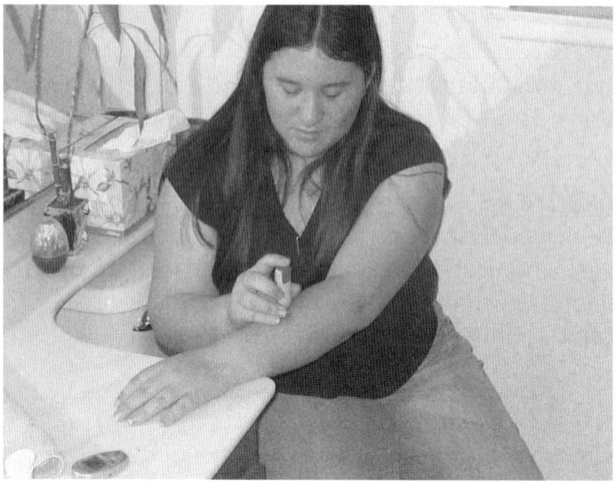

FIGURE 19-2
"Alternate site testing" (AST) or "off-site" testing locations can be used to obtain blood glucose sampling using several new devices available on the market.

Alert! *Alternate site testing is not as accurate as testing fingertips, heels, and toes when measuring hypoglycemia because the rate of blood flow to digits is faster than to alternate sites and the dermis does not have the vascularity that digits do; therefore, when glucose is changing rapidly, the digits are more accurate than alternate sites that lag behind. Alternate site testing is not recommended for people with hypoglycemia unawareness or those unable to verbalize symptoms of hypoglycemia. Discrepancies in blood glucose between fingertip and forearm during rapid changes in blood glucose have been reported, although these discrepancies may be due to patients not accurately following the manufacturer's instructions on the use of the measurement instrument.*

Steps	Rationale/Points of Emphasis
7. Wash the child's hands with warm water, or place a warm, wet cloth on the alternate site to be used for 1 minute. A heel-warming device can be used when testing on the foot. **Alert!** *Monitor the temperature of the warming device to avoid burns.*	Application of heat for 1 minute has been shown to promote vasodilation, which assists in obtaining an adequate-sized sample.
8. Place test strip into meter per manufacturer's instructions.	Prepares for testing.
9. Calibrate the meter by matching the code on the meter to the code on the test strip container according to manufacturer's instructions.	Matching codes ensures the reading is accurate.
10. Hold the child securely and place the puncture site in the appropriate position (e.g., place extremity in a dependent position).	Placing extremity in a dependent position facilitates blood flow to the area. **KidKare** If the child is anxious, place your nondominant hand against his or her body while performing the procedure so that the child will not be able to pull away as the lancet device is deployed. An infant may be swaddled, leaving the chosen extremity uncovered for access.
11. Wipe the puncture site with 70% alcohol or wash with soap and water. May need to wipe with sterile gauze pad to ensure all alcohol has dried.	Removes glucose from the skin, which gives a false reading. Wet alcohol can cause discomfort when the skin is pricked and can influence accuracy of results.

Steps	Rationale/Points of Emphasis
Alert! *Make sure the finger is completely dry before obtaining the sample, because alcohol stings if present when skin is punctured, and alcohol and soaps interfere with reagents on strips, giving an inaccurate reading. Fluid (water, alcohol) also dilutes the specimen, giving a false low reading.*	
12a. Hold lancet perpendicular to the skin and puncture site using the lancet device. 12b. Continue to position the site below the child's heart.	Allows for adequate skin penetration. Positioning the site below the heart allows gravity to help increase blood flow and obtain adequate-sized sample.
13. Ensure that an adequate-sized drop of blood is obtained before applying it to the kstrip/meter. Do not squeeze the site; if needed, many lancets can be used to apply pressure to the site.	Facilitates accurate test results. Too little blood may give a false low reading, may not start the test, or may give an error code, depending on the meter. Volume size required by the meter may range from 0.3 to 30 microliters. ***Alert!*** *Avoid squeezing the site excessively, because excessive squeezing can contaminate the sample with tissue fluid and cause hemolysis of sample and trauma to the site.*
14. Apply first drop of blood to the test strip.	All material manufacturers currently recommend using the first drop of blood. Check meter manual for verification; each meter is different. A "hanging drop" may be needed, and the finger may not touch the test pad. The meters have hematocrit and ambient temperature restrictions as well as substances in the bloodstream that may interfere with an accurate reading. In a child in shock or with severe dehydration, there will be a lowered result. The accuracy of results is dependent on proper technique. Clinical decision making is based on blood glucose result. ***Alert!*** *Follow the manufacturer's instructions completely when performing the test.*
15. Apply cotton ball or gauze to puncture site and apply pressure. Apply bandage if needed.	Minimizes bleeding at site. ***Alert!*** *If the child has a clotting problem, you may need to apply pressure for a longer time.*
16. Follow the manufacturer's directions regarding the developing time and method for reading and interpreting the results.	Proper developing time and use of the equipment are critical to achieving accurate test results. Ensures accuracy when making treatment decisions. **caREminder** *A reading from a blood glucose meter is not as accurate as a laboratory result and does not distinguish between true hypoglycemia and a low-normal reading. The diagnosis of diabetes or verification of hypoglycemia must be made using laboratory blood glucose results, not meter results. Venous and capillary blood glucose concentrations may differ, depending on how long after a meal the sample is collected. Plasma and serum readings may be 10% higher than whole blood.*

Continued

Steps	Rationale/Points of Emphasis
17. For a visual reading, find a good light source and compare the test and pad colors to the color scale on the bottle label from which the test strip was drawn.	Each bottle has a color chart that corresponds to the reaction characteristics of the test strips within that vial.
caREminder *To obtain an accurate value, follow the manufacturer's instructions for appropriate timing of steps.*	
18a. Dispose of equipment and waste in appropriate receptacles.	Standard precautions.
18b. If required, turn off meter and return to appropriate storage area.	Makes meter available for future testing.
19. Remove gloves and perform hand hygiene.	Reduces transmission of microorganisms.

CHILD AND FAMILY EVALUATION AND DOCUMENTATION

- Record test results in the child's chart and on the appropriate institutional forms.
- When appropriate, document blood glucose monitoring education and quality of child/parent's technique of blood glucose monitoring.
- Document results of quality control measures completed on the equipment.
- For a child with diabetes, start or maintain a record of blood glucose results for the child's diabetes records.
- Review present and recent blood glucose results and contact physician as required for hyperglycemia and hypoglycemia.
- For hypoglycemia, immediately treat with appropriate amount of carbohydrate.

COMMUNITY CARE

- For a child with diabetes, blood glucose monitoring will be continued in the community. Because the child may have a different blood glucose meter than the hospital meter, assess proper technique using the child's meter.
- The child may perform the procedure on himself or herself. Younger children, children using a new blood glucose meter, and children suspected of having hypoglycemia should be supervised when testing.
- The child's blood glucose meter may be assessed by comparing its readings with laboratory blood glucose readings, correcting for plasma and whole blood calibration. The child's meter should be within 20% of the laboratory result. Some meters are calibrated to plasma glucose, whereas others are calibrated to whole blood.
- Teach the child and parent to mark when to perform quality control on their meter so that the reading will not be factored into the memory of the meter; when downloaded will then be marked as a control, not an actual test.
- For concerns about the child's meter, refer to the instruction manual or call the manufacturer.
- In the community setting, some diabetes care providers may advise that children do not need to use alcohol with blood glucose monitoring but should wash hands to remove glucose from skin. In either case, the skin should be dry before puncturing.
- Review proper sharps disposal at home and school. The family should use a sharps container or should follow the local community's medical waste disposal guidelines.
- Review proper storage of strips at child's home (e.g., if strips are kept in a canister, the lid should always be kept closed).
- Follow the manufacturer's recommendation of ambient temperature necessary for meter accuracy.
- Provide family with instructions for home treatment of hypoglycemia or hyperglycemia.
- If the child attends school or day care, make provisions to educate the staff and develop a healthcare plan that includes contact numbers, diet, child's level of participation, blood glucose monitoring, specific emergency guidelines, and hypoglycemia treatment (glucagon availability and medications and food to administer).
- Instruct the family to contact the healthcare provider if
  - Child demonstrates signs of hypoglycemia or hyperglycemia and is unresponsive to recommended home treatments provided by physician
  - Child's blood glucose level cannot be maintained within designated parameters
  - Equipment is malfunctioning

Unexpected Situations

- *The finger is pricked for the blood sample, but even with squeezing of the finger, no blood drops are produced:* Feel the pad of the finger, assessing for calluses. Restick child using another finger. Before the stick, check the pad for calluses, place the extremity in a dependent position, and place a warm, wet cloth on the site as needed to enhance circulation.
- *Upon completing the finger stick and following the manufacturer's instructions for reading and interpreting results, you note the child has a glucose level of 300:* Assess the child for hyperglycemia. Complete another finger stick using new supplies and, if needed, a different blood glucose meter. If results remain elevated, contact healthcare prescriber immediately.

Bibliography

American Association of Diabetes Educators. (2000). Position statement: Management of children with diabetes in the school setting. *Diabetes Educator, 26,* 32–35.

American Diabetes Association. (2002). Bedside blood glucose monitoring in hospitals. *Diabetes Care, 25,* S110.

American Diabetes Association. (2004). Clinical practice recommendations 2004. *Diabetes Care, 27,* S5–S10.

Lock, J., Szuts, E., Malomo, K., & Anagnostopoulos, A. (2002). Whole-blood glucose testing at alternate sites: Glucose values and hematocrit of capillary blood drawn from fingertip and forearm. *Diabetes Care, 25,* 337–341.

Mensing, C. (2004). Helping patients choose the right blood glucose meter. *Nurse Practitioner, 29*(5), 43–46.

Perwien, A. R., Johnson, S. B., Dymtrow, D., & Silverstein, J. (2000). Blood glucose monitoring skills in children with type I diabetes. *Clinical Pediatrics, 39,* 351–357.

Reynolds, L., & Karounos, D. (2002), Emerging technology in diabetes mellitus: Glucose monitoring and new insulins. *Southern Medical Journal, 95*(8), 914–918.

Spollett, G. (2003, July/August). Choosing a blood glucose meter. *Diabetes Self-Management,* 99–106.

Tieszen, K., & New, J. (2003). Alternate site blood glucose testing: Do patients prefer it? *Diabetic Medicine, 20,* 325–328.

CHAPTER

20

Blood Product Administration

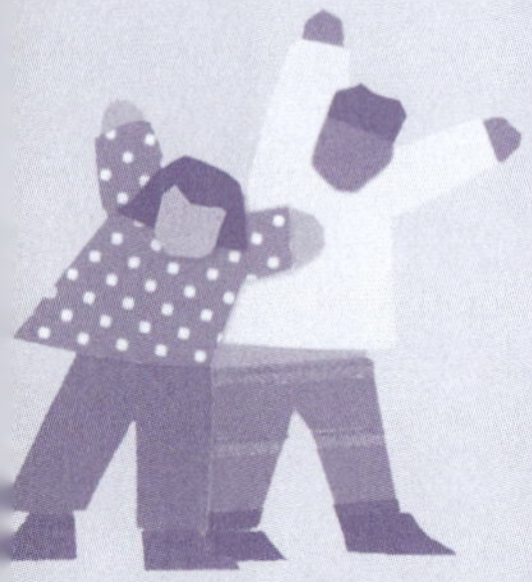

Clinical Guidelines

- A healthcare prescriber orders blood product administration. This order should include
  - Type of blood product
  - Amount to be given
  - Length of product administration time
  - Special instructions (e.g., washed cells, cytomegalovirus negative, irradiated, donor-directed blood)
- The registered nurse (RN) or physician is responsible for blood administration.
- A type and crossmatch is performed before administration of blood products to ensure that blood products given are ABO compatible and free of antigens that might react with the child's antibodies.
- Ensure adequate venous access (≥22 gauge is preferable; in neonates, because of vein size, 24 gauge is acceptable) before starting blood product administration.
- Obtain consent for transfusion from parent/guardian, unless an emergency situation.
- Donor and recipient blood types and groups must be verified by two personnel (RN or physician or qualified technician [per institutional policy]) before administration.

Equipment

- Blood component
- Infusion set
- IV-controlled infusion device (follow manufacturer's directions for use)
- Blood-warming coil and blood warmer, as indicated
- Nonsterile gloves
- Protective gear (mask with eye shield, gown)
- Normal saline
- Appropriate blood product filter (Table 20-1)
- Blood pressure cuff
- Stethoscope
- Thermometer

TABLE 20-1

Blood Product Administration Guidelines

Component	Description	Indication	Type of Filter	Dose	Rate	Administration	Special Considerations
Whole blood	Single-donor anti-coagulated blood	Massive blood loss Exchange transfusion Special procedures (ECMO to prime the circuit, apheresis)	Microaggregate filter	Massive blood loss—20 mL/kg initially Exchange transfusion: 2 times child's blood volume	As rapidly as necessary to reestablish blood volume 45–60 min (longer if hemodynamically unstable)		Always administer ABO group and Rh type specific
Packed red blood cells	Concentrated red blood cells with most plasma, leukocytes, and platelets removed	Severe anemia Surgical blood loss Suppression of erythropoiesis (e.g., thalassemia or sickle cell anemia) ECMO—blood loss from bleeding or multiple sampling for laboratory analysis	Microaggregate filter	10 mL/kg	5 mL/kg/hr		Administer ABO group and Rh type specific if possible. If not, group and type compatible can be transfused safely. May use O-negative uncrossmatched blood for infants up to 4 months of age Red blood compatibility: Recipient — Donor A — A,O B — B,O AB — AB, A,B,O O — O Rh+ — Rh+ Rh– — Rh– Undetermined — O
Saline-washed red blood cells	Red blood cells washed with normal saline, which removes 80% leukocytes	Children with history of repeated febrile transfusion reactions Immunocompromised patients	Same as packed red blood cells	Same as packed red blood cells	Same as packed red blood cells		Same as packed red blood cells
Frozen deglycerolyzed red blood cells	Specially processed red blood cells that can be stored for up to 3 yr	Rare blood types History of repeated febrile nonhemolytic reactions not	Same as packed red blood cells	Same as packed red blood cells	Same as packed red blood cells		Same as packed red blood cells

Continued

TABLE 20-1

Blood Product Administration Guidelines (continued)

Component	Description	Indication	Type of Filter	Dose	Rate	Administration	Special Considerations
		responsive to other leukocyte depletion methods Immunoglobulin A (IgA) deficiency with sensitivity to IgA					
Albumin	A plasma protein available in 5% and 25% solutions	5% Solution: hypoproteinemia, volume deficits 25% Solution: severe burns, cerebral edema		5%: Hypoalbuminemia or hypovolemia 10 mL/kg per dose 25%: 1 g/kg = 4 mL/kg	5%: 1–2 mL/min (60–120 mL/hr can be administered as fast as possible to correct shock) 25%: 0.2–0.4 mL/min (12–24 mL/h)		Needs no blood filter Only one person must identify product and patient Vital signs can be taken prn Compatibility testing not required 25% Albumin rapidly mobilizes large volumes of fluid into circulation (therefore, watch for pulmonary edema or other symptoms of fluid overload) Product is stored at room temperature and has very long shelf life Check expiration date before administering
Fresh frozen plasma	Contains all the clotting factors and some fibrinogen	Massive hemorrhage Hypovolemic shock Multiple clotting deficiencies	Standard blood filter or microaggregate filter	10–30 mL/kg	Hemorrhage—as indicated by patient's condition Clotting deficiency—over 2–3 h	Administer within 6 hr of thawing to preserve clotting factor activity	Donor's plasma should be ABO compatible with recipient's red blood cells. Rh compatibility not required because product does not contain red blood cells.

Platelets	Platelets suspended in a small amount of plasma	Severe thrombocytopenia (platelet count < 20,000) Platelet count < 50,000 in child who requires surgery or in child with hemorrhage or imminent bleeding Cardiac surgery with massive blood replacement Platelet count < 80,000–100,000 in child undergoing ECMO	Microaggregate filter	10 mL/kg or 1 random unit per year of age	Platelets may be given by IVP (5–10 min/U) if volume is a problem, transfuse total dose over 2–3 h using infusion pump.	Gently agitate bag even more often (every hour) than other blood products because platelets tend to clump; if giving pooled random platelets or platelet aliquots, notify the blood bank 60 min before anticipated transfusion time to allow for special handling.	Must be Rh compatible; ABO plasma compatibility preferred Available platelets include: • Random—different donors, not necessarily type specific • Type specific—blood type is the same as recipient • Single donor—pheresed platelets from single donor (1 pheresed platelet unit is equivalent to 8–10 random platelets) • HLA-pheresed—HLA testing has been done and matched to the recipient's HLA type. Platelets may be irradiated to inactivate donor lymphocytes that cause graft vs. host disease in immunocompromised patients. Premedicate as ordered, if patient has a history of reaction. If single-donor or HLA platelets are ordered, obtain a 1-h and a 24-h platelet count after transfusion to determine adequate platelet response.

Continued

TABLE 20-1

Blood Product Administration Guidelines (continued)

Component	Description	Indication	Type of Filter	Dose	Rate	Administration	Special Considerations
							Observe patient for transfusion reaction because platelets may be contaminated with some red blood cells.
Cryoprecipitate	A concentration of clotting factors VIII, XIII, fibrinogen and von Willebrand factor	Hemophilia A von Willebrand disease Hypofibrinogenemia Disseminated intravascular coagulation (DIC)	Standard blood filter or microaggregate filter	One bag per 5 kg, for mild bleed One bag per 2 kg, for severe life-threatening bleed Repeat every 12–24 h as necessary	May infuse as quickly as possible or be given by IVP Each bag contains about 15 mL	Neonates: Use syringe to draw cryo through filter. Infuse through syringe pump. Administer within 6 hr of thawing.	Monitor vital signs as instructed Administer ABO compatible Rh type (compatibility preferable, but not required).
Granulocytes	Infection-fighting white blood cells	Severe gram-negative infection or severe neutropenia unresponsive to routine forms of therapy in immunosuppressed patient Severe granulocyte dysfunction	Standard blood filter or microaggregate filter	10–15 mL/kg per dose	About 5 mL/kg/h	Granulocyte product must be irradiated (if so ordered) and infused within 24 h of donation, preferably within 6 h of donation.	Type and crossmatch needed before transfusion Mild fever and chills are a common reaction. Compress blood bag to mix the white cells periodically throughout the transfusion. Vital signs should be taken every 15 min × 4, then every hour during infusion. Amphotericin cannot be administered for 6 h before or after granulocyte transfusion.

Factor VIII concentrate	Sterile lyophilized powder containing the blood coagulation factor VIII, which is prepared from pooled human plasma	Hemophilia A	Filter needle provided with product	Minor bleed: 20 U/kg Severe bleed: 40 U/kg	Administer by IVP over about 5 min (2 mL/min max). If patient complains of headache, slow the rate because product is high in protein.	Reconstitute product per manufacturer instructions. Withdraw solution from vial using filter needle, then administer through syringe. Administer within 1 h of reconstitution.	Dose is ordered in units. No compatibility testing is required. Children on long-term therapy, if other than type O, should be monitored for hemolysis caused by isoagglutinins (anti-A and anti-B antibodies). Group-specific concentrates are available if needed.
Factor IX complex	Concentrated powdered blood coagulation factors II, VII, IX, and X	Congenital factor deficiency VII and X; acquired deficiency of factors II, VII, IX, and X	Filter needle provided with product		Administer by IVP over about 5 min. Maximum rates: Monoclate = 2 mL/min Humanate = 4 mL/min Others = 10 mL/min	Reconstitute product per manufacturer instructions. Withdraw solution from vial using filter needle, then administer through syringe.	No type or crossmatch required

ECMO, extracorporeal membrane oxygenation; IVP, intravenous pyelogram.

CHILD AND FAMILY ASSESSMENT AND PREPARATION

- Assess the cognitive level, readiness, and ability to process information of the child and family.
- Explain the procedure and the reason for blood administration to the child and family.
- Identify the child and family's religious beliefs and discuss the religious justification and ramifications associated with blood transfusion; some religions prohibit blood transfusion, so be sure to elicit the family's views.
- Discuss the risks and benefits of blood product administration with child and family.
- Assess the child's transfusion history for the presence of transfusion-related reactions. A direct relationship exists between the number of transfusions the patient has had and the likelihood of having a transfusion reaction. If the child has had previous transfusion reactions, question the child and family about which pretransfusion medications most effectively reduced symptoms in the child.
- Assess the child's vital signs (temperature, heart rate, respiratory rate, blood pressure) to establish a pretransfusion baseline.
- Assess need for use of blood warmer in infants, in children who are hypothermic, and in children in whom large amounts of blood are to be transfused.
- Obtain written consent for blood product administration from the parent/guardian or child, if emancipated.

PROCEDURE Administering a Blood Transfusion

Steps	Rationale/Points of Emphasis
1. Verify prescriber's order for transfusion. (See Table 20-1 for blood product selection and dose calculation.)	Safety measure to ensure that correct product and dose are administered, as required for transfusion therapy.
2. Ascertain if a specimen for typing and crossmatch is necessary or already available from blood bank. If necessary, draw a blood specimen from child and send to laboratory for typing and crossmatch.	Type and crossmatch specimens are typically usable for 48 hours, when drawn before blood product administration. Neonatal type and crossmatch are usable for 3 months.
3. Verify patency of IV infusion site.	Blood products must be hung within 20 to 30 minutes after leaving blood bank refrigerator to avoid deterioration of the product. If venous access must be reestablished, the blood product may be sitting too long.
4. Administer prescribed antihistamine or other medications if the child has a history of transfusion reaction.	Reduces occurrence of allergic reaction to blood products.
5. Obtain blood product from blood bank.	Administer blood products immediately upon receipt; do not store on unit where storage conditions may not be adequate to maintain integrity of blood products.
6. Visually inspect blood product for discoloration, separation of products, and signs of contamination.	If there are any inconsistencies, notify blood bank immediately and return blood product. Potential for lethal transfusion reactions increases with contamination.
7. With another RN, physician, or qualified technician (per institutional policy), check blood product label against the original order, transfusion record form, and child's identification band and any other patient identifier required by the institution, verifying the following: • Child's name and medical record number • Type of blood component • Patient's ABO group and Rh factor • Donor's ABO group and Rh factor • Blood product unit number • Expiration date of blood product • Special requirements, (e.g., cytomegalovirus negative)	Two qualified personnel verifying the information reduces the risk for incorrect administration.
8. Both inspecting personnel should then sign verification on transfusion record form.	Documents that proper verification was performed.
9. The individual beginning the transfusion should then perform hand hygiene.	Reduces transmission of microorganisms.
10. Don appropriate protective apparel: nonsterile gloves, mask with eye shield, gown.	Standard precaution to reduce transmission of microorganisms.

Steps	Rationale/Points of Emphasis
11. Open tubing infusion set and appropriate blood filter (see Table 20-1) and attach together.	Accesses equipment; prepares for administration.
12. Close all roller clamps and spike blood product with a direct upward motion using a filter and tubing infusion set; or for small amounts of blood, spike the bag with a blood filter attached to a syringe and aspirate blood into the syringe. Connect syringe to tubing and put syringe into syringe pump.	Prevents blood spills and accesses blood. If the bag is spiked at an angle, it pierces a hole in the bag. **KidKare** Blood products are kept refrigerated and therefore are usually very cold. Use blood-warming setup, following manufacturer's directions for infants and neonates, if necessary, or if signs of hypothermia appear: low temperature, chills, or irregular heart rate.
13. Open roller clamp between blood and drip chamber and fill drip chamber, covering blood filter.	Allows for filtering of blood product.
14. Open roller clamp on tubing infusion set and prime tubing.	Prevents air embolus.
15. Close roller clamp when tubing is primed and place tubing into IV-controlled infusion device.	Prevents blood spills and readies for administration.
16. Cleanse infusion port (per institutional policy) of child's venous access catheter and insert primed blood tubing.	Reduces transmission of microorganisms.
17. Set the rate of infusion on the controlled infusion device, open roller clamp, and begin transfusion.	Allows transfusion to proceed. ***Alert!*** *Start transfusion of blood products that contain red blood cells slowly. The transfusion rate should be selected by calculating 5% of the total product to be administered and then infusing this calculated amount over 15 minutes. This ensures that only a small amount of blood will have been transfused if a transfusion reaction occurs.*
18. Stay with the child and monitor continuously for signs of transfusion reaction for the first 15 minutes (Table 20-2). Explain to child and family signs of transfusion reaction and instruct them to notify healthcare provider if these occur.	Transfusion reactions usually occur within the first 15 minutes of infusion. Changes can be detected that indicate a transfusion reaction. ***Alert!*** *If a transfusion reaction occurs at any time, stop the transfusion immediately to minimize the amount of blood infused and potentially reduce the severity of the reaction. Notify the physician and blood bank, and return the unused portion of blood to the blood bank per institutional policy. Maintain the venous access catheter with normal saline infusion. Follow institution's policy regarding transfusion reaction and complete required interventions (e.g., blood cultures, urine specimen, vital sign monitoring).*
19. Obtain vital signs (temperature, heart rate, respiratory rate, blood pressure) every 15 minutes for 1 hour and every 30 minutes thereafter; compare vital signs to baseline. If no signs of a transfusion reaction occur within the first 15 minutes, adjust the rate to infuse blood as prescribed. Monitor for signs of fluid overload.	Enables early detection of complications.

Steps	Rationale/Points of Emphasis
20. Complete transfusion within 4 hours of transfusion initiation, faster if ordered.	Blood begins to clot after 4 hours, and the likelihood of bacterial contamination markedly increases after 4 hours.
21. At the completion of blood product administration, clamp the tube infusion set and venous access catheter and disconnect tubing.	Prevents blood spills.
22. Flush the venous access catheter with normal saline, and care for as specific to venous access line.	Prevents clotting and allows for later use. **caREminder** *Change tubing after each blood product is finished. When administering two or more blood products, change the tubing between the products; when administering two units of PRBCs, the tubing can be used for administration of two units.*
23. Dispose of equipment and waste in appropriate receptacle. Perform hand hygiene.	Standard precautions. Reduces transmission of microorganisms.

TABLE 20-2

Signs of Transfusion Reaction

	Hemolytic Reaction	Febrile Reaction	Allergic Reaction
Signs and symptoms	Fever Chills Urticaria Restlessness Headache Chest pain Abdominal/lower back pain Tachycardia Hypotension Oliguria Shock Laboratory findings Anemia Spherocytosis Disseminated intravascular coagulation (DIC) Hemoglobinemia Hemoglobinuria Positive Coombs' test	Fever Chills Diaphoresis	Rash Hives Urticaria Swelling Respiratory distress Anaphylaxis
Preventive measures	Type and crossmatch accurately. Use leukocyte-depleted blood products to help prevent alloimmunization.	Pretreat with antipyretic and corticosteroid. Use leukocyte-depleted blood products.	Pretreat with antihistamine and corticosteroid. Wash red blood cells.

CHILD AND FAMILY EVALUATION AND DOCUMENTATION

- Monitor the child's intake and output.
- Evaluate the child regularly to monitor patency of venous access catheter and for signs or symptoms of a blood-related reaction, which can include but are not limited to fever, chills, flank pain, red urine, urticaria, anaphylaxis, increased white blood cell count, and positive blood cultures.
- Evaluate the child for hyperkalemia and hypocalcemia because stored blood develops a high potassium level due to red blood cell lysis and because citrate ions in stored blood bind with calcium and are then excreted by the body.
- Evaluate the child's response to treatment, specifically hemoglobin and hematocrit levels, increased blood pressure, decreased heart rate, increased urine output, and improved oxygenation/respiratory status.
- Evaluate the child and family's understanding of the procedure and determine whether they have other areas of concern to discuss.
- Document the following on the appropriate institutional forms:
  - The pretransfusion assessment
  - Donor and recipient blood types and groups, blood product unit number of the administered blood product(s), and names of the two personnel verifying the information
  - Date and time transfusion was initiated and discontinued
  - Baseline and serial vital signs
  - Amount of blood product infused hourly
  - Type and amount of total blood product transfused
  - Child's response to the infusion
- Place transfusion record (along with blood product validation signed by two personnel) in the child's record.

COMMUNITY CARE

- Instruct family to keep a record of child's blood type with other medical records.
- Instruct the family to contact the healthcare provider if signs of delayed transfusion reaction occur, such as infection (jaundice, fever) or anemia.

Unexpected Situation

- *During transfusion, the child develops tachypnea, labored breathing, dry cough, and rales at lung bases, which are signs of fluid overload:* Slow infusion rate of blood product and notify physician.

Bibliography

American Association of Blood Banks (AABB). (2003). *Standards for blood banks and transfusion services* (22nd ed.). Bethesda, MD: Author.

Bratton, S. L., & Annich, G. M. (2003). Packed red blood cell transfusions for critically ill pediatric patients: When and for what conditions? *Journal of Pediatrics, 142*, 95–97.

Fergusson, D., Hebert, P. C., Lee, S. K., et al. (2003). Clinical outcomes following institution of universal leukoreduction of blood transfusions for premature infants. *JAMA: Journal of American Medical Association, 289*, 1950–1956.

Goldman, M., Savard, R., Long, A., Gelinas, S., & Germain, M. (2002). Declining value of preoperative autologous donation. *Transfusion, 42*, 819–823.

Hume, H. A., & Limoges, P. (2002). Perioperative blood transfusion therapy in pediatric patients. *American Journal of Therapeutics, 9*, 396–405.

Maier, R. F., Sonntag, J., Walka, M. M., et al. (2000). Changing practices of red blood cell transfusions in infants with birth weights less than 1000g. *Journal of Pediatrics, 136*, 220–224.

Murray, N. A., & Roberts, I. A. (2004). Neonatal transfusion practice. *Archives of Disease in Childhood: Fetal & Neonatal Edition, 89*, F101–F107.

Roseff, S. D., Luban, N. L., & Manno, C. S. (2002). Guidelines for assessing appropriateness of pediatric transfusion. *Transfusion, 42*, 1398–1413.

Rossetto, C. L., & McMahon, J. E. (2000). Current and future trends in transfusion therapy. *Journal of Pediatric Oncology Nursing, 17*, 160–173.

Whitsett, C. F., & Robichaux, M. G. (2001). Assessment of blood administration procedures: Problems identified by direct observation and administrative incident reporting. *Transfusion, 41*, 581–586.

CHAPTER

21

Bone Marrow Aspiration

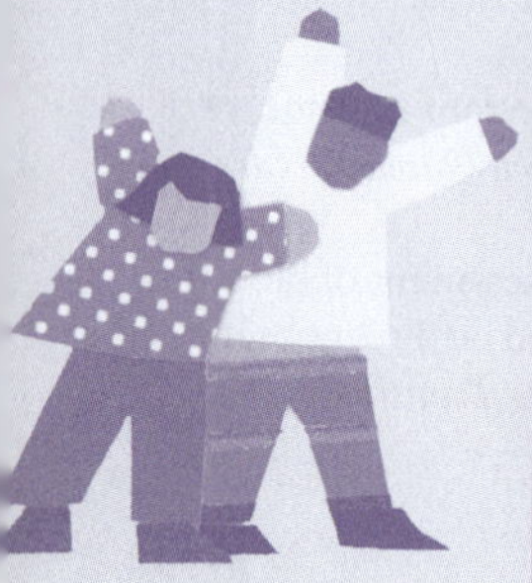

Clinical Guidelines

- Bone marrow aspiration is completed by a healthcare prescriber according to scope of practice.
- A healthcare prescriber, registered nurse (RN), or licensed practical nurse (LPN) assists with the procedure and participates in sedation procedures as ordered.
- If the child is receiving medication for sedation, nursing personnel remain present during the procedure to monitor the child, and sedation guidelines are used (see Chapter 105).
- Family members are permitted in the patient care area during invasive procedures.

Equipment

- Bone marrow tray, which includes
  - Three sterile cotton balls or gauze
  - Sterile forceps
  - Sterile bowl
  - Sterile drape
  - Gauze pads of various sizes
  - Two 10-mL syringes
  - Adhesive bandage or pressure dressing
  - Chlorhexidine solution
  - Sterile gloves (for practitioner performing procedure)
  - Bone marrow aspirate needle (may use a spinal needle), sized according to the child
  - Specimen containers/slides with labels, depending on diagnostic tests being completed
  - Tape
- Nonsterile gloves (for assistive personnel)
- Small sheet, rolled
- Anesthetic cream
- 1% lidocaine with syringe, if being used
- Pain/sedation medications as ordered
- Stethoscope
- Blood pressure monitoring equipment (as needed)
- Pulse oximeter (if child is sedated)
- Age-appropriate resuscitation equipment
- Age-appropriate diversional activities (music, guided imagery, hand-holding)

Child and Family Assessment and Preparation

- Assess child and family's readiness to learn.
- Explain to child and parents the use of the anesthetic cream, sedation medications, and NPO status, as needed.

- Explain the procedure to the child and the family. Reassure them that the procedure may be somewhat uncomfortable and that there will be some soreness for 1 or 2 days after the procedure that may be relieved with acetaminophen. No activity restrictions are required.
- Hydrate the child before the procedure whenever possible to facilitate bone marrow withdrawal. Providing twice the amount of maintenance intravenous fluid is preferable when physiologically possible.
- Assess the child's coagulation status to anticipate bleeding complications.

> **Alert!** *Prophylactic therapy with coagulation factor replacement is required before the procedure in patients with hemophilia (factor VIII or IX deficiency) and related bleeding disorders.*

- Show the child and family the procedure/treatment room.
- Assess the child for previously used comfort methods and diversional strategies. Reinforce these strategies or teach new methods (e.g., breathing techniques, music therapy).
- Verify that a legal consent form for the procedure has been obtained and signed by the parents or guardians.
- Assess the child for medication allergies if using anesthetic cream, lidocaine, or sedation/pain medication during the procedure.
- If using sedation, follow institution's policy regarding NPO status before the procedure and for monitoring the child's status before and after the procedure.
- Explain to the parents that their role during the procedure is to offer physical and verbal support to their child. Discuss with the parents ways they can provide diversionary activities for the child.

PROCEDURE Aspirating Bone Marrow

Steps	Rationale/Points of Emphasis
1. Apply anesthetic cream to site of aspiration at least 1 hour before procedure.	Anesthetic cream will help to decrease pain at the injection site.
2. Gather the necessary supplies.	Promotes efficient time management and provides an organized approach to the procedure. Preparation before the child is in the room can help to decrease the child's anxiety by limiting the length of time the child is in the treatment room.

> **Alert!** *Ensure age-appropriate resuscitation equipment is accessible to the treatment room, because children under sedation are at an increased risk for adverse events. Age-appropriate resuscitative equipment and personnel trained in pediatric resuscitation techniques should be available in the event of cardiovascular or respiratory complications.*

Steps	Rationale/Points of Emphasis
3. Perform hand hygiene.	Reduces transmission of microorganisms.
4. Set up sterile bone marrow tray.	Maintains sterility while setting up the supplies.
5a. Bring the child and family member (if available and willing to accompany child) into the treatment room. Place the infant or young child on the procedure table, keeping one hand on the child at all times to ensure safety. Permit the older child to climb on to the procedure table with minimal assistance (if not sedated).	Painful procedures are never completed in the child's own room; that area should remain a "safe haven." The child should not be left unattended on the procedure table because there is the potential to roll off or fall off the table.
5b. Show the family member where he or she can stand to be of most support and benefit to the child during the procedure.	Family presence during invasive procedures has been demonstrated to be beneficial to the child and the participating family members. Families perceive themselves as active participants, caring for the child with the staff. Families generally view their presence as a right, an obligation, and a natural event. Family presence is optional and their choice in this matter should be respected.

Continued

Steps	Rationale/Points of Emphasis
6. Assess the child's vital signs and comfort level. **Alert!** *Changes in vital signs may indicate bleeding or infection.*	Provides baseline for monitoring changes during and after the procedure.
7. Perform hand hygiene, and don gloves.	Standard precaution to reduce transmission of microorganisms. *Note:* The healthcare prescriber performing the procedure will be wearing sterile gloves. The nurse assisting in the procedure does not need sterile gloves unless their activities enter the sterile field.
8a. Administer pain management/sedation medications as ordered. 8b. If ordered, administer sedation. Monitor the child according to sedation guidelines (see Chapter 105).	Bone marrow aspiration is a painful procedure. Pulse and oxygen saturation monitoring should be used to assess the child's status because of the potential for decreased responsiveness and altered respiratory status during sedation. **KidKare** Effective pain management reduces deleterious effects of pain and enhances the child's coping with current and subsequent procedures.
9. Position the child according to the aspiration site selected by the healthcare prescriber: • Posterior iliac crest: prone with a small roll under the child's hips • Sternum or anterior iliac crest: supine • Vertebral: on one side, with knees and head tucked tightly together. • Tibia: supine with knee bent and supported by pillow or towel roll (Figure 21-1) **caREminder** *The most common sites in children are the anterior and posterior iliac crests. The tibia is sometimes used in infants. Spinous processes may be used when both bone marrow aspiration and lumbar puncture must be performed.*	Assists the healthcare prescriber in locating the correct landmark for the aspiration procedure. Decreases risk of complication by misplacement of needle. **KidKare** If the child is overweight, a pillow, folded towel, or blanket can be placed under the abdomen to elevate the hips and facilitate access to the posterior iliac crest.

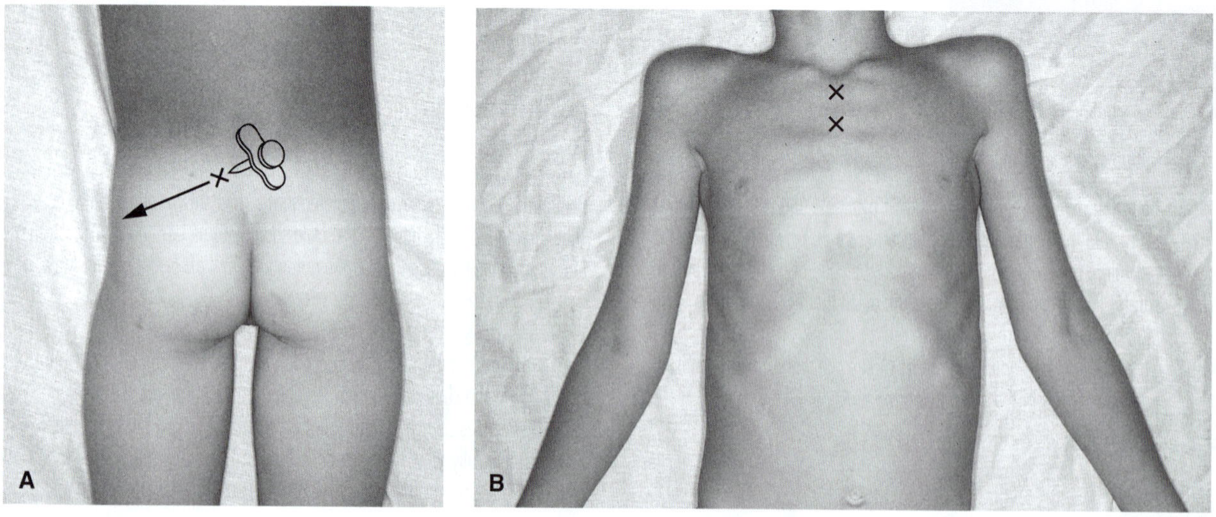

FIGURE 21-1
Aspiration sites for bone marrow include (**A**) posterior iliac crest, (**B**) sternum (**C**) anterior iliac crest, and (**D**) tibia.

Steps	Rationale/Points of Emphasis

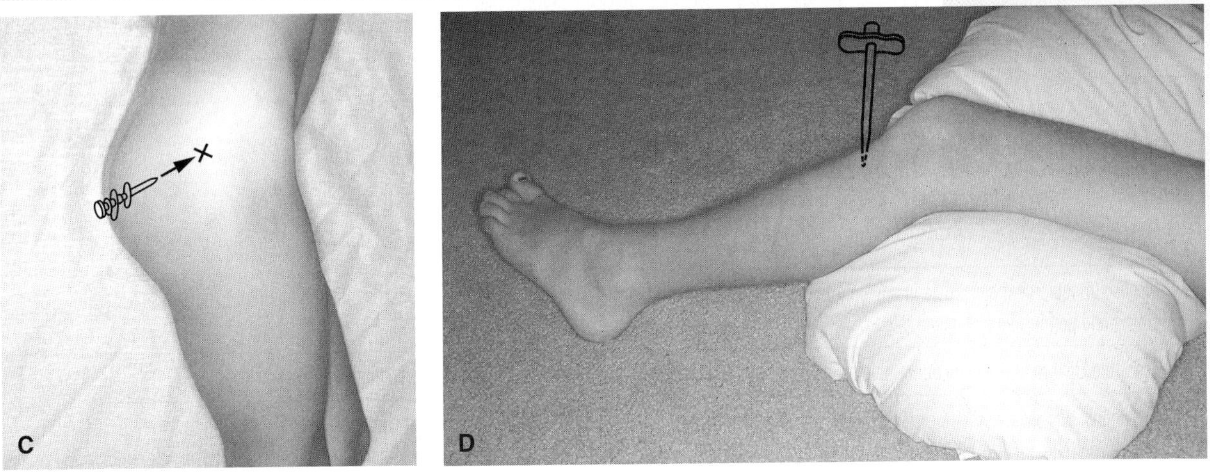

FIGURE 21-1
Continued.

Steps	Rationale/Points of Emphasis
10. Wipe the site with a clean cloth or gauze to remove the anesthetic cream.	Removes white cream for clear visualization of landmarks.
11a. The healthcare prescriber will perform the aspiration procedure using sterile technique. Several sites and attempts may be necessary to gather the needed amount of specimen.	The initial aspirate on a newly diagnosed leukemic child may be difficult to withdraw because the bone marrow is very hypercellular and packed with leukemic cells.
11b. The healthcare prescriber will drape the selected area with sterile towels and cleanse the site with a chlorhexidine solution.	Cleaning the site reduces transmission of bacteria.
11c. A surface anesthetic is injected at this time.	Surface analgesia aids in pain relief during the procedure.
12. Hold the child in place during the procedure.	Decrease in movement allows for the procedure to be completed with ease and prevents misplacement of the needle. Older children may be able to hold still with little need for physical restraint. Young children will require more physical restraint to maintain correct positioning during the procedure. **caREminder** *Parents should not be placed in a position to assist in restraining the child. Parents do not have training in proper restraint techniques and their role should be to offer love and support.*
13. During the procedure, use age-appropriate diversion and breathing techniques to distract the child. For instance, the older child may prefer to listen to music on headphones during the procedure.	May help distract and reduce child's perception of pain and help enhance the child's coping skills.
14. After the procedure is completed, remove the drapes and cleanse the chlorhexidine from the area.	Decreases the risk for skin irritation from the chlorhexidine.
15. Assess the bone marrow aspirate site for signs of bleeding and apply a dressing (using a gauze pad secured with tape) or an adhesive bandage.	Detects complication promptly. Reduces risk of bleeding. **Alert!** *Apply a pressure dressing to prevent bleeding if the child's platelet count is 50,000 or less.*

Continued

Steps	Rationale/Points of Emphasis
16. Label the specimens and send to the appropriate laboratory for examination. ***Alert!** The child should never be left unattended while on the procedure table. Attention to specimens and disposal of equipment may need to be delayed until the child is safely secured in the crib/bed with safety measures used (e.g., side rails up).*	Decreases the risk for error and loss.
17. Dispose of equipment and waste in appropriate receptacle. Remove gloves and perform hand hygiene.	Standard precautions. Reduces transmission of microorganisms.
18. Assist the child to return to a comfortable position and maintain diversion.	Promotes comfort and reduction of anxiety.
19. If sedation was used, assess the child until he or she is fully awake (which can take about 60 minutes from the time the medication was administered), because duration of medications administered for sedation may extend beyond length of time needed to complete the procedure.	Ensures early detection of cardiorespiratory compromise. Monitoring must be maintained until child reaches baseline premedicated cognitive state to ensure child's safety.
20. Assess the child for discomfort and medicate as ordered.	The child may have pain at the injection site for 1 to 2 days after the procedure.
21. Return the child to his or her room or discharge child home when stable.	Moving the child to a more comfortable and safe location will help alleviate the child's anxiety.

Child and Family Evaluation and Documentation

- Monitor the bone marrow aspiration site for signs and symptoms of bleeding and infection.
- Continue ongoing assessment of the child's pain and implement pharmacologic and nonpharmacologic interventions as needed.
- Document the following:
  - Location of bone marrow aspirate
  - Condition of the site at the end of the procedure
  - Type of dressing applied to site, and time dressing was applied
  - Child's status before, during, and after the procedure, including vital signs, oxygen saturation
  - Child's response to medications
  - Diversional activities provided during procedure and effectiveness of these interventions
  - Postprocedural instructions provided to the child and family

Community Care

- For pain relief, the child may use acetaminophen or ibuprofen. Aspirin should not be used because it may interfere with platelet aggregation.
- No restrictions on the child's activities are required after the procedure.
- Instruct the child and parent to remove the original dressing no earlier than 8 hours and no later than 24 hours after the procedure to prevent bleeding. Leaving the bandage in place for longer periods of time may predispose the immunocompromised child to infection.
- If the child is reluctant to have the bandage removed, suggest taking the bandage off during the child's bath because a wet bandage is easier to remove.
- Instruct the family to contact the healthcare provider if
  - The child develops a fever
  - The aspiration site becomes reddened or irritated or oozes any fluid or blood
  - The child complains of unmanageable pain

Unexpected Situation

- *Fifteen minutes after the completion of the bone marrow aspiration, you check the dressing site and find the dressing saturated with blood:* Wearing gloves, remove the dressing and apply pressure using sterile gauze to the site. Continue to apply pressure until bleeding ceases. Redress the site. Notify the healthcare prescriber. Evaluation of the child's platelet count may be warranted.

Bibliography

Association of Pediatric Oncology Nurses. (2002). *Nursing care of children and adolescents with cancer*. Philadelphia: W. B. Saunders.

Hodges, A., & Koury, M. (1996). Focus: Bone marrow. Needle aspiration and biopsy in the diagnosing and monitoring of bone marrow diseases. *Clinical Laboratory Science, 9*(6), 349–353, 363–365.

Malviya, S., Voepel-Lewis, T., Tait, A. R., & Merkel, S. (2000). Sedation/analgesia for diagnostic and therapeutic procedures in children. *Journal of Perianesthesia Nursing, 15*, 415–422.

McCarthy, A., Cool, V., Petersen, M., & Bruene, D. (1996). Cognitive behavioral pain and anxiety interventions in pediatric oncology centers and bone marrow transplant units. *Journal of Pediatric Oncology Nursing, 13*(1), 3–11.

Meyers, T., Eichhorn, D., Guzzetta, C., et al. (2004). Family presence during invasive procedures and resuscitation. *Topics in Emergency Medicine, 26*(1), 61–73.

Reeves, S., Havidich, J., & Tobin, P. (2004). Conscious sedation of children with propofol is anything but conscious. *Pediatrics, 114*(1), e74–e76.

Trewhitt, K. (2001). Bone marrow aspiration and biopsy: Collection and interpretation. *Oncology Nursing Forum, 28*(9), 1409–1415.

CHAPTER

22

Breast Milk: Handling and Storage of Expressed Human Milk

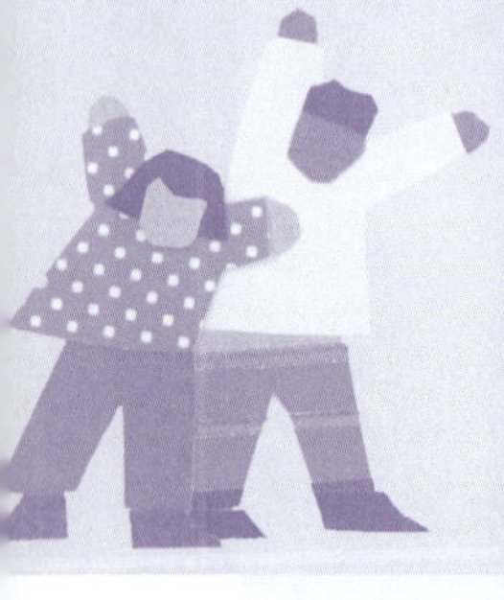

Clinical Guidelines

- After the mother pumps the milk, the mother, father, or any healthcare provider who is educated about the technique may label the milk containers.
- Only staff members may access the storage refrigerator/freezer to deposit or retrieve milk.
- Two persons must verify that the correct milk is to be fed to the correct infant. Any healthcare provider who is educated about the technique may verify; a parent may serve as the double check.
- Each mother–infant dyad should be educated, encouraged, and supported to breast-feed or to provide mother's milk, even in situations of illness, prematurity, hospitalization, or separation.
- Maternal contraindications to providing mother's milk in developed countries are few: positive HIV status, untreated tuberculosis, positive HTLV (human T-lymphoma virus), or active use of illicit drugs or pharmaceuticals that are contraindicated for breast-feeding.
- In situations where the infant is unable to breast-feed, expressed mother's milk should be safely stored for use.
- Donor human milk from a recognized human milk bank is a viable alternative for the mother who is unable to supply her own milk to her infant or child.
- Refrigerators and freezers for storing human milk should be labeled "For Human Milk Storage." Human milk is not a biologic hazard, and refrigerators and freezers need not be labeled as such.
- Refrigerators must be kept at 33° F to 39.2° F (>0°C to ≤ 4°C). Freezers must be kept at −4°F (−20°C) or lower.
- Refrigerators and freezers for storing human milk should be on emergency power circuits to prevent warming of milk to room temperature for greater than 4 hours or thawing and refreezing during power outages.
- Refrigerators and freezers storing human milk should have temperature alarms or a designated staff member must be responsible for documenting appropriate temperatures once every 24 hours.

EQUIPMENT

- Refrigerator/freezer or stand-alone units labeled for human milk storage
- Emergency power circuits for the refrigerator/freezer units
- Thermometer for checking refrigerator/freezer temperatures
- Individual storage bins or, for small quantities, gallon Zip-lock bags
- Clean food grade (hard) polypropylene plastic or glass containers

CHILD AND FAMILY ASSESSMENT AND PREPARATION

- Assess each mother's plans for infant feeding. What were her prenatal plans or goals? What would she like to do now? How has the infant been feeding at home before the hospitalization?
- Assess mother's need for education, equipment, and support related to breast-feeding or pumping and storage of her milk.
- Instruct each mother in appropriate hand hygiene and pump kit cleaning procedures to reduce risk of contamination of pumped milk, storage containers, and pumping kits. Human milk is not a sterile product, so sterile handling is not required. Teach the mother to clean all parts of the pump kit that come in contact with human milk after use with warm, soapy water, then rinsing thoroughly.
- Provide a comfortable private area where mother can breast-feed her infant or pump her milk.
- Provide guidelines for pumping and storage of mother's milk at your facility.
- Utilize board-certified lactation consultants as resources within your setting for education, support, and assistance with special needs.

PROCEDURE **Human Milk Storage in the Hospital Setting**

Steps	Rationale/Points of Emphasis
1. Perform hand hygiene.	Reduces transmission of microorganisms.
2. Ensure mother has needed equipment:	
• Personal pumping equipment	Reduces risk of cross-contamination.
• Clean containers of food grade polypropylene (hard) plastic or glass with hard spill-proof lids for storage of her expressed milk within the hospital setting	Human milk is not a sterile substance. Storage in clean but not sterile containers has not been shown to increase bacterial counts. Immunologic and nutritional properties are better maintained in these containers than in thinner polyethylene bags. Use of baby bottle nipples to cover stored milk provides a potential source of contamination due to the open nipple hole.
• Individually labeled bins or containers for placement in the refrigerator/freezer unit.	Facilitates easy identification of an infant's milk stores; externally labeled bins or containers lessen the risk of giving milk to the wrong infant. **caREminder** *Place "Name Alert" tags on each refrigerator/freezer and individual bin for similar or like names within the unit to help avoid storage of milk in the wrong bin or giving milk to the wrong infant.*
3. Have mother pump breasts.	Obtains milk.
4. Place freshly pumped milk in containers in quantities equaling no more than 24-hour feeding volumes.	Reduces waste; ensures that milk can be used or stored in quantities needed by the infant.
5. Ensure that each individual container of pumped milk is labeled with the infant's name, medical record or identification number, date of birth, and date and time the milk was pumped.	Assists in proper identification of each container of milk, and avoids giving to the wrong infant. Dating of each bottle allows the oldest milk to be used first.
6. Place milk in the labeled bin or container.	Facilitates easy identification of an infant's milk stores; externally labeled bins or containers lessen the risk of giving milk to the wrong infant.

Steps	Rationale/Points of Emphasis
7. Refrigerate or freeze freshly pumped milk as soon as possible unless it is to be used within 4 hours.	Fresh pumped milk may be at room temperature 77°F to 79°F (25°C to 26.1°C), slightly warmer than room temperature, for up to 4 hours without significant bacterial cell growth. Fresh milk offers the best nutritional and health benefits for the infant.
8. In hospital situations, fresh pumped human milk may be refrigerated for up to 48 hours but should be frozen by 48 hours if not used. Immediately freeze fresh pumped milk volumes if greater than anticipated feeding needs for 48 hours.	Reduces growth of microorganisms and helps preserve milk's nutritional and immunologic benefits.
9. Storage time guidelines: • Fresh pumped milk may be stored in freezers at −4°F (−20°C) for up to 12 months. For sick or preterm infants, use within 3 months is optimal. • Do not store milk in the door of the freezer.	Milk's nutritional and immunologic properties are reduced with long-term storage. Even so, human milk stored safely for longer periods has significantly more nutrients and immunologic value than artificial infant formulas currently offer. Helps maintain a stable temperature because temperature fluctuations are greatest in the door of the freezer.

PROCEDURE Preparing Milk for Feeding

Steps	Rationale/Points of Emphasis
1. Leave unfrozen milk in the refrigerator. Frozen human milk may be thawed by • Moving container to refrigerator for several hours • Sitting container at room temperature, or • Sitting container inside a clean glove submersed in warm water; avoid water directly touching the container or lid	Allows milk to avoid a warm environment where bacteria can thrive but to attain liquid properties. Water directly in contact with the container or lid may expose milk to water contaminants.
2. When milk is liquid but still chilled, label the container with date and time thawed and return to refrigerator until ready to use. Thawed milk must be used within 24 hours or discarded.	Identifies the milk to avoid feeding to wrong infant. Avoids pathologic growth of microorganisms.
3. Immediately before feeding, warm milk by again placing container inside glove in warm water bath or by holding under running warm tap water, keeping lid dry to avoid contamination.	Brings milk to physiologic temperature. Cold milk may reduce a preterm infant's temperature and increase their metabolic needs. ***Alert!*** *Never microwave human milk for defrosting or warming. Resultant "hot spots" from the microwave within the milk increases risks of burning the infant. IgA and other anti-infective properties are also reduced with microwaving.*
4. Before feeding, verify with another healthcare provider or parent the match between the labeled milk container and the infant's identification band by comparing the name and medical record or identification number and any other patient identifier required by the institution.	Ensures accurate identification of milk and infant to reduce risk of wrong milk being given to the wrong infant.
5. When using thawed human milk for continuous feedings in the hospital setting, replace the connecting tubing and syringe every 4 hours with new equipment.	Bacteria growth increases after 4 hours at room temperature with milk that has been previously frozen.

CHILD AND FAMILY EVALUATION AND DOCUMENTATION

- Note the amount of stored milk available for the infant. Notify the mother if supplies are low or inadequate for the needs of the day.
- Contact the lactation consultant for assistance with the mother who has low milk volume with pumping.
- Assess state of milk when brought from home—fresh, cold, or frozen—and store appropriately.
- Document the following:
  - Date and time milk was thawed on the individual container
  - Initials of healthcare providers and parents checking identification information on milk container and infant before feeding in the medical record

- Time, amount, route, and calories of maternal human milk fed to the infant
- Batch number if human donor milk is used

COMMUNITY CARE

- Teach parents to transport refrigerated or fresh pumped human milk in an insulated cooler or bag with frozen gel packs. Tightly pack frozen milk in a cooler or insulated bag with frozen gel packs and toweling, crumpled paper, or packing peanuts filling any empty air space to help maintain cold temperature. Frozen gel packs keep milk cold or frozen better than ice cubes, whose temperature is actually warmer than frozen milk, thereby hastening the thawing process.
- Human milk may be safely stored in home refrigerators and freezers for the infant.
- Home freezers that keep ice cream frozen hard are appropriate for milk storage. For the healthy infant, freshly pumped human milk may be safely stored and used for up to 8 days in the home refrigerator or for up to 12 months in a deep freezer (−4°F or −20°C).
- Day care settings have varying requirements for milk storage, labeling, and use, though generally not more stringent than hospital guidelines.
- If the mother has more pumped milk than her infant will be able to use, she may contact a local milk bank for information about donating her excess milk.
- Instruct the family to contact the healthcare provider if
  - Mother develops a fever or her breasts are red and painful
  - Mother's milk supply significantly decreases over usual volumes
  - Mother will be starting new medications

Unexpected Situations

- *Upon opening the container of thawed milk, the milk is foul-smelling:* Discard milk and use another container of milk; verify date and time the milk was collected, and milk/infant verification.
- *Pumped milk is red in color:* Nipple cracks or breast trauma may result in tissue bruising and open tissue that may introduce droplets of maternal blood into the pumped milk. Milk is not harmful to the infant as the blood protein is easily digested by the infant. Milk should not be discarded. Consult with lactation professional to determine cause of trauma and appropriate treatments.
- *An infant is fed the wrong milk:* Complete an institutional incident report. Refer to the Human Milk Banking Association of North America (Tully & Jones, 2005) for protocol to handle the specific situation. Then evaluate the situation in a nonpunitive way to identify circumstances causing the error and correct and educate to avoid future incidents.
- *A mother who has been pumping to provide breast milk for her infant is fully lactating at the time of the infant's death:* Encourage the mother to continue pumping during this early grieving period to avoid severe engorgement and mastitis. Gradual weaning is important. Many mothers appreciate the opportunity and desire to donate their milk to a donor milk bank so that another infant may benefit from her milk. Provide information to the mother about this option.

Bibliography

American Academy of Pediatrics, Section on Breastfeeding. (2005). Breastfeeding and the use of human milk. *Pediatrics, 115*, 496–506.

Askin, D. F., & Diehl-Jones, W. L. (2005). Improving on perfection: Breast milk and breast-milk additives for preterm neonates. *Newborn and Infant Nursing Reviews, 5*, 10–18.

Fenton, T. R., & Belik, J. (2002). Routine handling of milk fed to preterm infants can significantly increase osmolality. *Journal of Pediatric Gastroenterology and Nutrition, 35*, 298–302.

Gale, G., & Brooks, A. (2006). Implementing a palliative care program in a newborn intensive care unit. *Advances in Neonatal Care, 6*, 37–53.

Human Milk Banking Association of North America. (n.d.). *Donor human milk: Ensuring safety and ethical allocation.* Retrieved August 11, 2005, from http://www.hmbana.org/position-paper-safety-ethical.pdf

Nyqvist, K. H. (2005). Breastfeeding support in neonatal care: An example of the integration of international evidence and experience. *Newborn and Infant Nursing Reviews, 5*, 34–48.

Ovesen, L., Jakobsen, J., Leth, T., & Reinholdt, J. (1996). The effect of microwave heating on vitamin B1 and E and linoleic and linolenic acid and immunoglobulins in human milk. *International Journal of Food Sciences and Nutrition, 47*, 427–436.

Pessoa-Silva, C. L., Dharan, S., Hugonnet, S., et al. (2004). Dynamics of bacterial hand contamination during routine neonatal care. *Infection Control and Hospital Epidemiology, 25*, 192–197.

Pittard, W. B., Geddes, K. M., Brown, S., Mintz, S., & Hulsey, T. C. (1991). Bacterial contamination of human milk: container type and method of expression. *American Journal of Perinatology, 8*, 25–27.

Read, J. S., & Committee on Pediatric AIDS. (2003). Human milk, breastfeeding, and transmission of human immunodeficiency virus type-1 in the United States. *Pediatrics 112*, 1196–1205.

Spatz, D. L. (2004). Ten steps for promoting and protecting breastfeeding for vulnerable infants. *Journal of Perinatal & Neonatal Nursing, 18*, 385–396.

Tully, M. R., & Jones, F. (2005). *Best practice for expressing, storing, and handling human milk in hospitals, daycares, and homes.* Raleigh, NC: Human Milk Banking Association of North America.

Updegrove, K. (2005). Human milk banking in the United States. *Newborn and Infant Nursing Reviews, 5*, 27–33.

Warner, B. B., & Sapsford, A. (2004). Misappropriated human milk: Fantasy, fear and fact regarding infectious risk. *Newborn & Infant Nursing Reviews, 4*, 56–61.

CHAPTER

23

Cardiopulmonary Monitoring

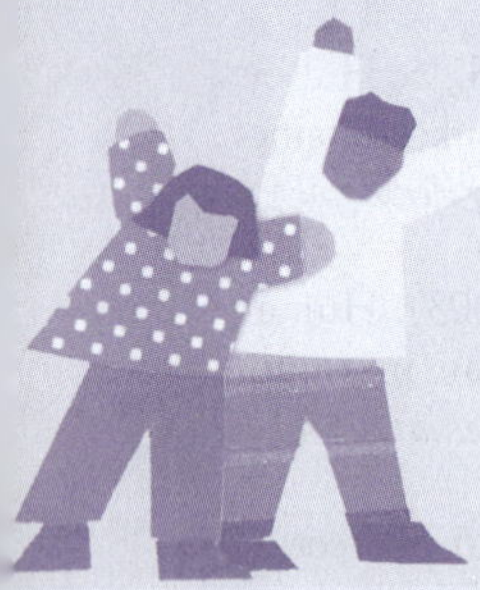

Clinical Guidelines

- Cardiopulmonary monitoring is implemented by a registered nurse (RN) or designee within institution guidelines for an acute evaluation of the child's heart rate and/or basic rhythm determination.
- A healthcare prescriber orders cardiopulmonary monitoring and the prescriber or unit policies specify frequency of assessment and alarm parameters.
- Cardiac monitoring is indicated for
  - Children in critical care areas or with known or suspected irregularities of heart or breathing patterns
  - Children who have undergone cardiac surgery
  - Children undergoing diagnostic/therapeutic procedures requiring conscious sedation or anesthesia
- All children receiving cardiopulmonary monitoring are assessed by an RN every 1 to 4 hours (per healthcare prescriber orders, unit policies, or patient status) or more frequently as indicated by the child's status. Assessment should include respiratory status, heart rate, skin color, peripheral pulse evaluation, and knowledge of child's baseline diagnosis and status.
- All children on cardiopulmonary monitoring will have appropriately sized oxygen delivery devices readily available (e.g., bag-mask, oxygen tubing, oxygen source).

Equipment

- Soap and water
- Washcloth
- Electrodes with attached wires or electrodes and cable with monitor wires
- Nonsterile gloves
- Hair clipper or blunt scissors (optional)
- Bedside oxygen delivery equipment including oxygen source, flowmeter, and bag-mask (size appropriate)

Child and Family Assessment and Preparation

- Explain purpose and demonstrate procedure on a teaching doll, taking into account the developmental age of the child.
- Assist child to feel comfortable with the equipment by having him or her feel the electrodes and touch the cables. Child may assist with placing electrodes on his or her chest.
- Explain the readout on the monitor, discuss range of age-appropriate normal values, and reinforce that alarms alert for abnormal parameters but that movement and disconnection also cause alarms.

- Explain to parents that false alarms may be common and that parents should focus on assessing and comforting child instead of assessing the monitor. If there is a change in child's status (e.g., color change, level of consciousness), the parents should notify the staff immediately.

PROCEDURE Monitoring Cardiopulmonary Status

Steps	Rationale/Points of Emphasis
1. Gather the necessary supplies. Check that cables and wires are in good condition and are connected correctly and securely.	Promotes efficient time management and provides an organized approach to the procedure.
2. Perform hand hygiene.	Reduces transmission of microorganisms.
3. Verify that monitor is plugged into an emergency power grounded plug.	Ensures that the monitor will continue to function during an emergency that affects the electricity.
4. Turn monitor on; set heart rate and respiratory alarms appropriate to age of child; silence alarm during application of electrodes.	Appropriate alarm settings minimize the number of "false" alarms.
5. Position child on his or her back. Have parents stay at bedside, if present. In an emergency situation, child may need to be placed on cardiopulmonary monitoring immediately without waiting for parental presence. Equipment and use should be explained to parents when they do arrive at child's bedside.	Electrode placement on the chest provides the most effective method of monitoring; if this area is not accessible, electrode placement may need to be modified. Parental presence will help reassure the child.
6a. Don gloves. Cleanse an area of the upper right chest, upper left chest, and abdominal area on left upper quadrant with soap and water using washcloth. 6b. Rinse well to remove soap residue. Remove gloves and dispose in appropriate receptacle.	Standard precaution to reduce transmission of microorganisms. Cleanses area and removes dead skin cells where electrodes will be placed. Soap leaves a film on the skin, interfering with contact between the electrode and the skin. Removal of body oils allows for optimum adhesion of electrodes. Skin preparation should not be used because it may decrease the transmission of impulses. **caREminder** *Alcohol should not be used on infants because their skin is sensitive and fragile. Adolescents may have chest hair that requires clipping before electrode application to facilitate electrode contact with the skin.*
7a. Place wires on electrodes and then apply electrodes (Figure 23-1); do not place directly over a bony prominence. 7b. Perform the following steps: • Remove backing from electrode. • Verify that conduction gel is moist. • Apply electrode by pressing on adhesive perimeter, not center. • Place the upper two electrodes far apart, with the path between them crossing over the heart. • Place the upper right electrode and abdominal electrode as far apart as possible. • For electrodes with attached wires: ▪ Place white wire on upper right chest. ▪ Place black wire on upper left chest. ▪ Place green/red wire on left abdomen or left thigh. • For electrodes with separate wires: ▪ Place electrodes on upper right chest, upper left chest, and left abdomen or left thigh. ▪ Clip cable wires onto electrodes, with the white wire to the upper right chest, the black wire to the upper left chest, and the green/red wire to the left abdomen or left thigh.	Snapping wires onto electrodes first prevents having to push on child's chest to connect the lead. Enhances detection of electrical impulse. Pressing on center pushes gel onto adhesive area and decreases adherence. The indicated positions enhance the monitor's capability to detect the heart rate and enhance the monitor's capability to detect the respiratory rate.

Continued

Steps	Rationale/Points of Emphasis

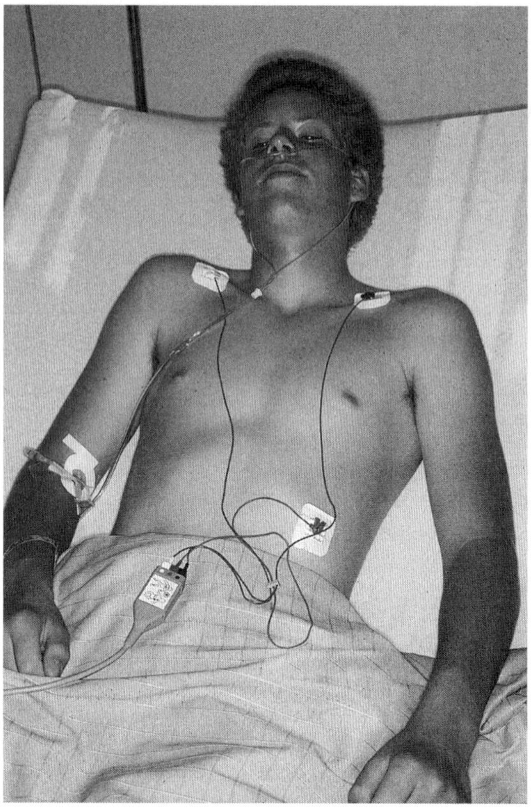

FIGURE 23-1
Electrode placement as follows: white, upper right chest; black, upper left chest; and green/red, left abdomen or left thigh.

- If child's trunk is unavailable for electrode placement:
  - Place appropriate electrode on shoulders or upper arms and abdominal electrode on thigh.

Steps	Rationale/Points of Emphasis
8a. Check monitor screen for correlating heart rate and respiratory rate. Adjust size of complex, sensitivities, and other adjustments as necessary. Leads I, II, and III are the more commonly used leads in children.	Adjustments may be needed to allow the monitor to detect the heart rate and respiratory rate correctly.
8b. Check manufacturer's manual regarding specifics on how to adjust the specific monitor.	Ensures appropriate use of equipment.
9. Verify that alarms are activated before leaving bedside and that audible tone is loud enough to alert staff.	Ensures notification when heart rate or respiratory alert rates are outside of acceptable values.
10. Perform hand hygiene.	Reduces transmission of microorganisms.
11. Inspect site daily and change electrodes as needed for infants and every 72 hours for older children and as needed. Assess skin for irritation. Rotate sites when applying new electrodes.	Conductive gel of electrodes may dry and decrease conductivity. Sensitivity to electrode gel or adhesive may cause skin breakdown.

caREminder

Use of cellular phones near external cardiopulmonary monitoring devices does not cause clinically significant interference. Researchers hypothesize that using cellular phones at a reasonable distance (at least 60 inches [1.5 meters]) from medical devices is not likely to cause serious malfunction.

TABLE 23-1

Normal ECG Parameters for Children by Age*

	0–1 d	1–3 d	3–7 d	7–30 d	1–3 mo	3–6 mo	6–12 mo	1–3 y	3–5 y	5–8 y	8–12 y	12–16 y
Heart rate/min	94–155 (122)	91–158 (122)	90–166 (128)	106–182 (149)	120–179 (149)	105–185 (141)	108–169 (131)	89–152 (119)	73–137 (109)	65–133 (100)	62–130 (91)	60–120 (80)
PR interval lead II, s	0.08–0.16 (0.107)	0.08–0.14 (0.108)	0.07–0.15 (0.102)	0.07–0.14 (0.100)	0.07–0.13 (0.098)	0.07–0.15 (0.105)	0.07–0.16 (0.106)	0.08–0.15 (0.113)	0.08–0.16 (0.119)	0.09–0.16 (0.123)	0.09–0.17 (0.128)	0.09–0.18 (0.135)
QRS interval lead V_5, s	0.02–0.07 (0.05)	0.02–0.07 (0.05)	0.02–0.07 (0.05)	0.02–0.08 (0.05)	0.02–0.08 (0.05)	0.02–0.08 (0.05)	0.03–0.08 (0.05)	0.03–0.08 (0.06)	0.03–0.07 (0.06)	0.03–0.08 (0.06)	0.04–0.09 (0.06)	0.04–0.09 (0.07)

*All values 2nd–98th percentile; numbers in parentheses are means.

Adapted from Drew, B., Califf, R., Funk, M., et al. (2005). AHA scientific statement: Practice standards for electrocardiographic monitoring in hospital settings. An American Heart Association scientific statement from the councils on cardiovascular nursing, clinical cardiology, and cardiovascular disease in the young. Endorsed by the International Society of Computerized Electrocardiology and the American Association of Critical-care Nurses. *Journal of Cardiovascular Nursing, 20*(2), 83.

CHILD AND FAMILY EVALUATION AND DOCUMENTATION

- Reinforce explanation of monitor readouts and expected ranges to child and family.
- Review with the family the nurse's response to the alarms and expected activities of nursing personnel.
- Evaluate the cardiac cycle, including heart rate, cardiac rhythm, P-wave configuration, PR interval, QRS duration, QT interval, ST segment, and T-wave configuration. Compare with age-appropriate norms (Table 23-1).
- Document the following when initiating cardiopulmonary monitoring:
  - Date and time that electrodes were applied
  - Any skin preparation performed before electrode placement
  - Where monitor alarm limits are set and that alarms are on
- Document the following when the child is on cardiopulmonary monitoring:
  - Heart rate
  - Respiratory rate
  - Quality of peripheral pulses
  - Skin color
  - Capillary refill
  - Evaluation of cardiac cycle
- Record a rhythm strip upon initiation of cardiac monitoring, every shift, and when arrhythmias are detected. Document on strip: lead, date and time, and initials. Post in medical record per institutional guidelines.
- Notify healthcare prescriber of any variations from child's normal cardiopulmonary status.

COMMUNITY CARE

- A full cardiopulmonary monitor is not typically used in the home setting; more frequently, apnea monitors are used for home monitoring.
- Instruct the family to contact the equipment vendor if equipment malfunctions or more supplies are needed.
- Instruct family to contact the healthcare provider if
  - Child is experiencing an increasing number of episodes during which the apnea monitor notes a decrease in heart rate below set parameters
  - Child requires an increase in stimulation efforts to return to baseline cardiac parameters

Unexpected Situations

- *It has been 24 hours since you applied the cardiac electrodes. You note that the waveform on the monitor is extremely weak:* The electrodes may be improperly applied or you may have wire or cable failure. Do one or more of the following: Reapply the electrodes, reset the gain so that the height of the QRS complex is more visible, try monitoring the child on another lead, and/or replace any faulty wires or cables.

- *The cardiac monitor display baseline is very fuzzy:* There may be monitor interference from other equipment in the room, improper grounding of the child's bed, or an electrode malfunction. Do one or more of the following: Ensure that all electrical equipment is attached to a common ground, check all three-pronged plugs to make sure none of the prongs is loose, ensure that the bed ground is attached to the room's common ground, and/or replace the electrodes.
- *Child has no baseline waveform:* Child is in asystole (there is no pulse); **this requires immediate initiation of basic life support and/or advanced life support protocols.** If child has a pulse, equipment malfunctions that can result in no waveform include improper electrode placement, electrodes disconnected, dry electrode gel, or wire/cable failure. Electrodes should be repositioned, replaced, or reconnected as needed. Faulty wires or cables should be replaced.

Bibliography

Drew, B., Califf, R., Funk, M., et al. (2005). AHA scientific statement: Practice standards for electrocardiographic monitoring in hospital settings. An American Heart Association scientific statement from the councils on cardiovascular nursing, clinical cardiology, and cardiovascular disease in the young. Endorsed by the International Society of Computerized Electrocardiology and the American Association of Critical-Care Nurses. *Journal of Cardiovascular Nursing, 20*(2), 76–106.

Jacobson, C. (2003). Bedside cardiac monitoring. *Critical Care Nurse, 23*(6), 71–73.

Jenkins, R. L., & Champion, V. (1999). Assessing parent apprehension related to apnea home monitoring. *Neonatal Intensive Care, 12*, 27–35.

Lund, C., Kuller, J., Lane, A., Lott, J. W., & Raines, D. A. (1999). Neonatal skin care: The scientific basis for practice. *Journal of Obstetric, Gynecologic and Neonatal Nursing, 28*, 241–254.

McKinley, M. G. (2001). Electrophysiologic monitoring: Hardwire and telemetry. In D. J. Lynn-McHale & K. K. Carlson (Eds.), *AACN procedure manual for critical care* (pp. 329–337). Philadelphia: W. B. Saunders.

Tri, J., Hayes, D., Smith, T., et al. (2001). Cellular phone interference with external cardiopulmonary monitoring devices. *Mayo Proceedings, 76*(1), 11–15.

CHAPTER 24

Cardiopulmonary Resuscitation

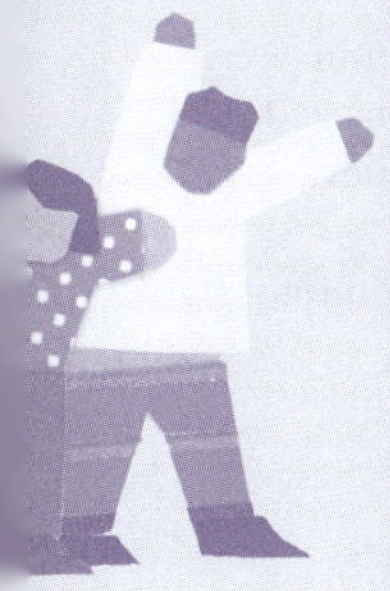

Clinical Guidelines

- All healthcare providers who are properly trained may perform cardiopulmonary resuscitation, including bag-mask ventilation and use of automated external defibrillators (AEDs).
- Cardiopulmonary resuscitation (CPR), or basic life support, is indicated in any situation in which breathing, heartbeat, or both are absent (Table 24-1).
- CPR must be initiated in all children who do not have a "do not resuscitate" (DNR) order.
- Newborn CPR guidelines are appropriate for newborns in the first hour after birth or at any time during the initial hospital admission (this time period could extend for a few days to months after the birth).
- Infant CPR guidelines are appropriate for victims younger than approximately 1 year of age.
- Child CPR guidelines are appropriate for victims from about 1 year of age to the onset of adolescence or puberty (about 12 to 14 years of age). However, the size of the child should be taken into consideration when deciding whether to use adult or child CPR techniques. Institution policy may designate the use of Pediatric Advanced Life Support Guidelines (PALS) to pediatric patients of all ages (generally up to about 16 to 18 years of age).
- For the purposes of this procedure, the term "child" is used to represent all newborn/infant/child CPR guidelines that are applicable to all three age groups. If guidelines are specific to a specific age group, this is so indicated by use of the term *newborns*, *infants*, or *children* (>1 year old).
- Age-appropriate resuscitation equipment should remain easily accessible in all areas of the healthcare facility where pediatric patients may be seen or treated.

Equipment

- Hard, flat surface, such as cardiac board or the headboard from the hospital bed
- Suction equipment
- Barrier or bag-valve mask device
- Oxygen source
- Automated external defibrillator
- Length-based resuscitation tape (eg., Broselow)
- Emergency medication and drip calculation sheet
- Emergency drugs
- Cardiac monitor and rhythm strips

TABLE 24-1

Basic Life Support Maneuvers by Healthcare Providers for Children, Infants, and Newborns

Maneuver	Child (Lay rescuers: 1 to 8 years; HCP: 1 year to adolescent)	Infant (<1 year of age)	Newborn (First hour of life or at any time during the initial hospital admission)
Activate	Activate after performing five cycles of CPR. For sudden witnessed collapse, activate after verifying the victim is unresponsive.	Same as child	Same as child
Airway	Head-tilt/chin-lift. Suspected trauma, use jaw-thrust.	Same as child	Head-tilt/chin-lift
Breathing: Initial	Two effective breaths at 1 second/breath	Same as child	Same as child
Rescue breathing without chest compressions	12–20 breaths/min (approximately 1 breath every 3–5 seconds)	Same as child	40–60 breaths/min
Ventilations during CPR with advanced airway	8–10 breaths/min (approximately 1 breath every 6–8 seconds)	Same as child	30 breaths/min
Foreign-body airway obstruction	Abdominal thrusts	Back slaps and chest thrusts	If meconium present, perform endotracheal suctioning immediately after birth only on infants who are not vigorous (strong respiratory efforts, good muscle tone and heart rate)
Circulation: Pulse check (≤10 sec)	Carotid or femoral	Brachial or femoral	Same as infant
Compression landmarks	Center of chest, between nipples	Just below nipple line (lower half of sternum)	Lower third of sternum
Compression method Push hard and fast Allow complete recoil	Two hands: Heel of one hand, with second hand on top One hand: Heel of one hand only	One rescuer: two or three fingers Two rescuers: two thumb-encircling hands	Two thumb-encircling hands
Compression depth	Approximately one third to one half the depth of the chest	Same as child	To one third of the depth of the chest
Compression rate	Approximately 100/min	Same as child	Approximately 90/min
Compression-ventilation ratio	One rescuer: 30:2 Two rescuers: 15:2	Same as child	3:1 (90 compressions and 30 breaths to achieve 120 events/min)
Defibrillation: AED	Use AED after 5 cycles of CPR (out of hospital). Use pediatric system for child 1–8 years old if available. For sudden collapse (out of hospital) or in-hospital arrest, use AED as soon as possible.	No recommendation for infants <1 year of age	No recommendation for newborns

From American Heart Association. (2005). AHA guidelines for cardiopulmonary resuscitation and emergency cardiovascular care. *Circulation, 112*, 12–18, 167–211.

- Pulse oximeter
- Nasogastric tube
- Intubation equipment
- Intravenous equipment and fluids
- Arrest documentation record

CHILD AND FAMILY ASSESSMENT AND PREPARATION

- The Pediatric Advanced Life Support (PALS) guidelines support the option of family presence during resuscitation. A person on the rescue team has a discussion with family members to determine how they would like to be involved and whether they want to be in the area in which the resuscitation efforts are being conducted.

caREminder

Family presence during invasive procedures has been demonstrated to be beneficial to the child and the participating family members. Family presence has been viewed by families as a right, obligation, and natural event.

- Assess the family's emotional needs and ensure support from an assigned volunteer, social worker, nurse, or chaplain. The patient's family should be that support person's sole focus (Chart 24-1).
- It is important to maintain frequent communication with the family during this stressful time and to allow the family to be with the child, regardless of the outcome of the resuscitation efforts.
- Optimally, the healthcare providers caring for the child will have assessed the child's clinical history and current physical status and be aware that the child is at risk for respiratory or cardiac arrest. Identified children at risk for respiratory or cardiac should be placed on a unit where access to resuscitation equipment and trained resuscitation personnel is immediately available.
- When breathlessness or pulselessness is noted, the healthcare provider should respond using "phone fast" or "phone first" guidelines:
  - *Phone fast* means to perform 1 minute of CPR before leaving the child to get help; this applies to children up to 8 years old.
  - *Phone first* means to immediately notify help and then initiate resuscitation efforts; this applies to children 8 years old and older and to children known to be at risk for ventricular fibrillation (VF) or ventricular tachycardia (VT) who experience sudden witnessed collapse.

CHART 24-1 Responsibilities of Support Staff Assigned to the Family During Resuscitation

- Discuss with family how they would like to be involved and whether they want to be present in the resuscitation room.
- Make final determination about family member's ability to be present without interference to healthcare interventions or danger to themselves (e.g., fainting).
- Establish boundaries or limits related to family member presence.
- Ensure all communication with the family from the healthcare team goes through the support staff person.
- If family members choose not to be present, support person provides ongoing updates of child's status to the family.
- Provide anticipatory guidance to the family in regards to general atmosphere, medical equipment, procedures, etc.
- Assist in debriefing the family after the resuscitation efforts are completed, whether successful or not.

PROCEDURE Assessing and Managing the Airway

Steps	Rationale/Points of Emphasis
1. Assess child's ability to respond. Gently tap the child on the shoulder to arouse him or her and loudly call for help.	Determine whether the child is sleeping or unconscious and in need of assistance. These actions may startle a conscious child.
2. If the child is unresponsive and you are alone, follow "phone fast": Start CPR immediately, continue for 1 minute, and then call for help. If the child (8 years of age or older) is unresponsive and you are alone, follow "phone first": call immediately for help and then begin CPR.	Most children arrest because of respiratory difficulties. Initiating CPR and opening the airway may be all that is necessary to revive the child. Older children may have a cardiac origin of arrest, and ensuring the quickest arrival of a defibrillator improves chance of survival.

Alert! *The "phone first" and "phone fast" sequences are applicable only when one rescuer is present. If two rescuers are present, one rescuer always stays with victim and initiates CPR while the other calls for help.*

Continued

Steps	Rationale/Points of Emphasis
3a. Place the child on a firm, flat surface, in a horizontal supine position, turning the body as a whole unit.	The child must be on his or her back for the rescuer to perform CPR. It is important to prevent movement of the head and neck when positioning the infant/child to prevent aggravation of possible neck injuries. A firm, flat surface is optimal for facilitating proper compression of the chest.
3b. If it is necessary to transport the newborn or infant in which trauma is not suspected, support the head and back with your hand and forearm. Keep your arm positioned so that the newborn's/infant's head is not above the feet.	The supine position facilitates blood flow to the brain.
4. Decide whether to open the airway with the head-tilt/chin-lift or the jaw-thrust method.	If neck or cervical spine injury is suspected, use the jaw-thrust method. **caREminder** *In an unconscious person, the tongue relaxes and falls against the back of the throat, blocking air to the lungs. Sometimes, just opening the airway is enough to get the infant or child breathing again.*
5a. To perform the head-tilt/chin-lift method, tilt the head back by gently pressing the forehead into a neutral position with the palm of your hand that is closest to the head (see "sniffing position," Figure 24-1).	Newborns and infants have small flexible airways, and hyperextending the head may occlude the airway.

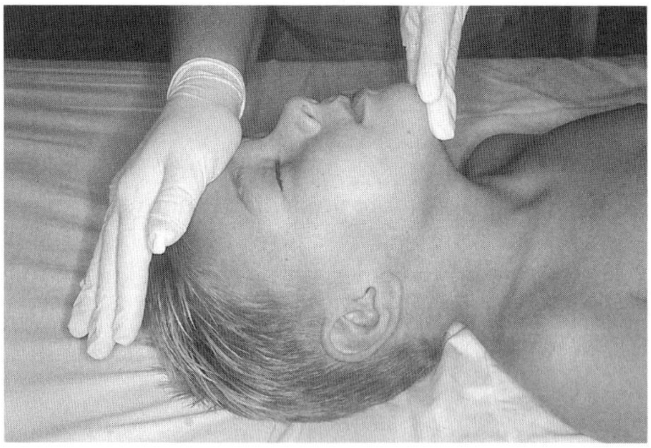

FIGURE 24-1
Head-tilt/chin-lift maneuver.

Steps	Rationale/Points of Emphasis
5b. Place your fingertips from the other hand on the bony part of the jaw near the chin and lift upward and outward.	Prevents fingers from pressing on the soft tissue under the chin and occluding the airway.
5c. If a foreign body or vomitus is visible, remove it. Use suction if available.	Do not perform a blind sweep of the mouth. This technique may push the foreign body further into the back of the throat.
6a. To perform the jaw-thrust method on infants and children (>1 year of age) who may have a neck or cervical spine injury, rest your elbows above the child's head on the hard surface and place two or three fingers under each side of the lower jaw at an angle and lift the jaw upward and outward. If a second rescuer is available, that rescuer should immobilize the spine (Figure 24-2).	This opens the airway by moving the tongue and epiglottis away from the back of the throat. **Alert!** *Do not close the mouth completely or press on the soft area under the chin. This may further occlude the airway.*
6b. If the jaw-thrust maneuver alone does not open the airway, a slight head-tilt maneuver may be added in patients with no evidence of cervical spine injury.	Minimizes the child's neck movements.
7a. To determine whether the child is breathing, place your ear near the child's mouth, face, and chest.	This enables you to feel any air movement.

Steps	Rationale/Points of Emphasis
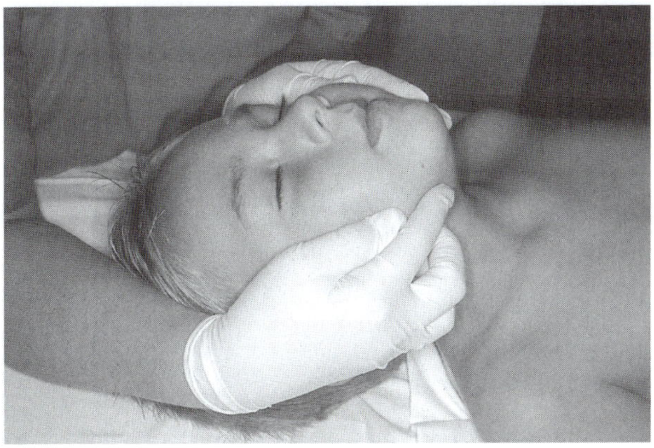 FIGURE 24-2 Jaw-thrust maneuver.	
7b. Look to see whether the chest and abdomen are moving; listen and feel for air movement from the mouth or nose.	The chest may be moving up and down, but there may not be any air movement into the lungs because of an obstruction.
7c. If the child is breathing, maintain the open airway and continue to monitor.	Giving breaths to a breathing child is unnecessary and could damage the child's respiratory tract.
7d. Check for breathing for 5–10 seconds.	Minimizes the time the child is without oxygen.
7e. Call for help.	Dial 911 to activate the EMS in your area or activate the emergency system in your institution.

PROCEDURE Implementing Rescue Breathing

Steps	Rationale/Points of Emphasis
1a. For a breathless child, use a barrier device or bag-mask and oxygen if available, delivering two slow breaths (1–1.5 seconds' duration for inspiration).	Delivering breaths provides oxygen to the child. Use a mouth-to-barrier device or bag-mask to avoid contact with body secretions.
1b. The volume of your breath should be adjusted to the size of the child.	Gastric distension may occur if the breaths are delivered too fast and the volume of air is too large for the size of the child.
1c. Watch for a normal chest rise with each breath and allow the chest to fall as the infant/child exhales between breaths.	The chest wall will rise if the breath was adequate enough to ventilate the infant/child. Pause between breaths to increase oxygen concentration and decrease carbon dioxide retention.
2a. In newborns/infants, make a seal by covering both the nose and mouth with your mouth or mask (Figures 24-3 and 24-4). Mouth-to-nose breathing is an acceptable alternative if the rescuer is unable to cover the newborn's/infant's mouth and nose simultaneously.	A complete seal must be maintained or you will not be able to ventilate the infant. Properly performed bag-mask ventilation has been shown to be an extremely safe and effective way of providing ventilation. It may be necessary to close the infant's mouth when providing mouth-to-nose breathing to prevent air from escaping.
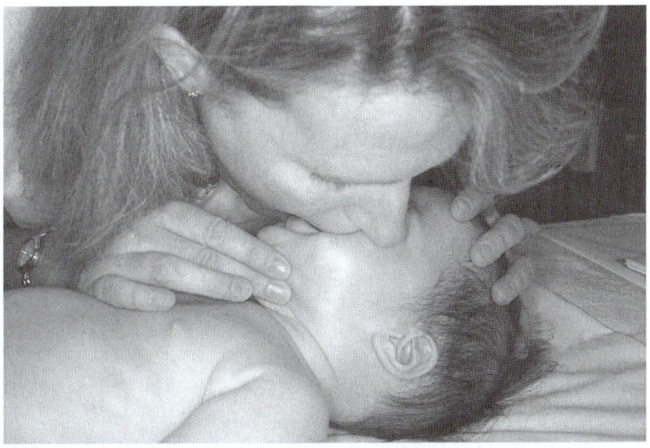 FIGURE 24-3 Infant mouth-to-nose rescue breathing.	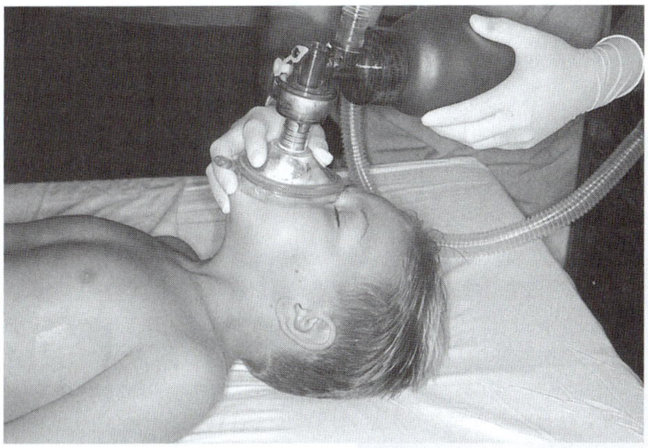 FIGURE 24-4 Use of a bag-mask to give rescue breaths.

Continued

Steps	Rationale/Points of Emphasis
2b. In children (>1 year old), use mouth-to-mouth breathing; pinch the nose and seal the mouth with your mouth (Figure 24-5). Inflate the lungs slowly.	You need to pinch the nose with your fingers or cover with the mask to prevent air from leaking. The mask must completely cover the mouth and nose without covering the eyes or chin. Note: If the child has a stoma, it may be possible to deliver breaths through the opening.

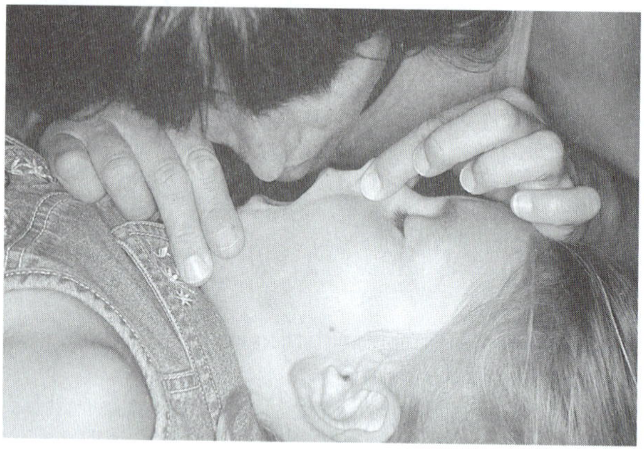

FIGURE 24-5
Child mouth-to-mouth rescue breathing.

PROCEDURE Managing Circulation

Steps	Rationale/Points of Emphasis
1. Check the pulse for 10 seconds.	
a. The brachial pulse (located on the inside of the upper arm between the elbow and shoulder) or femoral artery is used to check pulse in newborns and infants (Figure 24-6).	Newborns/infants have short necks, making it difficult to palpate the carotid artery; thus, the brachial artery is used.
b. The carotid artery (located on the side of the neck between the trachea and the sternocleidomastoid muscles) is used to check pulse in children (>1 year old) (Figure 24-7).	The carotid pulse is the most accessible pulse to find in children (>1 year old). Many healthcare providers palpate the femoral pulse in both infants and children in the hospital setting.

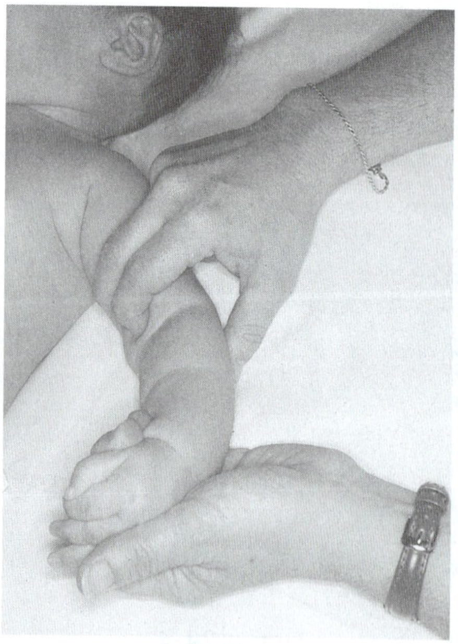

FIGURE 24-6
Palpating brachial pulse in an infant.

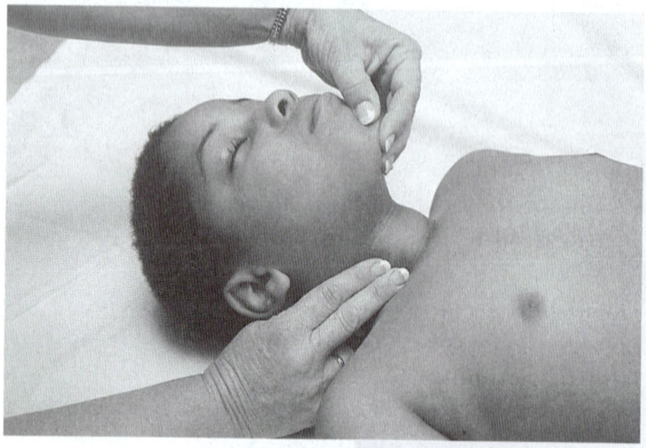

FIGURE 24-7
Palpating carotid pulse in a child.

Steps	Rationale/Points of Emphasis
2. If the pulse is present and the respirations are absent, give a breath at a rate of approximately 40 to go breaths/min for newborns and at a rate of 12 to 20 breaths/min for the infant and child (>1 year of age) as long as necessary.	Without breathing, the child will not be oxygenated, and his or her heart will soon stop. It is very important to maintain oxygenation to prevent cardiac arrest and decrease oxygen perfusion to the brain and other vital organs. This breathing rate is adequate for short-term oxygenation.
3a. If there is no pulse, you are uncertain a pulse is present, or the pulse is less than 60 beats/min with signs of poor perfusion, begin chest compressions.	If you are uncertain if a pulse is present and the child is not breathing, it is better to start chest compressions than omit them. Compressions provide blood to the vital organs, including the lungs and brain.
3b. Neonatal resuscitation should begin if the heart rate is 60 beats/min or less for more than 30 seconds despite adequate ventilation with supplementary oxygen for 30 seconds and stopped when the heart rate is >60 beats/min.	Prompt treatment of asphyxia can prevent tissue hypoxia, acidosis, poor cardiac function, and cardiac arrest.
3c. Place the child on a firm, flat surface.	Facilitates the effectiveness of compressions.
3d. Children (>1 year old) with no signs of circulation should be placed on an AED or cardiac monitor/defibrillator/pacer if available.	Children (>1 year old) are at greater risk of cardiac arrhythmia as the primary cause of cardiopulmonary arrest.
4. Perform newborn chest compressions (Figure 24-8).	
a. The two-thumb, encircling hands technique should be implemented to perform compressions. Place both thumbs side by side on the lower third of sternum and encircle the chest with your hands. Press straight down to a depth of one third the depth (anterior-posterior diameter) of the chest.	Proper placement facilitates adequate cardiac output and minimizes chances for injuries to the sternum and ribs. The chest of a newborn is smaller and more flexible than that of adults and does not require as much pressure to compress.
b. Compression with two fingers just below the nipple line with a second hand supporting the back may be used.	Data show that the two-thumb, encircling hands technique is recommended because this technique can provide better blood flow than two-finger compressions.
c. Release the pressure and allow the chest to expand fully.	Allows the heart time to refill.
d. Keep fingers in contact with the chest.	Maintains proper positioning and minimizes injury to the sternum and ribs.
e. Give rescue breaths at a 3:1 compression ventilation ratio (30 breaths/min). Each breath should take 2 seconds for inspiration in newborns, with exhalation occurring during the first compression after each ventilation.	Provides oxygen to the newborn.
f. Watch for normal chest rise while delivering a breath.	Ensures adequate ventilation of the newborn.
g. Compression rate is 90/min for newborns.	Provides perfusion to vital organs.
h. After 1 minute of CPR or 120 events (90 compressions and 30 breaths), stop for 5 seconds to recheck the pulse.	Determines whether there is a pulse present or if you need to continue CPR.
i. Call for help if alone.	The sooner the child can receive further treatment, the better are his or her chances of recovery.
j. If you must leave the child to get help, position the child on his or her side if there is no evidence of neck or back injury.	Prevents aspiration and helps keep the airway open.
k. Once calling for help has been initiated, if there is still not a pulse present, resume 3:1 cycles in newborn of compressions and ventilations.	Allows for oxygenation and ventilation at the proper ratios to maintain optimal recovery.
l. Repeat pulse check every few minutes and then continue CPR as indicated.	Determines resumption of spontaneous breathing and circulation and whether you need to continue CPR.

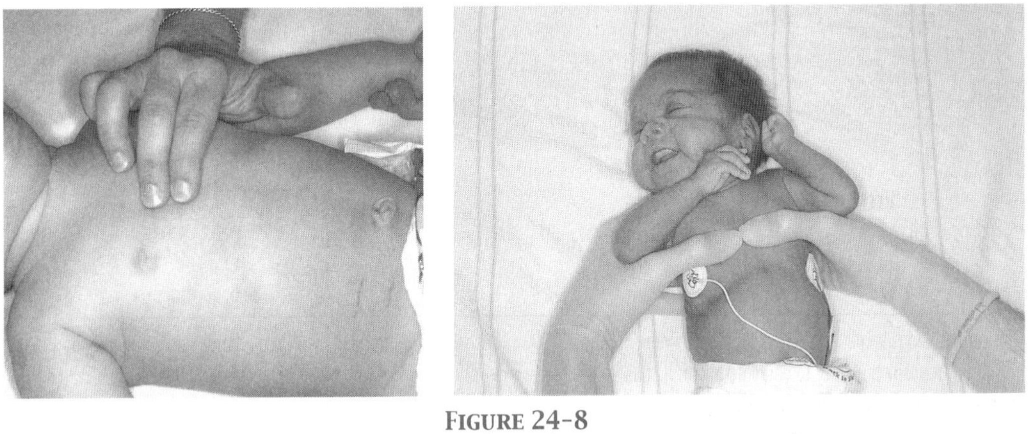

FIGURE 24-8
Locating proper finger position for cardiac compressions on an infant.

Continued

Steps	Rationale/Points of Emphasis
5. Perform infant chest compressions.	
a. For one rescuer, compress with two or three fingers just below the nipple line (lower half of the sternum). Press straight down to a depth of one third to one half the depth of the chest.	Proper placement facilitates adequate cardiac output and minimizes chances for injuries to the sternum and ribs. The chest of an infant is smaller and more flexible than that of adults and does not require as much pressure to compress.
b. For two rescuers, the two-thumb, encircling hands technique should be implemented to perform compressions. Place both thumbs side by side on the lower third of sternum and encircle the chest with your hands.	Most effective method of providing cardiac output.
c. Release the pressure and allow the chest to expand fully.	Allows the heart time to refill.
d. Keep fingers in contact with the chest.	Maintains proper positioning and minimizes injury to the sternum and ribs.
e. Give two rescue breaths. Each breath should take 1 second for inspiration (8–10 breaths/min) in infants.	Provides oxygen to the newborn.
f. Watch for normal chest rise while delivering a breath.	Ensures adequate ventilation of the infant.
g. Compression rate is 100/min for infant.	Provides perfusion to vital organs.
h. After 1 minute of CPR, stop for 5 seconds to recheck the pulse.	Determines whether there is a pulse present or whether you need to continue CPR.
i. Call for help if alone.	The sooner the child can receive further treatment, the better are his or her chances of recovery.
j. If you must leave the child to get help, position the child on his or her side if there is no evidence of neck or back injury.	Prevents aspiration and helps keep the airway open.
k. Once calling for help has been initiated, if there is still not a pulse present, resume 30:2 (single rescuer) or 15:2 (two rescuers) cycle of compressions and ventilations.	Allows for oxygenation and ventilation at the proper ratios to maintain optimal recovery.
l. Repeat pulse check every few minutes and then continue CPR as indicated.	Determines resumption of spontaneous breathing and circulation and whether you need to continue CPR.
6. Perform child (>1 year old) chest compressions (Figure 24-9).	
a. Place the heel of one hand over the lower half of the sternum between the nipples. Avoid compressing the xiphoid process.	Proper placement facilitates adequate cardiac output and minimizes chances for injuries to the sternum and ribs.
b. Press straight down to a depth of one third to one half the depth of the chest.	The chest of a child is smaller and more flexible than that of an adult and does not require as much pressure to compress.
c. Complete steps 5c through 5l. These steps are the same for the infant and the child.	
7. During the compression–ventilation cycle, if unable to ventilate the newborn/infant, reposition and try to ventilate again. If still unable, the airway may be obstructed with a foreign body.	Repositioning the head may be all that is necessary to open the airway.

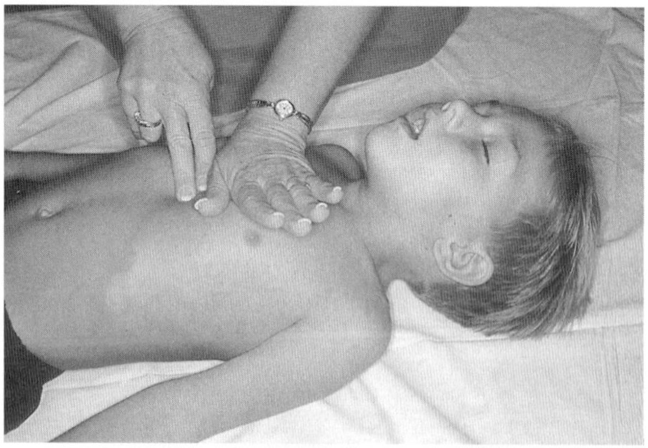

FIGURE 24-9
Locating proper hand placement for cardiac compression on a child.

Steps	Rationale/Points of Emphasis
8. For an obstructed airway in an infant (Figure 24-10):	
a. If a newborn's or infant's airway is obstructed with a foreign body, use a combination of five back slaps and five chest thrusts to dislodge the foreign body.	Chest thrusts are used to avoid trauma to the abdomen and internal organs.
b. For back slaps, place the newborn/infant on your forearm face down with head slightly lower than chest and his or her legs straddling your elbow.	The head should be lower than the chest so that the foreign body will move toward the mouth if dislodged.
c. The neck and head are supported by resting the chin in the curve between your thumb and index finger.	Remember to support the head and neck, especially if a head or neck injury is suspected.
d. Use the heel of your hand to deliver up to five forceful slaps to the infant's back between the shoulder blades.	Helps dislodge the foreign body.
e. Place the hand that you used for the back slaps behind the newborn's/infant's head and neck with your wrist and arm extending down the back. Turn the newborn/infant, carefully supporting the head and neck and rest your arm on your thigh with the newborn/infant slightly head down.	Ensures that the newborn's/infant's body remains in proper alignment and allows you to turn the body as a whole.
f. Use two fingers on the lower third of the sternum to apply up to five quick downward chest thrusts at a rate of one per second.	Chest thrusts are similar to chest compressions. Chest thrusts produce an "artificial cough" to dislodge the foreign body.
g. Remove the foreign body if you can see it. Do not perform a blind finger sweep.	Blind finger sweeps can further lodge the foreign body in the airway.

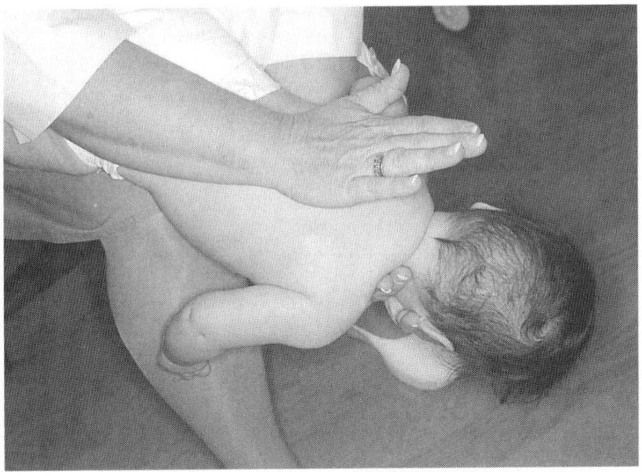

FIGURE 24-10
Technique to clear the airway in an infant.

Steps	Rationale/Points of Emphasis
9. During the compression–ventilation cycle, if unable to ventilate the child (>1 year old), reposition and try to ventilate again. If still unable, the airway may be obstructed with a foreign body (Figure 24-11).	
a. Make sure that the child is positioned on his or her back on a firm, flat surface.	A firm, flat surface facilitates the abdominal thrusts.
b. Grasp the child's lower jaw and lift away from the back of the throat. Depress the tongue with your thumb. If an object is visible, remove it. Do not do a blind finger sweep.	Allows a better view into the mouth and back of the throat so you can remove the foreign object if visible.
c. Open the airway with a head-tilt/chin-lift and attempt to give rescue breaths. If unable, reposition and reattempt ventilation.	Inability to provide rescue breaths confirms airway is obstructed.
d. Kneel down and straddle the child's legs.	Helps locate the proper position for your hands.
e. Place one hand directly over the other and place the heel of your hand in the middle of the abdomen a little above the navel.	Do not place the hands too high and cover the xiphoid or ribs because this may result in injuries.
f. Press quickly inward and upward into the abdomen toward the head five times in rapid succession.	The pressure of the abdominal thrusts may dislodge the foreign body.

Continued

Steps	Rationale/Points of Emphasis
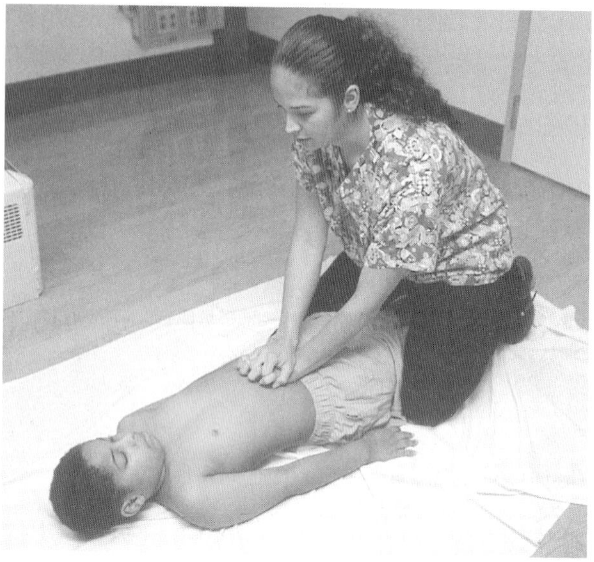 **FIGURE 24-11** Clearing obstructed airway in unconscious child lying on the ground.	
g. Foreign-body checks should be performed before delivering another breath.	The foreign body may have become dislodged by previous actions and if not removed may be pushed back by subsequent breaths.
h. Repeat sequence until object is expelled or rescue breaths are effective.	Foreign body may take more than one attempt to dislodge.
i. Once effective breaths are delivered, proceed with CPR sequence. If child demonstrates adequate breathing and circulation, place in the recovery position.	Ensures breathing and circulation are present.
10. For an obstructed airway in a conscious infant/child (>1 year old) (Figure 24-12)	
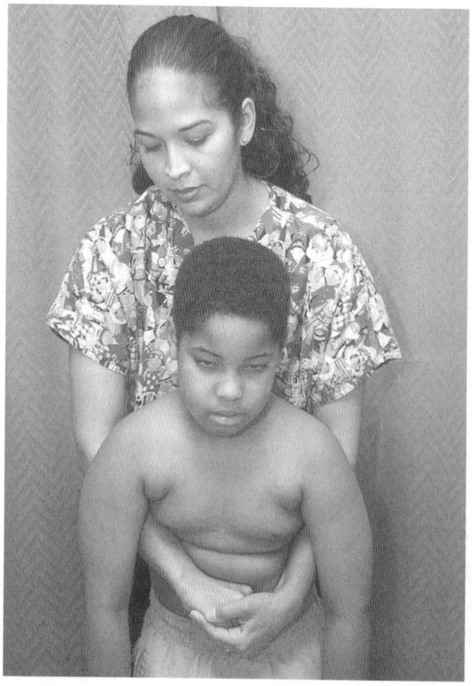 **FIGURE 24-12** Clearing obstructed airway in conscious child standing with support.	

Steps	Rationale/Points of Emphasis
a. Do not interfere if the child can cough forcefully, can respond when asked if he or she is choking, or if an infant can cry.	Infants/children (>1 year old) may be able to clear the airway with no interventions. Make sure that you stay with them until they can breathe normally or become unconscious, and then follow the procedure for the unconscious infant/child. Stay with the infant or child. Do not leave the room until the airway is clear. If the infant/child lapses into total airway obstruction, initiate sequence for breathing and circulation in the resuscitation cycle (see above)
11. For a conscious child (>1 year old), use the Heimlich maneuver. a. Stand or kneel behind child and place arms under the child's axillae and encircle the chest. b. Place the thumb side of one fist midline on the abdomen above the navel and below the xiphoid process. c. Grasp the fist with the other hand and thrust inward and up quickly five times. d. Continue doing series of five thrusts until a foreign object is expelled or child becomes unconscious.	**KidKare** The Heimlich maneuver for children is the same as for adults except less force is used for the thrusts. Do not touch the xiphoid process or lower rib cage to prevent damage to internal organs.
12a. Perform ongoing resuscitation efforts and stabilization of the child. Use Broselow tape and emergency medication and drip calculation sheets to guide calculations for ongoing resuscitative efforts.	Use of precalculated medication sheets prevents medication dosage errors. The Broselow tape can be used to calculate endotracheal tube sizes, amount of fluid for volume replacement, and drug dosages as needed.
12b. Frequent assessment and reassessment of cardiac and respiratory function must be performed to monitor for symmetric chest expansion, equal breath sounds, oxygenation, carbon dioxide elimination, color, and perfusion.	Detects deterioration of child's status promptly.
12c. Automated external defibrillation may be used in the treatment of cardiac arrest in children (>1 year old).	Pediatric ventricular fibrillation (VF) may be more common than previously suspected. Early defibrillation of VF and pulseless ventricular tachycardia (VT) are important and highly successful treatment measures. Ideally, the rescuer should use a pediatric dose-attenuating system.
12d. As soon as possible, the child should be transferred to an area with staff who are skilled in techniques that are required to continue advanced life support.	Staff specially trained in caring for pediatric emergencies is necessary in providing continued evaluation, stabilization, and treatment.
12e. The child should be placed on a cardiac/apnea monitor and an oximeter.	The pulse oximeter is a noninvasive technique used to measure arterial saturation and heart rate. The oxygen saturation reading may not be reliable if the heart rate does not correlate with the cardiac monitor or if the infant's/child's perfusion is poor.
12f. Continue to maintain normal ventilation without hyperventilation using bag-mask ventilation and compressions at the appropriate ratios.	Provides oxygenation for the vital organs. Bag-mask ventilation has been shown to be highly safe and effective. **Alert!** *Hyperventilation is not recommended to be used routinely. Hyperventilation reduces cerebral blood flow and may create cerebral ischemia.*
12g. Stabilization of the airway may require intubation and mechanical ventilation (see Chapters 59 and 126).	Tracheal intubation should be performed only by a healthcare provider who is well trained in and has frequently practiced this skill.
12h. Circulatory support is provided once IV access has been established. Fluids and emergency medications may then be administered.	Infants/children (>1 year old) in arrest are often hypovolemic and require rapid fluid boluses of isotonic crystalloid solution at a dose of 20 mL/kg. Several large-bore IV lines should be placed as rapidly as possible.
12i. If unable to insert a peripheral IV, an intraosseous line (IO) may be inserted for infants and children (see Chapter 65 for information on intraosseous infusions).	An IO line is a reliable route to infuse fluids, drugs, and blood products. There is no upper age limit on who can receive an intraosseous access route.
12j. If still unable to provide IV assess, several emergency medications can be given into the endotracheal tube. Epinephrine, atropine, naloxone, and lidocaine may be given by this route (see Chapter 62 for information on endotracheal medication administration).	A syringe can be attached to a suction catheter and then inserted into the endotracheal tube to ensure that the medication reached the end of the tube.

Continued

Steps	Rationale/Points of Emphasis
12k. All efforts should be made to maintain or provide a neutral thermal state.	Evidence suggests that mild hypothermia reduces damage from an ischemic insult, particularly when the hypothermia preceded the insult. Hyperthermia increases oxygen demand and should be corrected. Infants and children have a large surface area and less subcutaneous tissue and brown fat stores, which contributes to a decreased ability to produce heat. Infants have an immature nervous system that delays their response to thermal stress.
12l. Assess glucose levels to ensure that normal levels are maintained.	Hyperglycemia or hypoglycemia can have detrimental effects on the child, and alterations must be detected immediately.
12m. Perform brief neurologic examination to include level of consciousness and pupillary response.	Obtains baseline after arrest. Without sufficient cardiac output to provide oxygen, the brain will sustain injury.
13. Maintain ongoing resuscitation efforts as directed by the healthcare prescriber	Ongoing assessments and interventions will likely be necessary to ensure optimal health outcomes for the child.

CHILD AND FAMILY EVALUATION AND DOCUMENTATION

- Evaluate child's response to resuscitation efforts.
- Evaluate family's understanding of the situation, the need for resuscitation measures, the options for resuscitation (e.g., advance directives, DNR), and understanding of outcomes after resuscitation efforts.
- Documentation should be completed on an arrest record to include
  - Ongoing time documentation of events
  - Vital signs
  - Medications administered
  - Treatments
  - Responses to all resuscitation measures
  - Personnel present
  - Cardiac rhythm strips
- Document parental presence during procedure, noting supportive personnel to assist parents and parental response to resuscitation efforts.

COMMUNITY CARE

- All parents of newborns/infants discharged from a special care or neonatal unit and families with infants and children at risk for cardiopulmonary arrest should receive CPR instructions before discharge.
- Children who experience cardiopulmonary arrest in a community setting should be transported immediately to a healthcare facility for ongoing support and evaluation.
- Instruct family to call 911 if the child experiences loss of respirations or consciousness or if a heartbeat is not noted. Use the phone fast/phone first guidelines, depending on the child's age and any underlying medical conditions.

Unexpected Situation

- *During the resuscitation efforts, the parent, who is standing in back of the room, faints:* Optimally a family facilitator should be assigned to the family members at all times. If the facilitator is present, the team should not disrupt their resuscitative efforts and the family member should be attended to by the assigned facilitator. Removing the family member from the room as soon as possible provides optimal safety of the family member and of others in the room whose efforts to have access to the child may be impaired by the ill parent. If a family facilitator is not present, a member of the resuscitation team should assist the parent and/or retrieve an individual to assist the parent. The goal is to maintain an environment that is focused on treating the child and is free from overcrowding, impediments, and distractions.

Bibliography

American Heart Association. (2005). AHA guidelines for cardiopulmonary resuscitation and emergency cardiovascular care. *Circulation, 112*, 12–18, 167–211.

American Heart Association & American Academy of Pediatrics. (2006). 2005 American Heart Association guidelines for cardiopulmonary resuscitation (CPR) and emergency cardiovascular care (ECC) of pediatric and neonatal patients: Neonatal resuscitation guidelines. *Pediatrics, 117*(5), e1029–e1038.

Bauchner, H., Vinci, R., Bak, S., Pearson, C., & Corwin, M. (1996). Parents and procedures: A randomized controlled trial. *Pediatrics, 98*(5), 861–867.

Eppich, W., & Arnold, L. (2003). Family member presence in the pediatric emergency department. *Current Options in Pediatrics, 15*, 294–298.

Linder, C., Suddaby, E., & Moweey, B. (2004). Parental presence during resuscitation: Help or hindrance? *Pediatric Nursing, 30*(2), 126–127, 148.

McGahey, P. R. (2002). Family presence during pediatric resuscitation: A focus on staff. *Critical Care Nurse, 22*(6), 29–34.
Meyers, T., Eichhorn, D., Guzzetta, C., et al. (2004). Family presence during invasive procedures and resuscitation. *Topics in Emergency Medicine, 26*(1), 61–73.
Nibert, L., & Ondrejka, D. (2005). Family presence during pediatric resuscitation: An integrative review for evidence based-practice. *Journal of Pediatric Nursing, 20*(2), 145–147.
O'Brien, M. M., Creamer, K. M., Hill, E. E., & Welham, J. (2002). Tolerance of family presence during pediatric cardiopulmonary resuscitation: A snapshot of military and civilian pediatricians, nurses, and residents. *Pediatric Emergency Care, 18*(6), 409–413.
Samson, R. A., Berg, R. A., Bingham, R., et al. (2003). Use of automated external defibrillators for children: An update: An advisory statement from the Pediatric Advanced Life Support Task Force, International Liaison Committee on Resuscitation. *Circulation, 107*, 3250–3255.
Wiswell, T. (2003). Neonatal resuscitation. *Respiratory Care, 48*(3), 288–295.

CHAPTER

25

Cast Care

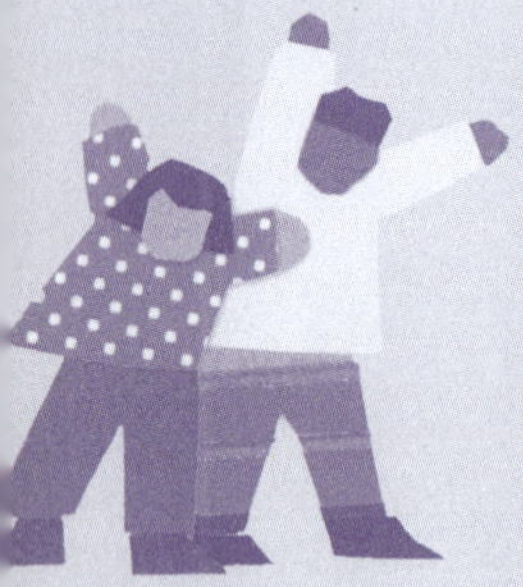

Clinical Guidelines

- The type of cast applied is determined by the physician. The registered nurse (RN) or licensed practical nurse (LPN) is responsible for daily care and management of the child in a cast.
- Assess neurovascular status every 4 hours for the first 48 hours after the application of a cast.
- Assess skin integrity every shift.
- Assess for pain every 2 to 4 hours during the acute phase and with vitals thereafter.
- Assess integrity and cleanliness of the cast every shift.

Equipment

- Nonsterile gloves (if indicated)
- Pillows or blankets
- Cold packs
- Pain medication
- Cloth tape or moleskin
- Blow dryer
- Diapers
- Sanitary napkins
- Plastic wrap
- Marking pencil
- Flashlight
- Baking soda
- Toothpaste or dry white cleanser
- Diversionary activities
- Crutches, sling, cast shoes, or wheelchair (if ordered)

Child and Family Assessment and Preparation

- Review chart to determine
  - The type of surgical or medical intervention completed on the child
  - History of increased temperature or heart rate. Elevations may indicate an infectious process is present.
  - Pain history and when child was last medicated for pain
- Determine the type of cast, style, and type of material used to make the cast (Figure 25-1).
- Assess child's vital signs to determine presence of fever or increased respiratory rate or heart rate that may indicate presence of infection.
- Assess child for pain and muscle spasms and provide interventions as indicated (see Chapter 7).

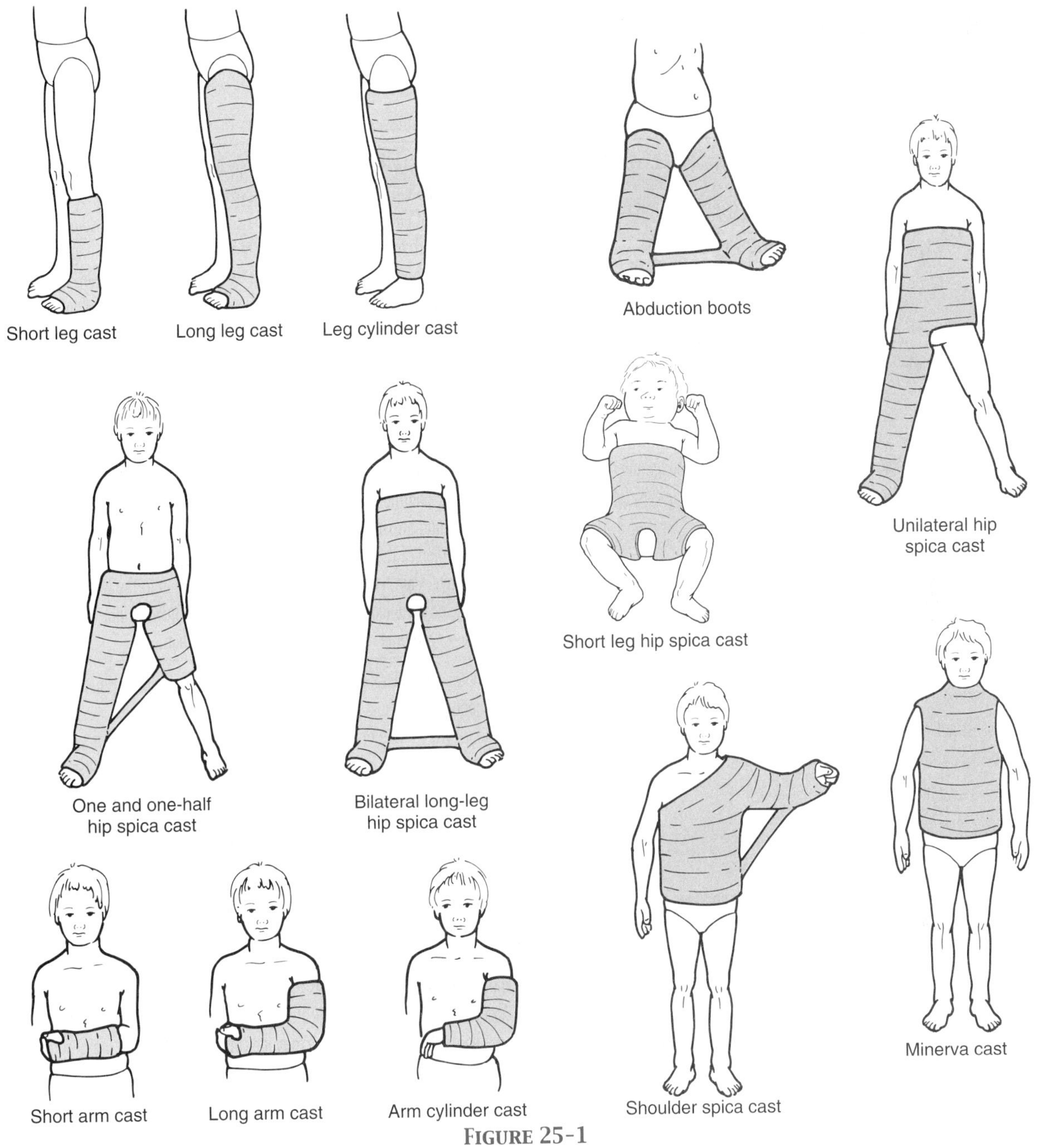

FIGURE 25-1
Types of casts.

- Administer pain medication when indicated 30 minutes before moving or assessing the patient.
- Use diversional activities and other nonpharmacologic interventions (e.g., music, stroking of unaffected extremities) to distract the child and assist in pain management during the procedure.
- Explain to the child the purpose of checking the cast and assessing the integrity of the skin and extremities near the cast.
- Encourage parents to be in the room during cast care to assist them in learning to complete care and assessment in preparation for discharge of the child to home.

PROCEDURE Cast Care and Assessment

Steps	Rationale/Points of Emphasis
1. Perform hand hygiene. Don gloves if necessary.	Reduces transmission of microorganisms.
2a. Assess the child for pain using an age-appropriate measure.	Pain assessment is completed concurrently with all other assessments to determine if palpation and movement of the extremity elicit verbal and nonverbal indications of pain. Age-appropriate measures are needed to ensure reliability of data acquired. Some pain at fracture site is normal. Pain or burning sensation distal to the fracture may be associated with tissue ischemia. Pain on passive movement may indicate compartment syndrome, a condition that involves the compression of nerves and blood vessels within an enclosed space. This leads to impaired blood flow and muscle and nerve damage. Extreme pain, especially on passive motion, is the most significant subjective sight of probable neurovascular deficiency of the extremity. The pain usually becomes more severe even with the use of narcotics.
2b. Use pharmacologic and nonpharmacologic pain management interventions (see Chapter 7).	Pain management techniques should not be limited to a single intervention. Combining pharmacologic relief with measures such as distraction, position changes, and massage will provide the most effective pain relief. Cold therapy and elevation of the extremity can reduce pain, especially after the child has been active. Pain that is progressive, out of proportion to the type of injury, or not relieved by analgesia or with ice and elevation may be indicative of compartment syndrome and requires immediate attention.
3a. Perform neurovascular assessment (see Chapter 77).	Promotes early identification of and intervention to compromised circulation and oxygenation of tissues.
3b. Assess pulses above and below the injured area.	Gradual weakening or absent pulse may indicate compartment syndrome. Absence of pulse is a late symptom. Subtle nagging change will often indicate an impending complication at its earliest stage. Neurovascular impairment is most often caused by pressure on the nerve or vascular supply to an extremity. Assessment of both extremities will give a baseline for comparison.
3c. Assess capillary refill by pressing on fingers and toes and observing time of capillary refill.	Normal capillary refill is 1 to 2 seconds. A delayed capillary refill may indicate insufficient circulation to the distal extremity and/or compartment syndrome. Greater than 3 seconds is indicative of inadequate arterial supply. A cool room may cause the fingers and toes to be cool to the touch.
3d. Determine sensation of extremities by gently touching the fingers and toes and by asking the child if he or she feels the sensation of your touch. Describe responses as absent, impaired, or normal.	Absence of sensation may indicate swelling beneath the cast or signs of a pressure sore. Changes in sensation may indicate paresthesia and are a sign of compartment syndrome. If a child's nerves are intact, he or she should feel your touch at areas of innervation above and below the injury. **KidKare** For the younger child, play a game like "Simon Says" to assess toe and finger sensation and mobility.
3e. Assess motor function by having child move the fingers and toes. Direct the child to demonstrate flexion, extension, abduction, and adduction, if possible.	Motion distal to the fracture would be documented as normal range of motion, impaired, or absent. Pain during motor function activities is also noted. Muscle weakness may be caused by pressure within the muscle compartment and may result in loss of movement. With nerve damage comes the loss of sensation and loss of motion, which can damage muscle tissue. After 4 to 12 hours of ischemia, permanent and irreversible muscle damage can occur.
4a. Perform skin assessment.	Promotes early identification of and interventions to disruptions to skin integrity.

Steps	Rationale/Points of Emphasis
4b. Assess and compare the color and temperature on both limbs; be sure to check above and below the injury site.	Skin that looks shiny and stretched or muscles that appear taut and bulging may indicate compartment syndrome. Tightness of the compartment may be experienced by the child and may also be palpated upon examination. Temperature of a limb may be affected by a cool room or decreased body temperature, vasoconstriction, or peripheral edema. A pale or white skin color may indicate inadequate arterial supply to the area.
4c. Assess swelling of fingers or toes distal to fracture or surgical site.	Swelling peaks within 24 to 48 hours. Swelling in the extremity may be indicative of inadequate venous return. Delay in attending to swelling, even for as little as 4 to 6 hours, can lead to compartment syndrome and full or partial paralysis.
4d. Assess skin areas around cast edges every shift for irritation, rash, or skin breakdown.	Area around cast edges can break down because of rubbing on rough edges of cast.
4e. Assess skin integrity over bony prominences for redness, tingling, and sensation.	Areas over the buttocks, back, and elbows are most vulnerable for any signs of skin irritation. Signs and symptoms of pressure sores include a burning sensation or pain, local heat, odor, staining through the cast, and pyrexia.
5a. Implement interventions to promote skin integrity as indicated.	Prevents skin breakdown.
5b. Petal cast edges with cloth tape or moleskin if they are rough (Figure 25-2). • Cut several strips of adhesive tape or moleskin 3 to 4 inches in length. Use 1-inch tape for smaller areas (e.g., adolescent's waist). • Round one end of each strip to keep the corners from rolling. • Apply the first strip by tucking the straight end inside the cast and by bringing the rounded end over the cast edge to the outside. • Repeat the procedure, overlapping each additional strip, until all rough edges are completely covered.	Decreases skin irritation and protects edges of casts from excessive wear. Tape or moleskin should not used on a fiberglass cast because they are unlikely to adhere for any significant length of time.

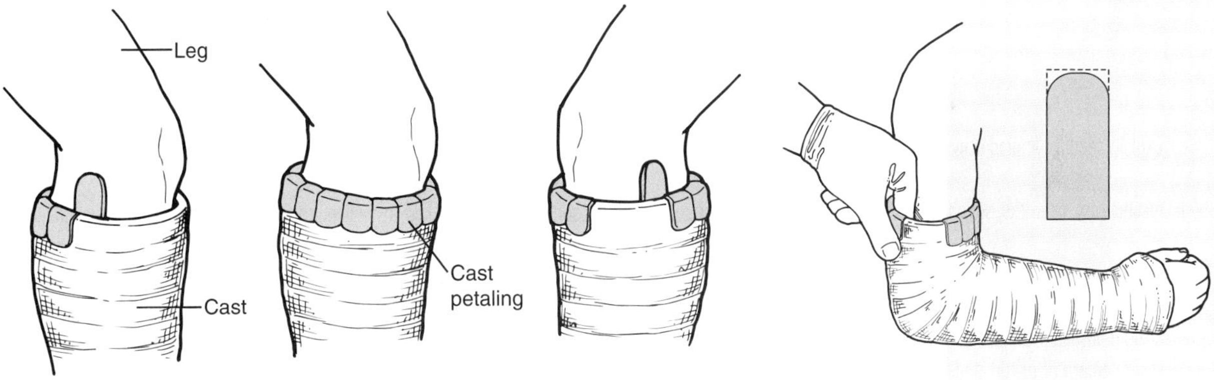

FIGURE 25-2
Petaling a cast.

Steps	Rationale/Points of Emphasis
5c. If itching occurs, instruct the child to use one of the following techniques to relieve the itching: • Blow cool air from a blow dryer into the cast • Rub the skin around the cast edges • Rub the opposite arm or leg • Tap on the cast over the itchy areas	The child should never put anything down the cast to try to scratch an area because these objects may become stuck underneath the cast.
5d. Provide daily tub bath or sponge bath. Wash fingers or toes near the cast with a damp washcloth.	Keeps accessible skin areas clean and may decrease skin irritation and itching.
5e. Provide peritoneal care for children with casts extending close to genital area.	The casted area around the genital area is at high risk for contamination with urine and feces.

Continued

Steps	Rationale/Points of Emphasis
5f. Use measures to protect cast from urine and feces. Place diapers under the cast edges and change the diaper every 1 to 2 hours while awake. At night, a sanitary napkin can be placed inside the diaper for more absorbency. Plastic wrap may be taped to the edge of the cast around the genital area to protect the cast.	In the young child, this area can become contaminated by urine and feces if care is not taken. A wet cast will irritate the skin, soften, and fail to hold the leg and hip in the correct position. For the infant, a one-piece T-shirt with snaps in the crotch can be used to hold diapers in place. **caREminder** *Do not cut a diaper to make it fit the groin opening of the cast; the raw edges of the diaper give off debris that can get under the cast and irritate the skin.*
6a. Assess integrity of the cast.	A cast that is not intact may impair healing.
6b. Expose wet cast to room air to dry, elevating cast on pillows up to 4 inches above the level of the heart, handling the cast with only the palms of the hands.	Plaster casts take 24 to 48 hours to dry. Synthetic casts dry within 30 to 60 minutes. The larger and thicker the cast, the longer the drying time. Soft flexible surfaces protect the cast from heat entrapment and from becoming dented or flattened and thereby prevent pressure on bony prominences. Ensure pillows are not covered in a rubber or plastic material. Placing the newly applied cast on disposable pillows allows the heat to dissipate and allows the cast to air dry. High elevation of the limb can be harmful in some circumstances (such as compartment syndrome). An elevation of 4 inches is unlikely to interfere with oxygenation unless the circulation is fragile. **KidKare** Having the child sit in a chair with his or her leg resting on a stool does not provide for adequate elevation of the leg above the heart. Using a bean bag chair with the injured leg elevated 4 inches above the level of the heart provides a comfortable seating alternative for the child.
6c. Explain need for limited activity while the cast dries.	Angles of the cast must be maintained during the drying process to prevent pressure on bony prominences.
6d. Inspect cast for cracks, softening, excessive flaking, or flattening.	A soft, flaking, or cracked cast will not give the needed support to maintain alignment of the fracture. Flaking and flattening of the cast can cause skin irritation and undue pressure on bony prominences.
6e. Inspect cast for signs of drainage or odor from wound underneath cast, using a flashlight as needed to view the areas more effectively. Mark the circumference of the drainage on the cast.	After a surgical procedure, drainage may occur. Drainage or odors may be indicative of infection or item under cast. Blood loss will stain a plaster cast. Marking the circumference provides a baseline parameter for future assessments. ***Alert!*** ***If the cast is synthetic, blood loss may not be apparent because of the nonabsorbent properties of the material. In this case, oozing may pool at the operative site or may not be present until it appears at the extremities of the cast.***
6f. Apply sodium bicarbonate (baking soda) to an odoriferous cast. Odor eaters can be taped to the cast to keep down odors.	Baking soda will help absorb body odors on cast.
6g. Check to see that the cast is not too tight by running your finger inside the cast.	Neurovascular compromise, skin breakdown, and malalignment can occur if the cast is not fitting properly. A well-fitted cast has approximately a finger's width of clearance between the cast and the child's skin.

Steps	Rationale/Points of Emphasis
6h. Clean the surface of the cast as needed. A cast made of plaster may be cleaned with a small amount of toothpaste or dry white cleanser on a slightly dampened cloth. Dry it with a hair dryer set on cool. Fiberglass casts can be cleaned with a damp cloth.	Keeps cast appearance clean. Use of a hair dryer on a hot setting can burn the skin.
6i. Instruct child not to put items down the cast and not to scratch under the cast with an object. ***Alert!*** *Do not put anything inside the cast. Do not use hangers, knitting needles, pens, pencils, or any other object to scratch under the cast. Do not put powder down a cast because it will become moist and pasty inside the confines of the cast.*	Items caught under the cast can lead to pressure sores.
7. Assist child to perform passive and active range of motion of all extremities at least every shift (see Chapter 101).	Prevents weakness in extremities and stiffness of joints. Assists to maintain functional ability of the extremities. With immobilization, there can be loss of muscle strength of up to 3% per day. Passive and active range-of-motion exercises should be completed three or four times a day. Exercises could include wiggling fingers/toes, bending elbow/knee, and moving the shoulders/hips.
8. Assist child to ambulate by the use of a walker, crutches, or walking boot. The walking boot should be worn during waking hours.	Children in casts should be encouraged to be up and out of bed once the cast has dried and pain is well managed. Some leg casts are made for weight bearing so that the child may walk with or without crutches. **KidKare** Reclining wheelchairs can be used to accommodate the child in a spica cast. Wagons can be used for smaller children to make them more mobile.
9. Collaborate with the technician to provide teaching about crutch walking to the child. ***Alert!*** *Do not allow the child or another person to lift, kick, or hit anything with the cast. The cast must be handled carefully because it can be cracked or chipped. Extreme or forceful movements of the cast may cause injury to the already impaired limb.*	Crutch teaching assists the child to learn correct method for using the equipment.
10. Provide diversional activities for the child on limited activity.	Activity level needs to be adjusted to the developmental level of the child.
11a. Position the child for comfort.	A limb in a cast will weigh more and should be positioned for comfort and to prevent swelling of the extremity. Once the cast is dry, use pillows or rolled blankets to support cast on leg. Use sling to support arm cast. Elevate the child's arm or leg no more than 4 inches above the level of the child's heart.
11b. Keep blankets from being pulled taut across an extremity.	Taut bed sheets can put pressure on the toes and cause poor mobility, circulation, and skin breakdown.
12. Complete interventions to prevent complications of immobility and promote healing.	Ongoing nursing activities focus on assessment and interventions for complications of immobility that include constipation, inadequate nutrition, and pulmonary stasis.
13. Notify physician of any abnormal findings.	Early identification of an abnormal finding is key in the prevention and treatment of complications of fractures. Subtle findings will often indicate an impending complication at the earliest stage.

CHILD AND FAMILY EVALUATION AND DOCUMENTATION

- Evaluate child and family's understanding of need for child to
  - Report sensations of discomfort and pain
  - Support environment where child is free from injury
  - Complete neurovascular and skin assessments
- Document the following:
  - Assessment findings, including vital signs, neurovascular, and circulation
  - Skin assessment findings and interventions to maintain skin integrity
  - Drainage noted on the cast
  - Integrity of cast and cast care given
  - Pain medication administration and child's response to pharmacologic and nonpharmacologic interventions
  - Teaching done with the family and educational materials provided to child and family

COMMUNITY CARE

- Evaluate the family's ability to perform needed assessment, knowledge of possible complications, and measures to use if complications should occur.
- For the child casted for an extended period of time, a referral to a physical therapist for range-of-motion exercises is recommended.
- For children with spica casts, a specially modified convertible car safety seat (the Spelcast) is available. The seat fits infants up to 20 pounds (rear-facing position) and toddlers up to 40 pounds (front-facing position). Contact numbers are 800-323-7698 and 561-747-8779.
- For older children, the E-Z-On vest is recommended. It is used with the normal car seats available in the car. Contact numbers are 800-336-7684 and 561-747-6920.
- Social services may need to be consulted to help the family with transportation concerns.
- Provide patient teaching related to care and management of the child in a cast (Chart 25-1).

CHART 25-1 TEACHING INFORMATION FOR THE CHILD WITH A CAST

Cast Care

- Cast must be kept dry. If a Gore-Tex lining was used to make cast, child can get cast wet. Water may cause the cast to soften and lose its shape.
- If an area of the cast becomes wet, a blow-dryer set on the "cool" setting will help dry the cast.
- To keep genitalia area of cast dry, tuck small diaper inside groin opening. At night, a sanitary napkin may be added inside the diaper to prevent leakage. Do not cut a diaper to make it fit the groin opening of the cast. The cut, unfinished edges of the diaper give off debris, which can get under the cast and irritate the skin.
- Cover the edges of the cast with clothing to prevent crumbs, toys, and other articles from getting inside the cast.
- Do not scratch inside the cast with anything.
- Clean soiled areas of the cast with a barely damp cloth. A small amount of white shoe polish can touch up a soiled white cast.
- A plastic bag may be taped over the cast to protect the cast while bathing.
- Do not paint or write on the entire surface of the cast because the cast needs to breathe.

Skin Care

- To decrease skin irritation and protect edges of the cast from excessive wear, petal the cast around the edges with moleskin and cover edges around the perineal area with waterproof tape. A fiberglass cast should have the perineal area petaled with moleskin first, then covered with waterproof tape.
- A persistent, foul odor could indicate an infection. Other signs include warmth over an area of the cast, drainage onto the cast, or development of a fever, lethargy, or complaints of discomfort.
- A daily tub bath or sponge bath is recommended to keep accessible skin areas clean.
- If itching occurs, try to divert the child's attention.
- Do not use lotion or powders on the skin around the cast edges or inside the cast.
- Inspect the skin daily for irritations.
- Alcohol applied 2 or 3 times a day under the edges of the cast can help toughen the child's skin. Do not use alcohol if the skin becomes cracked.

Toileting

- A bedpan or urinal may need to be used by the immobilized child.
- For girls, placing toilet paper inside the bedpan is helpful to prevent splashing of urine onto the cast.
- Plastic wrap can be tucked under the edges of the cast and funneled into the bedpan to prevent soiling of the perineal cast edges while using the bedpan.
- The neck of the urinal can be extended by placing a paper cup with the bottom cut out into the neck of the urinal.

Positioning

- Change the child's position at least every 4 hours while awake.

CHART 25-1 TEACHING INFORMATION FOR THE CHILD WITH A CAST (CONTINUED)

- The child in body cast can be on stomach with pillow under legs, or propped up on the side, or on the back at an angle of about 30 degrees with head up.
- The abduction stabilizer bar between the legs of the spica cast should not be used as a handle to help turn the child unless otherwise instructed by the ortho technician who has constructed the cast.
- Pillows or rolled blankets can be used to support the body and cast.
- Keep casted extremity elevated and supported with a pillow when not ambulating.

Neurovascular Checks

- Note color, sensation, motion, and temperature of involved extremities at least twice a day.
- Fingers and toes should be warm and pink.
- Squeeze the finger or toe until it turns white and then watch to see if it immediately turns pink after your release it.
- Ask the child if he or she feels any tingling, numbness, or pain in the extremity.
- Notify health care provider if there is a change in the neurovascular status.

Mobility and Transportation

- Keep toys, throw rugs, and small pets out of child's path.
- Use crutches as ordered to assist in ambulation.
- To allow play, the child in a spica cast can be seated in a beanbag chair with toys placed within reach.
- A reclining wheelchair can be used to allow the child with a spica cast to sit up or be transported.
- A prone cart or scooter can be used as a means of transportation for the child in a spica cast.
- The child who weighs less than 60 lb or is younger than 6 years of age must be restrained in a car seat. Special car seats can be ordered to accommodate the child in a cast.
- For the older child, a safety rest for the car restraint may be rented.
- Special wide ambulances may be needed to transport children in abduction casts.

Comfort

- Diphenhydramine may be ordered for severe itching.
- Children with cerebral palsy may need diazepam (Valium) as needed for muscle spasms that occur during cast wear.
- Acetaminophen can be administered to the child to ease discomfort.
- The child should not be extremely uncomfortable in the cast. If the child complains of pain in one specific spot, it may indicate a pressure sore, and it should be evaluated by a health care provider.

Clothing

- When in a body cast, girls can wear dresses or skirts. Boys and girls can wear shorts and pants that are cut down the side seam to accommodate the cast. The shorts can be pinned or fastened with Velcro strips.
- Clothing should be loose fitting (approximately two sizes larger than normal) and not have elastic around the hem, wrist, or ankle area.
- Clothing should be chosen to help the child stay as cool as possible because the cast will make the child's skin more sweaty.
- The lower extremities can be kept warm by wearing large socks over the feet and cast.

Nutrition

- Diet should be high in fiber, fresh fruits, and vegetables to prevent constipation.
- Small, frequent meals will decrease discomfort from abdominal distension.
- Fluid intake should be increased to prevent kidney stones and constipation.

Diversional Activities and Schooling

- Child can return to school if mobile and the cast is dry.
- A home tutor should be arranged for the child in a body cast.
- A daily schedule should include age-appropriate diversional activities.
- Visitors are encouraged.

- Instruct the family to contact the healthcare provider if the child exhibits:
  - Blue, cold, tingling, or very swollen fingers or toes in the affected extremity
  - Pain not relieved by oral analgesics
  - Burning sensation in extremities or under cast
  - Warmth over an area of the cast or drainage on the cast
  - Increased swelling above or below the cast
  - Odor or fluid coming from the cast or cast area
  - Lethargy or generalized discomfort
  - A soft or cracked cast

Unexpected Situation

- *A 10-year-old girl has been placed in a long leg cast after a skateboarding accident. She has been experiencing pain in the affected leg, unrelieved by analgesics. The skin on the exposed foot is shiny and stretched. The girl complains of numbness in her toes. Pedal pulses are weak. The unaffected leg is warm to touch with no swelling or change in sensation:* Compartment syndrome may be developing. Reposition the leg so that it is no higher than heart level. Contact the physician. The cast may need to be cut open (called "bivalving") to relieve the pressure.

Bibliography

Altizer, L. (2001). Neurovascular assessment. *Orthopedic Nursing, 20*(4), 48–50.

Altizer, L. (2004). Casting for immobilization. *Orthopedic Nursing, 32*(2), 136–141.

American Academy of Pediatrics Committee on Injury and Poison Prevention. (1999). Transporting children with special health care needs. *Pediatrics, 104*(4), 988–992.

McConnell, E. (2002). Assessing neurovascular status in a casted limb. *Nursing, 32*(9), 86.

Pifer, G. (2000). Casting and splinting: Prevention of complications. *Topics in Emergency Medicine, 22*(3), 48–54.

CHAPTER

26

Chemotherapy: Administration and Safe Handling

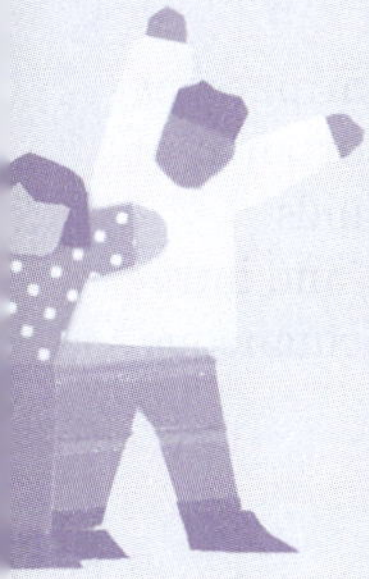

Clinical Guidelines

Personnel

- A healthcare prescriber orders chemotherapy medications.
- A pharmacist, physician, or registered nurse (RN) who has completed competency training in the administration and safe handling of chemotherapy may administer antineoplastic agents. These personnel must also be skilled in venipuncture, assessing and management of various types of central venous access devices (CVADs), and drug administration systems.
- The individual administering the chemotherapy is responsible for the prevention, early detection, and management of acute reactions associated with chemotherapy, including hypersensitivity, anaphylaxis, hypotension, extravasation, and nausea and vomiting.
- All personnel handling the transport of antineoplastic agents should have specific instructions related to hazardous waste and spill precautions.

Safe Handling

- All equipment used in drug preparation and any unused drugs are treated as hazardous waste and disposed of according to the institution's policies.
- The use of personal protective equipment (PPE) is one of the best ways for nurses to prevent occupational exposure to chemotherapy agents. The National Institute for Occupational Safety and Health (NIOSH) recommends reducing exposure by using the following PPE:
  - Gowns: Disposable, made of low-permeable fabric with a closed front, long sleeves, and tight-fitting cuffs. Laboratory coats and cloth patient gowns are not considered PPE.
  - Gloves: Disposable, powder free, nonlatex, at least 0.007 inches thick with long cuffs. Some acceptable products are nitrile, polyurethane, or neoprene. Latex gloves should be used with caution because of latex sensitivities.
  - Respirators and face masks: NIOSH-approved respirator or mask must be worn when cleaning cytotoxic spills.
  - Face shields or goggles: For protection if splashing or eye exposure is possible.

caREminder

Splashing can occur when child vomits, spits, or struggles when being given an oral cytotoxic medication.

Medication Preparation and Storage

- Storage and labeling of chemotherapeutic agents follow the institutional pharmacy guidelines. Family education is required when teaching about storage and labeling of chemotherapeutic agents in the home.
- According to NIOSH, cytotoxic drugs, including oral drugs that must be compounded or crushed, should be prepared in a biologic safety cabinet (BSC). Prime all tubing in the pharmacy with a solution that is not a chemotherapy solution (e.g., normal saline or the solution the chemotherapy is mixed in, such as D5W). Apply a label that says "Cytotoxic Agent" before transport for administration to patient.
- The BSC should provide vertical laminar airflow, eliminate exhaust with a Hepa filter, and have a continuously running blower. A class II type B or class III vertical airflow BSC is necessary to decrease exposure to cytotoxic agents during preparation.
- The room in which the BSC is located should be restricted to authorized personnel. Use of BSC does not eliminate the need for PPE.
- To prevent accidental ingestion of cytotoxic agents, it is prohibited to eat, drink, smoke, chew gum, apply cosmetics, or store food in areas where chemotherapy is prepared or administered.

Medication Administration

- Use aseptic technique in the preparation and administration of chemotherapy.
- A dose verification process is implemented by the institution to ensure safe administration of the correct type and dosage of the antineoplastic agent.
- Two chemotherapy-competent personnel should check the written orders and ensure that the correct drug, dose, time, route, and patient are identified and relevant test results are noted.
- All chemotherapy doses are calculated independently by the physician, the pharmacist, and the nurse.
- Verbal orders for chemotherapy administration are not acceptable.
- Administration of chemotherapy agents should be done through a central line if possible, especially if it requires continuous infusion.
- Intravenous (IV) access for chemotherapy administration is completed with minimal trauma, and repeated attempts are avoided. If repeated attempts are necessary, they should be done proximally to prevent leakage of the cytotoxic agent from previous needle insertion sites.
- An IV site for administration of chemotherapy should not be used if the site is more than 24 hours old.
- Optimal sites for IV insertion for administration of chemotherapy include large, healthy veins in the nondominant arm (e.g., upper extremities, especially veins of the forearms). The dorsum of the hand, foot, and antecubital fossa areas should not be used because of the increased risk for serious functional damage if infiltration occurs.
- Small-gauge (22- to 24-gauge) catheters are recommended. Catheters made of Teflon are preferred for longer infusions.
- If an IV needs to stay in for more than 1 hour, it is best to place an angiocath that will be less likely to infiltrate and will be less traumatic to the vein. If the patient is to receive only an injection of chemotherapy and IV antiemetics without hydration, a butterfly needle is preferred because it is easy to insert into small veins and is less traumatic due to the short duration of therapy.
- Insertion sites should be visible, secured, and stable at all times. Occlusive clear dressings are recommended for covering the site.
- Venous integrity will be assessed before each administration of chemotherapy to validate blood return and proper flow. For chemotherapy by push-pull method, blood return will be accessed every 1–2 mL. For longer infusions, blood return should be accessed every hour.
- The use of infusion pumps with high flow pressures are not recommended for peripheral line infusions.

EQUIPMENT

- Personal protective equipment (see Clinical Guidelines for specific details):
  - Gloves
  - Gown
  - Face shield or goggles
- Universal precautions door sign to inform persons involved with the child's care of the importance of handwashing and careful handing of body fluids
- Luer-Lok connections for needles, syringes, and intravenous lines if using these routes (IV, subcutaneous, intramuscular, or intrathecal)
- Chemotherapy medications
- Intravascular access administration setup
- Appropriate IV filters if using the side-port bolus administration technique
- Hard, plastic, puncture-resistant container that is disposable for any sharps, IV tubing, bags, bottles, needles, or syringes that are contaminated
- Body surface area (BSA) nomogram
- Extravasation kit (see Chapter 27)
- Chemotherapy spill kit:
  - Respirator mask (NIOSH approved)
  - Chemical splash goggles
  - Nonpermeable gown with cuffs and back closure
  - Shoe covers

- Utility gloves
- Plastic scraper
- Disposable dustpan
- Plastic-backed absorbent towels and/or spill control pillows
- Disposable syringes
- Sharps container
- Heavy-duty disposal bags
- Hazardous waste label

CHILD AND FAMILY ASSESSMENT AND PREPARATION

- Verify identification of child before medication administration.
- Assess the child's and family's readiness to learn.
- Verify that all necessary informed consents for treatment have been acquired.
- Determine child's previous experience with chemotherapy and chemotherapy-related side effects (e.g., nausea, vomiting).

KidKare Anticipate side effects from the chemotherapy and prepare for them; these include nausea and vomiting, anaphylaxis, diarrhea, and fever. The child may have a special toy, a clean toy animal, a clean blanket for security, an emesis basin, and medication to help alleviate some of the unwanted side effects.

- Teach the child and family about the medications to be administered, including
  - How antineoplastic agents work on cancer cells
  - Effects of chemotherapy on immune system functioning
  - Name of the antineoplastic agent
  - Route, frequency, and dose
  - Length of treatment
  - Anticipated side effects and possible adverse effects
  - Methods for preventing or managing adverse effects
  - Safe handling of chemotherapy
- Instruct the child and family that secretions, blood, urine, emesis, and stool are considered contaminated for 48 hours after the last dose of chemotherapy that was administered. Universal precautions should be used when handing diapers, emesis, or clothing containing body fluids.
- Teach the child and family age-appropriate relaxation and diversionary activities to use before, during, and after treatments as needed.
- Institute neutropenic and bleeding precautions.

PROCEDURE Administering Chemotherapy

Steps	Rationale/Points of Emphasis
1. Verify that the height and weight recorded and used for patient calculations are recent. Obtain BSA from BSA nomogram or using a BSA equation: BSA = Ht (cm) × Wt (kg) ÷ 3,600, then obtain the square root of the result.	Many chemotherapy agents are dosed per the child's BSA, not weight.
2. Assess the prescriber's order for appropriateness of the drug, dose, diluent, route, frequency, and duration of treatment. Calculate the amount of medication the child should receive. Recalculate the dose as ordered by BSA or mg/kg and check against child's BSA or mg/kg. Verify that findings are consistent with the prescriber's orders, dosage limits, and pharmacy preparation. Verify findings with a second person (nurse, physician, or pharmacist). **Alert!** *If the child is enrolled in a study protocol, review the protocol for correct dosing and schedule because these protocols often vary from the resource texts that are used. Ensure informed consent has been obtained for participation in the study.*	Ascertains that the child is receiving the correct treatment course. Verifying with a second person ensures accuracy of medication administration.
3. Ensure that the chemotherapy was prepared in a biologically safe hood or cabinet. The healthcare provider should wear a protective face shield/goggles, gown, and gloves to prevent inhalation, direct skin contact, or direct eye contact.	Reduces the opportunity for inadvertent ingestion, direct skin contact, or direct eye contact with the drugs by the healthcare provider or the patient.

Continued

Steps	Rationale/Points of Emphasis
4. Ensure that the chemotherapy is in a sealed container/bag.	Decreases risk for contamination to personnel or environment in case of accidental dropping.
5. Before administering the chemotherapy to the child, check the label to be sure it is the correct solution that was prescribed by the healthcare prescriber.	Decreases risk for error in administering the wrong medication. Also, recalculate the dose according to the protocol or reference material being used.
6. Gather the necessary supplies including emergency and extravasation supplies.	Promotes efficient time management and provides an organized approach to the procedure. Ensures supplies are available if child has a reaction to the chemotherapy administration. The nurse is responsible for the prevention, early detection, and management of acute reactions associated with chemotherapy.
7. If the child is to receive an agent that may cause a febrile or anaphylactic reaction, obtain a baseline set of vital signs.	Child must be monitored for signs of reaction to the chemotherapy throughout the therapy according to the institution's policy. Also, have therapy readily available in case of reaction.
8. Perform hand hygiene and don protective apparel.	Reduces transmission of microorganisms. Decreases risk for exposure to cytotoxic agents. According to the Occupational Safety and Health Administration (OSHA), safe levels of occupational exposure to cytotoxic agents cannot be determined. Therefore, it is imperative to adhere to practices designed to eliminate or reduce occupational exposure.
9. Use one of the following techniques to administer the medication: the two-syringe method, side-port bolus method, or infusion pump method.	Administration technique is influenced by rate by which medication can safely be administered.
a. *Two-syringe method* for intravenous (IV) bolus: Use one syringe to inject chemotherapeutic agent and the other syringe to check for blood return and IV patency. Drug bolus should be completed in 3 minutes or less, and blood return should be checked after every 1–2 mL of administered drug. Use the push-pull technique to administer a vesicant to a child. Push a very small amount, pull back on the plunger to obtain a blood return, and then push a small amount again; continue until the total amount has been administered. Blood return is assessed every 1–2 mL.	Slow intravenous push allows for continuous observation and immediate intervention if required.
b. *Side-port boluses* for peripheral IV sites: Prime the primary intravenous line with normal saline or the same solution the chemotherapy has been mixed in. Prime the secondary line with the antineoplastic agent, letting the vesicant run through the tubing and into gauze pad that is in a plastic bag; dispose of the gauze and the bag after the line is primed. Attach the secondary line into a side port of the primary line to allow free-flowing infusion of the chemotherapeutic agent.	This method is used for medication that must be administered over a longer period of time than can be given via the two-syringe method.
c. *Infusion pumps:* Prime the primary intravenous line with a normal saline or the same solution the chemotherapy has been mixed in. Prime the secondary line with the antineoplastic agent, letting the vesicant run through the tubing and into gauze pad that is in a plastic bag; dispose of the gauze and the bag after the line is primed. Attach the secondary line into a side port of the primary line and attach to a separate infusion pump, infusing at a rate consistent with the prescriber's orders. Access the central venous site per institution policy.	Infusion pumps with high flow pressures can increase the risk of injury and are not recommended for peripheral line infusions. For pediatric patients, all chemotherapy (except that given IVP) should be given using a volumetric pump. ***Alert!*** *The IV tubing should be primed with the same solution with which the agent is mixed. This reduces the chance of a spill that could occur if the chemotherapeutic agent was used to prime the tubing and avoids aerosolization of droplets.*
10. Assess the IV site. Gently draw back blood before starting to administer the drug through the tubing or a syringe.	Evaluates integrity of the IV line by validating presence of blood return and proper flow. ***Alert!*** *Never test the line with the cytotoxic agent.*

Steps	Rationale/Points of Emphasis
11a. Administer the chemotherapy by the prescribed route over the prescribed time frame.	Maintains safety and decreases risk for some side effects, especially anaphylaxis with some medications.
11b. Flush tubing or intravenous line upon completion of medication administration using normal saline or same solution that chemotherapy has been mixed in.	Avoids substance incompatibility.
11c. Remove and dispose of intravenous tubing and medication solution bag (see step 14).	New tubing will be used for administration of each chemotherapeutic agent.

Alert! ***If spills occur, follow institutional policy and NIOSH guidelines for managing spills. A large spill is one in which more than 5 mL of a chemotherapy agent is released (e.g., glass bottle of agent breaks). A small spill is one in which less than 5 mL of a chemotherapy agent is released (e.g., tubing becomes disconnected or dislodged). Large spills must be cleaned up using a chemotherapy spill kit; small spills may be cleaned using absorbent gauze.***

Steps	Rationale/Points of Emphasis
12. Monitor the child for potential side effects as needed during and immediately after administration. Take appropriate actions to treat allergic/hypersensitive responses and side effects.	Promotes comfort. The nurse is responsible for the prevention, early detection, and management of acute reactions associated with chemotherapy, including hypersensitivity, anaphylaxis, hypotension, extravasation, and nausea and vomiting.
13a. During chemotherapy administration, use measures to relax the child.	Measures include minimizing stimuli from noises, light, and odor.
13b. Monitor the child for effectiveness of measures to control nausea and vomiting.	If child can taste the chemotherapy agent, offer hard candy or gum. Antiemetics should be administered before initiation of emetogenic chemotherapy and continued at regular intervals.
14. After the chemotherapy has been administered, put contaminated items in a container that is puncture resistant, marked for "chemotherapy disposal only," seal the container, and follow institution's policy for disposal of hazardous substances. The items discarded should include any needles, syringes, intravenous tubing, bags, bottles, gowns, gloves, and face shields/goggles.	Reduces transmission of agents and cross-contamination to others. Dispose of all material that has come into contact with a cytotoxic drug by placing the material into a waste container designated for cytotoxic waste.
15. Perform hand hygiene.	Reduces transmission of microorganisms.

Alert! ***If the skin comes into contact with a chemotherapeutic agent, wash vigorously with soap and warm water to prevent a skin reaction.***

Steps	Rationale/Points of Emphasis
16. Child is now placed on chemotherapy precaution (Chart 26-1) for 48 hours after the last dose of chemotherapy was administered. Any secretion from the child is considered contaminated with the chemotherapy agent, and universal precautions are taken to decrease exposure by all caregivers to any secretions.	It is assumed that anything that is soiled with bodily secretions is contaminated with the chemotherapy agent, and taking caution in decreasing exposure to the agent decreases the risk for contaminating others with the agent. Comply with confidentiality rules to implement a strategy to alert other personnel that the child has received chemotherapy.

CHILD AND FAMILY EVALUATION AND DOCUMENTATION

- Evaluate child's response to chemotherapy, including presence of side effects.
- Evaluate child's and family's understanding of chemotherapy regimen, medication side effects, and measures to manage side effects.
- Document the following:
  - Type of medication and diluent
  - Dose
  - Site given
  - Time given
  - Appearance of access site
  - Presence/absence of adverse effects or side effects
  - Measures used to manage side effects

CHART 26-1 CHEMOTHERAPY PRECAUTIONS

- Wear gloves when handing diapers, urinals, urine hats, emesis basins, soiled clothes, or bed linens.
- Carry soiled items away from your body or place them in a pillowcase for transport.
- Label any linen that is soiled with the child's bodily secretions as needing chemotherapy precautions when handled.
- Label all specimens sent to the laboratory as being from a child undergoing chemotherapy.
- Instruct the child to flush the toilet twice after each use, with the lid down.
- Instruct family of additional measures to use at home:
  - Prelaunder contaminated lines before washing them with other clothes.
  - Protect mattresses and pillowcases using plastic covers.
  - Wash reusable items such as emesis basins every day with soap and water. Wear gloves while completing this task.
  - Wash hands after removing gloves.

- Child's tolerance of procedure
- Teaching completed with the child/family
- Family's participation in measures to relieve side effects and provide comfort to the child

COMMUNITY CARE

- To minimize side effects and complications of chemotherapy, teach child and family
  - To avoid use of aspirin or aspirin-containing products
  - Ways to prevent infection (e.g., using good handwashing techniques, avoiding crowds, practicing good hygiene)
  - Proper oral hygiene techniques
  - Use of oral nystatin suspension to control fungal infections (if ordered)
  - Signs and symptoms of stomatitis
  - Care of CVADs
  - How to maintain the diet ordered by the healthcare prescriber
  - To avoid hot and spicy food
  - To eat six small meals a day
  - To avoid temperature extremes and chemical treatments of the hair
  - To minimize sun exposure and use sunscreen
  - To wear protective mask if recommended by your healthcare prescriber
  - To avoid rectal temperatures, rectal suppositories, or rectal manipulation of any kind
  - That secretions, blood, urine, emesis, and stool are considered contaminated for 48 hours after the last dose of chemotherapy that was administered
  - Safe handling of chemotherapeutic agents
- Instruct the family to contact the healthcare provider if
  - Child develops fever or chills
  - Child experiences nosebleeds, excessive bruising, or tarry stools
  - Child develops mouth sores, especially if oral intake is compromised
  - Child loses appetite or refuses to eat for extended periods of time
  - Child experiences excessive nausea and vomiting or diarrhea

Unexpected Situations

- *During chemotherapy administration, the parent notices that the IV tubing has become disconnected:* The nurse should be notified immediately. The child's IV line should be clamped close to the IV access site. Don PPE. Disconnect child from wet chemotherapy IV tubing. Ensure patency of IV and take measures to maintain patency until chemotherapy administration can be resumed. Institute procedure to manage chemotherapy spills. Keep people away from the spill and keep child protected from any contact with hazardous agents.
- *While flushing the toilet after the child's use, fluid from the toilet splashes up into the mother's face:* Find the nearest source of water or an eye wash station and assist the mother to flush the eye with large amounts of water for 15 minutes. Contact physician/hospital administration per institution policy to notify them of the parent's exposure. Parent may be referred for physician observation. Complete institutional "Incident Report" forms. Ensure any fluid on floor has been cleaned following procedure for managing chemotherapy spills.

Bibliography

Cowan, E., Crouch, M., & King, M. (2000). Chemotherapy administration: Matching policy and practice. *Home Health Care Consultant,* 7(2), 1A–5A.

Ener, R. A., Meglathery, S. B., & Styler, M. (2004). Extravasation of systemic hematooncological therapies. *Annals of Oncology, 15,* 858–862.

Goodman, M. (2002). *Principles of chemotherapy administration: Administration policies and professional issues.* Retrieved September 1, 2004, from http://cancersourceRN.com

Goodman, M. (2002). *Principles of chemotherapy administration: Routes of drug administration.* Retrieved September 1, 2004, from http://cancersourceRN.com

Harris, D., & Knobf, M. (2004). Assessing and managing chemotherapy-induced mucositis pain. *Clinical Journal of Oncology Nursing, 8*(6), 622–628.

Hurst, S., & McMillan, M. (2004). Innovative solutions in critical care units. *Dimensions of Critical Care Nursing, 23*(3), 125–128.

Kassner, E. (2000). Evaluation and treatment of chemotherapy extravasation injuries. *Journal of Pediatric Oncology Nursing, 17*(3), 135–148.

Kline, N. (Ed.). (2004). *The pediatric chemotherapy and biotherapy curriculum.* Glenview, IL: Association of Pediatric Oncology Nurses.

Kloth, D. (2002). Prevention of chemotherapy medication errors. *Journal of Pharmacy Practice, 15*(1), 17–31.

Polovich, M., Blecher, C., Glynn-Tucker, E., McDiarmid, M., & Newton, S. A. (2003). *Safe handling of hazardous drugs.* Pittsburgh, PA: Oncology Nursing Society.

Polovich, M., White, J., & Kelleher, J. (Eds.). (2005). *Chemotherapy and biotherapy: Guidelines and recommendations for practice.* Pittsburgh, PA: Oncology Nursing Society.

The National Extravasation Information Service. *Extravasation risk factors.* Retrieved August 21, 2004, from http://www.extravasation.org.uk/Site.htm

CHAPTER

27

Chemotherapy: Management of Extravasation

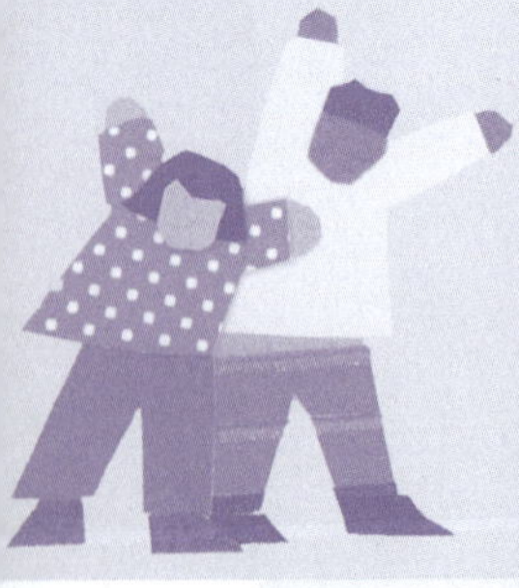

Clinical Guidelines

- Management of extravasation is performed by a registered nurse (RN) or healthcare prescriber with specialized training in the detection and treatment of extravasation.
- This procedure should be instituted immediately if extravasation of a chemotherapeutic agent with vesicant properties is suspected in order to minimize or prevent undue harm to the child undergoing chemotherapy.
- Extravasation is infiltration of a vesicant chemotherapy drug out of the blood vessel and into the soft tissue surrounding the injection delivery site. A vesicant is a drug that, if infiltrated, is capable of causing pain, ulceration, necrosis, and sloughing of damaged tissue (Chart 27-1).
- An extravasation kit should be readily available on a unit where chemotherapeutic agents are administered.

Equipment

- Extravasation kit:
  - Approved antidote for the chemotherapeutic agent (Table 27-1)
  - Ethyl chloride spray
  - Dimethyl sulfoxide (DMSO) 99% topical solution
  - Hydrocortisone 1% cream
  - Hyaluronidase
  - Sodium thiosulfate 25% injection, 10 mL
  - Gauze pads
  - 1-, 3-, and 10-cc syringes
  - 10 cc sterile water
  - 10 cc sterile saline
  - Needles of various sizes
  - Alcohol swab
  - Paper tape
- Measuring tape
- Warm and cold compresses
- Nonsterile gloves

CHART 27-1 SIGNS AND EFFECTS OF CHEMOTHERAPY INFILTRATION

- Local pain, burning sensation, swelling, or erythema at site
- Lack of blood return
- Immediate intense pain but may, on occasion, be painless
- Pain is usually followed by erythema and edema within hours and increased induration within days.
- Skin ulceration and skin necrosis may follow within weeks and can lead to necrosis. Ulcer progression becomes more prominent as the superficial edema decreases.
- Necrotic tissue of the underlying fascia, tendon, and periosteum can be seen by 7 days after infiltration.
- If not recognized early, wide surgical resection and débridement may be required.
- Severe permanent disability or even amputation of involved extremity may be necessary. Damage can be severe enough to result in physical deformity or a functional deficit, such as joint mobility, loss of vascularity, or loss of tendon function.

CHILD AND FAMILY ASSESSMENT AND PREPARATION

- Explain to child/family the hazards of chemotherapy administration before the initiation of therapy.
- Instruct child/family to report any changes at the IV site during or after administration of vesicant chemotherapy.
- Assess integrity of the venous infusion system before each administration of chemotherapy by validating blood return and ease when flushing the catheter.
- During the infusion, the IV site should be monitored frequently (at least hourly for continuous IV infusions).
- Assess the child for the following signs and symptoms:
  - Blotchy redness and subtle swelling at the catheter site
  - Increased warmth and pain at the catheter site
  - Change in infusion quality as indicated by absence of blood return (although not always present), difficulty flushing the catheter, or continuous alarming of the pump indicating an occlusion
  - Complaints of pain, pruritus, or unusual sensations such as burning or stinging

KidKare Listen to the child during the chemotherapy administration. The child may say the infusion

TABLE 27-1
Antidotes for Chemotherapy Extravasation

Antidote	Extravasted Agent	Treatment
Hyaluronidase	Plant alkaloids Vincristine Vinblastine Etoposide Teniposide	Immediately apply heat or warm soaks for 30–60 min. Then alternate with the heat on for 15 min, then off for 15 min, for 24 hr. (*Note:* if the medication was a vinca alkaloid [e.g., vincristine, vinblastine, vinorelbine], the healthcare prescriber may order and administer a local, subcutaneous injection of 1–6 mL of hyaluronidase. Continue to apply heat to activate the hyaluronidase.)
Dimethyl sulfoxide (DMSO)	Alkylating agents Mechlorethamine Cisplatin Carboplatin Ifosfamide DNA intercalating agents Doxorubicin Daunomycin Mitomycin C	Immediately apply ice for 30–60 min and then alternate on/off every 15 min for 24 hr. Elevate the affected area. Topical DMSO, 50%, should be applied to the affected area every 6 hr for 14 days. Allow the DMSO to air-dry and **do not** cover with a bandage. Side effects include mild tingling or burning, erythema, development of garlic-odor breath, headaches, dizziness, and sedation.
Sodium thiosulfate	Alkylating agents Mechlorethamine Cisplatin Carboplatin Ifosfamide	Remember that delayed treatment is ineffective, so the prescriber **must** be notified immediately of any suspicion of extravasation. **Do not** remove the infusion needle. Inject 5–6 mL sterile isotonic sodium thiosulfate intravenously through the **existing** site and also subcutaneously into the extravasated site. Use multiple injections, changing the needle for each new injection (see Fig. 27-2). • Apply ice to the site for 6–12 hr. • Do not apply pressure to the site. • Elevate the affected area. • Assess the site at least every hour for pain, erythemia, and induration or for early signs of tissue necrosis. Notify the prescriber if this occurs.

feels "different," "funny," "itchy," or "weird." If he or she complains about the IV site, do not take any chances. Stop the infusion immediately and report any concerns to the physician.

- Assess the child with a central venous catheter for these additional signs and symptoms:
  - Complaints of dull, aching pain in the shoulder area
  - Tingling, burning, or a sensation of warmth in the chest wall
  - Fever of unknown origin
- Explain to the child and the family why you are stopping the chemotherapy administration and the interventions you will be using to minimize tissue injury.

PROCEDURE **Managing Extravasation**

Steps	Rationale/Points of Emphasis
1. Follow guidelines for administering chemotherapeutic agents (see Chapter 26) (Figure 27-1).	Ensures safe administration of chemotherapeutic agents.
2. If extravasation is suspected, stop the administration of the chemotherapeutic agent immediately.	The degree of injury to local tissues is related to the vesicant properties, concentration, and amount of drug infiltrated. Most extravasation injuries are noticeable immediately after the event. However, induration and ulcer formation may be delayed. In some cases, continued tissue destruction may progress over several weeks to months. Visual inspection at the time of the injury will not determine the extent of the injury.
3. Leave the needle in place.	The Oncology Nursing Society (ONS) recommends leaving the IV catheter in place and attempting to aspirate residual drug. Antidote can then be administered through the existing line. If the IV needle has been removed, the antidotes can be injected subcutaneously, using a 25- to 26-gauge needle around the area of extravasation. **Alert!** *Do not apply pressure to the site. This could cause further dispersion of the vesicant.*
4. Gather the necessary supplies.	Promotes efficient time management and provides an organized approach to the procedure.
5. Perform hand hygiene. Don gloves.	Reduces transmission of microorganisms.
6. Immobilize and elevate the affected extremity. Instruct the patient to rest and elevate the site for 48 hours and then resume normal activity.	Reduces further dissemination of the vesicant.
7. For a peripheral extravasation, attempt to aspirate for blood and residual drug that may be in the IV tubing, the needle, and the suspected infiltrated site. Disconnect the IV tubing or syringe and attach an empty 1- to 3-cc syringe. For a central line extravasation, use a 10-cc syringe to aspirate. Attempt to aspirate any residual drug in the tubing and at the site.	Withdrawing as much drug as possible, combined with pharmacologic interventions, may interfere with the process of cellular destruction and minimize prolonged or permanent damage to the tissue and surrounding area.
8. Notify the healthcare prescriber.	Extravasation is likely to cause injury to the child and discontinuation of the chemotherapy administration at this time; thus the primary care provider needs to be notified of this incident as soon as possible.
9. Measure the size of the infiltration site and record on the extravasation report form.	Provides baseline data.

(Continued on page 202)

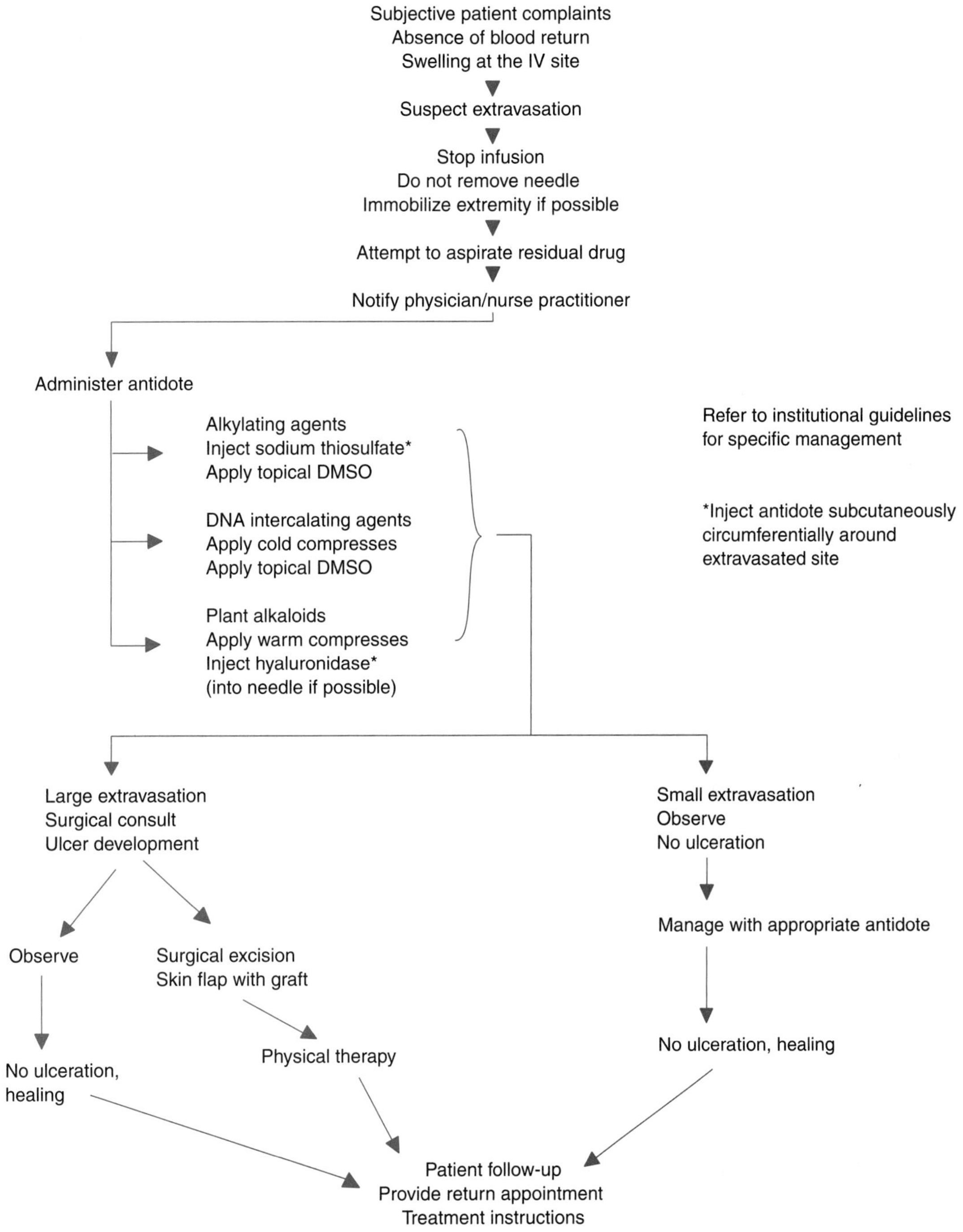

FIGURE 27-1
Treatment plan for extravasation management. (From Kassner, E. [2000]. Evaluation and treatment of chemotherapy extravasation injuries. *Journal of Pediatric Oncology Nursing, 17*[3], 135–148.) Used with permission.

Steps	Rationale/Points of Emphasis
10. Administer the antidote (Figure 27-2; see Table 27-1). It is recommended that the antidote be given using the original line and the surrounding tissue before discontinuing the line. The ONS recommends leaving the IV catheter in place and attempting to aspirate residual drug. Antidote should then be administered through the existing line and circumferentially around the site in a pincushion fashion using a 25-gauge needle.	When the antineoplastic drug infiltrates the interstitial tissue, DNA complexes form and cell death occurs. The newly formed complexes are released from dead cells and bind freely with DNA of surrounding tissues, resulting in persistent cellular death. Further tissue destruction occurs secondary to the formation of toxic oxygen free radicals. Extravasation antidotes are used to decrease tissue damage and reduce the chance of permanent disability or disfigurement.

Alert! *Cold applications are not indicated for injury caused by vinca alkaloid extravasation.*

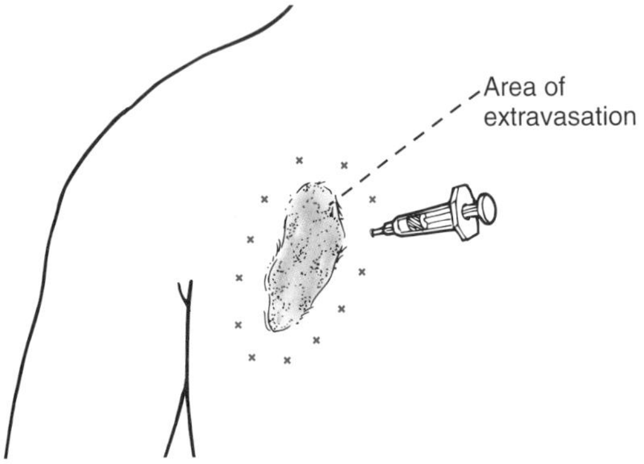

FIGURE 27-2
Sodium thiosulfate is given intravenously through the existing site and also subcutaneously into the extravasated site. Multiple injections are given around the periphery of the extravasated site, changing the needle for each new injection.

Steps	Rationale/Points of Emphasis
11. Apply warm or cold compresses as indicated. Apply warmth for 15 minutes four times daily for the first 24 hours for vinca alkaloids extravasation. Apply ice for 15 minutes every 3–4 hours for 24–48 hours for anthracycline extravasation.	Use of thermal interventions is controversial. Thermal manipulation of superficial skin is directed at decreasing local reaction and absorption. Heat applications are believed to induce vasodilation, which facilitates increased systemic absorption and distribution of the cytotoxic agent. Warm compresses may also help in the dispersion of the antidote. Cold applications are used to provide comfort measures, including the alleviation of local discomfort and irritation. It is also theorized that prolonged cold applications cause vasodilatory effects in tissues surrounding the extravasation. The increased blood flow further dilutes the cytotoxic agent and may decrease the damage to the tissues.
12. Cover affected area with gauze and paper tape as directed by the healthcare prescriber.	Protects site from further injury or infection. However, visualization of the site may necessitate leaving the area uncovered.
13. Remove gloves and perform hand hygiene. Dispose of equipment and waste in appropriate receptacle.	Reduces transmission of microorganisms. Standard precautions.

CHILD AND FAMILY EVALUATION AND DOCUMENTATION

- Complete risk management forms as required by the institution and submit to the appropriate administrative personnel.
- Observe for pain, erythema, induration, and necrosis every hour for the first 2 hours, then every 4 hours for the next 48 hours, and then every 8 hours.
- Evaluate child's level of pain and use pain management interventions as needed.
- Evaluate family's understanding of incident and provide further teaching as needed.

caREminder

Photographic documentation of the lesion is recommended. Follow up with serial photographs if possible.

- Document the following:
  - Date and time of event
  - Subjective complaints and reported symptoms made by the child/family
  - Insertion site and description
  - Size and type of needle or type of venous access device
  - Number of venipuncture attempts and locations
  - Drug administration technique and type of infusion device (if used)
  - Drug sequencing
  - Description of site appearance
  - Estimated amount of extravasated drug
  - Nursing interventions at the time of the incident
  - Healthcare prescriber notification, including name and time of notification
  - Surgical consult if initiated

COMMUNITY CARE

- Provide child and family with instructions for site care and follow-up appointment.

caREminder

With the family's consent, photograph the site at the time of the injury and on follow-up visits to create a visual record of the healing process.

- Observe for signs and symptoms of tissue damage that emerge over time:
  - After 24 to 48 hours: Dry desquamation of skin and ulcer formation begins.
  - By 7 days: Superficial edema resolves, ulcer progression becomes more prominent, necrotic tissue can be seen.

caREminder

Any extravasation site should be closely observed for up to 4 weeks after the incident.

- When tissue necrosis is observed, surgical intervention is required.
- Early intervention to prevent loss of movement or function should be initiated.
- A consult with a plastic surgeon may be warranted for a large extravasation, if the child experiences severe ongoing pain, or if minimal healing is evident 1–3 weeks after the initial injury.
- Instruct the family to contact the healthcare provider if
  - Child develops a fever
  - The site of the tissue damage begins to have a foul smell or a pus-colored discharge
  - Child experiences any changes in sensation or motion in the affected extremity
  - Family has any concerns about the appearance of the affected site

Unexpected Situation

- *Approximately 3 hours after chemotherapy administration, the child develops hives measuring less than 6 cm around the IV site:* These are signs of a localized allergic reaction to the chemotherapy. These are not indications of vesicant extravasation; therefore, extravasation measures should not be used. Notify the healthcare prescriber of the child's symptoms. The child's allergic reaction can be managed with an order of diphenhydramine (Benadryl).

Bibliography

Bertelli, G. (1995). Prevention and management of extravasation of cytotoxic drugs. *Drug Safety, 12*(4), 245–255.

Ener, R. A., Meglathery, S. B., & Styler, M. (2004). Extravasation of systemic hematooncological therapies. *Annals of Oncology, 15*, 858–862.

Goodman, M. (2001). *Principles of chemotherapy administration: Routes of drug administration.* Retrieved August 21, 2004, from http://cancersourcern.com

Hurst, S., & McMillan, M. (2004). Innovative solutions in critical care units. *Dimensions of Critical Care Nursing, 23*(3), 125–128.

Kassner, E. (2000). Evaluation and treatment of chemotherapy extravasation injuries. *Journal of Pediatric Oncology Nursing, 17*(3), 135–148.

Kline, N. (Ed.). (2004). *The pediatric chemotherapy and biotherapy curriculum.* Glenview, IL: Association of Pediatric Oncology Nurses.

Minter, B., Ryan, J., Barrett, K., et al. (1998). *Cancer chemotherapy.* Philadelphia: Association of Pediatric Oncology Nursing.

Polovich, M., White, J., & Kelleher, J. (Eds.). (2005). *Chemotherapy and biotherapy guidelines and recommendations for practice.* Pittsburgh, PA: Oncology Nursing Society.

CHAPTER

28

Chest Physiotherapy

Clinical Guidelines

- A registered nurse (RN) or a respiratory care technician may perform chest physiotherapy.
- Chest physiotherapy should facilitate the removal of excess secretions from the peripheral parts of the lung.
- Airway clearance is indicated for any patient whose condition alters mucous clearance (e.g., cystic fibrosis, dyskinetic cilia syndrome, bronchiectasis from any cause, pain secondary to surgical procedures, and atelectasis from mucous plugs, neuromuscular diseases, and hypersecretory states).
- The method of airway clearance selected is that which best fits child's needs (Figure 28-1).

KidKare Use of a mechanical vest, providing high-frequency chest wall oscillation, to deliver chest physiotherapy in older children allows greater independence for children in providing their own therapy rather than feeling dependent on assistance from others for this part of their care.

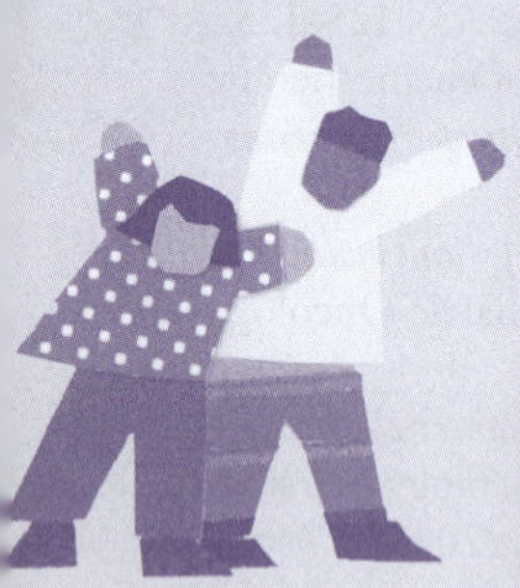

- Child's chest is covered with a t-shirt or blanket before chest physiotherapy to protect bare skin.
- Oxygen saturation levels are monitored during the procedure when indicated.
- Chest physiotherapy should not be performed for at least 1 hour after feedings/meals to prevent vomiting.
- Continuous drip feeds should be turned off at least 30 minutes before therapy to prevent vomiting and/or aspiration.
- The child with gastroesophageal reflux should be carefully monitored throughout therapy to ensure aspiration is avoided. Avoid Trendelenburg position.
- Chest physiotherapy is withheld when the child has episodes of hemoptysis, pulmonary hemorrhage, fractured ribs, vertebral compression fractures, or increased intracranial pressure.
- Implanted venous access devices (i.e., implantable ports) should be protected when performing therapy by using a handmade, donut-shaped, padded support. Do not percuss directly over device.
- If child requires oxygen, ensure that the nasal cannula remains in proper place during position changes.
- Percussion should not be performed directly over incisional areas; consider splinting for comfort.

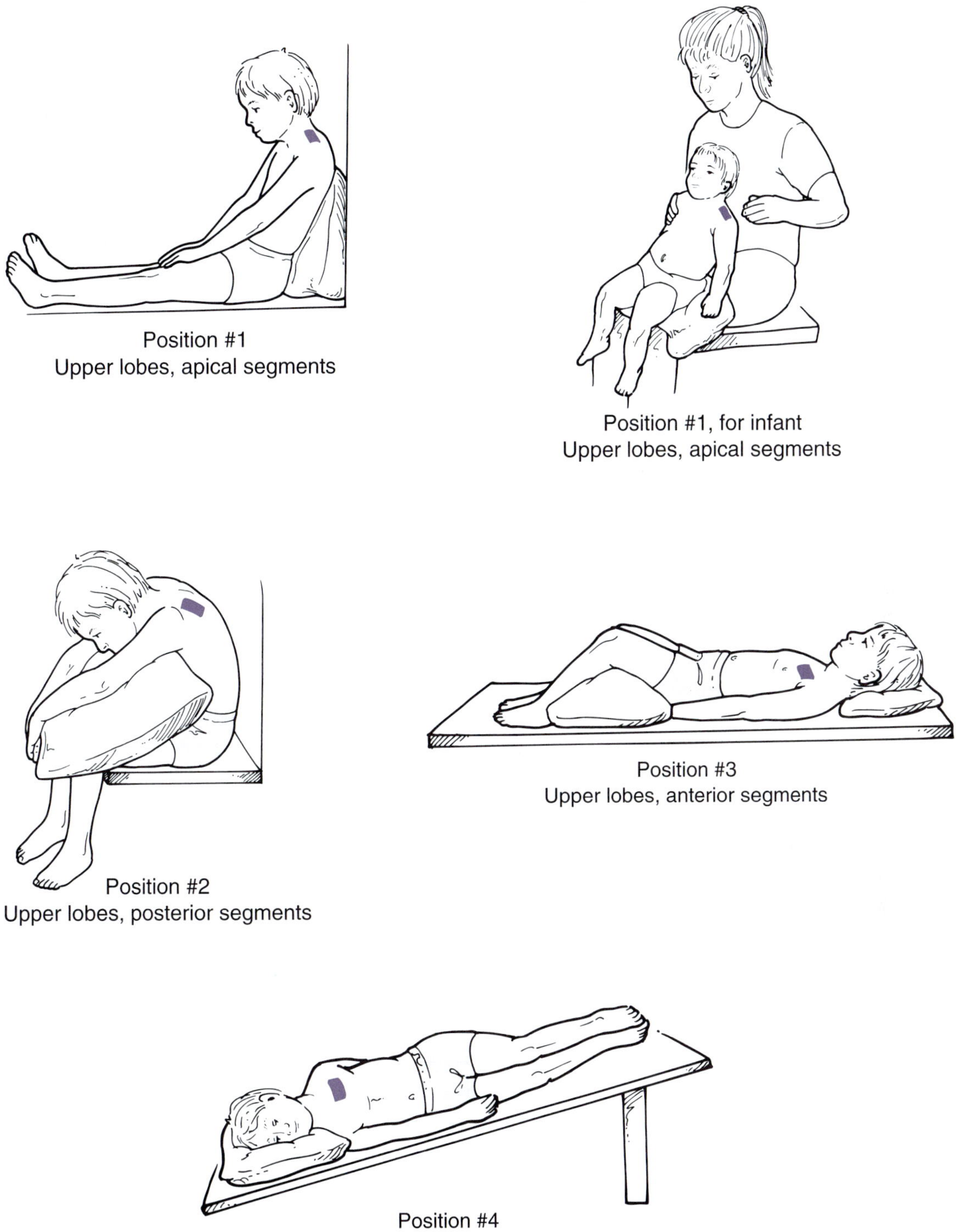

FIGURE 28-1
Positions for chest physiotherapy.

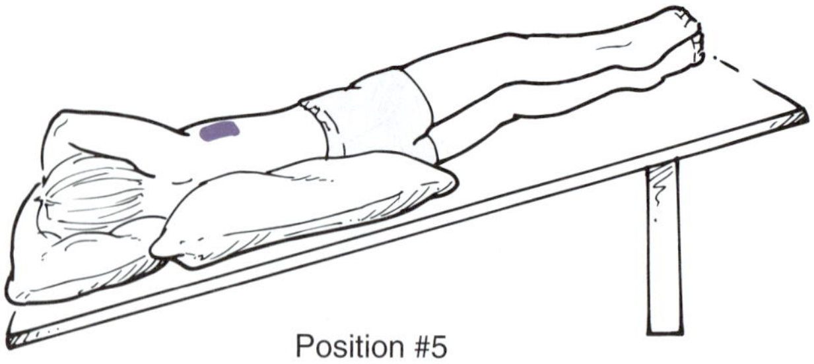

Position #5
Middle lobe

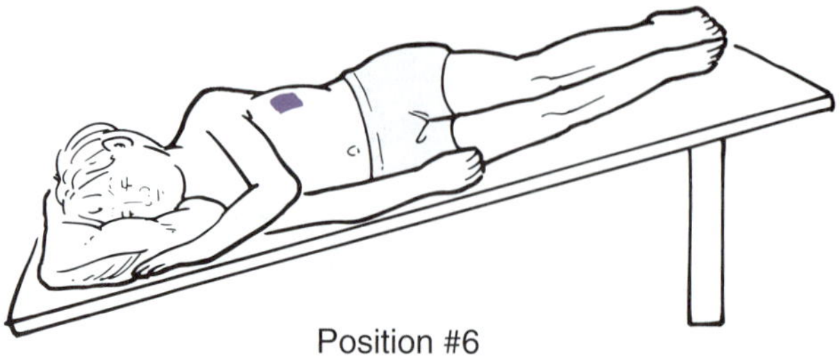

Position #6
Lower lobes, anterior basal segments

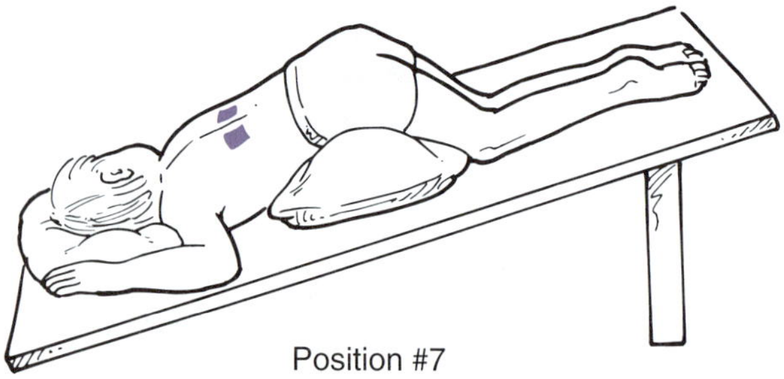

Position #7
Lower lobes, posterior basal segments

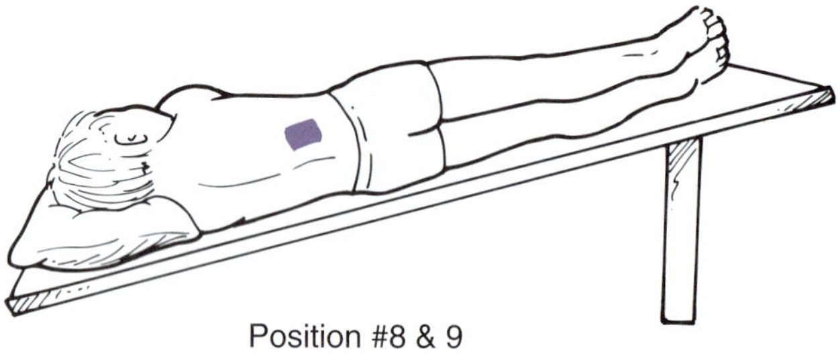

Position #8 & 9
Lower lobes, lateral basal segments

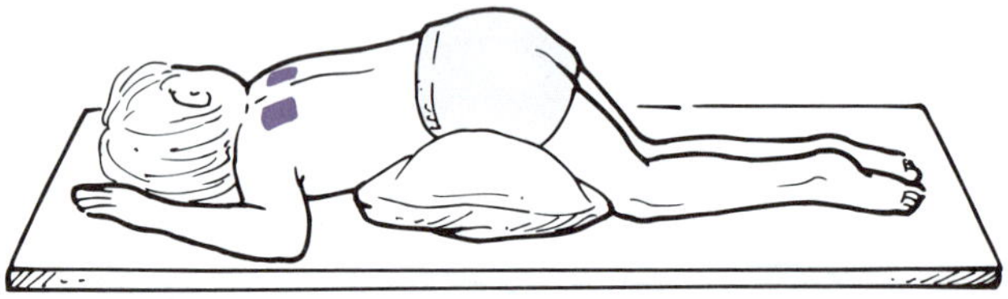

Position #10
Lower lobes, superior segments

FIGURE 28-1 (CONTINUED)
Positions for chest physiotherapy.

EQUIPMENT

- Stethoscope
- Blanket
- Pillows
- Mechanical percussor (if needed, padded electric toothbrush for neonates)
- Container for sputum
- Suction setup (if needed)
- Oxygen (if needed)
- Ambu-bag with oxygen setup (if needed)
- Diversional activities such as music therapy or videos (if needed)

CHILD AND FAMILY ASSESSMENT AND PREPARATION

- Determine when therapy was last given and child's response.
- Review the latest chest x-ray report or physician's orders to determine lung fields where therapy should be directed.

- Assess for other therapies/medications to be administered in conjunction with chest physiotherapy.

caREminder

Generally, bronchodilators and mucolytic medications are administered before chest physiotherapy procedures to assist with airway clearance, whereas inhaled corticosteroids and antibiotics are administered after airway clearance procedures to allow for maximal penetration of the medications into the lungs.

- Perform respiratory assessment using visual inspection of respiratory status and stethoscope for auscultation of breath sounds.
- Determine the last time child had oral intake.
- Determine time of analgesia administered when pain management is of concern. Administer pain medication before the procedure based on child's individual needs.
- Explain procedure to child and family.
- Initiate diversional activities before the procedure. Offer choices for distraction (e.g., favorite video, music).

KidKare When developmentally appropriate, help prepare child by demonstrating the procedure on a doll or stuffed animal. Demonstrate the sensation of cupping on child's leg. Offer to also demonstrate this on a parent's back. Reassure family and the child that child is not being "hit."

PROCEDURE Performing Chest Physiotherapy

Steps	Rationale/Points of Emphasis
1. Perform hand hygiene and gather the necessary supplies and equipment for the procedure.	Reduces transmission of microorganisms. Assembly of all necessary equipment ensures that chest physiotherapy will be completed efficiently and without unnecessary interruptions.
2. Position child in an upright sitting position with his or her back toward you.	Placing the body in an upright sitting position allows gravity to assist drainage of mucus from the lung periphery to the segmental bronchus and upper airway.
3. Using a mechanical percussor or with a cupped hand, percuss over the lung field in a successive rhythmic motion over each lung segment and in each diagrammed position (see Figure 28-1). Each position should be percussed for at least 3 to 10 minutes, based on child's tolerance and underlying disease process. Monitor for fatigue. **Alert!** *Postural drainage in the head-down position is contraindicated for infants because it increases gastroesophageal reflux.*	Percussion dislodges secretions from the bronchial wall. When a mechanical percussor is not available or preferred, a cupped hand creates an air cushion, which in turn vibrates through the chest wall. In conjunction with positioning, the secretions drain into the larger airways and are expectorated or swallowed, depending on the child's age. Percussing over bony prominences is not effective in vibrating the chest wall to loosen secretions.
4. Follow percussion procedure with vibration if percussion over each lobar area was completed using the hand technique. Using an open flat hand, provide a shaking motion on the chest wall, synchronized with exhalation to loosen the secretions.	This technique provides additional vibrations to loosen the secretions and assists with secretion mobilization. **caREminder** *If using a mechanical percussor, vibration is not necessary because mechanical percussors are more effective at loosening secretions than the hand technique.*
5a. After percussion and vibration, have the child sit up, take a deep breath, and cough up and spit out the mucus into a sputum container or tissue. 5b. If child is intubated or unable to generate an effective cough, perform suctioning as indicated.	Sitting up allows for maximal diaphragmatic excursion. Expelling mucus assists in clearing the airway. Mechanical removal of secretions is necessary when child is unable to cough or has an ineffective cough. **KidKare** Young children should be taught how to cough out their mucus into a tissue rather than swallowing it.

Continued

Steps	Rationale/Points of Emphasis
6. Reposition child in alternate positions (see Figure 28-1) and repeat percussion/vibration/cough therapy. Modifications may be necessary based on child's tolerance and condition. Be sure to allow child to rest, if needed, between positions. **caREminder** *Increased effectiveness of postural drainage has been identified using the following sequence of postures: supine, 45-degree rotative prone with left side up, 45-degree rotative prone with right side up, and return to supine. The positions of 10-degree right-side-up supine and 45-degree rotative prone with head raised 45 degrees have been noted to be helpful when added to the basic sequence.*	Performing the procedure in a systematic sequence establishes a pattern so that both the child and parents know what to expect. Systematically changing positions ensures that all segments of the lungs receive the needed therapy to loosen secretions.
7. Upon completion of therapy, assess child's respiratory status using visual inspection and auscultation techniques.	Provides evidence of effectiveness of therapy.
8. Return child to position of comfort, with side rails up. Assist child to brush teeth or rinse out mouth as needed.	Child may feel fatigued after chest physiotherapy and should be given an opportunity to rest. If child expectorated a lot of mucus, oral care is warranted to clean the mouth of microorganisms and increase the child's comfort.
9. Return equipment to appropriate storage area, and perform hand hygiene.	Ensures equipment can be easily located for subsequent procedures. Reduces transmission of microorganisms.

Child and Family Evaluation and Documentation

- Evaluate child's respiratory status, noting respiratory rate, breathing patterns, symmetric chest expansion, breath sounds, and skin color.
- Document the following:
  - Findings from respiratory assessment of child, before and after procedure
  - Completion of therapy and child's response to therapy
  - Adjunctive treatments given concurrently (e.g., nebulized or inhaled medication) and the child's response to these treatments
  - Education provided to parent
- If parents are learning to give this therapy, observe and evaluate their technique. Provide the family with feedback on their skills.

Community Care

- Provide the parent with a diagrammed procedure to follow for home care.
- Ask parents to demonstrate chest physiotherapy techniques to ensure that the hand is properly cupped with the correct positions.
- Assist parents/child to develop a schedule for chest physiotherapy that is optimal for the child in light of meal, sleep, play, and school activities.
- Instruct the family to contact the healthcare provider if
  - Child's respiratory condition worsens
  - Child develops bruising over areas of chest physiotherapy
  - Child complains of pain during the procedure

Unexpected Situations

- *A child with intracranial pressure monitoring demonstrates increased ICP readings during chest physiotherapy:* Stop the therapy immediately, returning child to his or her original resting position. Consult the physician.
- *Child vomits during the procedure:* Stop the therapy, clear the airway, and suction as needed. Administer oxygen while maintaining the airway. Return child to the previous resting position.
- *Child becomes hypoxic:* Oxygen should be administered in higher concentrations during the procedure if the potential for hypoxemia exists. If child becomes hypoxic during the treatment, administer 100% oxygen, stop the therapy immediately, and return child to the original resting position. Ensure adequate ventilation.

Bibliography

Button, B., Heine, R., Catto-Smith, A., Phelan, P., & Olinsky, A. (2004). Chest physiotherapy, gastro-esophageal reflux, and arousal in infants with cystic fibrosis. *Archives of Disease in Childhood, 89*(5), 435–439.

Davidson, K. L. (2002). Airway clearance strategies for the pediatric patient. *Respiratory Care, 47*(7), 823–828.

Fink, J. B. (2002). Positioning versus postural drainage. *Respiratory Care, 47*(7), 469–477.

Goodfellow, L. T., & Jones, M. (2002). Bronchial hygiene therapy from traditional hands-on techniques to modern technological approaches. *American Journal of Nursing, 102*(1), 37–43.

Hilling, L., Bakow, E., Fink, J., Kelly, C., Sobush, D., & Southorn, P. (1991). AARC clinical practice guideline: Postural drainage therapy. *Respiratory Care, 36*(12), 1418–1426.

Krause, M., & Hoehn, T. (2000). Chest physiotherapy in mechanically ventilated children: A review. *Critical Care Medicine, 28*(5), 1648–1651.

Rueling, S., & Adams, C. (2003). Close to the vest: A novel way to keep airways clear. *Nursing, 33*(12), 56–57.

Takahashi, N., Murakami, G., Ishikawa, A., Sato, T., & Ito, T. (2004). Anatomic evaluation of postural drainage of the lung with special reference to patients with tracheal intubation. *Chest, 125*(3), 935–944.

Wagener, J. S., & Headley, A. A. (2003). Cystic fibrosis: Current trends in respiratory care. *Respiratory Care, 48*(3), 234–247.

CHAPTER 29

Chest Tubes

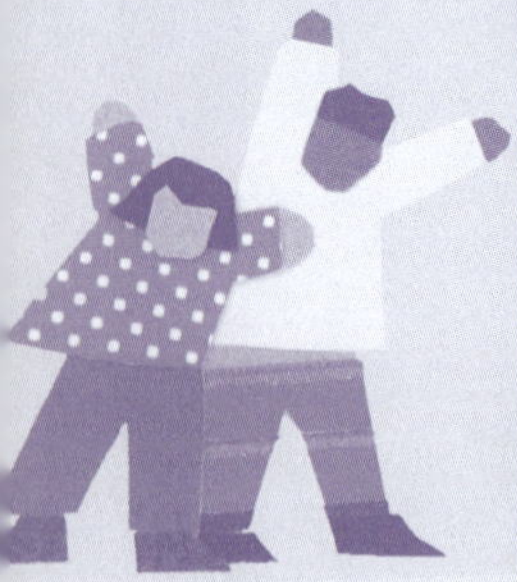

Clinical Guidelines

- Placement of a chest tube is a surgical procedure performed by a surgeon, intensivist, or emergency medicine specialist. Chest tube removal is the responsibility of the healthcare prescriber (i.e., nurse practitioner, advanced practice nurse, physician's assistant, or physician, according to scope of practice).
- The registered nurse (RN) is responsible to prepare and care for chest tube therapy, evaluate respiratory/thoracic assessments and vital signs that reflect effectiveness of therapy or impending complications, and know the appropriate interventions to make clinical decisions regarding changes in the child's therapy.
- Chest tube placement is used in children to provide for:
  - Removal of air or fluid (blood, pus, or nonbloody fluid) from the pleural cavity or mediastinum
  - Reexpansion of the lung
  - Restoration of negative pressure to the pleural space
  - Relief of respiratory distress associated with a collapsed lung
  - Improvement of ventilation and perfusion of the lung
- The water-seal chamber and suction level of the chest tube drainage system are assessed for bubbling and fluctuation every 4 hours or more often as symptoms warrant.

Equipment

For chest tube drainage system collection device:

- Single-use, disposable, sterile chest drainage collection unit (water-suction system or dry-suction system)
- Sterile water
- Suction source
- Wall regulator suction device
- Suction connection tubing
- Chest tube clamp (one per chest tube placed)

For chest tube insertion:

- Lidocaine (Xylocaine) local anesthetic (0.5% or 1%)
- Sterile gown, gloves, masks
- Protective eye gear
- Sterile drapes
- Sterile chlorhexidine prep swabs

- Sterile syringes (assortment of sizes: 3 mL, 5 mL, and TB)
- Sterile chest tube tray, which includes hemostats, trocar, scalpel, Kelly clamps, scissors, skin expanders, and sponges
- Sterile chest tube catheter (6 French for premature infants, up to 24 French for adolescents)
- Suture material (usually 2–0 to 3–0 silk)
- Sterile 5-in-1 connector, or Y connector for more than one chest tube
- 4 × 4, or 2 × 2 gauze dressing
- Tape
- Chest tube clamp (one per chest tube placed)
- 22- and 25-gauge needles
- Alcohol wipes
- Sterile transparent dressing (optional)
- Sterile petrolatum gauze (optional)
- Sterile nonadherent gauze (optional)
- Sterile water if infant

For drainage collection device replacement:

- Sterile gloves
- 4 × 4 gauze dressing
- Tape
- Chest tube clamp (one for each chest tube placed)
- Single-use, disposable, sterile chest drainage collection unit (institutional preference)
- Sterile water
- Suction source
- Suction connection tubing
- Sterile petrolatum gauze (optional)
- Sterile nonadherent gauze (optional)
- Sterile transparent dressing (optional)

For chest tube removal:

- Nonsterile gloves
- Sterile gloves
- 4 × 4 sterile gauze dressing
- Tape
- Chest tube clamp
- Topical analgesic cream
- Sterile petrolatum gauze (optional)
- Sterile nonadherent gauze (optional)

CHILD AND FAMILY ASSESSMENT AND PREPARATION

- Assess the cognitive level, readiness, and ability to process information of the child and family.
- Reinforce the need for chest tube placement, as appropriate, to both the child and family.
- Identify and discuss the risks and benefits of chest tube placement and chest tube removal. Amount of preparation of child and family may be dictated by the emergent nature of the chest tube insertion in some cases.
- Prepare the child for the procedure to include (but not limited to) positioning, sensations during insertion, and assessing and treating the child's pain.
- Assess child for signs and symptoms of respiratory distress, including tachypnea, decreased or absent breath sounds, dyspnea, cyanosis, asymmetric chest expansion, anxiety, restlessness, shortness of breath, tachycardia, hypotension, dysrhythmia, sudden sharp chest pain, or abnormal chest x-ray or blood gas results.
- Assess the child for history of previous chronic lung disease, spontaneous pneumothorax, and pulmonary disease or procedures that may have included the need for chest tube placement.
- In collaboration with the healthcare prescriber, provide pharmacologic and nonpharmacologic pain management options to the child during chest tube insertion, removal, and ongoing care.

PROCEDURE Chest Tube Drainage System Collection Device Setup

Steps	Rationale/Points of Emphasis
1. Gather the necessary supplies, and perform hand hygiene.	Promotes efficient time management and provides an organized approach to the procedure. Reduces transmission of microorganisms.
2. Open single-use sterile chest drainage unit. Fill the water-seal chamber to the specified level according to the manufacturer's instructions, using sterile water.	The water-seal chamber acts as a one-way valve to allow air to pass out of the lung, down through a narrow channel, and bubble out through the bottom of the water seal. Because air must not return to the child, a water seal is considered one of the safest means for protecting the child.
3. Maintain sterile patient connection tube, with cap in place, and set aside.	Allows for later connection of chest tube catheter to chest tube drainage system collection device.
4. Fill the suction-control chamber with sterile water to 20 cm of water or as ordered by the healthcare prescriber. If using a dry-suction chest drainage system, this step will not be necessary (Figure 29-1).	The addition of suction (10–20 cm of water) increases the negative intrapleural pressure and helps overcome air leakage by improving the rate of airflow out of the child as well as improving fluid removal. The dry-suction

Steps	Rationale/Points of Emphasis
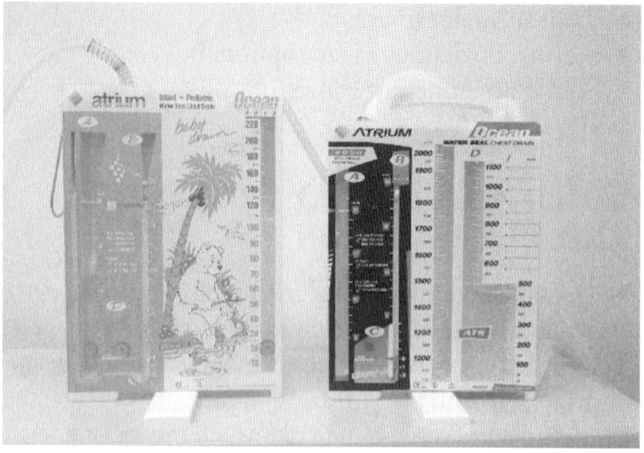 FIGURE 29-1 Left: Infant/pediatric sized dry chest drainage system. Note lack of water seal chamber to be filled. Right: Large child, adolescent, or adult sized dry chest drainage system.	systems use a bellows device and suction wheel to adjust amount of suction and do not require the addition of water to a suction control chamber. **Alert!** *The chest drain must be connected to the child first, before initiating suction. (Refer to following procedure for Chest Tube Insertion.)*
5. After chest tube drainage system has been connected to child's chest tube, connect the short end of the drainage collection system to the suction source and apply wall regulator chamber suction-to-suction outlet until gentle bubbling appears in the suction control chamber.	Connects the suction source to the water seal and activates suction.
6. Place the chest tube drainage collection device at the bedside, at least 1 foot (30 cm) below the child's chest in the upright position (Figure 29-2). 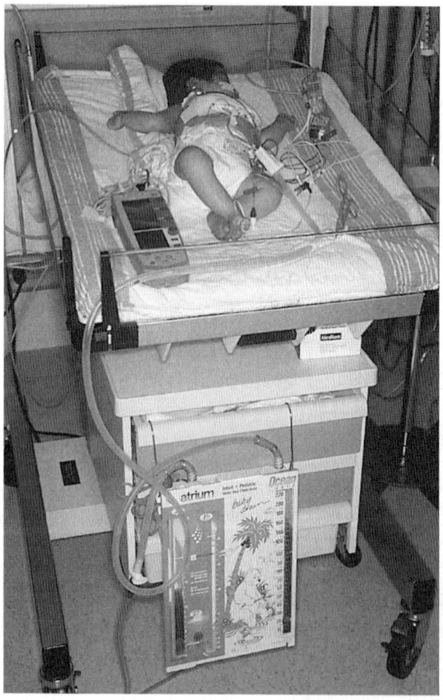 FIGURE 29-2 Place the chest tube device below the chest to allow gravity, in addition to negative pressure, to drain the tube for optimum results.	Placement of the device below the chest allows for gravity in addition to negative pressure to drain the tube for optimum results. **caREminder** *Avoid accidental knock-over of the device by hanging the system on the crib or bed frame with the hangers provided or by securing the base of the collection device to the floor with tape.*

PROCEDURE Chest Tube Insertion

Steps	Rationale/Points of Emphasis
1. Gather the necessary supplies, and perform hand hygiene.	Promotes efficient time management and provides an organized approach to the procedure. Reduces transmission of microorganisms.
2. Obtain baseline data (i.e., vital signs; respiratory rate, pattern, and effort; skin color; perfusion; level of consciousness; oxygen requirements; hemodynamic stability) of child.	This helps to identify and document any acute changes in child during and after procedure.
3. Administer sedation/pain medication per healthcare prescriber's orders.	The healthcare prescriber should request sedation (benzodiazepines) and opioid analgesia to reduce pain and help the child remain calm.
4. Don sterile attire, including eyewear.	Standard precautions for surgical sterile procedure.
5. Position the child for chest tube access by the healthcare prescriber, while maintaining sterile access for the healthcare prescriber.	Ease of access facilitates placement of a chest tube. **caREminder** *Generally, the healthcare prescriber places the chest tube in the midaxillary to anterior axillary line.* **KidKare** To expose the preferred site for chest tube placement, it is easiest to lay the child supine, using rolled towels/blanket to slightly rotate the upper body in a side lying position, with the arm of the affected side raised above head.
6. Restrain limbs as necessary to ensure sterility of procedure.	Keeps child from breaking sterile field required for chest tube placement.
7a. The healthcare prescriber will prepare a sterile field using sterile drapes. The healthcare prescriber will also complete a sterile prep of the child, using sterile towels and chlorhexidine swab stick to cleanse the insertion site. 7b. A local anesthetic is injected at the site.	Identifies access site. Reduces the risk for infection from microorganisms. In infants younger than 2 months of age, ensure that cleansing solution is removed with sterile water to prevent tissue damage. Reduces pain.
8. Healthcare prescriber makes a skin incision about 1 inch long and then inserts a hemostat through the opening to enter the pleural space. Using his or her finger, the prescriber creates a track for the chest tube. Then the prescriber clamps the tube with the hemostat and inserts the tube (size per healthcare prescriber choice), generally through the second intercostal space at the midclavicular line for pneumothoraces or the fifth to seventh intercostal space at the midaxillary line for fluid removal. Assist as needed while continually assessing child for any vital sign changes.	Air tends to collect in the apexes of the lung when the child is in a supine position, thus the high insertion point in the midclavicular line, whereas gravity pools fluid, warranting a lower insertion site. A drain of appropriate size in any position in the pleural cavity will restore negative pressure and allow for reexpansion of the lung, expelling excess pleural contents. The proximal end of the tube has several eyelets (small holes) to drain the air and fluid and prevent catheter occlusion. Prompt identification of any acute change in status can therefore be treated. **KidKare** Ask the child to take a deep breath just before tube insertion if age appropriate and child is able to cooperate. This displaces the diaphragm downward, minimizing risk for injury.
9. When chest tube insertion is completed and secured into place with suture material, assist the healthcare prescriber in attaching the disposable sterile chest drainage unit to the chest tube, using a 5-in-1 connector or, if more than one chest tube is placed, a Y connector.	Creates the drainage collection system. ***Alert!*** *Drain large effusions slowly. Rapid removal during the first 30 minutes after insertion may cause post-thoracentesis pulmonary edema.*

Steps	Rationale/Points of Emphasis
10. Healthcare prescriber may now request sterile petrolatum gauze to be wrapped around chest tube on skin.	This seals insertion site from any air entry or escape.
11. Assist in applying a gauze pressure dressing over chest tube insertion site and a semipermeable transparent dressing over gauze.	Protects site from microorganisms. **caREminder** *Time and date the dressing for change, if indicated.*
12. Tab-tape all connections with adhesive tape and ensure that all clamps are open.	Secures any loose connections and allows for sure flow of drainage.
13. Secure the chest tube and drainage tube so that there is no tension pulling on the insertion site.	Prevents accidental dislodgment of chest tube.
14. Ensure that the drainage tubing has a straight flow to chest tube drainage collection device and has no dependent loops or kinks. Connect chest tube drainage system to suction regulator as in step 5 of preprocedure setup.	If fluid collects in a loop in the tubing between the child and the collection device at a height greater than the suction control limit, the tube will be effectively sealed. This can lead to lung collapse as air and fluid again collect in the pleural space.

Alert! *Do not routinely "strip" (i.e., occlude the chest tube with one hand while quickly squeezing and moving the other hand down the tube to move fluid down the tube into the drainage chamber) a chest drain because intraluminal pressures can rise dangerously high, potentially converting simple pneumothoraces to life-threatening pneumothoraces and causing tissue trauma and unnecessary additional discomfort. Only in special circumstances, such as hemorrhaging, should the chest tube be stripped to maintain patency.*

Steps	Rationale/Points of Emphasis
15. Reassess child after the procedure. Obtain vital signs; respiratory rate, pattern and effort; skin color; perfusion; level of consciousness; oxygen requirements; hemodynamic stability; and comfort level/pain reassessment.	This will identify child's tolerance of procedure and response to chest tube placement.
16. Consult with the healthcare prescriber regarding an order for an x-ray, if necessary, after chest tube placement.	Chest tubes are normally radiopaque and should be visualized to ensure that they do not go further than the pleural space.
17. Dispose of equipment and waste in appropriate receptacle. Perform hand hygiene.	Standard precautions. Reduces transmission of microorganisms.

PROCEDURE Chest Tube Drainage Collection Device Replacement

Steps	Rationale/Points of Emphasis
1. Follow steps 1 through 6 as described in first procedure for Chest Tube Drainage System Collection Device Setup.	Sets up chest tube collection device.
2. Untape the connections from the old chest tube drainage system to the chest tube catheter.	Allows access to the chest tube catheter for drainage device replacement.
3. Instruct child to exhale and hold his or her breath if age appropriate.	Allows for maximum positive pressure in pleural space.

Steps	Rationale/Points of Emphasis
4. Clamp chest tube catheter (with padded clamp, so as not to rip or tear catheter), about 1½ to 2½ inches from the insertion site. Using two clamps will provide additional security and safety. **Alert!** *The clamp should only remain in place for several seconds, no longer. If clamps remain in place too long, air and fluid can accumulate in the pleural space or additional pneumothoraces could be caused.*	Minimizes dead space; stops air from entering or exiting catheter.
5. Don sterile gloves and, using aseptic technique, disconnect the old drainage system and connect the new one.	Standard precaution to reduce transmission of microorganisms and maintain asepsis. Creates the drainage collection system.
6. Remove the clamp(s) and instruct child to breathe normally.	Allows fluid and air removal to begin anew.
7. Tab-tape all connections with adhesive tape and ensure that all clamps are open.	Secures any loose connections and allows for sure flow of drainage.
8. Secure the chest tube and drainage tube so that there is no tension pulling on the insertion site.	Prevents accidental dislodgment of chest tube.
9. Ensure that the drainage tubing has a straight flow to chest tube drainage collection device and has no dependent loops or kinks. Make sure at this point that suction is connected to chest drainage device and turned on.	If fluid collects in a loop in the tubing between the child and the collection device at a height greater than the suction control limit, the tube will be effectively sealed. This can lead to lung collapse as air and fluid again collect in the pleural space.
10. Reassess child after the procedure. Obtain vital signs; respiratory rate, pattern, and effort; skin color; perfusion; level of consciousness; oxygen requirements; hemodynamic stability; and so forth.	This will identify child's tolerance of procedure and response to chest tube drainage device replacement.
11. Dispose of equipment and waste in appropriate receptacle. Remove gloves and perform hand hygiene.	Standard precautions. Reduces transmission of microorganisms.

PROCEDURE Chest Tube Removal

Steps	Rationale/Points of Emphasis
caREminder *The healthcare prescriber may elect to physiologically simulate tube removal by clamping the chest tube for 12 to 24 hours or place the tube to water seal before removal to evaluate child's tolerance. Clamping of the chest tube before removal is, however, not clinically necessary in many cases, and never done in the case of pneumothoraces.*	
1. Gather the necessary supplies, and perform hand hygiene.	Promotes efficient time management and provides an organized approach to the procedure. Reduces the transmission of microorganisms.
2. Apply topical anesthetic cream to chest tube wound site following manufacturer's instructions. With healthcare prescriber, assess the need for sedation and analgesia, in addition to local anesthetic, before chest tube removal.	Analgesia during chest tube removal reduces child's pain.
3. Position the child for chest tube removal by the healthcare prescriber, while maintaining sterile access for the healthcare prescriber.	Ease of access allows for swift removal of chest tube.

Continued

Steps	Rationale/Points of Emphasis
4. Don nonsterile gloves and remove old dressing from chest tube insertion site.	Standard precaution to reduce transmission of microorganisms. Allows access to the chest tube catheter for healthcare prescriber removal.
5. Clamp chest tube catheter (if not already done) about 1½ to 2½ inches from the insertion site.	Minimizes dead space; stops air from entering or exiting catheter.
6. Instruct child to exhale and hold his or her breath.	Allows for maximum positive pressure in pleural space. Recent studies indicate that discontinuation of chest tubes at the end of inspiration or at the end of expiration have similar rates of postremoval pneumothorax. Thus, healthcare prescriber preference may determine the point in the respiratory cycle at which the tube is removed.
7a. Remove nonsterile gloves. Don sterile gloves and prepare sterile dressing to be placed over insertion site and taped, using 4 × 4 gauze, as healthcare prescriber quickly and smoothly pulls out chest tube.	Wound care precautions to prevent contamination with microorganisms.
7b. Time, initial, and date the dressing.	Monitors dressing changes. **Alert!** *Healthcare prescriber may request sterile petrolatum gauze to be placed immediately over chest tube insertion site, followed by sterile 4 × 4 gauze, because this seals the insertion site from any untoward air entry.*
8. Instruct child to breathe normally.	Allows fluid and air removal to begin anew.
9. Closely monitor child after the procedure. Obtain vital signs; respiratory rate, pattern, and effort; color; perfusion; level of consciousness; oxygen requirements; hemodynamic stability; and chest x-ray, as ordered.	Identifies tolerance to procedure and response to chest tube removal. **Alert!** *Notify healthcare prescriber immediately if child develops any acute respiratory distress because a new chest tube may be indicated.*
10. Dispose of equipment and waste in appropriate receptacle. Remove gloves and perform hand hygiene.	Standard precautions. Reduces transmission of microorganisms.

PROCEDURE Chest Tube Maintenance and Troubleshooting

Steps	Rationale/Points of Emphasis
1. Maintain the sterility of the equipment and insertion site.	Prevents infection and transfer of microorganisms.
2. Check water seal for bubbling and fluctuation every 4 hours or more often as symptoms warrant.	Fluctuation of water in the water-seal chamber is a normal reflection of pressure changes in the pleural cavity during respirations. Bubbling indicates air leaving the system and is normal for the child with a pneumothorax, but it could indicate an air leak in a child without a pneumothorax. For the child on a ventilator with positive end-expiratory pressure (PEEP), continuous bubbling is typically seen because PEEP maintains positive pressure in the alveoli; thus air will continually flow through the lungs. It is also not abnormal to NOT have continuous bubbling for children on PEEP.
3. Observe the integrity of the drainage tubing and chest tube at least once every shift.	Ensures that the system is intact, with no air leaks, and helps to prevent kinks or clots from forming.

Continued

Steps	Rationale/Points of Emphasis
4. Check water seal and suction level every shift and maintain proper level.	Ensures that system is being used properly and maintains child safety while equipment is in use.
5. Keep chest tube clamps readily available at bedside (one for each chest tube in use).	Clamps are used to replace the drainage system or to locate the source of an air leak if bubbling occurs in the water-seal bottle while the system is on suction.
Alert! *Never clamp the tube to get the child out of bed or during transportation of the child. Whenever the chest tube is clamped, air or fluid cannot escape from the pleural space. This puts the child at risk for a tension pneumothorax.*	
6. Troubleshoot the system as needed when problems arise (Table 29-1).	Early and prompt attention to system or patient difficulties will minimize the child's complications.

TABLE 29-1

Troubleshooting Problems With Chest Tubes

Problem	Possible Causes	Intervention
1. Water level in the water-seal chamber does not rise and fall with breathing.	Clot in chest tubing or patient's chest	Gently pinch the tubing around the clot and gingerly milk fluid to move it into the collection chamber; repeat as needed. Unless absolutely necessary, do not strip the tubing because this creates high negative pressure and can damage lung tissue.
	Dependent loop or kink in patient tube with fluid occlusion	Straighten catheter and tubing along its length to its connection with the collection device.
	Dislodgment of catheter from patient	If tube accidentally pulls out, the insertion site should be immediately sealed with a sterile petroleum gauze dressing to prevent air from entering the pleural cavity; notify physician immediately.
	Disconnection of patient tube from chest tube connector	Always keep a chest tube clamp for each tube at the bedside. Quickly clamp the chest tube to prevent a sucking air injury and notify physician immediately.
	Patient tube clamp may be closed.	Clamp only when indicated; otherwise, leave tube open.
	Chest drain is not positioned sufficiently below patient's chest.	Lower chest tube to allow for gravity drainage.
	In-line connectors not properly secured, allowing for an air leak.	Ensure that in-line connectors are properly secured and sealed at all times; check for loose connections periodically.
2. There is constant bubbling in the water-seal chamber.	This confirms an air leak is present.	To determine source of an air leak (patient or catheter connection), momentarily clamp the chest tube close to the chest drain and observe the water seal. If the bubbling stops, the air leak may be from the catheter connections or the patient's chest. Check the catheter connections and patient dressing for a partially withdrawn catheter. If catheter is dislodged, follow procedure as above. If bubbling continues after temporarily clamping the patient's tube, this indicates a system leak requiring system replacement.
3. Overfilled water-seal level (water above 2 cm limit line) or over-filled suction control chamber	Too much water was added to the chamber.	Press and hold the negative-pressure relief valve at the top of the chest drainage system to vent excess negative pressure in the water-seal chamber. Release the valve when the level of the water returns to the 2-cm mark. To remove water from the suction control chamber, insert syringe and withdraw excess.

Continued

TABLE 29-1

Troubleshooting Problems With Chest Tubes (continued)

Problem	Possible Causes	Intervention
4. Not enough water in the water-seal or suction control chamber	Evaporation versus underfill or spillage	Add additional water to the suction control chamber by temporarily turning off the suction source, removing the rubber stopper, and adding water to the desired level. Additional water may be added to the water-seal chamber with a syringe by quickly and temporarily clamping the patient's tube and injecting water to the desired level.
5. Suction control chamber is not bubbling or is bubbling too vigorously.	Check suction source for disconnection or too much suction source pressure in the system.	Ensure that the suction tubing is connected and the suction source is turned on. A constant, gentle bubbling is the norm. Vigorous bubbling causes quicker evaporation. Adjust the suction control source for gentle bubbling.
6. Chest drainage system has accidentally been knocked over.	Human error	Set the system upright and check the fluid levels in the water-seal and suction control chambers for proper volumes. Adjust accordingly. Most units have a baffle system that prevents fluids from mixing between chambers, allowing for proper function after setting upright again.
7. Patient must be transported or leave the unit.	As the situation indicates (e.g., computed tomographic scan, surgery)	Do not clamp the catheter tubing; disconnect the suction tubing from the suction source. The system continues to collect fluid (by gravity) or air (by water seal).
8. Specimen collection required	Doctor's orders for laboratory analysis	Remove fluid with needle and syringe from the self-sealing portion of the drainage tubing after following hospital policy for cleaning the tubing fluid collection site.

CHILD AND FAMILY EVALUATION AND DOCUMENTATION

- Monitor the child's vital signs and note changes in respiratory rate, effort, or pattern, at least every 2 hours, on the appropriate institutional form.
- Evaluate system for water-seal bubbling or fluctuation every 4 hours or more as symptoms warrant; notify healthcare prescriber immediately of any unusual findings.
- Mark the drainage level on the disposable chest drainage collection device every 2 to 4 hours or as needed.
- Determine whether the child and family have other areas of concern to discuss.
- Document the following at the time of insertion:
  - Date and time of insertion
  - Who inserted the tube
  - Assessments
  - Insertion site position and placement (e.g., right upper chest)
  - Chest tube size used
  - Medications received during insertion
  - Amount of water-seal suction
  - The prescribed water level for suction or suction level on dial of dry suction
  - Child's response to the procedure
- Document the following every 2–4 hours:
  - Child's respiratory status
  - Child's vital signs
  - Amount of drainage and its color and consistency
- Document teaching provided to the family.

COMMUNITY CARE

- Instruct the family to notify the healthcare provider if
  - The child exhibits any signs or symptoms of infection at the wound site
  - The child experiences difficulty breathing (e.g., shortness of breath, chest pain)

Unexpected Situations

- *The chest tube becomes dislodged:* Immediately cover the site with a dry sterile dressing and call the healthcare prescriber. If you hear air leaking from the site, tape the dressing on only two or three sides to allow air to escape and to prevent a tension pneumothorax. Closely monitor the child and prepare for insertion of a new chest tube.
- *The chest tube becomes disconnected from the chest drainage system or the chest drainage system breaks:* Immediately submerge the chest tube's distal end in 1 inch of sterile 0.9% sodium chloride solution or sterile water in a sterile container. This creates a liquid seal until you can prepare and attach a new chest drainage system.

Bibliography

Atrium Medical Corporation. (2004). *A personal guide to managing chest drainage.* Hudson, NH: Author.

Bell, R., Ovadia, P., Abdullah, F., Spector, S., & Rabinovich, R. (2001). Chest tube removal: End-inspiration or end-expiration? *Journal of Trauma, 50*(4), 674–677.

Centers for Disease Control and Prevention. (2002). Guidelines for prevention of intravascular device-related infections. *MMWR, 51,* 1–29.

Gupta, N. (2001). Pneumothorax: Is chest tube clamp necessary before removal? *Chest, 119*(4), 1292–1293.

Laws, D., Neville, E. & Duffy, J. (2003). BTS guidelines for the insertion of a chest drain. *Thorax, 58*(Suppl. II), 53–59.

Lazzara, D. (2002). Eliminate the air of mystery from chest tubes. *Nursing, 32*(6), 36–43.

Rosen, D., Morris, J., Rosen, K., et al. (2000). Analgesia for pediatric thoracostomy tube removal. *Anesthesia and Analgesia, 90*(5), 1025–1028.

Waldhausen, J. H., Cusick, R. A., Graham, D. D., Pittinger, T. P., & Sawin, R. S. (2002). Removal of chest tubes in children without water seal after elect thoracic procedures: a randomized, prospective study. *Journal of the American College of Surgeons, 194*(4), 411–415.

CHAPTER

30

Child Abuse Reporting and Documentation

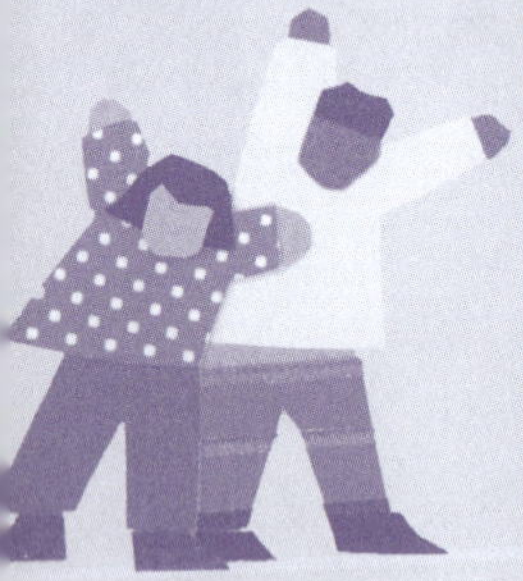

Clinical Guidelines

- All healthcare professionals are considered mandated reporters of suspected abuse. Mandated reporters must notify the appropriate Child Protective Services agency when they have reason to suspect that a child is being abused or maltreated in the course of their professional duties. All states have mandatory reporting laws based on public law.
- The purpose of the reporting statute is to identify abused and neglected children as soon as possible to protect them from further harm. By failure to report, mandated reporters may be guilty of a Class A misdemeanor and may be civilly liable for damage caused by such failure.
- All infants and children should be screened for possible abuse and neglect. Types of abuse that must be reported include physical abuse, physical neglect, sexual abuse, and emotional neglect. Another form of abuse that must be screened for is Munchausen syndrome by proxy (Chart 30-1).
- Child abuse reports remain confidential, and disclosure of this information is limited to official organizations designated to investigate child abuse. Privacy standards as outlined in the Health Insurance Portability Accountability Act of 1996 (HIPAA) must be followed to ensure confidentiality.
- Mandated reporters are provided immunity from civil and criminal liability as a result of making a report of known or suspected child abuse as long as the report was made in good faith and without malicious intent.
- No supervisor, administrator, or physician may impede or inhibit such reporting duties, and no person making such report shall be subject to any sanction for making such a report.

Equipment

- Scale
- Tape measure
- Sphygmomanometer
- Stethoscope
- Growth chart
- Patient gown
- Sheet
- Diapers
- Nonsterile gloves
- Specimen-collection materials
- Camera (35 mm or digital) or video equipment
- Colposcope (optional)

CHART 30-1 Definitions of Child Abuse

- *Physical abuse:* the nonaccidental physical injury of a child (younger than 18 years of age) inflicted by a parent or caretaker, ranging from superficial bruises and welts to broken bones, burns, serious internal injuries, and, in some cases, death
- *Physical neglect:* the withholding of, or failure to provide, adequate food, shelter, clothing, hygiene, medical care, education, or supervision needed for a child's normal growth and development
- *Sexual abuse:* the sexual exploitation of a child by a parent, relative, caretaker, or other person, which may range from nontouching offenses such as exhibitionism to fondling, intercourse, or use of a child in the production of pornographic materials
- *Emotional abuse:* acts or omissions that cause or could cause serious conduct, cognitive, affective, or other mental disorders as a result of such parent or caretaker behavior as torture or close confinement or the constant use of verbally abusive language to harshly criticize and denigrate a child; generally a result of the child's inability to meet unrealistic demands made by parents; also includes emotional neglect—the withholding of physical and emotional contact to the detriment of the child's normal emotional development, and, in extreme cases, physical development
- *Munchausen syndrome by proxy:* condition in which an adult, typically the mother, (a) fabricates a disease by indicating nonexistent or subjective symptoms; (b) creates wounds with instruments, including the hands or the mouth, hot liquids, or caustic substances; (c) creates objective signs of disease, such as vomiting, seizures, respiratory arrest, bleeding problems, and diarrhea; or (d) alters laboratory specimens

Child and Family Assessment and Preparation

- If abuse is suspected because of the child's report or a caregiver's report or because the history given does not correspond to the clinical presentation, a complete history and physical assessment of the child needs to be completed.

caREminder

All children should be screened for maltreatment because this is an essential action to assist in the prevention and early detection of child abuse and neglect.

- Obtain statements separately from the parent and the child. Interview with open-ended questions and with language developmentally appropriate for child.

Alert! ***Determine reliability of historian providing information about the child. It is very important in abuse cases to get an accurate history.***

- If language barrier makes it difficult to obtain history, make sure interpreter is not a family member if abuse is suspected.

caREminder

Objective and qualified interpreters need to be provided to those with limited English proficiency in accordance with Title VI of the Civil Rights Act of 1964. Qualified sign language interpreters and/or other auxiliary aids need to be provided for the hearing impaired according to the Americans with Disability Act (ADA).

- Have available age-appropriate toys or games to distract the child during the examination.
- Any person suspected of being involved in the abuse should not be present during the physical examination. Older children may prefer to be examined without the presence of their caregiver. The child's right to privacy needs to be respected. However, during any examination of the genitalia, a second healthcare provider should be in the room.
- The child should be allowed to remain fully clothed during history taking.
- Maintain privacy for the child.
- Explain to the child and family what to expect during the physical examination.
- Explain to child how any specimens may need to be obtained (e.g., if needed, show child swabs for cultures).
- Show equipment and let child handle, as appropriate, to familiarize himself or herself with it.

KidKare If a colposcope is used, explain to the child that it magnifies her "private area" like the otoscope magnifies "things inside your ear." Let her look through the colposcope and show how it magnifies a character in a book or whatever else is readily available.

caREminder

The delicate and sometimes difficult nature of investigating a possible abuse/neglect case makes it imperative that the nurse conduct herself or himself in a professional and caring manner. The parents may be angry and resentful once they find out that they may be under suspicion for child abuse. Care needs to be taken in these situations that everyone is kept safe and free from harm.

PROCEDURE **Conducting the Health History Interview and Physical Examination**

Steps	Rationale/Points of Emphasis
1. Obtain health history. See Table 30-1 for topics to be covered and key aspects to determine during the interview. Record information exactly as given by informant.	Make sure history is factual; record observations, not conclusions; and record direct quotes. Use quotations marks to denote exact words said by the parent, the caretaker, or the child.
2. Give child gown to put on and sheet to cover himself or herself.	Provides for privacy and modesty during examination.
3. Position for examination.	Helpful to have picture available to show the child various positions that he or she may need to be photographed in—knee–chest, frog-leg, and supine, and stirrups if needed. **KidKare** If the child is uncooperative, offer him or her the choice to sit on parent's lap for examination.
4. Perform hand hygiene. Don gloves.	Reduces transmission of microorganisms. Gloves should be worn for genital examination and specimen collection.
5. Complete physical examination. See Table 30-2 for summary of aspects that need to be evaluated and significance of the findings.	A thorough physical examination will assist in indicating the physical signs of trauma.
6. Document visible injuries with photography and/or videotaping. Individual facility policy regarding consent for these needs to be researched.	Photographs of the injuries assist in documenting extent of injuries. Photos may be used as evidence in court case against the abuser. **KidKare** Continuity of care should be provided by consistent nursing personnel staying with the child throughout the physical examination and any procedures.
7. Assist child to re-dress and place child back in bed or other place or position of comfort. Ensure child has favorite blanket or toy if desired.	Ensures child's privacy, modesty, and comfort are maintained.
8. Remove gloves and perform hand hygiene. Dispose of equipment and waste in appropriate receptacle.	Reduces transmission of microorganisms. Standard precautions.
9. Assist in notifying all appropriate healthcare and legal authorities of suspected abuse.	Actions required by public laws.

CHILD AND FAMILY EVALUATION AND DOCUMENTATION

- Evaluate child's and family's understanding of the examination and the next steps that will be taken.
- Document the following:
  - Results of child and family history
  - Results of physical assessment
  - All parent–child interactions
  - Notification to appropriate authorities regarding suspected abuse

COMMUNITY CARE

- Initiate appropriate referrals for counseling, parenting classes, and family support agencies.
- Initiate and review plan of care with child and family.
- Instruct the family to contact the healthcare provider if
  - Parents notice unusual bruises or other injuries on their child
  - Child displays sudden change in behavior (e.g., nightmares, afraid of certain people or places) or regressive behavior (e.g., enuresis).

TABLE 30-1

Components of the Health History

Assessment Parameter	Rationale
Prenatal history (prenatal infections, smoking, drug or alcohol abuse, planned pregnancy, when prenatal care started)	Important to note how mother cared for herself during pregnancy and her knowledge and care of her child. Children with parents who are substance abusers are at increased risk for abuse and neglect. Children of unwanted pregnancy or with health problems can be at risk for abuse and neglect.
Parental age at time of child's birth	Young parents are less prepared for parenting and report more social and developmental stresses related to their new role.
Neonatal history	History may suggest parental neglect or potential bonding problems because of parent–infant separation.
Childhood illnesses and surgeries	Stress related to not having the "perfect" child may lead to family discord and disappointment.
Previous hospitalizations, emergency room visits, and sources of past medical care	Recurrent visits may indicate previous child abuse incidents or unexplained injuries or simply lack of basic safety knowledge.
Current medications, treatments, allergies, and immunizations	Lack of immunizations suggests that well-child care is a low priority; this could reflect neglect or a family in crisis.
History of presenting complaint or symptom • Exact dates, times, and sequences of events • Interim of time from onset to seeking of medical attention • Identity of any witnesses • Identity of person responsible for child's care at time of incident • Identity of alleged perpetrator if known	Any injury without adequate explanation, especially in young children, raises concerns about either nonaccidental injury or neglect. Accounts that change often indicate nonaccidental injury. Delay in seeking medical care, especially for significant injury, needs to be carefully evaluated because it may indicate increased risk for abuse. In Munchausen syndrome by proxy, child's reported symptoms typically occur only when the parent is present and stop when the parent is not. Consider Munchausen syndrome by proxy when • Description of a prolonged, inexplicable illness that despite medical attention and therapies has not been resolved • Symptoms described by the parent are incompatible or inappropriate • Child's symptoms do not occur when others are present
Development • Age and developmental milestones achieved • Any developmental delays, chronic illness, or disability requiring special treatment or services from parent or other caretakers • Child behavior (e.g., likes to be alone; is aggressive, quiet, or unresponsive to pain)	Children with developmental delay are at increased risk for abuse and neglect. Important to note chronologic age-to-developmental age equivalent. Is child able developmentally to have incurred this injury to himself or herself? If developmental delay is inorganic in nature, this is an indicator that child is not receiving appropriate environmental stimulation.
Family history, including previous unexplained infant deaths	Previous abuse or neglect and stressful events can increase risk for abuse and neglect.
Health status of parents and other siblings • Medical problems of parents and other siblings • Stressful events in family • Coping strategies	Recent significant depression or emotional illness of parents suggests added family stress and may decrease their coping abilities.
Family personal/social history • Parents' education, occupation, and ages • Pets • Interests and hobbies • Child care • Religious/cultural practices	Single-parent households may suggest lack of economic support and assistance in parenting. Parents living alone or in unstable relationships are less likely to have optimum social support, and additional stress may be present. Low education may suggest limited cognitive and psychosocial skills. Occupation may cause economic stress. Folk remedies may expose the child to toxic substances or may appear to be maltreatment (e.g., coining, cupping).
Parental history of substance abuse or chemical dependency within past 6 months	Recent drug or alcohol abuse by the caregiver leads to high incidence of child abuse and neglect as a result of decreased parental capacity.

Continued

TABLE 30-1

Components of the Health History (continued)

Assessment Parameter	Rationale
Observe parent and child social interaction to include • Parents' response to child-initiated interaction • Child's response to parent(s) • Child's interaction with other people • Parents' discipline history toward child • Parents' beliefs regarding discipline	Attachment behavior is a predictor of protective behavior on the part of the mother. Parent may have unrealistic expectations for child's behavior.
History of home environment • Size of home • Whether the home is owned or rented • Sleeping arrangements • Safety, including access to open windows • Water supply	Physical neglect may be present if child is sharing quarters with multiple family members or is living in unsanitary conditions.
Nutritional status • Appetite, feedings, and calorie and fluid intake in 24 hours • History of feeding problems, vomiting, spitting with feedings • Child's ability to feed self • Family dietary practices, such as vegetarianism	Dietary history becomes very important in neglect and failure-to-thrive cases. It may help to distinguish organic from inorganic failure to thrive. Feeding problems suggest either a physiologic abnormality or a parent-mediated feeding problem.

TABLE 30-2

Physical Assessment Findings

Assessment Parameter	Alterations/Clinical Significance
General appearance, hygiene, emotional state and activity	Hygiene may indicate neglect. Emotional state and activity may indicate a flat affect or a very frightened child.
Growth percentiles for height, weight, and head circumference if younger than age 3 years	Need to plot on growth chart and include previous measurements to note any changes in growth patterns; for example, poor weight gain.
Vital signs (temperature, pulse, respirations, and blood pressure)	If blood loss, may see tachycardia; hypotension is an ominous late sign of hypovolemia.
Integumentary system • Absence or presence of any anomalies • Cuts, bruises, burns, welts, bites • Pain • Swelling, tenderness • Bleeding • Other signs of trauma	Bruises—need to note location, pattern size, and color. Bruises sustained over bony prominences are less likely to indicate abuse. Bruises on buttocks, hands, trunk, face, and on or behind ears are more likely to be the result of inflicted trauma. Size should include both horizontal and vertical length. Color can note age of bruise and if the color (age) corresponds to history of how the bruise occurred. Bites greater than 3 cm in diameter are usually inflicted by adults. Pattern description of burns may help note object used, such as cigarette, iron, and immersion burns from scalding.
Head and neck • Bruising • Hair loss • Changes in hair texture • Any difficulty in movement of neck	Patches of baldness may be a sign that the child was pulled by the hair.
Face, nose, and oral cavity • Note any swelling, asymmetry, ecchymosis • Other signs of trauma • Dental status	Lack of dental care may indicate neglect.
Eyes • Retinal changes • Blurred vision	Retinal hemorrhages are present (with few other external signs of abuse) in shaken baby syndrome.

TABLE 30-2

Physical Assessment Findings (continued)

Assessment Parameter	Alterations/Clinical Significance
Gastrointestinal • Nausea, vomiting • Constipation, diarrhea, encopresis • Rectal bleeding • Tenderness of abdomen, bruising, distention, or rigidity	Tenderness may indicate intra-abdominal bleeding or peritonitis caused by a blow to the abdomen.
Neuromuscular • Gait • Level of consciousness • Fatigability • Muscle wasting • Fontanel	Seizures, hyperirritability, poor feeding, and bulging fontanel in infants may indicate head trauma or shaken baby syndrome.
Genitourinary • Dysuria, enuresis • Vaginal discharge, urethral discharge, bleeding • Last menstrual period, if pubertal	Pelvic examination is necessary for pubertal girls and those with suspected internal injuries.
Musculoskeletal • Any deformity • Pain, swelling, and tenderness of an extremity	Twisting of an extremity may result in a spiral fracture or dislocation. Posterior rib fractures may be seen with shaken baby syndrome (anterior rib fractures are potentially seen after CPR).

- Child verbalizes that someone has inflicted actions against the child that may be considered physically or emotionally abusive

Unexpected Situations

- *Physical examination needs to be performed on the child and the parent who is the suspected perpetrator wants to remain during examination:* Neither the police nor child protective services would allow a suspected perpetrator to be present during the examination of the child. Inform the parent that it is in the child's best interest that the parent remains calm and respects the requests of the medical provider and the police in regards to not being present while the child is being examined. Reassure the parent that a nurse will be present and provide support to the child. Guide parent out of room. If parent becomes hostile, seek assistance of security personnel. If the parent is not suspect and the child is young, having the parent present would be helpful to alleviate the child's fears. You may want a separate time with the child without the parents to get the history of events.
- *Parent tries to leave with child before evaluation is completed:* You need to stress to the parent the importance of remaining for evaluation. If he or she is adamant about leaving, contact security (law enforcement if security not available) and child protective services in your community.

Bibliography

American Academy of Pediatrics. (1999). Guidelines for the evaluation of sexual abuse in children: Subject review. *Pediatrics, 103*(1), 186–191.

American Academy of Pediatrics. (2002). When inflicted skin injuries constitute child abuse. *Pediatrics, 110*(3), 644–645.

Barnes, M. (2001). Child abuse histories: What you need to know. *Patient Care for the Nurse Practitioner*, 7, 17–27.

Kellogg, N. (2005). The evaluation of sexual abuse in children. *Pediatrics, 116*(2), 506–512.

Meier, E. (2000). Children and international human rights abuses. *Pediatric Nursing, 26*(5), 545–546.

Mudd, S., & Findley, J. (2004). The cutaneous manifestations and common mimickers of physical child abuse. *Journal of Pediatric Health Care, 18*(3), 123–129.

Murry, S., Baker, A., & Lewin, L. (2000). Screening families with young children for child maltreatment potential. *Pediatric Nursing, 26*(1), 47–54.

Myer, J. E., Berliner, L., Briere, J., Hendrix, C. T., Jenny, C., & Reid, T. A. (2001). *The APSAC handbook on child maltreatment.* Thousand Oaks, CA: Sage Publications.

National Clearinghouse on Child Abuse and Neglect Information. (2003). *Recognizing child abuse and neglect: Signs and symptoms.* Retrieved September 21, 2006, from http://nccanch.acf.hhs.gov/pubs/factsheets/signs.cfm

National Clearinghouse on Child Abuse and Neglect Information. (2003). *About the federal child abuse prevention and treatment act.* Retrieved September 21, 2006, from http://nccanch.acf.hhs.gov/pubs/factsheets/about.cfm

Ramos, F. (2003). Legal update: HIPAA's new privacy rules. *ADVANCE for Nurse Practitioners, 11*(5), 24.

Reese, R. M., & Ludwig, S. (2001). *Child abuse medical diagnosis and management* (2nd ed.). Philadelphia: Lippincott Williams & Wilkins.

CHAPTER
31

Circumcision Care

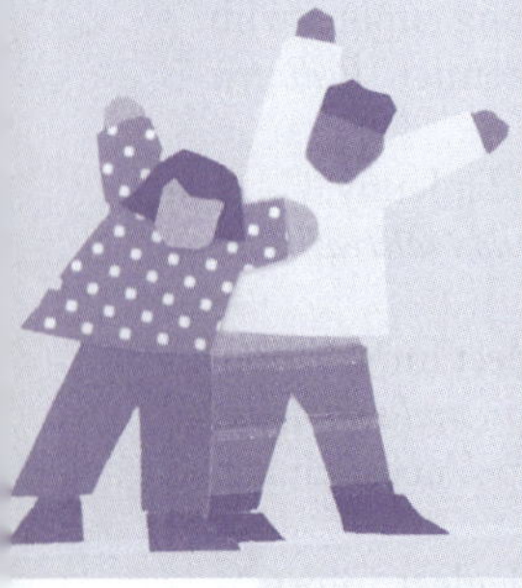

Clinical Guidelines

- Circumcision is performed by a healthcare prescriber.
- The registered nurse (RN), licensed practical nurse (LPN), or unlicensed assistive personnel (UAP) may assist the healthcare prescriber during the procedure. The RN or LPN is responsible for monitoring the postprocedural status of the infant.
- Informed consent must be obtained from the child's parents or legal guardian before performing the procedure.
- To ensure the newborn is stable, circumcision should not be performed until the infant is 12 to 24 hours old.
- Analgesia/anesthesia is used for the procedure: local plus adjuvant during the neonatal period, general anesthesia for older children.
- Circumcision is not performed on children with anatomic defects of the penis (e.g., hypospadias, epispadias) or on clinically unstable infants.
- Healthcare providers performing or assisting with this procedure should be familiar with religious beliefs regarding circumcision, the advantages and disadvantages of the procedure, and the American Academy of Pediatrics position regarding circumcision.

Equipment

- Disposable circumcision tray that includes sterile clamp
- Appropriate-sized bell or Plastibell (several sizes should be available)
- Circumcision restraining board
- Fluid-impervious gown
- Sterile gloves
- Sterile petroleum jelly or petroleum gauze packet
- Sterile 2 × 2 gauze
- Bulb syringe
- Chlorhexidine swabs
- Pacifier
- Sucrose (liquid solution)
- Acetaminophen, as prescribed
- Antibiotic ointment, as prescribed
- Sterile water

For dorsal penile nerve block or local anesthesia:

- 1% lidocaine without epinephrine buffered with sodium bicarbonate
- 27-gauge needle
- 1-mL syringe

For topical cream analgesia:

- EMLA cream and occlusive dressing

Optional equipment as requested by the healthcare prescriber:

- Needle holder
- Sutures
- Sheldon, Mogen, or Gomco clamp
- Plastibell and instruction card
- Topical adrenaline solution 1:1,000 or Gelfoam

CHILD AND FAMILY ASSESSMENT AND PREPARATION

- Evaluate parents' and older child's understanding of the procedure.
- Assess the genitalia before the procedure to detect the presence of visible anomaly (e.g., hypospadias, epispadias), a contraindication to circumcision because an intact foreskin may be required for later reconstructive surgery. Notify healthcare prescriber if anomaly is present.
- Before circumcision, review the chart and/or discuss with family to determine requests for ritualistic circumcision in accordance with the tenets of their religion (e.g., Jewish or Islamic faiths).
- Question parents about the existence of coagulation disorders in their family history. Monitor the infant for signs of a blood dyscrasia (e.g., the presence of unexpected ecchymotic spots or prolonged bleeding after newborn testing). Vitamin K may be administered before the procedure, depending on etiology of the dyscrasia.
- Before the procedure, if ordered, check bleeding coagulation time and notify healthcare prescriber of results.
- Healthcare prescriber must obtain consent for medical-surgical procedure. Authorization must be obtained from a parent and be witnessed.
- The infant may be allowed to eat if hungry, unless otherwise ordered.
- Assess infant for self-comforting behaviors, and identify these to the parents so that they can promote their use in the infant; provide the parents with information about other comfort measures, incorporating these measures during and after procedure.
- Discuss pain relief with healthcare prescriber (e.g., dorsal penile nerve block, EMLA) and prepare needed equipment.

KidKare Use a sucrose-coated pacifier and acetaminophen to augment the above measures.

PROCEDURE Providing Circumcision Care

Steps	Rationale/Points of Emphasis
1. Gather the necessary supplies.	Promotes efficient time management and provides an organized approach to the procedure.
2. Perform hand hygiene.	Reduces transmission of microorganisms.
3. Identify the infant using two different patient identifiers.	Reduces incidence of procedure being completed on wrong infant.
4. Prepare infant:	
a. If EMLA analgesia is used, apply EMLA cream at least 60 minutes before circumcision.	Provides adequate time for skin penetration of anesthetic.
b. Administer acetaminophen 30 minutes before procedure, as ordered.	Augments analgesia; provides time for adequate blood levels of medication.
c. Verify the infant's identification band and presence of signed consent with the healthcare prescriber.	Ensures that correct infant has procedure performed and consent has been obtained. **caREminder** *To detect potential for complications, assess infant for signs of blood dyscrasia, such as ecchymotic spots or prolonged bleeding, and report presence to healthcare prescriber.*
5. Place infant under radiant warmer or heat lamp on circumcision restraining board. Remove diaper and, if clean, place under the buttocks.	Prevents hypothermia and controls infant movement. Allows for complete visualization of the penis. The diaper provides area to collect drainage.
6. Dip pacifier in sucrose and offer to infant. Throughout procedure, check frequently to keep pacifier in infant's mouth.	Sucrose may be mediated through opioid receptors. Initiates some analgesia before procedure to augment, not replace, more potent pain prevention measures (e.g., dorsal penile nerve block, EMLA).

Steps	Rationale/Points of Emphasis
7. Don gloves.	Standard precaution to reduce transmission of microorganisms.
8. Cleanse penis, scrotal area, and groin with chlorhexidine. Remove gloves and perform hand hygiene.	Reduces transmission of microorganisms.
9. Assist in administration of subcutaneous ring block or dorsal penile nerve block. Wait 4–5 minutes.	Prevents pain. Subcutaneous ring block may be more effective than dorsal penile nerve block, which is more effective than EMLA. Waiting allows analgesia to occur.
10. Prepare equipment using aseptic technique:	
a. Open circumcision tray and sterile gloves.	Reduces chances of equipment contamination and transfer of microorganisms.
b. Place proper size of sterile clamp or Plastibell requested by healthcare prescriber on tray; have several sizes available.	Infants require different sizes of clamps or Plastibells.
c. Have bulb syringe readily accessible.	Prepares for suctioning in case of vomiting.
d. Dressing supplies (e.g., petroleum jelly and gauze) should be immediately accessible.	Dressing applied to site immediately after procedure prevents bleeding. Petroleum prevents gauze from sticking to wound and may promote healing.
11. Position light on groin area.	Enhances visualization of area.
12a. Monitor child's response and assist healthcare prescriber during procedure.	Ensures procedure is progressing without untoward effects.
12b. Provide soothing measures/pad restraint board if distress due to restraint; if distress is due to being exposed, cover with blanket or provide support by placing hands on infant to provide sense of containment.	Promotes atraumatic care. **caREminder** *If infant cries, evaluate cause. If due to pain, ensure that adequate time has elapsed for analgesia to take effect; recoat pacifier with liquid sucrose solution and reposition in infant's mouth.*
13. If foreskin tissue is being sent for evaluation, collect and handle tissue using aseptic technique. Place tissue in a sterile container labeled with infant's name, date, and time. Place specimen in biohazard bag and send to laboratory.	Ensures safe collection of tissue and that correct infant tissue is tested.
14a. At completion of procedure, don gloves and immediately apply dressing to penis using sterile petroleum jelly liberally applied around penis and then cover with sterile gauze, or use petroleum gauze packet if Gomco-type circumcision. If Plastibell type, apply antibiotic ointment as ordered by healthcare prescriber. Completely remove chlorhexidine solution with sterile water.	Controls bleeding and prevents diaper from adhering to surgical site. Chlorhexidine may cause tissue damage if left in contact with infant's skin. **Alert!** *Do not apply dressing if circumcision was performed using a Plastibell. In all cases, semipermeable dressings or large amounts of tape should not be used. Petroleum may cause Plastibell to loosen, and gauze may snag on Plastibell. Removing a semipermeable dressing or large amounts of tape can cause pain and irritation or can damage the infant's fragile skin.*
14b. Assess site for bleeding, and then loosely apply diaper. Comfort infant.	Detects complications. Circumcised area may ooze blood, but no frank bleeding should occur. Bleeding is the most common complication and usually is controlled well using local hemostatic measures. **Alert!** *If frank bleeding occurs, apply sterile pressure dressing using sterile gauze. Notify healthcare prescriber immediately.*
15. Wrap infant in blanket. Position infant on back.	Reduces risk of hypothermia. Decreases risk for sudden infant death syndrome and prevents placement of pressure on circumcision area.
16. Dispose of equipment and waste in appropriate receptacle. Remove gloves and perform hand hygiene.	Standard precautions. Reduces transmission of microorganisms.

CHILD AND FAMILY EVALUATION AND DOCUMENTATION

- Assess circumcision site every 30 minutes after the procedure for signs of frank bleeding for 2 hours, and then with every diaper change.
- Observe the infant for voiding. Assess adequacy of urinary stream and amount and presence of blood.
- Assess infant's level of comfort and administer analgesia as needed.
- Document the following:
  - Date, time, and method used for circumcision
  - The healthcare prescriber who performed the circumcision
  - The infant's tolerance of the procedure.
  - Any bleeding noted during and after the procedure and any medication given
  - Parent teaching regarding circumcision care

COMMUNITY CARE

- The infant must be monitored by healthcare provider for 1 hour after circumcision to monitor site for bleeding. The infant does not need to void before discharge.
- When making a home visit, assess circumcision site for signs of adequate healing or infection. Discuss with parents how site is healing (e.g., normal presence of penile swelling or mucous discharge over glans during healing).
- Reinforce parental teaching, as follows:
  - Administer acetaminophen every 4 hours for 24 hours as ordered.
  - Monitor voiding for first 8 hours after procedure; first-void urine may be tinged pink, but frank bleeding is abnormal.
  - Monitor for bleeding with every diaper change; apply petroleum dressing for 1 to 2 days.
  - Note that slight bleeding and red discoloration at the circumcision area may be normal.
  - Check site for signs of infection (i.e., foul-smelling drainage and swelling); as the penile head heals, there is usually a slight yellow plaque coloring, which is normal (do not try to wash this off).
  - If a Plastibell was used, it should fall off on its own within 3 to 4 days.
  - Tub baths may be started after 5 days if the infant's cord is off; if the cord is still present, no immersing of the umbilical site should occur.
  - Older boys should not ride straddle toys or play vigorously for 3 to 4 days.
- Provide written instructions, if not done previously.
- Instruct the family to contact the healthcare provider if
  - The child has not voided within 8 hours after the procedure
  - Increased redness, bleeding, swelling, or warmth at circumcision site is present
  - The infant develops a fever
  - The child seems to be in pain and cannot be consoled.

Unexpected Situations

- *While checking the circumcision site you note that the dressing is dry and has adhered to the penis:* Moisten the dressing with water and gently attempt to remove the dressing from the site. Redress the site with petroleum gauze.
- *While checking the circumcision site you notice the dressing is moist and reddened:* Remove the dressing to better assess the site. Apply pressure using sterile gauze. If bleeding continues, notify the healthcare prescriber because local hemostatic measures may need to be employed to stop the bleeding.

Bibliography

Alanis, M., & Lucidi, R. (2004). Neonatal circumcision: A review of the world's oldest and most controversial operation. *Obstetrical & Gynecological Survey, 59*(5), 379–395.

American Academy of Family Physicians. (2005). *Position paper on neonatal circumcision.* Retrieved April 29, 2005, from http://www.aafp.org/x1462.xml

American Academy of Pediatrics. (1999; reaffirmed 2005). Circumcision policy statement. *Pediatrics, 103,* 686–693.

American Academy of Pediatrics. (2000). Task force on circumcision: Circumcision debate. *Pediatrics, 105,* 641–642.

American Academy of Pediatrics. (2001). The assessment and management of acute pain in infants, children, and adolescents. *Pediatrics, 108,* 793–797.

Gray, D. T. (2004). Neonatal circumcision: Cost-effective preventative measure or "the unkindest cut of all?" *Medical Decision Making, 24*(6), 688–692.

Kaufman, G., Cimo, S., Miller, L., & Blass, E. (2002). An evaluation of the effects of sucrose on neonatal pain with 2 commonly used circumcision methods. *American Journal of Obstetrics & Gynecology, 186*(3), 564–568.

Kaufman, M., Clark, J., & Castro, C. (2001). Neonatal circumcision. *American Journal of Maternal Child Nursing, 26*(4), 197–201.

Lehr, V., Cepeda, E., Frattarelli, D., et al. (2005). Lidocaine 4% cream compared with lidocaine 2.5% and prilocaine 2.5% or dorsal penile block for circumcision. *American Journal of Perinatology, 22*(5), 231–237.

South, M., Strauss, R., South, A., Boggess, J., & Thorp, J. (2005). The use of non-nutritive sucking to decrease the physiologic pain response during neonatal circumcision: A randomized controlled trial. *American Journal of Obstetrics & Gynecology, 193*(2), 537–543.

Taddio, A., Pollock, N., Gilbert-MacLeod, C., Ohlsson, K., & Koren, G. (2000). Combined analgesia and local anesthesia to minimize pain during circumcision. *Archives of Pediatrics and Adolescent Medicine, 154,* 620–623.

CHAPTER

32

Cooling Measures, Use of

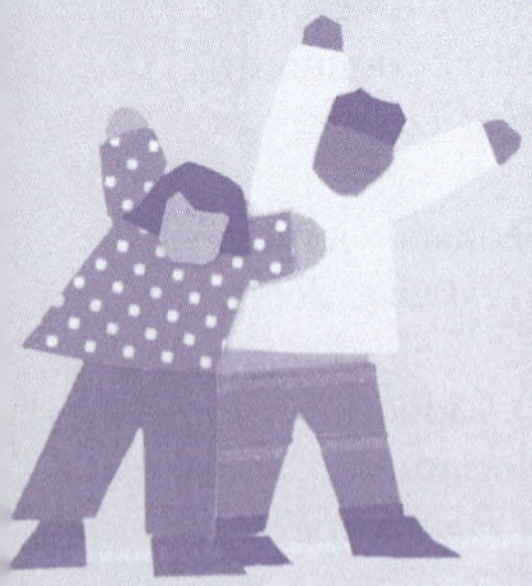

Clinical Guidelines

- A healthcare prescriber orders medications.
- Medications are administered by a registered nurse (RN), licensed practical nurse (LPN), physician, or parent who is knowledgeable about the medication and techniques of administering oral medications to a child.
- In the hospital, use of antipyretic medications and hypothermia blanket is implemented by the RN or LPN on the order of a healthcare prescriber.
- Basic cooling measures are administered by the RN, LPN, physician, or knowledgeable parent.
- Principles of pharmacologic management (see Chapter 6) are followed.
- Hyperpyrexia is defined as a temperature higher than 105.8°F (41°C) and is associated with severe infection, hypothalamic disorders, or central nervous system hemorrhage. It involves normal thermoregularity responses responding at a higher level. Hyperpyrexia responds best to central cooling interventions such as antipyretic therapy. Hyperpyrexia requires primary management by a healthcare prescriber because antipyretic therapy will need to be initiated.
- Hyperthermia exists when the set point is normal yet the child feels heated and overly warm (e.g., after increased physical exertion) with a higher body temperature. Hyperthermia involves a dysfunction of thermoregularity responses and responds best to physical cooling methods.
- Fever is defined as an elevation in set point such that body temperature is regulated at a higher level (e.g., as a result of a bacterial infection). Fever is considered an adaptive response and is one of many mechanisms to fight infection. There is evidence that various components of the immune system are enhanced at elevated temperatures. Fever is considered present when the child's temperatures are as follows:
  - Newborn: >99 to 100°F (37.4° to 37.8°C)
  - Older than 1 month of age: >101°F (38.3°C)
- Child's temperature is closely monitored during cooling measures and until the child's temperature has returned to within normal parameters.
- Tepid baths should not be administered. This method is not supported by research for fever management and is often uncomfortable to children and may produce little if any long-lasting effects to reduce fever.

Equipment

- Temperature measurement device (see Chapter 134 for types of temperature measurement devices).

- Cotton sheets (if needed, to replace flannel)
- Cotton blanket (if needed, to replace wool)

For administration of antipyretic medications:

- Medications as ordered
- See Chapters 70 and 72

For cooling blanket:

- Electronic cooling blanket
- Hypothermia machine preferably with thermometer probe
- Protective sheets

CHILD AND FAMILY ASSESSMENT AND PREPARATION

- Assess child for noninfectious reasons for an elevated temperature. The external environmental temperature and overbundling, recent administration of childhood immunizations, and some prescribed drugs may cause an elevation in temperature.
- Assess child's clinical history and related physical symptoms to determine reasons for an elevated temperature. Cooling measures may also be implemented in specific situations (e.g., after cardiac surgery or neurologic insult) to induce mild hypothermia and reduce metabolic demands.
- Explain to the child and parents what you will be doing to reduce child's temperature and to make the child more comfortable.
- Encourage parents to be present in the room.
- Use diversionary techniques if needed for cooperation.

PROCEDURE Preintervention Measures

Steps	Rationale/Points of Emphasis
1. Collect equipment to assess child's temperature.	Assembly of all necessary equipment ensures that the assessment can proceed in an efficient manner.
2. Perform hand hygiene.	Reduces transmission of microorganisms.
3. Determine child's temperature (see Chapter 134) and observe the child for clinical manifestations of fever or hyperthermia.	Normal body temperature is 98.6°F (37.0°C). Ranges vary with age (see Appendix D). Signs of fever include flushed skin, increased respiratory rate, increased heart rate, malaise, and "glassy" look of the eyes. In the absence of hyperemic insult, it is exceedingly rare for a child's temperature to exceed 107°F (41.7°C). **Alert!** *High fever and rapid rise in temperature in young children are associated with febrile convulsions.*
4. Notify healthcare prescriber of child's elevated temperature.	The child's therapy may need to be altered or additional laboratory tests required based on child's development of a fever.
5. Obtain diagnostic tests as ordered (e.g., complete blood count, blood culture, urine culture, spinal tap).	Laboratory analysis may identify bacterial agent causing fever. Such tests are not routinely recommended for all children exhibiting a fever; rather, careful evaluation of the child on a case-to-case basis must be made to determine the risks and benefits of testing. Testing may, in fact, do more harm than good to the child who is subject to such procedures.
6. Select intervention method to cool the child. Gather the necessary equipment to proceed with intervention measures. Follow manufacturer's instructions for initiating use of selected equipment (e.g., cooling blanket).	Cooling measures are selected based on child's temperature, age of the child, diagnosis, healthcare setting (emergency department, intensive care unit, general care unit, etc.), and resources available.
7. Perform hand hygiene before initiating interventions with the child.	Reduces transmission of microorganisms when initiating contact with the child.

PROCEDURE Basic Cooling Measures

Steps	Rationale/Points of Emphasis
1. Remove excessive clothing and blankets from child.	Excessive clothing and covering can result in elevation of body temperature.
2. Offer fluids to the child to drink.	Fever may cause diaphoresis that acts to dehydrate the child's body.
3. Ensure that child is laying on cotton sheets or other "breathable" material. Remove nonbreathable linens and replace with cotton.	Flannel or wool linens and blanket may feel warmer against the child's skin.

PROCEDURE Antipyretic Medications

Steps	Rationale/Points of Emphasis
1. Administer an antipyretic, as ordered, Follow guidelines in Chapter 70 for oral administration of medications or in Chapter 72 for rectal administration of medications.	Ibuprofen and acetaminophen are effective antipyretic agents in children, when used alone and in the appropriate dosing amounts.

Alert! *Alternating the use of acetaminophen and ibuprofen is common practice; however, there is a lack of evidence to support the efficacy and safety of this practice. In addition, inappropriate and liberal dosing of these medications places children at undue risk for antipyretic toxicity. Do not use aspirin for fever control in children because of the risk of Reye syndrome.*

caREminder

Antipyretic treatment alone has been demonstrated to have little or no preventive effect on reoccurrence of febrile seizures.

PROCEDURE Cooling Blanket

Steps	Rationale/Points of Emphasis
1. Obtain equipment and place in open area; do not cover with linen.	Reduces transmission of microorganisms. Unit needs to be ventilated.
2. Follow manufacturer's instructions for setting up equipment and ensure that equipment is in good working condition.	Ensures child safety during use of device.
3. Cover the hypothermia blanket with a sheet, position blanket either over or beneath child, and connect the blanket to the machine.	Protects the child's skin from frostbite and pressure areas and readies machine for use.

caREminder

Do not use safety pins because these will damage the thermal blanket and may injure the child.

Steps	Rationale/Points of Emphasis
4. If the automatic temperature control mode will be used, insert the temperature probe and secure as indicated (e.g., tape rectal probe to the child's buttocks).	Allows for constant monitoring of the child's temperature.

Alert! *Do not use rectal probes with children who have neutropenia, thrombocytopenia, a bleeding disorder, or rectal or bowel surgery.*

Continued

Steps	Rationale/Points of Emphasis
5. Set the machine to the manufacturer's suggested range (generally between 89.6°F and 95°F [32°C and 35°C]).	Allows the blanket to begin cooling.
6. Assess the child's temperature every 15 to 30 minutes. If using a rectal probe, periodically assess the child's temperature using an oral, axillary, temporal, or tympanic device.	Evaluates efficacy of interventions and alerts to change in child's status. Verification with alternate method helps to determine accuracy of rectal thermometer.
7. Position the child for comfort and turn every 1 to 2 hours.	Prevents tissue damage and promotes circulation.
8. Observe for sign of shivering, vasoconstriction, and goose bumps.	External cooling may also activate heat-conserving and heat-producing mechanisms that act to raise the body temperature. Shivering increases metabolic demands.
9. Turn off the machine when the child's temperature has reached desired temperature range.	Prevents child from becoming hypothermic.

CHILD AND FAMILY EVALUATION AND DOCUMENTATION

- Compare child's temperature with previous readings.
- Evaluate child's response to cooling measures.
- Evaluate parents' understanding of methods used to monitor and decrease child's temperature.
- Notify healthcare prescriber if the child's temperature does not decrease in response to the measures used.
- Assess child's ability to maintain normal body temperature after interventions are terminated.
- Document the following:
  - Child's vital signs before initiation of treatment measures, during treatment, and after treatment
  - Cooling measures initiated
  - Child's response to cooling measures
  - Education provided to the parents
  - Parent's participation in child's care
- Document that healthcare prescriber was notified of child's condition and chart specific orders given and completed at that time.

COMMUNITY CARE

- Assess parents' ability to measure the child's temperature and to read the device accurately.
- Educate parents about normal temperature and signs and symptoms of elevated temperature and that fever is the body's normal response to infection.
- Provide teaching instructions for cooling measures to include the following:
  - Dress child lightly.
  - Do not overbundle or use heavy blankets.
  - Encourage fluid intake.
  - Keep the temperature in the room at about 70°F (21°C).
  - Administer antipyretic as instructed.
  - Check child's temperature before administering the medication. If below indicated temperature, do not administer.
  - If the child is not taking medications by mouth, acetaminophen suppositories should only be given after discussion with the healthcare provider.

Alert! *Advise parents not to substitute alternative dosage forms, in particular, adult for pediatric preparations. Additionally, to avoid antipyretic toxicity, many cold, headache, and cough preparations may contain acetaminophen, and simultaneous use of more than one product containing acetaminophen may cause overdose. Advise parents to read medication labels for all over-the-counter products and make sure these contain no antipyretic medications. Advise if they have any doubts to contact healthcare provider.*

- Instruct the family to contact the healthcare provider if
  - A child younger than 6 months of age has a fever greater than 101°F (38.2°C) or a child older than 6 months of age has a fever greater than 104°F (40°C)
  - The fever persists for 2 additional days without other symptoms
  - The child develops symptoms such as a rash, trouble breathing, ear pain, headache, stiff neck, vomiting, diarrhea, joint swelling or pain, lethargy, or refusal of food and fluids

Unexpected Situation

- *Child is shivering, skin is mottled, and child says he or she is cold:* Obtain vital signs. Evaluate cooling measure(s) being used; if on hypothermia blanket, increase blanket temperature; evaluate time since last antipyretic medication and if another dose can be administered. If shivering is excessive or child's temperature is nearing desired measure, discontinue hypothermia blanket or other cooling measure. Notify the healthcare prescriber and document the event.

Bibliography

American Academy of Pediatrics. (2001). Acetaminophen toxicity in children. *Pediatrics, 108*, 1020–1024.

Axelrod, P. (2000). External cooling in the management of fever. *Clinical Infectious Diseases, 31*(Suppl. 5), S224–S229.

Carson, S. M. (2003). Alternating acetaminophen and ibuprofen in the febrile child: Examination of the evidence regarding efficacy and safety. *Pediatric Nursing, 29*, 379–382.

Creechan, T., Vollman, K., & Kravutske, M. E. (2001). Cooling by convection vs cooling by conduction for treatment of fever in critically ill adults. *American Journal of Critical Care, 10*, 52–59.

Crocetti, M., Moghbeli, N., & Serwint, J. (2001). Fever phobia revisited: Have parental misconceptions about fever changed in 20 years? *Pediatrics, 107*, 1241–1246.

Guy, E., & Bandi, V. (2002). Recognizing drug-induced hyperthermia syndrome: How to distinguish between the possible toxicities. *Journal of Critical Illness, 17*, 467–475.

Krantz, C. (2001). Childhood fevers: Developing an evidence-based anticipatory guidance tool for parents. *Pediatric Nursing, 27*, 567–571.

Watts, R., Robertson, J., & Thomas, G. (2003). Nursing management of fever in children: A systematic review. *International Journal of Nursing Practice, 9*, S1–S8.

CHAPTER

33

Developmental Care of the Neonate

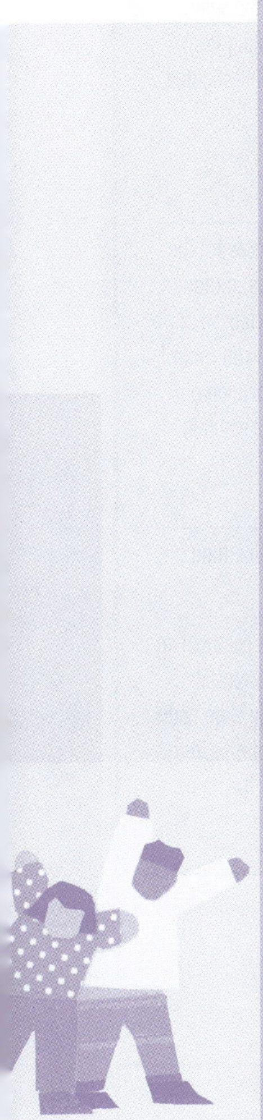

Clinical Guidelines

- Parents and healthcare providers modulate the environment to promote stabilization of neurophysiologic and behavioral systems that support and facilitate the infant's coping and development.
- Observations of the infant's behavior provide cues regarding the infant's organization and capacity for self-regulation and identify the infant's level of disorganization and threshold for stress.
- Families are taught the engagement–disengagement (approach–withdrawal) cues of the infant so they can fulfill their integral role in supporting and caring for their child.

Child and Family Assessment and Preparation

- Review with parents the concept of neurodevelopment of the neonate.
- Assess family's willingness and ability to participate in a developmental care approach to the infant's overall plan of care.
- Assess barriers that may affect the implementation of developmental care, including the following:
  - Environmental factors
  - Neonate's clinical condition
  - Parents' understanding of neonatal systems and developmental needs
  - Collaboration among healthcare team members to provide consistent developmental care

caREminder

Behaviors that indicate stress in the premature infant include facial grimace, yawning, tongue protrusion, hiccuping, finger splaying, gaze aversion, fussing, crying, and vomiting. Physiologic stress cues include changes in heart or respiratory rates (i.e., tachycardia, bradycardia, tachypnea, or apnea), grunting, gasping, cyanosis, and decreased blood oxygen levels (reflected in decreased oxygen saturation or transcutaneous oxygen [$TcPO_2$] levels). The infant exhibits these signs when the environment is stressful, such as in the presence of bright lights and loud noises or when handled excessively.

PROCEDURE Implement Environmental Modifications to Minimize Stimulation and Physiologic Stress to the Neonate

Steps	Rationale/Points of Emphasis
1. Use measures to decrease the intensity of light exposure to the neonate, to include • Dim lighting • Cycled lighting • Use of eye patches • Covers over the isolette • Minimal use of procedural lights • Use of window shades **Alert!** *Isolettes should never be covered if the neonate is unstable. This practice would obstruct ongoing assessment of the neonate.*	Primarily implemented to promote comfort, enhance preterm infants' rest and recovery, and assist in the development of rest–activity patterns. Findings from studies of the relationship between light exposure and retinopathy of prematurity are inconclusive. The use of continuous dim lighting, cycled lighting, eye patches, and covers over incubators has been implemented in many neonatal intensive care units (NICUs), with little research to support the effectiveness of these measures to prevent retinal injury. However, no adverse effect has been noted from using these measures. Cycled lighting has been found to be conducive to the development of rest–activity patterns that are in phase with the solar light–dark cycle. The retinal effects of short-term, high-intensity lighting from procedure lights and neighboring phototherapy lights has not been investigated.
2. Use measures to minimize extraneous environmental noise: • Eliminate bedside rounds, unless patient contact is needed • Minimize staff talking • Lower volume level on equipment alarms • Discourage loud talking and laughter in the unit • Avoid placing equipment on top of the isolette • Use electronic monitors to assess noise levels and make modifications to ambient noise levels as needed	Sudden and loud noise leads to physiologic and behavioral disturbances for the preterm and sick newborn. Adverse effects include sleep disturbances, motor arousals (e.g., startles and crying), hypoxemia, tachycardia, and increased intracranial pressure. In addition, careful attention to building design can control some transient sound. Careful placement of travel paths, size and location of bed spaces, and selection of equipment and communication systems result in decreasing the NICU background noises.
3. Use heated humidifiers instead of nebulizers in the NICU. When hoods are used, use those manufactured with noise-reduction features.	Heated humidifiers produce lower sound intensities and frequencies than nebulizers used with hoods.
4. Provide an environment with up to 95% relative humidity for all infants younger than 30 weeks' gestation, less than 1 kg birth weight, and during the first week of life. This can be done either by raising the level of ambient humidity inside the incubator or by creating a moist microenvironment using a waterproof covering over the infant.	Premature infants lose large amounts of heat by evaporation. Factors contributing to this condition include age (younger than 30 weeks' gestation), decreased amounts of subcutaneous fat, poorly developed epidermis, a relatively large body surface area, and frequently exposed body posture. By 2 weeks of age, the premature infant's epidermal barrier has matured in structure and functions similar to that of a term infant.

PROCEDURE Handle the Infant to Enhance Physiologic Stability and Motor Control While Minimizing Stress

Steps	Rationale/Points of Emphasis
1. Examine routine nursing procedures to evaluate what is essential and nonessential handling. When possible, eliminate unnecessary activities such that care is provided on an individualized basis to minimize stress to the newborn.	Handling of preterm infants leads to physiologic changes: decreased levels of oxygen in arterial blood (PaO_2) or $TcPO_2$, increased intracranial pressure, heat loss, tachycardia, tachypnea, and bradycardia. Many handling episodes are for nonessential care activities lasting less than 30 seconds. Whether the handling episode is a medical intervention or a soothing measure, handling, when poorly timed, stresses the vulnerable preterm infant.

Steps	Rationale/Points of Emphasis
2. Use kangaroo care (KC) regularly and consistently with medically stable premature infants and their parents. Consult guidelines provided in the literature to standardize selection criteria and intervention strategies.	Kangaroo care, or skin-to-skin contact, is safe, promotes parent–infant bonding, and positively affects infants' neurodevelopment. Research demonstrates mean cardiorespiratory and temperature outcomes remained within clinically acceptable ranges during KC. Apnea, bradycardia, and periodic breathing were absent during KC. **caREminder** *To increase reliability of monitoring periodic breathing and apnea during KC, place electrodes on the infant's back and monitor heart rate and oxygen saturation. When infants are placed in the KC position, the chest electrodes are in close contact with the paternal or maternal skin, and periodic breathing and apnea may not be detected.* **caREminder** *Offer all fathers the opportunity to participate in skin-to-skin holding. An optimal time for fathers to hold the infant may be right after delivery, keeping in mind that some fathers may want to wait until after the mother has first held the infant. Research shows that fathers hold premature infants significantly later than mothers despite the fact that fathers usually see the infants sooner than the mothers and their desire to hold the infants is equal to that of the mothers.*
3a. Position the neonate to enhance neurobehavioral states and to promote good body alignment.	Research supports the supine position as the optimal sleeping position for healthy term infants.
3b. For premature infants, the best position in an isolette is lying prone with the infant's pelvis slightly elevated, the lower limbs weight bearing through the anterior knee, and the hips not flexed greater than 90 degrees.	In premature infants, especially those experiencing respiratory distress, gastroesophageal reflux, or airway anomalies, the prone position is the position of choice. Improper infant positioning can contribute to long-term physical deformities such as bilateral head flattening, shoulder retraction, lateral flexion of the arms, and abnormal abduction of the hips, legs, and knees ("frog-leg" position). **caREminder** *If positioning is difficult due to medical condition, consultation with a physical therapist may be helpful.*
3c. Of the indirect positioning methods, gel pillows are the method of choice.	Research supports the use of indirect positioning methods (e.g., mattresses, supports) to promote vestibular stimulation, enhance neurobehavioral states, promote growth, prevent bilateral head flattening, and decrease episodes of apnea.
4a. Contain the neonate to minimize extraneous movements. Maintain contained position with use of blanket rolls or other developmentally supportive items alongside the infant.	Random movements by the infant may lead to inconsolability, alterations in vital signs, and increased consumption of oxygen and glucose. Containing an infant can lead to increased consoling behaviors and decreased extraneous movements of the extremities.
4b. Containment is achieved by placing the infant's arms and legs in a flexed midline position close to the infant's trunk with the infant in a supine position.	Stress responses in the newborn elicited by turning, moving, or painful procedures can be decreased by containing the infant's movements.

Continued

Steps	Rationale/Points of Emphasis
5. Per institutional guidelines, offer opportunity for co-bedding of twins. During co-bedding, use positioning and physical support of the newborns to enhance their ability to touch and hold each other while maintaining infants in supine position. Monitor the infants' temperatures and environmental temperature to avoid overheating the infants.	Co-bedding twins enhances extrauterine adaptation by allowing continued physical contact with the other twin and by supporting synchrony in caregiving and feeding of twins that may facilitate mutuality in their circadian rhythms and sleep–wake patterns. Co-bedding twins affects the environmental temperature requirements of the newborns when placed together or separated. Teaching of parents must convey that when infants go home, they may co-bed together; however, they may not co-bed with other children or adults because this places the infants at risk for suffocation. Some institutions may not allow co-bedding due to the unsubstantiated basis for this intervention.
6. Initiate non-nutritive sucking (NNS) with the infant before the onset of feedings. Introduction of the intervention 2, 5, and 10 minutes before feeding has proven to be beneficial to the infant. Although the optimal length of time of the intervention requires further investigation, careful monitoring of infant behavioral state assists the nurse in determining when the infant has achieved a quiet alert state and oral feedings may begin.	Medically stable infants provided with an NNS stimulus before feeding were more likely to be in transitional or alert states after the intervention and at the start of feeding. Infants who received NNS also have higher oxygen saturation rates during the intervention, faster first-suck onset during feeding, a significantly longer first-suck duration, and fewer behavioral state changes during feedings. They are also more likely to initiate nutritive sucking earlier. NNS does not have an overall effect on feeding time or on amount of formula consumed.
7. Structure the infant's 24-hour day such that care activities are clustered to allow for extended periods of uninterrupted sleep. Cover the isolette of the stable infant during scheduled naps while observing and monitoring the infant's status on a regular basis. Do not implement care and interventions during rest unless the infant requires emergency interventions or soothing activities to sleep.	Sleep–wake cycles of the preterm infant are affected by activities such as handling, routine nursing care, painful procedures, and interactions with family members. Inadequate periods of rest can slow weight gain growth and increase apneic episodes. Caregiving activities should be clustered, structured, and paced to promote adequate periods of rest; to avoid sudden disruptions in sleep or movement; and to ensure that maladaptive behaviors are not elicited during care and handling. Perform several procedures during a single contact with the infant if response is well tolerated, approach or arouse the infant in a soothing and calming manner, remain at the infant's bedside after interventions to ensure no maladaptive responses are present, and provide calming measures when maladaptive behaviors are demonstrated during or after care activities.

PROCEDURE Facilitate Interactions of the Infant With Family to Enhance Coregulatory Nurturance and to Support the Infant's Emerging Capabilities of Neurobehavioral Organization

Steps	Rationale/Points of Emphasis
1. Determine the type, sequence, and duration of infant stimulation by the infant's physiologic and neurobehavioral status as monitored before, during, and after intervention.	One type of stimulation does not appear to provide more benefit than another method in promoting infant development. Thus, the type of supplemental stimulation (e.g., visual, tactile) provided to the infant is less important than whether the intervention promotes state regulation.
2. Carefully use tactile stimulation measures with the neonate.	Tactile stimulation can produce undesired stress responses in the newborn, including tachycardia, hypoxia, and increased levels of intracranial pressure. Individualizing touch and handling based on the infant's responses, timing, and continuity needs as well as parent preference can be very beneficial for the infant. Stroking is not well supported in the literature as a consistently effective tactile stimulation method. Massage therapy has not been tested on fragile newborns and requires continuing investigation as to its effectiveness. Massage can produce both physiologic and behavioral disorganization, potentially adding to their distress. Gentle human touch can be implemented for short periods of time, three to five times per day, with positive behavioral outcomes for the infant.

Steps	Rationale/Points of Emphasis
3. Use auditory stimulation measures. Introduce the use of auditory stimulation provided by music, soothing environmental sounds, or fetal heart tones or the like on an individual basis to determine the optimal level and duration of the stimulation. Monitor the infant's motor, autonomic, and state-related responses to provide guidance to the individual appropriateness of auditory interventions.	The developing preterm infant is extremely sensitive and responsive to auditory stimulation. Premature infants exposed to controlled music stimulation have benefited by increased weight gain, reduced observed stress behaviors, increased oxygenation saturation levels, and reduced length of stay. These results appear to be more dramatic in girls. Intensity, timing, and duration of music exposure cannot be generalized to all infants.
4. Use demand-feeding protocols.	Demand-feeding protocols use infant feeding cues to indicate timing of feeding schedules. Infants who are fed when they display hunger cues can competently self-regulate their feeding schedule, have hiccups less often during their feeds, and require fewer feeds to be given through gavage. With demand feeding, infants generally need to be fed at intervals not more frequent than 2 hours and need to be gently awakened for feeds after a maximum of 5 hours.
5. Provide oral support during feedings. Oral support can be given during feeding by using the thumb and index finger to provide inward and forward support on the infant's cheek. The third finger is used to provide support under the mental protuberance of the mandible, giving a slight upward lift and stability. **Alert!** ***Do not use this method simply to promote faster or more effective bottle feeding because this type of coaxing can predispose the infant to longer apneic and bradycardic episodes.***	Oral support improves the sucking efficiency, as measured by volume intake, of preterm infants.
6. Encourage increased family involvement in the child's care.	Father interaction can be fostered by encouraging fathers access to their infant and involvement in all care and family teaching. Grandparents need information and support to help them cope and be supportive to the infant's parents.

CHILD AND FAMILY EVALUATION AND DOCUMENTATION

- Evaluate infant's behavioral cues before, during, and after initiating care procedures.
- Evaluate family members' ability to implement developmental care measures.
- Document the following:
  - Findings from evaluation of infant's behavioral cues
  - Measures used to support and enhance neurobehavioral integrity of the neonate
  - Family members' participation in care activities and the extent to which they are modifying their actions based on the infant's behavior

Unexpected Situation

- *The preterm infant is receiving daily care activities that are being "clustered," including repositioning, skin care, and suctioning. During these care activities, the oxygen saturation levels decrease significantly and the infant has two apneic episodes:* Not all infants can tolerate clustering of activities. Daily care interventions should be stopped for the time being and containment provided to "reorganize" the infant. Increase the oxygen support slightly (e.g., increase rate on ventilator, provide oxygen by blow-by). Once recovery has occurred, maintain containment and slowly reduce respiratory support to baseline parameters. If suctioning is required (to maintain the airway), defer other care activities until later and perform just that one procedure. Position prone with adequate containment supports. Consider that you may be moving through the care routine too quickly. Reevaluate the care routine. Consider that the infant may be more fragile than originally assessed and evaluate for other reasons the infant may be stressed (e.g., sepsis).

Bibliography

Als, H. (1997). *Program guide—newborn individualized developmental care and assessment program (NIDCAP): An education and training program for health care professionals* (Revision). Boston, MA: Children's Medical Center Corporation.

Als, H. (1998). Developmental care in the newborn intensive care unit. *Current Opinion in Pediatrics, 10*(2), 138–142.

Als, H., & Gilkerson, L. (1995). Developmentally supportive care in the neonatal intensive care unit. *Zero to Three, 15*(6), 2–10.

Als, H., Lawhon, G., Duffy, F., McAnnulty, G., Gibes-Gorssman, R., & Blickman, J. (1994). Individualized developmental care for the very low birthweight preterm infant: Medical and neurofunctional effects. *Journal of the American Medical Association, 272*(11), 853–858.

Beachy, J. (2003). Premature infant massage in the NICU. *Neonatal Network, 22*(3), 39–45.

Beckmann, C. (1997). Use of neonatal boundaries to improve outcomes. *Journal of Holistic Nursing, 15*(1), 54–67.

Bowden, V., Greenberg, C., & Donaldson, N. (2000). Developmental care of the newborn. *Online Journal of Clinical Innovations, 3*(7), 1–77.

Browne, J. (2000). Developmental care: Considerations for touch and massage in the neonatal intensive care unit. *Neonatal Network, 19*(1), 61–64.

Byers, J., Lowman, L., Francis, J., et al. (2006). A quasi-experimental trial in individualized, developmentally supportive family-centered care. *Journal of Obstetric, Gynecologic, and Neonatal Nursing, 35*, 105–115.

Byers, J., Waugh, W., & Lowman, L. (2006). Sound level exposure of high-risk infants in different environmental conditions. *Neonatal Network, 25* (1), 25–32.

Chou, L. (2003). Effects of music therapy on oxygen saturation in premature infants receiving endotracheal suctioning. *Journal of Nursing Research, 11*(3), 209–215.

Consensus Committee to Establish Recommended Standards for Newborn ICU Design. (1999). *Recommended standards for newborn ICU design.* Retrieved September 21, 2006, from www.nd.edu

Hayward, K. (2003). Cobedding of twins: A natural extension of the socialization process? *MCN, The American Journal of Maternal Child Nursing, 28*(4), 260–263.

Kledzik, T. (2005). Holding the very low birth weight infant: Skin-to-skin techniques. *Neonatal Network, 24*(1), 7–14.

Lee, Y., Malakooti, N., & Lotas, M. (2005). A comparison of the light-reduction capacity of commonly used incubator covers. *Neonatal Network, 24*(2), 37–44.

Ludington-Hoe, S., Anderson, G., Swinth, J., Thompson, C., & Hadeed, A. (2004). Randomized controlled trial of kangaroo care: Cardiorespiratory and thermal effects on healthy preterm infants. *Neonatal Network, 23*(3), 39–42, 43–48.

Martucci, M., & Lofgren, M. (2004). Foundations in newborn care: Considerations in planning a newborn developmental care program in a community setting. *Advances in Neonatal Care, 4*(2), 59–66.

McCain, G. (2003). An evidence-based guideline for introducing oral feeding to healthy preterm infants. *Neonatal Network, 22*(5), 45–50.

Rivkees, S., Mayes, L., Jacobs, H., & Gross, I. (2004). Rest-activity patterns of premature infants are regulated by cycled lighting. *Pediatrics, 113*(4), 833–839.

Sizun, J., & Westrup, B. (2004). Early developmental care for preterm neonates: A call for more research. *Archives of Disease in Childhood Fetal and Neonatal Edition, 89*(5), F384–F389.

Swinth, J., Anderson, G., & Hadeed, A. (2003). Kangaroo (skin-to-skin) care with a preterm infant before, during, and after mechanical ventilation. *Neonatal Network, 22*(6), 33–38.

Symington, A., & Pinelli, J. (2003). Developmental care for promoting development and preventing morbidity in preterm infants. *The Cochrane Database of Systematic Reviews*, (4), No. CD001814.

CHAPTER

34

Diapering

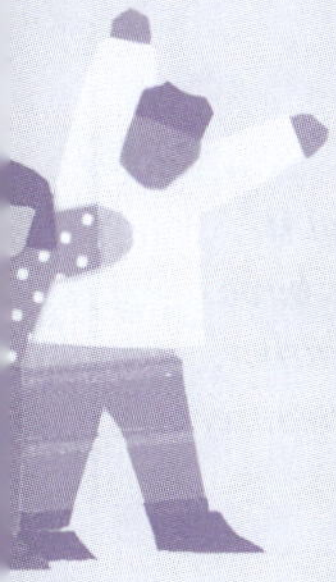

Clinical Guidelines

- Diapering is performed by parents or other family caregivers and/or any healthcare provider.
- Infant/child has diaper changed promptly after it is soiled.
- Umbilical cord stump is cleansed with each diaper change.
- Petroleum jelly is applied to the penis of the newly circumcised male infant with each diaper change.
- Infant/child's perineal area is monitored for redness, excoriation, and infection at each diaper change.

Equipment

- Diaper
- Nonsterile gloves
- Washcloth or diaper wipes (nonallergenic and nonscented)
- Mild soap
- Towel
- Cotton-tipped swab (for umbilical cord care)
- Petroleum jelly or petroleum jelly gauze (for newly circumcised infant with Gomco-type device)
- Barrier cream (such as petroleum or zinc oxide paste) if needed
- Topical anticandidal agent (Nystatin, Lotrimin, Micatin, Nizoral) if ordered for diaper dermatitis
- Low-potency, nonfluorinated, 1% hydrocortisone cream if ordered for severe inflammation due to diaper dermatitis

Child and Family Assessment and Preparation

- Instruct new parents on importance of prompt diaper changes to avoid skin irritation in the newborn.
- Involve parents and other care providers in care of the infant.

PROCEDURE Diapering

Steps	Rationale/Points of Emphasis
1. Perform hand hygiene. Don gloves.	Standard precaution to reduce transmission of microorganisms.
2. Place infant/child on firm clean surface, such as changing table or crib/bed mattress. Keep your hand on infant and do not turn away from infant during the procedure.	Prevents injury and falls.
3. Remove soiled diaper and assess contents of diaper for unusual appearance or odor of urine or stool.	The average newborn urinates about 20 times a day. Unusual characteristics of urine or stool may indicate a gastrointestinal or urinary disturbance. **caREminder** *If diaper sticks to circumcision site, use warm water to loosen diaper gently from area. Presence of a small amount of bloody discharge in the newly circumcised male may be normal. Excessive bleeding is abnormal. Female infants may have a small amount of vaginal, pink-tinged, mucoid discharge in the first several days after birth because of withdrawal of maternal estrogen.*
4. Assess infant/child's perineal area for redness, rash, or excoriation.	Prolonged contact with an irritant, most commonly feces, urine, soaps, detergents, ointments, or friction, is a major contributing factor in diaper dermatitis. Wet skin is more easily abraded and more permeable, and it has an increased microbial count. This situation can be exacerbated by alkaline soaps used to clean cloth diapers. The wet diaper also increases friction with the wet skin. Irritated, cut, or chapped skin is a contributing factor to diaper dermatitis. **Alert!** *When lesions or open wounds become infected, candidiasis may be a major culprit. Candida albicans can be cultured or recovered from the skin of 40% to 75% of infants with diaper dermatitis. It is rarely found in infants with healthy unbroken skin.*
5. Cleanse the skin with disposable wipes or a wet, warm washcloth with mild soap if necessary. Avoid soap contact with the newly circumcised glans penis as irritation may occur. Dry perineal area.	Cleanses perineal area of urine and feces and prevents skin irritation. **caREminder** *If the skin is clean underlying any diaper cream or ointments placed earlier on the child, the cream does not have to be removed completely with each diaper change; rather, lightly wiping the area with a washcloth and mild cleanser is sufficient.*
6. For the child with diaper dermatitis, consider one of the following: a. Apply a simple barrier cream (such as petroleum or zinc oxide paste) to the noninfected diaper rash. b. If candidal infection is present, apply topical anticandidal agent (Nystatin, Lotrimin, Micatin, Nizoral) to diaper area per healthcare prescriber's orders. c. If severe inflammation is present, per physician's orders, apply a topical, low-potency, nonfluorinated, 1% hydrocortisone cream to rash site for 7 to 10 days. d. Children with recurrent diarrhea may be prescribed an oral anticandidal agent (Nystatin) to sterilize the gastrointestinal tract and prevent systemic infection.	Barrier creams assist in preventing further breakdown due to the friction of the diaper against the sensitive skin. Medicated ointments may be used to treat infections that have developed on the genital and buttocks area. **Alert!** *All prescribed steroids should be of a low-potency (0.5% to 1%) nonfluorinated type. High-potency steroids are rapidly absorbed through the infant's thin skin and can cause systemic toxicity. Special care should be taken by the nurse to avoid combination products (e.g., antifungals and steroids) without verifying that the steroid is of the low-dose type.*

Steps	Rationale/Points of Emphasis
7. For the newborn, clean the umbilical area with soap and water. Observe umbilicus for redness or drainage. Lift cord and clean base; do not wet the umbilical cord. Rinse and dry the area. Leave site open to air; do not apply alcohol, antiseptics, or antibiotics to umbilical cord stump.	Promotes drying of the stump. Prevents infection (omphalitis) that can be life-threatening. Studies have shown that natural drying of the umbilical cord does not result in increased incidence of infection.
8. In the circumcised infant, a petroleum-coated gauze bandage or petroleum jelly should be applied to the tip of the penis if the circumcision was the Gomco type.	Keeps area moist, decreasing irritation of circumcision site and promoting healing.
9. Apply new diaper securely, folding front of diaper to avoid irritation of umbilical cord. Fold plastic away from skin.	Prevents accidental soiling and prevents unnecessary irritation of umbilical cord. Irritation to circumcised area can occur if diaper is secured too tightly.
10. Dispose of diaper and waste in appropriate receptacle. Remove gloves and perform hand hygiene.	Standard precautions. Reduces transmission of microorganisms.
11. Wrap infant in blanket and place in crib with side rails up. Return child to safe position in bed with side rails up.	Enhances infant thermoregulation and ensures patient safety.

CHILD AND FAMILY EVALUATION AND DOCUMENTATION

- Evaluate parental participation in care.
- Document the following:
  - Presence of urine and stool and characteristics
  - Appearance of umbilical cord
  - Appearance of circumcision site, noting any irritation, odor, or drainage
  - Appearance of skin on genitalia and buttocks area
  - Application of barrier cream or antibiotic or fungal cream

COMMUNITY CARE

Provide parental instruction in the following areas:

Use of Powders

- Infants do not need any powders on their diaper area. Use of baby powders containing "talc" or known as "talcum powder" can cause accidental aspiration, pneumonia, and death. In addition, when powders applied to the diaper area become moist (e.g., in humid climates and once the child has voided), the powder or cornstarch can clump and retain moisture on the skin, thus contributing to diaper dermatitis.
- If the parent still desires to use talcum powder or cornstarch, it should be applied by shaking it on the parent's hands first, as far away from the infant's head as possible.

> ***Alert!*** *Aspiration is predominantly caused when the infant receives a "puff of smoke" when the powder is shaken from the container directly onto the infant's skin.*

- All talcum powder containers should be closed and in a safe place, away from curious infants and toddlers.
- Lotions or creams (not alcohol-based products) should be substituted for powder to reduce diaper rash or other skin irritations.
- Parents should not use talcum powder on themselves in an infant's or toddler's presence.
- Use of baby powder should be discouraged in all individuals with asthma or reactive airway disease.

Use of Ointments

- If the diaper area is reddened:
  - Apply a simple barrier cream (such as zinc oxide paste) to the noninfected diaper rash.
  - Do not remove the paste with every diaper change so long as a layer of paste remains on the skin and the skin underneath is clean.
  - If the paste must be removed, use minimal amount of baby oil.

Diaper Wear

- Avoid airtight occlusive diapers or diaper covers on the child.
- Do not use plastic pants.
- Fasten the disposable diaper loosely.
- Brand-name disposable diapers can be altered to breathe better by snipping the elastic bands around the legs in a few places and cutting a few slits in the plastic diaper cover.
- Cloth diapers should always be washed in hot water with a mild soap and double-rinsed. Wash, rinse, and let the diaper soak in water with ammonia added for half an hour, and then rinse again.

- Use fabric softener when washing cloth diapers to help prevent skin friction and chafing. Be aware that some fabric softeners make fabrics nonabsorbent and thus should not be used.

Nighttime Care

- Apply creams liberally on diaper area before bedtime.
- Avoid plastic pants at night.
- Until rash improves, awaken the child at least once a night to change the diaper.

Prevention of Diaper Rash

- After the child's bath, let the child be diaper free for a period of time.
- Change diapers frequently. Never leave a child in a soiled diaper.
- Wash cloth diapers appropriately (see earlier).
- Instruct the family to contact the healthcare provider in the following cases:
  - Odor or drainage from umbilical cord is noticed.
  - Odor or drainage from site of circumcision is noticed.
  - Rash develops big blisters (more than 1 inch across), open sores, or boils.
  - Rash does not look better in 3 days.
  - Rash becomes solid and bright red.
  - Rash becomes raw and bleeds.
  - Rash causes enough pain to disrupt sleep.
  - Child develops temperature >99°F to 100°F (37.4°C to 37.8°C).

Unexpected Situation

- *During the diaper change on a 5 month-old child, you notice red, circular, open lesions on the buttocks area. The lesions are approximately ⅓ inch in diameter and appear randomly on the skin:* All lesions on a child's buttocks should be examined carefully to determine potential source of lesions. Open lesions from diaper dermatitis can become infected, with candidiasis as the major culprit. Lesions may also be caused by intentional harm that has been inflicted on the infant as a result of physical assault, burns, or scalding injury. The physician needs to be contacted immediately about the lesions to further assess potential causes and provide appropriate intervention and follow-up care. See Chapter 30 for more information about suspected child abuse.

Bibliography

Borkowski, S. (2004). Diaper rash care and management. *Pediatric Nursing, 30*(6), 467–470.

D'Alessandro, D., & Huth, L. (2002). *Diaper rash.* Retrieved July, 11, 2006, from http://www.vh.org/pediatric/patient/pediatrics/cqqa/diaperrash.html

Visscher, M., Chaterjee, R., Munson, K., et al. (2000). Development of diaper rash in the newborn. *Pediatric Dermatology, 17*(1), 52–57.

Zupan, J., Garner, P., & Omari, A. (2004). Topical umbilical cord care at birth. *The Cochrane Database of Systematic Reviews,* (3), No. CD001057.

C H A P T E R

35

Disaster Preparedness and Response

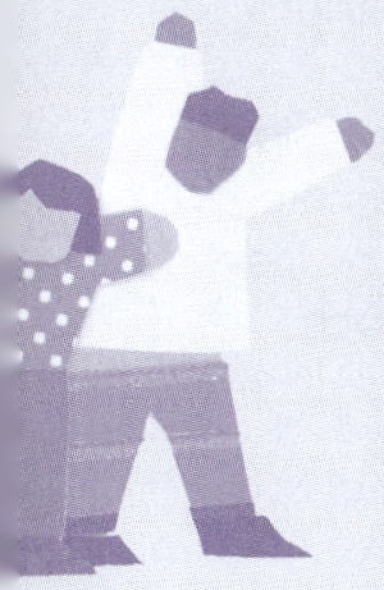

Clinical Guidelines

- The response to disaster varies based on the type of disaster (i.e., natural disaster vs. bioterrorist act); it is important to be knowledgeable regarding your own facility/community plan and its procedures.
- Key components of disaster preparedness are:
  - Describe the role of the facility during response to an emergency/disaster.
  - Locate and use the section of the hospital emergency response plan that applies to your department and position.
  - Describe your emergency response role and demonstrate it during drills or actual emergencies.
  - Demonstrate the use of emergency equipment (such as personal protective equipment) required by your emergency response role.
  - Describe your communication responsibilities and demonstrate them during drills or actual emergencies. Know the chain of command in a disaster, which may not be the same as the hospital organization structure.
  - Identify and describe the limits to your skills, knowledge, and authority.
  - Demonstrate flexible thinking and use of resources to solve problems that arise during emergency situations or drills. Routine resources may not be available (e.g., telephones, electrical power).
- Decontamination areas should have:
  - A water source
  - The ability to collect and contain large quantities of water
  - Soap available to remove the contaminant (water alone is not as effective)
  - Adequate lighting
  - Electricity
  - A conveyor system for nonambulatory patients
  - Provisions for patient privacy
  - Room for two to three personnel and family
- Special management plans should be in place to address the unique physical and psychological vulnerabilities of children (Chart 35-1). Ensure adequate supplies of antibiotics, antidotes, and vaccines in pediatric doses. Have ready access to a dosing guide, preferably in hard copy in the event of power loss.
- Keep family units together during a disaster whenever possible.

CHART 35-1 SPECIAL PEDIATRIC CONSIDERATIONS IN TERRORISM AND DISASTER PREPAREDNESS

Children are more vulnerable than adults.

- Children are particularly vulnerable to aerosolized biologic or chemical agents because they may breathe more times per minute than adults and they would get relatively larger doses of the substance in the same period of time. Also, because some such agents (e.g., sarin and chlorine) are heavier than air, they accumulate close to the ground (i.e., right in the breathing zone of children).
- Children are more vulnerable to agents that act on or through the skin because their skin is thinner and they have a larger surface-to-mass ratio than adults.
- Children are more vulnerable to the effects of agents that produce vomiting or diarrhea because they have less fluid reserve than adults, increasing the risk of rapid dehydration.
- Children have smaller circulating blood volumes than do adults; without rapid intervention, relatively small amounts of blood loss can quickly tip the physiologic scale from reversible shock to profound, irreversible shock or death.
- Children have significant developmental vulnerabilities not shared by adults. Infants, toddlers, and young children do not have the motor skills to escape from the site of a chemical, biologic, or other terrorist incident. Even if they are able to walk, young children may not have the cognitive ability to figure out how to flee from danger or to follow directions from others.
- Children are more susceptible to the effects of radiation exposure because they have a relatively greater minute ventilation compared with adults. They are likely to have greater exposure to radioactive gases, and because nuclear fallout quickly settles to the ground, children are exposed to a higher concentration of radioactive material because they are closer to the ground.

Children have unique treatment needs.

- Children's conditions can rapidly go from stable to life-threatening because they have less blood and fluid reserves, are more sensitive to changes in body temperature, and have faster metabolisms than adults.
- Children may struggle against the efforts of health-care workers because they do not understand what is going on or may be frightened by the appearance of workers in protective gear. Parents must approach the child in a developmentally appropriate manner.
- Children need different dosages or types of antibiotics or antidotes than do adults, not only because they are smaller, but because certain drugs and biologic agents may have effects on developing children that are not of concern in the adult population.
- Because children have smaller bodies, they require smaller equipment than do adults. Needles, tubing, oxygen masks, ventilators, imaging, and laboratory technology all need to be equipment that is specifically designed for children's size.
- Children require special consideration during decontamination efforts. Because children lose body heat more quickly than do adults, use heating lamps or other warming equipment to avoid hypothermia, and decontaminate children before adults if warm water is available but supply may be depleted.

Children have unique mental health needs.

- Children's reactions to situations beyond the usual scope of human experience, such as a terrorist attack or other disaster, vary greatly depending on their cognitive, physical, educational, and social development level and experience and requires a familiarity with age-appropriate interventions.
- Children are highly influenced by the emotional state of their caretakers. When the parents or other caretakers of a child are psychologically harmed by the events around them, it is likely to affect the psychological well-being of the child.

EQUIPMENT

- Personal protective equipment (gowns, gloves, masks, goggles/eyewear)
- Patient identification bands
- Decontamination kits for adults and children (gown, storage bag for contaminated clothing, soap for cleaning off the chemical contaminate, and tags for personal belongings)
- Emergency equipment as listed in Chapter 24
- Equipment to obtain vital signs as listed in Chapters 130, 131, 132, 133, and 134
- Equipment as needed to start an intravenous line, as listed in Chapter 55

CHILD AND FAMILY ASSESSMENT AND PREPARATION

- Assess type of disaster. Assessment of the child varies based on type of disaster, usually one of the following:
  - **Violence, explosions, or force from natural disaster:** Assess and prepare as any other trauma patient based on the nature of their injuries. Symptoms vary,

based on the area that is injured and the extent of the injury.

- **Nuclear/radiologic attacks:** Assess exposure and/or contamination. Symptoms vary from no obvious injury to deep burns. Some symptoms will develop over time because of a burn to the deep tissue.
  - External exposure: Assess if radiation was from a source distant or in close proximity to the body and if external radiation was to whole body or a local exposure.
  - Contamination: An unwanted radioactive material in or on the body.
- **Chemical attacks:** Assess for symptoms of hazardous chemical exposure:
  - Nerve agents (Sarin, VX): sudden loss of consciousness, seizures, apnea, and death
  - Vesicants (mustard agents): blistering and injury to the eyes, skin, airways, and some internal organs
  - Cyanide: hyperventilation, convulsions, asystole, and death
  - Pulmonary intoxicants (Phosgene, chlorine): cause life-threatening lung injury after inhalation, effects are usually delayed; irritation to the eyes and respiratory tract and severe pulmonary edema
  - Riot control agents (Mace, tear gas, pepper spray): tearing; eye, nose, mouth, and throat irritation
- **Biologic attacks:** Assess for signs of common diseases associated with bioterrorism:
  - Cutaneous anthrax (incubation period of 12 hours to 12 days): Initial lesion resembling a pimple or insect bite with surrounding erythema and often satellite vesicular or bullous lesions; by the fifth to seventh day the lesion becomes a painless black eschar.
  - Inhalation or pulmonary anthrax (incubation period 1 to 7 days, may be as long as 60 days): Nonspecific respiratory symptoms (cough with low-grade fever), fatigue, malaise, and muscle aches; respiratory distress becomes rapidly progressive and is often accompanied by a high fever and signs of systemic toxicity (sepsis or meningitis).
  - Smallpox (incubation period 7 to 17 days): Initial symptoms include high fever, fatigue, and head and backaches; synchronous vesicopustular eruption, predominately on face and extremities, follows in 2–3 days.
  - Plague (incubation period 2–8 days if due to flea-borne transmission, 1–3 days for pulmonary exposure): Febrile prodrome with rapid progression to fulminant pneumonia with bloody sputum, sepsis, and disseminated intravascular coagulopathy (DIC)
  - Tularemia (incubation period 1–14 days, average 3–5 days)
  - Pneumonic abrupt onset of fever, fulminant pneumonia
  - Typhoidal fever, malaise, abdominal pain
  - Botulism (incubation 1–5 days): Afebrile; descending flaccid paralysis; cranial nerve palsies, sensation and mentation intact
  - Viral hemorrhagic fevers (incubation 4–21 days): Febrile prodrome with rapid progression to shock, purpura, and bleeding diathesis

- Prepare the child and family for assessments and interventions using developmentally appropriate language and methods.

PROCEDURE Initial Steps

Steps	Rationale/Points of Emphasis
1. Perform hand hygiene and don appropriate personal protective equipment depending on the type of victim. Always use standard precautions; refer to levels of protection recommended by Local HazMat, Centers for Disease Control and Prevention (CDC) Guidelines, or Occupational Safety and Health Administration (OSHA) for specific guidelines based on exposure.	Reduces contamination and ensures compliance with standard precautions to reduce exposure to self and others. Helps prevent cross-contamination of the facility.
2. Perform the appropriate assessment based on the trauma primary (ABC) and secondary assessment or medical assessment if a biologic attack or illness from a natural disaster. Stabilize immediately.	Life-saving procedures must be implemented before decontamination.
3. Before bringing the child into the hospital, remove all clothing and personal items. Place identification band or other identifier on child and belongings. Proceed with decontamination procedures for the child if warranted by one of the following conditions: • Nuclear/radiologic exposure: Remove clothing and shoes, brush off loose particulate matter, wash uncovered skin and hair with soap and water.	Reduces in-facility exposure to contaminants. Identifies child, helps maintain consistency of treatment and chain of evidence (helps investigation into event and with matching patient with belongings).

Continued

Steps	Rationale/Points of Emphasis
• Chemical exposure: Many inhalation exposures are addressed by evacuation to a well-ventilated area; for liquid agents, immediately remove agent on skin and clothing with absorbent material, remove clothing, wash with soap and water. • Biologic exposure: Typically not indicated because exposure identification is often delayed and personal hygiene practices will have removed agent; also many agents not absorbed topically. If decontamination is indicated, use soap and water.	
4. Initiate treatment based on type of exposure (see below).	Treatment targets specific injury and needs.

PROCEDURE Treatment of Nuclear/Radiologic Exposure

Steps	Rationale/Points of Emphasis
1. Prevent and minimize internal contamination by initial decontamination (see Initial Steps, step 3).	Contamination can cause cellular damage and affect normal biologic processes; removal of agent reduces continued exposure.
2. Assess internal contamination and effectiveness of decontamination. A radiologic assessment should be done by a medical physicist under the supervision of medical personnel to include radiation measurements and collection of information relevant to the decontamination of the patient. An individual is considered to have internal contamination when radioactive material has gained access into the body through inhalation, ingestion, or absorption.	The better the decontamination is, the less cellular damage will occur, therefore causing fewer long-term complications.
3. Contain contamination and decontamination. Use soap and water to scrub the contaminated area. Collect, identify, seal, and store all clothes and personal gear from victim and healthcare personnel in a remote location. In the absence of contamination or after decontamination, the patient can be treated in any area of the emergency department.	Reduces exposure of others to contaminants.
4. Minimize external contamination to medical personnel: Wear personal protective equipment (gowns, rubber gloves, masks) at all times, wear radiation monitoring tag, contain and properly dispose of all items in contact with exposed child.	Once the medical personnel are considered contaminated, their services will be limited in helping others. They also may have cellular damage from the contamination and therefore have their own medical problems.
5. Reassess local radiation injuries/burns and flush if contaminated.	If contaminate is not removed, it continues to cause cellular damage.
6. Follow up on patients with significant whole-body irradiation or internal contamination.	Patients with significant whole-body irradiation or internal contamination will need to be followed over time to determine the extent of their injuries. These patients are at risk for further chronic illness and injury due to cellular damage, including such problems as cancer and genetic risks. In serious radiation exposures, the cells mutate; until these mutated cells multiply, the extent of the injury may be undetected.
7. Administer medications as ordered.	May reduce uptake or enhance removal of agents. For example, potassium iodide inhibits thyroid uptake of radioactive iodine, thus reducing risk of developing thyroid cancer; ferric ferrocyanide serves as an ion exchanger to help remove cesium, thallium, and rubidium; diethylenetriaminepentaacetic acid helps remove heavy metal isotopes such as plutonium.
8. Provide supportive care depending on injury and symptoms.	Most patients, after significant exposures, experience hematopoietic symptoms and need blood components to prevent bleeding and antibiotics to prevent/treat infection.

PROCEDURE Chemical Exposure

Steps	Rationale/Points of Emphasis
1. See Initial Steps, step 3 for decontamination. Administer antidote as ordered, if indicated.	Stops or reverses damage from agent. For example, nitrites and thiosulfates neutralize cyanide; oximines dislodge nerve agents from their bond with the enzyme and restore cholinesterase function.
2. Provide supportive care depending on injury and symptoms.	Supports body system functioning until recovery.

PROCEDURE Biologic Exposure

Steps	Rationale/Points of Emphasis
1. See Initial Steps, step 3 for decontamination. Treat exposure based on the agent: • Anthrax: ciprofloxacin, penicillin, doxycycline • Smallpox: smallpox vaccine, isolate • Plague: ciprofloxacin, gentamycin, doxycycline • Tularemia: ciprofloxacin, gentamycin • Botulism: antitoxin, supportive care • Viral hemorrhagic fevers: supportive care	Targets specific actions of the agent and increases efficacy of treatment.
2. Provide supportive care depending on injury and symptoms.	Supports body system functioning until recovery.

CHILD AND FAMILY EVALUATION AND DOCUMENTATION

- Evaluate the child's status and response to treatment.
- Follow through and document the completion of medical orders as written.
- Document all care given and resources utilized.
- Evaluate the child and family's understanding of the disaster and injury or illness.
- Document any referrals given to the family, especially as related to follow-up medical and psychological care.
- Notify the proper authorities (e.g., police, public health authority) if a bioterrorist attack or disease outbreak is suspected. In some cases the child and his or her belongings will be considered part of the investigation and must be treated in a forensic manner, keeping all contaminated clothing and personal belongings as evidence for the police. Document who was notified.

COMMUNITY CARE

- Counsel children and their family about potential long-term risks/effects. Instruct the family to follow up with the appropriate medical care as needed; provide written instructions.
- Give family referral for needed community mental health and social service resources.
- The following disaster planning is recommended to meet children's needs in the community:
  - Federal, state, and local disaster plans should include specific protocols for management of pediatric casualties.
  - Provide specialized areas for children, such as isolation zones and decontamination rooms.
  - Schools and child care and after-school care facilities must be prepared to evacuate children, take them to a safe place, notify parents, reunite children with their families, provide or arrange care for children whose parents are incapacitated or cannot reach them, and render first aid.
  - Government agencies should work to ensure that adequate supplies of antibiotics, antidotes, and vaccines are available to children; that they are safe and efficacious; and that pediatric doses are established. Resource allocation plans should ensure that these agents are readily available to pediatric healthcare sites and other locations where children congregate.
- Encourage families to develop a family disaster plan (postemergency phone numbers, include an out-of-state contact, assemble disaster supplies kits for each member of the household); review with children what to do in a disaster and practice emergency procedures (e.g., home fire drills). The best way to get the word out to families is through a working relationship between the hospital and the local schools as well as participation in Health or Injury Prevention Fairs.
- Discuss with parents, teachers, and day care providers normal responses of children and actions to minimize impact on children. Children who are not exposed or

injured also benefit from these interventions. Discuss how the responses of adults influence children: adult distress can increase the distress of children and positive emotional expressions seem to help children cope. Inform children about a disaster as soon as information is available; a child senses when a serious event occurs and often envisions something worse than the actual event. Encourage parents to maintain the child's routines as much as possible. Also, talk with the child, elicit his or her perceptions of the event, turn off the television—do not allow children to see repeated broadcasts of the event (they often believe it is happening repeatedly). Reassure children about their safety to the extent possible and tell them what steps are being taken to keep them safe. Keep the family together.

- Instruct the child and family to notify the healthcare provider if
  - Symptoms the child was treated for are not resolving
  - New symptoms appear
  - The child demonstrates dramatic changes in behavior

Unexpected Situation

- *A child presents in respiratory distress, fever of 104°F, looking toxic:* As you are stabilizing the child, you obtain a history of onset 2 days ago of cough, low-grade fever, fatigue, and muscle aches. You suspect pulmonary anthrax. Ensure all in contact with child follow standard precautions and respiratory precautions until the diagnosis is confirmed because many pathogens present with similar signs and symptoms. If anthrax is confirmed, follow standard precautions, administer antibiotic as ordered, and notify infection control in your facility and the public health department.

Bibliography

American Academy of Pediatrics (AAP). (2006). The pediatrician and disaster preparedness: Policy statement. *Pediatrics, 117,* 560–565.

Bernardo, L. M., & Kapsen, P. (2003). Pediatric implications in bioterrorism: Education for healthcare providers. *Disaster Management and Response, 1*(2), 52–54.

Cieslak, T., & Henretig, F. (2003). Bioterrorism. *Pediatric Annals, 32,* 154–165.

Fremont, W. P. (2004). Childhood reactions to terrorism-induced trauma: a review of the past 10 years. *Journal of the American Academy of Child and Adolescent Psychiatry, 43,* 381–392.

Gaines, S. K., & Leary, J. M. (2004). Public health emergency preparedness in the setting of child care. *Family & Community Health, 27,* 260–265.

Heymann, D. L. (Ed.). (2004). *Control of communicable disease manual* (18th ed.). Washington, DC: American Public Health Association.

Lynch, M. (2005). Atropine use in children after nerve gas exposure. *Journal of Pediatric Nursing, 20,* 477–484.

Lynch, E. L., & Thomas, T. L. (2004). Pediatric considerations in chemical exposures: Are we prepared? *Pediatric Emergency Care, 20,* 198–208.

Markenson, D., & Redlener, I. (2004). Pediatric terrorism preparedness national guidelines and recommendations: Findings of an evidenced-based consensus process. *Biosecurity and Bioterrorism, 2,* 301–319.

Markenson, D., Reynolds, S., Committee on Pediatric Emergency Medicine, & Task Force on Terrorism. (2006). The pediatrician and disaster preparedness: Technical report. *Pediatrics, 117,* e340–362. Retrieved July 12, 2006, from http://pediatrics.aappublications.org/cgi/reprint/117/2/e340

Martin, M. E., & Didion, J. (2003). The smallpox threat: the school nurse's role. *Journal of School Nursing, 19,* 260–265.

Mercuri, A., & Angelique, H. L. (2004). Children's responses to natural, technological, and na-tech disasters. *Community Mental Health Journal, 40,* 167–175.

National Center for Disaster Preparedness, Columbia University. (2003). *Pediatric preparedness for disasters and terrorism: A national consensus conference–Executive summary.* Retrieved July 12, 2006, from http://www.bt.cdc.gov/children/pdf/working/execsumm03.pdf

Rotenberg, J., Burklow, T. R., & Selanikio, J. S. (2003). Weapons of mass destruction: The decontamination of children. *Pediatric Annals, 32,* 260–267.

Rotenberg, J. & Newmark, J. (2003). Nerve agent attacks on children: Diagnosis and management. *Pediatrics, 112,* 648–658.

Tasota, F., Henker, R. A., & Hoffman, L. A. (2002) Anthrax as a biological weapon: An old disease that poses a new threat. *Critical Care Nurse, 22,* 21–35.

Veenema, T. G. (Ed.). (2003). *Disaster nursing and emergency preparedness for chemical biological, and radiological terrorism and other hazards.* New York: Springer.

Veenema, T. G., & Schroeder-Bruce, K. (2002). The aftermath of violence: Children, disaster, and posttraumatic stress disorder. *Journal of Pediatric Health Care, 16,* 235–244.

Yu, C. E. (2003). Medical response to radiation-related terrorism. *Pediatric Annals, 32,* 169–176.

Yu, C. E., Burklow, T. R., & Madsen, J. M. (2003). Vesicant agents and children. *Pediatric Annals, 32,* 254–257.

Other Resources

www.aap.org/terrorism
www.bioterrorism.slu.edu
www.bt.cdc.gov
www.bt.cdc.gov/children
www.cdc.gov
www.cdc.gov/HealthyYouth/terrorism/publications.htm
www.ems-c.org/disasters/framedisasters.htm
www.fema.gov/kids/dizkit.html

CHAPTER

36

Ear Irrigation

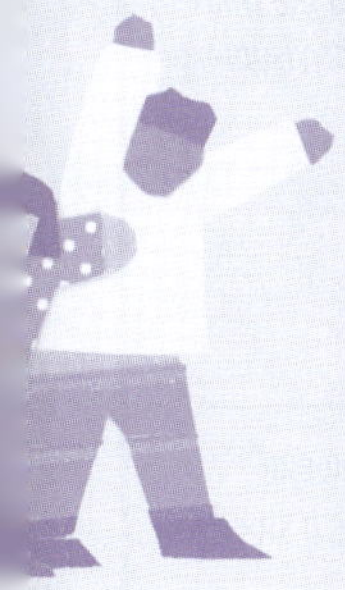

Clinical Guidelines

- A healthcare prescriber's order is required to complete this procedure in the clinical setting.
- A registered nurse (RN) or licensed practical nurse (LPN) may irrigate the ear per institutional policy.
- Ear irrigation is performed to remove material that blocks the external ear canal, to clean the ear canal of drainage, and to reduce local discomfort. Cerumen is the most common cause of ear pain and hearing deficits.

Equipment

- Otoscope
- Nonsterile gloves
- Cotton-tipped applicators
- Cotton balls
- Normal saline or mild antiseptic irrigating solution
- Bulb syringe or irrigating tip
- Emesis basin
- Waterproof pad
- Towel
- Blunt ear curette size 00 or wire curette/cerumen spoon (if needed)
- Blanket for mummy restraint (if needed)

Child and Family Assessment and Preparation

- Review child's history to determine prior and current ear pathology.
- Explain the procedure to the child and parent to prepare the child to anticipate effects of irrigation and to promote cooperation.

KidKare Explain to the child that the fluid placed in his or her ear will be warm and that it will feel the same as going under water.

PROCEDURE Irrigating the Ear

Steps	Rationale/Points of Emphasis
1. Gather the necessary supplies.	Promotes efficient time management and provides an organized approach to the procedure.
2. Prepare irrigating solution at a tepid temperature.	Solution should be body temperature because other temperatures stimulate the inner ear and can cause dizziness and nausea.
3a. Raise child's bed to working height or position the child on an examination table with the head of the bed elevated 45 degrees. The child may also sit in a chair or on the parent's lap for the procedure.	Raising the bed prevents back strain for the nurse.
3b. Have child sit up or lie with head tilted toward the side of affected ear.	Sitting up allows easier access to the child's ear and prevents dripping down the side of the face, neck, and back.
3c. Place a waterproof pad under the child's head. Have another towel available to dry the child's face, neck, and back as needed.	Waterproof pad prevents bed from becoming wet. **KidKare** Have an assistant immobilize the head and extremities as needed. The highly mobile or combative child may need to be further immobilized during the procedure to ensure safety. Use of blankets to apply a mummy restraint to the child can aid in immobilization. (See Chapter 102 on restraint techniques.)
4. Perform hand hygiene and don gloves.	Standard precaution to reduce transmission of microorganisms.
5a. Assess child's ear canal and pinna for redness, lesions, drainage, and pain.	Visual inspection of the ear is so obvious that it is frequently neglected.
5b. Use an otoscope to assess the inner canal and integrity of the tympanic membrane. Per institutional policy, this step may need to be completed by a healthcare prescriber.	Large accumulations of cerumen may not allow visualization of the tympanic membrane. Otitis media is present if the tympanic membrane is red and bulging and no light reflex is exhibited.
Alert! *If a foreign object is visualized in the ear canal or suspected to be in the ear canal, the procedure should not be attempted until the healthcare prescriber has been consulted.*	**Alert!** *If the tympanic membrane is not intact, do not irrigate the ear. This avoids transmission of fluid into the middle ear. Do not attempt irrigation if a foreign body is suspected or visualized until discussed with supervising provider.*
6. Clean outer ear if necessary using cotton swabs or a warm, wet washcloth.	Deters the spread of debris from outer ear into ear canal.
7. Place emesis basin below child's ear and fill bulb syringe/irrigating tip with solution.	Filling the syringe with fluid decreases the amount of air forced into the ear canal and the amount of noise the child is subjected to; it also provides a steady irrigating stream.
8. Pull the ear auricle down and back in child 3 years of age or younger and the ear auricle up and back in children over the age of 3 years. Keep the tragus forward in both groups (see Chapter 71, Figure 71-1).	This allows for maximum straightening of the ear canal. It also may provide a good view of the eardrum.
9. Place tip of bulb syringe/irrigating tip about 1 cm above opening of ear canal and gently squeeze syringe toward the roof of the ear. Do not "flood" the canal with fluid or occlude the canal with the irrigating nozzle. Allow the solution to flow out unimpeded. Continue slow stream of fluid until canal is cleansed or all solution has been used.	It is important to be gentle with the syringe in the ear because the epithelium lining the bony portion of canal is very thin and sensitive. Directing the solution at the roof prevents injury to the tympanic membrane. Obstructing the outflow fluid may cause the pressure to rise in the canal and on the eardrum, thus causing pain.

Steps	Rationale/Points of Emphasis
10. If a curette is needed to remove the cerumen, use a blunt ear curette size 00 or a wire curette (called a cerumen spoon). With an otoscope, visualize the ear and advance the curette beyond the point of the cerumen accumulation, resting medial to the occlusion. Pull cerumen toward the examiner.	Trauma risk to the eardrum and canal is high in children. The child's head must be immobilized to avoid nicking or irritating the tympanic membrane and canal.
caREminder *Per institutional policy, use of the curette may need to be completed by a healthcare prescriber.*	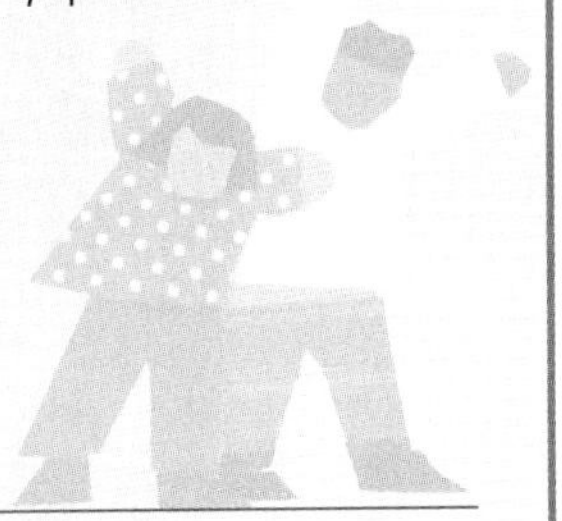
11. Dry child's outer ear and insert cotton ball loosely into canal opening. Instruct the child to lie on the affected side for a few minutes to continue the draining of the fluid.	A cotton ball absorbs fluid, and gravity allows the remaining solution in the canal to escape from the ear.
12. Repeat procedure on other ear if ordered.	Do not automatically irrigate both ears; only affected ears should be treated.
13. Clear away equipment and clean up area. Clean and dry the bulb syringe and allow it to air dry.	Decreases transmission of microorganisms.
14a. Remove gloves and perform hand hygiene.	Reduces transmission of microorganisms.
14b. Dispose of equipment and waste in appropriate receptacle.	Standard precautions.
15. Return child to position of comfort and lower bed to lowest position.	Promotes child's comfort and safety.

CHILD AND FAMILY EVALUATION AND DOCUMENTATION

- Ensure healthcare provider reassesses the ear using an otoscope to determine whether amount of cerumen has diminished.
- Document the following:
  - Color and amount of discharge
  - Type of solution used for irrigation
  - Child's tolerance to the procedure and current level of comfort
  - Findings from assessment of the ear before and after procedure

COMMUNITY CARE

- Ear irrigations using the bulb syringe can be completed in the home by the parent after doing a return demonstration of the previously described procedure.

Alert! ***Irrigations that require the use of a curette should not be attempted by the parent because of the potential of perforating the tympanic membrane.***

- Encourage parents to discuss use of over-the-counter medications to soften cerumen with healthcare prescriber; this might be safer and more comfortable for the child.
- Instruct the family to contact the healthcare provider if
  - Bleeding occurs during, or as a result of, the procedure
  - The child reports excessive pain
  - The child experiences hearing loss

Unexpected Situation

- *During the irrigation process the child begins to scream and complain of pain in the ear; bloody drainage is noted:* Stop the irrigation. Assess if pain continues when irrigating fluid is no longer being administered. Notify the healthcare prescriber of child's pain and bloody discharge.

Bibliography

Folmer, R. L., & Shi, B. Y. (2004). Chronic tinnitus resulting from cerumen removal procedures. *International Tinnitus Journal, 10*, 42–46.

Grossan, M. (2000). Safe, effective techniques for cerumen removal. *Geriatrics, 65*(1), 80–86.

Hand, C., & Harvey, I. (2004). The effectiveness of topical preparations for the treatment of earwax: A systematic review. *British Journal of General Practice, 54*, 862–867.

Roland, P., Eaton, D., Gross, R., et al. (2004). Randomized, placebo-controlled evaluation of Cerumenex and Murine earwax removal products. *Archives of Otolaryngology, Head and Neck Surgery, 130*, 1175–1177.

Whatley, V., Dodds, C., & Paul, R. (2003). Randomized clinical trial of docusate, triethanolamine polypeptide, and irrigation in cerumen removal in children. *Archives of Pediatric and Adolescent Medicine, 157*, 1177–1180.

CHAPTER

37

Enemas

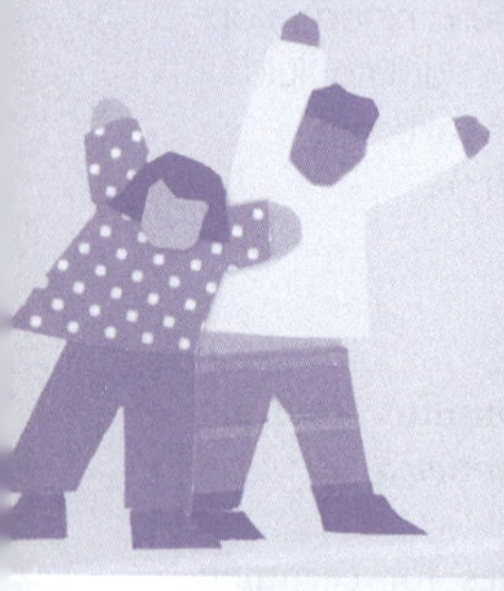

Clinical Guidelines

- A nurse practitioner (NP), registered nurse (RN), licensed practical nurse (LPN), or trained technician (with physician's orders) may administer an enema.
- An enema shall be administered for the purpose of instilling a solution into the large bowel to
  - Soften feces, assist peristalsis, and evacuate rectum and colon
  - Relieve distention and flatus
  - Prepare for diagnostic tests or surgical procedures
- The type and amount of enema solution to be instilled varies with the age and size of the child and with the reason for the enema (Chart 37-1 and Table 37-1).
- Administration of an enema is contraindicated for children with recent colon or rectal surgery, acute abdominal conditions, and/or a bleeding disorder or low platelet count.

Equipment

- Mineral oil or normal saline enema solution (amount varies by age and size of child; see Table 37-1) and bag with tubing and rectal catheter or manufacturer's prepackaged enema solution
- Protective pad
- Water-soluble lubricant
- Towels
- Toilet paper
- Bedpan
- Nonsterile gloves

Child and Family Assessment and Preparation

- Assess the child's health history and physical findings to determine timeframe and reason for previous enemas.
- Assess underlying factors that warrant this procedure (e.g., constipation, preparation for another procedure or for surgery).
- Review chart to determine whether colonic evacuation will be followed by laxative therapy.

caREminder

Research indicates that children with constipation who undergo some form of colonic evacuation followed by daily laxative therapy are more likely to respond to treatment.

CHART 37-1 Types of Enemas

Cleansing enema: Removes feces from the colon

Hypotonic or isotonic enema: Large-volume cleansing enema

Hypertonic enema: Small-volume cleansing enema

Oil retention enema: Lubricates the stool and intestinal mucosa, making defecation easier

Carminative enema: Helps to expel flatus from the rectum and relieve distention secondary to flatus

Medicated enema: Used to administer a medication rectally

Anthelmintic enema: Used to help destroy intestinal parasites

Nutritive enema: Replenishes fluids and nutrition rectally

Return-flow enema (Harris flush): Allows a small amount of solution to be administered and then allowed to return to the solution container. This process is repeated several times. Stimulates peristalsis to aid in expelling flatus.

- Assess psychosocial concerns of child and family in relation to administration of enema.
- Explain the procedure and the expected results to the child and the family. Use age-appropriate terminology.

KidKare An enema is a very private and scary experience for a child. The child's developmental level should be taken into consideration in regards to explanations of the procedure, parental presence, privacy concerns, and the degree to which the child assists in the procedure. In addition, the child's cultural needs must be considered to ensure sensitivity to cultural values is respected.

- Encourage the child to drink one to two glasses of water before the procedure.
- Ensure the child's privacy.

TABLE 37-1 Recommended Amount of Solution for Enema Administration

Age or Weight	Amount
Mineral Oil Enema	
2–6 yr	2.0 oz (½ enema)
>6 yr	4.5 oz
Phosphate Enema (Fleet's Enema)	
< 2 yr	Use not recommended
20 lb	1.0 oz
40 lb	2.0 oz
60 lb	3.0 oz
80 lb	4.0 oz
90+ lb	4.5 oz
Homemade Solution	
(2 level teaspoons table salt per quart of lukewarm water)	
2–6 yr	6.0 oz
6–12 yr	12 oz
> 12 yr	16 oz

PROCEDURE Administering an Enema

Steps	Rationale/Points of Emphasis
1. Perform hand hygiene. Gather the necessary supplies.	Reduces transmission of microorganisms. Promotes efficient time management and provides an organized approach to the procedure.
2. Prepare solution, select appropriate amount (Table 37-1), and warm to temperature of 100°F or 37.8°C.	Too much fluid can cause cramping and retention of fluids, leading to systemic absorption. Too little solution will lessen success of the procedure. Cold fluid may cause hypothermia and severe cramping. Hot fluids can burn the intestines.
Self-prepared solutions:	
a. Close the clamps on the enema bag tubing.	
b. Fill the bag with the warmed enema solution.	
c. Prime the tubing by opening the clamp and allowing the solution to free-flow through the entire length of the tubing.	Priming the tubing evacuates air from the tubing. If air enters the intestinal tract, it may produce abdominal cramping.
d. Close the clamp after all air has been removed from the tubing to prevent spilling.	
Prepackaged solutions:	
a. Open package, follow instructions from manufacturer for warming the fluid, and remove the cap on the enema tip.	

Continued

Steps	Rationale/Points of Emphasis
3. To provide the child with privacy, close curtains around the bed and drape towels over the child, exposing only the anal area.	Privacy can improve the child's comfort level during the procedure.
4. Don gloves.	Standard precaution to reduce transmission of microorganisms from potential contact with child's feces.
5. Place bed in high flat position and place the child in one of the following positions (Figure 37-1): a. On the left side in the lateral recumbent position with knees drawn up to the chest b. On back with the legs lifted to expose the anal orifice (best position for infants) c. A left Sims' position, with the right thigh flexed about 45 degrees to the body axis and positioned at the edge of the bed d. Knee–chest position with child balancing on knees and forearms, resting the head on a pillow so that the buttocks are angled upward off the bed	Elevated positions allow gravity to aid the flow of the solution into the descending colon. The knee–chest position helps to distribute the solution throughout the lower intestinal tract. **caREminder** *The child should be positioned in a manner that is most comfortable for him or her.*
6. Place waterproof protective pad under the child's buttocks.	Pad protects the bed.
7. Lubricate the rectal tube based on length of advancement (see step 8c).	Eases insertion of the tube and decreases rectal irritation.
8. Insert the rectal tube or enema tip: a. Separate the child's buttocks. b. Gently touch the anus, observing for anal contraction, followed by relaxation. c. Insert rectal tube (either of enema bag or tub of prepackaged container) with the tip pointing in the direction of the child's umbilicus to the appropriate length for advancement and hold in place. Recommended lengths of advancement are as follows: Infant (<22 lb) — 1 inch Small child (23–66 lb) — 2 inches Large child (67–110 lb) — 3 inches Adolescent (>110 lb) — 4 inches	 Relaxation of the anus will ease insertion of the tube. Inserting the tip toward the umbilicus decreases the chance of the tube scraping the rectal wall.

Alert! ***Never force the catheter into the anal canal. If a well-lubricated catheter does not advance easily, remove the tube and stop the enema. Forcing the tube may injure the intestinal mucosa wall.***

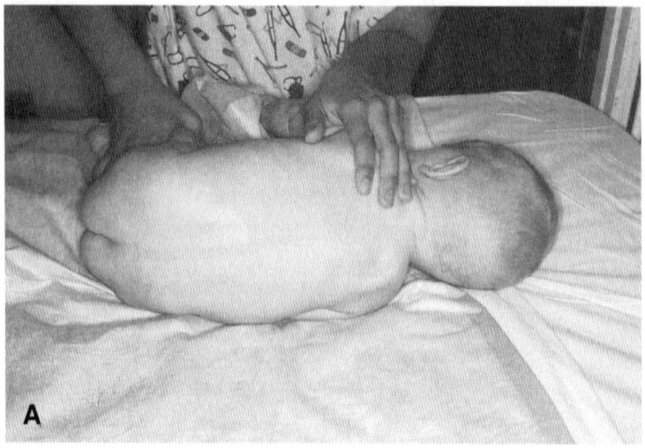

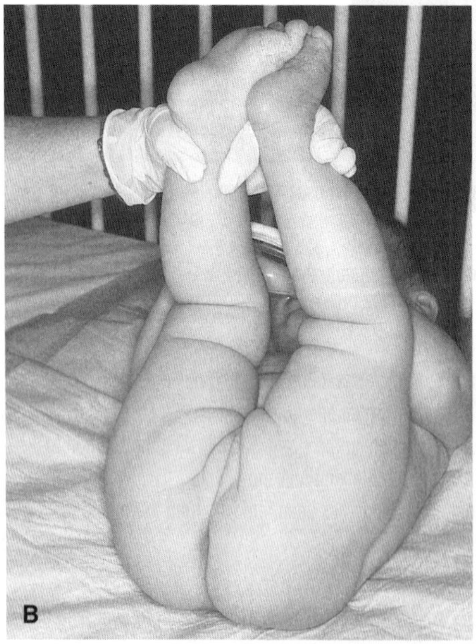

FIGURE 37-1
Positions for enema administration. (**A**) Left side lateral recumbent; (**B**) infant position; (**C**) Sims' position; and (**D**) knee–chest position.

Steps	Rationale/Points of Emphasis

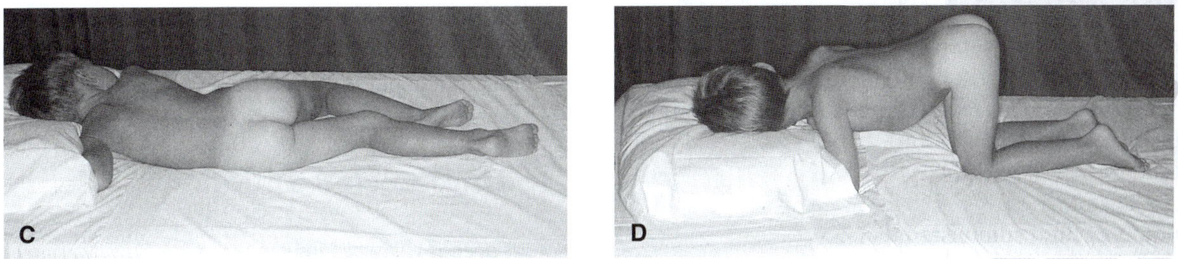

FIGURE 37-1
Continued.

Steps	Rationale/Points of Emphasis
9a. Elevate the solution bag about 10 cm (4 inches) above the anus, unclamp the tubing, and administer fluid as tolerated by child.	The height of the container determines the amount of pressure of the solution. Too much pressure may cause discomfort or premature expulsion of the solution.
9b. Squeeze and roll the prepackaged enema container toward the child's rectum until all the solution is administered.	Rolling the container assists in dispensing the solution into the intestines.
10. Techniques to reduce cramping during enema administration:	
a. Encourage child to relax, breathe deeply, and let his or her breath out rapidly through the mouth.	Promotes relaxation, distraction, and comfort.
b. For moderate cramping, pinch off the tube to temporarily interrupt the flow of the solution.	Permits pressure to equalize, thereby minimizing cramping.
c. For severe cramping, lower bag below the level of the bed.	Flatus pockets are often broken in this manner. **caREminder** *To ensure that the complete large bowel has been filled, do not end the enema until at least three fourths of the solution, or, if possible, the full amount of the solution, has been administered.*
11. Remove the rectal tube or container tip by pressing the buttocks together and quickly withdrawing the tube.	The urge to defecate is diminished with this approach.
12. Instruct the child to retain the solution as long as possible.	The evacuation reflex is stimulated by fluid retention. **KidKare** Holding the buttocks together of the infant or small child will assist him or her in retaining the solution.
13. Assist the child onto the bedpan or to the toilet.	An upright sitting position facilitates elimination of the solution and subsequent defecation.
14. Assist the child with hygiene as necessary. Return the child to a comfortable position.	Washing the child's buttocks decreases skin irritation and prevents the spread of microorganisms. **KidKare** Remind the child to always cleanse from front to back to prevent contamination of the urinary meatus.
15. Dispose of equipment and waste in appropriate receptacle. Remove gloves and perform hand hygiene.	Standard precautions. Reduces transmission of microorganisms.

CHILD AND FAMILY EVALUATION AND DOCUMENTATION

- Evaluate the child to determine presence of complications (e.g., excessive irritation of colonic mucosa, electrolyte abnormalities, arrhythmias due to vasovagal stimulation, water intoxication).
- Document the following:
  - Type of enema use
  - Amount of fluid administered
  - Approximate output
  - Child's response to treatment, including complaints by the child of unusual pain, symptoms of shock, or unusual reaction
  - Instructions provided to family about home care (e.g., enema use at home, use of laxatives).

COMMUNITY CARE

- If the procedure is to be completed at home, instruct the family about the following:
  - Where to purchase supplies
  - Type of enema solution (be sure to inform them to select only mineral oil or normal saline enemas for children)
  - Proper procedure for administering the enema
  - To administer one to two glasses of water to the child before the procedure
  - The importance of perineal hygiene and the use of anal rectal ointment or sitz baths to relieve any anal discomfort
  - To give the enema after the main meal of the day to take advantage of the gastrocolic reflex
  - To clean home enema equipment (nondisposable) in hot, soapy water; air-dry; and store in a plastic bag until next use
- Instruct the family to contact the healthcare provider if
  - The child remains constipated
  - The child complains of severe cramping that is not relieved after expulsion of the fluid from the enema
  - The child experiences rectal bleeding

Unexpected Situations

- *Resistance is met while inserting the tube:* Permit a small amount of solution to enter, withdraw the tube slightly, and then continue to insert the tube. Resistance may be due to intestinal spasms or failure of the internal sphincter to open. The solution may help to reduce the spasms and relax the sphincter. Ask the child to take deep breaths because this may also help relax the anal sphincter.
- *The child cannot retain the enema solution for an adequate amount of time:* The amount and length of administration may have to be modified. The child may need to be placed on a bedpan in the supine position while receiving the enema. Elevate the head of the bed 30 degrees to provide more comfort for the child.

Bibliography

Borowitz, S., Cox, D., Kovatchev, B., et al. (2005). Treatment of childhood constipation by primary care physicians: Efficacy and predictors of outcomes. *Pediatrics, 115*(4), 873–877.

Di Lorenzo, C., & Bennings, M. (2004). Pathophysiology of pediatric fecal incontinence. *Gastroenterology, 126*(1), S33–S40.

McKesson Corporation. (2004). *Enemas: How to give.* Retrieved April 26, 2005, from www.med.umich.edu/1libr/pa/pa_enemahom_hhg.htm

Schmelzer, M., Case, P., Chappell, S., & Wright, K. (2000). Colonic cleansing, fluid absorption and discomfort following tap water and soapsuds enemas. *Applied Nursing Research, 13*(2), 83–91.

CHAPTER

38

Enteral Tubes Placement and Management: Gastrostomy, PEG, Skin-Level Devices, and Jejunostomy

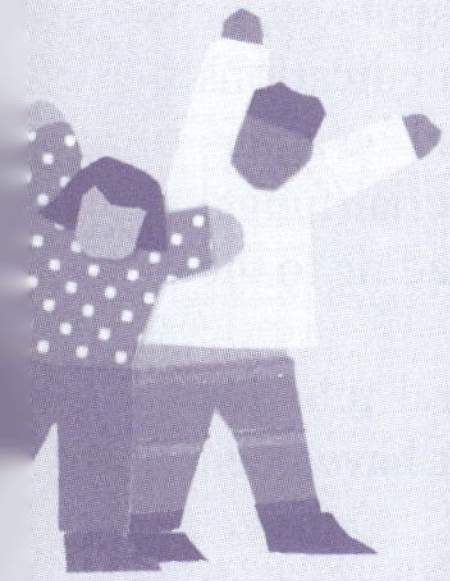

Clinical Guidelines

- Long-term enteral indwelling feeding tubes are placed by a physician. All long-term enteral indwelling feeding tubes must have an internal stabilizer to keep the tube from falling out. They must also have an external stabilizer to keep the tube in the correct position and prevent tube migration into the GI tract (Figure 38-1 and Table 38-1). The shapes of these stabilizers differ; care of the tube may need to be adjusted accordingly.
- Gastrostomy tubes (G-tubes) are placed either surgically, endoscopically, or, in some cases, by interventional radiology. Gastrostomy tubes are placed directly into the stomach. Percutaneous endoscopic gastrostomy (PEG) tubes are placed endoscopically. After an established G-tube tract is formed (about 6 weeks), a skin-level G-tube device can be placed. There are numerous devices available. The internal stabilizer for skin-level devices is either a balloon type or a mushroom type.
- Jejunostomy tubes (J-tubes) can be placed through similar procedures. The distal tip rests in the jejunum but may originate through the stomach (G-J) or directly into the jejunum. Skin-level devices are available.
- Tubes that originate in the oral cavity, oral-gastric (OG) nares, nasogastric (NG), or nasojejunal (NJ) are discussed in Chapter 39.
- If dislodgment of a newly placed tube occurs (usually less than 6 to 8 weeks after initial placement), reinsertion of the tube is performed by the physician.
- An RN, parent, or child trained in the balloon-type gastrostomy tube replacement can perform this task once the gastric tunnel and stoma are well established (usually within 6 to 8 weeks after initial placement of tube). These tubes include balloon-type G-tubes, skin-level devices, and/or a Foley catheter.
- If dislodgment of a jejunostomy tube occurs, a trained RN or primary caregiver/parent may insert a balloon-type replacement G-tube or Foley catheter into the stoma for the *sole* purpose of splinting open the stoma until the physician can replace the G-J or J-tube. Instructions must be given to not feed through the device until the transpyloric tube is in place.

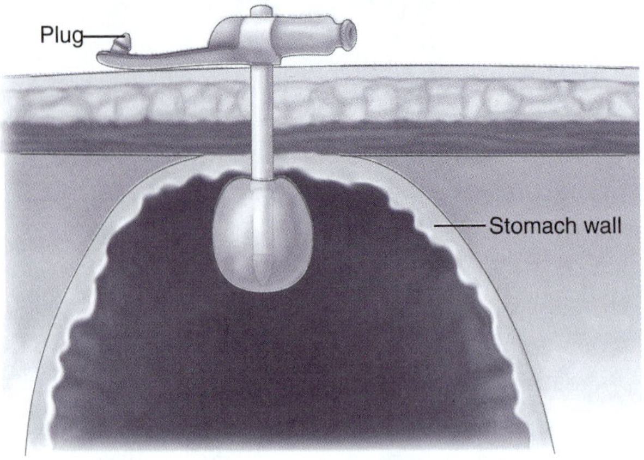

FIGURE 38-1
PEG gastrostomy tube. The internal, dome-shaped tip anchors tube in body and prevents tube from falling out. The cross-bar at skin level prevents internal tube migration.

- Children requiring enteral nutritional support for longer than 4 to 6 weeks should be considered candidates for long-term enteral tube access.
- Children with head or neck trauma or surgery, tumors of the esophagus, unrepaired cleft lip or palate, or neurologic deficit may be precluded from nasally placed enteral feeding tubes and would therefore benefit from placement of an enteral tube. Previous gastric resections, tumors blocking passage of an endoscope, ascites, morbid obesity, and esophageal or gastric varices may require a surgically placed tube.
- Jejunostomy tubes and G-J tubes, sometime referred to as transpyloric tubes, are indicated in children at increased risk for aspiration, who are unable to tolerate enteral feedings into the stomach, or who have significant altered motility.
- Indwelling enteral tube site care should be performed every day (during the bath is a convenient time) and as needed to maintain skin integrity.
- Indwelling enteral tubes are made of long-lasting material and should not require routine change unless they become accidentally dislodged or the integrity of the tube itself is breaking down. Follow manufacturer's instructions for routine time periods to replace enteral tubes in children receiving long-term enteral therapy.

EQUIPMENT

For Indwelling Enteral Tube Skin Care With Dressing Change

- Gauze
- 2 × 2 split gauze
- Water
- Cleansing solution (e.g., for newly placed tubes: sterile normal saline; for well-healed stomas: soap and water)
- Three cotton-tipped applicators
- Two small medicine cups
- Paper tape (1-inch)
- External anchor as needed (according to hospital policy)
- Skin barrier (optional)
- Antibiotic ointment (optional or as prescribed)
- Nonsterile gloves
- Tape measure

For Gastrostomy/Jejunostomy Tube Change or Replacement

- Foley catheter with a 5-mL balloon (sizes 8 to 18 French) or mushroom-type catheter and introducer
- Water-soluble lubricant
- Sterile water
- 5-mL syringe
- Catheter adapter (optional)
- Nonsterile gloves
- Tape
- Rubber band
- For external stabilizer: gauze and tape or 1-inch foam tape

CHILD AND FAMILY ASSESSMENT AND PREPARATION

- Assess the child for signs of poor wound healing, decreased muscle mass, and inadequate protein intake, which can be symptoms of poor caloric intake and may assist in determining need for long-term enteral therapy.
- Assess the need for long-term enteral access resulting from the child's inability to meet nutritional requirements and maintain body weight for longer than 2 weeks.
- Assess the skin and insertion site around the indwelling enteral tube for inflammation, tenderness, drainage, or breakdown. High-calorie formulas and medications mixed with high dextrose concentrations can be a perfect breeding ground for skin-surface bacterial/fungal infection at the tube insertion site or tract, leading to the gastrointestinal tract.
- Assess the patency of the indwelling enteral tube for clogging from formula or medications that have been administered through the tube.
- Assess the cognitive level, readiness, and ability to process information by the child and family. The readiness to learn and process information may be impaired as a result of age, stress, or anxiety. Explain the child's role in assisting with replacement of the tube or skin care (as age and developmentally appropriate).
- Reinforce the need for and identify and discuss the risks and benefits of tube replacement or skin care, as appropriate, to both the child and family.
- Explain the procedure, as appropriate, to both the child and the family.

(text continues on page 267)

TABLE 38-1

Comparative Chart of Gastrostomy Tubes in Children

				Skin Level G-Tubes	
Type	Traditional G-Tubes: Pezzar (Mushroom) Catheter	Percutaneous Endoscopic Gastrostomy (PEG)	Balloon-Type G-Tubes/ Foley Catheter	Button (Bard)	Balloon Type (e.g., MIC-Key)
Indications	• Surgically placed in conjunction with surgical emergency interventions of the newborn Frequently placed with Nissen fundoplication for GERD • Partial/total nutritional support	• Partial/total nutritional support	• Partial/total nutritional support • Replacement G-tube • Foley may be used for transition G-tube for dilatation of tract before skin level G-tube placement	• Partial/total nutritional support • Body image/personal preference/developmental • Usually can transition from PEG/traditional G-tube after 6–8 wk	• Partial/total nutritional support • Laparoscopic fundoplication • Body image/personal preference/ developmental • Usually can transition from PEG/traditional G-tube after 6–8 wk
Sedation/ preparation (Child life specialist can assist to prepare all children with age-appropriate strategies.)	• General anesthesia	• Moderate sedation with EGD • High-risk patients may need deep sedation or have it done in OR with anesthesia	• None used • Outpatient/bedside placement	• Sedation per patient need	• Sedation per patient need. • For laparoscopic fundoplication, in OR with general anesthesia outpatient/bedside placement
Device description	• Rubber latex • Internal stabilizer: "mushroom tip" • External stabilizer: placed by caregiver • No feeding port closure; use rubber band for closure	• Silicone • Internal stabilizer: dome shape • External stabilizer: crossbar • Has feeding port closure • Tract may need to be dilated with Foley to prep for skin-level G-tube	• Silicone or rubber latex • Internal stabilizer: 5-mL balloon • Foley requires external stabilizer	• Silicone • Has feeding port closure • Device is at skin level • One-way valve at base of device • Feeding attachments: bolus/continuous must match the FR size of the device • Internal stabilizer: mushroom tip	• Silicone • Has feeding port closure • Device is at skin level • One-way valve at top of device • Feeding attachments lock in place for bolus and continuous • Universal-size feeding attachments

Continued

TABLE 38-1

Comparative Chart of Gastrostomy Tubes in Children (continued)

Type	Traditional G-Tubes: Pezzar (Mushroom) Catheter	Percutaneous Endoscopic Gastrostomy (PEG)	Balloon-Type G-Tubes/ Foley Catheter	Skin Level G-Tubes: Button (Bard)	Skin Level G-Tubes: Balloon Type (e.g., MIC-Key)
	• Avoid use of clamps on tube 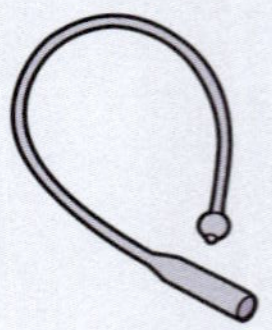	• Calibrations on external segment of tube 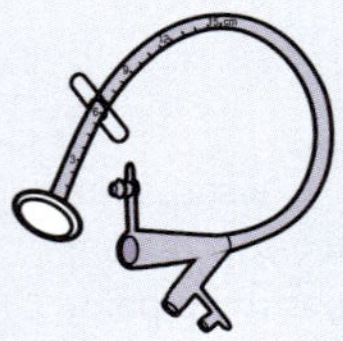	• No feeding port closure; use rubber band for closure 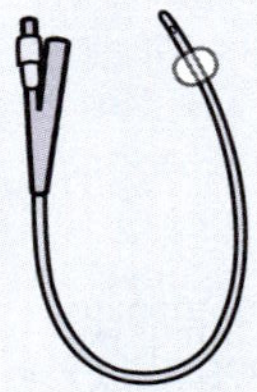 • Balloon-type G-tubes • Have an external stabilizer (e.g., disc shape) • Have feeding port closure 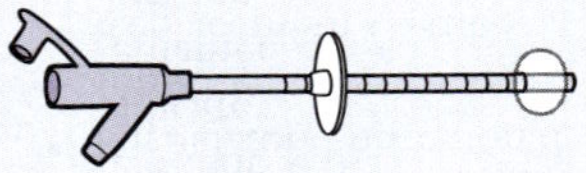 • Avoid use of clamps on both tubes	• Requires a special tubing for venting decompression 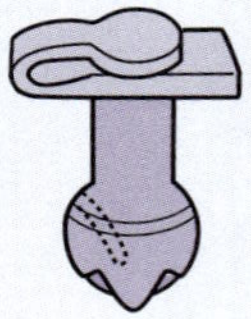	• Internal stabilizer: balloon: volume of H_2O: MIC-Key maximum is 10 mL 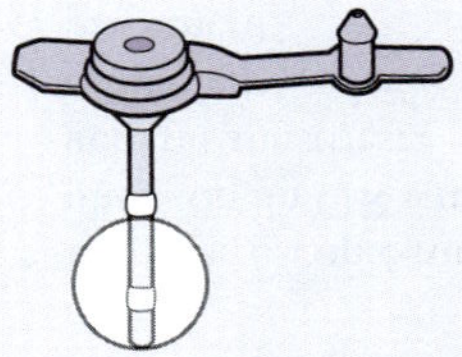
General information	• Sutures at stoma removed after 10–14 days	• No sutures • Do not change dressing during first 24 hr	• No sutures • No dressing • Tube can move freely in/out of stoma	• Requires a well-established G-tube tract • No dressing needed	• Requires a well-established G-tube tract • No dressing needed

	• After sutures removed, tube can move in/out of stoma freely • Vent stomach: after fundoplication: □ Before and after feeds □ Abdominal discomfort/distention □ Retching/gagging (must vent to maintain intact fundoplication)	• Minimal manipulation until well healed (10–14 days) • No ongoing dressing needed • Can vent stomach • The cm markings on external segment of tube help indicate that tube has remained in the initial position • Keep PEG tubing securely taped to abdomen for at least 3 days after initial placement	• Parent/caregiver can learn to replace • Balloon size can be adjusted for peristomal leakage • Balloon-type G-tube has cm markings on external segment that help to indicate that tube has remained in initial position • Foley catheter used as a replacement tube	• One-way valve allows gastric contents to remain in stomach when device is unplugged • Venting requires special decompression tubing	• One-way valve allows gastric contents to remain in stomach when device is unplugged • Can vent stomach by attaching the feeding tubing • Parent/caregiver can learn to replace with well-healed stoma • Postlaparoscopic fundoplication: sutures in place for several days to avoid accidental dislodgement
Skin care	• Initial: use normal saline • Stoma well healed: use soap and water • Apply external stabilizer: use “gauze bolster” or tape wrap to stabilize and correctly position	• Initial: use normal saline for 3 days • Stoma well healed: use soap and water • Check tension of external stabilizer: comfortably fit cotton-tipped applicator under external stabilizer • Rotate device during skincare	• Soap and water • For gauze external stabilizer: □ Change it with daily skin care □ Rotate it in a 3–6–9 o’clock fashion • For tape wrap: □ Increase the circumference of the tube at the skin level to avoid migration □ Pull tube back against stomach wall before wrapping tape □ Replace it as needed	• Soap and water • Rotate device during skin care	• Soap and water • Rotate device during skin care • Postlaparoscopic surgery: skin care may be ordered by surgeon. Can use sterile normal saline until sutures are removed

Continued

TABLE 38-1

Comparative Chart of Gastrostomy Tubes in Children (continued)

Type	Traditional G-Tubes: Pezzar (Mushroom) Catheter	Percutaneous Endoscopic Gastrostomy (PEG)	Balloon-Type G-Tubes/ Foley Catheter	Skin Level G-Tubes: Button (Bard)	Skin Level G-Tubes: Balloon Type (e.g., MIC-Key)
Flush*	• Routine flush with warm water • Flush after meds and feeds with water (3–5 mL)	• Routine flush with warm water • Flush after meds and feeds with water (3–5 mL)	• Routine flush with warm water • Flush after meds and feeds with water (3–5 mL)	• Routine flush with warm water • Flush after meds and feeds with water (3–5 mL)	• Routine flush with warm water • Flush after meds and feeds with water (3–5 mL)
Activity	• Bathe after stoma healed and sutures out • Secure tube to avoid dangling and tube dislodgment • May position prone as tolerates	• Bathe after stoma healed • Secure tube to avoid dangling and tube dislodgment • May position prone as tolerates	• Can bathe • Secure tube to avoid dangling and tube dislodgement • May position prone as tolerates	• Can bathe as usual • Better accepted for body image and increased activity • May position prone as tolerates	• Can bathe as usual; check with surgeon for postlaparoscopic surgery care • Better accepted for body image and increased activity • May position prone as tolerates

*For children at risk for fluid balance disturbance, adjust flush volumes individually.
EGD, esophagogastroduodenoscopy; G-tube, gastrostomy tube; GERD, gastroesophageal reflux disease.

PROCEDURE Indwelling Enteral Tube Skin Care and Dressing Change*

Steps	Rationale/Points of Emphasis
1. Perform hand hygiene.	Reduces transmission of microorganisms.
2. Gather the necessary supplies for skin site care and dressing change of long-term enteral tube.	Promotes efficient time management and provides an organized approach to the procedure.
3. Don gloves.	Standard precaution to reduce transmission of microorganisms.
4. Assist the child into a comfortable supine position.	Improves tolerance of procedure and allows for ease of access to skin at tube insertion site.
5. Remove old dressing, if used, and discard in appropriate waste receptacle.	Allows visualization of site; disposal follows standard precautions.
6. Prepare cleanser: for newly placed tube (under 5 days) pour sterile saline/water into a medicine cup; use soap and water for healed site.	Acts as cleansing agent to reduce microorganisms on skin that may cause breakdown of skin or infection.
7. For newly placed tube, saturate cotton-tipped applicator with sterile saline/water and cleanse around enteral tube insertion site, using a gentle rolling motion versus a scrubbing motion. Continue cleansing in the same manner with the remaining cotton-tipped applicators until all crusts and drainage have been removed. For established tube sites, wash with soap and water during the child's bath. **caREminder** *For tubes with external stabilizers (retaining rings or T bars) cleanse under the stabilizer with the cotton applicator using a gentle rolling motion. Do not use baby bottle nipples as anchors because they tend to seal in the moisture and decrease visualization of the site.*	Prevents infection and skin breakdown. **caREminder** *Avoid excessive pulling on the enteral tube; this can cause pain and irritation to the gastric mucosa.*
8. Dry insertion site with gauze. For skin-level G-tube devices, rotate device in full circle; refer to manufacturer's instructions. Rotating the J-tubes or G-J tubes is not indicated to avoid potential kinking of the tube.	Reduces moisture that could in turn promote bacterial growth. Rotation prevents device from adhering to gastric mucosal lining and skin.
9. (Optional or as prescribed.) Apply skin barrier and/or antibiotic ointment around site.	After the skin has healed, there should be very little, if any, discharge from the stoma, thus eliminating the need to apply ointment or a dressing. Recommendations vary on use of dressings, ointments, or skin barriers on skin as a part of the daily routine. Some success with the antibiotic or antifungal powders has been seen in preventing bacterial or fungal problems at the site. Should irritation occur at the stoma site, such irritations may respond best to exposure to air. If severe, skin barriers or ointments may be needed. These products protect against acidity that may leak out around tube insertion site and reduce skin flora that may promote growth of microorganisms.
10. When dressings are used, place a presplit 2 × 2 gauze dressing around tube over skin and secure loosely with tape. **caREminder** *Do not cut 2 × 2 to make dressing because threads adhere to stoma margins. When using dressing, assess frequently for the need to change the dressing.*	Not using a dressing leaves the site open to air, which may aid in maintenance of skin integrity. If a dressing is used, loose application promotes air circulation to the skin, thereby reducing moisture at the site, and dressing protects site from irritation.

*Dressings may be used per physician or institution preference.

Continued

Steps	Rationale/Points of Emphasis
11. For newly placed PEGs, secure a loop of tubing to abdomen.	Avoids tension, pressure, pulling, and accidental dislodgement at site, which would impair healing process. **caREminder** *Rotate site where tube is secured to the abdomen so that tension is distributed evenly around the stoma. An expandable tube-type dressing may be used to keep tube from dangling after stoma is well healed (e.g., burn net or surgi-net dressings). For infants, "onesies" are helpful.*
12. Dispose of equipment and waste in appropriate receptacle.	Standard precautions.
13. Remove gloves and perform hand hygiene.	Reduces transmission of microorganisms.

PROCEDURE Gastrostomy Tube Change or Replacement

Steps	Rationale/Points of Emphasis
1. Perform hand hygiene.	Reduces transmission of microorganisms.
2. Gather the necessary supplies for tube replacement.	Promotes efficient time management and provides an organized approach to the procedure.
3. Don gloves.	Standard precaution to reduce transmission of microorganisms.
4. Assist the child into a comfortable supine position.	Improves tolerance of procedure and allows for ease of access to skin at tube insertion site.
5. Remove old dressing, if used, and discard in appropriate waste receptacle.	Allows visualization of site; disposal follows standard precautions.
6. *Tube removal:* The physician removes old enteral tube with mushroom-type tip, PEG, and jejunostomy. The nurse, physician, or parent removes old enteral tube, balloon-type (e.g., MIC gastrostomy, MIC-Key, Foley, Corpak, Ross), if still in place, by connecting syringe to balloon port lumen and deflating balloon with appropriate-sized syringe (lumen size is usually labeled on the enteral tube). Pull tube out through stoma and discard.	Prepares for tube replacement.
7. Test balloon of new balloon-type tube by injecting designated amount of sterile water through balloon port lumen, and then deflate.	Ensures patency of new balloon before insertion. Replace old enteral tubes with like tube, if possible. Manufacturers recommend the use of sterile or distilled water for balloon inflation to maximize the life of the product. Tap water has minerals that may deteriorate the device material.
8. When using balloon-type (e.g., MIC gastrostomy tube, MIC-Key, Foley, Corpak, Ross) tubes, lubricate 3 to 5 cm of the distal tip of the new tube liberally with water-soluble lubricant and gently insert into stoma of abdomen until stomach contents drain out of open end. **caREminder** *When inserting a skin-level device, stomach contents will not be visible because of the one-way valve. In some products, if the feeding attachment is connected, then stomach contents will be observed.*	Use of water-soluble lubricant reduces friction, prevents trauma, and facilitates insertion.

Steps	Rationale/Points of Emphasis
9. Auscultate for bowel sounds after replacement of tube and secure in position with external anchor as appropriate, such as a gauze bolster or by increasing the diameter of the tube by wrapping foam tape around the tube at the skin level. This is usually needed when a Foley is used as a replacement G-tube. If in doubt that the tube is positioned properly, an x-ray may be indicated.	Facilitates early detection of complications. Anchor stabilizes tube, prevents excessive movement, and may reduce pressure and the potential of dislodgement of tube.
10. Inflate balloon of tube with appropriate amount of sterile water into balloon port.	Prevents tube from slipping out of place.
11. Gently pull back on tube until slight resistance is met for balloon-type tubes. G-tubes with a balloon have centimeter markings on the tube that allow for a baseline measurement. Measure external tube length for baseline measurement for an unmarked tube and Foley catheter.	Places balloon snugly against abdominal wall to prevent leakage of fluid. Indicates that tube has remained in the correct position.
12. Apply tube closure or insert catheter adapter and cap (optional).	Closes the feeding system and prevents leaks.
13. Clean and dress site as described above in previous procedure guidelines.	Maintains skin integrity.
14. Dispose of equipment and waste in appropriate receptacle.	Standard precautions.
15. Remove gloves and perform hand hygiene.	Reduces transmission of microorganisms.

CHILD AND FAMILY EVALUATION AND DOCUMENTATION

- Evaluate the child's bowel sounds at least every shift for motility. Gastrointestinal function affects the child's tolerance to enteral feedings.
- Evaluate the child for correct tube position at least once every shift. Tube malposition can be evidenced by tube length being shorter than baseline measurement, distended abdomen, high-pitched bowel sounds indicating obstruction, or blocked lumen of the bowel by the tube balloon.
- Monitor intake and output through the tube every hour or as determined by patient condition.
- Monitor the child's intake and output carefully.
- Evaluate the child for signs and symptoms of infection such as drainage, pus, inflammation, or tenderness at the tube insertion site.
- Document on the appropriate institutional forms:
  - Date and time of insertion or dressing change, assessments, size of tube used, the insertion site position and placement (e.g., left upper quadrant of abdomen), external tube length measurement, verification of placement, restraints used, medications, treatments applied, and child's response to the procedure
  - Intake and output and whether the tube is in use or clamped or to straight drainage
  - How tube is being used (e.g., for a G-J tube, medications are given through the gastrostomy port and feedings are administered via the jejunostomy port or G-tube port is used for decompression and the J-port is clamped)
  - Patency of feeding device status (intact, without leaks, kinks, or occlusion) at least once every shift (Table 38-2)
  - Child's weight and change trends (e.g., increasing or decreasing)
- Determine whether the child and family have other concerns.

COMMUNITY CARE

- If the child is to be discharged home with an enteral tube, initiate teaching plan for home care of the tube, including flushing of the tube and management if the tube becomes dislodged (see Tables 38-1 and 38-2).
- Discuss with family members the ways in which they can perform the procedure at home by using clean supplies (i.e., cotton-tipped applicators, water, and gauze) and by cleansing equipment in hot water and soap for reuse (i.e., syringes).
- Provide the family with a set of Foley catheters that are the same size and one size smaller than the gastrostomy or jejunostomy tube to use as a short-term replacement tube should the permanent tube become dislodged. Teach parents how to replace a dislodged tube. Some institutions will discharge a child with a balloon-type skin-level G-tube device with a device the same size as the child's placed tube and a smaller size replacement tube.
- Provide for a consultation with a nutritional support nurse specialist or dietitian to determine in-home feeding needs and equipment. Refer to Chapter 42 for more information on tube feedings.

(text continues on page 270)

TABLE 38-2

Troubleshooting Common Gastrostomy Tube Problems

Problem	Possible Causes and Interventions
Erythema	
Traditional G-tube types: Pezzar and balloon-type G-tubes (e.g., MIC-G and Foley)	• Determine where leakage is from and attempt to decrease it. • Adjust and secure tube position. • Assess for other signs of infection—swelling, tenderness, drainage, induration—and treat as indicated. • Notify physician. • Consider changing tension of external stabilizer. • Use of skin barrier may be of help. • Consider enterostomal nurse consult. • Avoid dangling tube; secure it to body. • If tube is immobile, consider that it has migrated into tract.
Percutaneous endoscopic gastrostomy (PEG)	• Assess date of PEG placement: if <6 wk since initial placement, consult gastroenterologist. • Consider cellulitis with newly placed tube. • Determine where leakage is from and attempt to decrease it. • Adjust and secure tube position. • Assess for other signs of infection—swelling, tenderness, drainage, induration—and treat as indicated. • Notify physician/APN. • Consider changing tension of external stabilizer. • If tube is immobile, consider that it has migrated into tract. • Avoid dangling tube; secure it to body.
Skin-level devices: button (Bard) and balloon type (e.g., MIC-Key)	• Check tube position: if device too loose, may build up device by placing gauze layers under flanges of device. • Assess volume of water in balloon: MIC-Key maximum is 10 mL. • Assess for other signs of infection—swelling, tenderness, drainage, induration—and treat as indicated. • If any device is too tight, contact gastroenterologist for evaluation or replacement for malfunction. • If tube is immobile, consider that it has migrated into tract.
Leakage	
Traditional G-tube types: Pezzar and balloon-type G-tubes (e.g., MIC-G and Foley)	• Check position of tube: ▫ Gently pull back until resistance is felt. ▫ Replace external stabilizer and secure tube to the body to avoid migration. • Observe/measure external length of tube, mark it, and record length. • Consider H_2 blocker. • Check volume in balloon: 5 mL is typical.
Percutaneous endoscopic gastrostomy (PEG)	• Assess duration of time of PEG placement: if PEG <6 wk old, consult gastroenterologist. • Assess tube position: ▫ Gently pull tube back until resistance is felt. ▫ Adjust external stabilizer for appropriate "fit." • Observe/measure external length of tube, mark it, and record length. • Consider H_2 blocker. • Notify gastroenterologist if problem persists.
Skin-level devices: button (Bard) and balloon type (e.g., MIC-Key)	• Determine if leakage is result of a valve malfunction or is from peristomal area. • Check tube position with child in both sitting and standing positions. • Contact gastroenterologist if device is too tight. • Assess valve for malfunction: keep feeding port extension tubing connected to tube if valve is leaking. Consult gastroenterologist for replacement device. • Assess volume of water in balloon: maximum is 10 mL. • Protect skin with skin barriers.
Vomiting and diarrhea	• Assess for tube position and dislodgment/migration. • Consider adjusting feeding. • Slow down/decrease the rate. • Ensure that feeding is at room temperature. • Adjust volume or administer via drip vs. bolus • Vent stomach. • Assess for other sources of illness

Continued

TABLE 38-2

Troubleshooting Common Gastrostomy Tube Problems (continued)

Problem	Possible Causes and Interventions
Tube migration	• Assess tube position: □ If tube is thought to have migrated into the tract or further in the GI tract, stop the feeding until correct tube position is confirmed. □ For "traditional-tube types" that have an external segment: gently pull tube up against abdominal wall. The tube should easily move up and down in tract. If immobile, the tube may have migrated *into* the tract. Consult gastroenterologist. □ If resistance is felt when pulled upward and external tube length is shorter than baseline, tube may have migrated through pylorus: reposition only if balloon-type tube and if tube has been in place for >6 wk. Re-stabilize tube with external stabilizer. • Consult gastroenterologist/PCP for further studies and interventions. • For skin-level devices: balloon type may be repositioned if tube is in well-healed tract (>6 wk). • For Bard button: device may appear elevated from the skin surface. Do not use tube. Consult gastroenterologist for further evaluation and interventions. • Increased drainage may be observed from the stoma. • The feeding may be slower than usual and the child may experience pain from the pressure of the feeding.
Bleeding	• Assess stoma condition. • Contact gastroenterologist to remove excess granulation tissue. • Topically treat infection; if child is immunosuppressed, may need intravenous antibiotics. • Stabilize tube to avoid increased irritation and chronic pulling at stoma level.
Blocked tube	• Prevention: □ Obtain order to use liquid medications as available/prescription for liquid medicines for home care. □ Flush tube after intermittent feedings and every 6 h during continuous feedings with 3–5 mL of warm water. □ For infants and children at risk for alterations in fluid balance, individually adjust flush volumes. □ Flush before and after medications and between multiple medications. □ Assess viscosity of formula and medications. □ Check tube position so that it is able to freely move in and out in the tract and is not migrated up into the tract. □ Consider daily flush of apple juice or cola (cola is not indicated for infants). • Declogging agents (require a healthcare prescriber order): □ "Clog Zapper" □ Sodium bicarbonate, 324 mg (crushed), and 1 capsule of Viokase (crushed) mixed with 25 mL warm water; administer 10 mL working the tube in and out with the solution to break down the occlusion. • Consult gastroenterologist; tube may need to be replaced.
Dislodged tube	• Consult medical record to determine if tube is newly placed or is an established G-tube tract: □ If G-tube is newly placed (<6 wk since initial placement), contact gastroenterologist or surgeon. □ If G-tube is >6 wk old, replace with Foley catheter of comparable size or balloon-type G-tube. If unable to insert comparable size, attempt to insert a smaller size to splint stoma/tract open.
Pain	• May be from gastric acid irritation from gastric contents (see erythema and leakage above). May benefit from topical treatment • Granulation tissue: treatment is to remove excess tissue with silver nitrate application; can try steroid cream for 10-14 days. • External stabilizer/crossbar too tight: treat by loosening the crossbar/external stabilizer on the tube. • Cellulitis: hallmark is induration around stoma; treatment depends on severity and patient condition: oral vs. IV antibiotics. • Retained suture on surgically placed tube: treatment is to remove suture, may need to change tube. • During feeding: consider feeding intolerance or tube malposition/dislodgement. Stop feedings and notify PCP. Consult gastroenterologist. • Tube is malpositioned in the G-tube tract (space between the skin surface and stomach): assess tube position, presence of induration or discharge; may need an EGD, an air contrast radiologic study, or other radiologic studies. Consult gastroenterologist to determine studies and replace tube as indicated. • Tube has migrated (see above).

APN, advanced practice nurse; EGD, esophagogastroduodenoscopy; G-tube, gastrostomy tube; GI, gastrointestinal; PCP, primary care provider
Courtesy of Karen Troutman, BSN, RN, GI Outpatient Nurse, and Linda Tirabassi, MN, RN, Clinical Nurse Specialist, Miller Children's Hospital, Long Beach, CA.

- Instruct the family to contact the healthcare provider if the child experiences
  - Signs and symptoms of intolerance to enteral feedings
  - Tube dislodgement or malposition
  - Mechanical tube problems
  - Stoma site problems

Unexpected Situation

- *The tube accidentally comes out:* If G-tube or J-tube is less than 6 weeks old, instruct to take child and tube to nearest emergency room and report that it is a newly placed G-tube. Some organizations may instruct the family to replace with balloon-type G-tube and contact physician. Emphasize to not use this tube until a physician can assess its position. If an established stoma tract for balloon-type tube exists, replace as in procedure above.

Bibliography

Burd, A., & Burd, R. S. (2003). The long road home. The who, what, why, and how-to guide for gastrostomy tube placement in infants. *Advances in Neonatal Care, 3,* 197–205.

Crawley-Coha, T. (2004). A practical guide for the management of pediatric gastrostomy tubes based on 14 years of experience. *Journal of Wound, Ostomy & Continence Nursing, 31,* 193–200.

Goldberg, E., Kaye, R., Yaworske, J., & Liacouras, C. (2006). Gastrostomy tubes: Facts, fallacies, fistulas, and false tracts. *Gastroenterology Nursing, 28*(6), 485–494.

Guerriere, D. N., McKeever, P., Llewellyn-Thomas, H., & Berall, G. (2003). Mothers' decisions about gastrostomy tube insertion in children: Factors contributing to uncertainty. *Developmental Medicine & Child Neurology, 45,* 470–476.

Leak, K. (2002). PEG site infections: A novel use for Actisorb Silver 220. *British Journal of Community Nursing, 7,* 321–325.

Lee, A., Carter, H., & Crabbe, D. (2003). Percutaneous endoscopic gastrostomy: Procedure in practice. *British Journal of Perioperative Nursing, 13,* 298–299, 301–302, 305.

Meert, K. L., Daphtary, K. M., & Metheny, N. A. (2004). Gastric vs. small-bowel feeding in critically ill children receiving mechanical ventilation: A randomized controlled trial. *Chest, 126,* 872–878.

Williams, T. A., & Leslie, G. D. (2005a). A review of the nursing care of enteral feeding tubes in critically ill adults: Part I. *Intensive & Critical Care, 20,* 330–343.

Williams, T. A., & Leslie, G. D. (2005b). A review of the nursing care of enteral feeding tubes in critically ill adults: Part II. *Intensive & Critical Care, 21,* 5–15.

C H A P T E R

39

Enteral Tubes: Naso/Orogastric Placement and Management and Nasojejunal Management

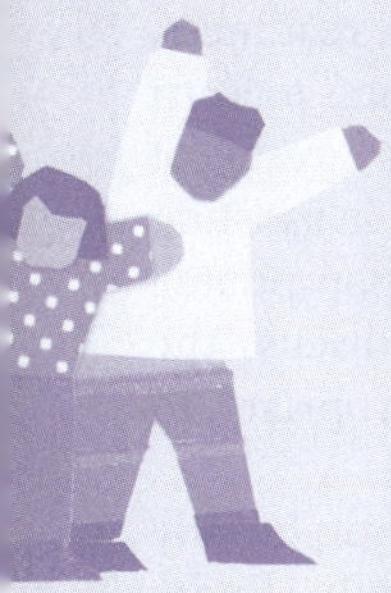

Clinical Guidelines

- A healthcare prescriber's order is required for enteral tube placement and discontinuation of the tube.
- The registered nurse (RN) or licensed practical nurse (LPN) accomplishes naso/orogastric enteral tube placement by passing a small-bore tube (which may have a weighted or non-weighted tip) through the nostril or mouth, into the oropharynx, and then through the esophagus to the stomach. Nasojejunal tubes, which originate at the nares and terminate in the jejunum, may be placed by physicians or skills-validated RNs.
- Nasogastric and orogastric enteral tube placement is used for both diagnostic and therapeutic purposes. Nasojejunal tubes are primarily used therapeutically for administration of nutrition. Enteral tubes are indicated:
  - To decompress the stomach and proximal small intestine
  - To evacuate blood, secretions, and ingested drugs or toxins
  - To control bleeding from gastric and esophageal therapies
  - To administer medications, fluids, or nutrition
  - To obtain samples of gastric contents
  - To administer lavage or irrigation
- Enteral tubes may have a single, double, or triple lumen, depending on their intended purpose (Chart 39-1).
- Intake and output through the enteral tube is monitored every hour or as determined by institutional policy or the child's condition.
- Enteral tube position and function are evaluated before use of the tube for diagnostic or therapeutic reasons.

CHART 39-1 ENTERAL TUBE NUMBER OF LUMENS

Tube Size	Purpose
Single-lumen weighted or nonweighted	Enteral or transpyloric tube feedings
Double-lumen nonweighted tube	Gastric decompression
Triple-lumen nonweighted tube	Gastric lavage

- At least once every shift, and before use for diagnostic or therapeutic reasons, the enteral tube is assessed to ensure proper position and function and the tube is patent without leaks, kinks, or occlusion.
- Enteral tube placement is changed every 3 to 7 days or as per institutional policy. Place the enteral tube in the other nostril when reinserted; this prevents necrosis of the nares tissue and ensures patency of the enteral tube. Nasojejunal tubes are not routinely changed unless the integrity of the tube is altered or occluded.
- Enteral tubes are irrigated with water as ordered by the healthcare prescriber every 4 to 6 hours to maintain patency. Some tubes may need to be flushed as often as every 2 hours.

EQUIPMENT

For Placement of the Enteral Tube

- Enteral tube of appropriate size, generally 5 to 8 French
- Topical anesthetic agent (as prescribed)
- Nonsterile gloves
- Emesis basin
- Water-soluble lubricant
- Tape or semipermeable, transparent dressing
- Cup of water with straw or ice chips (age appropriate)
- Tissues
- Towel
- Catheter-tip syringe
- pH tape
- Stethoscope
- Cup or basin of water

For Removal of the Enteral Tube

- Nonsterile gloves
- Adhesive remover (if necessary)
- Towel

CHILD AND FAMILY ASSESSMENT AND PREPARATION

- Assess child for history of nasal deformity, surgery, or trauma, which may provide information as to the patency of the nares, whether passage of the tube may be difficult or impossible, or whether tube may complicate breathing for the child.

Alert! *Nasogastric tubes are contraindicated in children with a basal skull fracture.*

- Assess the child for a history of varices or recent esophageal or gastric surgery, which may complicate placement of the enteral tube.
- Assess the child for signs and symptoms of gastric distention or irritation.
- Assess the child for presence of orthodontic appliances if tube is to be inserted through the mouth. Instruct the child to remove appliance because dislodgement during the procedure and possible aspiration may occur.
- Assess the child for a history of drug or toxin ingestion.
- Assess the child's potential for aspiration, secondary to accumulated gastric secretions and fluids or impaired gag reflex.
- Assess the child and family's cognitive level, readiness, and ability to process information. The readiness to learn and process information may be impaired as a result of age, stress, or anxiety. Explain the child's role in assisting with passage of the tube (as developmentally appropriate).
- Reinforce the need for, and identify and discuss the risks and benefits of, tube placement, as appropriate, to both the child and family.
- Explain the procedure, as age and developmentally appropriate, to both the child and the family. Invite the parents to remain with the child to provide comfort and/or diversionary measures.

PROCEDURE Placement of the Naso/Orogastric Enteral Tube

Steps	Rationale/Points of Emphasis
1. Perform hand hygiene.	Reduces transmission of microorganisms. If the child may cough and splash secretions, wear proper eye protection and a mask to provide further protection from potential droplets/secretions.

Steps	Rationale/Points of Emphasis
2. Collect all necessary equipment and supplies for tube placement. Use the smallest size small-bore feeding tube that will deliver the formula.	Promotes efficient time management and provides an organized approach to the procedure. The small diameter of the tube causes less gagging on insertion and is more comfortable once placed. The small diameter may also allow the child to continue oral intake and ingest food around the tube. This size tube is also indicated for transpyloric feedings because it must pass through the pyloric sphincter. These tubes are usually made of polyurethane or silicone and may have a weighted or nonweighted tip. If the child is likely to need gastric decompression, a larger bore tube would be indicated.
3. Position the child: • Infants/toddlers may need to be restrained in a supine position before the procedure begins, either with swaddle-type restraint or a second person securely holding the child. The older child may be placed in a sitting position for placement if the child can cooperate or if a second care provider can effectively support the child and keep him or her calm during the procedure. • If the child is in a supine position, arrange towels or pillows under the shoulders to initially slightly extend and elevate the head. • Older children may be placed in a sitting position with the head slightly extended.	Keeping the child's hands away from the tube helps prevent the child from pulling out the tube. Extending the nasal pharynx during initial tube insertion may help decrease the gag reflex. Once the catheter tip is passed distal to the pharynx, the head may be slightly flexed to anatomically direct the catheter insertion into the esophagus, enhance swallowing, and prevent passage into the trachea. **KidKare** Restraint may not be needed if the child can be effectively distracted using diversionary measures such as guided imagery and relaxation/breathing techniques.
4. Determine length of enteral tube to be inserted. Using the enteral tube, measure distance from tip of nose to the earlobe and from the earlobe to the tip of the xiphoid process and note mark on the tube, or mark the total length of tubing to be passed with a piece of tape on the tube (Figure 39-1). For weighted tubes measurement, consider where the formula ports are positioned versus the total tube length with the weight. Note the measured tube length that will remain external to assist in assessing proper tube position. 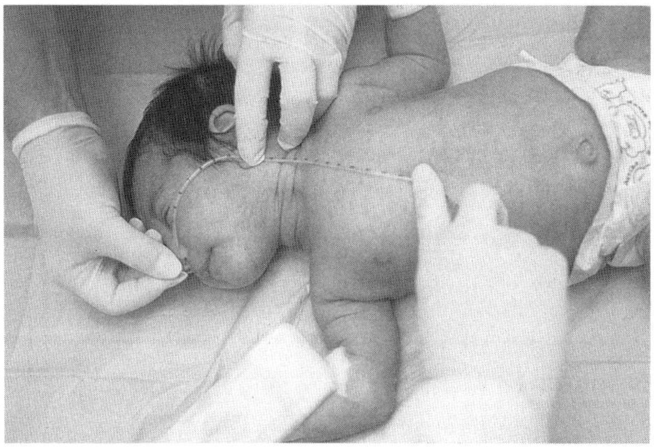 **FIGURE 39-1** To determine the length of tube to insert, measure from the tip of the patient's nose to the earlobe and from the earlobe to the tip of the xiphoid process and note mark on the tube, or mark the total length of tubing to be passed with a piece of tape on the tube.	Estimates the total length of tube to be passed.
5. Place emesis basin and tissues within easy access.	Allows for easier use, if needed during procedure.
6. Place towel over child's gown.	Protects clothing from emesis or secretions.

Continued

Steps	Rationale/Points of Emphasis
7. Don gloves.	Standard precaution to reduce transmission of microorganisms. If the child may cough and splash secretions, wear proper eye protection and a mask to provide further protection from potential droplets/secretions.
8. Many small-bore feeding tubes have a water-activated lubricant impregnated into the tube material. Dip the distal tip of the tube in water to activate the lubricant. The tube will feel slippery. If a water-activated lubricant is not a characteristic of the tube, lubricate the distal tip of the tube liberally with water-soluble lubricant. If a stylet is present, check that the stylet moves freely.	Reduces friction and prevents trauma to the area. If aspirated, water-soluble lubricant will not lead to pneumonia.
9. Gently insert tube into nostril or mouth, aiming down and back.	Aids enteral tube to follow the normal nasopharyngeal anatomy.
10. When enteral tube reaches the pharynx and the child gags, ask child to swallow or stimulate the swallow in the infant with a pacifier.	Swallowing promotes esophageal peristalsis, which facilitates passage of the enteral tube.
11. Allow the child to rest and resume insertion procedure.	Allows child to gain control of self again and allows the older child to be able to assist with procedure.
12. Continue to pass enteral tube until measured segment of tube is at the nares opening. Do not pass the enteral tube beyond the original mark until further assessment is made.	Advances enteral tube into the stomach. Inserting the enteral tube too far may result in looping the enteral tube in the stomach, causing ineffective drainage, kinking, or, in advancing the enteral tube into the duodenum, excessive removal of bile. Signs of respiratory distress indicate the enteral tube is in the respiratory tree. **Alert!** ***Remove enteral tube at once if there are signs of distress, coughing, gasping, or cyanosis.***
13. If an enteral tube with a stylet has been used, remove the stylet at this time. **caREminder** *Never reinsert the stylet into the enteral tube once the stylet has been removed.*	Reinsertion has the potential for puncturing the tube, resulting in perforation of the GI tract.
14. Temporarily secure tube to avoid accidental dislodgement until placement is verified using the "Verifying Enteral Tube Placement" procedure below.	Minimizes medical trauma by stabilizing tube while tube position can be properly verified.

PROCEDURE Verifying Enteral Tube Placement

Steps	Rationale/Points of Emphasis
1. Perform hand hygiene and don gloves, if not already on from placement of enteral tube.	Standard precaution to reduce transmission of microorganisms.
2. Check for proper tube placement: • For orogastric/nasogastric tubes, use a syringe to aspirate stomach contents, assess the characteristics of aspirate, and test acidity by pH tape (Table 39-1). Confirm that the external length of the tube is at baseline measurement. If unable to confirm placement after above steps, request order for abdominal x-ray. • For nasojejunal tubes, confirm placement by x-ray. Once placement is confirmed, measure the external length of the tube and mark it to have comparative measurements with baseline for further tube position confirmation.	Failure to obtain aspirate from an orogastric/nasogastric tube does not indicate that the enteral tube is placed improperly. There may be marginal stomach contents to aspirate, or the catheter may not be in contact with the gastric fluid. A pH level of 5 or less suggests gastric placement. A pH level of >5 may indicate respiratory, esophageal, or intestinal placement or may be present if the child is receiving acid suppression medications or continuous feedings. X-ray of the abdomen to verify placement is the most accurate verification method and may be indicated before instituting use of the enteral tube.

Steps	Rationale/Points of Emphasis
Alert! Tube placement errors are more likely to occur in the presence of an endotracheal tube, tracheostomy, or craniofacial trauma and in children who are uncooperative during insertion, disoriented, unconscious, or heavily sedated or have depressed gag and cough reflexes. Retching and vomiting may put the child at risk for displacement.	
3. After confirmation of proper tube placement, anchor the enteral tube to the child's face with tape or transparent dressing avoiding interference with the child's visual field, causing pressure, or irritating the nasal mucosa.	Maintains position of enteral tube to minimize potential for tube migration. Avoids skin breakdown from pressure of tube.
4. Connect or clamp the primary lumen, as prescribed (e.g., to suction, gravity drainage, enteral tube feeding).	Initiates therapy as prescribed.
5. Follow restraint policy, as necessary, to maintain position of enteral tube.	Provides for patient safety to protect from enteral tube dislodgment.
6. Dispose of equipment and waste in appropriate receptacle. Remove gloves and perform hand hygiene.	Standard precautions. Reduces transmission of microorganisms.

TABLE 39-1

Confirmation of Naso/Orogastric Tube Placement

Aspirate Location	Aspirate Characteristics	pH
Gastric	Clear, off white, grassy green, tan, brown-tinged if blood present	<5
Intestinal	Bile stained, light to dark golden-yellow or brownish green	>6
Pulmonary tracheobronchial	Watery, straw-colored mucus	>6

PROCEDURE Use of the Enteral Tube for Feedings, Medications, or pH Studies

Steps	Rationale/Points of Emphasis
Refer to Chapter 42: *Feeding, Enteral* Chapter 63: *Medication Administration: Enteral* Chapter 89: *pH Study*	Safe use of the enteral tube for diagnostic or therapeutic reasons should follow standard guidelines.

PROCEDURE Removal of the Enteral Tube

Steps	Rationale/Points of Emphasis
1. Perform hand hygiene and don gloves.	Standard precaution to reduce transmission of microorganisms.
2. Place towel over child's gown.	Protects clothing from emesis or secretions.
3. Position child in comfortable supine position with head of bed elevated or in sitting position. Ensure that the child is being held securely if there is a risk that he or she will resist the enteral tube removal.	Keeping the child's hands away from the tube helps prevent the child from pulling out the tube.

Continued

Steps	Rationale/Points of Emphasis
4. Remove tape or semipermeable transparent dressing. Use adhesive remover as needed to assist in tape removal and to provide patient comfort. **caREminder** *For neonates, remove adhesives with warm water and cotton balls; mineral oil or an emollient may also facilitate adhesive removal if reapplication of adhesives at the site of removal is not necessary.* **Alert!** ***Rapid removal of adhesive tape may cause damage to the skin of a neonate.***	Tape and dressings must be removed first to allow ease of tube removal.
5. Instruct the older child to breathe slowly through the mouth.	Provides a distraction that may help the child relax and prevents breath holding.
6. Kink the tube on itself and close the feeding and medication port. With a somewhat slow, smooth, steady movement pull the tube out of the nares or mouth.	Provides patient safety by preventing potential aspiration from leakage of residual formula/GI secretions in tube as tube is removed.
7. Remove towel and tube from the child's bed. Dispose of used equipment and waste in appropriate receptacle. If the tube is to be reused, irrigate the tube with water and cleanse the outside of the tube with soap and water. Dry reusable tube and place in secure location.	Standard precautions. Enteral tubes may be reused for another feeding. Enteral tubes with a water-activated lubricant should be replaced when the lubricant is not able to be effectively activated by water.
8. Remove gloves and perform hand hygiene.	Reduces transmission of microorganisms.

CHILD AND FAMILY EVALUATION AND DOCUMENTATION

- While tube is in place:
  - Verify tube placement and patency.
  - Evaluate integrity of skin around nares, areas where tape is placed, and of mucous membranes. Monitor intake and output as indicated.
  - Assess for signs of respiratory distress, especially in infants under the age of approximately 2 to 3 months who are obligate nose breathers and have varying ability to breath through their mouth.
  - Provide comfort measures as indicated.
- After insertion of the enteral tube, document the following:
  - Date and time of insertion
  - Size/length of enteral tube used
  - Origin of insertion site and verification of location
  - Verification method
  - Comfort/distraction and/or restraints used during placement
  - Child's tolerance of the procedure
- After removal of the enteral tube, document the following:
  - Date and time of removal
  - Comfort/distraction or restraints used during removal
  - Child's tolerance of the procedure
- While the enteral tube is in place, document the following:
  - Intake and output
  - Method of tube confirmation and patency (e.g., system is intact, without leaks, kinks, or occlusions) before each use
  - Tolerance to therapeutic interventions
  - Changes in the enteral tube placement
  - Flushing/irrigation volumes with sterile water to maintain patency and frequency
  - Condition of the skin around the nares, mouth, and cheek where the tube is secured
- Comfort measures:
  - Change tape as required; consider using skin barrier to protect skin surface from the irritating effects of tape.
  - Administer frequent oral care; offer throat spray for comfort or ice chips, unless contraindicated per diet orders.
- Determine whether the child and family have other areas of concern to discuss.

COMMUNITY CARE

- Enteral tube placement may be done in the child's home for feeding therapies or hospice care; if so, instruct the family how to perform the following:
  - Insert the enteral tube.
  - Verify placement of the enteral tube.
  - Secure the tube.

- Assess for signs and symptoms of respiratory distress (e.g., cyanosis, tachycardia, tachypnea, nasal flaring, retractions, expiratory grunting, wheezing, prolonged coughing, choking). Instruct family to stop insertion of tube or feeding if these signs or symptoms occur.
- Flush/irrigate the enteral tube.
- Administer medications and/or feedings via the enteral tube.
- Provide comfort measures for the child.
- Inspect nares for discharge and irritation and methods to avoid or address these effects:
  - Clean nares and enteral tube with cotton-tipped applicator moistened in water.
  - Apply a water-soluble lubricant to the nares if dry.
- Change skin barrier and/or tape.
- Provide oral care.
- Obtain order for local throat spray or ice/chips (as indicated).

- Instruct the family to contact the healthcare provider if
  - Child develops signs or symptoms of respiratory distress
  - Parents meet resistance in trying to insert and remove the enteral tube
  - Child experiences vomiting while tube in place
  - Child develops skin breakdown due to tube placement and use of tape or other dressings

Unexpected Situations

- *While inserting the enteral tube there appears to be an obstruction:* Do not use force. Try rotating the enteral tube while gently attempting to advance it. If still unable to pass the enteral tube, remove it and try the other nostril. Visually assess the mouth to see if the tube has coiled in the oral cavity.
- *While removing the enteral tube, resistance is encountered:* Rotate the tube and again attempt removal. Forcing an enteral tube to be removed may cause damage to the stomach or esophagus. If resistance continues to be met, stop procedure; location of the tube may need to be verified using x-ray.

Bibliography

Eisenberg, P. G. (1994). Nasoenteral tubes. *RN, 57*, 62–66, 68–70.

Ellett, M. L. C., Beckstrand, J., Flueckiger, J., Perkins, S. M., & Johnson, C. S. (2005). Predicting the insertion distance for placing gastric tubes. *Clinical Nursing Research, 14*, 11–31.

Gharpure, V., Meert, K. L., Sarnaik, A. P., & Metheny, N. A. (2000). Indicators of postpyloric feeding tube placement in children. *Critical Care Medicine, 28*, 2962–2966.

Hawes, J., McEwan, P., & McGuire, W. (2005). Nasal versus oral route for placing feeding tubes in preterm or low birth weight infants. *The Cochrane Database of Systematic Reviews*, (2), No. CD003952.

Huffman, S., Jarczyk, K. S., O'Brien, E., Pieper, P., & Bayne, A. (2004). Methods to confirm feeding tube placement: Application of research in practice. *Pediatric Nursing, 30*, 10–13.

Metheny, N., Eikov, R., Rountree, V., & Lengettie, E. (1999). Indicators of feeding-tube placement in neonates. *Nutrition in Clinical Practice, 14*, 307–314.

Metheny, N. A., & Meert, K. L. (2004). Monitoring feeding tube placement. *Nutrition in Clinical Practice, 19*, 487–495, 542.

Metheny, N. A., & Titler, M. G. (2001). Assessing placement of feeding tubes. *American Journal of Nursing, 101*(5), 36–45.

Nyqvist, K. H., Sorell, A., & Ewald, U. (2005). Litmus tests for verification of feeding tube location in infants: Evaluation of their clinical use. *Journal of Clinical Nursing, 14*, 486–495.

Phang, J. S., Marsh, W. A., Barlows, T. G., & Schwartz, H. I. (2004). Determining feeding tube location by gastric and intestinal pH values. *Nutrition in Clinical Practice, 19*, 640–644.

Tedeschi, L., Altimier, L., & Warner, B. (2004). Improving the accuracy of indwelling gastric feeding tube placement in the neonatal population. *Neonatal Intensive Care, 17*, 16–18.

Westhus, N. (2004). Methods to test feeding tube placement in children. *MCN: The American Journal of Maternal/Child Nursing, 29*, 282–287, 290–291.

CHAPTER

40

Exchange Transfusions

CLINICAL GUIDELINES

- A physician, nurse practitioner, or physician's assistant performs this procedure in accordance with state practice guidelines.
- A registered nurse (RN) assists the healthcare prescriber in the procedure of exchange transfusion.
- Informed consent to complete the procedure must be obtained.
- Exchange transfusion involves substituting donor red blood cells for recipient red blood cells. During exchange transfusion, small quantities of the recipient's blood are alternately removed and replaced with donor blood until the desired volume of blood has been exchanged. Exchange transfusions may be prescribed:
  - When the increased blood volume from a simple transfusion might not be tolerated (e.g., newborn at risk for fluid overload, child with severe anemia at risk for congestive heart failure)
  - To decrease the quantity of an abnormal element in the blood or to remove an excessive amount of a normal component (e.g., sickle cell crisis, polycythemia, hyperbilirubinemia)
- The infant/child undergoing an exchange transfusion is monitored in the intensive care unit with cardiopulmonary monitoring, pulse oximetry, and blood pressure monitoring.
- Clinical guidelines for blood product administration (see Chapter 20) must be maintained, including procedures for verifying prescriber's order, verifying blood product once delivered to the bedside, and reviewing patient history for transfusion reaction.

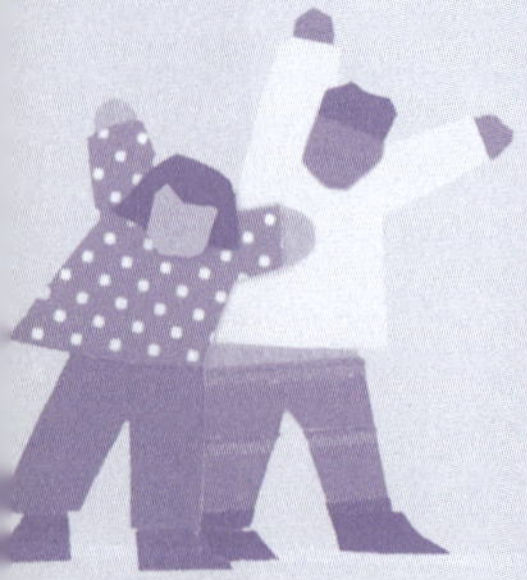

EQUIPMENT

- Open bed with radiant heat source (for infant), bed in ICU (for child)
- Cardiopulmonary monitor
- Pulse oximeter
- Noninvasive blood pressure monitor
- Soft restraints
- Freshly washed, cytomegalovirus-negative, irradiated whole blood
- Blood warmer with appropriate tubing
- Blood administration set
- Sterile gown
- Sterile gloves
- Mask/head cover
- Exchange transfusion tray with form
- Pretransfusion laboratory results
- Blood glucose monitoring equipment

- Laboratory specimen tubes with labels
- Umbilical catheterization tray (if large-bore catheter not already in place)
- Code cart, including age-appropriate code medications
- Sterile towels/drapes

CHILD AND FAMILY ASSESSMENT AND PREPARATION

- The individual performing the procedure explains the procedure to the parents, answering questions as necessary.
- Assess the parents' understanding of the procedure and reinforce information, as needed.
- Verify that informed consent for procedure and any state-mandated requirements for blood administration have been obtained.
- Verify orders with the blood bank for time frame for obtaining packed red blood cells.
- Obtain preprocedural laboratory tests, as ordered.
- Assess the child's history for clinical indications of need for exchange transfusion, history of previous transfusions, and relevant laboratory data (e.g., bilirubin levels in neonate).
- Ensure that all emergency equipment is in place and functioning. Code drug dosages should be calculated and posted for provision of immediate resuscitation, if necessary.
- Ensure that infant/child has been NPO for 3–4 hours before procedure to prevent aspiration of stomach contents during procedure.
- Verify intravenous fluid orders with healthcare prescriber and ensure separate IV access for fluid/dextrose maintenance and glucose and medications.

caREminder

Large-bore intravenous tubing and a large blood vessel is necessary to aspirate and inject increments of blood and to minimize damage to red blood cells.

PROCEDURE Administering Exchange Transfusions

Steps	Rationale/Points of Emphasis
1. Perform hand hygiene.	Reduces transmission of microorganisms.
2. Gather the necessary supplies.	Promotes efficient time management and provides an organized approach to the procedure.
3. Place infant supine on radiant warmer in servo-control mode, or place child supine in bed, attach cardiopulmonary monitor and pulse oximeter and apply noninvasive blood pressure monitor with set time intervals of 3 minutes. For the infant, secure arms/legs for procedure.	Prevents hypothermia that can result in apnea, increased caloric and oxygen requirement, acidosis, and stress. The warmer allows for easier access to infant. Monitoring provides for ongoing assessment of the infant. Securing of extremities prevents contamination of sterile field and dislodgment of catheter as the young infant moves.
4. Check blood products with two licensed personnel (e.g., two RNs, RN/MD) verifying crossmatch and child's identification (see Chapter 20).	Ensures proper identification and crossmatching.
5. Set up blood tubing and blood warmer as per package and manufacturer's direction. Prime tubing. Temperature of blood should not exceed 98.6°F (37.0°C).	Ensures appropriate use of equipment.
6. Assist healthcare prescriber with sterile gown and gloves as necessary. All personnel in the area must wear a mask. Open sterile towel on bedside stand to establish sterile working area for healthcare prescriber.	Minimizes contamination of area. Reduces transmission of microorganisms.
7. Open exchange transfusion tray; remove transfusion record form. Document pretransfusion vital signs and laboratory results.	Provides baseline data.
8. Connect tubing from exchange transfusion tray: a. Attach blood warmer tubing to side port of stopcock. b. Attach second extension tubing to top port of stopcock and place other end in blood discard bag. c. The healthcare prescriber will connect the stopcock to the child's IV access site. d. Release roller clamp.	Decreases chance of dislodgment and therefore contamination of personnel. The waste blood container should be below table level to allow gravity to assist with the drainage.

Steps	Rationale/Points of Emphasis
9. Monitor vital signs closely during procedure every 15 minutes. Document temperature, pulse, respiration, blood pressure, oxygen saturation, and blood aliquots in and out, maintaining ongoing total balance.	Ensures prompt detection of vital sign instability, which may occur because of too large an infusion or rapid speed of withdrawal; ensures detection of heart failure due to fluid depletion or overload (Chart 40-1).
10. The healthcare prescriber is responsible for performing aspirations/injections of blood aliquots, maintaining aseptic technique. a. Open stopcock to the child and withdraw desired amount of blood, continue monitoring infant/child, and record "blood out" amount. b. Assess vital signs to determine infant/child's tolerance to and amount and rate of blood withdrawal. c. Rotate stopcock to waste/discard tubing; expel contents of syringe. d. Rotate stopcock to warm blood tubing; fill with same increment as withdrawal amount. e. Rotate stopcock to child, infuse blood into child, and record "blood in" amount.	Equal amounts of blood in and blood discarded aid in maintaining homeostasis. This process completes one cycle of the exchange process.
11. Repeat step 10 as needed. Perform procedure over 1 to 4 hours.	
12. Obtain laboratory work during procedure as ordered; monitor blood glucose every 15 minutes or as ordered or if there are signs of hypoglycemia. **Alert!** *Citrate (as a preservative in the blood product) binds calcium and magnesium, resulting in decreased ionized calcium, which can lead to hypocalcemia.*	Continual monitoring is needed due to effects of anticoagulants and other additives used in the blood products (see Chart 40-1).
13. During procedure, gently invert blood bag every 15 minutes.	Keeps cells and plasma mixed.
14. Assist to obtain postprocedural laboratory tests as ordered.	Validates the effectiveness of the exchange as well as the need for any adjustment of fluids.
15. Upon completion of procedure, clamp blood tubing and disconnect from catheter. Flush intravenous line with normal saline and reconnect the ordered intravenous solution.	Maintains the line patency.
16. Dispose of equipment and waste in appropriate receptacle. Remove gloves and perform hand hygiene.	Standard precautions. Reduces transmission of microorganisms.

CHART 40-1 ADVERSE EVENTS ASSOCIATED WITH EXCHANGE TRANSFUSION*

Thrombocytopenia	Hypertension
Hypocalcemia	Respiratory distress
Metabolic acidosis	Vessel thrombus
Hypoglycemia	Seizures
Catheter malfunction	Sepsis
Apnea	Renal failure
Bradycardia	Omphalitis (neonate)
Hypotension	Necrotizing enterocolitis (neonate)

*These complications have been noted to occur within 7 days of a transfusion.

CHILD AND FAMILY EVALUATION AND DOCUMENTATION

- Evaluate vital signs every 15 minutes times 4 and then continue until infant/child returns to pretransfusion baseline vital signs to provide prompt detection of hemodynamic instability.
- Monitor glucose for the first 2 hours posttransfusion. Feedings can be attempted 2 to 4 hours after exchange transfusion.

Alert! ***Hypothermia and hypoglycemia are common adverse effects of an exchange transfusion.***

- Monitor laboratory values for complications of exchange transfusion and verification of effectiveness of therapy (e.g., bilirubin levels).
- Document the following:
  - Who performed the procedure
  - Time procedure started and finished
  - Infant/child's status before, during, and after procedure
- Complete institutional blood bank documentation, including time and amount of blood in and out.

caREminder

The exchange transfusion record becomes a permanent portion of the patient chart.

COMMUNITY CARE

- Ensure that parents have a record of the child's blood type for their home medical records.
- Instruct the family to contact the healthcare provider if
  - Infant/child shows signs of bruising or bleeding
  - Infant shows signs of delayed transfusion reaction, such as infection (jaundice, fever) or anemia

Unexpected Situation

- *During the procedure the infant's temperature decreases below 97.2°F (36.2°C):* Institute warming measures such as increasing the temperature of the radiant warmer or isolette. Ensure the blood being administered is warm.

Bibliography

American Academy of Pediatrics. (2004). Management of hyperbilirubinemia in the newborn infant 35 or more weeks of gestation. *Pediatrics, 114*, 297–316.

Ballas, S. (2002). Sickle cell anaemia: Progress in pathogenesis and treatment. *Drugs, 62*, 1143–1172.

Dennery, P. A., Seidman, D. S., & Stevenson, D. K. (2001). Neonatal hyperbilirubinemia. *New England Journal of Medicine, 344*, 581–590.

Lowe, E., & Werner, E. (2005). Thrombotic thrombocytopenic purpura and hemolytic uremic syndrome in children and adolescents. *Seminars in Thrombosis & Hemostasis. Thrombotic Thrombocytopenic Purpura-2005, 31*, 717–730.

Murray, N., & Roberts, I. (2004). Neonatal transfusion practice. *Archives of Disease in Childhood Fetal & Neonatal Edition, 89*(2), 101–107.

Patra, K., Storfer-Isser, A., Siner, B., Moore, J., & Hack, M. (2004). Adverse events associated with neonatal exchange transfusion in the 1990s. *Journal of Pediatrics, 144*, 626–631.

Porter, M. L., & Dennis, B. L. (2002). Hyperbilirubinemia in the term newborn. *American Family Physician, 65*, 599–606, 613–614.

CHAPTER 41

Fall Prevention

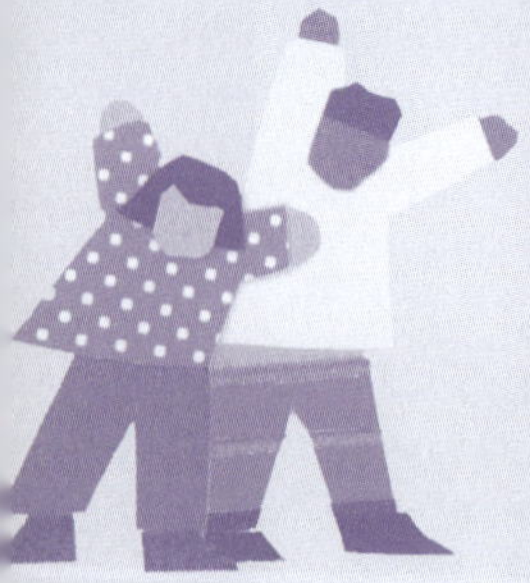

Clinical Guidelines

- Fall prevention measures are to be implemented by all healthcare providers, staff, and volunteers within the institution.
- A fall risk assessment will be completed on each child older than 8 months admitted to the institution. This assessment will be completed by a registered nurse (RN). All children less than 8 months of age are exempt.
- Reassessment of fall risk is completed when the child's condition changes, the child is moved to another level of care, or medications are ordered that may increase the risk for falling.
- *Falls* are defined as a patient on the floor secondary to an unplanned or unintended occurrence. *Developmental falls* are those occurring secondary to a child's developmental stage or age.
- Falls may be caused by:
  - An unsafe environment (crowded hallways and rooms)
  - Response to a medication (diuretics, anesthesia, analgesics, sedatives, etc.)
  - Developmental factors (toddlers learning to walk, running and playing in the hallways or playrooms)
  - Child's health status (cerebral palsy, muscular disorders, neurologic disorders)
  - Orthopedic diagnosis (fractures with/without casts, splints, external fixators)
  - Medical devices (IVs, nasogastric tubes, chest tubes, etc.)
- A fall prevention plan will include:
  - Providing a clean and safe environment (see Chapter 103)
  - Identifying children at risk for falls
  - Nonpunitive reporting of the circumstances of patient falls
  - Education and reeducation of staff
  - Implementation of a fall intervention strategy, flexible enough to meet individual needs

Equipment

- Fall risk assessment tool
- Fall reporting and documentation

Child and Family Assessment and Preparation

- Assess child's health history, age, height, weight, review of systems, physical examination, baseline laboratory values, presence of orthopedic devices or the need for such devices, and current home medications (Chart 41-1).
- Assess child's response to anesthesia, analgesics, and sedatives or diuretics if applicable.
- Assess child's developmental stage/age, noting acquisition of milestones that may impact incidence of falls (e.g., ability to crawl, walk).

CHART 41-1 FALL ASSESSMENT RISK FACTORS

Neurologic impairment
Seizures
Use of assistive devices
Ambulation with IV pole and/or oxygen
Impaired mobility or sensory deficit
History of falls during previous hospitalization
Administration of any of the following:
- Diphenhydramine
- Hydroxyzine
- Narcotic analgesics (e.g., acetaminophen with codeine, morphine, oxycodone)
- Benzodiazepine agents (e.g., alprazolam, clonazepam, clorazepate, lorazepam, etc.)
- Vinca alkaloid agent (e.g., vinblastine, vincristine, vinorelbine)

caREminder

Falls by toddlers and infants learning to walk are an expected occurrence and are not usually reported unless the child incurs an injury.

- Assess the child and family's understanding about medication uses and side effects and the affect they may have on the child's ability to ambulate safely.
- Assess the child and family's understanding regarding the orthopedic diagnosis and/or device and the affect it may have on the child's mobility.
- Assess the child's ability to ambulate with orthopedic devices and need for ongoing assistance and training, if applicable.
- Ensure child is oriented to unit environment. Falls can occur due to unfamiliarity with environment.

PROCEDURE Environmental Safety

Steps	Rationale/Points of Emphasis
1. Clear hallways and rooms of all unused equipment and unneeded furniture.	Uncluttered rooms and hallways reduce the risk of falls.
2. Clearly mark wet floors with signs until floor is dry. Whenever possible, clean one side of the hallway, leaving room for patients and families to safely walk on dry part of floor.	Clearly marked wet floors help reduce the risk of falls by alerting patients and families of the floor's condition.
3. Ensure that the patient has the proper footwear when ambulating. Shoes and/or socks with a rubberized sole should be worn.	Shoes with a slick sole (e.g., dress shoes) and socks without a rubberized sole are more likely to slip on hospital floors, thus increasing the risk for falls.
4. Ensure side rails are in a locked and in highest upright position when infant or child is in crib or bed. Ensure bed is maintained in lowest possible position (see Chapter 15).	Aids in prevention of falls from crib or bed.

PROCEDURE Personal Safety

Steps	Rationale/Points of Emphasis
1. Complete fall risk assessment tool on any child suspected to be at risk for falls.	Tools for use in the adult population such as the Morse scale are not published, valid, and reliable tools for the pediatric population at this time. There are at least two tools for pediatric patients that are currently awaiting publication. Neither tool has been tested for validity and reliability as of the date of this publication, but it is anticipated that they will be in the near future (Figure 41-1). Caution should be used when using a tool that has not been tested for validity and reliability. Tools that are based on sound research techniques must still be tested to be sure the tool is accurately measuring what it was developed to measure. If in doubt about the reliability and validity of any tool you may choose to use, contact the author of the tool and request confirmation of validity and reliability testing.

Steps	Rationale/Points of Emphasis

Date/Time: ____________________

Deficit	Evaluation	Score
1. **History of falls:** within 3 months	No = 0 Yes = 3	
2. **Physical alterations/Impairment:** surgery within admission, underlying medical conditions (seizure, history of vertigo or syncope, Guillain-Barré syndrome, multiple sclerosis, alteration in visual acuity)	No = 0 Yes = 3	
3. **Functional status:** altered mobility, gait/transferring problems, significant metabolic disturbances (hypotension, hypoxia, hypovolemia), use of ambulatory aids	None = 0 Weak = 1 Impaired or age specific (learning to walk) = 2 Crutches, walker, brace, orthostatic hypotension = 3	
4. **Equipment:** IV/Heparin lock, IV pole, or Foley catheter	No = 0 Yes = 2	
5. **Cognitive/Psychological:** impaired mental status, developmental delay, biobehavioral concerns (ADHD, depression, oppositional defiant behavior)	Oriented to own ability = 0 Neuro limitations due to illness or biobehavioral concerns = 2	
6. **Medications that alter equilibrium:** narcotics, anticonvulsives, antipsychotics, sedatives, chemotherapy, or hypotensive meds	No = 0 Yes = 3	
		Total =

Risk Level	PFAS Score	Action
No Risk	0	None
Low Risk	1–7	Use treaded socks. Teach parents/family to raise side rails or close isolettes when away from patient side. Implement frequent toileting and monitoring by staff, and clear patient environment of hazards/obstacles.
High Risk	8	All of the above plus apply orange "fall potential" band on same limb as name band, and family or staff to accompany patient with ambulation.

FIGURE 41-1
Pediatric fall risk tool. Used with permission of Phoenix Children's Hospital.

Steps	Rationale/Points of Emphasis
2. Assess patient for unsteadiness, dizziness, and so on whenever patient gets up for the first time after administration of anesthesia, analgesics, sedatives, or any other medication that might interfere with the patient's ability to stand or ambulate. Document findings on fall risk assessment tool.	Assessing the patient's response to the medication and assisting patient after the first dose and subsequent doses if necessary will reduce the risk of falls.
3. Obtain orders for physical therapy for anyone with a new orthopedic device, for help with ambulation, or for getting a patient out of bed after a long period of bedrest.	Specially trained team members can reduce the risk of falls by teaching and using correct techniques when assisting patients with special needs.

PROCEDURE Education

Steps	Rationale/Points of Emphasis
1. Educate child and family about fall prevention. a. Proper footwear (shoes or socks with rubberized soles) b. Parental involvement in care as applicable: • Assisting patient in and out of bed • Assisting patient to the bathroom • Assisting with ambulation • Side rails up on cribs when unattended by an adult • Notifying staff of unsafe environmental issues (wet floors, crowded rooms)	Ensures child and family are aware of measures to reduce falls. Parental presence helps prevent falls.
2. Ongoing training and vigilance by staff members to ensure a safe environment and fall prevention.	The Joint Commission on Accreditation of Healthcare Organization (JCAHO) 2006 National Safety Goals are to reduce the risk of patient harm resulting from falls and to have institutions implement a fall reduction program and evaluate the effectiveness of the program. Vigilance and training will reduce the risk of patient falls by ensuring that staff members and family are aware of the ongoing risk of falls in the hospital arena and that such falls can be prevented by using patient safety measures.

CHILD AND FAMILY EVALUATION AND DOCUMENTATION

- Evaluate the child's response to the medication (if applicable).
- Evaluate the child's response to orthopedic devices (if applicable).
- Evaluate the family's cooperation with plan of care and safety rules (e.g., crib rails must be up when child is unattended).
- Assess the child for injury with any fall.
- Document the following on all children:
  - Family presence and involvement in patient care
  - Family cooperation with safety issues
  - Child's response to medication (if applicable)
  - Child's ability to use the orthopedic device correctly (if applicable)
  - Patient's and family's understanding of education
- Document the following if a fall occurs:
  - Date and time of fall
  - How the fall occurred
  - Cause of fall (if applicable)
  - Who found the patient
  - Evidence of injury (level of consciousness, vital signs, pain, etc.)
  - Time doctor was called
  - Care given in response to fall (x-rays, surgery, sutures, dressings, etc.)
  - Who was with the patient at time of fall
  - Time family notified (if not with patient)

COMMUNITY CARE

- Encourage family presence while child is in the hospital.
- Encourage family involvement in all aspects of patient care.
- Empower patients and families to report unsafe environments and situations.
- Instruct the family to contact the healthcare provider if
  - A fall was sustained and the child continues to have ongoing pain or physical limitations related to the fall
  - The child has difficulty standing or ambulating after taking a medication
  - The child has difficulty standing or ambulating when these are developmental milestones that have been previously achieved

Unexpected Situations

- *A 13-year-old boy was admitted with a femur fracture and went to surgery immediately for placement of rods to repair the femur. He has to be non–weight-bearing on that leg for 12 weeks. Shortly after returning from postoperative recovery, while mom is down in the cafeteria for lunch, the patient has to go to the bathroom, but can't find the call light and can't wait any longer. He gets out of bed and subsequently is found on the floor crying:* Frequent monitoring of this child who is recovering from an anesthetic agent and who has a parent out of the room is warranted. Immediately check the child for injury. Assist the child back to bed. The call light should be within the reach of the patient and should be answered as quickly as possible. The urinal should be placed with in reach. Determine whether the child was instructed not to get out of bed and if he understood the instructions. Determine whether the mom let the staff know she would be out of the room, and ensure that such communication takes place in the future.

- *A 2-year-old girl is celebrating her birthday with her family in the play room. Upon opening a box containing a new pair of black patent leather shoes with big bows, she immediately puts them on and goes running out of the play room to show her favorite nurse her special new shoes. The housekeeper has just finished mopping the floor in front of the nurses' station and has placed a big yellow sign appropriately. Suddenly, the birthday girl is sitting on the floor:* Unless there is a way to keep this little girl's enthusiasm under control, there really is no way to prevent this fall. Perhaps a family member could have been holding her hand and walking her to the nurses' station. Determine whether the environment was unsafe. (The housekeeper placed the sign as she should, but a 2-year-old most likely can't read this sign.) Determine whether this is classified as a developmental fall. What was the girl's developmental stage? Was she stable on her feet? Did she need any assistance with mobility before this time? Determine whether this was a reportable fall. Was it a developmental issue? If so, did she injure herself? If it was not a developmental issue, then it should be reported.

Bibliography

Cummings, R. (2005). *Cummings pediatric fall assessment scale.* Unpublished scale. © Phoenix Children's Hospital, Phoenix, Arizona.

Graf, E. (2004). *Identifying predictor variables associated wit pediatric in-patient fall risk assessments.* Unpublished manuscript. © Children's Memorial Medical Center, Chicago, Illinois.

Graf, E. (2005). *General risk assessment for pediatric in-patient falls (GRAF PIF scale, 5 day version).* Unpublished scale. © Children's Memorial Medical Center, Chicago, Illinois.

Miranda, L. (2000). *Miami Children's Hospital patient falls indicator.* Miami, FL: Miami Children's Hospital.

Myers, H., & Nikoletti, S. (2003). Fall risk assessment: A prospective investigation of nurses' clinical judgment and risk assessment tools in prediction of falls. *International Journal of Nursing Practice, 9*(3), 158–165.

Sedman, A., Harris, J., Schulz, K., et al. (2005). Relevance of the Agency for Healthcare Research and Quality patient safety indicators for children's hospitals. *Pediatrics, 115*, 135–145.

CHAPTER 42

Feeding, Enteral

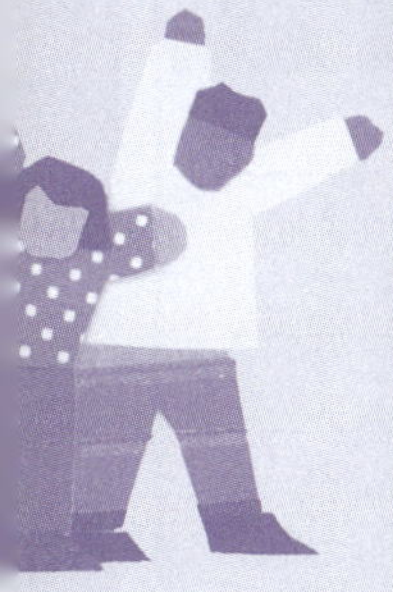

Clinical Guidelines

- Enteral feeding may be administered by a registered nurse (RN), licensed practical nurse (LPN), physician, or appropriately trained child or parent.
- A healthcare prescriber must order enteral tube feeding.
- Enteral feedings may be given by a number of routes, including nasogastric or orogastric tube placement, gastrostomy tube, PEG, skin-level G-tube devices (e.g., MIC-Key, BARD button), jejunal tube, or transpyloric tubes (G-J tube, skin-level G-J tube).
- Enteral feedings are indicated for children who are unable to ingest an adequate amount of nutrition orally. This may include children who are unconscious, ventilated, transitioning from parenteral nutrition, are unable to swallow, or have primary aspiration.
- Children who are comatose, are neurologically delayed, or otherwise have a decreased cough and gag reflex are at increased risk for aspiration with tube feedings and should therefore receive feedings that are transpyloric.
- The child receiving enteral nutrition must have a functioning gastrointestinal tract (e.g., audible bowel sounds and occurring peristalsis) for nutrition to be digested and absorbed.
- Feedings provided by way of the gastrointestinal tract promote gut barrier structure and function, are more cost effective than parenteral nutrition, provide the child with a much lower risk for complications (e.g., catheter sepsis, thrombophlebitis), and prevent the development or worsening of malnutrition.
- The most common method of enteral feeding delivery for children is an enteral feeding pump, which controls delivery. Feedings may be intermittent, also called a bolus, or by continuous drip or a combination of delivery methods that best meet the needs of the infant or child.
- Because jejunostomy tube placement is in the small intestine, high-osmolality formulas may not be tolerated well if they are given in bolus form; therefore, jejunostomy tube feedings should be administered through a continuous feeding via an enteral pump.
- Numerous commercially made formulas are available and are prepared to meet a variety of the child's needs, including nutritional and calorie requirements in relation to disease states.
- Children may require additional free water to be delivered through the feeding tube to prevent dehydration and a hyperosmolar state. However, some conditions place children at risk for fluid overload due to their underlying diagnosis and age.
- Placement of the enteral tube must be confirmed before administration of tube feedings. Most institutions require that tube placement be confirmed by x-ray to prevent aspiration.

EQUIPMENT

For intermittent or bolus feeds:

- Enteral tube (see Chapters 38 and 39)
- Towel or washcloth
- Nonsterile gloves
- 60-mL catheter-tip syringe
- Prescribed enteral formula
- Clean graduated measuring cup
- Stethoscope
- Pacifier (optional)

For continuous drip feeds:

- Enteral tube (see Chapters 38 and 39)
- Nonsterile gloves
- Towel or washcloth
- 5-mL catheter-tip syringe
- Stethoscope
- Prescribed enteral formula
- Enteral feeding bag and administration set
- Enteral feeding administration pump
- Intravenous (IV) pole
- Pacifier (optional)

CHILD AND FAMILY ASSESSMENT AND PREPARATION

- Refer to Chapters 38 and 39 for preliminary questions regarding child and family assessment and preparation.
- Assess the child for symptoms of malnutrition, including weight loss, muscle atrophy, edema, weakness, lethargy, failure to wean from ventilatory support, or poor wound healing, which may indicate the severity of malnutrition.
- Assess the child's gastrointestinal tract, auscultate for the presence of bowel sounds, and palpate the abdomen to ensure that it is soft, nondistended, and nontender.
- Obtain the child's baseline weight; note the presence or absence of edema. Note the child's weight from admission and track weight trends; this provides evidence of the effectiveness of nutritional support and the patient's response to the nutritional interventions.
- Assess the child for a history of cardiac, renal, hepatic, or pulmonary disease because these may limit the fluid volume or the type of formula the child can receive and the volume of flushes administered.
- Assess the child for conditions that increase metabolic demand and therefore increase caloric requirements.
- Assess the cognitive level, readiness, and ability to process information of the child and family. The readiness to learn and process information may be impaired as a result of age, stress, or anxiety.
- Reinforce the need and identify and discuss the risks and benefits of enteral tube feedings, as appropriate, to both the child and family.
- Explain the procedure, as appropriate, to both the child and family.

PROCEDURE Intermittent or Bolus Enteral Feeds

Steps	Rationale/Points of Emphasis
1. Perform hand hygiene.	Reduces transmission of microorganisms.
2. Gather the necessary supplies.	Promotes efficient time management and provides an organized approach to the procedure.
3. Don gloves.	Standard precaution to reduce transmission of microorganisms.
4. Place child in a supine position, before the procedure begins, with the head of bed up 30 degrees (if not otherwise contraindicated). Older children may be placed in a sitting position or a position of comfort.	Discourages aspiration of gastric contents by using positioning and gravity to keep formula down when feeding. **caREminder** *A semi-Fowler's, head-of-bed up, right side-lying position is best for promoting gastric emptying and peristalsis.*
5. Measure prescribed amount of enteral formula to be infused into clean graduated measuring cup or catheter-tip syringe.	Prepares formula for administration. Promotes safety for the delivery of the ordered volume of feeding.
6. Place a towel or washcloth under child's indwelling enteral tube or below chin and chest.	Protects clothing and linens from emesis or secretions.

Steps	Rationale/Points of Emphasis
7. To verify proper tube placement of nasogastric, orogastric, and nasojejunal tubes, refer to Chapter 39. With gastrostomy, jejunal, or PEG tubes, malposition may be evidenced by the external tube length being shorter than baseline measurement, distended abdomen, high-pitched bowel sounds indicating obstruction, or blocked lumen of the bowel by the tube balloon from tube migration. **Alert!** *Semicomatose and comatose (versus alert) children and those with either swallowing problems or vomiting are more likely to experience tube insertion and tube positioning errors.*	Avoids complications associated with inappropriate administration of feeding.
8. For skin-level devices, attach feeding tube extension to enteral device (as needed depending on type of enteral device) (Figure 42-1).	Skin-level devices require that a feeding tube be connected to the device to administer the feedings or medications.
9. Attach 60-mL catheter-tip syringe with plunger removed to the end of the enteral tube or the end of the feeding tube.	Syringe is used to administer bolus feeding.
10. Assess for residual fluid in gastrointestinal tract for gastrostomy tubes (this is not indicated for jejunal or transpyloric tubes) (Figure 42-2): • Nasogastric or orogastric tubes—use syringe to aspirate for residual fluid. • Gastrostomy tubes—use passive flow by positioning the tube with an open syringe attached (without the plunger) below the stomach level. • Low-profile gastrostomy tubes—use the manufacturer-recommended decompression/vent tube attached to an open syringe. Attach decompression/vent tube to low-profile gastrostomy tube and position the open syringe to assess residual. It may be necessary to gently aspirate the stomach contents by using the syringe plunger to determine entire residual.	Monitoring residuals aids in prevention of overfeeding and detecting early signs of feeding intolerance. Gastric residuals may be elevated because of formula intolerance, delayed gastric emptying, sepsis, or underlying gastrointestinal disease process.

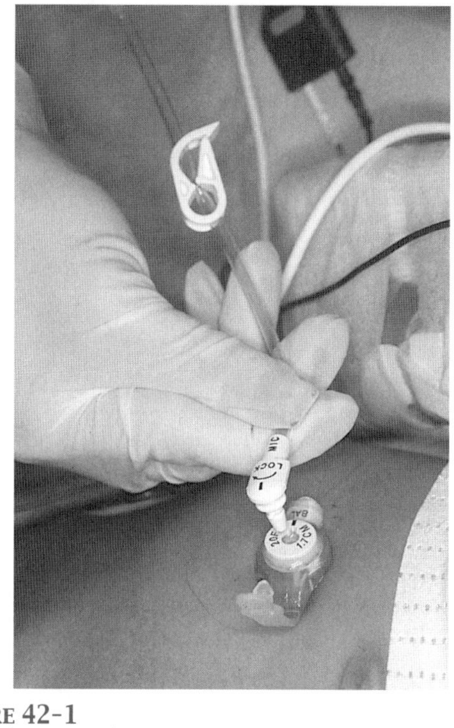

FIGURE 42-1
Enteral devices, such as the "button," require that a feeding tube be connected to the device to instill any medications or fluids.

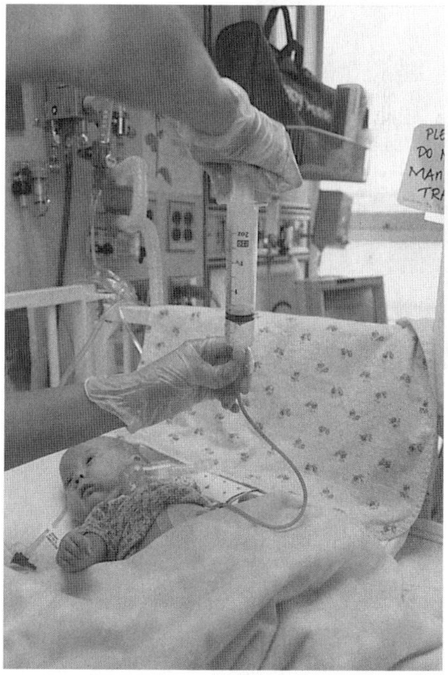

FIGURE 42-2
Before beginning the feeding, gently aspirate a gastrostomy tube for gastric contents or attach the barrel of a syringe to the tubing and gently palpate the child's abdomen. Note presence of gastric contents in syringe. Vigorous aspiration is avoided because it may pull gastric mucosa against the tube.

Continued

Steps	Rationale/Points of Emphasis
caREminder *The MIC-Key skin-level device has a one-way valve positioned at the top of the device that allows for aspiration of stomach contents and for venting of the stomach when feeding extension is connected. The Bard button has the one-way valve at the base of the device, requiring separate decompression/venting tubing.* • Manufacturer's recommendation is to not check residuals with jejunal or transpyloric tubes.	
11. If residual feeding is obtained and is greater than one half of the previous feeding volume, hold the present feeding, noting color and consistency, and notify the prescribing practitioner. If there is a small amount of residual, return the aspirate and continue with the enteral feeding procedure.	Continued feeding may cause negative vital sign changes, vomiting, and potential aspiration. Gastric aspirates contain enzymes, electrolytes, and secretions essential for digestion, so discarding aspirates repeatedly could lead to electrolyte imbalances.
12. Elevate catheter-tip syringe to a level to deliver the feeding over about 15 minutes, gradually adding the total feeding volume to the syringe. Allow feeding to flow slowly by gravity; raising or lowering syringe can adjust the rate of flow (Figure 42-3). The flow of feeding may need to be initiated by placing plunger into barrel of syringe and depressing slightly.	Gravity allows any back pressure to be released and avoids direct forceful pressure on gastric mucosa.

Alert! *Enteral feedings delivered too rapidly may interfere with peristalsis, causing abdominal distention, possible cramping, regurgitation, and/or diarrhea.*

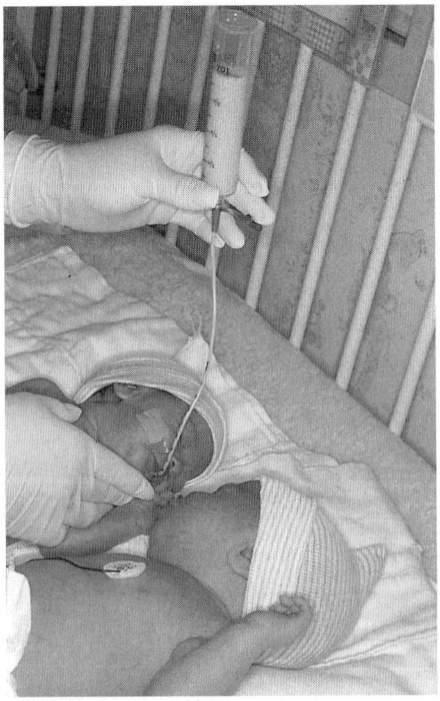

FIGURE 42-3
The enteral feeding should flow freely by gravity to administer the feeding over about 15 minutes, which is a typical time frame for a feeding.

Steps	Rationale/Points of Emphasis
13. Observe child during the feeding for intolerance and complications: elevated gastric residuals, emesis, abdominal distention, bradycardia, or apnea. In the sedated or comatose child, retching may not be observed (see Unexpected Situation).	Stimulation of the vagal nerve by the enteral tube can cause bradycardia or apnea. Feeding intolerance can occur with decreased gastric peristalsis secondary to underlying disease process, leading to inability to digest formula. **KidKare** Offer a pacifier to an infant during enteral feedings to promote secretion of digestive aids and stimulate oral motor muscles.
14. After feeding is complete, gently clear tubing and catheter-tip syringe with warm water flush.	Warm water prevents the tube from clogging. Depending on child's age and diagnosis, added free water may be needed to avoid potential dehydration that can result from high osmolality formulas. Free water may also place some children at risk for fluid overload. **KidKare** Infants and children may be fluid sensitive secondary to age, specific diagnoses (e.g., pulmonary, renal, and/or cardiac conditions), and acute illness. Free water may not be indicated for many of these children. Assess and monitor total volume of free water, including flush volumes.
15. If feeding tube is discontinued after each feeding, pinch or clamp the enteral tubing and withdraw the tubing with a slow, smooth, steady movement.	Avoids leakage of contents from tubing, preventing possible aspiration of contents during removal. Minimizes risk for vomiting.
16. Used supplies, such as catheter-tip syringe and feeding extension tubing, can have repeated use for up to 24 hours. Label administration set with date and time when first used; cleanse thoroughly with warm, soapy water and rinse well.	Changing enteral feeding set/disposable supplies every 24 hours prevents bacterial overgrowth in set. Date and time labeling indicates to parents and nursing staff when supplies should be changed.
17. Dispose of equipment and waste in appropriate receptacle.	Standard precautions.
18. Remove gloves and perform hand hygiene.	Reduces transmission of microorganisms.

PROCEDURE Continuous Drip Enteral Feeds

Steps	Rationale/Points of Emphasis
1. Perform hand hygiene.	Reduces transmission of microorganisms.
2. Gather the necessary supplies.	Promotes efficient time management and provides an organized approach to the procedure.
3. Affix enteral pump to IV pole and plug in to bedside electrical outlet.	Readies enteral pump for feeding.
4. Open sterile package of enteral feeding administration set and bag. Close clamp on tubing. Thread tubing through enteral pump per manufacturer's directions.	Readies feeding administration set for formula.
5. Pour premeasured 4-hour volume of formula into feeding bag and prime feeding administration set per manufacturer's recommendations; some can be primed while tubing is through pump, whereas others require priming before threading through the pump.	Decreases potential for bacterial overgrowth in formula by limiting volume. Priming the tubing minimizes delivery of air into the gastrointestinal tract.

Continued

Steps	Rationale/Points of Emphasis
6. Label administration set with date and time when first hung. Administration set and tubing can be used continuously for up to 24 hours.	Changing enteral feeding administration set every 24 hours prevents bacterial growth. Labeling with date and time indicates to nursing staff when set should be changed.
7. Don gloves.	Standard precaution to reduce transmission of microorganisms.
8. Place child in a supine position, before the procedure begins, with the head of bed up 30 degrees (if not otherwise contraindicated). Older children may be placed in a sitting position or a position of comfort. **Alert!** *Do not use the "blue-dye method" of tinting enteral feedings as a means for detection of aspiration. This method has not been adequately tested and its direct effects to the child are unknown.*	Discourages aspiration of gastric contents by using gravity to keep formula down when feeding.
9. Place a towel or washcloth under child's indwelling enteral tube or below chin and chest.	Protects clothing and linens from emesis or secretions.
10. To verify proper tube placement, refer to Chapter 39 for information on nasogastric, orogastric, or nasojejunal tubes. With gastrostomy, PEG, or jejunal tubes, malposition may be evidenced by tube length being shorter or longer than baseline measurement, distended abdomen, high-pitched bowel sounds indicating obstruction, or blocked lumen of the bowel by the tube balloon.	Avoids complications associated with inappropriate administration of feeding.
11. With gastric feedings (not transpyloric or jejunal), use a syringe to aspirate stomach contents. If greater than half of the previous hour's worth of continuous feeding are aspirated from the stomach, hold the present feeding, note color and consistency of gastric contents, and notify the prescribing practitioner.	Helps confirm tube placement and may indicate the need for further treatment or intervention before beginning feedings. Gastric residuals may be elevated because of formula intolerance, delayed gastric emptying, sepsis, or gastrointestinal disease.
12. If there is a small amount of gastric aspirate, return the aspirate and continue with the enteral feeding procedure.	Gastric aspirates contain enzymes, electrolytes, and secretions essential for digestion of formula.
13. Connect the end connector of the feeding bag administration set to the distal end of the enteral tube and tape the connections.	Prevents accidental disconnection of tubing.
14. Set the prescribed infusion flow rate on the enteral feeding administration pump, release all clamps, and begin infusion through the pump.	Initiates administration of feeding.
15. Observe child during the feeding for intolerance and complications: elevated gastric residuals, emesis, abdominal distention, bradycardia, or apnea.	Stimulation of the vagal nerve by the enteral tube can cause bradycardia or apnea. Feeding intolerance can occur with decreased gastric peristalsis secondary to disease or illness, leading to inability to digest formula. **KidKare** Offer a pacifier to an infant during enteral feedings to promote secretion of digestive enzymes and stimulate oral motor muscles for feeding.
16. If feeding through a jejunal tube, stop the feeding and flush the tubing with warm water every 4 to 6 hours.	Jejunal tubes are prone to occlusion, so flushing with warm water helps prevent the tube from clogging.
17. Dispose of equipment and waste in appropriate receptacle.	Standard precautions.
18. Remove gloves and perform hand hygiene.	Reduces transmission of microorganisms.

CHILD AND FAMILY EVALUATION AND DOCUMENTATION

- Evaluate enteral tube position and function every hour or as determined by institutional policy or the child's condition.
- Observe the enteral tube system to ensure the system is intact, without leaks, kinks, or occlusions, at least once every shift.
- Auscultate the child's bowel sounds every 4 hours for motility.
- Evaluate the child for gastric residuals every 4 hours while on feedings or as ordered by physician or advanced practice nurse. Note color, consistency, pH testing, occult blood testing, and whether the residuals were given back to the child or discarded. Hold feedings for 1 hour if residuals are greater than half of the previous intermittent feeding or greater than half of the previous hour's worth of continuous feeding. If feeding residuals continue after feeding is held for an hour, notify prescriber to obtain further orders.
- Evaluate child's intake, output, and tolerance to feeding. Monitor for decreased or increased urine output.
- Evaluate for diarrhea; consider diarrhea as a possible result of the use of hyperosmolar formula, lactose intolerance, prolonged use of antibiotics, or bacterial contamination of formula.
- Evaluate children experiencing persistent diarrhea on enteral tube feedings for any relation to formula rate and content. Review medications for those that may contribute to diarrhea. Obtain stool to check for *C. difficile.*
- Evaluate the child's weight pattern by weighing the child daily.
- Evaluate the need for in-home enteral nutritional support.
- Document the following:
  - Date and time of feeding administration
  - Type and size of enteral tube in use
  - Origin of enteral tube site and distal tip position (e.g., nasogastric, orogastric, gastrostomy tube)
  - Verification of method of placement
  - Verification of tube patency
  - Type of feeding, medication, or treatment administered through the enteral tube
  - Amount of intake (for continuous feedings document hourly), including flushes and output
  - Amount of gastric residuals, color and characteristics of residuals, results of any pH or occult blood testing, and whether the residuals were given back to the child or discarded.
  - Child's response to and tolerance of the procedure
  - Child's daily weight
  - Presence and quality of bowel sounds
- Determine whether the child and family have areas of concern to discuss.

COMMUNITY CARE

- Enteral tube feedings may be administered in the child's home for feeding therapies or hospice care.
- Instruct the family in
  - Tube insertions when appropriate
  - Evaluating tube patency and management
  - Initiating and discontinuing enteral feedings
  - Recognizing signs and symptoms of feeding intolerance
  - Safety and problem solving related to developmental level of child
- Encourage child and family questions to in-home feeding therapies and consult with a nutritional support counselor or nurse for discharge planning related to obtaining necessary equipment for in-home enteral feedings.
- For the child receiving tube feedings at home, instruct the family to contact the healthcare provider if
  - Child's abdomen becomes distended
  - Child vomits after feedings
  - Child has an increased residual from the previous feeding (parameters are established by the healthcare team)
  - Enteral tube becomes dislodged
  - Child develops a skin rash or redness at enteral tube placement site
  - Child has oozing of secretions or formula at the entrance site of the enteral tube
  - Mechanical tube problems (e.g., tube occlusion, altered tube integrity)

Unexpected Situation

- *Halfway through a feeding, the child vomits and becomes bradycardic, and you note that her abdomen is distended:* Stop the flow of feeding and vent the stomach through the tube. Remove the feeding tube if not contraindicated (e.g., do not remove long-term tubes or those placed during surgery). Provide basic life support as indicated. Auscultate bowel sounds. Notify the physician or advanced practice nurse. A larger-bore tube may need to be inserted to decompress the stomach.

Bibliography

Dautle, M., Wilkinson, T., & Gauderer, M. (2003). Isolation and identification of biofilm microorganisms from silicone gastrostomy devices. *Journal of Pediatric Surgery, 38,* 216–220.

Echeverria, P. (2003). Questioning the use of blue food dye in enteral tube feedings. *Support Line, 25*(2), 22–24.

Edward, S. J., & Methany, N. A. (2000). Measurement of gastric residual volume: State of the science. *MEDSURG Nursing, 9,* 125–128.

Evans, S., MacDonald, A., & Holden, C. (2004). Home enteral feeding audit. *Journal of Human Nutrition & Dietetics, 17,* 537–542.

Horn, D., & Chaboyer, W. (2003). Gastric feeding in critically ill children: A randomized controlled trial. *American Journal of Critical Care, 12*, 461–468.

Khair, J. (2003). Clinical nutrition: Managing home enteral tube feeding for children. *British Journal of Community Nursing, 8*, 116, 118–126.

Mahoney, J., Ryan, T., Brasel, K., et al. (2002). Food dye use in enteral feedings: A review and a call for a moratorium. *Nutrition in Clinical Practice 17*, 169–181.

Matlow, A., Wray, R., Goldman, C., et al. (2003). Microbial contamination of enteral feed administration sets in a pediatric institution. *American Journal of Infection Control, 31*, 49–53.

McClave, S. A., Lukan, J. K., Stefater, J. A., et al. (2005). Poor validity of residual volumes as a marker for risk of aspiration in critically ill patients. *Critical Care Medicine, 33*, 324–330.

McGuire, W., & McEwan, P. (2004). Systematic review of transpyloric versus gastric tube feeding for preterm infants. *Archives of Disease in Childhood–Fetal & Neonatal Edition, 89*, F245–F248.

Metheny, N. A., Schallom, M. E., & Edwards, S. J. (2004). Effect of gastrointestinal motility and feeding tube site on aspiration risk in critically ill patients: A review. *Heart & Lung, 33*, 131–145.

Premji, S. S. (2005). Enteral feeding for high-risk neonates: A digest for nurses into putative risk and benefits to ensure safe and comfortable care. *Journal of Perinatal & Neonatal Nursing, 19*, 59–73.

Williams, T. A., & Leslie, G. D. (2005a). A review of the nursing care of enteral feeding tubes in critically ill adults: Part I. *Intensive & Critical Care, 20*, 330–343.

Williams, T. A., & Leslie, G. D. (2005b). A review of the nursing care of enteral feeding tubes in critically ill adults: Part II. *Intensive & Critical Care, 21*, 5–15.

CHAPTER

43

Feeding, Infant: Breast-Feeding and Formula-Feeding

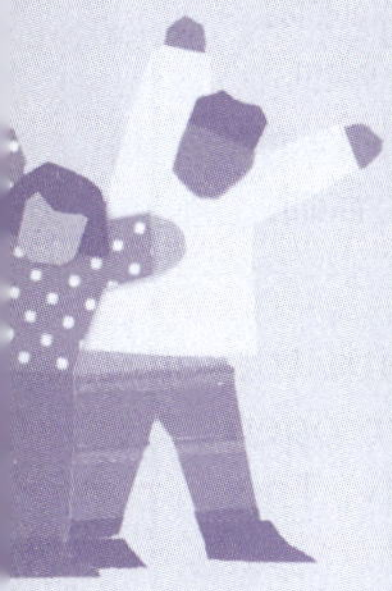

Clinical Guidelines

- Infant feeding is performed by family members or healthcare providers. Authorized volunteers working at the facility may participate in infant feeding when approved to do so by the registered nurse (RN) or licensed practice nurse (LPN) assigned to that infant.
- Infants must have adequate intake to maintain weight gain along their own growth curve.
- Infants are exclusively breast-fed or fed human milk for the first 4 to 6 months of life whenever possible. Contraindications to breast-feeding include galactosemia, maternal use of illegal drugs, untreated active tuberculosis, human immunodeficiency virus (HIV) infection, and administration of certain drugs (e.g., radioactive isotopes, antimetabolites, and cancer chemotherapy).
- Infants are fed human milk or iron-fortified infant formula for the first 12 months of life.
- If the infant has special needs requiring specific feeding interventions, referrals are made as indicated and parents are educated on specific feeding techniques for their child.
- Infants who are receiving adequate fluid and calories have at least six to eight thoroughly wet diapers a day, have a bowel movement with most feedings, nurse approximately 8 to 12 times a day, seem satisfied after nursing (e.g., not irritable or fussy), and gain approximately 1 ounce a day in the first 3 months of life.
- Guidelines for breast milk handing and storage are presented in Chapter 22.
- Prepared formula can be kept refrigerated for 24 to 48 hours, although it is safest to consume within the first 24 hours.
- Open cans of concentrated formula powder have a shelf life of 30 days.

Equipment

For breast-feeding:

- Nonsterile gloves
- Washcloth and soap (if needed)
- Pillow or blanket roll
- Drinking water for the mother

For formula preparation and bottle-feeding:

- Measuring cup (1 quart)
- Appropriate formula, either stored breast milk, powdered concentrated liquid, or ready-to-feed formula
- Scoop
- Bottled water
- Additives as prescribed by the healthcare prescriber (e.g., oil, Polycose)
- Long-handled spoon
- Bottles with appropriate nipples and rings or disposable bottle liners with nipple, rings, and support form

CHILD AND FAMILY ASSESSMENT AND PREPARATION

- Assess infant's general health status (including weight and length), developmental age, chronologic age, and previous feeding experiences.
- Assess infant's oral motor development, particularly if the infant has been intubated, was drug exposed in utero, or has a congenital defect (such as cleft lip or palate).
- Assess parents' preferences to breast-feed or bottle-feed. Explain merits of breast-feeding and the American Academy of Pediatrics support of this feeding method. Clarify any misconceptions regarding breast-feeding.
- Assess parents' level of comfort with feeding, knowledge about positioning infant with head slightly elevated during feeding, and level of knowledge regarding formula preparation and storage if bottle-feeding and maternal nutrition and fluid intake if breast-feeding.
- If using formula, determine type of formula per healthcare prescriber's orders, formula source (e.g., ready to feed, concentrated liquid, powdered), and calorie amount based on birth weight, history of prematurity, allergies, and presence of pathology.
- Assess financial resources of the family to purchase formula and equipment and whether a social service referral may be needed.
- Determine infant state before feeding and assist infant to achieve quiet alert state.
- Provide nursing mother or person feeding the infant with a relatively quiet environment that is as private as possible and free from interruptions. Assist the person feeding the infant to assume a position of comfort using a comfortable chair, pillows for arm support, and a footstool to support the feet and the infant.

PROCEDURE Breast-Feeding

Steps	Rationale/Points of Emphasis
1. Perform hand hygiene and don gloves.	Standard precautions to reduce transmission of microorganisms.
2. Assist nursing mother as needed to perform hand hygiene before feeding and wash and dry breasts if wearing perfume, oils, powders, or lotion other than lanolin cream.	Reduces transmission of microorganisms. Cleansing of the breasts removes perfume, lotion, or oils that may interfere with the infant accepting the breast. Removal of dried milk reduces potential irritation of the mother's nipples.
3. Position the infant close to the mother with head slightly elevated and abdomen turned in contact with mother's body. Infant should be lined up with mouth, chin, and umbilicus in a line. Infant should be able to latch onto the breast, taking the entire areola or as much of it as possible with his or her mouth wide open. The infant's nose and chin should touch the breast with equal pressure. Use pillows or blanket rolls as needed to assist in positioning the infant.	Promotes successful breast-feeding by making the milk flow better, stimulates a good milk supply, and helps prevent overly engorged breasts. If the infant latches on to just the nipple, pain or trauma may occur. Pillows and blanket rolls can help support the infant in a position of comfort for the mother and infant. **KidKare** "Tickling" the infant's cheek with the nipple of the breast encourages the infant to open his or her mouth wider to latch on properly. This elicits the rooting reflex.
4. The mother should rotate which breast the infant starts on with each feeding.	Infants are more awake and energetic at the beginning of the feeding and tend to empty the first breast more completely. By rotating, you avoid emptying the same breast every time.
5. Encourage mother to have infant nurse 10 minutes per side, burping the infant in between breasts and at the end of feeding.	A total feeding time of 20 to 30 minutes should adequately empty both breasts. Infants may continue to suckle at breast for comfort and non-nutritive sucking.
6. To break suction while infant is feeding, instruct mother to insert the tip of her little finger between the breast and the corner of infant's mouth and pull slightly downward.	Breaks the seal and prevents trauma to the nipple.

Steps	Rationale/Points of Emphasis
7. Offer mother water to drink during breast-feeding.	Inadequate maternal hydration slows milk production.
8. When done breast-feeding, assist the mother to place infant in safe and secure supine position in the crib (with side rails up) or bassinet. Assist mother as needed to re-dress and assume position of comfort.	Ensures safety of infant and mother. Supine position prevents aspiration.
9. Perform hand hygiene.	Reduces transmission of microorganisms.

PROCEDURE Infant Formula Feeding

Steps	Rationale/Points of Emphasis
1. Gather the necessary supplies.	Promotes efficient time management and provides an organized approach to the procedure.
2. Perform hand hygiene.	Reduces transmission of microorganisms before formula preparation.
3a. Prepare concentrated or powdered formula exactly as recommended.	
• Review directions for preparation listed on the label as specific for each type and brand of formula. Use boiled, "nursery," or distilled water.	Ensures appropriate preparation. City or well water directly from the tap may contain impurities, parasites, or additives that are not safe for an infant.
• Concentrated formula is usually a 1:1 dilution, and powdered is usually 2 oz of water to one level scoop of powder.	Using the appropriate measuring device ensures proper dilution and allows for preparation of multiple feedings.
• Using the quart measuring cup, measure the concentrated formula into the cup. If a scoop is provided, use the scoop as the unit of measure. Add the appropriate amount of bottled water; mix well with a long-handled spoon. Water may be warmed before mixing if the formula is going to be used immediately.	Extensively altering the formula mix by diluting or concentrating formula increases an infant's vulnerability to hyponatremic seizures if a large amount of additional water is fed or to constipation and hypernatremic dehydration if too little water is used. These consequences can cause permanent disability or death and often require hospitalization. Reconstituting formula with warm tap may increase the amount of lead in prepared formula. Infants who are fed reconstituted formula ingest a large quantity of water per unit of body weight, so that any lead in the water used to reconstitute formula is a concern.
• Add ordered additives at time of feeding, not before.	Additives such as Polycose or oil may separate or coagulate after a period of time. Adding cereal to formula is not recommended.
Alert! *Adding sweeteners to infant formula is not recommended; honey has been linked to infant botulism, and other sweeteners provide only empty calories and increase the risk of dental caries.*	
3b. Ready-to-feed formulas need only be lightly shaken before use.	Ingredients of formula may have "settled" in the container, so shaking slightly helps to redistribute all ingredients equally.
3c. Stored breast milk preparation must follow guidelines in Chapter 22.	Handing and use of stored breast milk requires that specific guidelines are followed to ensure safety.
4. Appropriately label and store formula that is not used immediately. Concentrated or powdered formula should not be prepared more than 24 hours in advance and should be refrigerated once prepared.	Reduces chance of bacterial overgrowth.
5a. Warm formula slowly to comfortable temperature.	Slow heating is recommended to avoid scalding contents or exploding bottles. Infant burns from overheated bottles can be severe enough to require hospitalization, and even amputations have been reported.

Continued

Steps	Rationale/Points of Emphasis
5b. Position supplies so that they are readily accessible to the feeder. **Alert!** *Never microwave a bottle because it will not heat evenly. In addition, steam building within the bottle can result in an explosion and spraying of hot liquid.*	Provides organized approach to the procedure.
6. Hold infant on the lap with head elevated and close to the parent's body.	Reduces chance of aspiration and otitis media. Facilitates bonding. **caREminder** *Never prop a bottle in an infant's mouth. Propping a bottle increases potential for aspiration. Putting an infant to bed with a bottle containing a liquid high in carbohydrate can cause dental caries in a pattern called "baby bottle tooth decay," which can be so extensive that extraction of teeth is required in children as young as 18 months.*
7. Tilt bottle to keep the nipple full at all times. The nipple should have a steady drip, but not a steady stream of flow.	Reduces the amount of air ingested and prevents the potential development of otitis media. Slow flow causes the infant to suck very hard and potentially tire quickly; too fast a stream increases the risk for aspiration.
8. Stimulate rooting reflex by rubbing nipple along lower lip or tickling side of cheek. Place nipple on top of tongue. See Table 43–1 for strategies to deal with the challenging feeder.	Encourages infant to open mouth. Positions nipple appropriately.
9. After 5 minutes or 1–2 ounces, stop and burp infant. Burp again at end of feeding.	Expels ingested air, allows infant to take more formula, and decreases potential for reflux and colic-like symptoms.
10. When feeding is to be discontinued, assist the mother/parent to place infant in safe and secure supine position in the crib or bassinet.	Ensures safety of infant, and prevents aspiration.
11. Discard bottle and formula remaining in bottle at end of feeding.	Formula may be contaminated with bacteria during feeding.
12. Perform hand hygiene.	Reduces transmission of microorganisms.

CHILD AND FAMILY EVALUATION AND DOCUMENTATION

- Evaluate family understanding of nutritional needs of an infant and formula preparation.
- Determine concerns of the parents regarding feeding.
- Evaluate infant's weight gain, and document serial measurements on standardized growth chart.
- Evaluate feeding behaviors and infant–parent interaction and attachment behaviors. Provide written instructions as needed.
- Document the following:
  - Time fed
  - Type of feeding (human milk or formula)
  - Method of feeding (breast or bottle)
  - If breast-fed, note which breast used, length of time on each breast, and any problems encountered
  - If bottle-fed, note amount, type of feeding (human milk or type of formula), and any problems encountered.

COMMUNITY CARE

- For the breast-feeding mother provide the following information:
  - Drink a glass of fluid with each breast-feeding time.
  - Avoid highly spiced or flavored foods and nicotine. The mother may note the infant reacts to certain foods eaten by the mother with increased fussiness, gas, diarrhea, or even increased nursing. With food reactions, the symptoms usually occur within 24 hours. Recommend mother stops eating the particular item that causes problems for infant.
  - Infants who breast-feed do not usually need water in between feedings. Water intake by infant may decrease milk production because the infant will not empty the breast, which stimulates continued milk production.
  - Breast-feed on demand. Infants who breast-feed often eat every 2 to 3 hours.

TABLE 43-1

Strategies for Dealing With the Challenging Feeder

Problem	Strategy	Rationale
Poor suck	a. Assess if nipple is correct, if bottle-fed: too hard, too big, or flow too slow.	a. Infant may be working too hard to initiate flow or unable to handle amount of flow.
	b. Assess infant state: • If infant is sleepy, talk with baby, change diaper, gently massage infant awake. • If infant is highly irritable, move to a quiet, dimly lit room.	b. Infant may be too sleepy to suck well or may be overstimulated and cannot focus on eating.
	c. Assess parent's anxiety level. Reassure parent frequently. Provide information materials (booklets, videos). Provide counseling support as needed.	c. Anxious parents may transfer anxiety to infant, and infant will not suck well.
	d. Assess infant's hunger level.	d. An overly hungry or satiated infant will not suck well.
Decreased motor postural control (e.g., children with cerebral palsy and neurodisabilities)	a. Ensure child is in upright position with good head–trunk alignment b. Use chin-tuck head posture (head is upright and midline with neck flexion so that the chin is directed slightly downward and inward).	a. Alignment and stability of oral structures for feeding and swallowing may be compromised by abnormal or weak muscle tone.
Gastroesophageal reflux (GER)	a. Assess if and how much infant regurgitates after feedings.	a. A wet burp occasionally after feeding is normal, but if amount of fluid is significant, projectile, or the occurrence is regular, the baby may have reflux.
	b. Elevate infant's head after every feeding.	b. GER is commonly seen in premature infants. Can be caused by positioning, formula intolerance, or medical conditions. Proper positioning may decrease incidence.
	c. Monitor amount of formula or breast milk the infant is taking.	c. It may be necessary to limit amount taken at any one feeding.
	d. Ensure the head of the infant is elevated while feeding.	d. Proper position can prevent reflux.
Cleft lip or palate	a. Assess extent of cleft lip or palate. If breast-feeding is not possible, modification of a nipple may be needed (Figure 43-1).	a. An infant with only a cleft lip may successfully breast-feed, if the mother prefers. If the child also has a cleft palate, breast-feeding may not be possible because of the inability to produce effective suction to extract the breast milk.
	b. Monitor weight gain carefully in an infant with cleft lip or palate.	b. Ensures good nutrition and hydration.
	c. Feed slowly, evaluating child's ability to suck and swallow using modified nipple.	c. Monitors for potential aspiration during feedings.

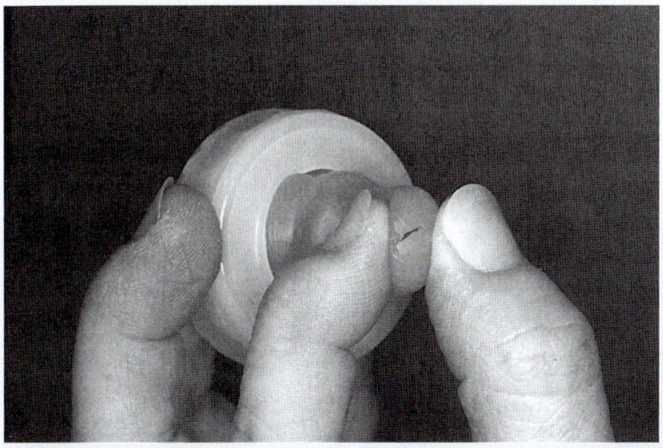

FIGURE 43-1
A crosscut bottle nipple can be used to feed a child with cleft palate. Note the crosscut is off center; when feeding, direct the cut down to the side of the mouth with the most intact palate.

   - Breast milk is easily digestible by the infant. Frequent feeding often prevents sore nipples, breast engorgement, and early weaning.
   - If breast milk is being expressed and stored for home use, review handing and storage procedures with family (see Chapter 22).
- Determine need for social services follow-up to assist with resource allocation.
- Refer to appropriate support group for emotional support if child has a specific problem, such as cleft lip or palate.
- Instruct family to contact the healthcare provider if
   - Infant has less than 6 wet diapers in a 24-hour period.
   - Urine is a color other than pale yellow beginning around the third or fourth day of life (not deep yellow or orange).
   - Infant is frequently fussy or irritable after feeding.
   - Infant does not show steady weight gain or starts losing weight after the first week of life.
   - Stools become extremely watery or are of increased frequency, or infant does not defecate for 48 hours or stools are very hard. Bowel movements of breast-fed babies usually smell "sweeter" than stools of formula-fed babies.

Unexpected Situation

- *During the feeding the infant vomits:* Determine the amount of emesis, evaluating color and consistency. A small amount may represent a "wet burp," indicating the child needs to burp more frequently during feeding. A projectile vomit that consists of undigested milk or formula may indicate pyloric stenosis. Emesis that is green or yellow contains bile. Emesis that is pink or red may contain blood. Do not attempt to feed the infant again immediately; allow him or her to rest and feed 1 to 2 hours later. Document the emesis. If this is a reoccurring event or reoccurs in a future feeding, notify the primary healthcare provider.

Bibliography

American Academy of Pediatrics. (1997). Breastfeeding and the use of human milk. *Pediatrics, 100*(6), 1035–1039.

American Academy of Pediatrics. (1999). Iron fortification of infant formulas. *Pediatrics, 104*(1), 119–123.

American Academy of Pediatrics. (2001a). The transfer of drugs and other chemicals into human milk. *Pediatrics, 108*(3), 776–789.

American Academy of Pediatrics. (2001b). WIC program, provisional section on breastfeeding. *Pediatrics, 108*(5), 1216–1217.

American Academy of Pediatrics. (2005). Dietary recommendations for children and adolescents: A guide for practitioners. *Pediatrics, 117*(2), 544–559.

Douglas, J. M., Douglas, A. B., & Silk, H. J. (2004). A practical guide to infant oral health. *American Family Physicians, 70*(11). Retrieved September 21, 2006, from www.AAFP.ORG/afp/20041201/2113.html

Fein, S., & Falci, C. (1999). Infant formula preparation, handling and related practices in the United States. *Journal of the American Dietetic Association, 99*(1), 1234–1240.

Humennick, S., & Gwayi-Chore, M. (2001). Leader or left behind: National and international policies related to breastfeeding. *Journal of Obstetric, Gynecologic, and Neonatal Nursing, 30*(5), 529–540.

Moreland, J. & Coombs, J. (2000). Promoting and supporting breast feeding. *American Academy of Family Physicians, 61*, 2093–2100, 2103–2104.

Redstone, F., & West, J. (2004). The importance of postural control for feeding. *Pediatric Nursing, 30*(2), 97–100.

Samour, P., & King, K. (2005). *Handbook of pediatric nutrition.* Sudbury, MA: Jones and Bartlett Publishers.

Shaker, I., Scott, J., & Reid, M. (2004). Infant feeding attitudes of expectant parents: Breastfeeding and formula feeding. *Journal of Advanced Nursing, 45*(3), 260–268.

CHAPTER

44

Growth Parameter Assessment

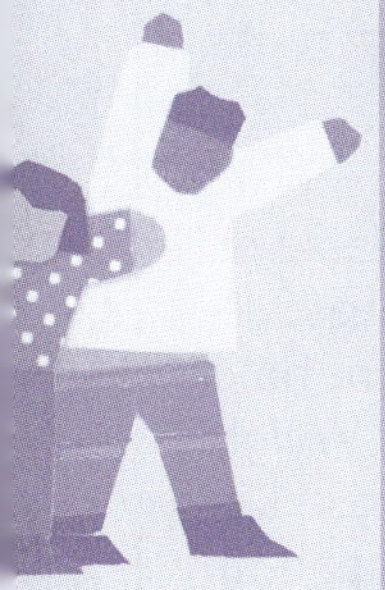

Clinical Guidelines

- Measurements of height, weight, and head circumference may be performed by a registered nurse (RN), a licensed practical nurse (LPN), or unlicensed assistive personnel (UAP) who have received education in the appropriate techniques for growth assessments.
- Growth parameter assessments are obtained at each visit to the healthcare provider, at each home visit by the healthcare provider, and on admission to the healthcare facility.
- Head circumference is assessed in all children younger than 36 months of age.
- Growth parameter assessment continues throughout the child's stay in the healthcare facility:
  - Daily weights should be obtained in infants as well as children admitted for renal disease, fluid and electrolyte imbalances, cardiac disorders, cystic fibrosis, anorexia, and failure to thrive.
  - Daily weights should be assessed at about the same time each day, ideally in the morning before breakfast.
- All clinicians in the same setting should use the same measurement techniques to ensure reliability of growth measurements and growth curves.
- The same growth should be used for each healthcare visit, thus providing an accurate growth history and illustration of growth trends.
- BMI (body mass index), an indicator that reveals body weight adjusted for height, is used to assess underweight, overweight, and risk for overweight in children and teens aged 2–20.

Equipment

- Small sheet or paper drape to cover scale
- Infant/toddler scale
- Adult scale
- Bed scale
- Paper measuring tape
- Flat surface or flat measuring board
- Measuring device affixed to a wall (stadiometer), height assessment rod attached to scale, or an electronic length measurement device
- Growth chart
- Calculator

CHILD AND FAMILY ASSESSMENT AND PREPARATION

- Assess child's previous growth pattern and most recent weight, height, and head circumference.
- Discuss with parents and child the rationale for growth assessment.
- Ensure that the room temperature is adequate for the comfort of the unclothed child.
- Select Centers for Disease Control and Prevention (CDC) growth charts that are age and gender appropriate for the child (available at http://www.cdc.gov/growthcharts). When the CDC growth charts were revised, data on low-birth-weight infants were included but not data on very-low-birth-weight infants (<1,500 g). Alternate charts are available to assess the growth of VLBW infants. Currently, the most appropriate to use are the Infant Health and Development Program (IHDP) charts. Growth charts are also available in French and Spanish. Growth charts that are specific to certain conditions such as Down syndrome, Prader-Willi syndrome, low-birth-weight/premature infants, and Turner syndrome are published by the Washington State Department of Health and are available at http://www.doh.wa.gov/cfh/documents/nutrition_interventions.pdf.

PROCEDURE Growth Assessment of the Infant/Toddler up to 24 Months of Age: Assessing Weight

Steps	Rationale/Points of Emphasis
1. Note child's previous weight, if available.	Serves as a baseline to detect weight changes.
2. Perform hand hygiene.	Reduces transmission of microorganisms.
3. Place light drape or paper on scale pan.	Provides comfort and protects from microorganism cross-contamination.
4. Calibrate scale to "0" position.	Negates weight of drape or paper.
5. Completely undress and safely place infant/toddler on scale.	Allows for accurate measurement of infant/toddler body weight. **caREminder** *Children aged 0 to 24 months should be weighed nude for accurate body weight determination.* **caREminder** *If available, use of in-bed scales with infants in special care units allows for accurate weight while keeping the infant in a safe temperature-controlled environment.*
6. Hold hand slightly above infant while on scale (Figure 44-1).	Prevents falls or potential injury. **KidKare** If infant/toddler scale is unavailable or child is extremely fearful or active, weight measurement may be accomplished by having a parent hold child in his or her arms on a stand-up scale. Weigh parent alone and then weigh parent holding child. To assess child's weight, subtract weight of parent alone from weight of parent and child together. **KidKare** NEVER turn your back to an infant on a scale.

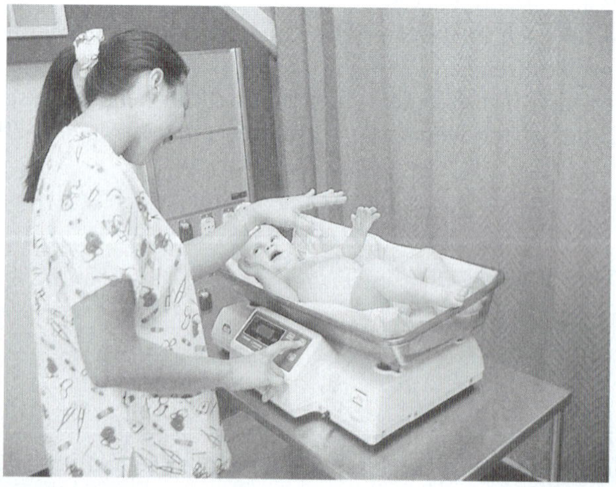

FIGURE 44-1
To prevent injury when weighing the infant, hold your hand slightly over infant and never turn your back on the child.

Steps	Rationale/Points of Emphasis
7. Note and record child's weight in kilograms on a notepad.	Allows accurate notation of weight. Weight in kilograms is used for accurate calculation of medication dosages.
8. Diaper infant. Carefully remove infant from scale, re-dress, and return infant to parent's arms or crib.	Places infant in secure location.
9. Dispose of paper on scale and disinfect scale per institutional policy. Perform hand hygiene.	Reduces transmission of microorganisms.
10. Document weight on child's growth chart and/or related records specific to care location.	Communicates findings to other members of the healthcare team.

PROCEDURE Assessing Length of Children Younger Than 2 Years of Age

Steps	Rationale/Points of Emphasis
1. Note child's age and previous length, if available. ***Alert!*** *A child's height is less than his or her length; if standing height/stature is plotted on a length chart, the perception is that the rate of growth has decelerated when, in fact, the issue is that the measurement has been plotted on an incorrect growth chart.*	Serves as a baseline and enables nurse to detect changes in child's length. Children younger than 2 years of age must be measured lying down because of the marked lordosis at that age and because the measurements will be recorded on length growth charts that are for children who are newborn to 24 months of age.
2. Perform hand hygiene.	Reduces transmission of microorganisms.
3. Place light drape or paper on flat surface or flat measuring board.	Provides comfort and protects from microorganism cross-contamination.
4. Lay infant/toddler in supine position, placing the vertex of the infant's head at the top of the board and the soles of the feet firmly against the footboard. ***Alert!*** *It is difficult to obtain reliable length measurements in term infants because of the natural flexion of the newborn infant and the cranial molding that takes place during the labor and delivery process. Clinicians should be aware of the magnitude of error in length measurements and interpret length measurements with caution.*	Allows for full extension of body for accurate length assessment. **caREminder** *Keep hand on infant/toddler at all times.*
5a. Hold child's head at midline point and extend legs fully.	Full body extension is required for accurate measurement. **KidKare** Having parent hold the child's head provides emotional comfort for the child and assists with full extension of body.
5b. For electronic length measurement devices, follow manufacturer's instructions for extending child's body and ensuring accuracy of measurement. For scales with length devices attached, hold the child's head against the head plate. The child should be supine with knees down and feet flexed against the movable footplate.	It is important to consider the differences in the various measuring devices.

Continued

Steps	Rationale/Points of Emphasis
6. Stretch a tape measure from crown of child's head to heel of child's foot, alongside child's body boundaries (Figure 44-2).	Denotes upper and lower body measurement. This is less accurate than length measuring boards and should only be used when these devices are unavailable.

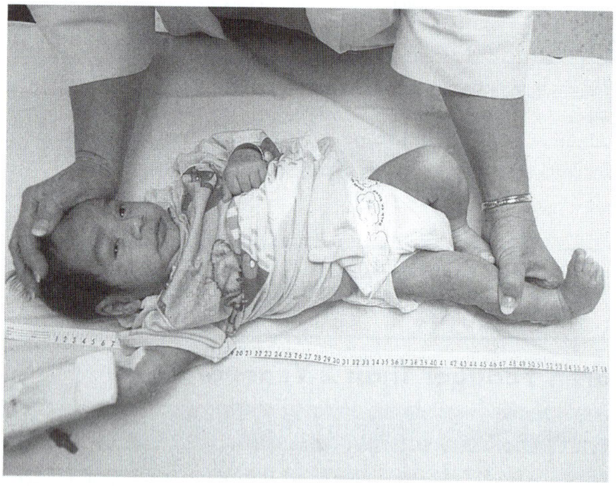

FIGURE 44-2
To measure an infant's length, stretch a tape alongside infant's body from crown of head to heel of foot, ensuring that the infant's leg is fully extended.

KidKare If it is difficult to use a tape measure with child in position, draw two pencil lines on the paper drape, one at the uppermost part of the child's head and one at the heel of the child's foot, or use an electronic length measurement device.

Steps	Rationale/Points of Emphasis
7. Note and record infant's length in centimeters on a notepad.	Allows accurate notation of length.
8. Carefully remove infant from flat surface and return infant to parent's arms or crib.	Places infant in secure location.
9. Perform hand hygiene.	Reduces transmission of microorganisms.
10. Document length on child's growth chart and/or related records specific to care location.	Communicates findings to other members of the healthcare team.

caREminder
Weight and length measurements should be shared with parents in kilograms and centimeters as well as in pounds and inches to assist parental understanding of growth.

PROCEDURE Assessing Head Circumference

Steps	Rationale/Points of Emphasis
1. Note child's last recorded head circumference, if available.	Serves as a baseline and enables nurse to detect changes in child's head circumference.
2. Perform hand hygiene.	Reduces transmission of microorganisms.
3. Place light drape or paper on flat surface.	Provides comfort and protects from microorganism cross-contamination.
4. Place infant/toddler in supine position or seated on paper drape.	Allows for accurate measurement of head circumference.

KidKare Head circumference of infant/toddler may be obtained with child sitting in parent's lap to decrease child's fear.

Steps	Rationale/Points of Emphasis
5. Place tape measure over the most prominent point of the occiput, around the head just above the eyebrows and pinna (Figure 44-3). Take two separate readings. If these measurements do not agree within 0.2 centimeters (¼ inch), reposition child and remeasure a third time. Use the average of the two measures in closest agreement.	This is point of largest head circumference.

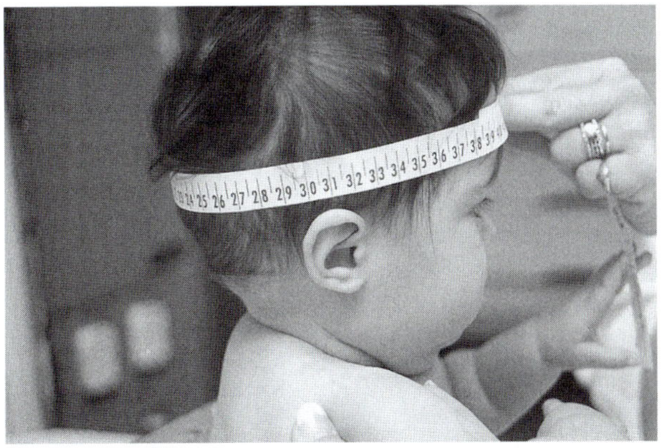

FIGURE 44-3
Measure head circumference by placing the paper tape over the eyebrows and around the occipital prominence.

Steps	Rationale/Points of Emphasis
6. Note and record infant's head circumference to the nearest 0.1 centimeter (⅛ inch) on a notepad.	Allows accurate notation of head circumference.
7. Carefully remove infant from flat surface and return infant to parent's arms or crib.	Places infant in secure location.
8. Perform hand hygiene.	Reduces transmission of microorganisms.
9. Document head circumference on child's growth chart and/or related records specific to care location.	Communicates findings to other members of the healthcare team.

PROCEDURE Growth Assessment of Older Ambulatory Child: Assessing Weight

Steps	Rationale/Points of Emphasis
1. Determine whether child is able to stand and balance on scale.	Assesses safety of use of stand-up scale.
2. Note child's previous weight, if available.	Serves as a baseline and enables nurse to detect changes in child's weight.
3. Place paper or drape on scale.	Provides comfort and protects from microorganism cross-contamination.
4. Calibrate scale to "0" position.	Negates weight of drape or paper.
5. Ask child to remove shoes and heavy clothing. Children older than 24 months of age may be weighed while wearing light clothing, unless otherwise specified.	Allows for accurate measurement of body weight.
6. Assist child to stand on scale.	Prevents falls or potential injury. **KidKare** Older toddlers and preschool-aged children may sit on scale.

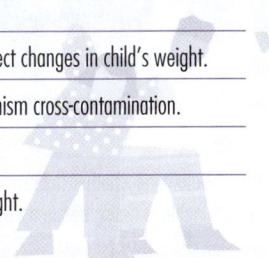

Continued

Steps	Rationale/Points of Emphasis
7. Have child place hands at side of body or hold belly (Figure 44-4). Ask child to be still.	Allows for accurate weight assessment. Newer scale models allow children to hold onto the scale, and the scales do not shake.

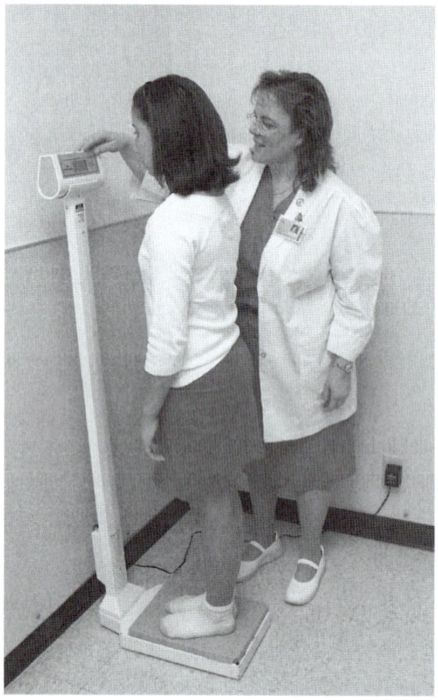

FIGURE 44-4
The ambulatory child should stand on the scale with arms at his or her sides for weight measurements.

Steps	Rationale/Points of Emphasis
8. Note and record child's weight in kilograms on a notepad.	Allows accurate notation of weight.
9. Assist child to step down from scale or proceed to height assessment.	Places child in secure location.
10. Document weight on child's growth chart and/or related records specific to care location.	Communicates findings to other members of the healthcare team.

PROCEDURE Growth Assessment of the Nonambulatory Child: Using a Bed Scale

Steps	Rationale/Points of Emphasis
1. Note child's previous weight and height, if available.	Serves as a baseline and enables nurse to detect changes in child's weight and height.
2. Determine whether child can assist with movement onto scale. If child is unable to assist, obtain assistance from another healthcare provider.	Provides safety for child and healthcare provider.
3. Bring bed scale to edge of child's bed.	Allows for easier transfer of child.
4. Lock brakes on bed and scale.	Prevents potential fall or injury.
5. Raise bed to height of scale.	Allows for easier transfer of child.
6. Perform hand hygiene.	Reduces transmission of microorganisms.
7. Place sheet or drape on scale.	Provides comfort and protects from microorganism cross-contamination.

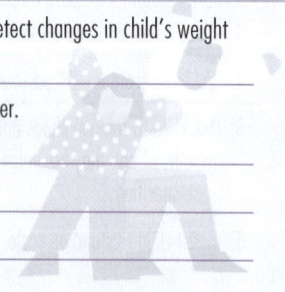

Steps	Rationale/Points of Emphasis
8. Assist child in removing most clothing.	Provides accurate weight of child.
9. Calibrate scale to "0" position.	Negates weight of sheet or drape.
10. Using proper body mechanics, transfer child onto weighing surface of bed scale. Note: If using hydraulic lift bed scale with soft litter, logroll child onto litter, attach hooks or straps securely to scale, and lift litter and child until litter is not in contact with bed surface (Figure 44-5).	Prevents injury of nurse or child and places child in correct position for weight determination.

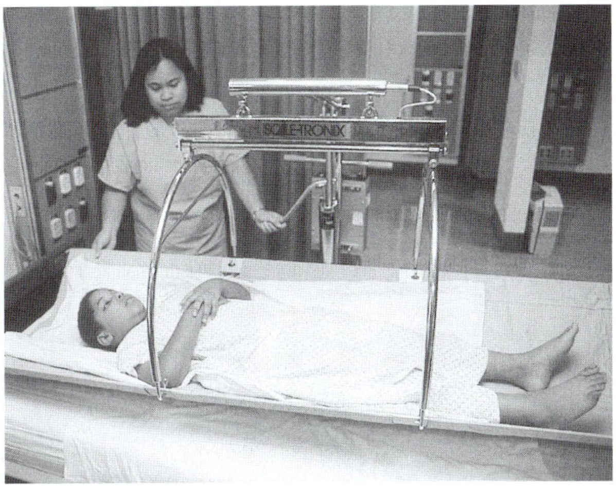

FIGURE 44-5
To weigh a nonambulatory child, logroll child onto litter, securely attach hooks or straps to scale, and lift litter and child until litter is not in contact with bed surface.

Steps	Rationale/Points of Emphasis
11. Ask the child to lie as still as possible.	Allows for accurate weight measurement.

> ***Alert!*** ***Infants and children being weighed with equipment (e.g., intravenous tubes, chest tubes) need to have their weights adjusted to deduct for the weights attributed to the equipment. Developing a unit-specific reference table for the weight of equipment items can assist in ensuring accuracy of weight measurement. Hold equipment off the child when possible (e.g., tubing).***

Steps	Rationale/Points of Emphasis
12. Note and record child's weight in kilograms on a notepad.	Allows accurate notation of weight.
13. If using hard-surface bed scale, height may be measured by extending child fully and measuring from crown of head to heel of foot held in dorsiflexion.	Allows determination of height during same procedure as weight.
14. Carefully transfer child back to bed. Note: If using hydraulic lift bed scale with soft litter, slowly lower litter back to surface of bed and logroll child from litter.	Prevents injury to self or child.
15. Document weight and height on child's growth chart and/or related records specific to care location.	Communicates findings to other members of the healthcare team.

PROCEDURE Assessing Height

Steps	Rationale/Points of Emphasis
1. Determine whether child is able to stand and balance on scale or move child to area where measure is attached to the wall.	Assesses safety of use of stand-up scale with height rod. Many stand-up scales move or shake and thus may be unstable for the young child to stand on to receive an accurate measurement.

Alert! *The measuring devices (arms) attached to a scale are inherently inaccurate because the arm is floppy and not a fixed right angle and the child is unable to stand against a flat surface. For increased reliability of height measurements, a wall tape measure or stadiometer is recommended.*

Steps	Rationale/Points of Emphasis
2. Note child's previous height, if available.	Serves as a baseline and enables nurse to detect changes in child's height.
3. Ask child to remove shoes. Child should not be wearing a hat or hair ornaments.	Allows for accurate measurement of body height.
4. Assist child to stand on scale with back to scale or place child with back to wall/stadiometer. The child's heels, buttocks, and shoulders should be in contact with the wall or height bar of the scale. The child should look straight ahead without tilting the head (Figure 44-6).	Prevents falls and places child in correct position for height determination.

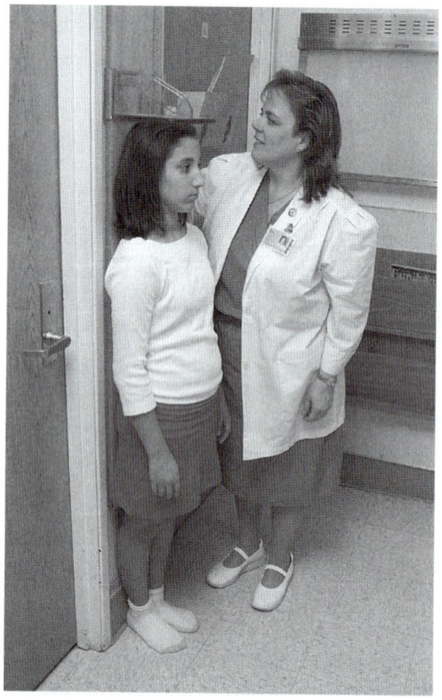

FIGURE 44-6
During height measurement, the child's heels, buttocks, and shoulders should be in contact with the wall or height bar of the scale.

Steps	Rationale/Points of Emphasis
5. Raise height rod and extend height assessment bar high over child's head.	Prevents injury.
6. Lower height rod to top of child's head.	Indicates child's height. Ensures accuracy of measurement.

caREminder
Ensure that height assessment bar is perpendicular to height rod.

Steps	Rationale/Points of Emphasis
7. With the examiner eye to eye with the child and with gentle traction applied to the jaw, note the height measurement and then record child's height in centimeters on a notepad.	Allows accurate notation of height.
8. Assist child to step down from scale or proceed to weight assessment.	Places child in secure location.
9. Document height on child's growth chart and/or related records specific to care location.	Communicates findings to other members of the healthcare team.

PROCEDURE Calculating Body Mass Index (BMI)

Steps	Rationale/Points of Emphasis
1. Obtain accurate weight and height measurements using procedures above.	Allows for accurate calculation of BMI.
2. Calculate BMI using one of the following formulas: *English formula:* *BMI = [weight in pounds ÷ height in inches ÷ height in inches] × 703* *Metric formula:* *BMI = weight in kilograms ÷ [height in meters]^2* or *BMI = [weight in kilograms ÷ height in centimeters ÷ height in centimeters] × 10,000* **caREminder** *Online calculators are available to determine BMI through the Centers for Disease Control and Prevention at http://www.cdc.gov/nccdphp/dnpa/bmi/calc-bmi.htm and through Shape-Up America at www.shapeup.org/oap/entry.php*	BMI calculation provides a numbered indicator that is used to determine whether an individual's weight is appropriate for his or her height. A child with a BMI measurement between the 85th and 95th percentile is classified as at risk of being overweight; a child with a measurement higher than the 95th percentile is overweight. A child with a BMI measurement lower than the 5th percentile is considered underweight.
3. Record BMI on appropriate BMI chart for child's gender and age.	Communicates findings to other members of the healthcare team.

CHILD AND FAMILY EVALUATION AND DOCUMENTATION

- Evaluate family knowledge regarding child's growth progress.
- Document the following:
  - Child's exact chronologic age (e.g., 5 years 4 months or 5$\frac{4}{12}$)
  - Child's weight, height and/or length, and head circumference on child's growth chart and/or related records specific to care location
- Track child's growth parameters on standardized growth charts. Growth charts are available online at http://www.cdc.gov/growthcharts.
- Compare parents' and siblings' growth patterns with child's measurements.
- Discuss findings of all growth parameter assessments with age-appropriate child and child's parents.
- Assist parents to interpret findings and to discuss possible causes for dramatic changes in growth parameters or significant deviations above or below age-appropriate norms. Discuss what it means to be outside norms.
- Provide teaching, follow-up referrals, and monitoring for children above or below norms for age.

COMMUNITY CARE

- Infant/toddler scales carried and used by visiting home care providers should be recalibrated before each weight because transport of scales from location to location may lead to scale fluctuations.
- Bathroom scales in the home may be used to weigh older children.
- Assist family in maintaining records of child's growth patterns.

- Teach family about interpretation of findings based on norms.
- Instruct the family to contact the healthcare provider if
  - Parents or the child are concerned about atypical growth patterns (e.g., too slow or too rapid).
  - Child does not appear to be attaining weight and height parameters consistent with other children of the same age.

Unexpected Situations

- *The 2-year-old child is uncooperative during weight assessment, refusing to stand on the scale:* Encourage the child to sit on the scale to measure weight. If this is not successful, have the parent hold the child while standing on the scale. Weigh parent without child and deduct weight from first measurement to obtain child's weight.
- *The child you need to weigh is in the intensive care unit, with ventilator tubing, Foley catheter, intravenous lines, and several monitors attached to the child:* Weigh the child at the same time each day. If the child has an in-bed scale, this is the preferred method of measurement. Otherwise, use the sling scale, removing all nonessential equipment if possible. Once the child is position on the scale and ready to obtain the reading, support the tubings and equipment slightly above the child so it is not touching the scale and therefore adding artificial weight to the final measurement.

Bibliography

Barlow, S. E., & Dietz, W. H. (1998). Obesity evaluation and treatment: Expert committee recommendations (electronic article). *Pediatrics, 102*(3), e29. Retrieved September 27, 2006, from http://pediatrics.aappublications.org/cgi/content/full/102/3/e29

Corkins, M., Lewis, P., Cruse, W., Gupta, S., & Fitzgerald, J. (2002). Accuracy of infant admission lengths. *Pediatrics, 109*(6), 1108–1111.

Guo, S. S., Roche, A. F., Chumlea, W. C., Casey, P. H., & Moore, W. M. (1997). Growth in weight, recumbent length, and head circumference for preterm low-birthweight infants during the first three years of life using gestation adjusted ages. *Early Human Development, 47*, 305–325.

Hench, K., Shults, J., Benyi, T., et al. (2005). Effect of educational preparation on the accuracy of linear growth measurement in pediatric primary care practices: Results of a multicenter nursing study. *Journal of Pediatric Nursing, 20*(2), 64–74.

Johnson, T., Engstrom, J., Warda, J., Kabat, M., & Paters, B. (1998). Reliability of length measurements in term infants. *Journal of Obstetric, Gynecologic, and Neonatal Nursing, 27*, 270–276.

Legler, J., & Rose, L. (1998). Assessment of abnormal growth curves. *American Family Physician.* Retrieved September 27, 2006, from http://www.aafp.org/afp/980700ap/legler.html

Lipman, T., Hench, K., Logan, J., DiFazio, D., Hale, P., & Singer-Granick, C. (2000). Assessment of growth parameter by primary care providers. *Journal of Pediatric Healthcare, 14*, 166–171.

Miller, K. (2001). Evaluating growth in children: Distinguishing between normal and worrisome. *Advance for Nurse Practitioners, 4*(11), 42–49.

National Centers for Health Statistics, Centers for Disease Control and Prevention. (2000). 2000 CDC growth charts: United States. Retrieved September 27, 2006, from http://www.cdc.gov/growth charts

Ogden, C. L., Kuczmarski, R. J., Flegal, K. M., et al. (2002). Centers for Disease Control and Prevention 2000 growth charts for the United States: Improvements to the 1977 National Center for Health Statistics version. *Pediatrics, 109*(1), 45–60.

Roche, A., & Guo, S. (2001). The new growth charts. *Pediatric Basics, 94*, 2–13.

Spence, K., Smith, J., & Peat, J. (2003). Accuracy of weighing simulated infants with in-bed and freestanding scales while connected and disconnected to a ventilator. *Advances in Neonatal Care, 3*(1), 27–36.

Washington State Department of Health. (2002). *Nutrition interventions for children with special healthcare needs.* DOH Publication Number 961-158. Retrieved September 27, 2006, from www.doh.wa.gov

CHAPTER 45

Hearing Screening

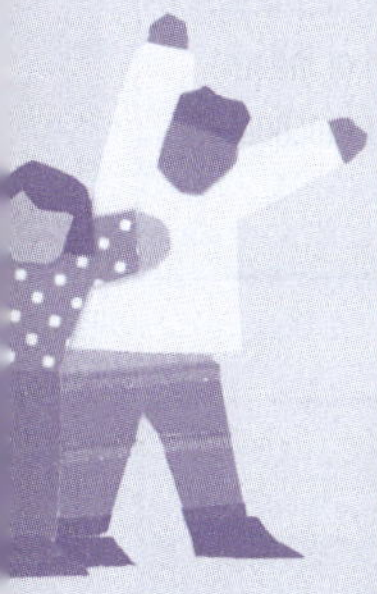

Clinical Guidelines

- The purpose of hearing screening is early identification of auditory dysfunction that causes developmental delay in speech and language. The American Academy of Pediatrics (AAP) reports that 1 to 6 per 1,000 newborns who have significant hearing loss would be identifiable through newborn and infant screening. However, some congenital cases do not become evident until later in childhood. AAP recommends not only the screening of newborns but also continued screening in infancy, childhood, and through adolescence using age-appropriate screening methods:
  - Birth to 9 months—automated auditory brainstem response (ABR) or otoacoustic emissions (OAE), which tests for auditory pathway structural integrity but does not actually test hearing. Tests may be performed by audiologists, nurses, physicians, and other staff who have received appropriate training in accordance with state laws.
  - 9 to 12 months—conditioned oriented responses (COR) or visual reinforced audiometry (VRA), which conditions the child to associate speech or frequency-specific sound with a reinforcement stimulus, usually performed by an audiologist in a soundproof room.
  - 2 to 4 years—play audiometry, which conditions the child to respond to an auditory stimulus through play, such as dropping a block or other interesting object into a bowl or similar container when a sound is heard through the earphones. May be performed by physicians, audiologists, nurses, and personnel who have received appropriate training
  - 4 years and older—identification audiometry. May be performed by physicians, audiologists, nurses, and personnel who have received appropriate training, in accordance with state laws
- Newborn or infant screening is best performed in the hospital before discharge to home. Check your state requirements to verify if hospital newborn hearing screening programs are state mandated and in place.
- Hearing screening with the use of identification or play audiometry is carried out in two stages: (1) sweep screening, which identifies those with a hearing deficit; and (2) threshold test, which determines the level of hearing loss.
- When screening is performed in the school setting, the school nurse may need a certification for school audiometrist from the state; check your state and local district policy.

Equipment

- Audiometer with headset/earphones, calibrated annually
- Blocks, bears, or equivalent
- Basket, bowl, or equivalent

- Source of electricity: 110 volts AC
- Report sheet, documentation form
- Pen
- A quiet room, a desk, two chairs

CHILD AND FAMILY ASSESSMENT AND PREPARATION

- If the parents or the caregivers are concerned about a child's hearing, assume they are correct until proven wrong. It has been shown that parents were as much as 12 months ahead of physicians in the identification of their child's hearing loss.
- Explain to the parent and to the child what procedure is being performed and what is expected of the child. Avoid the word "test" because of the anxiety associated with it. "Hearing check" may be substituted for "hearing test."
- Tell the child, "You will be wearing earphones. You will be hearing some soft sounds through the earphones so you will have to listen very carefully. As soon as you think you can hear the sound, you need to raise your hand and keep it up as long as the sound is heard and put it down when the sound is gone." Instruction is modified in play audiometry as discussed below.
- Ensure the parent and the child that the procedure is painless.

PROCEDURE Preparation

Steps	Rationale/Points of Emphasis
1. Perform hand hygiene.	Reduces transmission of microorganisms.
2. Select a quiet room. Set up the audiometer. Place the audiometer on top of the desk. Plug it in and switch to on. Check the cords, switches, dials, and headset. Make sure the indicator light is on. Perform a dry run or a practice test.	Noise affects screening results. Setting up the audiometer takes time and may create unnecessary anxiety for the child. Ensures proper functioning of equipment.
3. Bring the child into the room. If accompanied by a parent, allow the parent to watch the procedure.	Younger children are more comfortable in the presence of their parents.
4. Seat the child slightly behind the audiometer. Position him or her so that you can see most of the face.	Prevents the child from seeing you operate the interrupter switch while allowing you to observe his or her facial reactions.
5. Have the child remove eyeglasses, headband, hair clips, and earrings.	External objects may make it uncomfortable for the child to wear the earphones.

> **Alert!** *Do not test the child if discharge from the child's ear is present; refer the child for medical care.*

Steps	Rationale/Points of Emphasis
6. Smile while placing the earphones on the child according to manufacturer's instructions (e.g., red ear phone over the right ear and the blue ear phone over the left ear). Adjust the headband so the earphone fits snugly.	An aura of assurance may comfort the child who may sense confusion or indecision and may refuse to wear the earphone. Ensures proper equipment function to obtain accurate results.

PROCEDURE Sweep Screening

Steps	Rationale/Points of Emphasis
1. Set the frequency dial at 1,000 Hz and the tone at 50 dB.	At 50 decibels, the tone is loud enough such that both ears are able to hear the tone even if the tone is only introduced to one ear. This is possible because of bone conduction via the skull.
2. Test the right ear first.	Establishes routine.
3. Depress the interrupter switch one or two times for about 1 to 2 seconds and then release. Watch for the child's hand to go up as you depress the switch.	This orients the child to the type of sound that he or she is supposed to hear and assures you that he or she understands the instruction.
4. Set at the desired hearing level; verify your state recommendations for settings (e.g., 25 dB); use this setting throughout the sweep screening.	Standardizes testing. A hearing loss of 30 dB and greater in the 500- to 4,000-Hz range interferes with normal speech and language development.

Steps	Rationale/Points of Emphasis
5. Test the right ear at 1,000, 2,000, and 4,000 Hz by depressing the interrupter switch in each of these frequencies. Observe response. **caREminder** *Present tones in an irregular pattern; do not create any pattern when depressing the switch. Do not look up, move your head, make facial expressions, or create eye movements each time you present a tone. Be familiar with your equipment so you can operate the dials without looking at the equipment and keep your eyes on the child. If you must look at your equipment, lower your eyes to see the audiometer controls and watch the child with your peripheral vision. If the child notices a pattern of tone presentation or movements by the examiner, he or she might respond even though he or she does not actually hear a tone.*	These frequencies are essential for speech and language development because speech sounds occur in these frequencies.
6. Leave the frequency at 4,000 and switch the tone to the left ear. Test the left ear at 4,000, 2,000, and 1,000 Hz.	Establishes a pattern. By doing it this way, the dial is always set at 1,000 Hz in the beginning of a screening. If in doubt as to which ear has already been screened, check at which frequency the dial is set. If it is at 4,000 Hz, then you know that you have yet to check the left ear.
7. Record the result in each ear as either "pass" or "fail." If a child passes, the screening is complete. If the child fails, immediately perform a threshold test.	Passing is consistent response at all tone presentations in both ears. Failing means that the child did not respond to at least one of the tones presented in either ear.

PROCEDURE Threshold Test

Steps	Rationale/Points of Emphasis
1. Set the frequency selector at the failed frequency and set the hearing level dial at 40 dB. **caREminder** *The first threshold test is used to confirm the screening results. Screen the child on the frequency that was failed. For example, if he or she did not respond to the tone at 1,000 and 2,000 Hz in the right ear, resulting in failing the sweep screen, only perform a threshold test on the right ear at 1,000 and 2,000 Hz.*	The goal is to introduce a sound that is loud enough to elicit a response but not too loud so sound is transmitted to the ear that is not being tested.
2. Depress the interrupter switch for 1 to 2 seconds and then release. Observe for child's response.	Presents tone and allows time to elicit a response.
3. If the child responds, consider this as his or her upper threshold. If the child does not respond, set the hearing level at 50 dB and present the tone again. If necessary, increase the hearing level 10 dB at a time until the child responds. At the level at which a response is noted, increase by 10 dB one more time.	This determines the upper limit of the child's threshold. Increasing the level by 10 dB one more time ensures that the child is able to hear the tone well. The upper threshold level means that his or her hearing is not worse than that level.
4. Once you have the upper threshold, decrease the level from that point by 10 decibels. If the child responds, continue decreasing the level by 10 dB	Establishes the child's lower threshold. This means that his or her hearing level is not better than this level.

Continued

Steps	Rationale/Points of Emphasis
until the child does not respond. The last level at which the child responds is his or her lower threshold.	**caREminder** *Establishing the upper and lower limits brackets the child's threshold; the actual threshold is some level between these two.*
5. Starting with the lower limit, increase the intensity by 5 dB until the threshold is reached.	The child's threshold is the lowest hearing level at which the subject responds at least 50% of the time.
6. Repeat the previous step and compare results. They should not differ by more than 5 dB in either direction. If there is a difference of 10 dB or more between the two tests, verify that the child understands the instructions and repeat the threshold test on the ear.	Ensures reliability of test result.
7. Record results. Advise the parent and child that a second screening is needed in 2 to 6 weeks.	A child may fail a hearing screening for numerous reasons, such as otitis media, nasal congestion, sinusitis, or allergic reaction. If the child passes the second screening, referral is not indicated. If the child fails the second screening, refer the child to an audiologist, audiometrist, or other hearing specialist.

PROCEDURE Play Audiometry

Steps	Rationale/Points of Emphasis
1. Set up equipment and position the child as for a sweep or threshold screening but do not place the earphones on the child. Inform the child that the two of you will be playing a game. Set the hearing level at 90-dB tone and the frequency at 4,000 Hz; hold the earphones or place them on table, present the tone, and respond in an exaggerated animated manner.	Presenting the screening as a game makes it fun for the child and optimizes response. Set the tone at 90 dB so that both you and the child can hear the beep without the earphone. **KidKare** Play audiometry is the preferred method when testing a developmentally delayed or a non-English-speaking child, no matter what the age. In screening a child with a disability such as poor muscle control (e.g., cerebral palsy) or lack of extremity (congenital anomaly), a verbal response can be elicited instead. The child may say "yes" or "I hear it" every time the beep is heard, instead of raising his or her hand.
2. Place the empty bowl on the table in front of the child; keep all the blocks on your side of the table. Give both the child and yourself a block. Explain the game: "When you hear the beep, put the block in the bowl."	Keeps the instruction short and simple to facilitate understanding: beep . . . block . . . bowl.
3. Depress the interrupter switch and as the beep goes off, put a block in the bowl. The child automatically copies you and places the block in the bowl. If the child does not do it, gently direct the child's hand to the bowl and help him or her drop it in. Respond to the child's attempts with enthusiasm and animated facial expressions.	Orients the child to the appropriate response. Positive reaction to the child's responses helps keep the screening interesting and rewarding for the child.
4. Play the game again and let the child "win" by letting him or her put the block in first and then put your block in. Make a big deal about the child winning the game.	This keeps the child excited and motivates him or her to keep playing the game. **KidKare** Give the child one block at a time, before presenting a tone. Giving all the blocks before the screening may confuse the child.

Steps	Rationale/Points of Emphasis
5. Play the game again, but this time, do not join the game. Give the child a block but do not take one for yourself. Respond very positively and enthusiastically.	Evaluates the child's understanding of the desired response and keeps him or her enthused.
6. Set the hearing level to 50 dB and place the earphones on the child. Give him or her a block. Play the game again.	The audiometer is set, initially, to a louder level to ensure that the child can easily hear the sound.
7. Set the intensity to 25 dB and continue screening using play audiometry following the procedures in the identification audiometry.	The only difference is that the child puts a block in the bowl instead of raising his or her hand.
8. Record results.	Results obtained may vary with the child's developmental level.

CHILD AND FAMILY EVALUATION AND DOCUMENTATION

- Sweep screening results are reported as either "pass" or "fail."
- Document threshold screening results by filling out a report form or data sheet specifically used for hearing screening that details result for each ear in each tone/intensity and frequency.
- Children who fail must be rescreened in 2 to 6 weeks before referral to an audiologist is made. Ensure follow-up for these children.

COMMUNITY CARE

- Rescreen children who fail the initial screening and refer those who fail the second screening to a hearing specialist.
- Advise the parent and the child to avoid exposure to loud noise; hearing loss associated with noise exposure can occur at any age. Advise teenagers to avoid risk factors for hearing loss such as exposure to high-intensity sound sources.
- Ensure that the audiometer is calibrated annually per manufacturer's instructions.
- Instruct the family to contact the healthcare provider if
  - Child with a normal hearing suddenly appears to be having difficulty following directions
  - Child complains of pain in the ear or if there is visible drainage from the ear

Unexpected Situation

- *The child does not respond during play audiometry on the right ear:* Perform test on the left ear. If there is still no response, remove the earphones and play the game as above to verify that the child understands the directions. If he does not respond when the earphones are on, then he fails the test.

Bibliography

American Academy of Pediatrics. (2003). Hearing assessment in infants and children: Recommendations beyond neonatal screening. *Pediatrics, 111*, 436–440.

California Department of Health Services. (2005, September). *Manual for the school audiometrist.* Children's Medical Services Branch, Department of Health Services, Health and Welfare Agency. Retrieved August 21, 2006, from http://www.dhs.ca.gov/pcfh/cms/publications/pdf/audmanschool.pdf.

Helfer, T., Lee, R., Maris, D., & Shields, A. (2003). Wanted: A national standard for early hearing detection and intervention outcomes data. *American Journal of Audiology, 12*, 23–30.

Kemper, A. R., Fant, K. E., Bruckman, D., & Clark, S. J. (2004). Hearing and vision screening program for school-aged children. *American Journal of Preventive Medicine, 26*, 141–146.

Sabo, D., Paradise, J., Kurs-Lasky, M., & Smith, C. (2003). Hearing levels in infants and young children in relation to testing technique, age group, and the presence or absence of middle-ear effusion. *Ear & Hearing, 24*, 38–47.

Welham, N., & Flynn, M. (2002). Developing, implementing, and evaluating a hearing screening programme in the speech-language pathology clinic setting. *Advances in Speech-Language Pathology, 4*, 23–31.

CHAPTER

46

Hemodynamic Monitoring: Central Venous Pressure

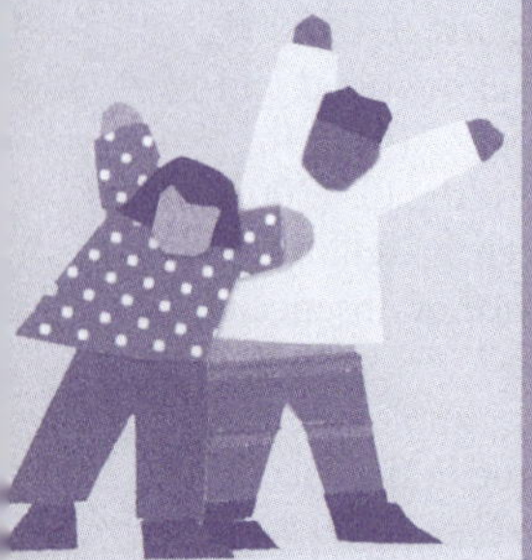

Clinical Guidelines

- Central venous pressure (CVP) monitoring is ordered by the healthcare prescriber for the purpose of assessing the critically ill child by providing information about the body's fluid volume status and right heart function.
- The registered nurse (RN) caring for the child should have a good understanding of
  - Principles of hemodynamic monitoring
  - Cardiac anatomy and physiology
  - Physiology of fluid and electrolyte balance and imbalance
  - Pathophysiology of heart disease and hemodynamic alterations expected with cardiac interventions and surgery
- The nurse caring for the child is competent to prepare and care for hemodynamic monitoring equipment, evaluate waveforms and their data, and make clinical decisions regarding changes in the child's therapy.
- CVP is the pressure measured at the tip of a catheter that is centrally placed within the right atrium of the heart. The insertion of such a centrally placed catheter can be performed at the bedside under surgical sterile conditions.
- CVP catheter insertion sites can include femoral, antecubital, jugular, subclavian, umbilical, or transthoracic placement.
- The child undergoing CVP monitoring is maintained in an intensive care setting.
- Informed consent to complete the insertion of the central line is obtained. Such consent may be incorporated into the general consent for treatment in the intensive care setting.
- Sedation and pain management of the child with CVP monitoring are implemented on an individual basis according to the child's needs.

Equipment

Refer to Chapter 47, as the following equipment should already be at bedside:

- Sterile single-, double-, or triple-lumen catheter for central venous placement (healthcare prescriber or institutional preference)
- A 250-mL bag of normal saline (with or without 1 unit of heparin per milliliter of normal saline, as prescribed by healthcare prescriber placing catheter)
- Pressure bag or intravenous (IV) pump
- Transducer holder on an IV pole or other holding device

- Disposable pressure transducer system (per institutional preference)
- Individual institution monitoring system and equipment (i.e., module, bedside monitor, cable, and hookup)
- Syringe pump or microinfusion pump (for severely fluid-restricted children)
- Carpenter's level
- Sedation and pain medications (as ordered)

CHILD AND FAMILY ASSESSMENT AND PREPARATION

- Assess the cognitive level, readiness, and ability to process information of the child and family.
- In collaboration with other healthcare team members, identify and discuss the risks and benefits of monitoring with the family.
- Assess the child for significant past medical history (i.e., heart, lung, liver, or renal disease, infections or sepsis) and past surgical history.
- Assess the child for history of any previous CVP catheter placement or any other catheter that may be present within the central venous system. Inform the healthcare prescriber of the location of the previous hemodynamic monitoring site and intravascular or intracardiac shunts. Assess for any complications that may have occurred during any previous procedures for catheter placement.
- Assess for signs of fluid deficit (i.e., sunken fontanel, lethargy, poor skin turgor, tachycardia, dry mucous membranes, dark and sunken orbits, decreased urine output).
- Assess for signs of fluid overload (i.e., wet and congested breath sounds, bulging fontanel, fluid intake greater than output, excessive weight gain, dependent edema).
- Assess the child's need for sedation and pain management.

PROCEDURE **Central Venous Pressure Monitoring**

Steps	Rationale/Points of Emphasis
1. Proceed with catheter placement as described in Chapter 47. Confirm proper placement with chest x-ray after CVP line insertion.	Placement of a CVP catheter is used to monitor and obtain hemodynamic readings for evaluation of intravascular volume status, venous return, and right heart function. **caREminder** *When using double- or triple-lumen central venous catheters, the distal lumen (closest to the RA) is recommended for CVP monitoring. The "pigtail" connected to each lumen is color-coded with the gauge and the location (proximal, medial, distal) printed on it.*
2. Review baseline data—vital signs, level of consciousness, hemodynamic stability—of the child.	Assists in identifying any acute changes in child. Fluid volume deficit usually corresponds with a decreased CVP, and this should be noted when considering the child's overall clinical status. Fluid volume overload usually corresponds with an increased CVP, and this should be noted when considering the child's overall clinical status.
3. Assess sedation and pain management needs of the child in collaboration with the healthcare prescriber. Administer sedation and pain management medications as indicated.	Ensures child's comfort during the procedure.
4. Observe and assess the IV pressure bag infusion device used to maintain patency of the CVP catheter by infusing heparinized normal saline or D5W. Ensure 300-mm Hg inflation pressure on the attached manometer. Reinflate as necessary by turning stopcock open to inflation and squeezing air into balloon hand pump. If using IV pump, ensure flow rate is correct. ***Alert!*** *Neonates and infants or children who are severely fluid restricted may require placement of the CVP infusion fluid using a syringe pump or microinfusion device to limit the flow of infused fluid. Flow rate amounts are variable and are dictated by patient size and fluid restriction. Tubing is available that is capable of delivering as little as 0.3 mL/hr.*	Pressure is required for most flush devices to avoid blood backup and to maintain line patency. When inflated to 300 mm Hg of pressure, most flush devices deliver 3 mL/hr of fluid. The amount of pressure in the infusion device decreases naturally over time because fluid infuses and must be reinflated periodically.

Steps	Rationale/Points of Emphasis
5. Maintain the position of the transducer stopcock on the IV pole level with the child's right atrium. While using the carpenter's level, move the air–fluid interface of the disposable pressure monitoring system, up or down, along the IV pole, so that the chamber is level with the right atrium of the child's heart, usually at the fourth intercostal space, midaxillary line (phlebostatic axis).	Ensures accuracy of readings by eliminating hydrostatic forces on the transducer (see Figure 47-1 in Chapter 47).
6. Zero-balance and calibrate the transducer at the start of each shift by turning the stopcock above the transducer off to the patient line and by opening the stopcock on the transducer to air, and then pressing the 0 (zero) button on the bedside monitor.	By opening the stopcock to air, the monitor uses atmospheric pressure as a reference for zero. Pressing the zero button negates the effects of atmospheric pressure, so that the pressure values reflect only that of the patient.
7. Return transducer stopcock back to monitoring open position to start pressure monitoring. Check that the stopcock above the transducer is now open to monitoring.	Pressure monitoring cannot occur if stopcocks are not in the correct positions. (Refer to manufacturer's system instructions for correct stopcock placement.)
8. CVP waveform and mean reading should be continuously monitored and interpreted, along with electrocardiogram (ECG) and other monitor tracings (Figure 46-1). See Chart 46-1 to assist in identifying and managing problems with the CVP equipment and waveform.	A continuous waveform and readout is provided at the child's bedside monitor along with ECG and other monitor tracings, which allows the nurse to identify any acute or gradual changes and make clinical decisions based on these changes.

caREminder

The normal mean CVP reading in children is 5 to 15 mm Hg. Normal waveform components of the CVP include the A wave (mechanical atrial systole), c wave (increase in RA pressure from closure of the tricuspid valve), and V wave (mechanical atrial diastole).

***Alert!** Appropriate pressure alarms should be on at all times during monitoring to provide an alert to clinical changes in the child's condition or equipment malfunction.*

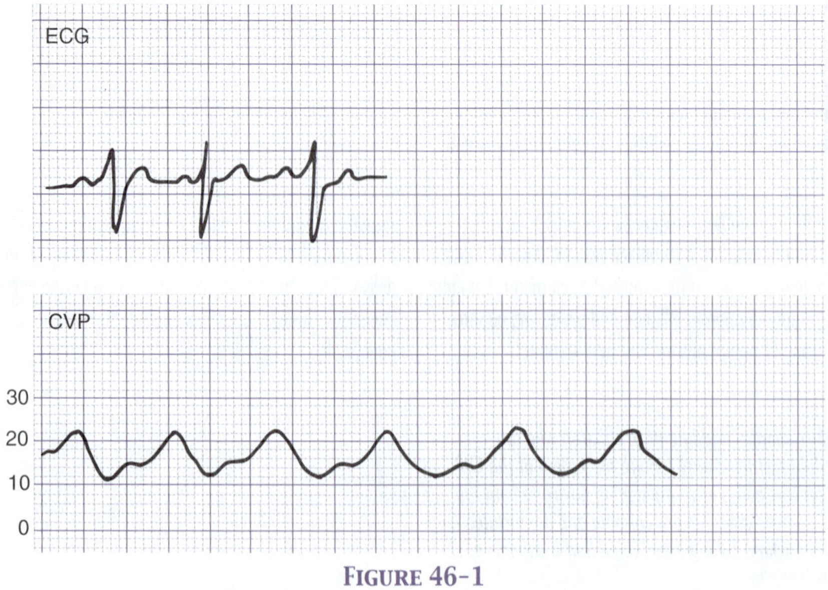

FIGURE 46-1
Typical central venous pressure waveform.

CHART 46-1 TROUBLESHOOTING THE CVP LINE

Problem	Management and Rationale
Absent or dampened waveform	• Assess child and ensure there has not been a change in condition resulting in fall in CVP. Onset of hypovolemia or shock could lead to fall in CVP that mimics dampened waveform. • Ensure that all stopcocks are open to the monitoring transducer with dead-end caps (not vented caps) in place. Improper stopcock positioning prevents waveform transmission to the monitor. Vented caps allow air entry into the system—replace all vented caps with dead-end caps (refer to manufacturer's system instructions for correct stopcock placement). • Check throughout the course of the tubing for air bubbles and ensure that no air bubbles are present. Air can dampen the transmission of the actual waveform and result in falsely low values. • Ensure that transducer is securely plugged in to monitor and bedside monitor is on. Monitor must be on and plugged in to function properly. • Ensure that the correct scale on bedside monitor has been chosen in relation to pressure being monitored (i.e., 30-mm Hg scale for CVP monitoring). A large scale may cause the waveform to be much smaller; therefore, it may not be visible on bedside monitor. • Ensure that transducer and accompanying cable is not faulty. Replace if necessary. A faulty transducer or cable results in an absent waveform. • Ensure that pressure bag is inflated to 300 mm Hg and that infusion device is functioning properly. Low pressure may result in dampened waveform or clotted catheter. • Check that all connections of CVP transducer tubing are tight, without leaks. Loose connections can allow air into the tubing. • Ensure blood can aspirate through catheter. A clotted catheter has no waveform and cannot draw blood.
Blood backing up into catheter	• Ensure that all connections are closed to air and are tight. Blood may exert a backpressure on system on flow back to open stopcocks. • Ensure pressure bag is inflated and IV-controlled infusion device is infusing. Low backpressure may result in blood backup.
Excessively peaked waveform	• Ensure placement of CVP catheter in right atrium. Obtain chest x-ray as necessary to confirm proper placement. If CVP catheter has migrated into right ventricle of heart, the healthcare prescriber will pull back line as necessary. • Ensure that CVP catheter is in vein and not artery. Obtain blood gas from line and assess for arterial parameters. Discontinue line if necessary (per institutional policy).
Lack of blood return from catheter when aspirating	• Blood should aspirate easily from catheter lumen. Follow institutional protocols for line flushing as indicated. Inform the healthcare prescriber if a lumen does not show blood return with aspiration. A chest x-ray may be ordered to evaluate catheter position. Lack of blood return when aspirating may indicate clotting of the catheter lumen, catheter against the vessel wall, or catheter malposition.

CHILD AND FAMILY EVALUATION AND DOCUMENTATION

- Evaluate the child regularly for potential complications of central venous catheters, which can include venous air embolism, vessel wall perforation, pneumothorax, dysrhythmias, catheter-related thrombosis, and catheter-related infections. Inform the healthcare prescriber immediately if any complications occur.
- Evaluate the child regularly for signs or symptoms of fluid imbalance. Include intake and output at least every 2 hours on the child's record.
- Ensure that appropriate alarms are set and kept on at all times. Document alarm settings and that alarms are on.
- Evaluate the CVP system setup regularly for air bubble formation because they can be potentially lethal if infused into the child. Remove air emboli by flushing through a system stopcock.

- Evaluate the child regularly for signs or symptoms of a catheter-related infection, which can include but are not limited to fever, chills, tachycardia, increased white blood cell counts, redness or swelling at catheter insertion site, and positive blood cultures.
- Document the following:
  - Catheter insertion site, position, placement, catheter size, skin assessment at insertion site, type and amount of flush solution per hour, and amount of heparin (e.g., a right antecubital 7-French triple-lumen catheter, cutdown for CVP placement, infusing 1 unit of heparin per milliliter of normal saline at 3 mL/hr; insertion site clean and dry without inflammation or infiltrate and with sutures intact; chest x-ray reveals catheter tip in right atrium)
  - Color, warmth, and pulse strength of the extremity, distal to the catheter insertion site, every 2 to 4 hours, on the appropriate institutional form
  - Cardiopulmonary assessment and vital signs of the child, along with the CVP reading, at least every 2 hours. Mount a readout strip of the CVP into the child's record at the beginning of each shift. Assess waveform for changes and troubleshoot the line, as necessary.
  - Pain assessment, need for sedation, and all interventions (pharmacologic and nonpharmacologic) used to maintain the child's comfort
  - Dates and times that monitoring lines are changed along with catheter site dressing change dates and times. Dressing changes should be done per institutional protocols.
- Determine whether the child or family has any other concerns to discuss. Document educational and supportive interventions related to child or family concerns.

COMMUNITY CARE

- If the child is to be discharged home soon after removal of a CVP catheter, instruct the child and family to observe the insertion site for signs and symptoms of drainage, redness, swelling, or fever.
- Instruct the family to contact the healthcare provider if
  - Catheter site shows signs of drainage, redness, or swelling
  - Child develops a fever
  - Child develops any motor or sensory changes in the catheterized limb

Unexpected Situation

- *Blood is backed up in the pressure tubing:* Ensure that all connections are closed to air and are tight. Ensure pressure bag is inflated and IV-controlled infusion device is infusing. Flush tubing slowly to reinsert blood back into the child. Tubing may need to be replaced if blood residue remains.

Bibliography

American Association of Critical Care Nurses. (2006). *Core curriculum for pediatric critical care nursing.* Philadelphia: W. B. Saunders.

Cartwright, D. (2004). Central venous lines in neonates: A study of 2186 catheters. *Archives of Disease in Childhood–Fetal & Neonatal Edition, 89*, F504–F508.

Darovic, G., & Zbilut, J. (2002). Fluid-filled monitoring systems. In G. Darovic (Ed.), *Hemodynamic monitoring: Invasive and noninvasive clinical applications* (3rd ed.). Philadelphia: W. B. Saunders.

McGee, D. C., & Gould, M. K. (2003). Preventing complications of central venous catheterization. *The New England Journal of Medicine, 348*, 1123–1133.

Metz, L. C., & Whitford, K. (1996). Fluid delivery by pressure monitoring systems in the pediatric intensive care unit: A retrospective comparative analysis of two systems. *American Journal of Critical Care, 5*, 66–67.

Tibby, S. M., & Murdoch, I. A. (2003). Monitoring cardiac function in intensive care. *Archives of Disease in Childhood, 88*, 46–52.

Vettukattil, J., Thomas, E., & Salmon, A. (2003). Safe retrieval of impacted central venous line. *Archives of Disease in Childhood, 88*, 630–631.

CHAPTER

47

Hemodynamic Monitoring: Insertion and Setup for Central Venous Pressure and Intraarterial Blood Pressure Monitoring

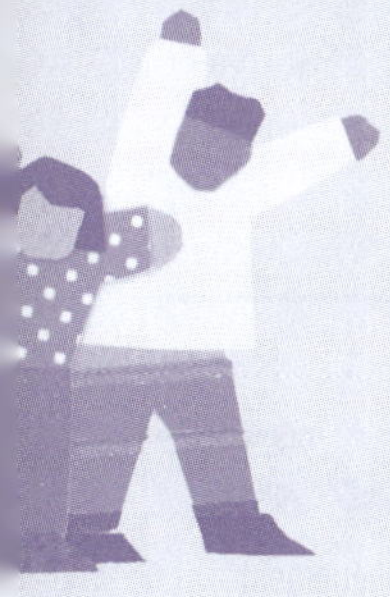

CLINICAL GUIDELINES

- Hemodynamic monitoring is ordered by the healthcare prescriber for the purpose of assessing the critically ill child by
  - Early identification of life-threatening conditions
  - Evaluating immediate responses to therapies
  - Assisting in medical diagnosis determination
- The registered nurse (RN) caring for the child is competent to prepare and care for hemodynamic monitoring equipment, evaluate waveforms and their data, and make clinical decisions regarding changes in the child's therapy.
- The child with hemodynamic monitoring is maintained in an intensive care setting.
- Informed consent to complete this procedure is obtained. Such consent may be incorporated into the general consent for treatment in the intensive care setting.
- Sedation and pain management of the child with hemodynamic monitoring is implemented on an individual basis according to the child's needs.

EQUIPMENT

- Several masks, caps, protective eyewear, sterile gloves, and gowns
- Clean, dry bedside table
- Disposable pressure transducer system (per institutional preference)
- 250-mL bag of normal saline (with or without 1 unit heparin per milliliter of normal saline, as prescribed by healthcare prescriber placing catheter)
- Flush tubing
- Pressure bag or intravenous (IV) pump
- Syringe pump or microinfusion pump (for severely fluid-restricted children)

- Transducer holder on an IV pole or other holding device
- Individual institution monitoring system and equipment (i.e., module, bedside monitor, cable, and hookup)
- Sterile towels
- Antiseptic solution (chlorhexidine is preferred)
- Several sterile normal saline vials
- Sterile syringes (assortment of sizes: 3, 5, and 10 mL, and tuberculin)
- Lidocaine (Xylocaine) local anesthetic (0.5% or 1%)
- Sterile catheter for arterial placement (healthcare prescriber or institutional preference) *or*
- Sterile single-, double-, or triple-lumen catheter for central venous placement (healthcare prescriber or institutional preference)
- Suture material (per healthcare prescriber preference)
- Sterile transparent dressing
- Carpenter's level
- Surgical light (optional for healthcare prescriber)
- Sedation and pain medications (as ordered)
- Armboard or limb-immobilization device (if needed)

CHILD AND FAMILY ASSESSMENT AND PREPARATION

- Assess the cognitive level, readiness, and ability to process information by the child and family.
- Reinforce the need for device placement, as appropriate, to both the child and family.
- In collaboration with other healthcare team members, identify and discuss the risks and benefits of monitoring with the family.
- Ensure that informed consent has been obtained as needed per institutional policy.

CHART 47-1 HOW TO PERFORM THE ALLEN'S TEST

The test is used to determine the integrity of the blood supply to the hand.

- With the hand elevated, both the ulnar and the radial arteries are occluded, which leads to blanching of the hand.
- Then, one of the arteries is released; normally, the blanching disappears over the whole of the hand. Failure of the blood to diffuse into the hand when opened indicates that the artery not compressed is occluded.
- This is repeated with both arteries. If the hand remains pale, the blood is often collected from another artery, usually in the groin or elbow crease.

- Observe child for signs and symptoms of gradual or acute hypotension/hypertension, dysrhythmias, circulatory collapse, cardiac arrest, hemorrhage, hypoxemia, metabolic acidosis/alkalosis, fluid imbalance, diminished mental status, or laboratory abnormalities.
- Assess the child for history of any previous hemodynamic catheter placement. Inform the healthcare prescriber of the location of the previous hemodynamic monitoring site and of any complications that may have occurred during any previous procedures.

caREminder

Allen's test should be performed before radial artery insertion of an intraarterial catheter (Chart 47-1).

PROCEDURE Inserting and Setting Up for Hemodynamic Monitoring

Steps	Rationale/Points of Emphasis
1. Perform hand hygiene. Gather the necessary supplies.	Reduces transmission of microorganisms. Promotes efficient time management and provides an organized approach to the procedure. **caREminder** *This is a sterile procedure. Reduce traffic in the area as much as possible during the procedure.*

Steps	Rationale/Points of Emphasis
2. Obtain baseline data—vital signs, level of consciousness, hemodynamic stability—of child.	Assists to identify any acute changes in child during and after the procedure. Prompt treatment of critical illness is associated with improved chances of survival. The earlier signs and symptoms of critical illness are identified, the sooner a hemodynamic monitoring device can be placed for patient assessment and monitoring.
3. Assess sedation and pain management needs of the child in collaboration with the healthcare prescriber. Administer sedation and pain management medications as indicated.	Ensures child's comfort during the procedure.
4. Open prepackaged pressure transducer system and secure any loose connectors.	Prepackaged systems often have loose connections for sterilization purposes. Loose connections or vented caps provide an entry for bacteria, microorganisms, and air. **caREminder** *All air must be expelled from the system because this can affect the waveform and can be potentially lethal to the child if air bubbles enter the bloodstream, causing air emboli.*
5. Spike the 250-mL bag of normal saline with the flush tubing, open the roller clamp, and gravity purge the normal saline throughout the flush tubing and disposable pressure tubing system, including all stopcocks. Replace any vented caps with dead-end Luer-Lok caps. **Alert!** *Neonates and infants or children who are severely fluid restricted may require placing the 250-mL bag of normal saline to a syringe pump or microinfusion device to limit the flow of infused fluid.*	Accesses IV flush solution, primes the drip chamber, and flushes tubing and the pressure tubing system. This eliminates air from the system and provides a column of fluid needed to transmit pressure waveforms.
6. Place the normal saline bag within the IV pressure bag and inflate pressure bag to 300 mm Hg. If using a pump, validate the flow rate.	Pressure is required for most flush devices to avoid blood backup and to maintain line patency. When inflated to 300 mm Hg pressure, most flush devices deliver 3 mL/hr of fluid. **KidKare** Flow rates are variable and are dictated by patient size and fluid restriction. Tubing is available that is capable of delivering as little as 0.3 mL/hr.
7. Attach disposable pressure transducer to holder/manifold that is secured to an IV pole or other device. Note that the tubing to deliver the flush is positioned pretransducer and is soft and compliant; the tubing that transmits the pressure wave from the patient to the transducer is hard and noncompressible.	Secures transducer to pole and ensures easy repositioning of the transducer for correct leveling during position changes. Noncompressible tubing, located post-transducer to the patient, ensures that external pressure (e.g., kinking) cannot falsely influence pressure readings.
8. Turn on institutional bedside monitoring device, plug in transducer cabling, set program monitor for the appropriate pressure to be measured (i.e., arterial line reading or central venous pressure reading), and plug monitoring cable into disposable pressure transducer system (Figure 47-1).	Allows for signal transmission to monitor along with waveform display and pressure readings.

Continued

Steps	Rationale/Points of Emphasis

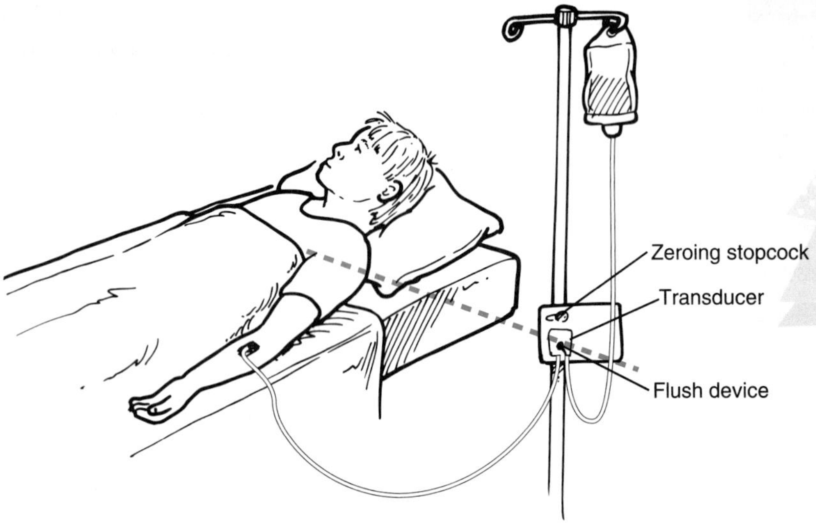

FIGURE 47-1
Place the hemodynamic monitoring transducer level with the right atrium of the child's heart.

Steps	Rationale/Points of Emphasis
9. Position the child for catheter access by the healthcare prescriber, while maintaining sterile access for the healthcare prescriber.	Facilitates ease of access for catheter placement.
10. Restrain limbs as necessary to ensure sterility of procedure.	Keeps child from moving and violating sterile field required for catheterization. **caREminder** *Depending on where the catheter is placed, an armboard or limb-immobilization device may be required.*
11. Don sterile attire.	Standard precaution for surgical sterile procedure.
12. Assist the healthcare prescriber with sterile placement of the catheter line. The healthcare prescriber will obtain a sterile field and sterile prep of the child, using sterile towels and chlorhexidine to cleanse the insertion site.	Identifies access site. Reduces the risk for infection from microorganisms. **caREminder** *The healthcare prescriber may request additional sedation for the child during the procedure. Have sterile normal saline, syringes, lidocaine (Xylocaine), and sutures available and ready during catheter insertion.*
13. Assist the healthcare prescriber as needed throughout the procedure and continually assess child for any changes in vital signs, level of consciousness, or hemodynamic status.	Provides baseline for ongoing assessment and monitoring.
14. When catheter insertion is completed and secured into place, assist the healthcare prescriber in attaching the disposable transducer monitoring system to the catheter.	Allows hemodynamic waveform to be continuously monitored along with electrocardiogram and other monitor tracings.
15. Recheck system for tight connections and absence of any air bubbles.	Identifies any loose connections or potential sites for infection or air emboli.
16. Assist in placing a semipermeable transparent dressing over the catheter insertion site. Label dressing with date and time.	Protects the site from microorganisms and allows for continuous visualization of the insertion site if it becomes infected or inflamed.
17. Position the child in bed after catheter insertion, and, using the carpenter's level, move the air–fluid interface of the disposable pressure monitoring	Ensures accuracy of readings by eliminating hydrostatic forces on the transducer. If the transducer is lower than the RA, pressure readings will be falsely

Steps	Rationale/Points of Emphasis
system up or down along the IV pole, so that the chamber is level with the right atrium of the child's heart, usually at the fourth intercostal space, midaxillary line (phlebostatic axis).	elevated; if the transducer is higher than the RA, pressure readings will be falsely lowered.
18. Turn the stopcock above the transducer off to the patient line. Zero-balance and calibrate the transducer by opening the stopcock on the transducer to air, removing the dead-end cap, and then pressing the zero button on the bedside monitor. When completed, the monitor will display a message that indicates zeroing is completed.	By opening the stopcock to air, the monitor uses atmospheric pressure as a reference for zero. Pressing the zero button negates the effects of atmospheric pressure, so that the pressure values reflect only that of the patient.
19. Return transducer stopcock back to the monitoring position and replace the dead-end cap to start pressure monitoring. Check that the stopcock above the transducer is now open to monitoring.	Pressure monitoring cannot occur if stopcocks are not in the correct positions. (Refer to manufacturer's system instructions for correct stopcock placement.)
20. Consult with healthcare prescriber whether an order for an x-ray is necessary to check catheter placement.	Central venous catheters are normally radiopaque and should be visualized to ensure they are correctly placed. Chest x-ray ensures correct placement and can identify complications (e.g., pneumothorax) that can occur during placement.
21. Dispose of equipment and waste in appropriate receptacle. Perform hand hygiene.	Standard precautions. Reduces transmission of microorganisms.

CHILD AND FAMILY EVALUATION AND DOCUMENTATION

- Monitor the child's vital signs and note trends in pressure wave readings, at least every 2 hours, on the appropriate institutional form. Correlate pressure readings with the child's clinical condition and hemodynamic responses to therapies.
- Evaluate the child regularly for signs or symptoms of a catheter-related infection, which can include but are not limited to fever, chills, tachycardia, increased white blood cell counts, redness or swelling at catheter insertion site, and positive blood cultures.
- Document the following:
  - Date and time of insertion, assessments, the insertion site position, and placement (i.e., right antecubital cutdown), catheter size used, type of flush solution (and amount of heparin, if any), and child's response to the procedure on the appropriate institutional forms
  - Color, warmth, and pulse strength of the extremity, distal to the catheter insertion site, every 2 to 4 hours, on the appropriate institutional form
  - Amount of flush solution infused hourly, on the appropriate institutional form
  - Pain assessment, need for sedation, and all interventions (pharmacologic and nonpharmacologic) used to maintain child's comfort

COMMUNITY CARE

- If the child is to be discharged home soon after removal of a central venous pressure (CVP) catheter or arterial line, instruct the child and family to observe the insertion site for signs and symptoms of drainage, redness, swelling, or fever.
- Instruct the family to contact the healthcare provider if
  - Catheter site shows signs of drainage, redness, or swelling
  - Child develops a fever
  - Child develops any motor or sensory changes in the catheterized limb

Unexpected Situation

- *The CVP waveform becomes dampened:* Assess tubing for air bubbles. Assess pressure of IV pressure bag. Assess tubing connections and stopcock position. Ensure transducer is plugged in and monitor is on. Zero-balance and recalibrate the transducer.

Bibliography

American Association of Critical Care Nurses. (2006). *Core curriculum for pediatric critical care nursing.* Philadelphia: W. B. Saunders.

Darovic, G., & Zbilut, J. (2002). Fluid-filled monitoring systems. In G. Darovic (Ed.), *Hemodynamic monitoring: Invasive and noninvasive clinical applications* (3rd ed.). Philadelphia: W. B. Saunders.

Infusion Nurses Society. (2002). *Policies and procedures for infusion nursing* (2nd ed.). Cambridge, MA: Author.

McGee, D. C., & Gould, M. K. (2003). Preventing complications of central venous catheterization. *The New England Journal of Medicine, 348*(12), 1123–1133.

O'Grady, N. P., Alexander, M., Dellinger, E. P., et al. (2002). *Guidelines for the prevention of intravascular catheter-related infections.* Atlanta, GA: Centers for Disease Control and Prevention.

Tibby, S. M., & Murdoch, I. A. (2003). Monitoring cardiac function in intensive care. *Archives of Disease in Childhood, 88,* 46–52.

CHAPTER

48

Hemodynamic Monitoring: Intraarterial Pressure

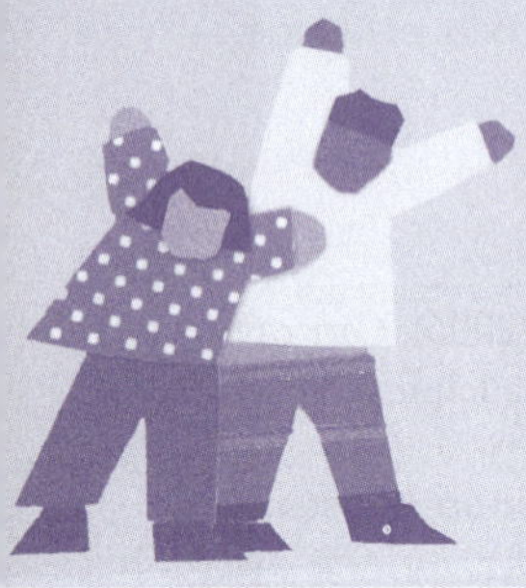

Clinical Guidelines

- Intraarterial pressure monitoring is ordered by the healthcare prescriber for the purpose of assessing the critically ill child by providing information about the arterial blood pressure (ABP).
- The registered nurse (RN) caring for the child has a good understanding of
  - The principles of ABP monitoring
  - Cardiac anatomy and physiology
  - Physiology of fluid and electrolyte balance and imbalance
  - Pathophysiology of heart disease and heart hemodynamic alterations expected with cardiac interventions and surgery
- The nurse caring for the child is competent to prepare and care for intraarterial monitoring equipment, evaluate waveforms and their data, and make clinical decisions regarding changes in the child's therapy.
- The nurse caring for a child with an intraarterial catheter plays an important role in preventing catheter complications with their inherent health risks. These may include
  - Infection at the insertion site, which can spread into the bloodstream
  - Clot formation within the catheter, which can then be carried into the general circulation
  - Catheter perforation of the vessel wall, which can be associated with excessive bleeding and extravasation of flush solution into the surrounding tissue
  - Impaired circulation to the extremity distal to the catheter insertion site, which, if not treated promptly, can cause loss of tissue or, ultimately, loss of limb
- Intraarterial monitoring in children is a particularly sensitive indicator of changes in cardiac output and blood volume.
- The insertion of arterial catheters can be performed at the bedside under sterile surgical conditions by the healthcare prescriber.
- Arterial catheter insertion sites can include placement in the radial (most common), dorsalis pedis, axillary, posterior tibial, umbilical, and femoral arteries.
- The child with intraarterial pressure monitoring is maintained in an intensive care setting.
- Informed consent to complete this procedure is obtained. Such consent may be incorporated into the general consent for treatment in the intensive care setting.
- Sedation and pain management of the child with intraarterial pressure monitoring is implemented on an individual basis according to the child's needs.

EQUIPMENT

Refer to Chapter 47, as the following equipment should already be at the bedside:

- Arterial pressure catheter, labeled as arterial line (to avoid confusing arterial line with an intravenous line)
- A 250-mL bag of normal saline (with or without 1 unit of heparin per milliliter of normal saline, as prescribed by healthcare prescriber placing catheter)
- Pressure bag or intravenous (IV) pump
- Transducer holder secured on an IV pole or other holding device
- Disposable pressure transducer system (per institutional preference)
- Individual institution monitoring system and equipment (i.e., module, bedside monitor, cable, and hookup)
- Syringe pump or microinfusion pump (for severely fluid-restricted children)
- Carpenter's level

CHILD AND FAMILY ASSESSMENT AND PREPARATION

- Assess the cognitive level, readiness, and ability to process information of the child and family.
- In collaboration with other healthcare team members, identify and discuss the risks and benefits of monitoring with the family.
- Assess for signs that may warrant the use of intraarterial pressure monitoring (e.g., children at risk for circulatory collapse, cardiac arrest, hemorrhage, hypertensive crisis, shock, neurologic injury, postoperative complications, trauma, respiratory failure, or sepsis).
- Assess the child for significant past medical history (i.e., heart, lung, liver, or renal disease; infection or sepsis; diabetes; hypertension; and peripheral vascular disease).
- Assess the child for history of any previous intraarterial pressure catheter placement. Inform the healthcare prescriber of the location of the previous hemodynamic monitoring site and of any complications that may have occurred during any previous procedures.
- Assess for signs of fluid deficit (i.e., sunken fontanel, lethargy, poor skin turgor, tachycardia, dry mucous membranes, dark and sunken orbits, and decreased urine output).
- Assess for signs of fluid overload (i.e., wet and congested breath sounds, bulging fontanel, fluid intake greater than output, excessive weight gain, and dependent edema).
- Assess for hypotension/hypertension and causes of ABP alterations (i.e., changes in cardiac output, heart rate, stroke volume, and systemic vascular resistance).
- Assess the child's need for sedation and pain management.
- Instruct the child and family about the possibility of the use of restraints, sedation, or a limb-immobilization device.

PROCEDURE Monitoring Intracranial Pressure

Steps	Rationale/Points of Emphasis
1. Proceed with catheter placement as described in Chapter 47.	An intraarterial catheter is used to monitor and obtain hemodynamic readings for evaluation of blood pressure (systolic, diastolic, and mean) for cardiovascular monitoring of acutely ill children.
2. Review baseline data—vital signs, level of consciousness, hemodynamic stability—of child.	Assists to identify any acute changes in child during and after the procedure. Prompt treatment of critical illness is associated with improved chances of survival.
3. Assess sedation and pain management needs of the child in collaboration with the healthcare prescriber. Administer sedation and pain management medications as indicated.	Ensures child's comfort during the procedure.
4. Immobilize intraarterial catheter insertion site with the use of an armboard or limb restraint. Keep the catheter site visible at all times—do not allow linens to cover site.	Holds intraarterial catheter in place, helps prevent dislodgment of catheter with child movement, and helps prevent intraarterial catheter from lacerating internal vessel. The risk of an intraarterial line becoming dislodged leads to a high risk for exsanguination (in the pediatric/neonatal population, this can take place in a very short period of time and can be fatal). Overcoming a child's and family's fears and anxiety is important in repeatedly explaining the necessity of a device.

Steps	Rationale/Points of Emphasis
5. Observe the IV pressure bag and maintain inflation to 300 mm Hg; reinflate as necessary. If using a pump, validate the flow rate.	Pressure is required for most flush devices, and when inflated to 300 mm Hg of pressure, most flush devices deliver 3 mL/hr of IV fluid.
Alert! *Children who are severely fluid restricted may require placement of the 250-mL bag of normal saline to a syringe pump or microinfusion device to limit the flow of infused fluid. Flow rate amounts are variable and are dictated by patient size and fluid restriction. Tubing is available that is capable of delivering as little as 0.3 mL/hr.*	
6. Level the position of the transducer stopcock on the IV pole or other holding device, with the child's right atrium. While using the carpenter's level, move the air–fluid interface of the disposable pressure monitoring system up or down along the IV pole so that the chamber is level with the right atrium of the child's heart, usually at the fourth intercostal space, midaxillary line (phlebostatic axis).	Ensures accuracy of readings by eliminating hydrostatic forces on the transducer.
7. Zero-balance and calibrate the transducer at the start of each shift by turning the stopcock above the transducer off to the patient line and by opening the stopcock on the transducer to air and then pressing the 0 (zero) button on the bedside monitor.	By opening the stopcock to air, the monitor uses atmospheric pressure as a reference for zero. Pressing the zero button negates the effects of atmospheric pressure, so that the pressure values reflect only that of the patient.
8. Return transducer stopcock back to monitoring position to resume pressure monitoring.	Pressure monitoring cannot occur if stopcocks are not in the correct position. (Refer to manufacturer's system instructions for correct stopcock placement.)
9. Arterial blood pressure waveform and mean reading should be continuously monitored and interpreted, along with electrocardiogram (ECG) and other monitor tracings.	A continuous waveform and readout is provided at the child's bedside monitor along with ECG and other monitor tracings, which allows the nurse to identify any acute or gradual changes and make clinical decisions based on these changes.
Alert! *Appropriate pressure alarms should be on at all times during monitoring to provide an alert to clinical changes in the child's condition or equipment malfunction.*	
10a. Frequently assess that the pressure bag is inflated to 300 mm Hg.	Appropriate inflation is necessary for proper function of flush device to deliver 3 mL/hr of fluid and to prevent blood from back-flowing into the catheter.
10b. At least once per shift, ensure that there is flush solution in IV bag.	Continuous flush is necessary to keep the intraarterial catheter from clotting off.
10c. Continuously observe arterial waveform quality as viewed from monitor. Compare intraarterial pressure with cuff BP (should be within 10 mm Hg). A normal waveform has a peak systole, clear dicrotic notch, and end diastole.	Ensures accuracy of pressure waveform and detection of changes in child's hemodynamic status.
11. Troubleshoot the ABP waveform as problems occur. Notify healthcare prescriber as appropriate. If the intraarterial waveform suddenly becomes dampened:	
a. Check the child.	A sudden hypotensive episode can look like a dampened waveform on the monitor and can be potentially life-threatening if not treated properly.
b. Check the arterial line insertion site for catheter position.	For peripheral insertion of a catheter, movement of the child can cause kinking or dislodgment, resulting in dampened waveform.
c. Attempt to aspirate and flush the catheter.	Clots can form at the catheter tip and obstruct flow, causing a dampened waveform or emboli. Aspirate to pull back and dislodge the potential clot formation.

CHILD AND FAMILY EVALUATION AND DOCUMENTATION

- Evaluate the child regularly for potential complications of ABP catheters that can include air embolism, vessel wall perforation, exsanguination, catheter-related thrombosis, and catheter-related infections. Inform the healthcare prescriber immediately if any complications occur.
- Evaluate the configuration of the arterial waveform continuously because this can identify early dampening or changes and can alert the nurse to accidental disconnection or decreased cardiac output.
- Compare ABP pressure with cuff BP at least once per shift and record variance.
- Evaluate the child regularly for signs and symptoms of fluid imbalance, including intake and output, at least every 2 hours, and document on the child's record.
- Evaluate the ABP system setup regularly for air bubble formation; remove air emboli by flushing through a system stopcock because they can be potentially lethal if infused into the child.
- Evaluate the child regularly for signs and symptoms of a catheter-related infection, which can include but are not limited to fever, chills, tachycardia, increased white blood cell counts, redness or swelling at catheter insertion site, and positive blood cultures.
- Ensure that appropriate alarms are set and kept on at all times. Document alarm settings and that alarms are on.
- Document the following:
  - Catheter insertion site, position, and placement; catheter size; and type and amount of flush solution per hour and amount of heparin, if any (e.g., left radial 22-gauge arterial catheter, in place for continuous ABP readings; infusing 1 unit of heparin per milliliter of normal saline at 3 mL/hr)
  - Color, warmth, pulse strength, and capillary refill of the extremity, distal to the catheter insertion site, every 2 to 4 hours, on the appropriate institutional form
  - Cardiopulmonary assessment and vital signs of the child, along with the ABP reading, and record at least every 2 hours. At least once per shift, mount a readout strip of the ABP along with the continuous ECG strip and other hemodynamic waveforms into the child's record.
- Document the dates and times that monitoring lines are changed along with catheter site dressing change dates and times.
- Determine whether the child or family has any other concerns to discuss. Document educational and supportive interventions related to child or family concerns.

COMMUNITY CARE

- If the child is to be discharged home soon after removal of an intraarterial catheter, instruct the child and family to observe the insertion site for signs and symptoms of drainage, redness, swelling, or fever.
- Instruct the family to contact the healthcare provider if
  - Catheter site shows signs of drainage, redness, or swelling
  - Child develops a fever
  - Child develops motor or sensory changes in the catheterized limb

Unexpected Situation

- *The child is oozing blood from the arterial catheter site and the extremity is edematous with poor peripheral infusion:* The catheter may be dislodged or clotted. Check patency of the catheter to determine whether the catheter needs to be removed. If the catheter is patent, elevate extremity on pillow and re-secure site so that child's movements do not cause dislodgement.

Bibliography

American Association of Critical Care Nurses. (2006). *Core curriculum for pediatric critical care nursing.* Philadelphia: W. B. Saunders.

Darovic, G., & Zbilut, J. (2002). Fluid-filled monitoring systems. In G. Darovic (Ed.), *Hemodynamic monitoring: Invasive and noninvasive clinical applications* (3rd ed.) Philadelphia: W. B. Saunders.

Mims, B. C., Toto, K. H., Luecke, L. E., et al. (2004). *Critical care skills: A clinical handbook* (2nd ed.). Philadelphia: Elsevier.

Tibby, S. M., & Murdoch, I. A. (2003). Monitoring cardiac function in intensive care. *Archives of Disease in Childhood, 88,* 46–52.

CHAPTER 49

Heparin Lock/Flush

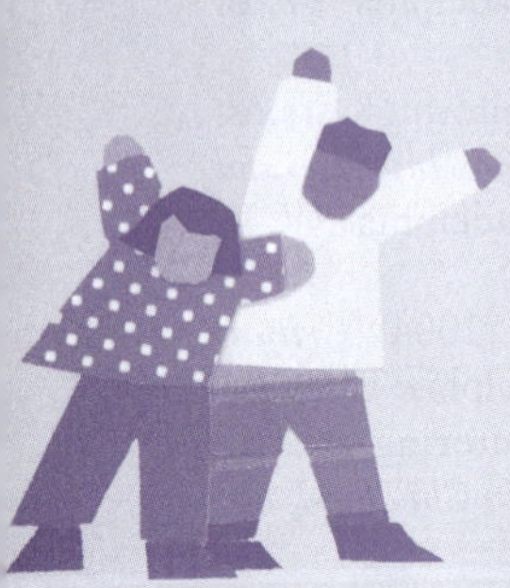

Clinical Guidelines

- The healthcare prescriber must order heparin locks and flushes.
- A physician, registered nurse (RN), or licensed practical nurse (LPN) may administer heparin flushes per state practice act.
- Children who do not require continuous intravenous (IV) infusion yet but may still require IV access for intermittent IV medication administration are considered candidates for a heparin lock.
- Heparin flushes and assessment of the IV site must be completed every 6 to 8 hours as ordered for optimal catheter maintenance.
- Flush peripheral catheters with heparin using the following:
  - Children and infants: 10 U/mL preservative-free normal saline
  - Neonates:
    - Weight <800 g: 2 U/mL in 5% dextrose solution
    - Weight 800 g to 1.5 kg: 2 U/mL preservative-free half-normal saline
    - Weight >1.5 kg: 10 U/mL preservative-free normal saline
- See Chapters 56, 57, and 58 for recommendations regarding heparin flushing of other types of IV access devices.
- Saline flushes may be considered a safe and effective alternative to heparin flushes. Research has supported the efficacy of saline flushes to maintain the patency of an intermittent IV access site for children of all ages, including neonates, using catheters of 24 gauge and larger (see Chapter 104). Heparin continues to be used based on physician preference and when cannula size is less than 24 gauge.

Equipment

- Nonsterile gloves
- Alcohol swabs
- Heparin pre-prepared 10-U/mL syringe with injection cartridge *or* vial of heparin solution, 10 U/mL, and a 3-mL needleless syringe
- Needleless male adapter (injection cap), if converting an IV continuous infusion to a heparin lock
- Vial of saline sterile solution 0.9%, if converting heparin lock to primary continuous infusion

Child and Family Assessment and Preparation

- Assess the cognitive level, readiness, and ability to process information by the child and family. The readiness to learn and process information may be impaired as a result of age, stress, or anxiety.

- Reinforce the need for, and identify and discuss the risks and benefits of, heparin lock placement, as appropriate, to both the child and family. Explain the signs and symptoms that may indicate the need for IV catheter site change should the heparin lock become infiltrated or clotted. This enables the patient and family to recognize when the IV is not functioning properly and to know when to notify the nurse.
- Explain the procedure, as appropriate, to both the child and the family. Use therapeutic play as indicated.

KidKare Be honest; never say "It won't hurt." In this case, the heparin solution may "sting" when being put in the line.

- Assess the IV site for signs of infiltration, irritation, or phlebitis.

PROCEDURE Flushing a Heparin Lock

Steps	Rationale/Points of Emphasis
1. Check healthcare prescriber's orders and medication administration records for time intervals to be administered.	Flushing of the IV cannula with heparin at the prescribed intervals improves the duration of catheter patency. Studies indicate that catheters flushed every 6 to 8 hours remain patent significantly longer than catheters flushed at 4-hour intervals.
2. Perform hand hygiene and gather the necessary equipment and supplies.	Reduces transmission of microorganisms. Promotes efficient time management and provides organized approach to the procedure.
3. Use a commercially available syringe of heparin solution or draw up from a vial a solution of heparin and NS and label with patient's name and name of medication.	Using a commercially available prefilled syringe reduces medication error. Labeling syringe provides for safe administration of right drug to right patient.
4. Identify the child using two different patient identifiers.	Reduces incidence of treatment being administered to wrong child.
5. Don gloves.	Standard precaution to reduce transmission of microorganisms.
6. Assess IV site.	The IV site should be free from signs of infection or infiltration before heparin is administered.
7. To convert a primary continuous infusion to a heparin lock: • Clamp T-connector tubing closest to catheter hub. • Remove the IV administration set tubing from the T-connector tubing or from the hub on the catheter cannula (if no T-connector tubing is present). • Attach a needleless male adapter (injection cap) to the end of the T-connector tubing or to the hub on the catheter cannula.	This is done to keep the IV line available in case it is needed later or to keep the line open for administration of IV medication. With a pediatric patient, it may be hospital policy to keep the IV site patent until the child is discharged.
8. Flush lock with heparin solution.	
a. Cleanse needleless male adapter (injection cap) with alcohol pad for at least 3 seconds or per institutional policy.	Reduces presence of microorganisms.
b. Insert needleless syringe with heparin solution into injection cap. Unclamp white side clamp on T-connector tubing if necessary.	The type of solution used to cleanse the site is according to hospital policy.
c. Gently pull back to check for blood flow.	Lack of blood flow is not an accurate determination of cannula placement because a fibrin shield may have formed at the tip of the cannula.
d. Gently inject heparin solution into catheter while assessing for resistance.	Resistance may mean the catheter is blocked or otherwise not functioning properly. If resistance is felt, never continue to apply force. Stop and evaluate cause.
e. Inject last 0.1 mL while removing the syringe tip or closing white side clamp on T-connector tubing (positive fluid displacement).	Provides positive pressure as syringe tip is being removed. Prevents blood from accumulating at IV catheter tip.
f. Close the clamp.	Positive fluid displacement must be maintained within the cannula lumen during and after a flush to prevent reflux of blood into the lumen.

Steps	Rationale/Points of Emphasis
9. To convert a heparin lock to a primary continuous infusion:	
a. Cleanse injection cap with alcohol.	Reduces presence of microorganisms.
b. Insert needleless syringe with saline solution into injection cap. Unclamp T-connector if necessary. Gently inject 1 mL saline while assessing for resistance or signs of swelling.	Ensures patency of access site before starting a continuous infusion of fluids. If resistance is felt, never continue to apply force. Stop and evaluate cause. If swelling occurs, stop flush because this indicates an infiltration.
c. Attach an IV administration set tubing to the injection cap.	
d. Start infusion. Monitor for infiltration.	
10. Assess IV site after manipulation of the catheter.	Check for infiltration at the cannula site of insertion.
11. Dispose of the syringe in appropriate needle receptacle. Remove gloves and perform hand hygiene.	Promotes needle safety. Reduces transmission of microorganisms.

CHILD AND FAMILY EVALUATION AND DOCUMENTATION

- Document the following:
  - Date, time, concentration, and amount of heparin flush solution used
  - Presence or absence of blood return and any resistance to flushing
  - Site appearance (presence or absence of redness, swelling, drainage, tenderness, or streaking)
  - Steps taken to intervene if complications are present (see Chapter 55, Table 55-1)
- Evaluate the IV site every 8 hours for complications and discontinue the catheter as necessary.
- Change the IV access site dressing per type of catheter (e.g., tunneled, PICC, peripheral) requirements and if dressing becomes damp, loosened, or soiled or when inspection of the catheter site is necessary. Use aseptic technique, while observing proper wound site care. Label the dressing with the time, date, and initials when reapplied to ensure proper change times.
- Determine whether the child and family have other areas of concern to discuss.

COMMUNITY CARE

- If the child is to be discharged home with a heparin lock and orders for intermittent IV infusions or medications, begin discharge planning with a home health nurse as early as possible.
- Communicate with the home care provider the type of catheter, including manufacturer and size if known; date of insertion; dressing change and flush protocol taught in healthcare setting; and any complications after placement.
- Instruct parents in hand hygiene techniques; dressing changes; flushing the heparin lock; medication administration and syringe pump use, as applicable; disposal techniques for syringes; and age- and developmentally appropriate methods to maintain the heparin lock.
- Before discharge, have the family repeat what they've learned about the most common complications of IV therapy (i.e., sepsis and accidental removal), what to look for, and actions to take in the event of complications to ensure they understand the information.
- Instruct the family to contact the healthcare provider if
  - The IV insertion site is reddened, swollen, or oozes fluid or blood
  - The IV becomes dislodged
  - The child develops a fever

Unexpected Situation

- *While administering the heparin flush, the child complains of acute pain at the IV insertion site:* Slow down the rate of heparin infusion. If the child continues to complain, stop the heparin flush. Slowly flush the lock with normal saline. If the child continues to complain of pain during the saline flush, stop the flush. Assess for infiltration and irritation at IV insertion site. Discontinue the IV catheter. Record your findings. Evaluate need for continued IV therapy and if needed insert new catheter.

Bibliography

Beecroft, P., Bossert, E., Chung, K., et al. (1997). Intravenous lock patency in children: Dilute heparin versus saline. *Journal of Pediatric Pharmacology Practice, 2*(4), 211–223.

Campbell, S., Trojaniwski, J., & Ackroyd-Stolarz, S. (2005). How often should peripheral intravenous catheters in ambulatory patients be flushed? *Journal of Infusion Nursing, 28*(6), 399–404.

Crews, B. E., Gnann, K., Rice, M., & Kee, C. (1997). Effects of varying intervals between heparin flushes on pediatric catheter longevity. *Pediatric Nursing, 23*(1), 87–91.

Gyr, R., Smith, K., Pontius, S., et al. (1995). Double blind comparison of heparin and saline flush solutions in maintenance of peripheral infusion devices. *Pediatric Nursing, 21*(4), 383–389, 366.

Hanrahan, K., Kleiber, C., & Berends, S. (2000). Saline for peripheral intravenous locks in neonates: Evaluating a change in practice. *Neonatal Network, 19*(2), 19–24.

Heilskov, J., Kleiber, C., Johnson, K., & Miller, J. (1998). A randomized trial of heparin and saline for maintaining intravenous locks in neonates. *Journal of the Society of Pediatric Nurses, 3*(3), 111–116.

Infusion Nurses Society. (2006). Infusion nursing: Standards of practice. *Journal of Infusion Nursing, 29*(1S), S1–S92.

Knue, M., Doellman, D., & Jacobs, B. (2006). Peripherally inserted central catheters in children: A survey of practice patterns. *Journal of Infusion Nursing, 29*(1), 28–33.

Kyle, L., & Yurner, B. (1999). Efficacy of saline versus heparin in maintaining 24-gauge intermittent intravenous catheters in a rabbit model. *Neonatal Network, 18*(6), 49–54.

LeDuc, K. (1997). Efficacy of normal saline solution versus heparin solution for maintaining patency of peripheral intravenous catheters in children. *Journal of Emergency Nursing, 23*(4), 306–309.

Mudge, B., Forcier, D., & Slattery, M. (1998). Patency of 24-gauge peripheral intermittent infusion devices: A comparison of heparin and saline solutions. *Pediatric Nursing, 24*(2), 142–146.

O'Grady, N. P., Alexander, M., Dellinger, E. P., et al. (2002). Guidelines for the prevention of intravascular catheter-related infections. *MMWR, 51*(RR-10), 1–29.

Pandurengan, A., Chandler, J., & Klein, A. (2005). A national telephone enquiry into the use of heparinised saline in flush systems of intravascular cannulae. *Anaesthesia, 60*(3), 314–315.

Shah, P., Ng, E., & Sinha, A. (2002). Heparin for prolonging peripheral intravenous catheter use in neonates. *Cochrane Database System Reviews*, (4), No. CD002774.

CHAPTER

50

Immunizations

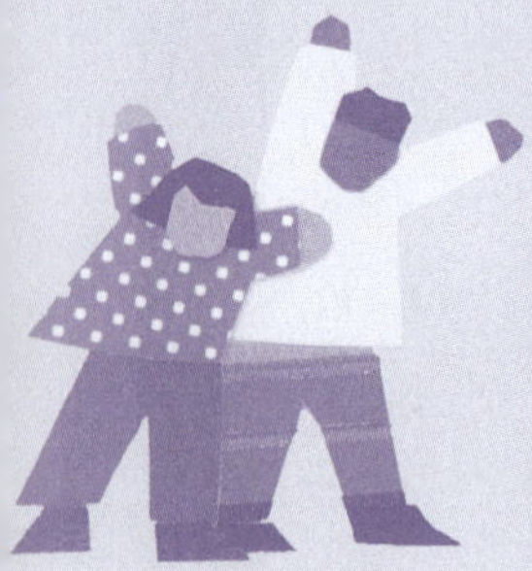

Clinical Guidelines

- A healthcare prescriber orders vaccination administration according to the Centers for Disease Control and Prevention (CDC) and American Academy of Pediatrics (AAP) guidelines.
- A registered nurse (RN) or licensed practical nurse (LPN) may administer immunizations.
- All children in the United States should be vaccinated per the schedule approved by the Advisory Committee on Immunization Practice (ACIP), the AAP, and the American Academy of Family Physicians (AAFP). The schedule can be found at www.cdc.gov/nip/recs/child-schedule.htm or www.aap.org/. For vaccinations for teenagers, see www.cdc.gov/nip/recs/teen-schedule.htm.
- Children who are not immunized starting in the first year of life should have immunizations started immediately after the catch-up schedule.
- Minimum age and minimum immunization interval requirements should follow the CDC guidelines.
- Immunization guidelines set forth by the AAP and the U.S. Public Health Service should be followed for travel to foreign countries.
- Children born prematurely should receive immunizations at the appropriate chronologic age, not the adjusted age.
- In compliance with the National Childhood Vaccine Injury Act (NCVIA), a vaccine information statement (VIS) will be provided to the vaccine recipient and his or her parent or legal guardian before administration of vaccines containing diphtheria, tetanus, pertussis, polio, measles, mumps, rubella, hepatitis B, *Haemophilus influenzae* type B (HIB), varicella, pneumococcal, meningococcal, influenza, hepatitis A, and others less commonly administered (e.g., anthrax, rabies, encephalitis, etc.). A VIS must be given with every vaccination, including each dose in a multidose series.
- VISs are available in non-English versions through your state health department or from the CDC. See www.cdc.gov/nip/publications/vis.
- Informed consent must be obtained from the parent or legal guardian before administering a vaccine (see Chapter 53).
- Measles-mumps-rubella (MMR) vaccine, although a live vaccine, is usually administered to children who are immunosuppressed because of the potential severity of the measles illness should it be contracted by an immunosuppressed child. Varicella vaccine should also be considered.

Equipment

- Vaccine information statement
- Health department or institution-specific documentation records
- Child's immunization record

Note: For equipment needed to administer vaccine, see Chapters 64 and 73.

Child and Family Assessment and Preparation

- Before teaching, assess parent's readiness to learn and barriers that would affect teaching, including communication barriers and cultural beliefs and practices.
- Obtain child's immunization record from parent. If child does not already have an immunization record, provide one to the family.
- Provide the parent with verbal and written information about the vaccines to be administered.
- Teach the parent about the recommended immunization schedule necessary for children and the rationale for administration, routes of administration, immunizations required for school entry, possible adverse reactions, and side effects.
- Assess the child's previous vaccine history.
- Assess the child's allergy history, including latex allergy.
- Assess the child for presence of fever, illness symptoms, known allergies, and pregnancy; assess the immunocompromised status of child and family.
- Obtain informed consent from the parent or legal guardian to administer the immunization.

caREminder

High body temperature and severe illness are reasons to delay immunization until the child has recovered from the acute stage of the illness. Minor illnesses, such as a cold, otitis media, and mild diarrhea without fever, are not contraindications to immunization.

PROCEDURE Administering Vaccines

Steps	Rationale/Points of Emphasis
1. If needed, review vaccine information with the parent and answer questions regarding the immunizations to be given. Provide the following information to the parent: purpose of the vaccination, its route of administration, care of the child after administration, and possible side effects.	Assists parent in understanding the benefits and possible side effects of vaccines. Prepares parent to assist with vaccine administration and to comfort child. Giving discharge instructions before administration of vaccine allows the parent to dedicate his or her attention to comforting the child afterward. **caREminder** *Redness and tenderness at the site of injection, crankiness, and a low-grade fever are the most common side effects of vaccine delivery.*
2. Encourage the parent to comfort child during and after immunization administration.	Ensures parent has active positive role in the child's healthcare.
3. When time allows, institute pain relief measures using a topical anesthetic according to manufacturer's instructions (e.g., EMLA, LMX4, vapocoolant, iontophoresis) (see Chapter 7).	Pain management measures reduce distress and trauma for the child.
4. Perform hand hygiene.	Reduces transmission of microorganisms.
5. Gather and prepare all needed supplies (e.g., draw up and label vaccine, open adhesive bandage) before entering the child's room.	Labeling the vaccine ensures correct vaccine given by the correct route, particularly when multiple vaccines are administered. Preparing ahead of time ensures that the nurse can administer the vaccination quickly after entering room, which, in turn, can decrease child and parent anxiety.
6. Don gloves and administer vaccines via route indicated on immunization schedule; follow procedures as outlined in Chapters 64 and 73.	Standard precaution to reduce transmission of microorganisms. Vaccine must be administered via indicated route to elicit immune response. **caREminder** *IPV, MMR, and Varivax vaccines are given subcutaneously. Hepatitis, HIB, DaPT, dT, influenza, pneumococcal conjugate, and meningococcal vaccines are given intramuscularly.*

Continued

Steps	Rationale/Points of Emphasis
7. If the child requires multiple injections, administer the injections in different extremities. If multiple injections must be given in the same extremity, leave at least 1 inch between the injection sites. Attempt to give the injections that have the greatest chance of local irritation (e.g., pneumococcal conjugate) in an extremity without another injection. **Alert!** *As with any medication, rare severe systemic reactions such as anaphylaxis or generalized urticaria are possible. Because of the potential for anaphylaxis with the administration of a vaccine, any child receiving a vaccine should be observed for several minutes after the vaccine is given for signs of immediate allergic or anaphylactic reaction.*	Allows for optimal absorption of vaccine and decreases irritation at sites of injection and overlapping local reactions.
8. Apply adhesive bandages to immunization sites as needed. Evaluate necessity of adhesive bandage use in young children as it may present a choking hazard.	Aids in stopping bleeding and provides comfort measure for child.
9. Dispose of equipment and waste in appropriate receptacles.	Standard precautions.
10. Provide parent with information about time frame for child's next scheduled immunizations.	Reinforces immunization schedule to improve compliance.

CHILD AND FAMILY EVALUATION AND DOCUMENTATION

- Document vaccine administration in child's medical record. Documentation should include the following:
  - Name and title of provider administering vaccine
  - Type of vaccine, vaccine manufacturer, and lot number of vaccine
  - Route of vaccine administration
  - Sites of injection
  - Adverse reactions
  - Distribution and review of VIS (note the publication date of the VIS given)
- Document the vaccine administration in the child's home immunization record. Documentation should include the following:
  - Name of immunization
  - Initials of provider who administered vaccine
  - Date of administration
  - The provider's name and address
- Evaluate child for immediate response to vaccine administration, noting immediate reaction, presence of local irritation at injection sites, and presence of any symptoms indicating anaphylactic reaction.

Alert! *Initiate immediate emergency intervention should the child experience signs of an anaphylactic reaction (e.g., respiratory distress or decreased respiratory effort, change in responsiveness, hives).*

COMMUNITY CARE

- Instruct parent about care of the child after immunizations:
  - For discomfort, apply a cool, clean washcloth to injection sites for 24 hours, followed by warm compresses.
  - Acetaminophen may be administered as needed.

Alert! *Children should not be given aspirin. Aspirin administration in children has been associated with Reye syndrome.*

- Instruct family to contact the healthcare provider or seek immediate medical care if the child experiences
  - Body temperature higher than 105°F (40.6°C)
  - Seizure
  - Persistent or inconsolable crying lasting more than 3 hours
  - Change in level of consciousness
  - Collapse or shock-like state
- Identify children in need of immunizations and refer them to an appropriate healthcare provider to ensure that immunizations are given as required.
- Report adverse reactions to vaccines, as appropriate, using the Vaccine Adverse Report System (VARS). Forms can be obtained by calling the VARS hotline at 1-800-822-7967, or they can be found in the back of the *Physician's Desk Reference* (*PDR*).

- Take every opportunity to immunize! Assess immunization needs at each encounter, whether well child or acute care interaction.
- Vaccine recommendations are continuously reviewed and updated by the CDC and other organizations such as the AAP. For the most current recommendations, consult your state health department and the current Red Book published by the AAP. The Immunization Action Coalition (www.immunize.com) also provides up-to-date information.

Unexpected Situation

- *After administration of the vaccine, the child develops acute respiratory distress:* Immediately initiate supportive or rescue measures for airway management. Assess severity of respiratory compromise. Activate emergency response system if indicated. As with any medication, rare severe systemic reactions such as anaphylaxis or generalized urticaria are possible. Because of the potential for anaphylaxis with the administration of a vaccine, any patient receiving a vaccine should be observed for several minutes after the vaccine is given for signs of immediate allergic or anaphylactic reaction.

Bibliography

Abdel Salam, H., & Sokal, M. M. (2004). Accuracy of parental reporting of immunization. *Clinical Pediatrics, 43*, 83–85.

American Academy of Pediatrics. (2006). *Red book: Report of the Committee on Infectious Diseases* (27th ed.). Elk Grove Village, IL: Author.

Farren, E., & McEwen, M. (2004). The basics of pediatric immunizations. *Newborn and Infant Nursing Reviews, 4*(1), 5–14.

National Immunization Program. (n.d.). *Standards for pediatric immunization practices.* Retrieved September 9, 2004, from http://www.cdc.gov/nip/recs/rev-immz-stds.htm#child

National Immunization Program. (2004). *Recommendations and guidelines to contraindications to vaccinations.* Retrieved September 9, 2004, from http://www.cdc.gov/nip/recs/contraindications.htm

National Vaccine Advisory Committee. (2003). Standards for child and adolescent immunization practices. *Pediatrics, 112*, 958–963.

Raucci, J., Whitehill, J., & Sandritter, T. (2004). Childhood immunizations, part one. *Journal of Pediatric Health Care, 18*, 95–99.

Schuval, S. (2003). Avoiding allergic reactions to childhood vaccines (and what to do when they occur). *Contemporary Pediatrics, 20*(4), 29–30, 33–34, 37–38.

Whitehill, J., Raucci, J., & Sandritter, T. (2004). Childhood immunizations, part two. *Journal of Pediatric Health Care, 18*, 192–197.

Wroe, A. L., Turner, N., & Salkovskis, P. M. (2004). Understanding and predicting parental decisions about early childhood immunizations. *Health Psychology, 23*, 33–41.

CHAPTER

51

Incentive Spirometry

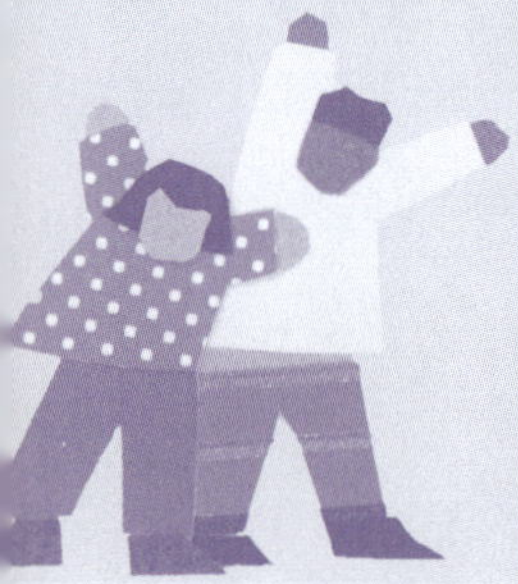

Clinical Guidelines

- A registered nurse (RN), licensed practical nurse (LPN), respiratory therapist, or physician initiates use of incentive spirometry to enhance voluntary deep breathing.

caREminder

For reimbursement purposes, a healthcare prescriber order must be obtained when this treatment is initiated.

- Incentive spirometry may be incorporated into routine postsurgical care in addition to deep breathing, coughing, turning, positioning, and early mobilization and ambulation.
- The objectives of this procedure are to increase transpulmonary pressure and inspiratory volumes, improve inspiratory muscle performance, and reestablish or stimulate the normal pattern of pulmonary hyperinflation and promote expectoration.

caREminder

There is no evidence that the use of incentive spirometry is associated with any harmful side effects. However, recent evidence does not support the use of incentive spirometry for decreasing the incidence of postoperative pulmonary complications after cardiac or upper abdominal surgery in adults.

- Children may perform the procedure while supervised by a trained staff member or other adult (e.g., parent who has been trained on the procedure). Direct supervision of the child performing the procedure is not necessary once the child has demonstrated mastery of the technique.
- The child should use the spirometer five to ten breaths per session at a minimum of every hour while awake.

Equipment

- Incentive spirometer
- Pillows or folded bath blanket (if needed); can use stuffed animal instead of pillow
- Tissues

Child and Family Assessment and Preparation

- Obtain baseline respiratory assessment, including
  - Previous incentive spirometry measurements obtained to use as a guide for current treatment goals
  - Arterial blood gas results, if available; not necessary
- Assess both child and family readiness to learn and determine whether any barriers to learning exist. Determine whether child and family can learn to perform the treatment independently.

- If the child is a surgical candidate, provide preoperative instruction to the child and family to facilitate use of the incentive spirometer postoperatively.

KidKare Send incentive spirometer home with the child before surgery to provide a time for practice. Both child and parent will have an opportunity to become comfortable with the instrument and the technique during this time.

PROCEDURE **Assisting With Incentive Spirometry**

Steps	Rationale/Points of Emphasis
1. Collect equipment. Assemble device, if necessary, and label it with child's name.	Ensuring that the device is used only by the child whose name appears on the device prevents nosocomial transmission of respiratory infections.
2. Perform hand hygiene.	Reduces transmission of microorganisms.
3. Assess the child's comfort level, and use pain management interventions as needed.	Appropriately managing the child's pain level enhances the child's ability to follow directions and participate in the procedure with more effective inspirations.
4. Raise the bed to a comfortable working level, and lower the side rails, if appropriate.	Decreases the potential for back injury.
5. Position child in a semi-Fowler's or a high-Fowler's position.	Allows for maximum lung expansion.
6. Demonstrate the breathing techniques the child should use to perform the procedure (see steps 8 and 9).	Prepares child for participation in the activity.
7. If child has an abdominal incision, have the child splint the abdomen with a pillow or bath blanket.	Allows for support and comfort of incision area while simultaneously allowing for maximum expansion of chest and lungs. **KidKare** The child can also be encouraged to hold a favorite stuffed animal in place to splint the abdomen.
8. Have the child exhale "until there is no more air to come out," and then direct the child to place the mouthpiece of the device in his or her mouth, sealing the lips around the mouthpiece.	Exhaling purges the lungs of air before sustained maximum inhalation. Effectiveness of the incentive spirometer is enhanced when an adequate seal is made around the mouthpiece, thus preventing leakage of exhaled air.
9. While ensuring that the child maintains the seal around the mouthpiece, direct the child to inhale slowly and deeply through the mouthpiece (without using his or her nose) and watch the indicator on the device.	During inhalation, the child's goal should be to keep the ball or indicator in the optimal region on the device or to move the ball or indicator to its highest level (depending on the device used at your institution). Inhaling through the nose or mouth and nose diminishes the child's ability to move the indicator to the highest level (Figure 51-1).

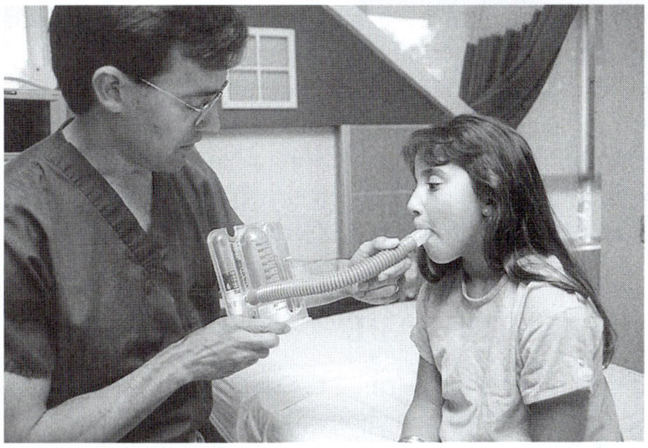

FIGURE 51-1
The child is instructed to place his or her mouth over the mouthpiece of the device so there is a good seal over the mouthpiece.

Continued

Steps	Rationale/Points of Emphasis
10. Instruct the child to hold his or her breath for 3 to 5 seconds, remove the mouthpiece, and then exhale normally in a slow and even fashion.	Holding the breath ensures optimum lung expansion by allowing the alveoli to reexpand. Normal slow exhaling prevents collapse of the alveoli.
11. Note the highest level the volume indicator reaches. Mark this on the device. Volume on incentive spirometry should increase with practice as the child reaches maximum lung capacity.	Marking the baseline assists the child as he or she seeks improvement during future attempts.
12. Direct the child to take two to four normal breaths and then repeat the process five to ten times per session, at a minimum, every hour while awake. If appropriate, encourage the child to perform the procedure independently, with new and increasing volumes established each day. Have tissue available and encourage child to cough as needed.	When the procedure is repeated on a regular basis, airway patency is maintained, and lung atelectasis can be prevented or reversed. Procedure facilitates expectoration of secretions.
13. Monitor the child for any untoward effects, such as dizziness, hyperventilation, or shortness of breath.	Hyperventilation, exacerbation of bronchospasm, and extreme fatigue may occur. If such symptoms occur, stop the procedure and notify a physician.
14. When the session is complete, return the child to a comfortable position, and return the bed to its lowest position. Assess child's safety and raise side rails, if appropriate.	Ensures child's comfort and safety.
15a. Remove the mouthpiece from the spirometer and rinse with soap and water as needed. 15b. Reattach the mouthpiece and store the unit at the child's bedside within easy reach of the child.	Removes sputum from device and reduces transmission of microorganisms during future use. Allows child easy access to the spirometer.

CHILD AND FAMILY EVALUATION AND DOCUMENTATION

- Evaluate the child's respiratory status, sputum production, and level of comfort.
- Document the child's ability to correctly use the device, and evaluate ability of child or family to perform the procedure independently.
- Document completion of the procedure on the nursing flow sheet each time it is carried out by the child.
- Summarize the following information in the medical record at least once per shift:
  - Child's respiratory status before and after procedure
  - Sputum production (if any)
  - Number of repetitions performed by the child
  - Frequency of the repetitions
  - Volume level achieved during inhalations
  - Any untoward affects, such as hyperventilation, dizziness, exacerbation of bronchospasm, or extreme fatigue

COMMUNITY CARE

- If the child will be learning the skill preoperatively and taking the instrument home, provide instructions on the following:
  - Use of the device
  - Demonstration and return demonstration of the procedure
  - Frequency of sessions and volumes desired
  - Cleaning and storage of the device
- Instruct the family to contact the healthcare provider if
  - Child experiences shortness of breath, dizziness, extreme exacerbation of coughing, or extreme fatigue associated with use of the incentive spirometer

Unexpected Situation

- *The child becomes light-headed during the process:* Tell the child to stop and take a few normal breaths before resuming incentive spirometry.

Bibliography

Brenner, Z. R. (1999). Preventing postoperative complications: What's old, what's new, what's tried-and-true. *Nursing1999, 29*(10), 34–40.

Brooks-Brunn, J. (1995). Postoperative atelectasis and pneumonia. *Heart and Lung, 24*(2), 94–115.

Gosselink, R., Schrever, K., Cops, P., et al. (2000). Incentive spirometry does not enhance recovery after thoracic surgery. *Critical Care Medicine, 28*(3), 679–683.

Hilling, L. (1991). AARC clinical practice guidelines: Incentive spirometry. *Respiratory Care, 36*, 1402–1405.

Lezon, K. (1999). Teaching incentive spirometry. *Nursing1999, 29*(1), 60–61.

Overend, T., Anderson, C., Lucy, D., et al. (2001). The effect of incentive spirometry on postoperative pulmonary complications: A systematic review. *Chest, 120*(3), 971–978.

Pasquina, P., Tramer, M., & Walder, B. (2003). Prophylactic respiratory physiotherapy after cardiac surgery: Systematic review. *British Medical Journal, 327*(7428), 1379.

Pullen, R. L. (2003). Clinic do's & don'ts: Teaching bedside incentive spirometry. *Nursing, 33*(8), 24.

Traver, G. (1985). Ineffective airway clearance: Physiology and clinical application. *Dimensions in Critical Care, 4,* 198–208.

CHAPTER 52

Infection Control and Standard Precautions

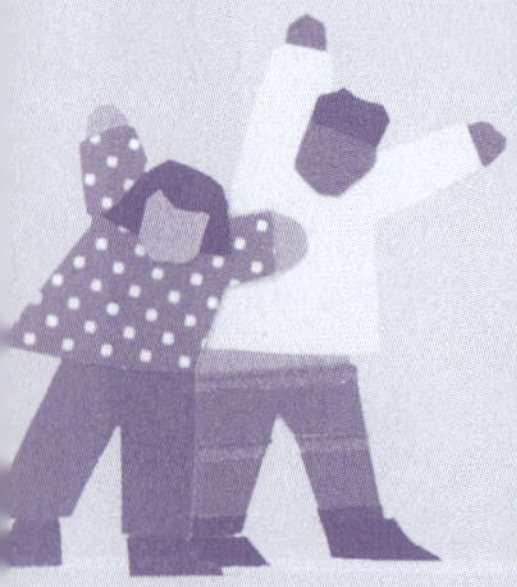

Clinical Guidelines

- Standard precautions for infection control must be implemented by all healthcare providers, staff, and volunteers within the institution.
- Standard precautions are applied to all children at all times and assist in infection prevention.
- Standard precautions indicate a philosophy of providing patient care whereby the healthcare provider selects barriers (gloves, gowns, mask, goggles) to wear based on the interaction with the patient, not on the patient's diagnosis.
- Transmission-based precautions are additional safeguards to standard precautions, used to prevent transmission of specific microorganisms. Transmission-based precautions include
  - Contact precautions (for both direct and indirect transmission)
  - Droplet precautions
  - Airborne precautions
- Goggles or facial shields are used when splashing or aerolization is likely and with a mask during intubation procedures
- Transmission-based precautions are applied to children when so determined by the primary care physician or consulting infection control healthcare practitioner (Table 52-1).
- When transmission-based precautions are to be applied, signs are posted outside the child's room and on the child's medical record to inform healthcare providers of the safeguards that must be implemented when providing care to the child.
- Use latex-free products to implement standard or transmission-based precautions in all cases in which the child or the nurse has known or potential latex allergies.

Hand Hygiene

- Perform hand hygiene before and after each patient contact, before and after using gloves, between caring for children, after eating or using the toilet, and whenever hands are soiled.
- Hand hygiene between tasks on the same child may be necessary to prevent cross-contamination of different body sites.
- An antimicrobial soap product is recommended for use with hand hygiene before and after participating in an invasive procedure and after exposure to blood or body fluids.
- The length of the scrub varies based on need.
- An alcohol-based hand disinfectant solution is recommended for use with hand hygiene before and after all contacts with patients.
- Healthcare providers' nails are kept short and hands, including the nails and surrounding tissue, must be kept free of inflammation.

TABLE 52-1

Classification of Transmission-Based Infection Control Precautions

	Contact Precautions	Droplet Precautions	Airborne Precautions	Neutropenic Precautions
Purpose	Used for children known or suspected to be infected or colonized with epidemiologically important microorganisms that can be transmitted by direct contact with the child or indirect contact with environmental surfaces of patient care items in the child's environment	Used for children known or suspected to be infected with microorganisms transmitted by droplets (large particles) that can be generated by the child during coughing, sneezing, talking, or the performance of procedures	Designed to reduce the risk for airborne transmission of infectious agents through dissemination of droplet nuclei (small particle residue of evaporated droplets that may remain suspended in the air for long periods of time) or dust particles containing the infectious agents	Initiated to protect the child who is immunosuppressed from exposure to personnel and environmental contagions
Environment and supplies	• Private room or cohort with child with similar microorganism • Gown and glove when entering child's room and remove before leaving. • Do not allow hands or clothing to touch potentially contaminated surfaces or items in child's room. • Dedicate noncritical patient care equipment to single child. • Clean and disinfect reusable equipment before use on another child. • May require mask (e.g., with methicillin-resistant *Staphylococcus aureus* [MRSA]).	• Private room or cohort with child with similar microorganism • If above not possible, maintain spatial separation of at least 3 feet between infected child and other patients and visitors. • Wear regular mask if within 3 feet of the child. • Child's door may be open; no special air handling or ventilation is required. • Limit transporting child from room for essential purposes only. If child is transported, have child wear mask to minimize dispersal of droplets.	• Private room • Special air handling and ventilation required (monitored negative air pressure in relation to surrounding areas). • Keep room door closed and child in the room. • Use of N95 mask or other special masks is required for pulmonary tuberculosis. • For people immune to rubeola or varicella, no mask required when visiting patients with these; only immune healthcare workers and family or visitors are allowed in room; if susceptible workers must enter room, they should wear masks. • Limit transporting child from room for essential purposes only. If child is transported, have child wear mask to minimize dispersal of droplets.	• Private room • Place in physical location with other noncontagious children. • Enforce strict handwashing by all healthcare workers, family members, and visitors. • Neutropenic child may wear mask outside of room to protect against environmental exposures. • Child's activities need not be limited; see institutional policies for specific recommended activity for children with neutropenia (e.g., school attendance, play room visits).

Continued

TABLE 52-1

Classification of Transmission-Based Infection Control Precautions (continued)

	Contact Precautions	Droplet Precautions	Airborne Precautions	Neutropenic Precautions
Examples for use	• Children younger than 6 years of age or anyone with poor hygienic practices (e.g., developmental delay). • Initial workup for diarrhea (*Clostridium difficile*, rotavirus, vancomycin-resistant enterococcus) • Respiratory syncytial virus • Parainfluenza virus • Herpes simplex virus • MRSA • Impetigo • Cellulitis • Pediculosis and scabies • Staphylococcal furniculosis	• Invasive *Haemophilus influenzae* type B disease • Invasive *Neisseria meningitides* disease • Children with meningitis, influenza, pneumonia, and sepsis until causative organism is determined and need for precautions eliminated • Diphtheria • Mycoplasma pneumonia • Pertussis • Streptococcal pharyngitis • Adenovirus • Mumps • Parvovirus B19 • Rubella • Scarlet fever	• Pulmonary tuberculosis • Measles (rubeola) • Chickenpox (varicella)	• Child with cancer who develops fever (>38.3°C or 101°F). • Child with neutropenia (absolute neutrophil count <500/mm³).

Data from Nettina, S. (2005). *The Lippincott manual.* Philadelphia: Lippincott Williams & Wilkins.

- Artificial nails (any material applied to the nail for the purpose of strengthening or lengthening) cannot be worn and nails cannot have chipped nail polish when providing patient care.

Gloves

- Gloves are worn to provide a protective barrier of the hands of the healthcare provider and to reduce transmission of microorganisms from the care provider to the child.
- Wearing gloves does not replace the need for hand hygiene before and after the removal of the gloves.
- Gloves must be changed between caring for different children to prevent infections.
- Doubling gloving and changing gloves often are recommended for lengthy and high-risk procedures and surgeries.

Gowns

- Gowns are worn to prevent contamination of clothing and to protect the skin of the healthcare provider from blood and body fluid exposures.
- Impermeable gowns, leg coverings, and boots or shoe coverings are worn when the healthcare provider is at risk for coming into contact with splashes or large quantities of infected materials.
- Gowns are worn during care of children with pathogens that can be transmitted by contact with the pathogen (either from the child or items in the environment) to other children or other personnel in the setting.
- Gowns are removed before leaving the child's environment and hands are washed.

Masks, Goggles, and Face Shields

- Masks, goggles, and/or face shields are worn to protect the mucous membranes of the eyes, nose, and mouth during care of the child when there is a likelihood of splashes or sprays of blood, body fluids, or secretions.
- Masks are worn to provide protection to the healthcare provider against the spread of infectious large-particle droplets during contact with the child who is on airborne or droplet precautions.
- Masks may be worn by the immunosuppressed child vulnerable to direct or indirect exposure to pathogens in the environment.

Air Filters

- When caring for a child with known or suspected tuberculosis, the healthcare provider wears a N95 respirator, a high-efficiency particulate air (HEPA) filter respirator, or a powered air-purifying respirator (PAPR).

Care of Equipment

- Sterile packaging is inspected before use and returned to central supply if wet or torn or if the barrier is compromised in any way.
- Linens and patient care equipment that are soiled with blood, body fluids, secretions, or excretions are handled and transported in a manner that avoids transmission of microorganisms to the child, family members, and healthcare personnel.

Needle and Sharps Disposal

- All sharps are discarded in impervious containers marked as biohazardous waste, located as close as possible to the area of use.
- Used needles are not recapped, removed from syringes, bent, or broken.

Child Placement

- Private rooms are recommended for children and families with poor hygienic practices or with highly transmissible or epidemiologically significant microorganisms.
- When a private room is not available, two children infected with the same organisms can share a room (cohorting).
- Children with microorganisms spread by airborne transmission are placed in a private room that has monitored negative air pressure in relation to the surrounding areas.
- Children who are immunosuppressed are placed in private rooms. Staff assignments should be made such that personnel caring for highly transmissible or epidemiologically significant microorganisms are not caring for immunosuppressed children.

Employee Safeguards

- All employees are periodically screened for communicable diseases as a component of the infection prevention and control program.
- The Exposure Control Plan developed by the facility designates how exposure to blood should be handled, including delineation of employees at greatest risk.
- All healthcare workers who have potential exposure to bloody body fluids are recommended to receive the hepatitis B immunization.
- Healthcare workers who are susceptible (e.g., pregnant women, nonimmunized staff) should not enter the rooms of children known or suspected to have measles (rubeola) or chickenpox (varicella). If susceptible individuals must enter the room, a surgical mask should be worn.

CHILD AND FAMILY ASSESSMENT AND PREPARATION

- Review child's medical record to determine whether the child is a source of infection or at risk for infection and assess need for transmission-based precautions.
- Assess child and family's understanding of standard precautions.
- Explain, in developmentally appropriate terms, the need for standard and transmission-based (if applicable) precautions (e.g., "I'm wearing this mask so I won't breathe on you"). Use resource personnel (child life specialist, infection control nurse) to assist in teaching process.
- Teach child the importance of hand hygiene and how and when to perform.
- Secure isolation gloves, gowns, and masks as needed and place on a cart outside the child's room.
- Place transmission-based precaution signs on entryway to child's room to alert healthcare providers, family members, and visitors of the need for protective apparel or isolation.
- Teach family members and visitors about the proper use of gowns, gloves, and masks.

CHILD AND FAMILY EVALUATION AND DOCUMENTATION

- Evaluate child and family's understanding of need for standard precautions and transmission-based precautions.
- Evaluate child and family's integration of standard or transmission-based precautions into care practices for the child.
- Document the following:
  - When standard or transmission-based precautions are implemented
  - Teaching provided to the family about these precautions

COMMUNITY CARE

- Stock home health bag with gloves, disposable gown, paper towels, soap, and waterless hand sanitizer to be prepared for no running water and no disposable towels in a home.
- Provide family with community vendors to obtain disposable gloves, needle disposal containers, and other equipment as needed.

- Instruct day care workers to use gloves when changing diapers, dispose of soiled diaper immediately, wash hands after glove removal, and disinfect the diapering area after each diapering.
- Instruct the family to contact the healthcare provider if
  - Additional teaching is needed regarding standard or transmission-based precautions
  - New information arises that may change need for infection control practices, such as a new disease in family member or close contact with someone who has a contagious condition

Unexpected Situation

- *Frequent handwashing with soap causes breaks and bleeding of the skin of the healthcare provider:* Soaps and detergents are damaging to the skin when applied on a regular basis. Alcohol-based formulations for hand disinfection are less irritating than antiseptic or nonantiseptic agents. Alcohol-based solutions with added emollients are recommended and may protect against cross-infection by keeping the skin flora intact. Hand lotions help protect the skin and reduce microbial shedding. While the skin breaks are healing, the healthcare provider should wear gloves during all patient contacts.

Bibliography

Committee on Infectious Diseases and Committee on Hospital Care. (1998). The revised CDC guidelines for isolation precautions in hospitals: Implications for pediatrics. *Pediatrics, 101*(3), e13.

Committee on Infectious Diseases and Committee on Practice and Ambulatory Medicine. (2000). Infection control in physician's offices. *Pediatrics, 105*, 1361–1369.

Gupta, A., Della-Latta, P., Todd, B., et al. (2004). Outbreak of extended-spectrum beta-lactamase–producing *Klebsiella pneumoniae* in a neonatal intensive care unit linked to artificial nails. *Infection Control and Hospital Epidemiology, 25*, 210–215.

Hedderwick, S., McNeil, S., Lyons, M., & Kauffman, C. (2000). Pathogenic organisms associated with artificial fingernails worn by healthcare workers. *Infection Control and Hospital Epidemiology, 21*(8), 505–509.

Kellerman, S. E., Simonds, D., Banerjee, S., et al. (1998). APIC and CDC survey of mycobacterium tuberculosis isolation and control practices in hospitals caring for children. I. Patient and family isolation policies and procedures. *American Journal of Infection Control, 26*, 483–487.

Korniewicz, D., Garzon, L., & Plitcha, S. (2003). Health care workers: Risk factors for nonlatex and latex gloves during surgery. *AIHA Journal, 64*(6), 851–855.

Larson, E. (2001). Hygiene of the skin: When is clean too clean? *Emerging Infectious Diseases*, 7(2), 225–230.

Larson, E., Albrecht, S., & O'Keefe, M. (2005). Hand hygiene behavior in a pediatric emergency department and a pediatric intensive care unit: Comparison of use of 2 dispenser systems. *American Journal of Critical Care, 14*(4), 304–312.

Lawson, L. (2001). Handwashing: A neonatal perspective. *Journal of Neonatal Nursing*, 7(2), 42–46.

McNeil, S., Foster, C., Hedderwick, S., & Kauffman, C. (2001). Effect of hand cleansing with antimicrobial soap or alcohol-based gel on microbial colonization of artificial fingernails worn by health care workers. *Clinical Infectious Diseases, 32*, 367–372.

Pittet, D. (2001). Improving adherence to hand hygiene practice: A multidisciplinary approach. *Emerging Infectious Diseases*, 7(2), 234–240.

Pottinger, J., Burns, S., & Manske, C. (1989). Bacterial carriage by artificial versus natural nails. *American Journal of Infection Control, 17*, 340–344.

Preston, R. (2005). Infection control nursing: Aseptic technique. Evidence-based approach for patient safety. *British Journal of Nursing, 14*(10), 540–542, 544–546.

Roberts, L., Jorm, L., Patel, M., et al. (2000). Effect of infection control measures on the frequency of diarrheal episodes in child care: A randomized, controlled trial. *Pediatrics, 105*, 743–746.

Ward, D. (2001). The role of the school nurse in infection control. *Primary Health Care, 10*(10), 37–39.

CHAPTER 53

Informed Consent

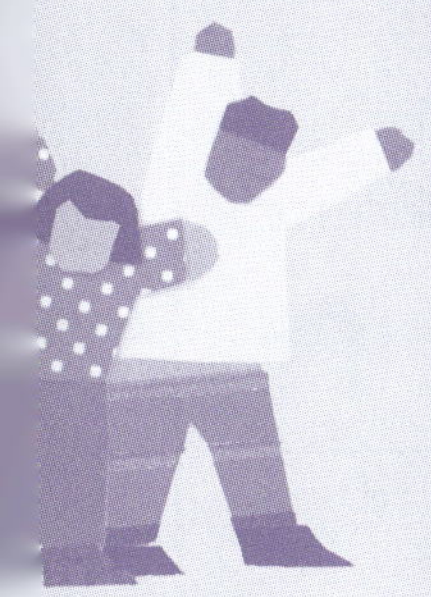

Clinical Guidelines

- The healthcare provider performing the procedure is responsible for discussing the procedure with the child and family and for obtaining informed consent before implementation of any surgery, research protocol, procedures, or treatments that warrant informed consent.
- Informed consent must be obtained from parents or legal guardians and children who are cognitively able in order to respect the right to self-determination in decision making.
- Only patients who have appropriate decisional capacity and legal empowerment can give their informed consent to medical care. In all other situations, parents or surrogates provide informed permission for diagnosis and treatment of children, with assent of the child whenever appropriate.
- Healthcare providers should seek parent permission in most situations. However, they must focus their goal on providing appropriate care and be prepared to seek legal intervention when parent refusal places the child at clear and substantial risk.
- Privacy standards as outlined in the Health Insurance Portability Accountability Act of 1996 (HIPAA) must be followed to ensure confidentiality.
- The process of informed consent must minimally address the following:
  - A full explanation of the condition
  - An explanation of the procedure or therapy to be used in terms appropriate to the parent or child's level of understanding provided by the person performing the procedure or therapy
  - A description of alternative treatments or therapies available
  - A description of benefits to be expected from the treatment or therapy
  - A description of risks associated with the treatment or therapy
  - Sufficient time and encouragement to answer the parents' and child's questions
  - Discussion that is free from any coercion, unfair persuasions, or other inducements to comply with the treatment being discussed
- In emergency care situations when the need for treatment is immediate or the child has lost any decision-making capacity, consent is then implied. Consent is considered with regard to what the child or parents would have wanted to approve had they been present or mentally capable of making the decision.
- When the child is a minor, all attempts should be made to attain assent for a procedure or research. Information presented in attaining assent should be limited to the child's level of understanding. Assent would be the child's permission to proceed.
- Minors are deemed emancipated and treated as adults for all purposes, including informed consent, if the minor is any of the following:
  - Self-supporting and/or not living at home
  - Married

- Pregnant or a parent
- In the military
- Declared to be emancipated by a court

In addition, many states give decision-making authority (without the need for parental involvement) to some minors who are otherwise unemancipated but who have decision-making capacity or are seeking treatment for certain medical conditions, such as sexually transmitted diseases, pregnancy, and drug or alcohol abuse.

- Legal statutes preclude obtaining informed consent from anyone younger than the age of 18 years. Researchers, however, are encouraged by institutional review boards to obtain assent from anyone older than 7 years of age. This legal mandate may need to be adapted for the adolescent who can clearly participate in his or her own decision making.

EQUIPMENT

- Consent document if required for the particular procedure. Some procedures are covered by the general consent-to-treat form that was signed upon admission to a healthcare facility or upon initial treatment.
- Indelible-ink pen.
- Dependent on the procedure or treatment to be discussed, the following may be helpful in aiding the parent or child's understanding of care:
  - Various forms of learning material addressing the parent or child's learning style and literacy skills (e.g., written pamphlets, videos, picture boards, anatomic models)
  - Teaching mannequins for the parent or child to have a visual hands-on experience

CHILD AND FAMILY ASSESSMENT AND PREPARATION

- Provide as private an environment as possible to protect confidentiality of patient information and to limit distractions during the informed consent process.
- If not previously done, assess the child and family's learning style. In an emergency situation, assessment will have to be rapid based on the person's response and questions about explanations of treatment plan.
- Assess the parent or child's ability to make informed decisions.

PROCEDURE Obtaining Informed Consent

Steps	Rationale/Points of Emphasis
1. Gather consent form (if used), along with necessary equipment and supplies needed to provide child and family with clear explanation and demonstration of the procedure to be performed.	Form is essential for legal medical record. Having needed supplies readily available facilitates flow of the explanation/demonstration.
2. The person completing the procedure or intervention provides a verbal explanation of the procedure or treatment to the child and the family. This should be done in understandable language and must include the nature of the condition, propose steps of the treatment, probability of success, potential benefits and risks involved, and any alternatives to the proposed treatment. Arrange for translator services if needed.	Full disclosure of this information is essential in meeting the criteria of the informed consent process. Appropriate translator services allow the child and family to better communicate their concerns and understand the explanations of healthcare providers.
3. Assure the parent and child, within clinical feasibility, that they have the right to refuse any treatment or seek care elsewhere.	There should be neither coercion to comply with care nor any evidence of inducements or unfair persuasions.
4. Throughout the explanation of the treatment and at the end of the session, elicit questions from the parent and child.	It is essential for the parent and child to feel free to ask questions that may aid in the interpretation of the information they are being told.
5. Assess the parent's or child's understanding of the information. This can be accomplished through having the parent or child repeat back what the procedure is to entail.	Determines what, if any, further explanation or alternative methods of teaching are necessary. **KidKare** It may be useful to have a doll available for the child to use as a vehicle for pointing concerns out and asking questions.

Steps	Rationale/Points of Emphasis
6a. Obtain appropriate personnel to witness the signatures of the family. The witness should be someone who is not related to the child and not involved in giving care during the procedure.	The witness validates that he or she has seen the child or family sign the consent form. Healthcare providers assisting in the procedure cannot serve as witnesses to the informed consent signing because of potential conflict-of-interest concerns.
6b. Obtain informed signed consent. Consent should be obtained from the parent or guardian and the child if cognitively able.	Avoid violating the right to self-determination whenever possible.

caREminder

After family members sign the consent, they have the right to cancel the procedure at any time.

CHILD AND FAMILY EVALUATION AND DOCUMENTATION

- Evaluate the parent's or child's understanding of the informed consent process.
- Determine whether or not the parent or child has any other concerns or questions at this time.
- If the child is to participate in a research study, there should be documented evidence of informed consent or assent within the record.
- Signed consent forms should be placed in the child's medical record. A copy of the form must be given to the parent, legal guardian, or child.
- Nursing documentation should reflect methods used in explaining the procedure, the procedure's risks and benefits, and any questions or concerns the family had and what was done to clarify those concerns.

COMMUNITY CARE

- The same standards of informed consent apply to the community setting as to the acute care setting.
- Consent obtained outside the acute care setting is relevant if it is the same provider who is to perform the procedure and the consent is less than 24 hours old.

Unexpected Situation

- *The signed consent form is missing from the medical record:* The appropriately obtained signed consent must be physically available and immediately retrievable from the child's current medical record before the consented procedure. If the previously signed consent cannot be located, a new consent must be obtained.

Bibliography

American Academy of Pediatrics. (1995). Informed consent, parental permission, and assent in pediatric practice. *Pediatrics, 95*, 314–317.

American Academy of Pediatrics, Berger, J. E., & Committee on Medical Liability. (2003). Consent by proxy for nonurgent pediatric care. *Pediatrics, 112*, 1186–1195.

American Academy of Pediatrics, Committee on Bioethics. (1994; reaffirmed January 2004). Guidelines on forgoing life-sustaining medical treatment. *Pediatrics, 93*, 532–536.

American Academy of Pediatrics, Committee on Pediatric Emergency Medicine. (2003). Consent for emergency medical services for children and adolescents. *Pediatrics, 111*, 703–706.

Fisher, C. B. (2004). Informed consent and clinical research involving children and adolescents: Implications of the revised APA ethics code and HIPAA. *Journal of Clinical Child & Adolescent Psychology, 33*, 832–839.

Kanner, S., Langerman, S., & Grey, M. (2004). Ethical considerations for a child's participation in research. *Journal for Specialists in Pediatric Nursing, 9*, 15–23.

Kopelman, L. M. (2004). Minimal risk as an international ethical standard in research. *Journal of Medicine & Philosophy, 29*, 351–378.

Lashley, M., Talley, W., Lands, L. C., & Keyserlingk, E. W. (2000). Informed proxy consent: Communication between pediatric surgeons and surrogates about surgery. *Pediatrics, 105*, 591–597.

Runeson, I., Elander, G., Hermeren, G., & Kristensson-Hallstrom, I. (2000). Children's consent to treatment: Using a scale to assess degree of self-determination. *Pediatric Nursing, 26*, 455–458, 515.

CHAPTER

54

Intracranial Pressure Monitoring, Assisting in Placement and Care of

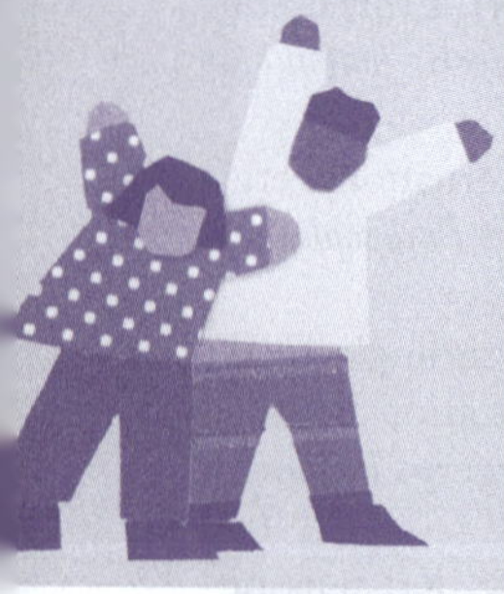

Clinical Guidelines

- Placement of an intracranial pressure (ICP) monitor is a surgical procedure performed by a physician, and the removal of such a device is the responsibility of the physician. Informed consent to complete the procedure must be obtained.
- The registered nurse (RN) is responsible for monitoring the child and system; monitoring takes place in an intensive care setting.
- Sedation and pain management of the child with ICP monitoring are implemented on an individual basis according to the child's diagnosis and unique healthcare needs.
- The accuracy of the monitoring system is assessed at least once a shift by zero-balancing the ICP system, checking the status of system alarms, assessing the level of the transducer, and assessing device placement.

Equipment

Setup and Placement

- Surgical examination light (if needed by physician)
- Several disposable razors
- Sterile povidone-iodine prep swabs
- Sterile gowns, gloves, masks, and caps
- Sterile drapes or towels
- Lidocaine (Xylocaine) local anesthetic (0.5% or 1%)
- Sterile syringes (assortment of sizes: 3- and 5-mL, and tuberculin)
- Needles (22- and 25-gauge)
- Cranial drill and bit
- Alcohol wipes
- Scalpel
- Sterile retractor
- Forceps
- Sterile scissors
- Hemostats
- Subarachnoid bolt or silastic intraventricular catheter (institutional preference)

- Suture material (usually 2–0 to 3–0 nylon/silk)
- Gauze dressing (4 × 4)
- Sterile transparent dressing (if needed)
- Gauze dressing roll (3-inch)
- Hypoallergenic knitted tape (1-inch)
- Preservative-free sterile normal saline for injection
- Individual institution monitoring system and equipment (i.e., ICP module, microsensor control unit, transducer, cable, and hookup)
- Level to check height of transducer
- Sedation and pain medications (as ordered)
- Antibiotics (as ordered)

Daily Care

- Latex-free sterile gloves
- Sterile povidone-iodine prep swabs
- Alcohol wipes
- Gauze dressing (4 × 4)
- Sterile transparent dressing (if needed)
- Gauze dressing roll (3-inch)
- Hypoallergenic knitted tape (1-inch)
- Preservative-free sterile normal saline for injection
- Level to check height of transducer

CHILD AND FAMILY ASSESSMENT AND PREPARATION

- Assess the child's and family's cognitive level, readiness, and ability to process information.
- Assess child for signs and symptoms of increased ICP, including altered or decreased level of consciousness, anxiety, restlessness, irritability, agitation, lethargy, confusion, drowsiness, headaches, seizures, posturing, inappropriate motor function or dysfunction, widened pulse pressure, bradycardia, altered respiratory pattern, and pupillary dysfunction. An infant may also display tense or bulging fontanels, separated cranial sutures, increased head circumference, projectile vomiting, high-pitched "neuro" cry, or "sunset" eyes.
- Ensure that informed consent has been obtained and that the appropriate documents are signed and present in the child's medical record.
- Reinforce the need for device placement, as appropriate, to both the child and family.
- Reinforce the physician's explanation of the risks and benefits of monitoring.
- Discuss with parents the need to talk to the child and provide physical comfort, even while child is sedated.

PROCEDURE Setup for Bedside Insertion of ICP Monitoring by Physician

Steps	Rationale/Points of Emphasis
1a. Perform hand hygiene.	Reduces transmission of microorganisms.
1b. Gather the necessary equipment, personnel, and supplies for device placement.	Assembly of all necessary equipment promotes efficient time management and provides an organized approach to the procedure. Note that two healthcare personnel will be needed to assist physician in placement of catheter device: one person positions and holds the child in place while assessing the child's condition during the procedure and the other provides and gathers equipment as needed. **caREminder** *This is a sterile procedure. Reduce traffic in the patient area as much as possible during the procedure.*
2. Obtain the following baseline data: • Vital signs • Level of consciousness • Pupil response • Skeletal motor function • Sensory function	Having baseline data facilitates identification of any acute changes in the child's condition during and after procedure. The earlier that signs and symptoms of brain injury are identified, the sooner treatment can begin to improve outcome.
3a. Assess sedation and pain management needs of child in collaboration with the physician. Administer sedation and pain management medications as ordered.	ICP placement is a painful procedure. The child's comfort will be enhanced by administration of medications to manage pain and sedation.
3b. The physician may elect to administer IV antibiotics to the child during preparation and after catheter insertion.	Antibiotic therapy may assist in preventing infections that may occur secondary to this invasive procedure.
4. Perform hand hygiene.	Reduces transmission of microorganisms.

Steps	Rationale/Points of Emphasis
5. Assemble ICP pressure monitoring system to interface with the institutional monitor (i.e., ICP module, transducer, cable, and hookup) (Figure 54-1) and prepare catheter, if needed, per manufacturer's instructions (e.g., some systems need to be primed with preservative-free, sterile, normal saline and the catheter wrapped in sterile gauze soaked in preservative-free sterile normal saline to a depth of 5 cm below catheter tip, calibration may be required; other systems come precalibrated and the neurosurgeon will prime the system when placing the catheter).	Ensures proper setup and facilitates procedure. Priming line avoids introducing air into the ventricular or subdural spaces. The preservative in saline may cause cortical necrosis.

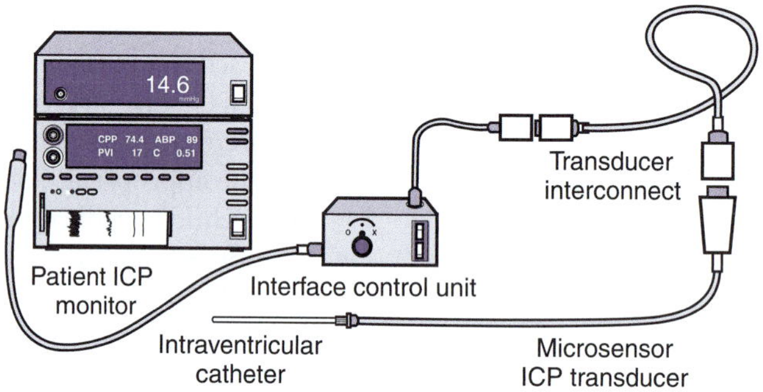

FIGURE 54-1
Intracranial pressure monitoring equipment.

Steps	Rationale/Points of Emphasis
6. Prepare sterile field and place instruments on field.	Maintains aseptic technique.
7. Don sterile attire.	Standard precautions for surgical sterile procedure.
8. Position the child for access by the physician (this may include turning the child so that the head is at side of the bed horizontally) and hold the child's head securely in midline position throughout procedure, while maintaining sterile access for physician.	Facilitates ease of access, and assists with catheter insertion.
9. Restrain the child's limbs as necessary to ensure sterility of procedure.	Keeps child from moving and possibly breaking sterile field required for catheter insertion.
10. Assist physician in identifying area on scalp for device placement. The left frontal/temporal scalp area is the most preferred access point for most physicians. Follow institution policy and procedure for ensuring preoperative verification process is completed, appropriate operative site is marked, and "time out" is completed before start of procedure.	Identifies access site. "Time-out" implements Universal Protocol for Preventing Wrong Site, Wrong Procedure, Wrong Person Surgery.
11. Assist the physician in shaving the scalp and prepping the area with sterile povidone-iodine scrub. Shave an area large enough to accommodate the transparent dressing that will be placed over the site at the end of the procedure.	Visualizes insertion site; prevents hair from falling into and thereby contaminating sterile field. Transparent dressing will not secure well if attached to hair. **KidKare** Child's hair should be kept and placed in a plastic bag. Parents may wish to keep the child's hair.
12. Assist physician in draping head in sterile fashion.	Protects insertion site from contamination.
13. After applying the subcutaneous lidocaine (Xylocaine), the scalp and the skull are incised by the physician, using the hand drill and scalpel.	Lidocaine anesthetizes the site. Allows for insertion of ICP monitor.

Steps	Rationale/Points of Emphasis
14. Using sterile technique assist the physician as needed throughout the procedure, and continually assess the child for changes in neurologic and vital sign status.	Ongoing monitoring of the child facilitates early detection of problems.
15. Once the catheter is in place (Figure 54-2), attach the microsensor control unit cable to the ICP device.	Provides interface between bedside monitor and child's ICP system.

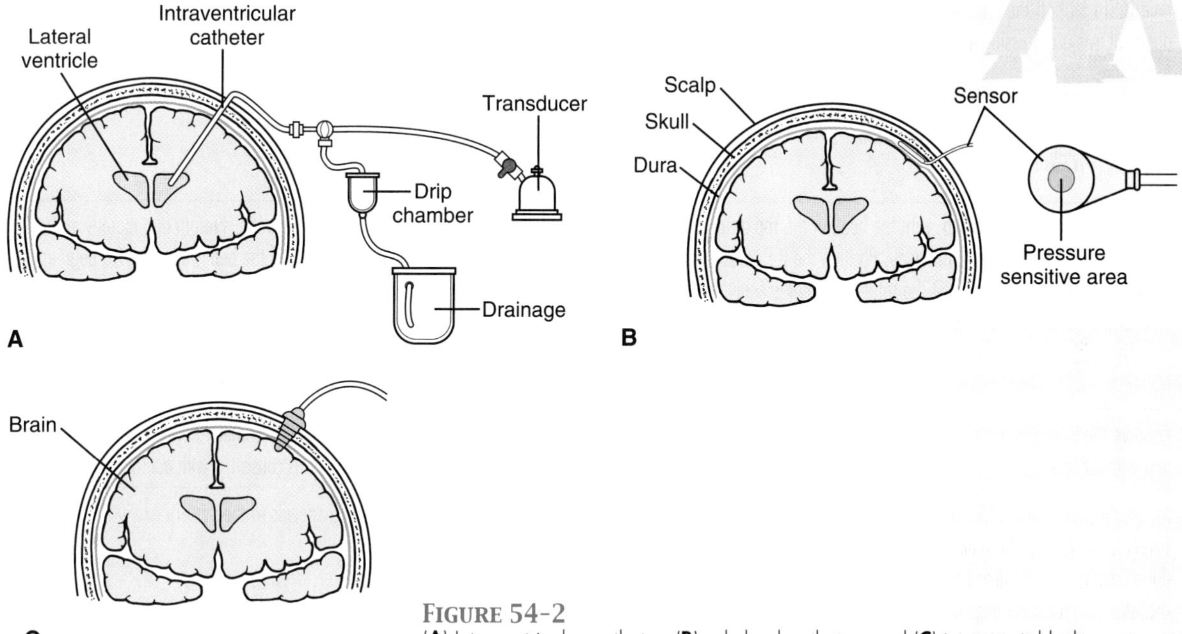

FIGURE 54-2
(**A**) Intraventricular catheter, (**B**) subdural catheter, and (**C**) intracranial bolt.

Steps	Rationale/Points of Emphasis
16. When the ICP device is in place, assist in placing semipermeable transparent dressing over the catheter insertion site on the child's scalp.	Protects the site from microorganisms.
17. Zero-balance the fiberoptic system with bedside monitoring system. a. Depress zero control until the number "0" appears. b. Continue to press zero control while pressing zero at bedside ICP monitor. c. When the number "0" appears on the bedside monitor, release the zero control on the microprocessor.	Allows waveform to be viewed with electrocardiogram and other pressure tracings. Zero-balancing and calibrating system provides more accurate measurements.
18. If requested by the physician, assist in dressing the entire scalp with gauze and Kerlix dressing.	Further protects the site from contamination or from accidental disconnection of device by child.
19a. Reposition the child upright in bed with the head at the top of the bed in a midline position to the rest of the body. 19b. Position the child and equipment to keep the ICP transducer at the foramen of Monro. Anatomically, the reference point is equivalent to the level of the ear or the outer canthus of the eye.	Flexion or rotation of the head can obstruct venous return and thereby increase ICP. Positioning the child so that the head of the bed is elevated 30 degrees promotes venous return. Flexion or rotation of the neck can obstruct venous return. Transducer placement at a point above or below the anatomically correct position will result in false readings.
20. Dispose of equipment and waste in appropriate receptacles.	Standard precautions.
21. Remove gloves and perform hand hygiene.	Reduces transmission of microorganisms.

PROCEDURE Daily Care of the Child With a Pressure Monitoring Device

Steps	Rationale/Points of Emphasis
1a. Validate the accuracy of the system setup by zero-balancing and assessing the level of the transducer and device placement.	Zero-balancing and calibrating system provides more accurate measurements.
1b. Ensure that alarms are set appropriately.	Appropriate alarm parameters aid in early detection of problems.
2. Maintain the sterility of the equipment and insertion site and observe the insertion site and sterile dressing for signs of drainage or cerebrospinal fluid (CSF) leak. If the dressing is wet, notify physician. After physician approval, replace dressing if wet, soiled, or dislodged, using sterile technique. **Alert!** *CSF drainage is more likely to occur if the child's ICP is elevated.*	System integrity must be maintained because of the potential for infection into the central nervous system. Report the occurrence of drainage immediately to the physician because subsequent permanent neurologic impairment may occur.
3. Position the child upright in bed, with the head at the top of the bed in a midline position to the rest of the body. Position the ICP transducer at the foramen of Monro. Anatomically, the reference point is equivalent to the level of the ear or the outer canthus of the eye.	Flexion or rotation of the head can obstruct venous return and thereby increase ICP. Positioning the child so that the head of the bed is elevated 30 degrees promotes venous return. Flexion or rotation of the neck can obstruct venous return. Maintaining the proper position of the ICP transducer ensures accurate waveform and pressure data. Transducer placement at a point above or below the anatomically correct position will result in false readings.
4. Observe the tubing and catheter system to ensure that the system is intact and without kinks.	Decreases the risk for increased ICP related to catheter flow and drainage. Ensures accurate pressure readings and waveforms consistent with neurologic assessment.
5. Assess for mechanical difficulties specific to the monitoring system, for example, kinking of the tubing, accidental disconnection from the transducer monitor, electrical interference, false readings from a nonfunctioning catheter, and false readings from a catheter that has been clamped off.	Identifies the need for interventions specific to the system.
6. Observe for and identify changes in stimuli that could cause an increase in ICP (i.e., suctioning, repositioning, coughing, pain, straining, or agitation).	Seek to avoid prolonged elevations of ICP. Identify the need for changes in interventions, sedation, positioning, or stimulation.
7. Observe and monitor the ICP reading and notify the physician immediately of any untoward increase in the child's ICP.	Changes in ICP or changes in ICP waveform require prescribed physician orders.
8. Administer sedation and pain medication to the child as ordered.	Promotes comfort and facilitates effective pain management of child. An agitated child may contaminate the ICP device insertion site or dislodge the catheter.

CHILD AND FAMILY EVALUATION AND DOCUMENTATION

- Monitor the baseline and ongoing neurologic assessments, including ICP, pressure waveform, cerebral perfusion pressure, level of consciousness, respiratory pattern, and vital signs. Note trends and response to therapeutic interventions, at least every 2 hours, and document on the appropriate institutional form.
- Observe the drainage tubing to ensure the system is intact, without leaks, kinks, or clots, and document at least once every shift.
- Evaluate for and document the potential of infection related to device placement, including temperature, white blood cell count, CSF cultures, device cultures (if obtained), inflammation at the insertion site, and signs or symptoms of meningitis; notify the appropriate physician immediately if signs of infection are present.
- Document the following on the appropriate institutional forms:
  - Date and time of device insertion, assessments, the insertion site position and placement (e.g., intraventricular, intraparenchymal), catheter size used, medications, and child's response to the procedure
  - The amount of drainage, color, and consistency of the CSF, every 2 to 4 hours
- Document administration of sedation or pain medication or any other measures, including diversionary activities, used to provide pain management and comfort and child's response to these measures.
- Determine whether the child and family have other areas of concern to discuss.

COMMUNITY CARE

- Assure the child and the parents that the child's hair will regrow at the site it was shaved off for catheter placement.
- Instruct the family to contact the healthcare provider if
  - Child has signs of infection at the ICP insertion site, such as redness, drainage, or swelling
  - Child develops a fever
  - Child exhibits changes in neurologic status, such as changes in level of consciousness, headache, irritability, onset of high-pitched cry (infants), and bulging fontanel (in infants)

Unexpected Situations

- *The catheter becomes dislodged from the insertion site:* Apply pressure to the insertion site with sterile gauze, and immediately notify physician. Assess for changes in child's neurologic status. Continuously observe and assess child for signs and symptoms of increased ICP until catheter is replaced or other appropriate intervention is initiated.
- *The integrity of the catheter or drainage tubing is compromised:* A break or other compromise in the catheter or tubing should be immediately secured by occluding the damaged area with sterile gauze. Notify the physician to assess for catheter repair, replacement, or other intervention.

Bibliography

American Association of Neuroscience Nurses (2005). *Guide to the care of the patient with intracranial pressure monitoring.* Glenview, IL: Author.

Downard, C., Hulka, F., Mullin, R. J., et al. (2000). Relationship of cerebral perfusion pressure and survival in pediatric brain-injured patients. *Journal of Trauma, 49*, 654–659.

Fan, J. (2004). Effect of backrest position on intracranial pressure and cerebral perfusion pressure in individuals with brain injury: A systematic review. *Journal of Neuroscience Nursing, 36*, 278–288.

Hickey, J. V. (2003). Intracranial hypertension: Theory and management of increased intracranial pressure. In J. V. Hickey (Ed.), *The clinical practice of neurological and neurosurgical nursing* (5th ed., pp. 285–318). Philadelphia: Lippincott Williams & Wilkins.

Joint Commission on Accreditation of Healthcare Organizations (JCAHO). (n.d.). Universal protocol for preventing wrong site, wrong procedure, wrong person surgery. Retrieved July 12, 2006, from http://www.jcipatientsafety.org/show.asp?durki=11517

March, K. (2000). Intracranial pressure monitoring and assessing intracranial compliance in brain injury. *Critical Care Nursing Clinics of North America, 12*, 429–436.

Ng, I., Lim, J., & Wong, H. B. (2004). Effects of head posture on cerebral hemodynamics: Its influences on intracranial pressure, cerebral perfusion pressure, and cerebral oxygenation. *Neurosurgery, 54*, 593–597.

Palmer, J. (2000). Management of raised intracranial pressure in children. *Intensive and Critical Care Nursing, 16*, 319–327.

Price, A. M., Collins, T. J., & Gallagher, A. (2003). Nursing care of the acute head injury: A review of the evidence. *Nursing in Critical Care, 8*, 126–133.

CHAPTER

55

Intravascular Therapy: Peripheral Catheters

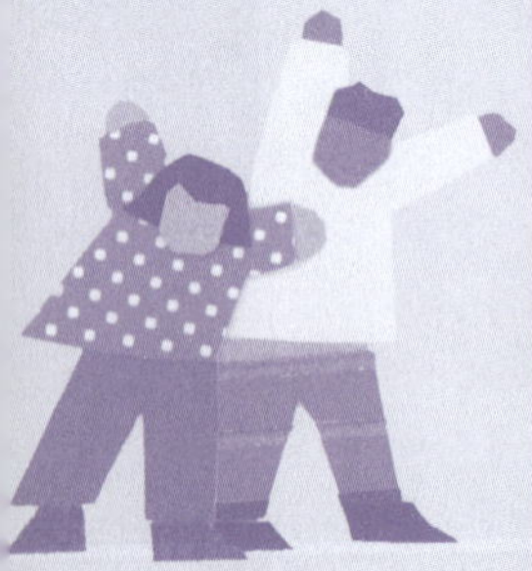

Clinical Guidelines

- Initiation of intravascular therapy (calculation based on age, height, weight, or body surface area) is on order of a physician or healthcare prescriber.
- Peripheral intravenous (IV) catheters are placed by a physician, registered nurse (RN), licensed practical nurse (LPN), or appropriately certified technician.
- Placement is accomplished by cannulating a superficial vein with a sterile needle/catheter. Peripheral IV catheters are used for direct administration of primed IV fluids, intermittent use with medications and blood products, parenteral nutritional supplement, and occasional venous blood draws for laboratory analysis (see Chapter 5).
- Peripheral IV catheters in children may remain in place as long as there are no signs of complications; they do not need to be changed on a routine basis.
- Disposable catheters of various lengths and sizes are available from several manufacturers. Infants and children with small veins may tolerate large-volume IV rates with small-bore (20- to 24-gauge) catheters.
- The practitioner placing the IV catheter is knowledgeable regarding normal anatomy and physiology of children and selecting appropriate sites (Figure 55-1). The choice of access depends on the hemodynamic status of the child, the expertise of the nurse, the availability of supplies, the general condition of the vasculature, and the nature of the fluid being infused.
- The practitioner placing and monitoring the IV catheter is knowledgeable regarding complications associated with IV lines, including infiltration, hematoma, phlebitis, thrombosis, bacteremia, septicemia, nerve damage, and mechanical problems.
- Local anesthesia is used for catheter placement in nonemergent situations (see Chapter 7).

Equipment

- Local anesthetic: topical agents (e.g., EMLA cream, LMX4, Numby Stuff iontophoresis) or injectable buffered lidocaine for nonemergent insertion
- IV catheter of appropriate size and length
- Tourniquet or rubber band
- Nonsterile examination gloves
- Antiseptic swabs or pads: 2% chlorhexidine-based preparation is preferred, tincture of iodine, an iodophor (e.g., povidone-iodine), or 70% alcohol can be used.

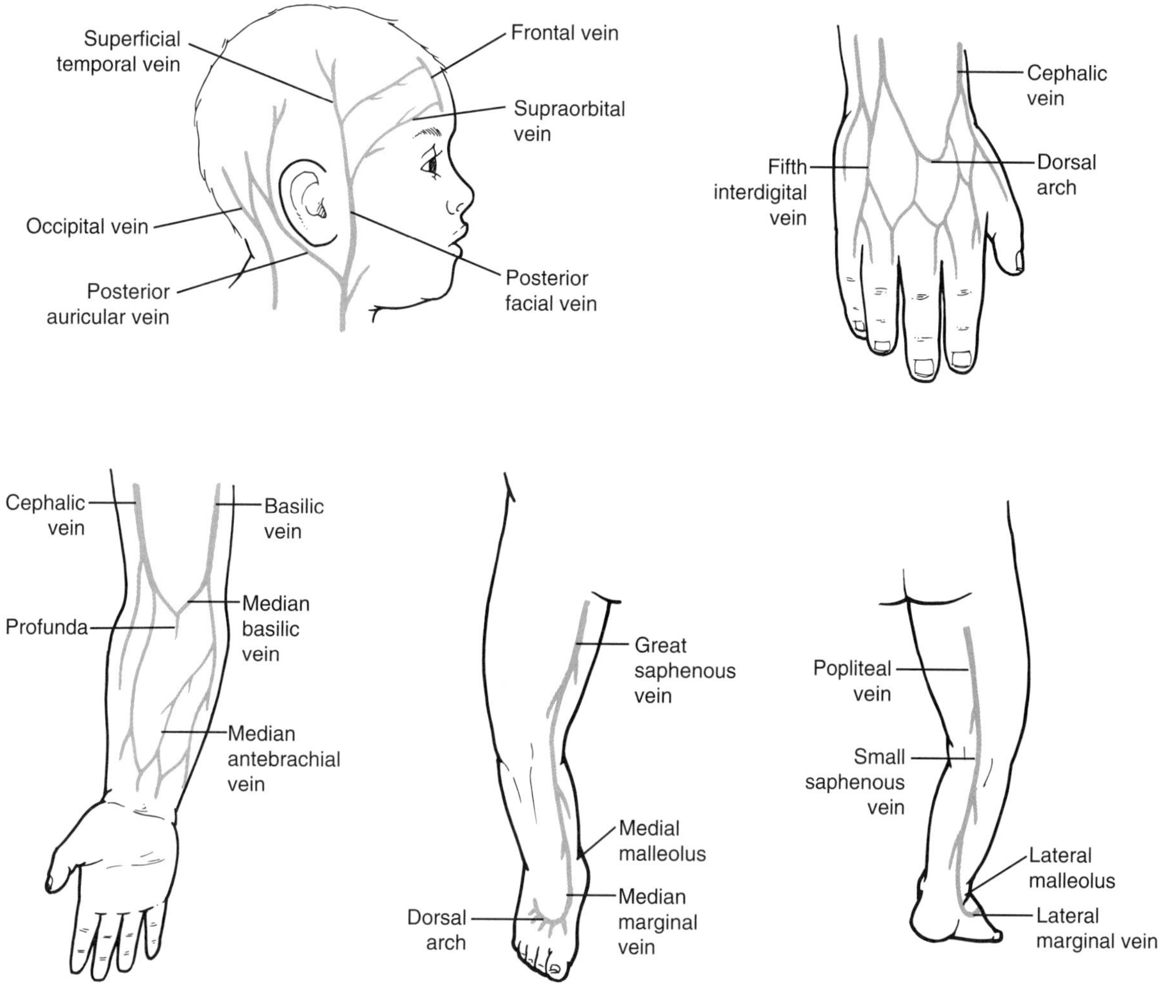

FIGURE 55-1
Potential sites of peripheral IV access include the scalp, the back of the hand, the arm (including the antecubital fossa), the foot, and the leg.

caREminder

The CDC makes no recommendation for the use of chlorhexidine (CHG) in infants aged <2 months. AWHONN neonatal skin care guidelines recommend either CHG or povidone-iodine. The use of CHG in infants weighing <1,000 grams has been associated with contact dermatitis and should be used with caution in this population (INS, 2006; AWHONN, 2006).

- Sterile, saline-filled, 3-mL syringe
- Short T-infusion primer set
- Dressing materials: cotton or gauze and tape or semipermeable transparent dressing
- Heparinized saline as ordered, if IV is to be clamped and not used for continuous infusion
- IV fluid as prescribed
- IV administration tubing
- IV controlled infusion device (follow manufacturer's directions for use)
- Material to secure line: tape, secure-lock device, surgical netting, armboard

CHILD AND FAMILY ASSESSMENT AND PREPARATION

- Assess the cognitive level, readiness, and ability to process information of the child and family. Readiness to learn and ability to process information may be impaired as a result of age, stress, or anxiety.
- Discuss the purpose of venipuncture; reinforce the need for and identify and discuss the risks and benefits of IV placement with the child and family.
- Assess for chlorhexidine allergy; if present, use alternative antiseptic agent.
- Assess presence of or risk factors for latex allergy; if present, implement latex precautions (see Chapter 60).
- Elicit the child's input (as developmentally appropriate) in IV site selection, avoiding dominant hand (if appropriate). Explain the amount of discomfort the child can expect with IV insertion and encourage cooperation and understanding.

KidKare Stress the importance of holding still during the catheter placement because this facilitates insertion. Children identify needles as the most painful and scary part of any hospitalization. Include a child life specialist, if available, to assist with distraction techniques.

- Explain to parents what they can do to comfort and support child during the procedure (see Chapter 7).
- Explain the signs and symptoms that may indicate the need for IV catheter site change after the original catheter is placed. This enables the patient or family to recognize when the IV is not functioning properly and when to notify the nurse.
- Assess the child's age, general size, and overall skin condition. Observe for peripheral skin grafts or shunts, cellulitis, vascular surgeries, thrombosis, or peripheral vascular disease, which aid in the selection of an appropriate IV site for the child. Identify the catheter insertion site before beginning the procedure.
- Apply topical or local anesthetic agent before IV insertion.

PROCEDURE Insertion of Peripheral IV Catheter

Steps	Rationale/Points of Emphasis
1. Identify vein and insertion site. If a topical anesthetic agent is to be applied, choose the IV insertion site and allow the agent to remain on the skin for appropriate length of time (e.g., 1 hour for EMLA cream, about 15 minutes for iontophoresis) (see Chapter 7). Remove topical anesthetic cream with soft cloth before beginning procedure. If using buffered lidocaine, inject and wait 1 minute before catheter insertion.	Reduces pain during insertion. **caREminder** *Obtain the assistance of an additional person to hold the child securely to prevent unnecessary attempts and to prevent dislodging the catheter as needed.*
2. Gather necessary equipment and supplies for IV catheter placement; select catheter size based on assessment of identified insertion site. Perform hand hygiene.	Promotes efficient time management and provides an organized approach to the procedure. Reduces transmission of microorganisms.
3. Open and prepare all supplies. Prime short T-infusion primer set with sterile normal saline and leave saline-filled syringe attached to primer set.	Readies supplies for ease of insertion.
4. Don gloves.	Standard precaution to reduce transmission of microorganisms and maintain asepsis.
5. Apply tourniquet above the proposed IV puncture site.	Increases venous pressure and allows better visualization of vessel to be cannulated. **caREminder** *For scalp veins in infants and neonates, a large rubber band works well around the head, with a gauze pad under the rubber band to grasp and pull up once the IV is inserted; the band is then cut in two to release. Touching of a child's head by strangers may be offensive to some Asians. Explain the need to touch the child's head to the parents before starting the IV.*
6a. Cleanse the skin over the chosen insertion site with antiseptic swab: 2% chlorhexidine or other appropriate antiseptic swab, working from the center outward in a circular motion and allow area to dry for 30 seconds. 6b. For neonates, remove antiseptic solution with sterile saline or water.	Decreases number of organisms on the skin. Prevents further absorption of antiseptic solution and tissue damage.

Steps	Rationale/Points of Emphasis
7. Hold extremity of insertion site with nondominant hand. Using dominant hand, remove the protective sheath over the catheter and puncture the skin of the IV insertion site at a 45-degree angle with the bevel of the catheter needle up, parallel to the vein.	Holds extremity steady and causes the least amount of discomfort during insertion. **caREminder** *When placing IV lines in extremities, access the most distal site first, using the nondominant hand. Do not use the antecubital veins until other sites have been exhausted because catheters in the antecubital region, or any joint, can be easily disturbed by joint flexion and the immobilization required may cause joint stiffness and pain. Allow an older child a choice of catheter placement sites.*
8. Reduce the angle of the catheter needle and insert ⅛ to ¼ inch into the vein until retrograde blood flow appears in the catheter.	Allows for insertion into the vein lumen without puncturing the posterior wall of the vein.
9. Release tourniquet.	Prevents rupture of vein as needle is advanced into vein lumen.
10. Advance catheter into vein while gently removing inner needle from catheter, leaving only catheter sheath in place.	Establishes catheter in vein.
11. Stabilize catheter in place with nondominant hand and connect primed short T-infusion set to catheter hub.	Provides direct entrance for IV fluids to flow through catheter, while assessing patency of catheter.
12. Initiate flow of saline through the catheter and assess for signs of infiltration.	If needle of catheter has punctured the vein wall, fluid will fill into surrounding tissue, causing localized edema or hematoma formation.
13. Secure catheter in place with gauze and tape dressing or semipermeable transparent dressing to site so that it is covered occlusively (Figure 55-2).	Prevents catheter movement and accidental dislodgment. Transparent dressings provide greater visualization of site.

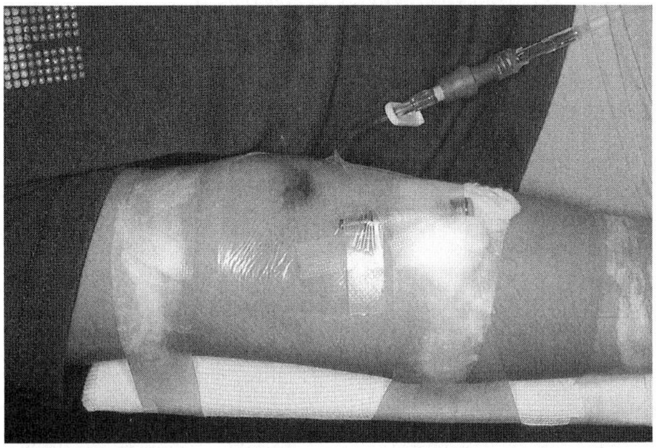

FIGURE 55-2
The insertion site is taped securely and covered with semipermeable transparent dressing so that the site is occlusively covered.

Steps	Rationale/Points of Emphasis
14. Begin IV fluids as prescribed and regulate IV infusion or place catheter to "heparin or saline lock" for intermittent infusions, as prescribed.	Provides fluid delivery as prescribed. **caREminder** *Although saline locks are common practice in adults, evidence in pediatrics is contradictory and does not support discontinuing use of heparin. This may be related to the smaller lumen sizes of catheters used.*

Continued

Steps	Rationale/Points of Emphasis
15. Secure the line with additional tape and armboard as needed to prevent accidental removal (Figure 55-3).	Secure connections may prevent air embolizations or migration of the catheter.

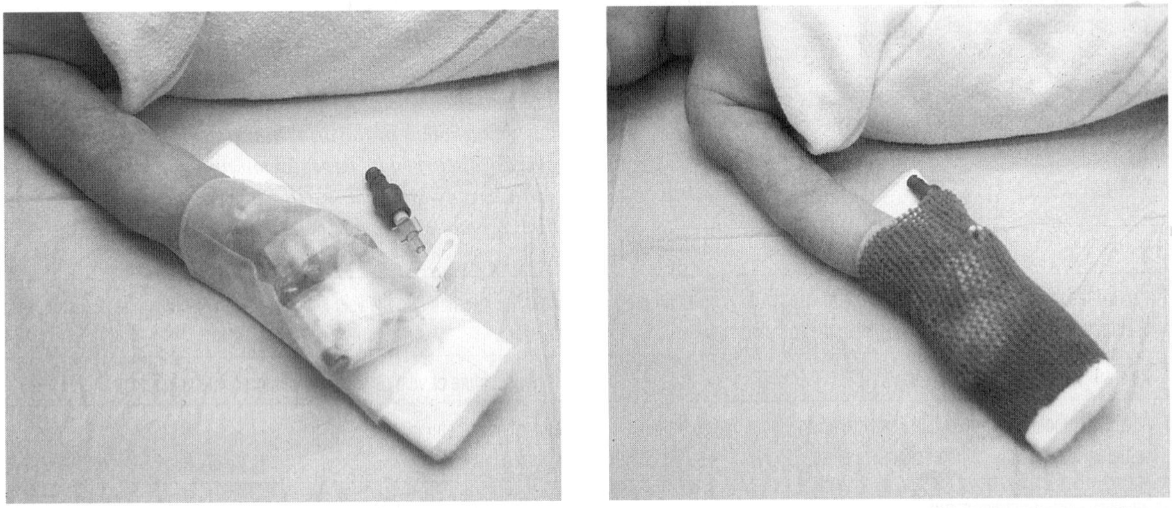

FIGURE 55-3
The IV site is secured with additional tape, an armboard, and surgical netting as needed.

Steps	Rationale/Points of Emphasis
	KidKare In the young child, cover the insertion site with surgical netting to keep out of sight. Use armboard as needed to prevent excessive movement.
16. Discard used supplies.	Standard precautions.
17. Perform hand hygiene.	Reduces transmission of microorganisms.

PROCEDURE Maintenance of Infusion

Steps	Rationale/Points of Emphasis
1. Assess the IV site every hour for complications (Table 55-1); discontinue the IV as indicated.	Ensures prompt detection of complications.
2. Hang no more than 4 hours' worth of IV fluid at any one time during fluid infusion or infuse fluid via a controlled infusion device. For peripheral IV catheters not used for continuous infusion, refer to Chapter 49 or Chapter 104.	Prevents accidental fluid overload and reduces complications from IV infiltration.
3a. Change the IV tubing using aseptic technique no more frequently than every 72 hours or when contamination occurs or is suspected.	Limits bacterial contamination of infusion tubing.
3b. Label the IV tubing with time, date, and initials of person who hung tubing.	Identifies proper change times.
4a. Change the IV access site dressing when the site appears soiled, damp, or loose, using aseptic technique, while observing proper wound site care.	Limits bacterial contamination.
4b. Label the dressing with the time, date, and initials of the person who reapplied.	Identifies last dressing change and personnel responsible.

TABLE 55-1

Complications of Intravascular Therapy: Peripheral Access

Problem	Intervention
Bacteremia: Indicates presence of bacteria in the blood and possible contamination of the IV system.	• Do not apply compresses because this may potentiate infection. • Notify healthcare prescriber and obtain orders for antibiotics.
Bleeding: Mild bleeding at IV insertion site may occur for first 24 hours after placement.	• Apply gauze dressing after initial placement of IV and change first dressing in 24 hours. • Limit movement of extremity using armboard as necessary. • If bleeding increases or persists past first 24 hours, notify healthcare prescriber.
Infiltration: Infiltration is the unintended administration of medication or solution into the interstitium and tissue surrounding the vein. An increase in circumference of the extremity may indicate an infiltration is present. Treatment of an infiltration is dependent on the properties of the infiltrated medication or solution, the manufacturer's guidelines for that agent, and the severity of the infiltration.	• IV site checks are to include assessment along the path of the catheter. • Measure the circumference of the extremity above the IV site and compare serial measurements. • If infiltration occurs, discontinue infusion. Notify healthcare prescriber of infiltration, solution, or medications infusing at time of infiltration, and site appearance. • Obtain healthcare prescriber order for agent to treat infiltration of a vesicant as needed. • Immediately elevate extremity to promote venous return; maintain elevation for 24 to 48 hours.
Hematoma: Indicating undue trauma to the vessel wall or extravasation of blood into the extravascular space.	• Apply warm compress to extremity for discomfort. • If symptoms increase, discontinue IV use at the site.
Mechanical: Can be indicated by catheter migration, breaks in the catheter or connective tubing, or accidental catheter removal.	• May be caused by excessive movement, loose tape, or excessive amount of give in the IV tubing. • Encourage limitation of limb or extremity movement. • Place IV site extremity on an armboard and securely fasten catheter and tubing.
Nerve damage: Indicates trauma to adjacent nerve during insertion of IV.	• May be caused by excessive movement.
Phlebitis: An inflammation of the vein usually caused by mechanical irritation from catheter trauma or early signs of infection. Some catheter materials are associated with increased risk for phlebitis. An increase in circumference of the extremity may indicate an infiltration is present.	• Apply warm compress to extremity to ease discomfort. • If symptoms increase, if there is streak formation, or if palpable cord is present, notify healthcare prescriber.
Septicemia: Indicates systemic infection related to presence of blood-borne infection.	• Do not apply compresses because this may potentiate infection. • Notify healthcare prescriber and obtain orders for antibiotics.

PROCEDURE Removal of Peripheral IV Catheter

Steps	Rationale/Points of Emphasis
1. Perform hand hygiene and gather the necessary supplies.	Hand hygiene reduces the transmission of microorganisms. Assembly of all necessary equipment facilitates quick and efficient removal of the IV catheter.
2. Don gloves.	Standard precaution to reduce transmission of microorganisms and maintain asepsis.
3. Close clamp on IV administration set and turn IV controlled infusion device off; ensure that IV short T-infusion set is clamped.	Stops flow of fluids and prevents potential infiltration while removing peripheral catheter.

Continued

Steps	Rationale/Points of Emphasis
4. Remove old tape and dressing from around insertion site.	Allows access to insertion site.
KidKare Use of an adhesive remover may ease the trauma of tape removal. In preterm infants, slow careful removal with warm water and cotton balls is recommended. Mineral oil or emollients may facilitate adhesive removal; do not use if reapplication of tape is necessary.	
5. Using gauze pad or cotton ball, apply slight pressure over insertion site while withdrawing peripheral IV catheter.	Facilitates removal of catheter.
6. Continue holding pressure at insertion site for 1–2 minutes.	Applying pressure prevents bleeding while clotting occurs.
7. Remove gauze or cotton ball; assess insertion site for continued signs of bleeding, infection, infiltration, or phlebitis.	Ensures prompt detection of complications.
8. Apply bandage over insertion site.	Standard precautions. Reassures child that procedure is complete.
9. Discard used supplies.	Standard precautions.
10. Perform hand hygiene.	Reduces transmission of microorganisms.

CHILD AND FAMILY EVALUATION AND DOCUMENTATION

- Evaluate the IV site every hour for site appearance and signs of complications: note presence or absence of redness, swelling, drainage, tenderness, or streaking; initiate steps to intervene if complications are present (see Table 55-1); and document this assessment.
- Label the IV tubing with time, date, and initials when it is hung to ensure proper change times.
- Label the IV site dressing with time, date, and initials when it is applied.
- Document the following:
  - Date and time of IV insertion, insertion site, type and gauge of catheter used (e.g., butterfly catheter, Quik catheter), any difficulty in placing the catheter, number of attempts, child's tolerance of the insertion, and identification of the person inserting the device
  - Date, time, type, and amount of flush solution used; presence or absence of blood return; and any resistance to flushing
  - Teaching provided regarding potential complications associated with treatment
- Determine whether the child and family have other areas of concern to discuss.

COMMUNITY CARE

- If the child is to be discharged home with an IV, begin discharge planning with a home health nurse as early as possible.
- Communicate to the home care provider: type of line (including manufacturer and size if known), date of insertion, dressing change and flush protocol taught in healthcare setting, and notification of any complications after placement.
- Instruct parents in handwashing, dressing changes, flushing the IV line, medication administration and syringe pump use as applicable, disposal techniques for syringes, and age and developmentally appropriate methods to maintain the IV line.
- Before discharge, the family should verbalize knowledge of the most common complications of IV therapy (i.e., sepsis and accidental removal), what to look for, and actions to take in the event of complications.
- Instruct the family to contact the healthcare provider if
  - IV insertion site remains reddened or oozes fluid or blood
  - IV becomes dislodged
  - Child develops a fever

Unexpected Situation

- *The IV-controlled infusion device is alarming, indicating occlusion. You check the IV site and the tape is tight and the area looks puffy and feels taut:* Remove the IV because it has infiltrated. Collaborate with prescriber about need for continuing IV therapy.

Bibliography

AWHONN (Association for Women's Health, Obstetric and Neonatal Nurses). (2001). *Neonatal skin care: Evidence based clinical practice guidelines.* Glenview, IL: Author.

Centers for Disease Control and Prevention. (2002). *Guidelines for prevention of intravascular catheter-related infections.*

Retrieved August 15, 2006, from http://www.cdc.gov/mmwr/preview/mmwrhtml/rr5110a1.htm

Eichenfield, L. F., Funk, A. F. F., Cunningham, B., & Bari, B. (2002). A clinical study to evaluate the efficacy of ELA-Max (4% liposomal lidocaine) as compared with eutectic mixture of local anesthetics cream for pain reduction of venipuncture in children. *Pediatrics, 109*, 1093–1099.

Fetzer, S. J. (2002). Reducing venipuncture and intravenous insertion pain with eutectic mixture of local anesthetic: A meta-analysis. *Nursing Research, 51*, 119–124.

Infusion Nurses Society. (2006). Infusion nursing. Standards of practice. *Journal of Infusion Nursing, 29*(Suppl. 1S), S1–S92.

Krzywda, E. A., & Andris, D. A. (2005). Twenty-five years of advances in vascular access: Bridging research to clinical practice. *Nutrition in Clinical Practice, 20*, 597–606.

Lininger, R. A. (2003). Pediatric peripheral IV insertion success rates. *Pediatric Nursing, 29*, 351–354, 360–361.

Mermel, L. A., Farr, B. M., Sheretz, R. J., et al. (2001). Guidelines for the management of intravascular catheter-related infections. *Journal of Intravenous Nursing, 24*, 180–205.

Montgomery, L. A., Hanrahan, K., Kottman, K., et al. (1999). Guideline for IV infiltrations in pediatric patients. *Pediatric Nursing, 25*, 167–169, 173–180.

Moureau, N., & Zonderman, A. (2000). Does it always have to hurt? Premedications for adults and children for use with intravenous therapy. *Journal of Intravenous Nursing, 23*, 213–219.

Oishi, L. A. (2001). The necessity of routinely replacing peripheral intravenous catheters in hospitalized children: A review of the literature. *Journal of Intravenous Nursing, 24*, 174–179.

Shah, P. S., Ng, E., & Sinha, A. K. (2004). Heparin for prolonging peripheral intravenous catheter use in neonates. *The Cochrane Library, 4*, CD002774.

CHAPTER 56

Intravascular Therapy: Peripherally Inserted Central Catheters

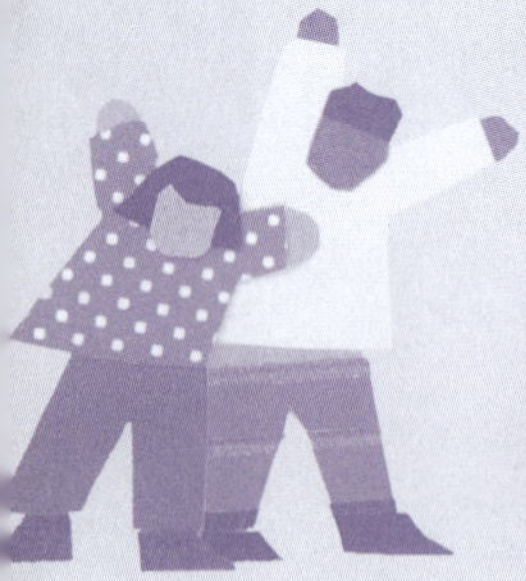

Clinical Guidelines

- A physician, interventional radiologist, or registered nurse (RN) specially trained in peripherally inserted central catheter (PICC) placement performs insertion and removal of PICCs.
- PICC access, site care, and infusion may be performed by an RN, physician, or appropriately trained child or parent. The RN is responsible for monitoring the site and the status of the child after PICC placement, particularly when anesthetic/sedation measures were used.
- A PICC is a catheter that is inserted percutaneously into a peripheral vein with the tip residing in the lower one third of the superior vena cava, to the junction of the superior vena cava and right atrium. Centrally placed catheters are associated with fewer complications in infants and children. Location of the catheter tip must be confirmed radiographically before use. Midline catheters are 3- to 8-inch peripheral catheters with tip placement outside the central veins, below the axillary level and distal to the shoulder.
- There are two types of PICCs: open ended and Groshong, which has a three-way valve at the tip to prevent backflow of blood that opens with negative pressure for blood aspiration and positive pressure for infusions and is in the neutral position when not in use.
- A topical/local anesthetic agent, such as lidocaine cream, may be applied to the insertion site before catheter insertion. Sedation may be required in the young and/or fearful infant or child for successful placement.
- Indications for PICC placement include intermediate to long-term intravenous (IV) access for antibiotics, pain medications, chemotherapy or other vesicants, parenteral nutrition (PN) or other hyperosmolar solutions, or blood products. The early use of PICCs may also spare peripheral veins and the pain of repeated needle sticks, which can be traumatic to children. PICCs are not intended for central venous pressure monitoring, hemophoresis, or hemodialysis.
- Contraindications to PICCs include inadequate veins, bleeding disorders, trauma to involved extremity, severe burns or skin infections, severe immunosuppression, patient noncompliance, and lack of follow-up care.
- Blood pressure cuffs and/or tourniquets should not be applied over the site of the PICC but may be placed distal to the catheter's location.
- All add-on devices shall have a Luer-Lok design.

- To minimize the associated risk for infection, aseptic technique must be used when caring for a PICC. Maximum barrier precautions must be followed during PICC placement and include the use of mask, protective eyewear, sterile gown, cap, powder-free sterile gloves, and large sterile drapes and towels.

EQUIPMENT

For PICC dressing change:

- Antiseptic applicators/swabs/pads: One 2% chlorhexidine-based preparation (preferred antiseptic; see Table 57-1) *or* three iodophor (e.g., 10% povidone-iodine) or 70% alcohol preparations can be used.
- Dressing materials: semipermeable, transparent dressing, or gauze and tape
- Tape measure
- Nonsterile gloves and sterile gloves
- Catheter stabilization device
- Material to secure IV tubing/line: tape or surgical netting

For flushing and locking PICC:

caREminder

Refer to the manufacturer's recommendation for size of syringe to use for flushing a specific type of line. Manufacturers believe that a smaller syringe exerts too much pressure on the PICC tubing, possibly causing a rupture in the catheter. The size of the syringe used for flushing thus varies based on construction of the catheter (polyurethane versus Silastic) and the amount of pressure the line can sustain.

- 5- or 10-mL syringes
- Alcohol swabs or pads
- Heparinized saline per healthcare prescriber's order (preservative-free in neonates)
- Preservative-free 0.9% sodium chloride
- Sterile needleless connector/catheter cap
- Soft jaw clamp (depending on the manufacturer)

CHILD AND FAMILY ASSESSMENT AND PREPARATION

- Determine the child's and family's understanding of the need for the PICC and the importance of site care and infection control.
- Assess the need to provide developmentally appropriate material to the child to explain the mechanics of the PICC. Therapeutic play may also be beneficial.
- In general, to maintain good blood flow around the catheter, children are encouraged to use the arm as usual where the PICC is placed, rather than guard it. Very active children are at greater risk for breaking or dislodging a PICC. Immobilization of the extremity may be necessary in these children, and this should be explained to the child/family with appropriate range of motion provided at regular intervals.

PROCEDURE **PICC Site Care and Dressing Change**

Steps	Rationale/Points of Emphasis
1. Gather the necessary supplies and obtain the assistance of an additional person as needed. Involve parent in comforting child during procedure. Have child assume a comfortable position with arm well supported.	Promotes efficient time management and provides an organized approach to the procedure. Assistance may be required to hold child securely to prevent dislodging catheter or breaking the sterile field.
2. Perform hand hygiene and don gloves. Remove old dressing carefully to avoid dislodging catheter. Discard old dressing in trash receptacle and remove gloves.	Standard precautions to reduce transmission of microorganisms. **caREminder** *To facilitate removing transparent dressing, pull edges first in outward direction, parallel to the skin surface. This releases the adhesive bonds of the dressing and lifts it off the skin, decreasing skin trauma.*
3. Apply new sterile gloves and a mask; inspect site for redness, inflammation, drainage, tenderness, or streaking (Figure 56-1).	Aseptic technique helps decrease risk of infection in central venous catheters with extended dwell times.
4. If external segment of catheter is visible, measure from the exit site to the hub of catheter and document, being careful to maintain sterility. Compare with the baseline external length documented at time of PICC insertion. The PICC may have external centimeter markings on it which can be used to determine the length.	Comparison will allow for monitoring of catheter migration. A discrepancy of more than 2 cm in length should be reported to the healthcare prescriber.

Continued

Steps	Rationale/Points of Emphasis
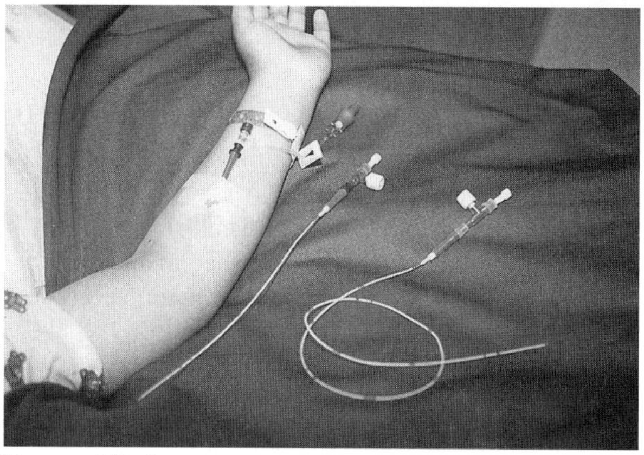 **FIGURE 56-1** The PICC catheter is inserted percutaneously into a peripheral vein, with the tip of the catheter residing in the superior vena cava, a central vein.	
5. Cleanse around exit site with antiseptic applicator, swab, or pad.	Cleanses microorganisms from exit site.
a. If using 2% chlorhexidine applicator, scrub in back-and-forth motion using friction for 30 seconds. Only one applicator is required with this product. Allow site to air-dry; do not fan or blow on skin. Remove antiseptic from skin of neonates with sterile water or sterile saline using sterile gauze.	Antiseptics must be applied with sufficient friction to ensure that the solution reaches into the cracks and fissures of the skin. Chlorhexidine requires 30 seconds with friction scrub for antiseptic effectiveness. Fanning or blowing may introduce contaminants and hasten drying, reducing antimicrobial action.
b. If using 10% povidone-iodine solution, use one swab to cleanse, beginning at the PICC exit site and working outward in a circular pattern, cleansing an area the size of the dressing that will be applied; do not return to an already cleaned area with the same swab. Repeat twice more with a new swab for a total time of 2 minutes. Allow site to air-dry; do not fan or blow on skin. Remove povidone-iodine solution from skin after air-drying.	Povidone-iodine must remain on the skin for 2 minutes and dry to be most effective; thus, three swabs are used. It has been thought that working from the center outward moves microorganisms away from the exit site, although there is no research to support this. Working outward does allow area to dry, facilitating antiseptic effectiveness. One swab can be used, using a slower cleansing technique to cleanse for 2 minutes.
c. Do not use antimicrobial ointment in routine site care.	Use of polyantibiotic ointments may increase the risk for *Candida* colonization.
KidKare Some infants and children have sensitivity to iodine products, which may also affect the neonatal thyroid. These products should not remain on the skin. Also, use of chlorhexidine may be associated with contact dermatitis in low-birth-weight neonates.	
6. Ensure that any external catheter present is looped away from the antecubital fossa and secured before applying dressing.	Avoiding the antecubital fossa prevents kinking of the catheter during infusions.
7. Apply chlorhexidine patch (optional) and semipermeable transparent dressing to site so that it is covered occlusively. Change transparent dressings at least every 7 days or more frequently if wet, soiled, or loose, as needed.	Added antiseptic action from chlorhexidine patch may provide protection from microorganisms. The use of chlorhexidine gluconate in infants weighing <1,000 g has been associated with contact dermatitis and should be used with caution in this population (Association for Women's Health, Obstetric and Neonatal Nurses, 2001; Infusion Nurses Society, 2006a). Studies demonstrate no clinically substantial differences between gauze and transparent dressings in either the incidences of catheter-site colonization or phlebitis. Transparent dressings provide greater stabilization of the catheter and visualization of site. The transparent dressing holds the PICC in place, because most PICCs are not sutured in place in children.

Steps	Rationale/Points of Emphasis
8. Secure hub and extension tubing of PICC to skin with a catheter securement device (preferable), Steri-Strips, or tape. All connections should be Luer-Loked. Secure the IV tubing with additional tape as needed to prevent pulling and inadvertent removal.	Inadvertent dislodgement is one of the most frequently reported complications in children. **KidKare** In the young child, cover the PICC line with surgical netting to keep out of sight. Use armboard as needed to prevent excessive movement. Dislodging the line is possible when tubing is changed at hub. There is no increased risk for infection provided that extension tubing is attached under sterile conditions.
9. Change primary and secondary intravenous (IV) tubing every 72 hours or per institutional policy, except for intralipid tubing, which should be changed every 24 hours. PICC IV tubing is changed up to the extension set.	Prevents microorganisms from growing in IV tubing. Exposure to lipids has been identified as an independent risk factor for bloodstream infections.

PROCEDURE Maintaining Patency of the PICC

Steps	Rationale/Points of Emphasis
1. When infusion is discontinued or PICC is used intermittently, apply heparin or saline lock, depending on the type of PICC catheter (open or valved tipped) by flushing catheter after each use or once daily (see Chapters 49 and 104).	Maintains patency of catheter.
2. Follow manufacturer's recommendations to select syringe size for this procedure. **Alert!** *Smaller diameter syringes create higher internal pressure with little manual force. Excessive pressures can cause catheter rupture.*	
3. Cleanse needleless connector/catheter cap with alcohol using friction and allow it to dry.	Reduces risk for infection from microorganisms.
4. Attach syringe and apply clamp, if appropriate. Flush PICC with heparinized saline/0.9% sodium chloride as per healthcare prescriber order using a push-pause method. For Groshong catheters with valved distal tips, use a saline flush. **Alert!** *Use at least twice the volume capacity of the catheter and add-on device as the minimum volume of the flush solution (Infusion Nurses Society, 2006a.)*	Although use of saline locks is common practice in adults, evidence in children is contradictory and does not support discontinuing the use of heparin. This may be related to the smaller lumen sizes. It also relates to the type of catheter and the type of needleless connector used. Push-pause method creates mild turbulence, which may prevent clots from forming on catheter wall.
5. Use saline/antibiotic/saline/heparin (SASH) technique if there is incompatibility between a medication and heparin. Use the saline/antibiotic/saline (SAS) method when the catheter does not require heparin.	SASH/SAS may prevent formation of precipitations that can occlude the PICC.
6. Continue to apply pressure as you withdraw the syringe and clamp the catheter. Follow manufacturer's directions for completion of flushing with specific needleless connectors.	This prevents backflow of blood and potential clot formation.

CHILD AND FAMILY EVALUATION AND DOCUMENTATION

- Evaluate site appearance and line patency; note presence or absence of redness, swelling, drainage, tenderness, or streaking. Troubleshoot as needed (Chart 56-1). If appropriate, culture the site. Notify the healthcare prescriber of any signs of skin breakdown, infection, infiltration/extravasation, or catheter migration or occlusion.
- Evaluate child's and parent's readiness to learn about care of the PICC. Involve family in hands-on care as early as possible.

CHART 56-1 TROUBLESHOOTING A PICC

If unable to flush or draw blood:

- Examine catheter to ensure that clamps (if used or may be part of an extension tubing) are open and catheter is not kinked.
- If sutures are present, ensure they are not causing obstruction.
- Assess other etiologies for catheter occlusion: medication profile/compatibilities, position of patient. Occlusions may occur as a result of external or internal mechanical obstruction (kinked catheter under dressing, catheter migration, precipitations, thrombosis); nonthrombotic occlusions, such as drug precipitates (internal); or thrombotic occlusions due to fibrin deposits or blood clots (internal). Thrombosis may cause partial or complete occlusion. Catheter pinch-off (internal cause of occlusion) may be caused by an area of compression between the first rib and clavicle. Continued compression can lead to thrombosis or shearing of line. Note when catheter was last functioning and when last blood return was documented.
- Reposition child (i.e., extend or raise arm over head). If catheter remains positional, notify healthcare prescriber. Radiograph may be needed to determine tip placement.
- If occlusion from precipitation is suspected, attempt to aspirate to clear catheter. If successful, flush with preservative-free 0.9% sodium chloride saline between all medications. If unsuccessful, obtain healthcare prescriber's order for agent to treat precipitate. Consult with pharmacy and check the organizational policy on who may perform this procedure. The instilled volume of the solution to clear precipitates should not exceed the internal volume of the catheter to avoid IV administration. Instillation, aspiration, and flushing should be done using a method that does not exceed the catheter manufacturer's maximum pressure limits to avoid line rupture.
- If occlusion is due to thrombosis, obtain healthcare prescriber's order for thrombolytic declotting agent; follow manufacturer's recommendations and check the organizational policy for who may do this procedure.

If infiltration or extravasation is suspected/occurs:

- Extravasation is the unintended administration of a vesicant medication or solution into the tissue surrounding the vein. Infiltration is the unintended administration of a nonvesicant medication into the surrounding tissue. Infiltration/extravasation associated with a central venous catheter may be difficult to detect.
- Always include assessment along the path of the catheter when performing IV site checks.
- Measure the circumference of the extremity above the exit site and compare with the baseline measurement obtained when the PICC was placed; an increase in circumference of the extremity and/or complaints of pain/discomfort may indicate infiltration/extravasation.
- If infiltration/extravasation occurs, discontinue infusion but do not remove PICC.
- Notify healthcare prescriber of infiltration/extravasation, solution or medications infusing at time of infiltration, and site appearance.
- Obtain healthcare prescriber's order, in collaboration with pharmacy, for agent to treat infiltration/extravasation. Treatment is dependent on the properties of the infiltrated medication or solution, the manufacturer's guidelines for that agent, and the severity of the problem. It is recommended to remove the PICC.

If phlebitis occurs:

- Phlebitis is an inflammation of the vein usually caused by mechanical irritation from the catheter. Some catheter materials are associated with increased risk for phlebitis.
- Encourage limitation of movement at site.
- Apply warm, moist soak to extremity to ease discomfort.
- If symptoms increase or if streak formation or palpable cord is present, notify healthcare prescriber.
- Phlebitis may necessitate removal of PICC line when pain at access site with erythema and/or edema is present.

If catheter migration is suspected/occurs:

- Suspect migration of PICC distally if the child complains of chest pain or hears a noise during flushing

Continued

CHART 56-1 TROUBLESHOOTING A PICC (CONTINUED)

of the PICC. Catheter migration may be caused by excessive sneezing, coughing, or vomiting. Report to healthcare prescriber if external PICC migration is greater than 2 cm.

- Notify healthcare prescriber to obtain order for radiograph to confirm tip placement.
- External migration may necessitate replacement of a PICC or a change in therapy. Internal migration requires manipulation/removal.

If the catheter is leaking, damaged or broken:

- Clamp and secure the catheter to prevent migration and possible embolization of catheter fragment. Catheter embolization is an emergency and may require surgical intervention.
- Determine extent and location of damage.
- Repair of the PICC line may be done by an RN competent in this procedure using the manufacturer's repair kit and guidelines. Not all PICC manufacturers provide repair kits; repair with other materials may lead to catheter separation and migration or embolization.
- Inability to repair necessitates removal of the PICC.
- Report a defective catheter per institutional policy.

If bleeding is present:

- Apply gauze dressing after initial placement of PICC and change first dressing in 24 hours. Mild bleeding at site may occur for the first 24 hours after PICC placement.
- Limit movement of extremity using armboard as necessary.
- If bleeding increases or persists past first 24 hours, notify healthcare prescriber.

- Document the following:
  - Type, size, length of catheter, date, time, and initials of person completing the dressing change on the dressing and in the patient record
  - Site appearance, noting presence or absence of redness, swelling, drainage, tenderness, or streaking
  - Date, time, type, and amount of flush solution used, presence or absence of blood return, and any resistance to flushing
  - Pain due to PICC placement or associated with use; interventions and child's response

COMMUNITY CARE

- If the child is to be discharged home with a PICC, begin discharge planning with a home care company as early as possible. The use of a doll with a PICC for teaching may be less intimidating to the child and family initially as they begin to learn the skills needed for home care.
- Include in communication with the home care provider the type of PICC, including manufacturer and size if known; internal and external length; date of insertion; practitioner(s) responsible for line placement and follow-up care; last dressing change with dressing/flush protocol taught in healthcare setting; and notification of any complications that occurred after placement.
- Instruct parents in hand hygiene/infection control, dressing changes, flushing, medication administration and flow control device/syringe pump use as applicable, disposal techniques for syringes, and age/developmentally based safety methods to secure the PICC.
- Before discharge, parents should verbalize knowledge of infection control, safety, and the most common complications of PICCs (i.e., sepsis and inadvertent removal), what to look for, and actions to take in the event of complications.
- Provide parents with the PICC repair kit supplied by the manufacturer and instruct them to take the kit with them to nearest healthcare facility in the event of leakage or catheter damage.
- Booklets are provided by the PICC manufacturers for family education. Another source that can be accessed for PICC information is the website www.cc.nih.gov/ccc/patient_education/pepubs/piccsicc.pdf
- Instruct the family to contact the healthcare provider if
  - Child has a fever
  - PICC insertion site remains reddened or oozes fluid or blood
  - Mechanical problems occur, such as inability to flush, leaking, or unintended dislodgement

Unexpected Situation

- *While dressing is being changed, the PICC is inadvertently withdrawn a small amount:* If the catheter is not totally removed, measure from exit site to the hub of the catheter, reapply a sterile dressing to protect the site, and note the difference of the external length of the PICC compared with the baseline measurement. Notify healthcare prescriber. A chest radiograph may be ordered to determine PICC tip position.

Bibliography

Association for Women's Health, Obstetric and Neonatal Nurses. (2001). *Neonatal skin care: Evidence-based clinical practice guidelines.* Glenview, IL: Author.

Carson, S. M. (2004). Chlorhexidine versus povidone-iodine for central venous catheter site care in children. *Journal of Pediatric Nursing, 19,* 74–80.

Centers for Disease Control and Prevention. (2002). *Guidelines for prevention of intravascular catheter-related infections.* Retrieved August 15, 2006, from http://www.cdc.gov/mmwr/preview/mmwrhtml/rr5110a1.htm

Frey, A., & Schears, G. (2001). Dislodgement rates and impact of securement methods for peripherally inserted central catheters (PICCs) in children. *Pediatric Nursing, 27,* 185–189.

Golombek, S. G., Rohan, A. J., Parvez, B., Salice, A. L., & LaGamma, E. F. (2002). "Proactive" management of percutaneously inserted central catheters results in decreased incidence of infection in the ELBW population. *Perinatology, 22,* 209–213.

Gorski, L. A., & Czaplewski, L. M. (2004). Peripherally inserted central catheters & midline catheters for the home care nurse. *Journal of Infusion Nursing, 27,* 399–409.

Infusion Nurses Society. (2006a). Infusion nursing: Standards of practice. *Journal of Infusion Nursing, 29*(Suppl. 1S), S1–S92.

Infusion Nurses Society. (2006b). *Policies and procedures for infusion nursing* (3rd ed.). Norwood, MA: Author.

Krzywda, E. A., & Andris, D. A. (2005). Twenty-five years of advances in vascular access: Bridging research to clinical practice. *Nutrition in Clinical Practice, 20,* 597–606.

Sherrod, J., Warner, B., & Altimier, L. (2004). Designing and monitoring an RN-based PICC team. *Neonatal Intensive Care, 17,* 19–21.

C H A P T E R

57

Intravascular Therapy: Totally Implantable Devices

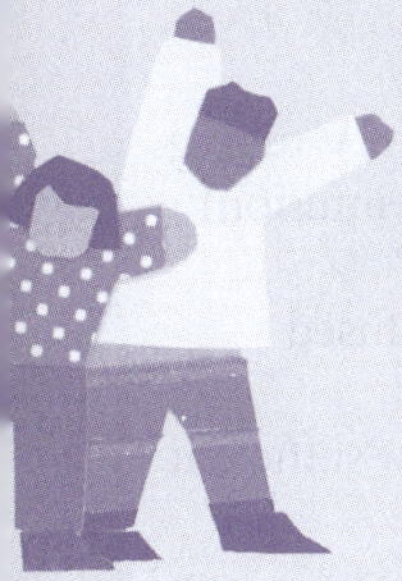

Clinical Guidelines

- Long-term central venous catheters, placed to reduce the trauma of repeated venipuncture in the child, are surgically inserted and removed by a physician under sterile conditions. They are used for direct administration of intravenous (IV) fluids; for intermittent use with medications, chemotherapy, blood and blood products, and parenteral nutrition; or for venous blood draws for laboratory analysis. They may be used in the home setting for parenteral therapies, thereby improving the child's quality of life.
- TID access, site care, and infusion may be performed by a registered nurse (RN), physician, or appropriately trained child or parent.
- There are basically two types of long-term venous access devices. The first type is the totally implantable device (TID); examples of brand names are Port-a-Cath (Figure 57-1), Infuse-A-Port, P.A.S. Port, or Chemo-Port. The second type is the right atrial Silastic catheter, which is sometimes called a *tunneled catheter* or is named for its manufacturer (e.g., Broviac or Hickman) (see Chapter 58). The underlying condition of the child, the indication for use, and the capability of the family or child to perform self-care for home maintenance help determine which venous access device is appropriate for that child. TIDs are better suited for prolonged (6 months or more) intermittent IV therapy. However, because of size restrictions, they may not be available for use in neonates and small infants. Low-profile devices may be placed in younger children, according to the surgeon's preference.
- Access to a TID reservoir is accomplished with a noncoring needle (e.g., Huber) because a standard needle will damage the self-sealing silicone septum. Noncoring needles come in varying lengths and sizes; however, the most commonly used size for children is a 22-gauge right-angle needle with a variable length to accommodate the depth of subcutaneous tissues (Figure 57-2).
- Topical anesthetic agents are an option for comfort with noncoring needle insertion in nonemergent situations, based on child preference.
- Aseptic technique is used when caring for or using long-term venous access devices to minimize the associated risk for infection.
- A 2% chlorhexidine-based preparation is the preferred solution for skin antisepsis. Tincture of iodine, an iodophor (e.g., povidone-iodine), or 70% alcohol can be used.
- Follow manufacturer's instructions for the specific venous access devices.
- When the TID is used daily, the noncoring needle remains in place and is changed weekly with the dressing.

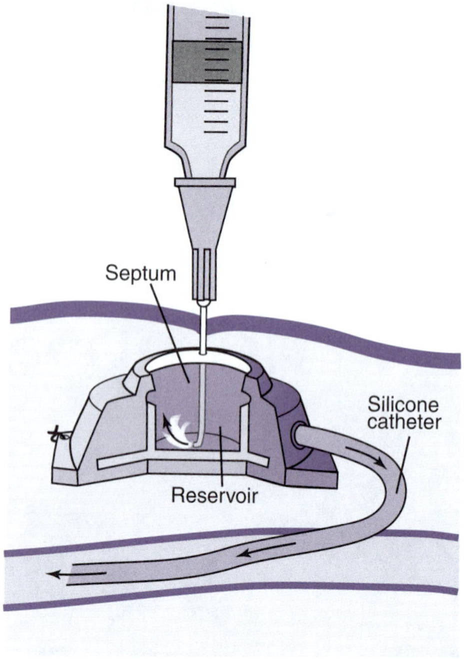

FIGURE 57-1
Schematic of an implanted port with noncoring needle inserted.

- Monthly flushes with sterile heparin are required to maintain patency when the TID is not in use and the port reservoir is deaccessed.
- All add-on devices have a Luer-Lok design.
- Intravenous fluids are administered via a flow-controlled infusion device.
- Care and management techniques vary based on the procedure being performed per institutional policies and include
  - Sterile technique (sterile dressings and sterile gloves)
  - Modified clean technique (nonsterile gloves and sterile dressings)

EQUIPMENT

For access and administration of solutions through a TID:

- Sterile drape
- Two pairs of sterile gloves
- Two sterile 10-mL syringes
- Two sterile needleless access devices (per institutional policy)
- Appropriate-sized right-angle noncoring needle with attached extension tubing
- Sterile needleless connector/catheter cap (to attach to noncoring needle extension tubing)
- Antiseptic solution (Table 57-1)
- Three alcohol prep pads or swabs, if povidone-iodine antiseptic is used
- Sterile preservative-free 0.9% sodium chloride (20 mL) for injection
- Prescribed fluid for administration, along with administration set
- One-inch tape
- Steri-Strips
- Dressing materials: sterile, semipermeable, transparent dressing

For flushing and heparin locking an accessed TID:

- Nonsterile gloves
- Two sterile 10-mL syringes
- Sterile needleless system/blunt cannulas (per institutional policy)
- Heparin: 1–10 units/mL (per healthcare prescriber order, usually 5 mL)
- Three alcohol prep pads
- Sterile needleless connector/catheter cap (to attach to extension tubing of the noncoring needle)
- Sterile preservative-free 0.9% sodium chloride (20 mL) for injection
- Sterile male catheter cap/adapter (to attach to IV tubing to maintain sterility if disconnecting from an infusion)

For removing the noncoring needle from a TID and for site care and maintenance of an accessed TID:

- Nonsterile gloves
- Two sterile 10-mL syringes
- Sterile needleless access devices (per institutional policy)
- Sterile preservative-free 0.9% sodium chloride (20 mL) for injection
- Heparin: 1–10 units/mL (per healthcare prescriber order, usually 5 mL)
- Three alcohol prep pads
- Sterile 2 × 2 gauze
- Band-aid

For blood withdrawal through a TID:

- Nonsterile gloves
- Sterile needleless system/blunt cannulas (per institutional policy)
- Three alcohol prep pads
- Sterile male catheter cap/adapter (to attach to IV tubing to maintain sterility if disconnecting from an infusion)
- A 10-mL sterile syringe
- Heparin (10 units/mL), if blood will be reinfused
- Sterile needleless connector/catheter cap
- Sterile syringe of appropriate size to withdraw sufficient blood for ordered tests
- Specimen tubes for ordered labs
- Biohazard bag
- Specimen labels and requisition
- Ice, if needed for blood specimen

CHILD AND FAMILY ASSESSMENT AND PREPARATION

- Discuss the purpose of a TID and the intended reason for its use with the child and parents. Reinforce the purpose, and discuss the risks and benefits of long-term total implanted venous access device. Assess the cognitive level,

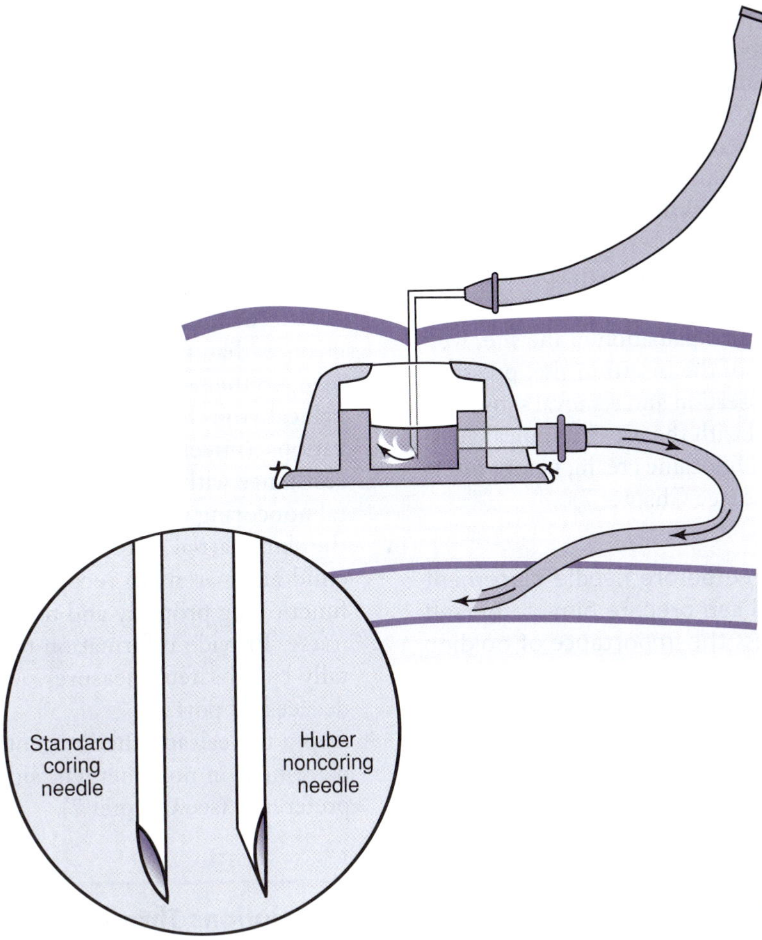

FIGURE 57-2
Note the difference between a noncoring needle with the lumen on the side versus a standard needle with the lumen at the end. This design avoids shearing of the material of the port septum when accessing the implantable device and maintains integrity of the septum.

TABLE 57-1
Skin Antisepsis

Age	Solution	Cleansing Method
Older than 2 months	Chlorhexidine gluconate solution (CHG)	Using one applicator, clean with repeated back-and-forth strokes of the sponge: For a dry site (e.g., abdomen, arm), cleanse for 30 sec. For a moist site (e.g., inguinal fold, neck), cleanse for 2 min.
Younger than 2 months/ neonate*	10% povidone-iodine (PI)	Start at the intended insertion site (e.g., septum of the port) and work outward in a circular pattern to an area at least the size of the dressing (2–4 inches [5–10 cm]). Use one swab for 30 sec. Repeat two more times using a new swab each time. Do not return to cleaned area with the same swab. Remove antiseptic with sterile water or sterile saline.

*The Centers for Disease Control and Prevention makes no recommendation for the use of chlorhexidine in infants aged < 2 months. The Association for Women's Health, Obstetric and Neonatal Nurses neonatal skin care guidelines recommend either CHG or PI. The use of CHG in infants weighing < 1,000 grams has been associated with contact dermatitis and should be used with caution in this population (Association for Women's Health, Obstetric and Neonatal Nurses, 2001; Infusion Nurses Society, 2006).

readiness, and ability to process information by the child and family. Readiness to learn and process information may be impaired as a result of age, stress, or anxiety.

- Explain that the TID is completely contained underneath the child's skin; therefore, when not in use, it is fairly inconspicuous (seen only as a bump under the skin) and has a greatly reduced risk for infection compared with a tunneled catheter.
- Explain the procedure, as appropriate, to both the child and parents. To help reduce anxiety, describe the sensations the child can expect: palpation of the site, wetness from the cleansing of the insertion site, pressure, and noncoring needle insertion and removal sensation. Explain comfort control with the use of a topical anesthetic agent, such as 4% lidocaine cream, before insertion of noncoring needle (see Chapter 7).

KidKare Count to three before needle placement and removal so the child can prepare him- or herself and is not surprised. Stress the importance of holding still during the noncoring needle placement to facilitate insertion. Children identify needles as the most painful and scariest part of any hospitalization. Involve a child life specialist, if available, to assist with preparation and distraction techniques.

- Assess the skin overlying the TID and the tissue surrounding the port. Observe for signs of infection or thrombosis. Insertion of the noncoring needle should not be undertaken if any of the following signs are present: erythema, inflammation, exudate, supraclavicular swelling, or venous distention.
- Obtain the child's baseline weight and height to aid in determining amount of heparinized normal saline to use for flushing and locking.
- Assess the child's baseline vital signs and observe for changes that may indicate a local or systemic infection (e.g., erythema, fever).
- Educate the child and parents about potential complications (infection, mechanical problems, including resistance with flushing, breaks, displaced or accidental noncoring needle removal, port extrusion through the skin, partial or total occlusions). This enables the child and parent to recognize when the TID is not functioning properly and to know when to notify the nurse. Provide information to promote developmentally based safety measures of child with accessed or deaccessed port.
- Apply topical anesthetic agent for noncoring needle placement in nonemergent situations, based on child preference (see Chapter 7).

PROCEDURE Access and Administration of Solutions Through a TID

Steps	Rationale/Points of Emphasis
1. Perform hand hygiene and gather all necessary supplies. Involve family in comforting child during procedure.	Reduces the transmission of microorganisms. Promotes efficient time management and provides organized approach to the procedure. **caREminder** *Obtain the assistance of an additional person as needed to hold child securely to prevent contamination of the sterile field.*
2. Remove child's top/clothing and locate the TID by palpating it under the skin.	Verifies proper position of TID.
3. Remove topical anesthetic cream, if used.	Allows for evaluation of effectiveness of topical anesthetic and prepares skin for cleansing.
4. Palpate/locate the silicone septum of the port reservoir within the perimeter of the TID under the skin.	Establishes landmarks of the septum and identifies where noncoring needle will be inserted.
5. Repeat hand hygiene.	Reduces the transmission of microorganisms.
6. Establish a sterile work area with the sterile drape; open supplies aseptically and drop them on the sterile field. Don sterile gloves.	Maintaining sterile precautions decreases the introduction of microorganisms.
7. Draw up 20 mL of sterile preservative-free 0.9% sodium chloride. Connect the filled syringe to the noncoring needle extension tubing and prime the extension tubing and noncoring needle. Close the clamp on the extension tubing and return noncoring needle with attached syringe to the sterile field.	Prepares syringe for use. Clears the noncoring needle and extension tubing of air before port access.

Steps	Rationale/Points of Emphasis
8. Prep the skin over the port septum and surrounding area to the same size of the dressing with appropriate antiseptic. Children with TID placed are typically older; thus the antiseptic of choice is chlorhexidine gluconate.	Cleanses microorganisms from insertion site.
9. Allow site to air-dry. Do not blot, fan, or blow on site.	Allows antimicrobial action of antiseptic. Blotting, fanning, or blowing may introduce contaminants and hasten drying, reducing antimicrobial action.
10. If a povidone-iodine–based antiseptic was used, remove the solution from the skin using an alcohol swab or pad. Start at the septum of the port and work outward in a circular pattern as the same size of the dressing. Repeat two more times with a new alcohol swab each time.	Removes povidone-iodine solution from the skin. Some children have sensitivity to iodine products; do not allow it to remain on the skin.
11. Don a new pair of sterile gloves, if nonsterile items were handled.	Maintains sterile technique.
12. With the nondominant hand, stabilize the TID reservoir between the thumb and the forefinger on the overlying skin.	Stabilizes the TID from moving or slippage due to the firm pressure required to access the silicone septum.
13. Grasp the noncoring needle with the dominant hand, using the forefinger to support the needle or the butterfly wing set. Insert the noncoring needle directly perpendicular to the septum of the TID; continuously apply steady pressure until you feel the needle touch the back base of the reservoir.	Prevents deflection of the needle into outlying skin. First step of confirming correct noncoring needle placement. **Alert!** *Do not access the TID septum through the same needle site that was previously used because of the potential for skin breakdown and potential abscess formation. The septum can typically withstand approximately 2,000 noncoring needle insertions.*
14. Pull back on syringe plunger until blood is aspirated.	Second step of confirming correct noncoring needle placement into TID reservoir. **caREminder** *Blood return may be brown with fibrin clots when the catheter has not been in use for some time. If this is the case, continue to aspirate blood until it is bright red, and then detach the syringe in use and replace with a new 20-mL saline-filled syringe. If no blood return is obtained and needle placement is correct, do not proceed with fluid administration and notify the healthcare prescriber immediately to ensure prompt intervention to reduce complications.*
15. Using small pulses of fluid, infuse the 20 mL of sterile preservative-free 0.9% sodium chloride and clamp when completed.	Flushing is the third step in confirming correct noncoring placement. Flushes any blood from the TID reservoir/catheter and prevents occlusion. Children who require fluid restriction (e.g., those with renal or cardiac conditions) may not tolerate 20 mL. Less flush volumes may be determined in conjunction with the healthcare prescriber (i.e., use 10 mL if it clears the line). **Alert!** *Observe for signs of extravasation, such as swelling in the reservoir pocket, or complaints of discomfort/pain, which indicate incorrect noncoring needle placement.*

Continued

Steps	Rationale/Points of Emphasis
16. Remove the syringe and apply the primed sterile needleless connector/catheter cap. Maintaining sterility, connect prescribed fluid by connecting the IV infusion directly to the needleless connector/catheter cap of the noncoring needle extension tubing. Open clamp and begin IV fluids as prescribed or place catheter to "heparin lock" for intermittent infusions by administering the prescribed heparin flush. Close clamp on extension tubing when system is heparin locked.	Provides fluid delivery as prescribed or maintains patent system for use. A closed clamp is a backup to prevent inadvertent communication into the vascular system.
17. Apply Steri-Strip over noncoring needle and a semipermeable sterile transparent dressing over the TID, noncoring needle, and the upper portion of the extension tubing. May place sterile gauze under device wings to prevent rocking motion of needle within the port.	Maintains sterility of system and allows for assessment of needle position and skin. Stabilizes needle in position. **Alert!** *Use of a 2 × 2 gauze to stabilize the noncoring needle does not constitute a gauze dressing if the insertion site is visible (Infusion Nurses Society, 2006a).*
18. Remove sterile gloves and secure the line with additional tape or Steri-Strips.	Prevents accidental dislodgment, tugging, or pulling at the noncoring needle site.
19. Replace the child's clothing over TID.	Maintains body image.
20. Dispose of equipment and waste in appropriate receptacle.	Standard precautions.
21. Perform hand hygiene.	Reduces transmission of microorganisms.
22. Ensure that fluid is infused via a flow-control infusion device and that no more than 4 hours worth of IV fluid (or refer to organizational policy) is allowed to hang at any one time. Change IV tubing using aseptic technique every 72 hours or when contamination occurs or is suspected, except for intralipid tubing, which should be changed every 24 hours. Label the IV tubing with time, date, and initials when hung.	Infusing using a flow-control infusion device and limiting amount of fluid hanging can prevent potential accidental fluid overload and complications from IV infiltration. Changing tubing at routine intervals reduces risk of microorganisms from growing in IV tubing. Labeling tubing aids in identifying proper change times.

PROCEDURE Flushing and Heparin Locking an Accessed TID*

Steps	Rationale/Points of Emphasis
1. Perform hand hygiene and gather all necessary equipment and supplies. Involve family in comforting child during procedure. **caREminder** *Obtain the assistance of an additional person as needed to hold child securely to prevent contamination of supplies.*	Reduces the transmission of microorganisms. Promotes efficient time management and provides an organized approach to the procedure.
2. Establish a clean work area; open supplies aseptically and drop them onto the clean work area.	Decreases the chance of microorganisms.
3. Don nonsterile gloves.	Standard precaution to reduce transmission of microorganisms.
4. Draw up 20 mL of sterile preservative-free 0.9% sodium chloride, label and return the filled syringe to the work area.	Prepares syringe for use.

Steps	Rationale/Points of Emphasis
5. Draw up 5 mL, as prescribed, of sterile heparin into syringe for flush, label and return to the work area. If only saline flush is prescribed, omit this step.	Prepares syringe for use. **caREminder** *Label the syringe that contains the sterile preservative-free 0.9% sodium chloride and the syringe that contains the heparin. Saline and heparin must be given in proper order to ensure the heparin dwells within the TID system when not in use.*
6. Locate noncoring needle extension tubing/IV tubing junction under child's clothes/shirt.	Establishes ease of access.
7. For an infusing IV solution: Cleanse the IV/needleless connector/catheter cap junction with the alcohol swabs (at least 10 strokes per swab). Close clamp on extension tubing, stop infusion, and disconnect the IV tubing, maintaining sterility. Cover IV tubing end with a sterile connector/cap for next IV infusion.	Reduces the transmission of microorganisms. Do not use povidone-iodine because it is not an effective antimicrobial on inanimate objects.
8. Cleanse the needleless connector/catheter cap with alcohol and connect it to the needleless system. Open the clamp.	Allows for infusion of flush solution.
9. Pull back on syringe plunger to visualize a flash of blood aspirate.	Verifies noncoring needle placement and patency of system before administering solutions/medications.
10. Once there is confirmation of a patent system, use small pulses of fluid to infuse the sterile saline solution. If unable to aspirate a blood return to confirm needle placement, have child change positions by raising arms overhead and cough to increase intrathoracic pressure to increase yield for blood return. If unable to obtain blood return and confirm noncoring needle placement, problem solve according to organizational policy.	Obtaining a blood aspirate confirms noncoring needle position before use. Preservative-free 0.9% sodium chloride flush clears blood and any medication from the port reservoir and ensures patency of the TID system. Use of positive pressure technique when completing the flush or a positive pressure displacement catheter connector helps avoid reflux of blood into the catheter tip.
11. Remove the preservative-free 0.9% sodium chloride syringe and connect the prescribed heparin syringe.	Allows for infusion of heparin solution.
12. Using small pulses of fluid, infuse the prescribed heparin.	Provides fluid delivery as prescribed.
13. Reapply the catheter clamp to the noncoring needle extension tubing.	Prevents accidental infusion of unwanted fluid and places the TID system to "heparin-lock."
14. Remove gloves and secure the line with additional tape.	Prevents accidental dislodgment, tugging, or pulling at the noncoring needle site.
15. Replace child's clothing over TID.	Prevents body image disturbance.
16. Dispose of equipment and waste in appropriate receptacle.	Standard precautions.
17. Perform hand hygiene.	Reduces transmission of microorganisms.

*If noncoring needle is not already in place, first follow procedure for Access and Administration of Solutions Through a TID.

PROCEDURE Removing the Noncoring Needle From a TID

Steps	Rationale/Points of Emphasis
1. Perform hand hygiene and gather all necessary equipment and supplies. Involve family in comforting child during procedure.	Reduces the transmission of microorganisms. Promotes efficient time management and provides an organized approach to the procedure.

Continued

Steps	Rationale/Points of Emphasis
	caREminder *Obtain the assistance of an additional person as needed to hold child securely to provide safety.*
2. Establish a clean work area; open supplies aseptically and drop them onto the clean work area.	Minimizes the risk of microorganisms introduced into the TID.
3. Don nonsterile gloves.	Standard precaution to reduce transmission of microorganisms.
4. Draw up and label 20 mL of sterile preservative-free 0.9% sodium chloride for flushing with needleless system and return to the clean work area.	Prepares syringe for use.
5. Draw up 5 mL (as prescribed) of sterile heparin and label for flushing and return the filled syringe to the clean work area.	Prepares syringe for use. **caREminder** *Be sure to label the syringe that contains the sterile preservative-free 0.9% sodium chloride and the syringe that contains the heparin. Flushing must be done in proper order to ensure the heparin dwells within the TID system to maintain patency when the TID is not in use.*
6. Locate noncoring extensions tubing/IV junction under child's clothes/shirt and establish ease of access. a. For an infusing IV: Cleanse junction of IV tubing and needleless connector/catheter cap (at least 10 strokes per swab). Clamp the extension tubing. Stop infusion and disconnect IV. b. For a heparin-locked system: Cleanse the surface area of the needleless connector/catheter cap with the alcohol swabs (at least 10 strokes per swab).	Reduces the transmission of microorganisms.
7. Connect the preservative-free 0.9% sodium chloride saline syringe to the needleless connector/catheter cap and open the clamp.	Allows for infusion of flush solution.
8. Aspirate for blood return if child was heparin locked. Using small pulses of fluid, infuse the sterile preservative-free 0.9% sodium chloride.	Blood aspirate confirms noncoring needle placement before flushing. Preservative-free 0.9% sodium chloride flush clears any medications from the port reservoir and ensures patency of the TID.
9. Remove the preservative-free 0.9% sodium chloride syringe and connect the prescribed heparin syringe.	Allows for infusion of heparin solution.
10. Infuse the prescribed heparin using small pulses of fluid.	Provides fluid delivery as prescribed.
11. Close the clamp to the extension tubing.	Places the TID system to "heparin-lock." Clamping before noncoring needle removal prevents inadvertent leakage of fluid as the noncoring needle is removed from the reservoir.
12. While stabilizing the TID with noncoring needle, carefully remove existing semipermeable transparent dressing.	Prepares the noncoring needle for removal. Provides for visual inspection of needle insertion site. **caREminder** *To facilitate removal of transparent dressing, pull edges first in outward direction, parallel to the skin surface. This breaks the adhesive bond and releases the dressing from the skin surface, resulting in less skin irritation.*

Steps	Rationale/Points of Emphasis
13. Visually inspect needle insertion site and surrounding skin. ***Alert!*** *Report signs of infection or skin breakdown immediately to the healthcare prescriber.*	Detection of impaired skin integrity is key to maintaining TID free from sepsis and complications.
14. With the nondominant hand, stabilize the TID reservoir between the thumb and the forefinger on the overlying skin.	Firm pressure is required to keep it from moving or slipping, which will prevent damage to the skin or septum, from movement of the noncoring needle.
15. Grasp the noncoring needle with the dominant hand, holding the hub of the needle between the thumb and forefinger. Withdraw the needle at a perpendicular angle to the skin. If the noncoring needle has wings, squeeze them together while pulling up for deaccessing.	Stabilizes the TID while deaccessing the reservoir.
16. Blot needle insertion site with sterile 2×2 gauze and apply sterile cover to absorb any oozing from needle site; apply adhesive bandage as needed or if child prefers.	Protects skin from organisms as noncoring needle site heals.
17. Replace child's clothing over TID.	Protects privacy of child.
18. Dispose of equipment and waste in appropriate receptacle.	Standard precautions.
19. Perform hand hygiene.	Reduces transmission of microorganisms.

PROCEDURE Site Care and Maintenance of an Accessed TID

Steps	Rationale/Points of Emphasis
1. Perform hand hygiene.	Reduces the transmission of microorganisms.
2. When TID is accessed and in continuous or intermittent use, assess the noncoring needle insertion site for signs of erythema, condition of dressing (dry and intact), and palpate the area for any swelling, assessing for fluid extravasation hourly or per institution policy and procedure.	Close observation allows for immediate interventions to avoid complications.
3. When TID is accessed and used intermittently, follow procedure for Flushing and Heparin Locking an Accessed TID, above.	Flushing and locking the TID system maintains patency for intermittent and long-term use.
4. When TID is accessed and in continuous use, the noncoring needle and dressing is changed weekly. Follow procedure for Access and Administration of Solutions Through a TID, above. The needleless connector/catheter cap is changed with administration set change.	Routinely changing the noncoring needle, semipermeable transparent dressing, and needleless connector/catheter cap minimizes the potential for infectious complications and increases preservation for long-term venous access use.
5. When TID is not accessed with the noncoring needle, it must be accessed and flushed every month. Follow the procedure for Access and Administration of Solutions Through a TID, above.	Monthly accessing and flushing the TID maintains patency for long-term venous access use.

PROCEDURE Blood Withdrawal Through a TID

Steps	Rationale/Points of Emphasis
1. Determine whether "discard" blood is to be reinfused or discarded.	Infants and children who are critically or chronically ill and undergoing frequent blood withdrawal are at risk for iatrogenic anemia. When discard blood is reinfused, blood loss is minimized.

Continued

Steps	Rationale/Points of Emphasis
2. Calculate minimum blood required to perform ordered tests.	Minimizes blood loss of child.
3. Follow steps 1 to 7 of procedure for Flushing and Heparin Locking an Accessed TID. Additionally, if discard blood sample is to be returned, prepare a heparinized syringe by drawing heparin (10 units/mL) into a 10-mL syringe, pull plunger to 10-mL mark, and then push plunger to base of syringe to empty syringe.	A heparinized syringe helps prevent blood clotting for return of discard blood sample while in the syringe during the time it takes to obtain the actual blood sample for testing.
4. Clean the needleless connector/catheter cap with alcohol. Connect a sterile syringe (use heparinized syringe if discard blood sample is to be returned) and unclamp.	Prepares for withdrawal of blood.
5. Gently pull plunger to withdraw 5 mL blood into syringe.	Clears port of residual fluid in reservoir (saline, heparin) and blood.
6. Remove the syringe containing discard fluid and place on clean work area if discard blood sample is to be returned.	Maintains sterility.
7. Apply sterile syringe of appropriate size to withdraw sufficient blood for ordered tests. Gently withdraw amount of blood required for ordered laboratory testing and remove syringe.	Obtains blood samples for testing.
8. If discard blood sample is to be returned: • Visually examine sample for evidence of clot formation; if none, connect syringe to needleless connector/catheter cap and slowly reinfuse. • Connect sterile preservative-free 0.9% sodium chloride syringe, infuse, and clamp extension tubing. If discard is not to be reinfused: • Connect sterile preservative-free 0.9% sodium chloride syringe, infuse saline, and clamp extension tubing.	Avoids infusion of clotted blood. Clears line of blood and prepares for desired use.
9. Change needleless connector/catheter cap if residual blood is present.	Reduces risk for infection.
10. Place blood in appropriate tubes for ordered tests.	Provides proper medium for ordered tests.
11. Follow: • Procedure for Access and Administration of Solutions Through a TID, steps 16 to 21, to commence fluid administration, *or* • Procedure for Flushing and Heparin Locking an Accessed TID, steps 11 to 16, if TID is to be placed to "heparin-lock."	Prepares line for desired use.
12. Prepare blood specimen for testing:	
a. Label specimen with child's name, medical record number and the date, time of collection, and collector's initials.	Ensures that correct specimen is tested for the right patient.
b. Transport specimen to laboratory if necessary. Provide appropriate environment for transport (e.g., ice, refrigeration).	Reduces degradation of specimen before analysis.
13. Perform hand hygiene.	Reduces transmission of microorganisms.

CHILD AND FAMILY EVALUATION AND DOCUMENTATION

- Evaluate site appearance and line patency; note presence or absence of redness, swelling, drainage, or tenderness. Troubleshoot as needed (Chart 57-1). If appropriate, culture the site. Notify the healthcare prescriber of any signs of skin breakdown, infection, infiltration/extravasation, or occlusion.
- Evaluate child and parent's readiness to learn about care of the TID as early as possible.
- Determine whether the child and parents have other areas of concern to discuss.
- Document the following:
  - Date and time of noncoring needle insertion, insertion site, type of needle used (e.g., right angle vs. straight), gauge and length (e.g., 22 g × ¾ inch), any difficulty in placing the needle, the number of

CHART 57-1 TROUBLESHOOTING A TID

If unable to flush or draw blood:

- Examine line for mechanical obstruction; ensure that clamps are open and noncoring needle extension tubing/IV tubing is not kinked.
- Always assume that the inability to irrigate or withdraw from the TID is caused by a malpositioned or occluded noncoring needle. If after the noncoring needle is changed flushing is still not possible, there is a high probability of occlusion.
- Occlusion may occur as a result of external or internal mechanical obstruction, including nonthrombotic occlusions such as drug precipitates or thrombotic occlusions due to fibrin deposits or blood clots. Thrombosis may cause partial or complete occlusion.
- If occlusion from precipitation is suspected, attempt to aspirate to clear TID system. If successful, flush with sterile preservative-free 0.9% sodium chloride between all medications. If unsuccessful, obtain healthcare prescriber order for appropriate nonthrombolytic agent to dissolve precipitate. Once drug crystals have lodged within the TID reservoir/catheter lumen, they are very difficult to dissolve. The instilled volume of the solution to clear precipitates should not exceed the internal volume of the TID system in order to avoid IV administration.
- If occlusion is due to thrombosis, attach a 10-mL syringe filled with 5 mL of heparin and alternately flush and aspirate using a push-pull technique. If unsuccessful, obtain healthcare prescriber order for a thrombolytic agent and use per the manufacturer's recommendations.
- If the child complains of pain or if complete resistance is met, discontinue flush procedure. Confer with healthcare prescriber regarding dye study to further define the problem. Refer to institutional policy for who has skill validation to perform declotting of central venous devices.

If infiltration or extravasation occurs:

- Extravasation is the unintended administration of a vesicant medication or solution into the tissue surrounding the TID. Infiltration is the unintended administration of a nonvesicant medication into the surrounding tissue.
- Always first assume that extravasation is caused by a malpositioned or occluded noncoring needle. Consider separation of catheter from TID reservoir.
- Assess extent of problem.
- Stop infusion immediately.
- Verify correct noncoring needle placement. Apply direct pressure on the needle until contact is made with the back base of the port reservoir.
- Aspirate for blood return.
- If unable to feel base of reservoir *or* unable to aspirate blood, notify healthcare provider.
- If unable to verify needle placement, remove existing needle and reaccess with new needle according to procedure, only if there is not evidence of infiltration/extravasation but complaints of discomfort that may indicate a possible problem.
- If swelling exists over port, remove noncoring needle and DO NOT attempt reaccess until problem is treated appropriately and swelling is resolved. The action taken with this situation depends on the severity of the incident. Consult the healthcare prescriber and Clinical Pharmacy as indicated.
- If the TID is thought to be damaged, report to healthcare prescriber. Damage of the port septum can be confirmed by an x-ray and/or radiographic dye study through the device.
- Consult reference source (pharmacist, policy and procedure, healthcare prescriber) to determine whether cold or warm compresses should be applied based on extravasated solution.
- Confirm plan to administer appropriate antidote and obtain order.

If local infection occurs:

- Local infection is indicated by an alteration in the skin integrity overlying the TID.
- Assess skin surrounding TID and noncoring needle for erythema, inflammation, tenderness, or exudate or skin breakdown.
- Evaluate child's temperature and vital signs.
- Notify healthcare prescriber for symptoms of localized infection.
- Obtain blood cultures, as ordered, only if a noncoring needle is already in place at the time the infectious process is noted. Do not access an erythematous site.

If systemic infection occurs:

- Systemic infection is blood-borne infection.
- Evaluate child's temperature and vital signs.
- Notify healthcare prescriber for symptoms of systemic infection.
- Blood cultures may be obtained from implanted venous access device if signs and symptoms do not appear for a localized infection at the noncoring needle insertion site. The healthcare prescriber will determine whether the TID requires removal.

If extrusion occurs, evidenced by the metal or plastic port reservoir extruding and visible through the child's skin:

- Repeated access through the skin may cause loss of integrity, especially in the case of children with chemotherapy-related skin breakdown.
- Notify healthcare prescriber to determine whether the TID requires removal.

attempts, and the type or topical anesthetic agent used
- Date, time, and initials of person completing the noncoring needle and dressing change and cap change on the dressing and in the patient record
- Date, time, type, and amount of flush solution used; presence or absence of blood return; and any resistance to flushing and, if present, what interventions were implemented
- Site appearance: presence or absence of redness, swelling, drainage, tenderness, or streaking
- Amount of blood drawn
- Child's tolerance of and response to the procedure

COMMUNITY CARE

- If the child is to be discharged home with a TID, begin collaboration with a home health nurse as early as possible, for discharge planning.
- Include in communication with the home care provider the type of TID, including manufacturer and size if known; date of insertion; surgeon's name and follow-up care; noncoring needle size with dressing change and flush protocol taught in healthcare setting; and notification of any complications after placement.
- Instruct parents in TID observation for signs of infection. If TID access and dressing changes or parenteral therapy will be done at home, teach hand hygiene; TID access and dressing and needleless connector/catheter cap changes; administration of flushes; medication and flow control infusion device, as applicable; disposal techniques for syringes; and age/developmentally based safety methods to secure the TID extension tubing.
- Before discharge, parents should verbalize knowledge of the most common complications of a TID (i.e., sepsis and accidental dislodgment of noncoring needle), what to look for, and actions to take in the event of complications.
- Educate the child and parents about the necessity for monthly heparin flush of the TID when not in use and stress the importance of follow-up visits with the healthcare professional.
- Instruct the family to contact the healthcare provider if
  - TID site is reddened or oozes fluid or blood
  - Child has signs of local or systemic infection (fever)
  - Unable to flush the TID system
  - TID extrudes through the skin
  - Any other concerns related to the TID

Unexpected Situations

- *Area around TID begins to swell when flushing:* Stop flushing. Aspirate for blood return to verify correct needle placement. Slowly begin to flush again. If swelling continues, stop flushing and notify healthcare prescriber. Assess comfort level of child, presence of erythema, and degree of swelling.
- *TID does not flush:* Check clamp to ensure it is opened. Verify correct needle placement by aspirating for blood return. Consider problem may be from an occluded noncoring needle. Change noncoring needle and reassess. Notify healthcare prescriber if inability to flush continues.

Bibliography

Association for Women's Health, Obstetric and Neonatal Nurses. (2001). *Neonatal skin care: Evidence based clinical practice guidelines.* Glenview, IL: Author.

Camp-Sorrell, D. (Ed.). (2004). *Access device guidelines: Recommendations for nursing practice and education* (2nd ed.). Pittsburgh, PA: Oncology Nursing Society.

Carson, S. M. (2004). Chlorhexidine versus povidone-iodine for central venous catheter site care in children. *Journal of Pediatric Nursing, 19,* 74–80.

Centers for Disease Control and Prevention. (2002). *Guidelines for prevention of intravascular catheter-related infections.* Retrieved August 15, 2006, from http://www.cdc.gov/mmwr/preview/mmwrhtml/rr5110a1.htm

Fisher, A. A., Deffenbagh, C., Poole, R. L., Garcia, M., & Kerner, J. A. (2004). The use of alteplase for restoring patency to occluded central venous access devices in infants and children. *Journal of Infusion Nursing, 27,* 171–174.

Harris, J. L., & Maguire, D. (1999). Developing a protocol to prevent and treat pediatric central venous catheter occlusions. *Journal of Intravenous Nursing, 22,* 194–198.

Infusion Nurses Society. (2006a). Infusion nursing: Standards of practice. *Journal of Infusion Nursing, 29*(Suppl. 1S), S1–S92.

Infusion Nurses Society. (2006b). *Policies and procedures for infusion nursing* (3rd ed.). Norwood, MA: Author.

Krzywda, E. A., & Andris, D. A. (2005). Twenty-five years of advances in vascular access: Bridging research to clinical practice. *Nutrition in Clinical Practice, 20,* 597–606.

Mayo, D. J. (2000). Current treatment options for catheter-related thrombosis. *Journal of Vascular Access Devices, 5,* 10–20.

McCloskey, D. J. (2002). Catheter-related thrombosis in pediatrics. *Pediatric Nursing 28,* 97–105.

Munro, F. D., Gillett, P. M., Wratten, J. C., et al. (1999). Totally implanted central venous access devices for pediatric oncology patients. *Medical and Pediatric Oncology, 33,* 377–381.

Orr, M. E. (2002). The peripherally inserted central catheter: What are the current indications for its use? *Nutrition in Clinical Practice, 17,* 99–104.

Vanek, V. W. (2002a). The ins and outs of venous access. Part I. *Nutrition in Clinical Practice 17,* 85–98.

Vanek, V. W. (2002b). The ins and outs of venous access. Part II. *Nutrition in Clinical Practice 17,* 142–155.

CHAPTER

58

Intravascular Therapy: Tunneled Catheters

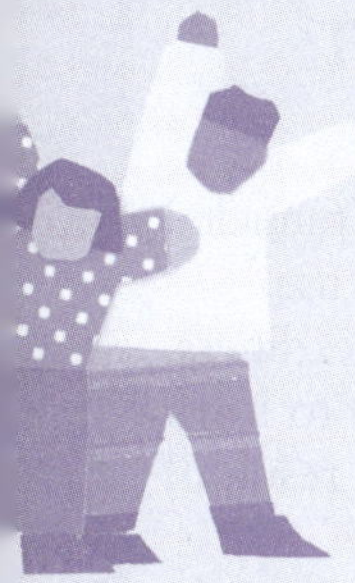

Clinical Guidelines

- Long-term central venous catheters, placed to reduce the trauma of repeated venipuncture in the child, are surgically inserted and removed by a physician under sterile conditions and are used for direct administration of intravenous (IV) fluids, intermittent medications/therapies, blood products, parenteral nutritional, and venous blood sampling for laboratory analysis. They may be used in the home setting for continuous infusion of medications, chemotherapy, and parenteral nutrition and therefore contribute to the improvement of the child's quality of life.
- Tunneled catheters may be accessed and site care or infusion given by a registered nurse (RN), physician, or appropriately trained child or caregiver.
- There are basically two types of long-term venous access catheters: the totally implantable device (TID) (see Figure 57-1 in Chapter 57), and the right atrial Silastic catheter, also called a tunneled catheter (Figure 58-1). Hickman or Broviac tunneled catheters have an open-ended tip, whereas the Groshong catheter (available as a tunneled catheter or implanted device) has a three-way valve at the tip to prevent back-flow of blood. The underlying condition of the child, the indication for use, and the capability of the family or child to perform self-care of the long-term catheter necessary for home maintenance help determine which catheter is appropriate for a specific child. TIDs are better suited to children requiring prolonged (6 months or more) or intermittent IV therapy without periods of severe immunosuppression. However, because of size restrictions, they are not available for use in neonates and small infants. Tunneled catheters are better suited to very small children, infants, and neonates.
- Use aseptic technique when caring for or using long-term venous access catheters to minimize the associated risk for infection.
- Follow manufacturer's instructions for the specific catheter.
- Change the dressing when it becomes loosened, damp, or soiled, or when inspection of the site is necessary.
- Change the needleless connector/catheter cap weekly or if residual blood remains after blood is drawn. All add-on devices have a Luer-Lok design.
- Intravenous fluids are administered via a controlled infusion device.
- When not in use, place an open-ended catheter (e.g., Hickman or Broviac) to heparin lock (saline lock in Groshong catheters); then cap and secure with tape to the chest under the child's clothing. When the catheter is used as a heparin-lock device, flush the line after each use or at least once daily. The healthcare prescriber must order the frequency of flush and the amount of solution used.

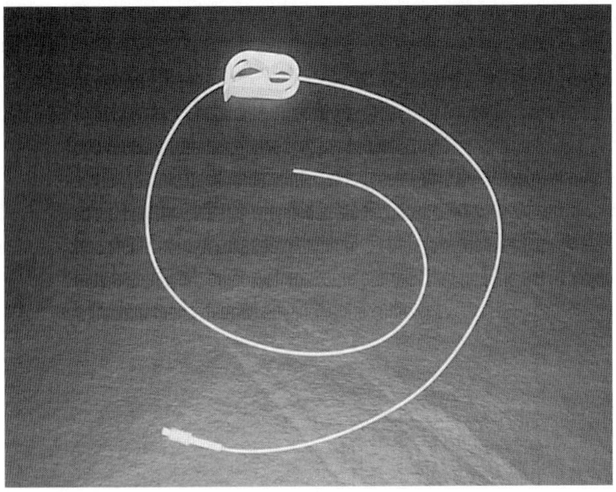

FIGURE 58-1
The right Silastic catheter is tunneled through the vein until the tip reaches the right atrium of the heart.

- Care and management techniques vary based on the procedure being performed (per institutional policies) and the setting in which the procedure is being performed in (e.g., hospital versus home):
  - Sterile technique (sterile dressings and sterile gloves)
  - Modified clean technique (nonsterile gloves and sterile dressings)

EQUIPMENT

For access and flushing/locking a tunneled catheter:

- Nonsterile gloves
- Soft jaw clamp (if catheter does not already have clamp preattached)
- Sterile 3-mL syringe
- Sterile needleless connector/blunt cannulas (per institutional policy)
- Sterile preservative-free 0.9% sodium chloride (10 mL) for injection
- Three alcohol pads
- Prescribed fluid for administration, metered volume container (e.g., Soluset, Buretrol), and IV flow control infusion device (follow manufacturer's directions for use)
- Tape
- Flush solution
  - For open-ended catheters: heparinized saline, 10 units/mL (per healthcare prescriber's order, preservative-free in neonates); and sterile preservative-free 0.9% sodium chloride (10 mL) for injection
  - For Groshong-type catheters: sterile preservative-free 0.9% sodium chloride (10 mL) for injection

For site care and maintenance of a tunneled catheter:

- Nonsterile gloves
- Sterile gloves
- Sterile towel
- Antiseptic swabs: one 2% chlorhexidine-based preparation is preferred, three tincture of iodine, an iodophor (e.g., povidone-iodine), or 70% alcohol can be used.
- Three alcohol prep pads or swabs, if iodine antiseptic is used
- Dressing materials: sterile semipermeable transparent dressing or sterile 2 × 2 gauze and 1-inch tape
- Sterile needleless connector/catheter cap

For blood withdrawal through a tunneled catheter:

- Nonsterile gloves
- Soft jaw clamp (if catheter does not have a preattached clamp)
- Three alcohol pads
- Two sterile 3-mL syringes
- Three sterile 5-mL syringes
- Appropriate syringes, number and size determined by blood specimens needed
- Sterile needleless access devices (per institutional policy)
- Flush solution:
  - For open-ended catheters: heparinized saline, 10 units/mL (per healthcare prescriber order, preservative-free in neonates); and sterile preservative-free 0.9% sodium chloride (10 mL) for injection
  - For Groshong-type catheters: sterile preservative-free 0.9% sodium chloride (10 mL) for injection
- If blood is to be re-infused, heparinized saline, 10 units/mL (preservative-free in neonates)
- Tape
- Specimen tubes for ordered laboratory tests
- Biohazard bag
- Ice, if needed for blood specimen
- Specimen labels and requisitions

CHILD AND FAMILY ASSESSMENT AND PREPARATION

- Discuss with the child and family the purpose of tunneled catheter placement and the intended reason for use.
- Assess the child's and family's cognitive level, readiness, and ability to process information. Readiness to learn and process information may be impaired as a result of age, stress, or anxiety.
- Explain the procedure, as appropriate, to both the child and the family.
- Reinforce the need, and identify and discuss the risks and benefits of long-term IV catheter placement, as appropriate, to both the child and family.
- Obtain the child's baseline weight and height because this will aid in determining how much heparinized preservative-free 0.9% sodium chloride will be used for irrigation and locking.
- Assess the child's baseline vital signs and observe for changes that may indicate a local or systemic infection. Infection may occur as a result of the presence of a for-

eign body in the subcutaneous tissue; accessing the catheter, which may introduce bacteria into the catheter; bacterial contamination at the exit site from loss of intact skin protection; and the necessity of long-term venous access and home maintenance procedures, which also may increase the risk for infection.

- Assess the child's age, general size, and overall skin condition. Observe for peripheral skin grafts or shunts, cellulitis, vascular surgeries, thrombosis, or peripheral vascular disease, which may limit the dwell time of the tunneled catheter. Assess the skin surrounding the catheter for pain, swelling, venous distention, or development of collateral circulation, because this may aid in detection of venous thrombosis.
- Explain the symptoms that may indicate complications and the need for catheter removal and having a new catheter placed. This enables the child and family to recognize when the catheter is not functioning properly and when to notify the nurse. Complications associated with long-term venous access catheters include infection, phlebitis, thrombosis, catheter occlusions, and mechanical malfunctions.

PROCEDURE Accessing, Flushing, and Locking a Tunneled Catheter

Steps	Rationale/Points of Emphasis
1. Perform hand hygiene and collect all necessary supplies. Involve caregiver in comforting child during procedure.	Reduces the transmission of microorganisms. Promotes efficient time management and provides an organized approach to the procedure. **caREminder** *Obtain the assistance of an additional person as needed to hold child securely to prevent contamination of the sterile field.*
2. Establish a sterile working area; open supplies aseptically and drop them on the sterile field.	Decreases the chance of microorganisms being introduced into the catheter by maintaining sterile precautions.
3. Locate catheter under child's clothes/shirt and establish ease of access. Atraumatically apply catheter clamp to the reinforced area of the external catheter.	Prevents blood loss and extravasation when the catheter is entered. Catheter padding prevents damage to the friable Silastic material. **caREminder** *If the catheter does not have a reinforced area or a preapplied clamp, wrap a piece of gauze around the catheter and clamp over the gauze material. Change the location of the gauze and clamp every time to avoid repeated wear in the same area of the catheter. Groshong catheters do not require clamping as they have an internal valve that opens during infusion and closes when not in use.*
4. Don gloves.	Standard precautions.
5. Depending on the child's size and the size of the catheter, draw up between 3 and 5 mL of sterile preservative-free 0.9% sodium chloride and return the filled syringe to the sterile work area.	Prepares syringe for use.
6. Cleanse the surface area of the needleless connector/catheter cap of the tunneled catheter with the alcohol swabs (at least 10 strokes per swab); allow to dry.	Reduces the transmission of microorganisms. Povidone-iodine is not an effective antimicrobial on inanimate objects.
7. Insert/connect the saline-filled syringe into the needleless connector/catheter cap and unclamp.	Prepares for infusion of irrigation solution.
8. Aspirate for a blood return. If no blood return, problem-solve according to organizational policy	Confirms patency of the catheter.

Continued

Steps	Rationale/Points of Emphasis
9. If a blood return is present, using a push–pause method, infuse the sterile saline solution.	Push–pause method creates mild turbulence, which may prevent clots from forming on catheter wall. Positive fluid displacement within the lumen of the catheter should be maintained to prevent reflux of blood.
10a. To connect to an IV infusion: Remove the syringe and connect the prescribed IV fluid directly to the needleless connector/catheter cap of the tunneled catheter and begin IV fluids as prescribed via flow control infusion device. Ensure that no more than 4 hours' worth of IV fluid is allowed to hang at any one time or that fluid is infused via a flow control infusion device. Change IV tubing using aseptic technique every 72 hours or when contamination occurs or is suspected, except for intralipid tubing, which should be changed every 24 hours. Label the IV tubing with time, date, and initials when hung.	Provides fluid delivery as prescribed. Limiting hanging fluid to 4 hours' worth can prevent potential accidental fluid overload and complications from IV infiltration. Changing tubing at routine intervals reduces risk of microorganisms from growing in IV tubing. Labeling tubing aids in identifying proper change times.
10b. To place catheter to "heparin lock" for intermittent infusions or for daily maintenance flushing to an open-tipped catheter: • Remove the saline syringe. • Connect the prescribed heparinized saline syringe. • Use a push–pause method to infuse the heparinized normal saline. • If the child has a double or triple-lumen catheter, each lumen must be flushed once a day. • Reapply the catheter clamp to the reinforced area of the external catheter.	Although saline locks are common practice in adults, evidence in pediatrics is contradictory and does not support discontinuing use of heparin. This may be related to the smaller lumen sizes of catheters used. Allows for infusion of heparin solution. Daily flushing with heparin of each lumen is routine and maintains patency of catheter with intermittent use. Clamping prevents inadvertent infusion of unwanted fluid and places the catheter to "heparin lock."
10c. To place a Groshong catheter to "saline lock" for intermittent use or to keep patent: • Flush the catheter with the preservative-free 0.9% sodium chloride using the push–pause method. • Reapply the catheter clamp to the reinforced area of the external catheter.	Preservative-free 0.9% sodium chloride is used with Groshong catheters; heparin is not contraindicated but is not needed due to the three-way valve distal tip. Clamping prevents inadvertent infusion of unwanted fluid and places the catheter to "saline lock."
11. Remove gloves and secure the catheter with additional tape.	Prevents accidental dislodgment, tugging, or pulling of the catheter.
12. Replace child's clothing over catheter.	Helps maintain body image.
13. Dispose of equipment and waste in appropriate receptacle.	Standard precautions.
14. Perform hand hygiene.	Reduces transmission of microorganisms.

PROCEDURE Site Care and Maintenance of a Tunneled Catheter

Steps	Rationale/Points of Emphasis
1. Perform hand hygiene and collect all necessary supplies. Involve caregiver in comforting child during procedure.	Reduces the transmission of microorganisms. Promotes efficient time management and provides an organized approach to the procedure. **caREminder** *Obtain the assistance of an additional person as needed to hold child securely to prevent contamination of the sterile field.*
2. Establish a sterile work area with the sterile towel; open supplies aseptically and drop them on the sterile field.	Decreases the chance of microorganisms being introduced into the catheter by maintaining sterile precautions.
3. Locate catheter under child's clothes/shirt and remove clothing covering insertion site. Ensure that the catheter is clamped.	Provides accessibility and visualization of catheter insertion site.

Steps	Rationale/Points of Emphasis
4. Don gloves.	Standard precautions.
5. While stabilizing the catheter, carefully remove old dressing and discard in appropriate waste container.	Provides visualization of skin at catheter insertion site. **KidKare** To facilitate removal of transparent dressing, pull dressing edges first in outward direction, parallel to the skin surface. This releases the adhesive bonds of the dressing and lifts it off the skin, decreasing skin trauma.
6. Visually inspect catheter exit site and surrounding skin.	Detection of impaired skin integrity is key to maintaining a catheter free from sepsis.
7. Remove gloves and repeat hand hygiene.	Gloves are contaminated by old dressing.
8. Don sterile gloves.	Standard precautions; reduces transmission of microorganisms.
9a. Cleanse around exit site with a 2% chlorhexidine or other appropriate antiseptic swab or pad. • For povidone-iodine, start at the catheter exit site and work outward in circular pattern for several inches. Repeat two more times with a new swab each time. Use friction to enhance the antifungal and antibacterial effects of the cleansing swab. Do not return to cleaned area with the same antiseptic. • For chlorhexidine, clean the site with a back-and-forth motion to get into the skin crevices. Clean the dry areas for 30 seconds; clean wet areas for 2 minutes (e.g., groin, neck, chest).	Cleanses microorganisms from insertion site.
9b. Allow site to dry; allow povidone-iodine to remain on the skin for at least 2 minutes, or longer if it is not yet dry before insertion. Do not fan or blow on site. For neonates, remove antiseptic with either sterile normal saline or sterile water.	Allows antimicrobial action of antiseptic. Fanning or blowing may introduce contaminants and hasten drying, reducing antimicrobial action.
10. If an iodine-based antiseptic was used, remove the solution from the skin using a sterile alcohol prep pad or swab (sterile saline or sterile water for neonates). Start at the catheter exit site and work outward in circular pattern to cover the same area as the size of the dressing. Repeat two more times with a new alcohol prep pad or swab each time.	Some infants/children have sensitivity to iodine products, which may also affect the neonatal thyroid; do not allow it to remain on the skin.
11. Allow site to air-dry.	Wet dressings can promote an environment for bacterial growth. **caREminder** *Do not use antimicrobial ointment in routine site care. Use of polyantibiotic ointments may increase the risk for* Candida *species colonization.*
12. Dress site by applying an air-permeable transparent dressing over the catheter at the exit site or by placing a sterile 2 × 2 gauze over the catheter exit dressing site and apply tape around all four edges, being careful to touch only the outer edges of either dressing.	Maintains sterility of the dressing that touches the catheter at the exit site. **caREminder** *Gauze and tape dressing are changed every 48 hours. Air-permeable dressings are changed every 7 days or when the dressing is loose, soiled, or wet.*

Continued

Steps	Rationale/Points of Emphasis
13. Loosely loop a portion of the external catheter and secure with tape to the child's skin.	Prevents inadvertent dislodgment, tugging, pulling, or kinking of the catheter at the exit site.
14. At least once weekly, change the catheter cap as follows: • Apply friction in a back-and-forth motion with an alcohol swab between the catheter cap and the catheter itself. • Repeat this procedure twice more with the other alcohol swabs. • Twist off the old needleless connector/catheter cap counterclockwise, set aside, and twist on the new sterile cap.	Reduces the transmission of microorganisms. Maintains closed system to prevent infection.
15. Remove sterile gloves.	Maintains sterile field.
16. Replace child's clothing over catheter.	Maintains body image.
17. Dispose of equipment and waste in appropriate waste receptacle.	Standard precautions.
18. Perform hand hygiene.	Reduces transmission of microorganisms.

PROCEDURE Blood Withdrawal Through a Tunneled Catheter

Steps	Rationale/Points of Emphasis
1. Determine whether "discard" blood is to be reinfused or discarded. Generally, blood is reinfused in children who are critically or chronically ill and undergoing frequent blood withdrawal, in infants, or in anemic children.	These children are at risk for anemia, and blood loss must be minimized.
2. Calculate minimum blood required to perform ordered tests.	Minimizes blood loss of child.
3. Follow Access/Flush and Locking a Tunneled Catheter Procedure, steps 1 to 7. Additionally, if discard blood is to be reinfused, prepare a heparinized syringe by drawing heparin (10 units/mL) into a 5-mL syringe, pull plunger to 5-mL mark, and then push plunger to base of syringe to empty syringe.	A heparinized syringe helps prevent clotting of discard blood that will be reinfused in the syringe while obtaining remainder of blood for testing.
4. Attach a 5-mL sterile syringe (use heparinized syringe if blood is to be reinfused) to the needleless connector/catheter cap and remove the clamp.	Prepares for withdrawal of blood.
5. Gently pull plunger to withdraw 3 to 5 mL of blood into syringe. For Groshong catheter: aspirate 1 to 2 mL, then pause for 2 seconds to allow catheter valve to open, then slowly aspirate for a total of 3 to 5 mL.	Clears catheter of residual fluid (saline, heparin) and accesses undiluted blood.
6. Remove the syringe containing discard fluid and place on sterile work area if blood is to be reinfused.	Maintains sterility.
7. Apply sterile syringe of appropriate size to withdraw sufficient blood for ordered tests. Gently withdraw amount of blood required for ordered laboratory testing and remove syringe.	Obtains blood for testing. **caREminder** *If blood withdrawal is sluggish, ask child and caregivers what facilitates blood withdrawal. To shift catheter position if it is lodged against wall of the vein, have the child take a deep breath or cough, perform Valsalva maneuver, change position, or raise arms overhead or lower arms.*

Steps	Rationale/Points of Emphasis
8. If discard blood is to be reinfused: a. Visually examine discard sample for evidence of clot formation; if none, apply syringe to needleless connector/catheter cap and slowly reinfuse discard volume. b. Apply sterile saline syringe; using a push–pause method, infuse 3 mL of saline and clamp catheter. It is not necessary to clamp Groshong catheter. If discard blood is not reinfused, perform Step 8b only.	Avoids infusion of clotted blood. Clears line of blood.
9. Place blood in appropriate tubes for ordered tests.	Provides proper medium for ordered tests.
10. Follow Access/Flush and Locking a Tunneled Catheter procedure, steps 10 to 14; follow step 10a to commence fluid administration or step 10b if catheter is to be placed to "heparin lock" or step 10c if catheter is to be placed to "saline lock."	Prepares line for desired use.
11. Prepare blood sample for testing: a. Label specimen with child's name, medical record number and unit, date and time of collection, and collector's initials. b. Transport specimen to laboratory if necessary. Provide appropriate environment for transport (e.g., ice, refrigeration).	 Ensures that correct specimen is tested for the right patient. Reduces degradation of specimen before analysis.
12. Remove gloves and perform hand hygiene.	Reduces transmission of microorganisms.

Child and Family Evaluation and Documentation

- Evaluate child and family's readiness to learn about care of the tunneled catheter. Involve family in hands-on care as early as possible.
- Evaluate site appearance for presence of redness, swelling, drainage, tenderness, or streaking. If appropriate, culture the site. Notify the healthcare prescriber of any signs of skin breakdown or infection.
- Evaluate line patency; troubleshoot as needed (Chart 58-1).
- Determine whether the child and family have other areas of concern to discuss.
- Document the following:
  - Date, time, and initials of person completing the dressing change on the dressing and in the patient record
  - Site appearance, noting presence or absence of redness, swelling, drainage, or tenderness
  - Date, time, type, and amount of flush solution used; any resistance to flushing; and, if present, what interventions were implemented
  - Amount of blood drawn
  - Child's tolerance of and response to the procedure

Community Care

- If the child is to be discharged home with a tunneled catheter, discharge planning with a home health nurse should begin as early as possible. Using a doll with a tunneled catheter to teach may be less intimidating to the child and family as they begin to learn the skills and gain mastery of their home care.
- Communication with the home care provider should include type of catheter, with manufacturer and size if known; date of insertion; position of catheter tip; and any complications after placement.
- Instruct family in hand hygiene/infection control; dressing changes and flushing the catheter per healthcare prescriber orders and home care agency policy; medication administration and flow control infusion device, as applicable; disposal techniques for sharps and biohazards; and developmental safety with appropriate methods to secure the tunneled catheter.
- Before discharge, the family should verbalize knowledge of the most common complications of tunneled catheter lines (i.e., sepsis, occlusion, and inadvertent removal); what to look for; actions to take in the event of complications; and whom to contact.
- Provide the family with the tunneled catheter repair kit supplied by the manufacturer, and instruct them to take kit with them to nearest health care facility in event of catheter damage.
- Tunneled catheter manufacturers provide booklets for family education. An online source of line information is www.cc.nih.gov/ccc/patient_education.
- Instruct the family to contact the healthcare provider if
  - Child has a fever
  - Exit site remains reddened or oozes fluid or blood
  - Tunneled area is red, swollen, and tender

CHART 58-1 TROUBLESHOOTING A TUNNELED CATHETER

If unable to flush line or draw blood:

- This may occur due to external or internal mechanical obstruction, nonthrombotic occlusions such as drug precipitates, or thrombotic occlusions due to fibrin deposits or blood clots. Thrombosis may cause partial or complete occlusion.
- Examine line to ensure that clamps are open and catheter is not kinked. If sutures are present, ensure that they are not causing obstruction.
- Reposition child (i.e., extend or raise arm over head). If catheter remains positional, notify healthcare prescriber. An x-ray may be needed to determine line placement. Catheter compression may occur; continued compression can lead to thrombosis or shearing of the line.
- If occlusion from precipitates is suspected, attempt to aspirate to clear line. If successful, flush with saline or sterile water between all medications. If unsuccessful, obtain healthcare prescriber order for lytic agent to dissolve precipitate. The instilled volume of the solution to clear precipitates should not exceed the internal volume of the catheter to avoid intravenous administration.
- If occlusion is due to thrombosis, obtain healthcare prescriber order for lytic agent and use following manufacturer's recommendations. Instillation, aspiration, and flushing should be done using a method that does not exceed the catheter manufacturer's maximum pressure limits.

For infiltration:

- Infiltration is the unintended administration of medication or solution into the tissue surrounding the vein. Infiltration associated with a central line is more difficult to detect. An increase in the size of the right anterior chest wall may indicate an infiltration is present.
- IV site checks are to include assessment along the path of the catheter.
- If infiltration occurs, discontinue infusion, but do not remove catheter. Notify healthcare prescriber of infiltration, solution or medications infusing at time of infiltration, and site appearance.
- Obtain healthcare prescriber's order for agent to treat infiltration of a vesicant as needed.
- Treatment of an infiltration is dependent on the properties of the infiltrated medication or solution, the manufacturer's guidelines for that agent, and the severity of the infiltration. The tunneled catheter may be used to instill medication ordered to treat infiltration of a vesicant.

For catheter migration:

- The Dacron cuff implanted under skin may not be fully engrafted. Catheter migration may be caused by excessive sneezing, coughing, or vomiting and lack of tissue adherence to the catheter.
- Suspect migration if the child complains of chest pain or feels the flush of a tunneled catheter.
- Notify healthcare prescriber to obtain order for x-ray to confirm placement.
- Migration may necessitate replacement or repositioning of the tunneled catheter.

For damaged or broken catheter:

- Clamp and secure the catheter to prevent migration and possible embolization of the catheter fragment. Catheter embolization is an emergency and may require surgical intervention.
- An RN trained in this procedure using the manufacturer's repair kit and guidelines may perform repair of the tunneled catheter. Not all tunneled catheter manufacturers provide repair kits; repair with other materials may lead to catheter separation and migration or embolization.
- Inability to repair line necessitates removal of the tunneled catheter.
- A defective catheter should be reported per institutional policy.

For bleeding:

- Apply gauze dressing after initial placement of tunneled catheter and change the first dressing in 24 hours. A semipermeable transparent dressing may be used at this time. Change dressings no more frequently than once per week until the insertion site is healed. The need for any dressing on well-healed exit sites of long-term tunneled venous access catheters is an unresolved issue.
- Mild bleeding at site may occur for first 24 hours after tunneled catheter placement. If bleeding increases or persists past first 24 hours, notify healthcare prescriber.

For local infection (as noticed by an alteration in the skin integrity overlying the implanted venous access device):

- Assess skin surrounding catheter for erythema, inflammation, tenderness, or exudate.
- Evaluate patient temperature and vital signs. Notify physician of symptoms of localized infection.
- Obtain skin cultures at catheter exit site.
- Blood cultures may be obtained from the tunneled catheter at the time the infectious process is noted.

For systemic (blood-borne) infection:

- Evaluate child's temperature and vital signs. Notify healthcare prescriber of symptoms of systemic infection.
- Antibiotics may be administered through the tunneled catheter to try clearing the catheter of infection. The healthcare prescriber determines whether the indwelling catheter requires removal.

- Child complaints of pain or irritability/crying with flushing
- Tunneled catheter is inadvertently pulled with concerns of cuff or catheter dislodgement
- Inability to flush the tunneled catheter or inability to obtain a blood aspirate
- Family has other concerns related to the tunneled catheter

Unexpected Situation

You are unable to flush catheter: Check catheter for kinks and check clamp to ensure that tubing is open. Have child change position or put his or her ipsilateral arm over the head. Attempt to aspirate the catheter using a method that does not exceed the catheter manufacturer's maximum pressure limits. If still unable to flush catheter, remove the needleless connector/ catheter cap and attach the syringe directly to the hub of the catheter, attempt to aspirate blood again, and flush. If still unable to flush catheter, notify healthcare prescriber.

Bibliography

AWHONN (Association for Women's Health, Obstetric and Neonatal Nurses). (2001). *Neonatal skin care: Evidence based clinical practice guidelines.* Glenview, IL: Author.

Carson, S. M. (2004). Chlorhexidine versus povidone-iodine for central venous catheter site care in children. *Journal of Pediatric Nursing, 19,* 74–80.

Centers for Disease Control and Prevention. (2002). Guidelines for prevention of intravascular catheter-related infections. Retrieved August 15, 2006, from http://www.cdc.gov/mmwr/preview/mmwrhtml/rr5110a1.htm

Fisher, A. A., Deffenbagh, C., Poole, R. L., Garcia, M., & Kerner, J. A. (2004). The use of alteplase for restoring patency to occluded central venous access devices in infants and children. *Journal of Infusion Nursing, 27,* 171–174.

Fitzpatrick, L. (1999). Care and management issues regarding central venous access devices in the home and long-term care setting. *Journal of Intravenous Nursing, 22*(6S), S40–S45.

Gordon, K., & Lloyd, A. (2003). An exploration of the possible causes of occlusion problems in skin-tunneled catheters used in paediatric oncology. *NT Research, 8,* 380–388.

Harris, J. L., & Maguire, D. (1999). Developing a protocol to prevent and treat pediatric central venous catheter occlusions. *Journal of Intravenous Nursing, 22,* 194–198.

Infusion Nurses Society. (2006). Infusion nursing: Standards of practice. *Journal of Infusion Nursing, 29*(1S), S1–S92.

Infusion Nurses Society. (2006). *Policies and procedures for infusion nursing* (3rd ed.). Norwood, MA: Author.

Krzywda, E. A., & Andris, D. A. (2005). Twenty-five years of advances in vascular access: Bridging research to clinical practice. *Nutrition in Clinical Practice, 20,* 597–606.

McCloskey, D. J. (2002). Catheter-related thrombosis in pediatrics. *Pediatric Nursing 28,* 97–105.

CHAPTER 59

Intubation

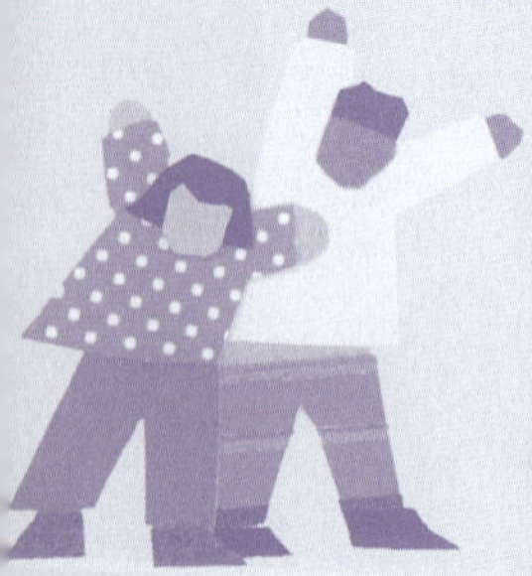

CLINICAL GUIDELINES

- A physician, nurse anesthetist, or nurse practitioner performs intubation. In some states, a trained respiratory therapist, paramedic, or emergency medical technician may perform intubation.
- A registered nurse (RN) or licensed practical nurse (LPN) with Pediatric Advanced Life Support training may assist in this procedure by providing support to the individual who will be intubating the child and being responsible for monitoring the status of the child before, during, and after the procedure.
- Intubation is a means to provide a patent airway to facilitate mechanical ventilation and to facilitate pulmonary toilet.
- Intubation is indicated when an infant or child experiences actual or potential loss of a patent airway, is in danger from aspiration, has no spontaneous respiration or inadequate ventilation or oxygenation, is in respiratory distress or failure, or is having surgery requiring anesthesia.

EQUIPMENT

- Intravenous (IV) access
- Sedatives and paralytics as ordered by a healthcare prescriber
- Cardiac and apnea monitors
- Pulse oximeter
- Stethoscope
- Gloves, masks, gowns, and goggles for standard precautions
- Length-based resuscitation tape
- Water-soluble or anesthetic jelly (lidocaine [Xylocaine] 2%)
- Endotracheal tubes (ETTs) of various sizes, cuffed and uncuffed (Table 59-1)
- Laryngoscope with curved and straight blades (see Table 59-1)
- Extra lightbulbs for laryngoscope
- Self-inflating resuscitation bag with mask connected to oxygen tubing and flow meter and oxygen source (must be capable of delivering 100% oxygen)
- McGill forceps (for nasotracheal intubation only)
- Stylet
- Water-soluble lubricant
- Soft restraints or safety devices
- Suction with Yankauer or large, rigid suction catheter
- Securement device or tape cut for securing the tube
- Tincture of benzoin

TABLE 59-1

Guidelines for Laryngoscope, Endotracheal Tube, and Suction Catheter Sizes

Age	Laryngoscope Blade	Endotracheal Tube I.D. (mm)	Suction Catheter (F)
Premature infant	00	2.5, 3.0 uncuffed	5–6
Term to 3 mo	0–1	3.0, 3.5 cuffed* or uncuffed	6–8
6 mo	0–1	3.5, 4.0 cuffed or uncuffed	8
1 yr	1	4.0, 4.5 cuffed or uncuffed	8
2 yr	2	4.5, 5.0 cuffed or uncuffed	8
4 yr	2	5.0, 5.5 cuffed or uncuffed	10
6 yr	2	5.5 cuffed or uncuffed	10
8 yr	2	6.0 cuffed or uncuffed	10
10 yr	2	6.5 cuffed or uncuffed	12
12 yr	3	7.0 cuffed	12
Adolescent	3	7.0, 8.0 cuffed	12

F, French; I.D., inner diameter. *Cuffed tubes are not recommended for newborns.

- Oropharyngeal airway (if needed)
- CO_2 detector
- Ventilator
- Nasogastric tube

CHILD AND FAMILY ASSESSMENT AND PREPARATION

- If possible, given the child's condition, discuss the process of intubation with the child and parent. Discuss suctioning, the inability to talk, and that the child will be restrained to prevent him or her from pulling out the tube. If this is a nonemergent situation, discuss an alternative means of communication while the child is intubated. Picture boards or alphabet charts may be used to help the child communicate.

caREminder

Explanations should be given in all situations but should not compromise resuscitation efforts; in an emergency situation, explanations can be given as the procedure is being performed. Children may hear even if unresponsive.

- If family members are not present during the procedure, communicate with them immediately after the intubation and reassure them about the status of the child. Allow the family to return to the child's bedside as soon as possible.
- If parents stay with their child during the procedure, explain intubation purpose and process. If possible, assign a staff person to support the family throughout the procedure. Allow family members to comfort the child even if the child is in a nonresponsive state.
- Before intubation, assess the child's mouth for loose teeth. Teeth may become dislodged during the procedure and become a potential risk for aspiration.
- Obtain vascular access before initiating the procedure. If vascular access is not possible to obtain, intraosseous access should be secured (see Chapters 55 and 65).

Alert! *Airway control is the first priority in an emergency situation. In such cases, obtaining airway access should not be delayed while attempts to start an IV are being made.*

PROCEDURE **Preparing for Intubation**

Steps	Rationale/Points of Emphasis
1. Notify the appropriate personnel of the necessity for the procedure. A respiratory therapist, an RN, and the healthcare provider intubating the child should be present.	Performance of the procedure by qualified personnel increases successful outcomes. The physician, nurse anesthetist, or nurse practitioner performs the procedure; the respiratory therapist assists in managing the airway; and the nurse monitors the child's status and suctions and tapes the endotracheal tube.
2. Verify that the child has a patent IV line for administration of sedatives, paralytics, and emergency drugs.	IV access is needed should the child experience cardiac arrest during intubation. Emergency medications can also be delivered by the interosseous route or by the endotracheal tube once it is verified to be in place.

Continued

Steps	Rationale/Points of Emphasis
3. Perform hand hygiene.	Reduces transmission of microorganisms.
4. Connect the child to cardiac/apnea monitors and pulse oximeter. Monitor the child's heart rate, respiratory status, and oxygenation status before, during, and after the procedure.	Allows ongoing assessment of the child for any changes in heart rate, respiratory rate or function, oxygen saturation, or level of consciousness.
5. Gather and assemble equipment, and check all equipment before the intubation procedure to ensure proper function.	Promotes efficient time management and provides an organized approach to the procedure.
a. Turn the suction on to between 80 and 100 mm Hg, and connect the Yankauer.	Suction equipment should be readily available to manage aspiration and to assist in visualization of the vocal cords.
b. Connect the self-inflating bag to an oxygen source with the flowmeter at 10 to 15 L/min of 100% oxygen.	The self-inflating bag should have the ability to deliver 100% oxygen to oxygenate the child effectively. Neonatal-sized (250-mL) resuscitation bags are discouraged except for use with premature infants. A bag with a volume of at least 450 L/min is recommended for term neonates and infants. An oxygen flow rate of at least 10 L/min is required with the pediatric resuscitation bag and 15 L/min with the adult-sized bag.
c. Select O_2 mask to use for bag-valve mask ventilations.	Bag-valve mask ventilations are necessary before the intubation procedure and possibly during the procedure if the intubation attempt is lengthy and the child requires oxygenation. Maintaining an appropriately sized mask at the bedside also is needed in the event of accidental extubation.
d. Attach the laryngoscope blade to the handle and check that the light bulb is tightly attached and functional (see Table 59-1).	A light source is needed to ensure good visualization of the esophagus and vocal cords.

caREminder

Curved or straight laryngoscope blades can be used. Ask the intubating practitioner which he or she prefers (Figure 59-1).

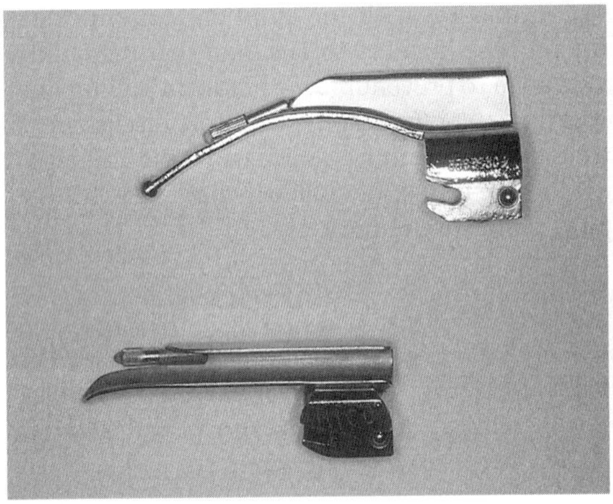

FIGURE 59-1
Laryngoscope blades may be either curved or straight.

Alert! ***A lightbulb that is not screwed in tightly may detach from the blade during the procedure.***

Steps	Rationale/Points of Emphasis
e. Obtain a McGill forceps for nasopharyngeal intubation.	The McGill forceps is used to advance the endotracheal tube from the back of the throat during a nasal intubation.

Steps	Rationale/Points of Emphasis
6. Select an uncuffed or cuffed age-appropriate ETT per the intubating provider's orders (see Table 59-1). Several methods can be used to select the size, including use of a length-based resuscitation tape or a standard tube size table.	If the ETT is too large and an air leak is not present, damage may occur to the surrounding tissues from excessive pressure.
a. The following is a quick formula for determining tube size for children older than 2 years of age: $$ETT = \frac{Age\ (yr)}{4} + 4$$	This is a very rough estimate for selection of an ETT and should only be used in emergency situations.
b. A quick visual estimation for tube selection is a tube that is the same diameter as the child's little finger.	This is an instantaneous guide for determining the child's airway size based on body size and can be used in emergencies where length-based tapes or other endotracheal tube size guides are not available.
c. Cuffed ETTs are not generally used for children younger than 8 years of age. A cuffed tube may be requested for a younger child in instances in which an air leak is not desirable.	The smallest part of the child's airway is the cricoid ring, which functions as a natural cuff, therefore requiring no cuff on the tube. A tube that is too large (preventing an air leak) may cause damage to the child's fragile airway.
d. If a cuffed tube is selected, inflate the cuff to make sure it assumes a symmetric shape and holds the volume without leaking and then deflate maximally.	Malfunction of the cuff must be determined before tube placement occurs.
e. The correct size of an uncuffed ETT should allow for an air leak.	Absence of an air leak may indicate that the tube is too large, that the cuff is inflated excessively, or that a laryngospasm is occurring around the endotracheal tube. These conditions may lead to excessive pressure on surrounding tissue. A tube that is too small in diameter will allow too much air leakage around the tube and thus provide ineffective ventilation of the child.
7. Lubricate the distal end of the ETT with sterile water, water-soluble lubricant, or lidocaine jelly (as ordered).	A lubricated ETT allows for ease in tube advancement. Lidocaine jelly provides an anesthetic effect in the mouth, nose, and throat.
8. Lightly lubricate the stylet with a water-soluble lubricant. Insert the stylet into the ETT, ensuring the tip does not extend past the distal end of the tube. With the stylet in place, the tube can be shaped into the desired configuration.	The stylet supports the tube, making it firmer and easier to insert and direct. Lubricating the stylet facilitates its withdrawal once the tube is positioned. Damage to the vocal cords can occur if the stylet protrudes from the distal end of the tube.
9. Cut tapes for securing the ETT after insertion or obtain appropriately sized securement device.	Having the equipment ready in advance prevents unnecessary delays during the procedure.
10a. Administer sedatives or paralytics as ordered immediately before the intubation.	The child should be kept quiet and still during the procedure to prevent additional injuries. If paralytics are used, an experienced practitioner in intubation techniques should be present.
10b. Atropine may also be given before treatment to reduce the incidence of reflex bradyarrhythmias.	Mechanical stimulation of the airway or hypoxemia may induce bradyarrhythmias in the infant and young child.

PROCEDURE Intubation

Steps	Rationale/Points of Emphasis
1. Don goggles or face shield, gowns, and gloves.	Splashing of secretions during intubation frequently occurs. Standard precautions should be maintained by all involved or assisting in the procedure to prevent contact with child's secretions.
2. Position the child's head as close to the edge of the bed as possible. If child's cervical spine is not injured, hyperextend the neck using a small towel roll placed under the shoulder blades.	Ensures good body mechanics.

Continued

Steps	Rationale/Points of Emphasis
a. For the child younger than 2 years of age, place a small pad under the body to keep the chest on an even level with the head and neck. Place the child on a flat surface with the chin in the sniffing position. Keep the neck midline and in a neutral position. Open the airway with jaw-thrust or chin-lift method.	Maintains proper alignment of mouth, pharynx, and trachea. The head is large and heavy, causing extension of the neck naturally when the head is placed on a flat surface. Infants have large tongues that may occlude the airway once they are sedated.
b. For the child 2 years of age or older, place the occiput of the head on a small pad and extend the head and neck. Keep the neck in a midline position.	The older child may require some anterior displacement of the cervical spine to obtain optimal airway patency.

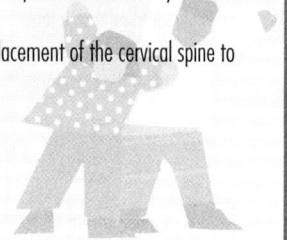

Alert! *Only use the positions described if there is no indication of cervical injury.*

Steps	Rationale/Points of Emphasis
3. Maintain good head alignment and manually ventilate the child with a self-inflating bag and mask and 100% O_2 until the provider intubating is ready to intubate.	Proper head alignment opens the airway, providing optimal oxygenation and perfusion to the brain. Ventilation is needed because preintubation medications cause respiratory suppression or cessation.
4. Immediately before intubation procedure, suction the back of the airway with a rigid large-bore Yankauer catheter or other large-bore catheter.	Suctioning clears the airway of secretions for better visualization of the ETT and prevention of aspiration.
5. Apply gentle cricoid pressure (Sellick's maneuver) as required during the procedure (Figure 59-2).	Pressure occludes the esophagus, thereby preventing aspiration of gastric contents. May facilitate visualization of the glottic opening.

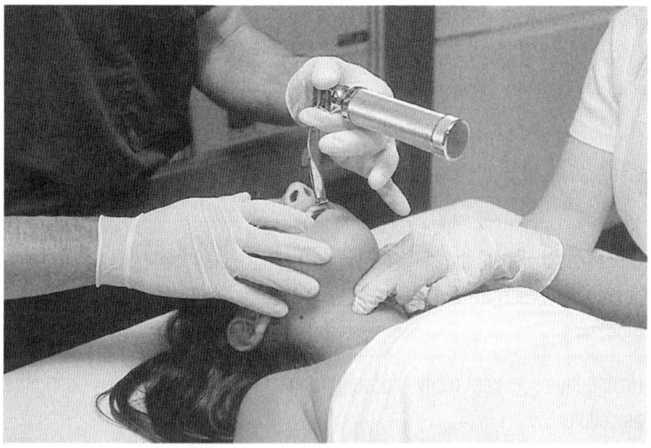

FIGURE 59-2
Applying cricoid pressure occludes the esophagus, thereby preventing aspiration of gastric contents.

Alert! *If the intubation is difficult or bradycardia occurs, interrupt the procedure and manually ventilate the child with 100% oxygen. Intubation attempts lasting longer than 30 seconds may produce profound hypoxemia. The small lung volumes and increased oxygen requirements of children rapidly consume oxygen reserves.*

Steps	Rationale/Points of Emphasis
6a. After insertion, hold the ETT in place while breath sounds are checked bilaterally and over the stomach and inspect for symmetric chest expansion. Breath sounds should be absent over the abdomen. Do not tape ETT in place until proper position of the tube has been initially evaluated.	Assessment validates the tube is in the correct position. Condensation in the tube indicates pulmonary placement, but lack of condensation does not necessarily indicate incorrect placement. If no breath sounds are heard on the right side but are heard on the left, the tube probably was inserted too far. Pull the tube back gently (while listening with a stethoscope) until breath sounds return on the right side. If the tube is not placed correctly and cannot be adjusted to be placed correctly, it must be removed, and the child needs to be reintubated.
6b. Connect CO_2 detector as an initial verification of tube placement and deliver four to six breaths. Read CO_2 detector according to manufacturer's instructions.	Exhaled CO_2 is a particularly reliable indicator of tube placement if the child has a perfusing cardiac rhythm present. A low end-tidal or exhaled CO_2 detector can mislead the provider into mistakenly suspecting an esophageal intubation in children with cardiac arrest even though the tube is in the trachea.

Steps	Rationale/Points of Emphasis
7. Continue to manually ventilate and maintain the stability of the tube until it is secure. Use a commercial securement device or tape to secure the tube in place. Measure the distance from the edge of the lip or naris to the end of the tube. Document the distance on the flow sheet or emergency sheet. If tape is used to secure the ETT	Provides optimal oxygenation and maintains proper tube placement. Commercial devices have been developed to hold the tube in place. This decreases the need for tape on the face, which can lead to dermal stripping upon removal. Baseline measurement of external length provides comparison to detect tube movement.
a. Cut two pieces of tape the same length as the distance from the edge of the mouth or nose to the base of the ear. Split the tape lengthwise halfway.	Prepares tape to secure ETT in place; some facilities use a premanufactured device to secure the endotracheal tube.
b. Apply an adhesive under the area where the tape would be placed.	The tape will adhere to the face more securely.
c. Again, measure the distance from the lip or naris to the end of the tube just before applying the tape.	Documentation of the length of the tube is necessary to ensure proper placement at all times.
d. Secure tape to the cheek and wrap one strand around the tube. The other strand should lay flat above the lip or across the bridge of the nose.	Provides stabilization of the ETT.
e. Follow the same procedure with the second piece of tape but wrap it in the opposite direction.	This method stabilizes the tube from the opposite direction, applying traction to maintain the tube more securely.
f. Measure the distance from the lip or naris again.	The ETT may slip in or out while the tape is being applied.
8. Suction (if needed) and continue to manually ventilate the child.	Removes excess secretions and increases oxygenation. **Alert!** *Do not hyperventilate. Hyperventilation reduces cerebral blood flow and may create cerebral ischemia.*
9. Verify tube placement with a secondary confirmation technique (chest x-ray).	Most accurate method to verify tube placement.

PROCEDURE After Intubation

Steps	Rationale/Points of Emphasis
1. Connect the ETT to the ventilator and assess the child's respiratory status on the ventilator.	Establishes baseline lung sounds and air leak once on the ventilator. Ensures tube has not become dislodged when transferring from bag-valve ventilation to a ventilator.
2. Remove gloves, mask, gown, and goggles and perform hand hygiene.	Reduces transmission of microorganisms.
3. Apply restraints or safety devices to the extremities if the child is not sedated (see Chapter 102).	Keeps the child safe from attempting to pull out the ETT.
4. Dispose of intubation equipment and waste in appropriate receptacle. Place laryngoscope and blades in area for cleaning and sterilization.	Reduces transfer of microorganisms.
5. Insert an oral airway into the mouth (if ordered) and secure with tape. The airway should fit into the mouth but not reach the back of the throat.	The oral airway prevents the child from biting on the ETT. An airway that is too long causes increased gagging and may cause aspiration with vomiting.
6. Place a nasogastric tube in the child (see Chapter 39).	For gastric decompression, which can assist ventilation.
7. Continue to assess cardiac and respiratory status and to evaluate the child's comfort level.	It may be necessary to remedicate the child to prevent him or her from fighting the ventilator.

Continued

Steps	Rationale/Points of Emphasis
8. Evaluate for complications (Figure 59-3).	Complications may include swelling of the airway, increased airway resistance, mucus plugging, pneumothorax, and dislodgment of the tube.

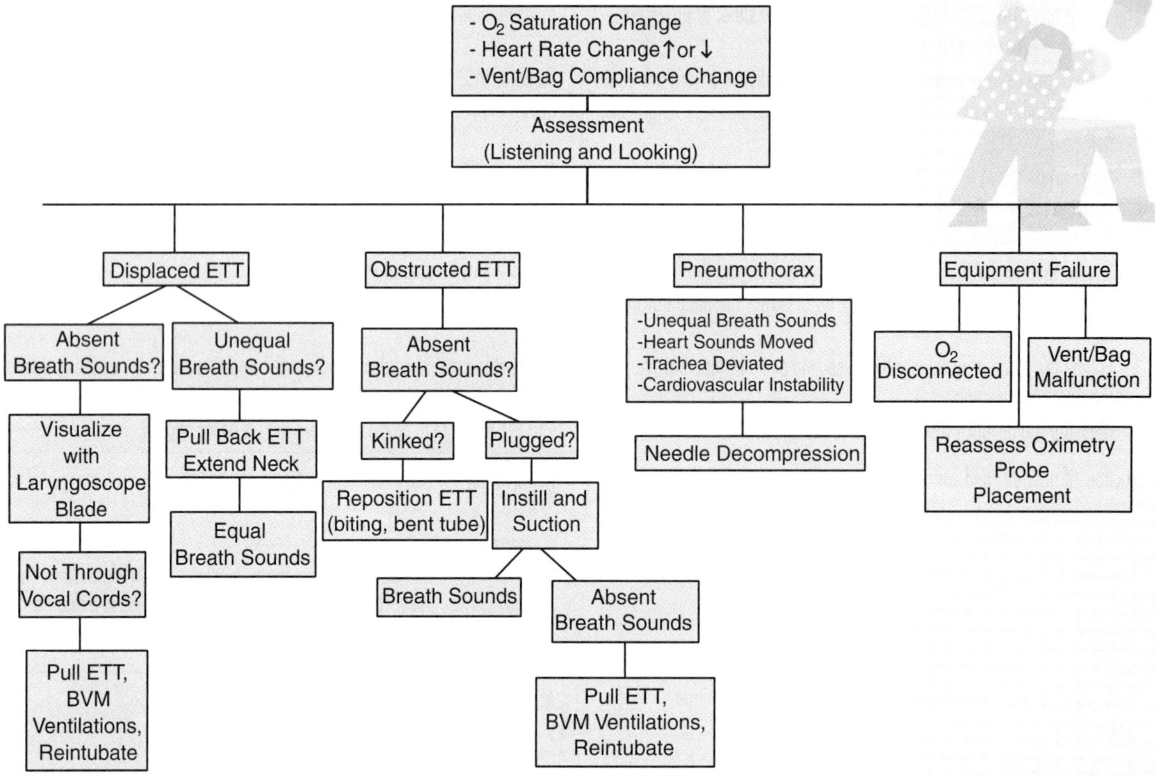

FIGURE 59-3
An algorithm for intervening in endotracheal tube complications. ↑, increase; ↓, decrease; ETT, endotracheal tube; BVM, bag-valve mask.

Steps	Rationale/Points of Emphasis
9. Ensure that the ETT cuff, if present, continues to be inflated.	Deflation may lead to dislodgment of the tube. The cuff should only be deflated during intubation, extubation, and tube repositioning.
10. Check ETT placement every shift and when the child's respiratory status changes.	Confirm placement and check that the ETT is in the same place each time it is reevaluated.

CHILD AND FAMILY EVALUATION AND DOCUMENTATION

- Document the following:
  - Tube size and centimeter level of insertion at the nares or teeth and gum
  - Whether the tube is cuffed or uncuffed. If it is a cuffed tube, record the amount of air used to inflate the cuff.
  - Any medications administered during the procedure and any side effects from them
  - Child's response to the intubation, noting if there was an improvement in respiratory status or comfort with breathing
  - Amount and type of secretions that were suctioned from the ETT
  - Response to sedation

COMMUNITY CARE

- After extubation, the child's throat may be sore. Ice packs may be applied to the throat to provide comfort.
- Instruct the family to contact the healthcare provider if
  - Child experiences difficulty swallowing that does not resolve within a few days
  - Child experiences difficulty breathing
  - Child complains of sore throat that does not resolve within 1 week after intubation

Unexpected Situations

- *During intubation the child becomes bradycardic and cyanotic:* If intubation can proceed quickly or epiglottal penetration has occurred, complete the procedure and quickly perform bag-valve ventilation to the ETT, which should improve the aforementioned conditions. However, if the intubation procedure is taking longer than expected (due to the difficulty of the situation), remove the laryngoscope and provide bag-valve mask ventilation until the parameters return to prior status and then attempt repeat.
- *You notice that the measurement markings on the ETT have changed from those noted when the chest x-ray to confirm tube placement was performed:* Assess the child. Notify the physician or advanced practice nurse immediately if signs of tube displacement (unequal or absent breath sounds, asymmetric chest expansion, abdominal breath sounds) or respiratory compromise are present.
- *During intubation you notice the child's abdomen becomes distended and tympanic:* Complete intubation and then place a nasogastric tube for gastric air decompression.
- *During intubation the child vomits:* Remove the laryngoscope and turn the child's head to the side. Suction the gastric contents and decompress the stomach by passing a suction catheter into the stomach. Provide bag-valve mask ventilation until the situation is stabilized and then attempt intubation.

Bibliography

American Heart Association. (2005a). Part 6: Pediatric basic and advanced life support [electronic version]. *Circulation, 112*(22 S), III-73–III-90. Retrieved August 21, 2006, from http://www.circulationaha.org

American Heart Association. (2005b). Part 12: Pediatric advanced life support [electronic version]. *Circulation, 112*(22 S), IV-167–IV-187. Retrieved August 21, 2006, from http://www.circulationaha.org

DeBoer, S., & Sever, M. (2004). End-tidal CO_2 verification of endotracheal placement in neonates. *Neonatal Network—Journal of Neonatal Nursing, 23*(3), 29–38.

DeBoer, S., Sever, M., & Arndt, K., (2003). Verification of endotracheal tube placement: A comparison of confirmation techniques and devices. *Journal of Emergency Nursing, 29*, 444–450.

Lane, B., Finer, N., & Rich, W. (2004). Duration of intubation attempts during neonatal resuscitation. *Journal of Pediatrics, 145*, 67–70.

Lucier, M. M., & Brisson, D. (2003). Extubation of pediatric patients by PACU nurses. *Journal of Perianesthesia Nursing, 18*, 91–95.

Marvez, E., Weiss, S. J., Houry, D. E., & Ernst, A. A. (2003). Predicting adverse outcomes in a diagnosis-based protocol system for rapid sequence intubation. *American Journal of Emergency Medicine, 21*(1), 23–29.

Mencke, T., Echternach, M., Kleinschmidt, S., et al. (2003). Laryngeal morbidity and quality of tracheal intubation: A randomized clinical trial. *Anesthesiology, 98*, 1049–1056.

Newth, C., Rachman, B., Patel, N., & Hammer, J. (2004). The use of cuffed versus uncuffed endotracheal tubes in pediatric intensive care. *Journal of Pediatrics, 144*, 333–337.

Orf, J., Thomas, S. H., Ahmed, W., et al. (2000). Appropriateness of endotracheal size and insertion depth in children undergoing air medical transport. *Pediatric Emergency Care, 16*, 321–327.

Ridling, D., Lynn, M. D., & Bratton, S. L. (2003). *Endotracheal suctioning with or without instillation of isotonic sodium chloride solution in critically ill children.* Retrieved October 8, 2003, from http://www.findarticles.com/cf_0/m0NUB/3_12/101414603/print.jhtml

Spence, K., Gilles, D., & Waterworth, L. (2003). Deep versus shallow suction of endotracheal tubes in ventilated neonates and young. *Cochrane Database of Systematic Reviews, 3*, No. CD003309.

Sullivan, K. J., & Kissoon, N. (2002). Securing the child's airway in the emergency department. *Pediatric Emergency Care, 18*, 108–121.

CHAPTER

60

Latex Precautions

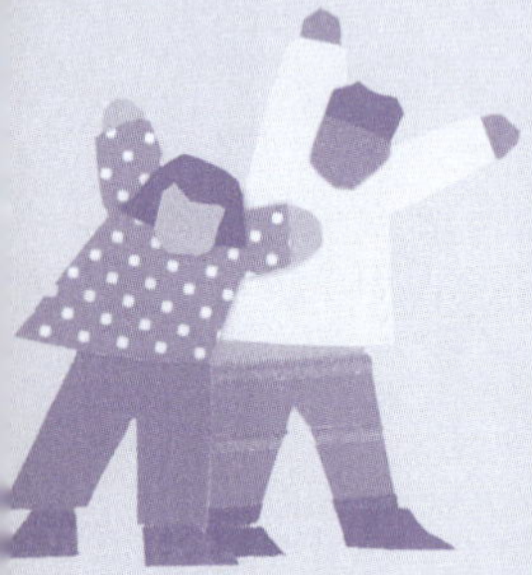

Clinical Guidelines

- The registered nurse (RN), licensed practical nurse (LPN), or unlicensed assistive personnel (UAPs) screens for presence of, or risk for, latex allergy.
- All children are screened for risk of latex allergy to identify those with known latex allergy and those who are at risk for latex allergy.
- All children who have known latex allergy or are at risk for latex allergy are
  - Provided with a care environment that is as latex free as possible
  - Identified by signage on identification band, at the bedside, and on the medical record
  - Given standing orders for emergency medications
- All healthcare providers shall wash their hands after latex glove use.

Equipment

- Latex-free supply cart containing but not limited to
  - "Latex Allergy" or "Latex Precautions" signage for the room's door
  - Latex-free gloves: sterile and nonsterile
  - Masks and bonnets with strings, not elastic banding
  - Latex-free stethoscope
  - Plastic tape
  - Plastic stopcocks
  - Webril bandage and stockinette
  - Latex-free tourniquet
  - Transport basket of latex-free supplies
- List of latex alternatives available within the facility
- Latex-free resuscitation equipment

Child and Family Assessment and Preparation

- Assess for any history of latex allergy, diagnosed by healthcare provider, and any high-risk factors for developing latex allergy:
  - History of neural tube defect (spina bifida) or congenital urologic conditions (particularly bladder exstrophy)
  - Frequent latex catheterizations
  - Previous surgeries, particularly genitourinary surgeries
  - History of environmental allergies
  - History of reactions or allergies to cross-reactive foods: predominantly banana, kiwi, avocado, chestnut, papaya, passion fruit, grapes, pineapples, peaches, and cherries

- History of reactions to rubber latex products in the environment (e.g., balloons, gloves, diapers, socks)
- Unexplained allergic reactions during a medical or dental procedure

- Identify the child who has a known or suspected allergy to latex with "Latex Allergy" on records and charts.
- Identify the child who has no symptoms upon exposure to latex but who is at risk for developing an allergy with "Latex Precautions."
- Explain goals of a latex-safe environment to child and family. Provide reassurance to child and family about a latex-safe environment. Emphasize that all healthcare personnel implement standard precautions by wearing gloves but that they wear nonlatex gloves when treating child.

PROCEDURE Preventing Latex Allergies

Steps	Rationale/Points of Emphasis
1. Provide the latex-allergic child with a latex-safe room. • Cover all cords in room with gauze or other nonlatex wrap. • Remove latex-containing items from room. • Cover the mattress completely with sheets or blankets. • Obtain latex-free supply cart and list of latex-containing and alternative products. • Do not use latex products for other patients in these rooms.	Aerosolized latex particles may provoke an inhalation-triggered or touch-transfer allergic response. **KidKare** Emphasize, and give permission, to child and family to be proactive with self-care by confirming knowledge of latex precautions and freely questioning healthcare personnel about gloves and supplies that are used. This helps to reduce anxiety for latex-allergic children and their families, empowers children and families to participate in self-care activities, and provides an additional alerting mechanism for patient safety.
2. Contact physician or advanced practice nurse (APN) to inform of latex risk status as indicated by history. Obtain orders indicated from history to implement latex precautions. Consider request for an allergy consult for at-risk children.	Screening may reveal patients at risk. Epicutaneous skin testing is used to identify latex-specific IgE antibodies; the proper precautions can then be initiated.
3. Apply identification band to child indicating "Latex Allergy" or "Latex Precautions."	Properly identifies the allergic or at-risk child.
4. When hospitalized, orient child and family to their room as well as supplies, resource list of latex-free supplies, and alternative products.	Decreases anxiety by helping patient and family become familiar with surroundings. Promotes family-centered care by encouraging child and family to participate.
5. Post "Latex Allergy" or "Latex Precautions" signs and labels outside patient's room, on medical record, and on all laboratory and diagnostic requisitions, including x-ray. Enter "Latex Allergy" or "Latex Precautions" in the facility computer system, when available. Notify interfacing departments/contacts (e.g., Child Life, nutrition services, pharmacy, schoolteacher) of child's latex allergy or latex precautions status.	Reduces the risk for exposure to latex through proper identification of precautions to be implemented by healthcare personnel.
6. Obtain order from healthcare prescriber to have emergency medications available, including diphenhydramine, epinephrine, and methyl prednisone.	Ensures that emergency medications are immediately available for administration in the event of an allergic reaction.
7. Schedule all diagnostic and surgical procedures, including dental procedures, as first-in-the-morning procedures.	Reduces the undue exposure to aerosolized latex glove powder (antigen avoidance) from personnel having used latex gloves with previous patients.
8. Perform hand hygiene and don gown before entering child's room if latex products were used before entering the room of the child on latex precautions.	Reduces potential exposure to latex powder.

Continued

Steps	Rationale/Points of Emphasis
9. When medications are administered, use latex-free products whenever possible. Check with manufacturer or with the materials distributor medication about the product's latex content and alternative products.	Eliminates latex exposure because anaphylactic reactions from systemic bolus of latex during IV administration have occurred.
a. Avoid use of latex-containing nipples; silicone nipples are an alternative.	
b. Draw up and give all medications immediately after preparation.	Reduces the direct exposure or time available to leech latex protein from the rubber syringe plunger.
c. Use latex-free plastic or glass syringes. Avoid the use of preloaded syringes with latex rubber plungers.	
d. Use medication from glass vials instead of multidose vials unless labeled by manufacturer that the stopper is not rubber.	Avoids introducing latex from the stopper into the solution in the vial.
e. Use latex-free IV tubing and supplies. Flush all tubing before use. If latex-free IV tubing is unavailable, cover all ports with tape. Use a 0.45-µm filter just proximal to the patient's IV connection. Add stopcocks at connection sites and use for medication administration.	Filter provides an added barrier. **Alert!** *Do not inject through rubber ports on tubing. Monitor child during medication administration for allergic response such as wheezing, dyspnea, generalized urticaria, tachycardia, and bronchospasm to ensure prompt detection of reactions.*
10. Use latex alternatives, such as silk or plastic tape or gauze, instead of adhesive bandages. Use a latex-free glove for a tourniquet if a nonlatex tourniquet is unavailable. When equipment must be used that contains latex, cover it before using (e.g., cover stethoscope tubing with stockinette); place a nonlatex transparent dressing (e.g., Tegaderm, 3M Health Care, St. Paul, MN) over the digit before placing the pulse oximeter probe; apply blood pressure cuff over gown or wrap area in gauze. Use silastic Foley catheters in place of gastrostomy tubes, urinary catheters, and enema inducers.	Adding a physical barrier to an unavoidable latex-containing product decreases or prevents direct latex exposure. **caREminder** *A list of latex alternatives can be obtained from the supply manufacturers. In addition, the Spina Bifida Association of America maintains a list of latex alternatives that is updated semiannually.*
11a. When hospitalized, encourage child and family to bring familiar latex-free items from home. These may include toys, favored objects such as blankets, and pajamas (with no elastic in waistband).	Provides comfort to the child in unfamiliar surroundings. Promotes safety with known latex-free items.
11b. Label all items brought from home.	Reduces the risk for loss of favorite items during hospitalization.
12. Provide developmentally appropriate education to the child and family as discussed under Community Care.	Reduces the potential for inadvertent exposure to latex and potentially decreases subsequent allergic reactions.
13. For the child at risk for latex allergy by history, maintain ongoing monitoring for development of latex allergy.	Provides prompt detection of allergy development so that more stringent latex avoidance measures can be implemented.
14. If a latex reaction occurs, remove the offending agent. Contact the physician or APN. Monitor for serious reactions.	Decreases ongoing exposure to the offending agent. Obtain further orders from the physician or APN to intervene appropriately.

CHILD AND FAMILY EVALUATION AND DOCUMENTATION

- Evaluate child and family's understanding of latex-safe environment.
- Solicit questions or concerns.
- Review the resources for latex-free products (Chart 60-1).
- Document the following:
  - Implementation of latex precautions
  - Placement of "Latex Allergy" or "Latex Precautions" identification band
  - Communication of latex precautions to appropriate departments
  - Family education regarding latex avoidance and latex-free alternatives

CHART 60-1 LATEX ALLERGY RESOURCES

ALERT, Inc.: 888-972-5378

American Latex Allergy Association: http://www.latexallergyresources.org/

Canadian Latex Allergy Association: 905-885-9708

Latex Allergy Information Service: 800-482-6869

Spina Bifida Association of America: 800-621-3141; http://www.sbaa.org

U.S. Food and Drug Administration Latex Allergy Hotline: 301-594-3060

COMMUNITY CARE

- Collaborate with health team for follow-up plan of care.
- Educate the child and family:
  - Discuss the process of latex sensitization.
  - Emphasize the importance of avoiding exposure to latex.
  - Review household products that contain latex (e.g., balloons, toys, chewing gum, rugs with nonskid backing, disposable diapers, elastic in waistbands, socks, condoms; refer to Spina Bifida Association of America list).
  - Provide and review list of latex-free alternatives.
  - Reinforce with family that the label "hypoallergenic" does not mean latex free. Read product labels to identify latex presence.
  - Increase awareness of restaurants that prepare foods while wearing latex gloves and avoid these establishments.
- Discuss symptoms of latex allergy that range from mild local reactions to life-threatening systemic anaphylaxis:
  - Red watering eyes, runny nose
  - Rash, hives, itching
  - Facial swelling, scratchy throat
  - Nausea, vomiting
  - Wheezing, coughing, difficulty breathing
  - Shock
- Provide list of latex allergy resources (see Chart 60-1).
- Advise that child wear a Medic Alert bracelet or that the parent carry an identification card for an infant.
- Advise parents to carry nonlatex gloves in case they are needed.
- Advise parents to carry an EpiPen or EpiPen Jr. and have available at school for children who have experienced a previous serious reaction; teach them to use it.
- Notify all healthcare providers, including pharmacists, of latex allergy and request latex-free alternatives. Advise parents to schedule first-morning appointments for child. Monday mornings are optimal for dental and surgical procedures.
- Avoid ingestion of cross-reactive foods.
- Provide information about alternative latex-free products to out-of-home care providers, school, and camp.
- Teach family and all care providers actions to be taken in allergic events:
  - Evaluate severity of reaction and institute supportive measures.
  - For mild local reactions: eliminate offending agent, administer an oral antihistamine (diphenhydramine or chlorpheniramine) and apply steroid cream to area if appropriate
  - For serious systemic and anaphylactic reactions: use EpiPen *and* call 911.
- Ensure that follow-up agencies (healthcare agencies, day care, and schools) have notice of child's latex allergy status.
- Provide follow-up agencies with appropriate resources to maintain continuity of care.
- Initiate referrals for education on latex-safe environments as indicated (e.g., home health or school nurse, out-of-home care).
- Instruct the family to contact the healthcare provider if
  - Child has a serious allergic reaction
  - Child has a mild reaction that does not respond to prescribed treatments
  - Child has an increased incidence of allergic reactions

Unexpected Situation

- *After completion of a procedure, the child develops respiratory distress, with wheezing, coughing, and cyanosis. The child is tachycardic and has delayed capillary refill. You notice some facial edema and rhinitis:* Immediately initiate supportive or rescue measures for airway management. Assess severity of cardiorespiratory compromise. Activate emergency response system if indicated; administer medications as ordered. Use a latex-free resuscitation bag, oxygen mask, and supplies and create a latex-safe environment.

Bibliography

American College of Allergy, Asthma, and Immunology. (1996). *Guidelines for the management of latex allergies and safe latex use in health care facilities.* Retrieved August 21, 2006, from http://www.acaai.org/public/linkpages/latex.htm

AORN. (2004). AORN latex guideline. *AORN Journal, 79,* 653–672.

Becker, H. (2000). An analysis of the epidemiology of latex allergy: Implications for primary prevention. *MEDSURG Nursing, 9,* 135–143.

Binkley, H. M., Schroyer, T., & Catalfano, J. (2003). Latex allergies: A review of recognition, evaluation, management, prevention, education, and alternative product use. *Journal of Athletic Training, 38,* 133–140.

Burh, V. (2000). Screening patients for latex allergies. *Journal of the American Academy of Nurse Practitioners, 12*, 380–383.

Centers for Disease Control and Prevention. (1998). *Latex allergy: A prevention guide.* Retrieved August 21, 2006, from http://www.cdc.gov/niosh/98-113.html

Emergency Nurses Association. (1998). Emergency Nurses Association position statement: Latex allergy. *Journal of Emergency Nursing, 24*, 29A–30A.

Hourihane, J. O., Allard, J. M., Wade, A. M., McEwan, A. I., & Strobel, S. (2002). Impact of repeated surgical procedures on the incidence and prevalence of latex allergy: A prospective study of 1263 children. *Journal of Pediatrics, 40*, 479–482.

Kimata, H. (2004). Latex allergy in infants younger than 1 year. *Clinical and Experimental Allergy, 34*, 1910–1915.

Muller, B. A. (2003). Minimizing latex exposure and allergy. How to avoid or reduce sensitization in the healthcare setting. *Postgraduate Medicine, 113*, 91–97.

Nakamura, C. T., Ferdman, R. M., Keens, T. G., & Davidson Ward, S. L. (2000). Latex allergy in children on home mechanical ventilation. *Chest, 118*, 1000–1003.

National Association of Neonatal Nurses. (1999). *Position statement on latex allergy (#3016a).* Glenview, IL: Author.

Perkin, J. E. (2000). The latex and food allergy connection. *Journal of the American Dietetic Association, 100*, 1381–1384.

Sparta, G., Kemper, M. J., Gerber, A. C., Goetschel, P., & Neuhaus, T. J. (2004). Latex allergy in children with urological malformation and chronic renal failure. *Journal of Urology, 171*, 1647–1649.

Taylor, J. S., & Erkek, E. (2004). Latex allergy: Diagnosis and management. *Dermatologic Therapy, 17*, 289–301.

Thomsen, D. F., & Burke, T. G. (2000). Lack of latex allergen contamination of solutions withdrawn from vials with natural rubber stoppers. *American Journal of Health-System Pharmacy, 57*(1), 44–47.

CHAPTER

61

Lumbar Puncture

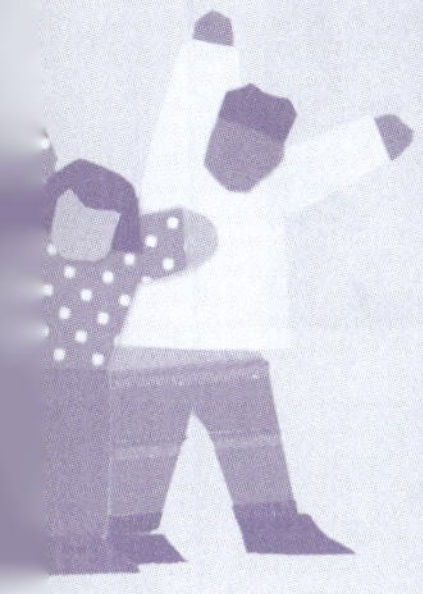

Clinical Guidelines

- A physician, nurse practitioner (NP), or physician's assistant (PA) performs this procedure.
- A registered nurse (RN) or licensed practical nurse (LPN) is present during the procedure to assist in positioning the child and in assessing the child's status.
- The procedure is performed in a treatment room, unless the child is in an emergency room or intensive care unit and should not be moved from the bed because of his or her condition.
- Informed consent must be obtained before the procedure.
- The procedure is carried out under aseptic technique.

Equipment

- Sterile disposable pediatric lumbar puncture tray to include
  - Sterile drapes
  - A 3-mL syringe with 25-gauge needle
  - Three-way stopcock
  - Adhesive bandage
  - Three to five fluid collection tubes
  - Povidone-iodine swabs
  - Spinal fluid pressure monometer (optional)
- Two lumbar puncture needles
- Ampule of 1% lidocaine
- Sterile gloves
- Labels with child's name for specimen tubes
- Anesthetic cream (optional)

Child and Family Assessment and Preparation

- Assess the pertinent history and physical findings for signs of increased intracranial pressure.
- Assess the age, developmental level, and coping strategies of the child.
- Discuss with the child and parents distraction techniques that may be useful during the procedure (e.g., imagery, focused breathing).
- Assess the child's and parents' knowledge of the reasons for the procedure, expected outcomes, and potential adverse reactions.
- Discuss role of the parent to provide support to the child if the parent will be present during the procedure.
- Ensure that written consent has been obtained to perform the procedure.
- Apply topical anesthetic to lumbar puncture site if using agent that requires advanced time for complete activation.

PROCEDURE Assisting With Lumbar Puncture

Steps	Rationale/Points of Emphasis
1. Perform hand hygiene.	Reduces transmission of microorganisms.
2. Set up equipment using aseptic technique.	Maintains sterile integrity of environment, promotes efficient time management, and provides an organized approach to the procedure.
3. Airborne and/or contact isolation precautions may be needed. Don gown, gloves, and mask as needed if the procedure is being performed on a child with a potential infection.	Meningococcal meningitis is highly contagious and is an airborne contaminant. Unprotected staff exposed to this organism by the child will have to undergo prophylactic treatment measures.
4. Verify child's identity and transport child to treatment room (unless procedure is to be done at the bedside). If not already completed, apply anesthetic cream to site; transport child to treatment room after the agent has been applied for the period of time recommended by manufacturer.	Helps ensure correct patient, correct procedure. Painful procedures should not be performed at the child's bedside unless absolutely necessary because of the child's critical condition. The child's hospital room should remain a safe haven where intrusive procedures are not completed. By applying anesthetic cream at this point, the site will be desensitized by the time procedure is performed.
5. Position child on the treatment table in one of the following ways:	
a. Knee–chest position (Figure 61-1). With back rounded and parallel to side of treatment table, place child on side with lumbar area exposed. Hold small infant in position by placing one hand over his or her neck and the other hand over the buttocks. Bend the child's back to the desired position.	Best position for infant. Maximizes separation of the vertebral bodies. The L3–L4 interspace is the preferred site for a lumbar puncture, but the L2–L3 and L4–L5 interspaces can also be used.
b. Recumbent position (Figure 61-2). Hold older infant or child in position by placing one hand behind child's neck or one arm around neck and grasping child's legs behind the knees. Place the other arm around child's buttocks and grasp his or her hands. Put pressure on neck and legs to bend child's body as necessary.	Best position for older infant or young child to maximize separation of vertebral bodies. **Alert!** *Modification of the positions may be necessary if the child is intubated or has fractures.*

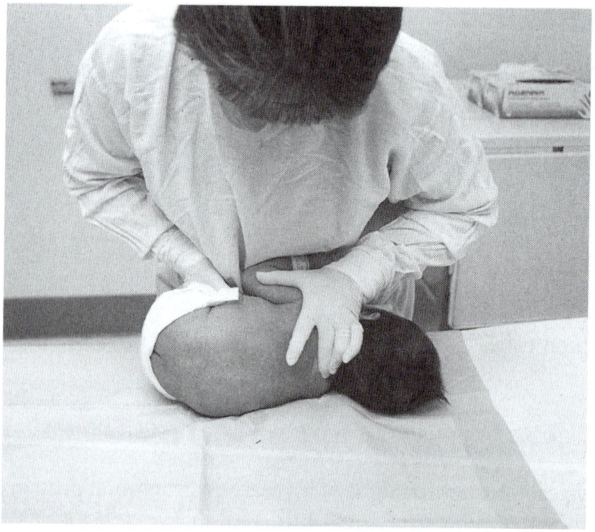

FIGURE 61-1
Knee–chest position.

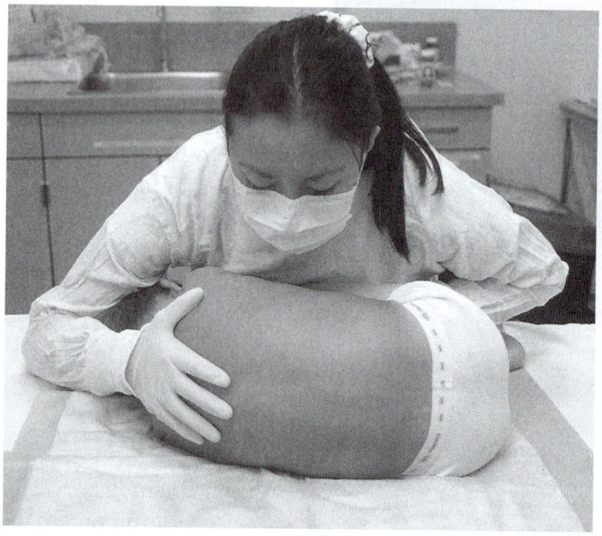

FIGURE 61-2
Recumbent position.

Steps	Rationale/Points of Emphasis
c. Sitting position (Figure 61-3). Support the child in position by having the child sit at edge of the table with shoulders and head bent forward. Elbows should be placed on the knees and the back arched.	This may be a comfortable position for the older child who is able to cooperate without restraint. An assistant must hold infants placed in this position in the sitting position.

Steps	Rationale/Points of Emphasis
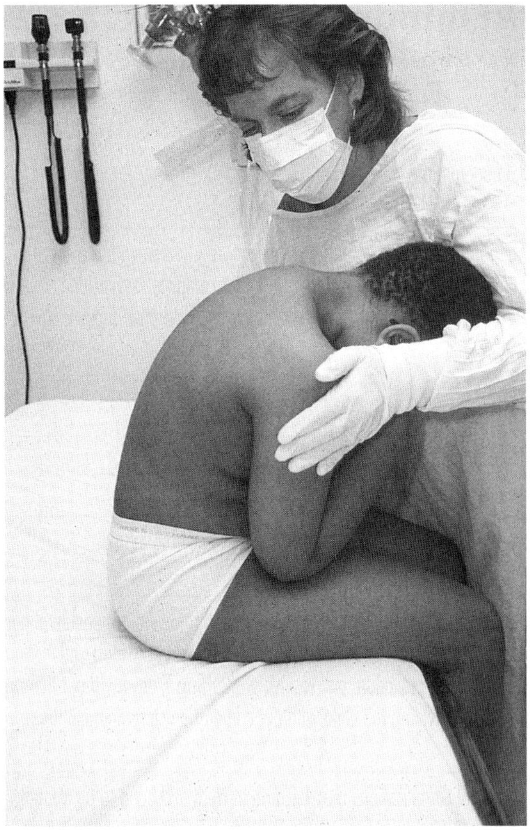 **FIGURE 61-3** Sitting position.	**KidKare** A pillow or large stuffed animal can be placed in front of the chest with the child instructed to grasp it.
6a. When the child is in position, the sterile drapes are placed over the back to expose the puncture area only.	Aseptic technique is used to decrease exposure to microorganisms during this invasive procedure.
6b. The child is instructed to stay as still as possible while the assistant continues to hold the child securely in position. The assistant or parent present in the room initiates distraction measures.	Research supports that parental presence decreases child fear and anxiety and that parents can use a variety of comforting and distracting strategies to support their child during the painful procedure.
7. Follow institution policy and procedure for ensuring preoperative verification process is completed, appropriate operative site is marked, and "time out" is completed before start of procedure. The healthcare provider performing the procedure identifies the puncture area and scrubs the area with povidone-iodine. Tell the child he or she will feel a cold sensation on the back during the cleansing.	Implements Universal Protocol for Preventing Wrong Site, Wrong Procedure, Wrong Person Surgery and follows the Joint Commission on Accreditation of Healthcare Organizations (JCAHO) National Patient Safety Goals 2004: (1) Improve the accuracy of patient identification; and (4) Eliminate wrong site, wrong patient, wrong procedure surgery. Decreases microorganisms at site. Telling the child what sensations they will feel may help them cope.
8. The healthcare provider performing the procedure instills lidocaine (Xylocaine) intradermally around the area of the puncture site.	Provides local anesthesia to the site.
9a. The healthcare provider performing the procedure inserts needle and stylet into the subarachnoid space. When the needle is in position, a free drip of cerebrospinal fluid (CSF) is established, and spinal pressure may be assessed using the spinal pressure manometer. The monometer is attached to the spinal needle by means of a three-way stopcock.	When CSF fluid fills the manometer, CSF pressure can be monitored. Normal pressure in the relaxed patient is 50–80 mm in children (Table 61-1). Each heartbeat creates a fluctuation of 2–5 mm and each respiration a fluctuation of 4–10 mm. Increased CSF pressure may be present with meningitis and other neurologic conditions that cause increased intracranial pressure.
9b. When the measurement is completed, the stopcock is turned to allow the CSF fluid to be collected in three to five sterile specimen tubes. CSF color and turbidity are noted at this time.	Normal CSF fluid is clear. Red fluid can indicate intracranial hemorrhage or a traumatic tap. Cloudy turbid fluid indicates infection. Yellow fluid indicates hyperbilirubinemia or hemolyzed red blood cells.

Continued

Steps	Rationale/Points of Emphasis
	caREminder *Number the collection tubes in the order in which they were filled.*
9c. Before removing the needle, the healthcare provider performing the procedure may choose to use the manometer to measure closing CSF pressure.	Assists in appropriate collection of results.
10. Throughout the procedure, the assistant monitors for complications such as • Decreased responsiveness • Tachycardia or bradycardia • Sluggish or unequal pupil reaction • Abnormal breathing due to positioning • Complaints of severe pain	Brainstem herniation is a potential complication. Children with increased intracranial pressure are at greatest risk. Other complications include penetration of a nerve and breakage of the needle (in an uncooperative moving child).
11. Spinal needle is withdrawn, the child's back is wiped clean of wet fluids, and an adhesive bandage is placed over the puncture site.	Protects the puncture site.
12. Dispose of equipment and waste in appropriate receptacle. Perform hand hygiene.	Standard precautions. Reduces transmission of microorganisms.
13. Return child to his or her own bed, making child comfortable lying flat in the bed. The child should remain lying flat for at least 1 hour after the procedure.	Despite a lower incidence than is seen in the adult population, postdural puncture headaches do occur in children. The headaches usually start within 48 hours after the procedure and resolve within 5 to 7 days without therapy. Lying flat and providing the child with good hydration can minimize the risk for headaches.
14. Continue to monitor the child for the complications noted in step 10.	Postprocedural complications may become evident and need to be treated.
15. Ensure that specimens are correctly labeled and sent to the laboratory immediately.	Prompt distribution of the specimens will assist in early diagnosis of the child's condition.

TABLE 61-1

Analysis of Cerebrospinal Fluid for Central Nervous System Infections

	Pressure	Appearance	Leukocyte (m^3)	Protein (mg/dL)	Glucose (mg/dL)
Normal cerebrospinal fluid	60–160 mm H_2O	Clear	0–5	10–30	40–80
Bacterial meningitis	Increased	Turbid, cloudy	Increased, 100–60,000; polymorphonuclear cells predominate	Increased, 100–500	Decreased
Aseptic meningitis	Normal or slightly increased	Clear	10–1,000	50–200	Normal to low, <40
Tuberculosis meningitis	Increased	Clear	10–500	100–500	<50
Brain abscess	Increased	Clear	Increased, 10–200	Increased, 75–500	>50

CHILD AND FAMILY EVALUATION AND DOCUMENTATION

- Document the following:
  - Time and duration of procedure
  - Name of healthcare provider performing procedure
  - Color and character of fluid withdrawn
  - Date and time that specimens were sent to the laboratory for analysis
- Evaluate response of the child during and after the procedure. Document findings in the medical record.

COMMUNITY CARE

- Encourage the child to drink plenty of fluids.
- Explain to child and parent the need to have child remain on bed rest for 1 hour after the procedure to decrease incidence of headaches. Although less frequently seen in the pediatric population, headaches are generally noted to start within 48 hours of the procedure, usually resolving within 5 to 7 days without therapy.
- Instruct the family to contact the healthcare provider if
  - Child has a severe headache
  - Child exhibits changes in neurologic status, such as changes in level of consciousness, irritability, onset of high-pitched cry (infants), and bulging fontanel (infants)
  - Child has bleeding or leaking of fluid from the puncture site
  - Redness or irritation develops at puncture site
  - Child develops a fever
  - Child complains of numbness in the legs

Unexpected Situations

- *The child moves unexpectedly during procedure:* The various holding positions used to facilitate lumbar puncture can be challenging to adequately execute. The child must remain in the correct position throughout the procedure to sufficiently expose the L2–L5 interspaces. For the safety of the child, the nurse must ensure a sustainable hold, regardless of which holding position is used, throughout the procedure. If the child moves, the provider performing the procedure will evaluate needle position, and the holder reestablishes the hold and the child's position.
- *The child experiences respiratory distress during the procedure:* The holding positions used for lumbar puncture may decrease lung excursion or compromise the upper airway. Ensure that the child's airway is not occluded during the procedure. Assess and remain alert to the child's baseline respiratory status. Noninvasive monitoring equipment, such as a pulse oximeter, may be useful in continuous assessment of the child's respiratory status during the procedure if underlying respiratory disease is a concern. If respiratory distress continues the procedure may need to be terminated.

Bibliography

Chordas, C. (2001). Post-dural puncture headache and other complications after lumbar puncture. *Journal of Pediatric Oncology Nursing, 18*, 244–259.

Ebinger, F., Kosel, C., Pietz, J., & Rating, D. (2004). Strict bed rest following lumbar puncture in children and adolescents is of no benefit. *Neurology, 62*, 1003–1005.

Ebinger, F., Kosel, C., Pietz, J., & Rating, D. (2004). Headache and backache after lumbar puncture in children and adolescents: A prospective study. *Pediatrics, 113*, 1588–1592.

Evans, R., Armon, C., Frohman, E., & Goodin, D. (2000). Assessment: Prevention of post-lumbar puncture headaches. Report of the Therapeutics and Technology Assessment Subcommittee of the American Academy of Neurology. *Neurology, 55*, 909–914.

Hickey, J. V. (2003). Diagnostic procedures and laboratory tests for neuroscience patients: Cerebrospinal fluid and spinal procedures. In J. V. Hickey (Ed.), *The clinical practice of neurological and neurosurgical nursing* (5th ed., pp. 102–103). Philadelphia: Lippincott Williams & Wilkins.

Janssens, E., Aerssens, P., Alliet, P., Gillis, P., & Raes, M. (2003). Post-dural puncture headaches in children: A literature review. *European Journal of Pediatrics, 162*, 117–121.

Joint Commission on Accreditation of Healthcare Organizations. (2004a). *National Patient Safety Goals 2004*. Retrieved September 10, 2004, from http://www.jcaho.org/accredited+organizations/patient+safety/npsg.htm

Joint Commission on Accreditation of Healthcare Organizations. (2004b). *Universal Protocol for Preventing Wrong Site, Wrong Procedure, Wrong Person Surgery™*. Retrieved September 10, 2004, from http://www.jcaho.org/accredited+organizations/patient+safety/universal+protocol/index.htm and http://www.jcaho.org/accredited+organizations/patient+safety/universal+protocol/universal+protocol.pdf

Kaur, G., Gupta, P., & Kumar, A. (2003). A randomized trial of eutectic mixture of local anesthetics during lumbar puncture in newborns. *Archives of Pediatrics & Adolescent Medicine, 157*, 1065–1070.

Tan, M., Tan, H., Büyükavci, M., & Karakelleoglu, C. (2004). Parents' attitudes toward performance of lumbar puncture on their children. *The Journal of Pediatrics, 144*, 400–402.

CHAPTER

62

Medication Administration: Endotracheal

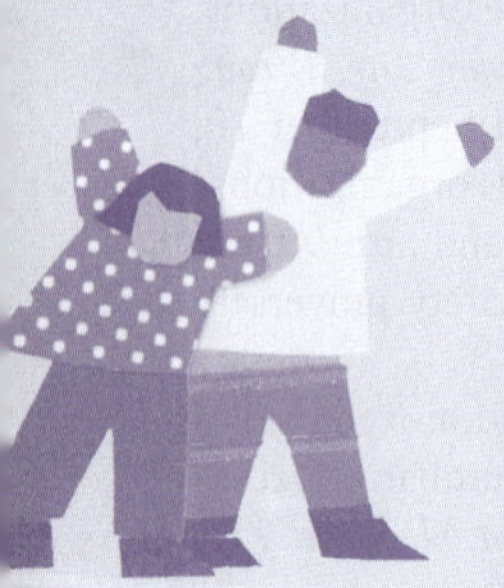

Clinical Guidelines

- A healthcare prescriber orders medications. If a prescriber is not available, medications are administered following Pediatric Advanced Life Support (PALS) protocol.
- Medications are administered by a physician, registered nurse (RN), or pharmacist who is knowledgeable about techniques of administering endotracheal medication to a child as well as the particular medication being used and its possible effects on the child.
- In most emergent hospital situations when a child requires endotracheal medications, a number of healthcare professionals are involved, each with specific responsibilities. Typically, a code leader (physician or advanced practice nurse) manages the situation; licensed nurses monitor vital signs and suction, perform chest compressions, prepare and administer medications (within their scope of practice) (one nurse may prepare the medications, while another nurse actually delivers the medications), perform or assist with procedures, record and document, and assist the family; a respiratory therapist assists in managing the airway; and a pharmacist may also prepare and administer medications (within their scope of practice). The staff member who is with the family should elicit information about the child's drug and latex allergies.
- Principles of pharmacologic management (see Chapter 6) are followed.
- Medication administration guidelines are followed, including correct patient, medication, dose, route, time, and approach to child.
- Because it is more efficacious, the intravenous (IV) route is the preferred method of administration of emergency medications. If, however, an emergent situation develops and IV or intraosseous access is not established within 3 to 5 minutes, there are four medications for children that can be administered through the endotracheal tube: lidocaine, epinephrine, atropine, and naloxone. These can be remembered by the mnemonic "LEAN."
- When drugs are administered by the endotracheal route, they should be diluted to a minimum volume of 3 to 5 mL with normal saline and then instilled into the endotracheal tube. To be absorbed, however, endotracheal medications must be delivered beyond the endotracheal tube into the tracheobronchial tree. Therefore, instill 5 mL of normal saline and deliver five breaths with a manual resuscitation bag to the endotracheal tube after drug instillation to encourage distribution of the drug into the tracheobronchial tree.

Equipment

For intubated patient:

- Length-based resuscitation tape
- Nonsterile gloves and goggles

- Manual resuscitation bag
- Oxygen
- Suction setup and equipment
- Several 1-, 3-, and 5-mL syringes and needles or needleless access devices
- Sterile normal saline
- Lidocaine, epinephrine, atropine, naloxone (as prescribed)
- Code blue/emergency/cardiopulmonary resuscitation (CPR) documentation record (institutional form)

CHILD AND FAMILY ASSESSMENT AND PREPARATION

- The need for emergent use of endotracheal medications means that IV access has not been established in a timely manner. This limits the amount of preparation that the child and family can receive with regard to endotracheal medications.
- Endotracheal medications are administered in emergency high-stress situations. Notify the family immediately of the seriousness of the situation and explain what is happening. The family's ability to process information may be impaired as a result of stress or anxiety related to the situation. Support the family of the child in dealing with this situation; a licensed care social worker, clinical psychologist, grief counselor, or chaplain may also provide support. If the family has a religious preference, notify the proper cleric.
- Determine the child's weight. Accurate determination of weight ensures correct dosage of medications. If the child's weight cannot be determined in an emergent situation, a length-based resuscitation tape (device developed applying length-based averages of a child) can be used to estimate the child's weight.
- Allow family members to stay with the child during resuscitation if they desire. If parents choose to be with their child during the procedure, explain the procedure to them so they know what to expect, and identify a staff member to be responsible for the family's needs. Position family members so they are out of the way but able to be reassured and comforted. If the parents opt to leave the room, allow them to return to the child's bedside as soon as possible.
- While the medications for endotracheal administration are being drawn up, if the child is not already intubated, follow Chapters 24 and 59.

PROCEDURE Administering Endotracheal Medications

Steps	Rationale/Points of Emphasis
1. Gather the necessary supplies. Perform hand hygiene and don nonsterile gloves and other protective wear as appropriate.	Promotes efficient time management and provides an organized approach to the procedure. Reduces transmission of microorganisms and protects against contact with body secretions.
2. Determine the child's weight or use length-based resuscitation tape to assist in determining emergency medication dosages.	The amount of endotracheal medication given is based on milligrams per kilogram of body weight.
3. Obtain order (it may be a verbal order in this case) for the medication and dosage of medication to be given or follow PALS protocol if no prescriber is present.	A healthcare prescriber's order is required for medication administration; PALS protocol may be accepted as standing orders. **caREminder** *Document verbal orders given during a code situation on the code blue/emergency/CPR record. This is a legal document and replaces the doctor's order form. All healthcare personnel involved in the emergency situation must sign the record.*
4. Obtain medication and read the label to verify that it is the same medication as prescribed in the order.	Ensures that the correct medication is being given.
5. Determine the amount (in milliliters) of medication to be given based on the order for milligrams per kilogram of body weight and draw up the correct amount into an appropriately sized syringe.	Ensures that the correct dosage is given.
6. Have another healthcare provider ensure that the endotracheal tube is free and clear of secretions. He or she should suction the endotracheal tube, as necessary, to ensure a clear airway.	Excessive amounts of secretions can block the airway passage and decrease the amount of medication that can be absorbed into the tracheobronchial tree.

Continued

Steps	Rationale/Points of Emphasis
7. Draw up 3 to 5 mL of normal saline solution into a separate syringe.	Provides diluent.
8. Dilute prescribed medication in normal saline diluent syringe.	Dilutes medication to proper volume for endotracheal administration.
9. Draw up 5 mL of normal saline flush into a syringe	This flush is used to follow endotracheal medication into the endotracheal tube to help spread the medication further throughout the tracheobronchial tree.
10. To confirm proper placement of endotracheal tube, auscultate the lungs bilaterally, listen over the stomach, assess for equal chest rise, and use an end-tidal CO_2 detector; if still in doubt that the tube is correctly positioned, a provider proficient in airway management should confirm correct tube placement by direct laryngoscopy.	Ensures safe and accurate drug administration into the tracheobronchial tree. Breath sounds should be absent over the stomach. During CPR, the absence of exhaled CO_2 may be due to low pulmonary blood flow, not incorrect tube placement.
11. Provide five to six ventilations through the bag-valve device immediately before administering medication.	Ensures preoxygenation of patient before delivery of medication.
12. Discontinue manual ventilation momentarily and instill the diluted medication into the endotracheal tube. While administering medication, state the medication's name and dose to transcribing RN.	Delivers medication into endotracheal tube while ensuring appropriate medication documentation. Noting the time the medication was given helps determine time the next dose of medication should be given, if necessary.
13. Follow instilled administration of medication with 5 mL of normal saline flushed into endotracheal tube.	Flush helps spread the medication further throughout the tracheobronchial tree.
14. Follow endotracheal drug administration with several quick positive-pressure manual ventilations in a row and resume resuscitation ventilation rate.	Pushes and distributes endotracheal medications through the tracheobronchial tree to aid in absorption.
15. Repeat endotracheal drug administration as necessary, following steps 3 to 14, until IV access is achieved or emergency has subsided.	Once vascular access is achieved, medications should be delivered through an IV. The venous system is the preferred and most effective route for drug administration in emergencies.
16. When emergency has subsided, dispose of equipment and waste in appropriate receptacle. Remove gloves and perform hand hygiene.	Standard precautions. Reduces transmission of microorganisms.

CHILD AND FAMILY EVALUATION AND DOCUMENTATION

- Evaluate the child for any change in vital signs, hemodynamic status, oxygen saturation, and so forth after medication administration. The practitioner who managed the code should notify the family of the outcome of resuscitation. Involve support personnel (i.e., social services, psychology, clergy) as much as possible in assisting the family.
- Document in the code blue/emergency/CPR record:
  - Airway type and size (e.g., no. 4.0 endotracheal tube, no. 3.5 fenestrated trachea tube); whether airway is cuffed or uncuffed; ETT landmark, if orally placed then landmark at gums or teeth, if nasally placed then landmark at nares (e.g., ETT taped at 10 at the gum); and tube location (i.e., oral, nasal, tracheal)
  - Date and time of suctioning; color, amount, and consistency of secretions; presence of blood; and any effects on the child
  - Date, time, type, dose, and route of the drug administered
  - Vital signs, hemodynamic status, oxygen saturation
  - Any other procedure occurring at the time
  - Child's response to instillation of medication
  - Laboratory work obtained and results
  - Interactions and discussions with family
- Obtain signatures of all healthcare personnel involved in emergency situation on the child's code blue/emergency/CPR record. It is the responsibility of both the nurse drawing up the medication and the nurse administering the medication to sign the record as documentation that the drug was given. It is the responsibility of the physician ordering the medication to sign the record to document that the drug was ordered.
- Determine whether or not the family has additional areas of concern to discuss.

COMMUNITY CARE

- Children are not discharged home receiving medications via the endotracheal route.

Unexpected Situations

- *Higher pressures are required to ventilate the child:* Assess breath sounds; if not present and equal with equal chest expansion, the endotracheal tube may need to be repositioned. Assess for abdominal distention; if present insert an orogastric or nasogastric tube to decompress the stomach.
- *Despite your best efforts, the child dies:* Briefly explain to the parents/family what was done to try to resuscitate the child. Offer to each parent, separately, to hold the child if they wish. Arrange unit so that family can say their good-byes to the child in a private area, taking as much time as they need. Create a memories box with hand or footprints of the child, a lock of hair, and photographs, as appropriate.

Bibliography

American Heart Association. (2005a). Part 8: Interdisciplinary topics [Electronic version]. *Circulation, 112*(22 S), III-100–III-108. Retrieved August 21, 2006, from http://www.circulationaha.org

American Heart Association. (2005b). Part 12: Pediatric advanced life support [Electronic version]. *Circulation, 112*(22 S), IV-167–IV-187. Retrieved August 21, 2006, from http://www.circulationaha.org

American Heart Association. (2005c). Part 13: Neonatal resuscitation guidelines [Electronic version]. *Circulation, 112*(22 S), IV-188–IV-195. Retrieved August 21, 2006, from http://www.circulationaha.org

Eichhorn, D. J., Meyers, T. A., Guzzetta, C. E., et al. (2001). During invasive procedures and resuscitation: Hearing the voice of the patient. *American Journal of Nursing, 101*(5), 48–55.

Hazinski, M. F., Zaritsky, A. L., Nadkarni, V. M., et al. (Eds.). (2002). *PALS provider manual.* Dallas, TX: American Heart Association.

Kattwinkel, J. (Ed.). (2000). *Textbook of neonatal resuscitation* (4th ed.). Elk Grove Village, IL: American Academy of Pediatrics and American Heart Association.

Niemann, J. T., & Stratton, S. J. (2000). Endotracheal versus intravenous epinephrine and atropine in out-of-hospital "primary" and postcountershock asystole. *Critical Care Medicine 28*, 1815–1819.

CHAPTER

63

Medication Administration: Enteral

Clinical Guidelines

- A healthcare prescriber orders medications.
- Medications are administered by a registered nurse (RN), licensed practical nurse (LPN), physician, or family member who is knowledgeable about the medication and techniques of administering enteral medications to a child.
- Principles of pharmacologic management (see Chapter 6) are followed.
- Medications are given by nasogastric (NG), gastrostomy, nasoduodenal, nasojejunal, or jejunostomy tube when the gastrointestinal (GI) tract is functional but the oral route is unavailable. The GI tract provides a vast absorptive area for medications. Absorption, distribution, metabolism, and elimination from the GI tract differ with maturation and some disease states. Factors such as gastric pH, gastric emptying time, motility, absorptive area, enzyme activity, and dietary factors affect GI absorption.
- For enteral administration, the medication must be in liquid form when passed through the enteral tube so as not to obstruct the tube.
- Administer enteral medications through oral or catheter-tipped syringes only. Use the largest syringe size that is practical—larger syringes generate less p.s.i. (pounds/square inch) than smaller syringes, thus reducing the potential of tube rupture. Do not use Luer-Lok–tipped syringes to avoid inadvertent intravenous or intramuscular administration of medication because needles cannot be attached to oral or catheter-tipped syringes.
- Medications are administered within 1 hour of prescribed time.

Equipment

- Prescribed medication
- Individual pill crusher or mortar and pestle, if needed for crushing pills
- Pill cutter, if needed to cut pills
- Medication cup
- Water or other appropriate diluents
- Syringes, oral, or catheter-tipped (appropriately sized for drawing up prescribed medication and flushes, 10–50 mL unless small volume of medication to be administered)
- Catheter-tip adapter (if catheter-tipped syringes are unavailable)
- Nonsterile gloves and goggles
- Disposable waterproof pad

CHILD AND FAMILY ASSESSMENT AND PREPARATION

- Refer to Chapters 38 and 39 for assessment and preparation for enteral tube use.
- Determine the child's height and weight. Accurate determination of weight ensures correct dosage of medications.
- Assess the child's and family's previous experience with enteral medications.
- Prepare the child, as appropriate to cognitive level, and parents before administration.
- Provide therapeutic play as indicated, or involve a child life specialist, to allow the child to work through his or her fears and master control of the situation (see Chapter 4).
- Explain the medication's actions and side effects and administration procedure.
- Teach parents how to administer medications to the child, if necessary, in preparation for discharge from the hospital.
- Assess for drug and latex allergies; if present, implement latex precautions (see Chapter 60) and notify healthcare prescriber of drug allergy. Label child's record and apply identification band indicating allergies.

PROCEDURE Administering Enteral Medications

Steps	Rationale/Points of Emphasis
1. Verify the order with the child's medical record, including calculation of appropriate dose. Check for allergy to drug; if present, do not administer drug and notify prescriber. Determine whether the prescribed drug should be given on full or empty stomach. Determine compatibility of drug–food–route interactions when giving medication through the enteral tube (Table 63-1).	Verifies correct drug, dose, route, time, and patient. Allergic reactions to medications may be life threatening. Provides best absorption of drug and avoids adverse outcomes such as congealing and possible tube obstruction.
2. Perform hand hygiene and gather necessary equipment and supplies.	Reduces transmission of microorganisms. Promotes efficient time management and provides an organized approach to the procedure.
3. Obtain medication and read the label to verify with the order. Check for expiration date; if expired, do not administer.	Route, dose, frequency, and time to be administered must be verified each time a medication is given. Expired medications may not give the intended effect. ***Alert!*** *Check institutional policy for automatic discontinuation of oral and enteral medications after surgery; check NPO status and postoperative orders to verify if the child is to continue to receive the medications.*
4. Prepare the medication for administration. Remove the cap from the medication container or open the unit dose package. If the medication is dispensed as a liquid, it is in a form ready for administration. Medications in pill or capsule form must be modified to liquid; follow steps 5 to 9 below.	Facilitates medication administration.
5. Score the tablet properly or pour the correct number of tablets into pill crusher or clean mortar.	To avoid contaminating the medication with previously crushed drugs, thoroughly wash and dry the individual pill crusher or mortar and pestle before and after each use.
6. Crush solid medications that are not sustained-release preparations into a fine powder with the pestle or pill crusher.	Medications in powdered form dissolve more thoroughly than those that are solid. ***Alert!*** *Check with the pharmacist or current drug manual before crushing tablets to ensure that it is not contraindicated. Enteric-coated or extended-release tablets are coated to release the medication appropriately over time in the gut; crushing destroys this protection and causes medication to be released all at once and may result in toxic levels of the drug.*

Continued

Steps	Rationale/Points of Emphasis
7. Pour the powder into a small medication cup.	The cup is used to aid in mixing the medication with the diluent.
8. Draw up 1 to 10 mL of warm diluent solution (e.g., formula, water) into a syringe and mix into medicine cup to dissolve the medication.	Provides diluent. Thoroughly dissolving the medication prevents pieces of medication from obstructing the gastric tube.

caREminder

When choosing amount of diluent, consider the child's clinical status (e.g., infants and children with some medical diagnoses are at higher risk for fluid overload), size of tube lumen, amount of medication that must be diluted, number of medications and flushes given daily, and 24-hour fluid intake. Consideration of these multiple factors when selecting amount of diluent may reduce the incidence of adverse events.

Steps	Rationale/Points of Emphasis
9. Draw up the medication from the cup into a syringe, and clear the syringe of excess air. Label syringe appropriately.	Instilling excess air into the stomach may cause flatus, cramping, and abdominal discomfort.
10. Draw up a small amount of diluent flush solution, 1 to 10 mL, depending on gastric or intestinal tube size, child's fluid status (e.g., potential for fluid overload), institutional policy, and manufacturer recommendation, into a separate syringe and label appropriately.	Provides flush solution so that the medication reaches the stomach.
11. Verify medication with electronic record or take the medication, the flush solution, and the medication record to the child to administer. Verify the child's identity by comparing name on medication (if verified electronically) or on medication record with child's identification band and any other patient identifier required by the institution. Also verify which tube port the medication is to be administered through (e.g., a feeding tube may have both a gastrostomy tube port and jejunostomy tube port).	Ensures proper identification of the child and proper administration site.
12. Don appropriate protective wear.	Standard precaution to reduce transmission of microorganisms.
13. Elevate the head of the bed 30 to 45° (unless elevation is contraindicated by the child's condition).	Aids in preventing aspiration and increases absorption.
14. Place a waterproof pad between the gastric tube and the child's bed and clothing.	Protects the linen and clothing from becoming damp or soiled.
15. Unclamp the gastric tube (if not in continuous use) and verify placement and patency of gastric tube (see Chapters 38 and 39).	Medications or other substances instilled down an improperly positioned tube could be aspirated.
16. Attach syringe to desired tube port and instill the diluted medication into the gastric tube by slowly and steadily pushing on the plunger.	Delivers medication.
17. Follow instilled administration of medication with 1 to 10 mL of diluent flush. Air may be used to flush if potential for fluid overload exists (e.g., small infants).	The diluent flushes the medication through the tube into the child's stomach and prevents the tube from becoming obstructed with medication.

caREminder

When multiple medications are administered at one time, it is desirable to flush with water or saline between medications to help reduce potential drug interactions. Calculate total fluid intake to avoid fluid overload. If air is used, it is especially important to verify compatibility of medications because air may not clear the line as completely as fluid.

Steps	Rationale/Points of Emphasis
18. Clamp the gastric tube for approximately 30 minutes after medication administration if the tube is not in continuous use.	Allows time for the medication to be absorbed.
19. Dispose of equipment and waste in appropriate receptacle.	Standard precautions.
20. Remove gloves and perform hand hygiene.	Reduces transmission of microorganisms.

TABLE 63-1

Incompatibility of Medications Administered Enterally

Type of Incompatibility	Characteristics	Known Incompatible Medications	Actions to Prevent Incompatibility
Pharmaceutical	Alteration of the form of dosing is contrary to the designed dosage form (i.e., crushing coated tablets).	• Enteric-coated tablets • Sublingual tablets • Sustained-release preparations • Extentabs	• Use an alternate dosage form. • Use an alternate route of administration. • Use a therapeutic equivalent. • Use an adjunct medication to treat adverse effect.
Physical changes	Noted visible changes when the drug is mixed with formula, water, or other diluent	• Water in oil preparations mixed with formula • Acidic syrups mixed with formula • Antacids, cimetidine, sulcrafate coagulate after mixing with liquid	• Do not mix medication with incompatible formula/diluent. • Check with pharmacist or current drug manual for food/drug incompatibilities. • Use alternate dosage form or alternate route.
Pharmacologic	Mechanism of action of drug alters GI tolerance or gastric motility.	• Narcotics • Anticholinergics • Antineoplastic agents	• Use a therapeutic equivalent. • Use an adjunct medication to treat adverse effect.
Physiologic	Diarrhea GI tract irritation	• High-osmolality medications (e.g., KCl elixir; elixirs with sorbitol, e.g., acetaminophen, theophylline) • Iron preparations • Aspirin	• Use an alternate dosage form. • Use an alternate route of administration. • Use a therapeutic equivalent. • Use an adjunct medication to treat adverse effect. • Dilute medication.
Pharmokinetic	Formula or diluent alters bioavailability, distribution, metabolism, or elimination of the medication.	• Dilantin • Digoxin • Morphine • Lasix	• Do not mix medication with incompatible formula/diluent. • Check with pharmacist or current drug manual for food/drug incompatibilities. • Use an alternate dosage form. • Use an alternate route of administration. • Use a therapeutic equivalent. • Alter feeding schedule to allow maximum amount of medication to be absorbed and re-adjust feeding rate (consult with registered dietitian).

CHILD AND FAMILY EVALUATION AND DOCUMENTATION

- Observe the child after medication administration for potential side effects or adverse events. Evaluate the child for change in vital signs, hemodynamic status, and other signs as appropriate after medication administration to assess the effects of the medication.
- Evaluate child's response to the procedure and comfort as needed.
- Evaluate child's and family's understanding of medication. Determine whether the child and family have additional areas of concern to discuss.
- Document the following:
  - Date and time administered
  - Type of medication
  - Dose
  - Route given (e.g., NG tube, gastrostomy tube, jejunostomy tube)
  - Presence or absence of adverse effects and notification of physician of such
  - Child's response to and tolerance of procedure
  - Teaching and information given to child and parents

COMMUNITY CARE

- If the child is to be sent home with an enteral tube in place, refer to Chapters 38 and 39 for discharge planning needs.
- When enteral medications are to be given in the home, teach the family the following:
  - Methods to prepare and administer enteral medications for administration and how to prevent complications such as aspiration or obstruction of the tube
  - Potential side effects and signs of adverse reaction
  - Storage of medication
  - Safe storage of supplies
  - Safe disposal or methods of cleaning for reuse of equipment
- When enteral medications are to be given in the home, ensure that the family has
  - Equipment to measure doses of liquid medications or crush tablets
  - Refrigeration (if needed to store medication)
  - Healthcare prescriber consent if child is to be given medication at school
- Identify problems that may prevent the family from obtaining the medications (e.g., inability to pay, lack of transportation in picking them up) and involve social services or support groups as necessary.
- Ensure that all medications have childproof caps and are kept beyond reach of children.
- Advise family members of guidelines such as whether they can still give medication if child vomits immediately after medication administration or if they forget to give a dose, to not give two doses together, and to call the healthcare prescriber or pharmacist if they have questions about dosing.
- Instruct the family to contact the healthcare provider if
  - Problems occur providing medication
  - Child has adverse reaction to medication
  - Condition for which medication is given is not controlled or eliminated

Unexpected Situation

- *When administering medication via the NG tube, the tube becomes clogged:* Remove the syringe with medication and attach a 60-mL syringe to the NG tube port. Aspirate gently and then apply light pressure to the plunger; repeat a few times. If this does not dislodge the medication and clear the tube, remove the NG tube. Replace NG tube, unless contraindicated (e.g., GI surgery). Attempt to identify why the tube clogged to avoid repeating the process and to avoid trauma to the child (e.g., If the medication was not in liquid form, was it crushed adequately? Was the medication incompatible with the diluent? Was the tube flushed adequately when previous medications were administered? Was there a food–medication interaction? Was there a drug–drug interaction?)

Bibliography

Crawley-Coha, T. (2004). A practical guide for the management of pediatric gastrostomy tubes based on 14 years of experience. *Journal of Wound, Ostomy, and Continence Nursing, 31*, 193–200.

Khair, J. (2003). Managing home enteral tube feedings for children. *British Journal of Community Nursing, 8*, 116–126.

Lee, A., Carter, H., & Crabbe, D. (2003). Percutaneous endoscopic gastrostomy: Procedure in practice. *British Journal of Perioperative Nursing, 13*, 298–289, 301–302, 305.

McConnell, E. A. (2002). Administering medications through a gastrostomy tube. *Nursing2002, 32*(12), 22.

C H A P T E R

64

Medication Administration: Intramuscular

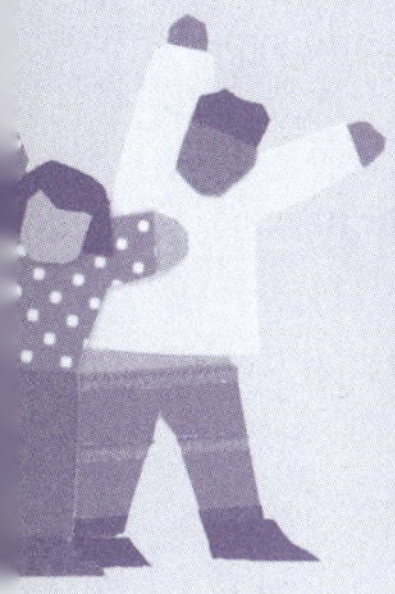

Clinical Guidelines

- A healthcare prescriber orders medications.
- Medications are administered by a registered nurse (RN), a licensed practical nurse (LPN), or physician who is knowledgeable about the medication and techniques of administering an intramuscular injection to a child.
- Principles of pharmacologic management (see Chapter 6) are followed.
- Medications are given intramuscularly (IM) for rapid drug absorption because muscle has a rich blood supply. The IM route is more painful than other routes because muscle has more nerves.
- Medications are administered through the least traumatic route when possible. Consider oral or intravenous access, when available, or alternative less painful routes over IM administration.
- Medications are administered within 1 hour of prescribed time.

Equipment

- Correct medication
- Syringe, appropriate size
- Needle, appropriate gauge and length (Table 64-1)
- Nonsterile gloves
- Alcohol swab
- Cotton ball or gauze
- Adhesive bandage
- Fun bandages (optional)
- Stickers (optional)

Child and Family Assessment and Preparation

- Assess the child's previous experience with receiving injections.
- Prepare the child, as appropriate to cognitive level, and parents for the injection before administration.
- Provide therapeutic play as indicated, or involve a child life specialist, to allow the child to work through any fears of injections and master control of the situation (see Chapter 4).
- Explain the medication's actions and side effects.

TABLE 64-1

Intramuscular Administration*

Site	Age	Needle Length (inches)	Volume (mL)	Insertion Angle (degrees)	Comments
Vastus lateralis	Infant	⅝	0.5	72–90	Recommended by AAP for infants younger than 7 months of age
	Toddler	⅝–1	0.5–1		Relatively free from major nerves and blood vessels
	Preschool-aged	1	1		Muscles easy to identify
	School-aged	1	1.5–2		Easy site to access and secure More painful than other sites
Ventrogluteal	Infant	⅝	0.5	72–90, directed toward iliac crest	Research suggests may be appropriate site for infants, recommended for infants older than 7 months of age
	Toddler	⅝–1	1		Free from major nerves and blood vessels
	Preschool-aged	1	1.5		Less subcutaneous tissue so that injection into muscle is more likely
	School-aged	1–1.5	1.5–2		
Deltoid	Infant, not recommended				
	Toddler, preschool-aged	⅝–1	0.5	72–90, pointed slightly toward acromium	Muscle mass limited Avoid irritating solutions and repeated injections in site
	School-aged	⅝–1	0.5–1		More rapid medication absorption than gluteal regions Radial nerve lies under the deltoid muscle.
Dorsogluteal	Infants, toddlers, preschool-aged, **not recommended**				Site not well developed. Should not be used in children younger than 5 years of age
	School-aged	½–1½	1.5–2	Perpendicular to the surface on which the child is lying	Can accommodate larger injectant volumes than other muscles Close to sciatic nerve and superior gluteal artery

*These are general recommendations. The nurse must evaluate the child's size, muscle mass, skin condition, age, and medication to be injected to determine site, needle length, volume of injectant, and adequate restraint of child before giving an injection.
AAP, American Academy of Pediatrics.

- Assess for allergies. If latex allergies are present, implement latex precautions (see Chapter 60). Notify healthcare prescriber of any drug allergy. Label child's record and apply identification band indicating allergies.
- Assess child's age, muscle mass, and other physical limitations that will impact choice of site for IM injection.
- Use a topical anesthetic (e.g., EMLA, LMX4, vapocoolant), when time allows, to reduce pain and trauma of injection (see Chapter 7).
- Assess the need for restraint and obtain additional help to support the child, as indicated.

KidKare Tell the child that his or her job is to stay as still as possible but that it is okay to yell or cry. Enlist the child's cooperation by having the child hold the bandage.

PROCEDURE **Administering Intramuscular Injections**

Steps	Rationale/Points of Emphasis
1. Verify the order with the medical record.	Detects possible transcription errors.

caREminder

Question whether another less traumatic route than IM injection is equally effective and can be used.

Steps	Rationale/Points of Emphasis
2. Perform hand hygiene.	Reduces transmission of microorganisms.
3. Obtain medication and read the label to verify with the order. Check for expiration date; if expired, do not administer.	To decrease chance of medication error, patient, route, dose, frequency, and time to be administered must be verified each time a medication is given.

caREminder

Bring medication to room temperature before administration. Cold medication causes increased discomfort when injected.

Steps	Rationale/Points of Emphasis
4a. Check the amount of medication to be administered to determine syringe size and appropriateness for the child. Limit volume according to the age of the child and the size of the muscle used (see Table 64-1).	Large volumes of medication injected into a small muscle can result in leakage of medication out of the muscle and muscle atrophy.
4b. Use a low-dose 1-mL syringe to give volumes of less than 0.5 mL.	Ensures dosage accuracy.
5. Choose appropriate needle length for the site and muscle size (see Table 64-1). Select gauge based on what is available for the appropriate needle length for the child and medication viscosity. Usually, a 22- or 23-gauge needle is appropriate, but viscous medication requires a larger bore/smaller gauge needle.	The needle must be long enough to enter the muscle mass. Minimizes injury to the tissue and leakage into the subcutaneous tissue. Larger gauge needles have a narrower bore and thus produce a jet under higher pressure, which causes more damage to the tissue.
6a. Draw up the medication in the medication room. Draw up correct amount of medication into the syringe.	The sight of the needle can increase the child's anxiety.
6b. If there is a large volume of medication, more than one injection may need to be given.	Medications must be measured accurately because a small error in amount could result in dangerous dosage variation.

Alert! *Do not draw up additional air into the syringe because clearing the needle of air can affect dose administered.*

caREminder

Use a filter needle to draw medication up from an ampule or rubber-topped vial and change to appropriate-sized needle before injection. This prevents small particles such as glass or other substances from entering the syringe.

Steps	Rationale/Points of Emphasis
7. Don gloves.	Standard precaution to reduce transmission of microorganisms.
8. Verify medication with electronic record or take medication record and syringe with medication to the child to administer. Verify the child's identity by comparing name on medication (if verified electronically) or on medication record with child's identification band and any other patient identifier required by the institution.	Ensures proper identification of the child.

Continued

Steps	Rationale/Points of Emphasis
9. Evaluate the child's muscle mass and choose the most appropriate site (Figure 64-1). If multiple injections are to be given, rotate injection sites.	Decreases risk for complications associated with giving IM injections, which may result from inappropriate site selection. Rotating sites reduces potential of tissue damage.

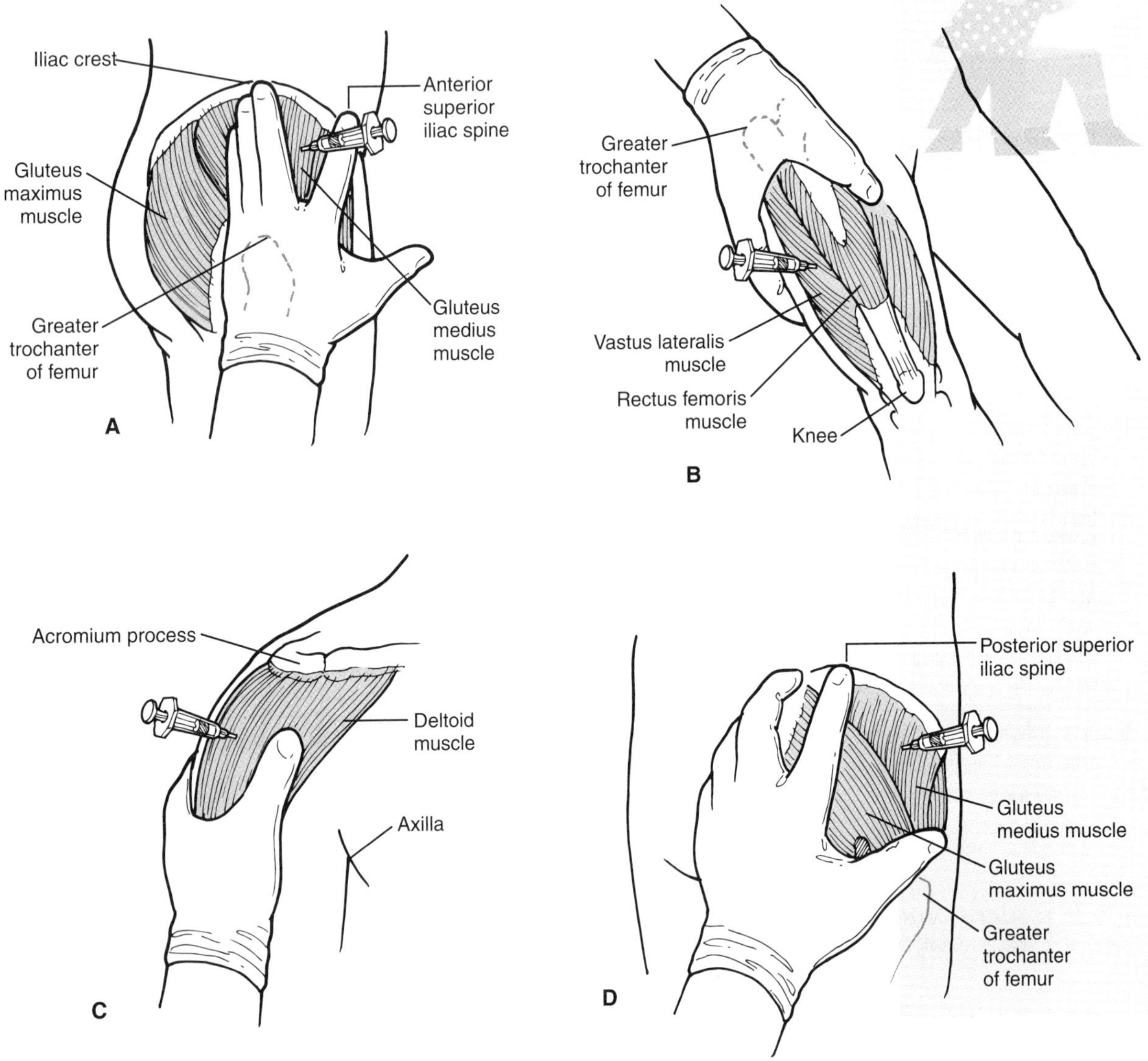

FIGURE 64-1
Steps for locating intramuscular injection sites in children. (**A**) Ventrogluteal. Place your index finger on the anterior superior iliac spine, middle finger on the superior iliac crest, and your palm on the greater trochanter (use your right hand for the child's left hip and vice versa). Inject into center of the "V" formed by the index and middle fingers. (**B**) Vastus lateralis. First, identify the middle third of the femur. Next, identify the area between two imaginary lines drawn from the greater trochanter to knee—one line midanteriorly and one midlaterally. Injection site is located between the lines in the middle third of the midlateral anterior thigh. Flexing the knee may promote relaxation of the muscle. (**C**) Deltoid. Identify site about two fingerbreadths below acromial process and just above axilla. Inject into upper third of deltoid muscle. (**D**) Dorsogluteal. Not recommended in children younger than 5 years of age or those with insufficient muscle mass. Place child on abdomen and have him or her point the toes inward. Draw an imaginary line between the posterior superior iliac spine and the greater trochanter. Inject in the upper outer region above this line into the gluteus medius muscle.

Steps	Rationale/Points of Emphasis
Alert! *Vastus lateralis is the preferred site for children younger than 7 months of age. For children older than 7 months, consider the ventrogluteal. Do not give in operative sites, wounds, or an extremity that has a pathologic process. The vastus lateralis is a relatively large muscle in infants, free from major blood vessels and nerves. The ventrogluteal muscle has a fairly consistent layer of adipose tissue (increasing deposition of medication into the muscle) and is free from nerves and major blood vessels. Avoiding areas of impaired tissue integrity avoids further tissue damage or potential spread of infection.*	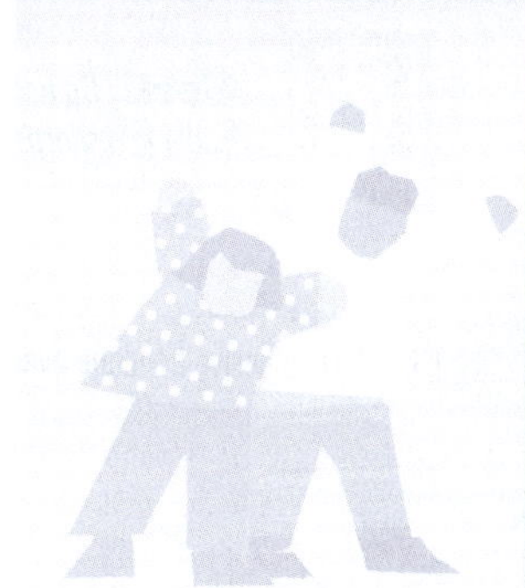 **KidKare** Give the child choices of the injection site, as appropriate (e.g., which leg or side), to help give the child some control of the situation. Evaluate the use of nonpharmacologic interventions: distraction (storytelling, blowing bubbles), cold therapy, manual pressure (apply with noninjection hand thumb for 10 seconds before injection), and other means that may help decrease perception of pain sensation (see Chapter 7).
10. Position and restrain the child securely.	Positioning may help relax the muscles, causing less pain (e.g., for ventrogluteal injection, place child on his or her side with upper leg flexed and over top of lower leg). Restraint decreases chance of injury from child's movement; even cooperative children have a tendency to move during injections. **caREminder** *Parents should not be responsible for securing the child but may remain to give support.*
11. Cleanse the site with alcohol wipe and allow to dry.	Decreases microorganisms and minimizes pain at the site of injection.
12a. Insert the needle quickly at a 72- to 90-degree angle. Aspirate to check for blood; if present, remove needle, replace with a sterile one, and start over. Slowly inject the medication. Withdraw the needle and apply pressure over the site with a dry cotton ball or gauze.	Facilitates needle entry into the muscle. Aspiration prevents intravenous or intraarterial administration. Slow injection may reduce local damage and pain. Alcohol over an injection site may sting and prolong bleeding. **caREminder** *For caustic medication, such as iron, use the Z-tract method, which helps prevent leakage of medication into subcutaneous tissue, decreasing pain and other complications.*
12b. To inject using the Z-track method: Use a new sterile needle. Pull the skin with your nondominant hand laterally or downward away about ½ inch (1.25 cm) from the injection site; insert the needle into the muscle at a 90-degree angle at the site where you initially placed your finger to displace the skin. Aspirate for blood return; if blood is aspirated discontinue the procedure; if no blood appears, inject the drug slowly. Wait 10 seconds, if possible, before withdrawing the needle; withdraw the needle slowly. Release the displaced skin and subcutaneous tissue to seal the needle track.	Using a new needle avoids medication being on the outside of the needle and coming in contact with tissue as the needle is inserted. Pulling the skin and subcutaneous layers displaces them out of alignment with the underlying muscle to trap the drug in the muscle after the structures return to their normal position. Aspiration prevents intravenous or intraarterial administration. Waiting before withdrawing the needle after injection helps ensure dispersion of the medication.

Continued

Steps	Rationale/Points of Emphasis
Alert! *Do not recap needle; dispose of syringe and needle in a sharps container to reduce chance of needle-stick injuries.*	
13. Place adhesive bandage over site.	Young children may feel that their insides will leak out the injection site if a bandage is not used. **KidKare** Use character or fun bandages to comfort the child.
14. Remove gloves and perform hand hygiene.	Reduces transmission of microorganisms.
15. Comfort the child and have the parent comfort the child after the injection.	Promotes positive relationship and decreases long-term negative effects of painful procedures. **KidKare** Giving the child a sticker or other reward can help promote comfort.
16. Return to the room a short time later for positive interaction with the child. Assess for signs of adverse reaction to medication.	Playing or other fun activities will help the child not associate the nurse with only painful procedures. Provides opportunity to further evaluate the child's physical and emotional response to the procedure.

Child and Family Evaluation and Documentation

- Healthcare provider must monitor child for 15 minutes after IM injection of drugs that may potentially cause a reaction for side effects or allergic reactions (e.g., respiratory distress). Evaluate the child for change in vital signs, hemodynamic status, and other signs as appropriate after medication administration to assess the effects of the medication.
- Evaluate child's response to the procedure and what comfort techniques were used.
- Evaluate child and family's understanding of medication. Determine whether the child and family have additional areas of concern to discuss.
- Document the following:
  - Date and time administered
  - Type of medication
  - Dose
  - Route and site given
  - Adverse effects, if any, and, if so, notification of physician
  - Child's response to and tolerance of procedure
  - Teaching and information given to child and parents

Community Care

- Provide parents instructions about expected response to IM medication administration (e.g., diphtheria, tetanus, pertussis [DTaP] may cause pain and swelling at the injection site) and self-management techniques (e.g., acetaminophen).
- If IM medications are to be given in the home, teach the family the following:
  - Sites for IM administration
  - Method to draw up medication
  - Technique to administer medication
  - Signs of adverse reaction
  - Storage of medication
  - Safe storage of supplies (including putting needles and syringes out of reach of small children)
  - Safe disposal of needles and syringes
- If IM medications are to be given in the home, ensure that family has
  - Name of medical supply vendor to obtain necessary equipment
  - Needle disposal container
  - Refrigeration (if needed to store medication)
  - Healthcare prescriber consent if child is also to be given medication at school

- Identify problems that may prevent the child from obtaining the medications (e.g., inability to pay for medications, lack of transportation to pick them up). Assist family to resolve identified problems or refer to social services (e.g., apply for public health insurance [Medicaid], identify vendors who deliver).
- Ensure that all medications have childproof caps and are kept beyond reach of children.
- Advise family members of guidelines regarding when they can still give medication if they forget to give a dose, to not give two doses together, and to call the physician or pharmacist if they have questions about dosing.
- Encourage selection of medications that can be given in the fewest number of doses per day to decrease potential of missed doses.
- Instruct the family to contact the healthcare provider if
  - Child develops rash over body
  - Child develops fever
  - IM site becomes hard, reddened, weeping, or tender to pressure/movement
  - Child has other reactions during therapy

Unexpected Situations

- *The child has a decreased amount of subcutaneous tissue:* Administer the IM injection utilizing a small-bore (25- to 27-gauge), short (no more than ½- to ⅝-inch) needle.
- *The child pulls away unexpectedly just as the needle touches the skin:* Even children who appear relaxed can lose control under stress of the procedure. Have someone available to help restrain the child if needed. Have an extra needle available so that delay is minimized, exchange new needle for the contaminated one, and complete the procedure as soon as possible.

Bibliography

Chung, J. W. Y., Ng, W. M. Y., & Wong, T. K. S. (2002). An experimental study on the use of manual pressure to reduce pain in intramuscular injections. *Journal of Clinical Nursing, 11*, 457–461.

Diggle, L., & Deeks, J. (2000). Effect of needle length on incidence of local reactions to routine immunisation in infants aged 4 months: Randomised controlled trial. *British Medical Journal, 321*, 931–933.

Gabhann, L. M. (1998). A comparison of two depot injection techniques. *Nursing Standard, 12*(37), 39–41.

Greenway, K. (2000). Using the ventrogluteal site for intramuscular injection. *Nursing Standard, 18*(25), 39–42.

Groswasser, J., Kahn, A., Bouche, B., et al. (1997). Needle length and injection technique for efficient intramuscular vaccine delivery in infants and children evaluated through an ultrasonographic determination of subcutaneous and muscle layer thickness. *Pediatrics, 100*, 400–403.

Hicks, J., Charboneau, J., Brakke, D., & Brakke, B. (1989). Optimum needle length for diphtheria-tetanus-pertussis inoculation of infants. *Pediatrics, 84*, 136–137.

Katsma, D., & Katsma, R. (2000). The myth of the 90°-angle intramuscular injection. *Nurse Educator, 25*(1), 34–37.

Mark, A., Carlsson, R.-M., & Granstrom, M. (1999). Subcutaneous versus intramuscular injection for booster DT vaccination of adolescents. *Vaccine, 17*, 2067–2072.

Nicoll, L. H., & Hesby, A. (2002). Intramuscular injection: An integrative research review and guideline for evidence-based practice. *Applied Nursing Research, 16*, 149–162.

Rodger, M. A., & King, L. (2000). Drawing up and administering intramuscular injections: A review of the literature. *Journal of Advanced Nursing, 31*, 574–582.

Sparks, L. (2001). Taking the "ouch" out of injections for children. *MCN. The American Journal of Maternal Child Nursing, 26*(2), 72–78.

CHAPTER

65

Medication Administration: Intraosseous

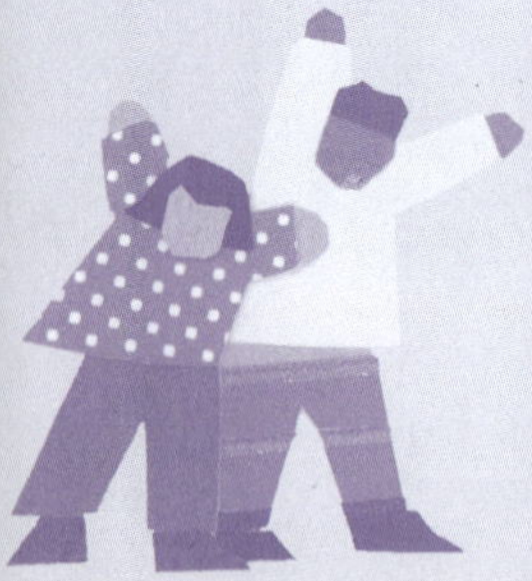

Clinical Guidelines

- A physician, registered nurse (RN), paramedic, or other healthcare professional trained in the insertion technique may perform intraosseous (IO) insertion. Who can perform IO insertion may vary according to local and state guidelines.
- A healthcare prescriber orders medications.
- Principles of pharmacologic management (see Chapter 6) are followed.
- Medication administration guidelines are followed, including correct patient, medication, dose, route, time, and approach to child.
- IO infusion is indicated for short-term fluid and drug therapy until intravenous (IV) access can be established.
- IO access should be initiated after three unsuccessful attempts or 90 seconds of IV access attempts in emergency situations. Vascular access may be accomplished through the IO route without first attempting IV access.
- IO access may be performed in children of any age. In newborns, IO access should be established if umbilical venous access cannot be established. Preferred site is the flat portion of the proximal tibia, about 1–3 cm below and slightly medially from the tibial tuberosity. After age 5 or 6 years, the bony cortex may be difficult to penetrate and alternate IO sites may be needed, such as the distal tibia, sternum, or other bones.
- The IO is discontinued as soon as a suitable vascular access route is established, or the child is able to tolerate oral intake.

Equipment

For needle insertion:

- IO needle
  - Children younger than 18 months old: 18- to 20-gauge needle (or a spinal needle may be used)
  - Older children: 13-, 15-, or 18-gauge needle
- Antiseptic solution (chlorhexidine or povidone-iodine)
- Lidocaine 1%, syringe, and 25-gauge needle
- Sterile gauze
- Nonsterile gloves
- Sterile normal saline (10 mL) for injection (preservative-free in neonates)
- Short T-infusion intravenous primer set

- Intravenous tubing and fluid
- Sandbag, folded towel, or IV bag to support the child's leg
- Gauze pads (4 × 4)
- Tape

For medication administration:

- Correct medication and fluids
- Syringe
- Alcohol pads or swabs
- Nonsterile gloves
- Normal saline (0.9% sodium chloride)

CHILD AND FAMILY ASSESSMENT AND PREPARATION

- Assess child's heart rate, respiratory rate, blood pressure, temperature, and neurovascular status of the extremity to obtain baseline values.
- Assess the child's medical history and site for the following contraindications to IO:
  - Presence of osteogenesis imperfecta, osteopetrosis, trauma, or fracture of the extremity (which may result in fluid infiltration into the subcutaneous tissue)
  - Presence of cellulitis, burns, or skin infections over the site (which increase the risk for infectious complications)
  - Previous attempts at IO insertion in the same bone
- Assess for drug and latex allergies; if present, implement latex precautions (see Chapter 60) and notify healthcare prescriber of drug allergy. After initial resuscitation, label child's record and apply identification band indicating allergies.
- Have a support person (e.g., social services, clergy, RN, psychologist) available for the family during resuscitation and stabilization of the child. If support person cannot provide explanations of medical care, a nurse or physician should explain procedure to family as soon as possible.
- If the child is aware, explain the procedure to the child as appropriate to the child's cognitive level.

caREminder

Explanations should be given in all situations but should not compromise resuscitation efforts; in an emergency situation, explanations can be given as the procedure is being performed. Children may hear even if unresponsive.

- Measure the leg circumference just below the knee to obtain baseline to evaluate potential infiltration.

PROCEDURE Insertion of Intraosseous Needle

Steps	Rationale/Points of Emphasis
1a. Gather the necessary supplies and equipment.	Promotes efficient time management and provides an organized approach to the procedure.
1b. Check needle package for instructions regarding recommended insertion technique.	Ensures proper insertion technique is used, because techniques may vary.
2. Perform hand hygiene, and don nonsterile gloves.	Reduces transmission of microorganisms.
3. Identify site for cannulation. Preferred site is the flat portion of the proximal tibia, about 1–3 cm below and slightly medially from the tibial tuberosity. If necessary, alternate sites such as the distal tibia, distal femur, or the sternum may be used.	The proximal tibia provides a stable access site that does not interfere with airway maintenance or chest compressions. This site also avoids major blood vessels, nerves, and muscles. The distal tibia and distal femur can also be used; in large adolescents, the sternum may be used.
4a. To insert in the proximal tibia, position the child supine with the leg externally rotated and the knee slightly bent and place a sandbag, rolled towel, or IV bag under the knee (or position the child as appropriate to site being accessed).	Stabilizes site.
4b. Support leg on firm surface. Have assistant hold child's lower leg to stabilize it; make sure the assistant is not holding the portion of the leg immediately behind the point of insertion.	Prevents needle-stick injury to assistant.
5. Cleanse site with antiseptic agent.	Reduces transmission of microorganisms.
6. If not an emergent situation, inject 1% lidocaine into skin down to periosteum.	Provides anesthesia.
7. Check IO needle to verify that bevels of the outer needle and inner stylet are aligned.	Ensures proper insertion.

Continued

Steps	Rationale/Points of Emphasis
	caREminder *Smaller needles have a greater tendency to bend on insertion, so the nurse needs to be extra careful.*
8. Grasp child's thigh and knee with nondominant hand.	Further stabilizes leg.
9a. Confirm site landmarks and insert the needle through the skin vertical to the long axis of the bone or 90 degrees to the tibia in a caudal direction.	Provides access to bone marrow. Directing the needle slightly toward the toes avoids the epiphysial plate.
9b. Apply firm downward pressure with a slight twisting motion until a decrease in resistance is felt (Figure 65-1).	Enables access to bony cortex. (Note: A pop may be felt as the needle penetrates the bony cortex.)

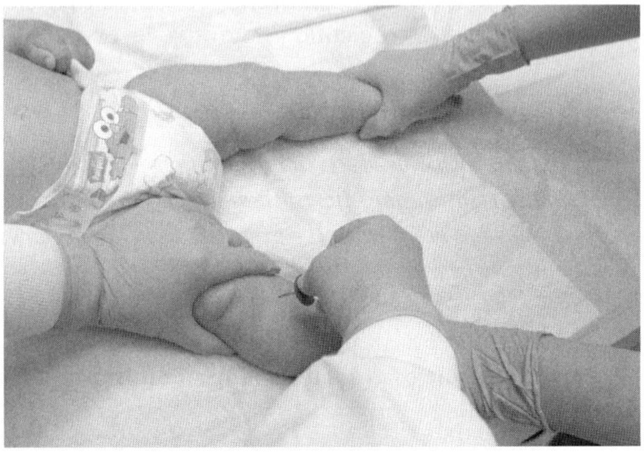

FIGURE 65-1
Placement of the intraosseous needle.

Steps	Rationale/Points of Emphasis
10. Remove the needle stylet, connect a syringe to the needle, and attempt to aspirate bone marrow. (Note: If able to aspirate bone marrow, inject into appropriate sample tubes so that samples can be used for laboratory studies.)	Confirms placement of needle in marrow; bone marrow may not be aspirated, even if properly placed. **caREminder** *The needle should stand securely without support. If the needle is loose or is able to move, suspect improper placement. Aspirating bone marrow into the needle is not always done, because it sometimes clogs the needle.*
11. Remove syringe and connect a new syringe with 10 mL of normal saline. Inject saline and monitor for the following signs of infiltration: • Increased resistance to injection • Increased circumference of the calf • Increased firmness of soft tissue of calf • Leaking of fluid around the site	Detects incorrectly positioned needle. If the needle is properly positioned, it should flush easily.
12. After needle placement is confirmed, remove syringe with saline and connect needle to intravenous infusion, as ordered.	Maintains needle patency.
13a. Anchor the needle by screwing the depth guard (if present) down until it is flush with the skin. Secure needle with tape, and place 4 × 4 gauze pads around needle base for support, if needed. For neonates, remove antiseptic solution with sterile water or saline.	Stabilizes needle and prevents dislodgment. Prevents further absorption of antiseptic solution and tissue damage.
13b. Loop and secure tubing with tape.	Avoids pulling tubing and placing tension on the needle.
14. Dispose of equipment and waste in appropriate receptacle.	Standard precautions.
15. Remove gloves and perform hand hygiene.	Reduces transmission of microorganisms.

PROCEDURE Medication Administration by the Intraosseous Route

Steps	Rationale/Points of Emphasis
1. Verify the medication order and medical record for drug allergy.	Detects possible transcription errors.
2a. Gather and assemble necessary equipment. 2b. Perform hand hygiene.	Promotes efficient time management and provides an organized approach to the procedure. Reduces transmission of microorganisms.
3. Obtain medication and read the label to verify that it is the same medication as prescribed in the order. Check for expiration date; if expired, do not administer.	Ensures that correct medication is being given. **caREminder** *Document verbal orders given during a code situation on the code blue/emergency/CPR record. This is a legal document and replaces the doctor's order form. All healthcare personnel involved in the emergency situation must sign the record.*
4. Verify patient, medication administration route, dose, frequency, and time to be administered.	Reduces risk of medication error.
5. Confirm that the needle is correctly placed in the bone marrow; see steps 10 and 11 under Insertion of Intraosseous Needle.	Prevents most common complications of subcutaneous and subperiosteal infusion.
6. Ensure that the needle is secured to the leg and the leg is immobilized. Immobilization can be done with pillows, sandbags, or leg restraints.	Minimizes risk of accidental dislocation of the needle.
7. Attach an IV short infusion set to the needle, if not already present.	IV tubing allows for easier administration of medication and fluids.
8a. Wipe injection port of IV tubing with alcohol swab and then administer medication as ordered. 8b. Follow medications with flush of 5 mL of normal saline.	Any medication or fluid required during resuscitation that can be administered by the IV route can safely be given by the IO route. Drug should be given in the equivalent dose as IV administration. Flushing ensures that medication reaches central circulation. **caREminder** *Strongly alkaline and hypertonic solutions must be diluted, because complications such as osteomyelitis are associated with these solutions.*
9. Monitor for the following signs of infiltration: • Increased resistance to infusion • Increased circumference of the calf • Increased firmness of soft tissue of calf • Leaking of fluid around the site	Detects infiltration promptly. **caREminder** *To overcome the resistance of the IO placement, administer all fluids and medication required for rapid administration or viscous medications under pressure using a syringe or pressure bag. IV pumps may not work because of their built-in pressure limits.*
10. After child has been stabilized, IV access should be achieved. Limit IO infusion to no longer than 8 to 12 hours.	IO access is for short-term use only. Limiting the time of access helps prevent complications, such as the following: • Iatrogenic fractures • Infiltration • Cellulitis • Osteomyelitis

Continued

Steps	Rationale/Points of Emphasis
	• Subcutaneous access • Compartment syndrome
11a. When ready to discontinue IO infusion, don gloves; remove the tape, dressing, and IO needle.	Discontinues IO infusion.
11b. Apply pressure to site with sterile gauze until bleeding has stopped (approximately 5 minutes).	Minimizes risk of bleeding from site.
12. Apply sterile dressing to the site.	Minimizes risk of infection.
13. Dispose of equipment and waste in appropriate receptacle.	Standard precautions.
14. Remove gloves and perform hand hygiene.	Reduces transmission of microorganisms.

CHILD AND FAMILY EVALUATION AND DOCUMENTATION

- Assess site for signs of bleeding, edema, pain or erythema, and infiltration of fluids (increasing calf circumference, discoloration, leakage of fluid, or a change in skin temperature); pay particular attention to the dependent area of the extremity where fluid will pool.
- Assess child's heart rate, respiratory rate, blood pressure, and temperature and neurovascular status of the extremity and compare to baseline values.
- Document the following:
  - Assessments of vital signs, neurovascular status, and appearance of site
  - Number and location of IO placement attempts, personnel who inserted
  - Location of IO infusion
  - Type of needle inserted
  - Time of insertion
  - Fluid type and amount; medication dose, concentration, route, and date and time infused
  - Presence or absence of adverse effects
  - Child's response to and tolerance of procedure

COMMUNITY CARE

- IO access is implemented under the direct supervision of healthcare personnel trained in the technique.
- Determine whether or not the child (if appropriate) and family have additional areas of concern to discuss.
- Instruct family to contact healthcare provider if
  - Child complains of pain at site of IO infusion
  - Child develops reddened hard area at site of IO infusion

Unexpected Situation

- *The IO needle was placed 1 hour ago and the child has been receiving fluid boluses. As you prepare to administer a medication, you notice that the area under the child's leg is wet:* Assess the IO needle for stability and movement, visualize needle insertion site for fluid leakage, and evaluate calf of that leg for increasing circumference or firmness. Assess perfusion distal to needle insertion site (e.g., pulses, capillary refill) to facilitate detection of circulatory compromise (fluid leakage into muscle may result in this). If these signs do not indicate needle malposition, use a saline flush to assess for increased resistance to infusion. If signs of needle malposition are present, attempt IV access again; fluid resuscitation may facilitate success at this time.

Bibliography

American Heart Association. (2005a). Part 6: Pediatric basic and advanced life support [Electronic version]. *Circulation, 112*(22 S), III-73–III-90. Retrieved August 21, 2006, from http://www.circulationaha.org

American Heart Association. (2005b). Part 12: Pediatric advanced life support [Electronic version]. *Circulation, 112*(22 S), IV-167–IV-187. Retrieved [month, day, year] from http://www.circulationaha.org

Atkins, D. L., Chameides, L., Fallat, M. E., et al. (2001). Resuscitation science of pediatrics. *Annals of Emergency Medicine, 37*(4 Suppl), S41–S48.

Bowley, D. M. G. (2003). Tibial fracture as a complication of intraosseous infusion during pediatric resuscitation. *Journal of Trauma: Injury, Infection, and Critical Care, 55*, 786–787.

Brown, B. W., & Altimier, L. (2003). Intraosseous infusion: A new option for neonates. *Neonatal Intensive Care, 16*(6), 44–46.

Hazinski, M. F., Zaritsky, A. L., Nadkarni, V. M., et al. (2002). *PALS provider manual.* Dallas, TX: American Heart Association.

LaRocco, B. G., & Wang, H. E. (2003). Intraosseous infusion. *Prehospital Emergency Care, 7*, 280–285.

CHAPTER

66

Medication Administration: Intravenous

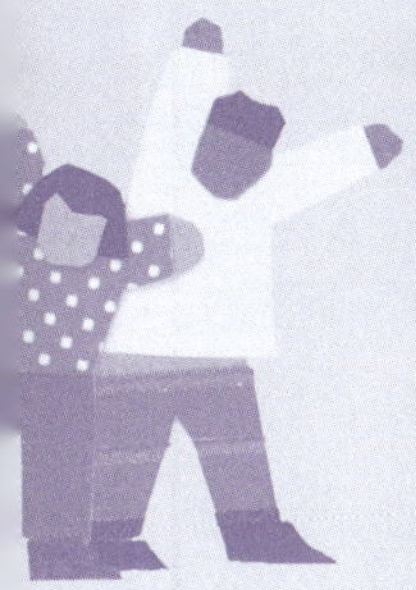

Clinical Guidelines

- A healthcare prescriber orders medications.
- Medications are administered by a registered nurse (RN) or physician who is knowledgeable about the medication and techniques of administering intravenous medications to a child, based on type of medication and scope of practice as defined by the Practice Act of each discipline.
- Principles of pharmacologic management (see Chapter 6) are followed.
- Medications are given by the intravenous (IV) route for rapid drug absorption when an IV line is in place. The IV route is less traumatic than other routes when an IV line is in place.
- Medications are administered within 1 hour of prescribed time.

Equipment

- Existing intravenous access (if not present, see Chapter 55)
- Correct medication
- Syringe, as needed
- Needleless access device
- Alcohol pad or swab
- Gloves
- IV tubing with volume-control chamber or piggyback setup
- IV pump or syringe pump
- IV tubing cap, as needed to maintain sterility of tubing

Child and Family Assessment and Preparation

- Assess child's height, weight, age, and hydration status, factors to consider when calculating medication dosage and fluid requirements.
- Assess child's previous experiences with receiving IV medications.
- Assess child's and parents' understanding of the need for the IV medications that will be administered.
- Prepare the child, as appropriate to cognitive level, and parents before medication administration. Explain the medication's actions and side effects.
- Utilize therapeutic play, as indicated, to allow the child to work through his or her fears and master control of the situation (see Chapter 4).

KidKare When the child has an established intravenous access, intravenous medication is less traumatic than subcutaneous or intramuscular injection. However, the use of the needle and syringe may create similar fears for the child; preparation of the child and parents and use of needleless systems may alleviate much of this.

- Assess for allergies. If latex allergies present, implement latex precautions (see Chapter 60). Notify healthcare prescriber of drug allergy. Label child's record and apply identification band indicating allergies.
- Assess existing vascular access for patency and signs of complications with line (e.g., redness, swelling, fluid leaking from site indicating phlebitis or infiltration). If line is not patent or signs of complications exist, establish vascular access before administering medication (see Chapter 55).

PROCEDURE Administering Intravenous Medications

Steps	Rationale/Points of Emphasis
1. Verify the medication order with the medical record.	Detects possible transcription errors.
2. Perform hand hygiene.	Reduces transmission of microorganisms.
3. Obtain medication and read the label to verify with the order. Check for expiration date; if expired, do not administer.	To decrease chance of medication error, check patient, route, dose, frequency, and time to be administered each time a medication is given.

caREminder

Bring medication to room temperature before administration. Cold medication increases discomfort of the infusion.

Steps	Rationale/Points of Emphasis
4. Prepare the medication in the medication room. Draw up correct amount of medication into the syringe; reconstitute powders as indicated.	The sight of the needle can increase the child's anxiety. Medications must be measured accurately because a small error in amount could result in dangerous dosage variation.

caREminder

Use a filter needle to draw medication up from an ampule or rubber-topped vial to prevent small particles of glass or other substances from entering the syringe. To reconstitute powdered medication, review manufacturer's recommendations or reference manual for type and amount of fluid to dilute with. Some medications must be diluted in specific solutions to avoid incompatibility or specific fluid amounts to obtain the correct dosage.

Steps	Rationale/Points of Emphasis
5. Determine the best method of IV administration for the medication and child. Whatever method is used, the medication must be completely infused within 1 hour unless otherwise specified.	The method of administration is determined by the volume to be infused, amount of time for infusion, infusion site, and size of the child (Table 66-1). Medications must be administered within 1 hour to maintain therapeutic drug levels and to ensure that the medication does not degrade before administration.

caREminder

The rate of infusion is determined by the medication; verify with reference source. This minimizes adverse effects associated with high serum drug levels.

Steps	Rationale/Points of Emphasis
6. Verify the medication with the electronic medication record or take the medication record and syringe with medication and any other IV equipment needed (e.g., IV pump) to the child to administer. Verify the child's identity by comparing name on medication (if verified electronically) or on medication record with child's identification band and any other patient identifier required by the institution.	Ensures proper identification of the child.
7. Explain to the child and family that you are going to administer the medication, as previously explained.	Keeps family members informed of therapy; may help reduce their anxiety.
8. Verify that IV access is patent and without complications (e.g., edema, redness, tenderness).	Ensures IV access without infiltration.
9. If the child has an intermittent lock:	
a. Cleanse the needleless injection cap with 70% alcohol.	Reduces transmission of organisms.
b. Insert the syringe with normal saline using appropriate needleless system adapter.	Accesses system.
c. Slowly infuse 1 mL of normal saline.	Flushes the tubing and verifies IV patency.
d. Connect medication; follow step 10, 11, 12, or 13 as appropriate for selected method.	Initiates medication infusion.
10. For medication administration through IV push:	
a. Cleanse the top of the needleless injection cap with 70% alcohol.	Reduces transmission of organisms.
b. Insert the syringe with medication, using appropriate needleless system adapter if required, into the port closest to the IV insertion site.	Using the port closest to the insertion site allows medication to be administered in the proper amount of time. Using a site high up on the IV tubing may result in the infusion taking place an hour or more later for a slowly infusing IV.
c. Inject the medication slowly over the time specified.	Injecting the medication slowly reduces pain and decreases adverse reactions.
11. For medication administration through a volume-control chamber (Figure 66-1):	
a. Fill the container using fluid from hanging IV bag, with amount of fluid required for dilution; calculate in the fluid volume of medication itself (e.g., if medication is to be diluted in 50 mL and was dispensed in 5 mL, add 45 mL of IV fluid to volume-control chamber).	Medication that is too concentrated may damage the vein and increase pain during infusion. Mixture of incompatible medications and IV solutions may result in a precipitate forming. When calculating dilution amounts, consider the child's 24-hour requirements, fluid status, hourly rate, number of other medications, and flushes required; use the minimum amount of fluid for dilution in children at risk for fluid volume overload. **caREminder** *Check reference source for minimum dilution amount and compatibility of the medication with diluents, IV solutions, and other medications to be administered. If medication is not compatible with infusing fluids, do not administer through this line and consider alternative method (e.g., small-volume IV-controlled infusion device).*
b. Cleanse the diaphragm used for medication administration located on the top of the chamber with 70% alcohol.	Reduces transmission of organisms.
c. Inject the medication into the chamber.	Makes medication available for infusion. **caREminder** *Label the chamber, to indicate that medication is infusing, with medication, dose, date, time, and initials of person hanging medication.*

Continued

Steps	Rationale/Points of Emphasis
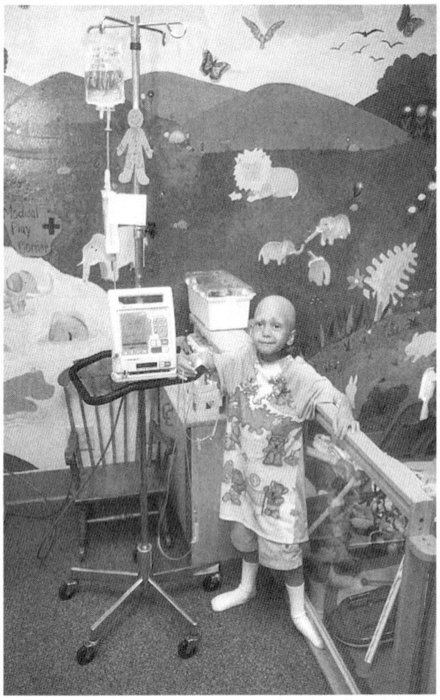 FIGURE 66-1 Proper labeling assists in identifying when medications have been placed in the IV volume control chamber.	
d. Set the infusion rate to infuse medication volume and flush over the desired time (antibiotics are usually given over 30 to 60 minutes) and start infusion.	Minimizes adverse effects associated with high serum drug levels if infused too rapidly.
12. For medication administration through a small-volume container:	
a. Cleanse the container diaphragm used for medication insertion with alcohol.	Reduces transmission of organisms.
b. Inject the medication into the bag/bottle or obtain premixed medication bag/bottle.	Ensures correct medication for infusion.
c. Connect administration tubing to small-volume bag/bottle (flush line with fluid if not already primed).	Allows means of medication administration.
d. Cleanse the port closest to the IV insertion site with 70% alcohol and connect medication administration tubing to main IV at Y connector closest to IV site.	Infusing into port closest to child allows quicker infusion into the child; prevents further dilution of the medication. **caREminder** *If infusing IV fluid is incompatible with medication to be infused, flush IV line from medication insertion point to child with compatible fluid before connecting medication to IV line to prevent incompatible medications and fluids from contacting each other.*
e. Set the infusion rate to infuse medication volume and flush over the desired time (antibiotics are typically given over 30 to 60 minutes) and start infusion.	Minimizes adverse effects associated with high serum drug levels if infused too rapidly. **caREminder** *To indicate medication is infusing, label the chamber with medication, dose, date, time, and initials of person hanging medication.*

Steps	Rationale/Points of Emphasis
13. For medication administration through a syringe pump (Figure 66-2):	
a. Obtain syringe of medication as dispensed from pharmacy or dilute medication (if necessary) in the appropriately sized syringe.	Children can develop fluid overload if too much fluid is used.
b. Prime infusion tubing, if needed, and attach infusion tubing to the syringe.	Removes air from tubing and provides means of infusion.
c. Attach the syringe to the IV-controlled infusion device.	Allows for small fluid volumes to be infused over a specified amount of time.
d. Cleanse the port closest to the IV insertion site with 70% alcohol and connect medication administration tubing to main IV at Y connector closest to IV site.	Reduces transmission of microorganisms. **caREminder** *If infusing IV fluid is incompatible with medication to be infused, flush IV line from medication insertion point to child with compatible fluid before connecting medication to IV line to prevent incompatible medications and fluids from contacting each other.*
e. Set the IV-controlled infusion device to infuse medication volume and flush over the correct time and start infusion.	Minimizes adverse effects associated with high serum drug levels if infused too rapidly.

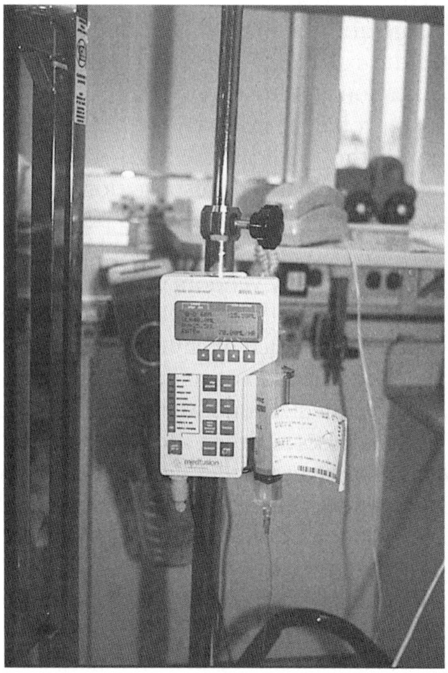

FIGURE 66-2
Infusion using a syringe pump.

Steps	Rationale/Points of Emphasis
14. Dispose of equipment and waste in appropriate receptacle. Perform hand hygiene.	Standard precautions. Reduces transmission of microorganisms.
15. Monitor the child initially and every 15 minutes during the infusion for adverse reactions such as respiratory distress, change in vital signs, hemodynamic status, and so on.	IV medication enters the vascular system rapidly. Monitoring provides early detection of adverse reactions. Onset of anaphylaxis or toxic side effects may occur at any time.
16. Flush medication from tubing at the completion of administration; flush amount is dependent on tubing volume. After infusion of medication and flush is complete, disconnect infusion tubing. Attach sterile tubing cap to end of infusion tubing.	Facilitates infusion of all medication into the child so none is left that could interact with other medications or solutions. Maintains sterility of tubing until next infusion of medication. Tubing used for intermittent infusions should be replaced when the main line tubing is changed or whenever the integrity of either line is compromised.

TABLE 66-1

Methods to Administer Intravenous Medications

Method	Indications for Use
IV push	Used with small volumes that are injected over a relatively short period of time, usually 1–5 min
Volume control chamber (Soluset, Buretrol, Volutrol)	Used when the medication can be diluted in the established IV fluids; volume for dilution is usually restricted to 150 mL or less
Small-volume container (IV bag/bottle containing small volumes)	Pharmacy may dispense in small-volume container if child can tolerate larger amounts of fluid; an option when the dilution fluid must be different from the established infusing IV fluids and a small-volume IV-controlled infusion device is unavailable
Syringe pump	Used to infuse medication over a specified period of time using smaller volume infusion tubing, which requires less fluid to get medication to child. May be used with intermittent IV locks or piggybacked into an existing IV

Child and Family Evaluation and Documentation

- Provide parents instructions on expected response to IV medication administration.
- Evaluate child's response to the procedure, monitoring for potential side effects or adverse reactions. Discontinue medication infusion immediately if infiltration occurs or child displays allergic reaction to medication, and notify healthcare prescriber.
- Evaluate child and family's understanding of medication. Determine whether the child and family have additional areas of concern to discuss.
- Document the following:
  - Type of medication
  - Dose
  - Route given
  - Date and time administered
  - Dilution and flush fluid amounts; include these amounts in the calculation of the child's 24-hour fluid intake
  - Appearance of access site
  - Child's response to and tolerance of procedure
  - Presence or absence of adverse effects and notification of healthcare prescriber of such
  - Teaching and information given to child and parent

Community Care

- When intravenous medications are to be given in the home, teach the family the following:
  - Assessment of intravenous access site
  - Method to draw up medication
  - Technique to administer medication
  - Signs of adverse reaction
  - Storage of medication
  - Safe storage of supplies (including putting needles and syringes out of reach of small children)
  - Safe disposal of needles and syringes
- When intravenous medications are to be given in the home, ensure that family has
  - Name of medical supply vendor to obtain necessary equipment
  - Needle disposal container
  - Refrigeration (if needed to store medication)
  - Healthcare prescriber consent if child is to be given medication at school
- Identify problems that may prevent the family from obtaining the medications (e.g., inability to pay for medications or lack of transportation to pick them up). Assist family to resolve identified problems or refer to social services (e.g., apply for public health insurance [Medicaid], identify vendors who deliver).
- Ensure that all medications have childproof caps and are kept beyond reach of children.
- Advise family members of guidelines regarding when they can still give medication if they forget to give a dose, to not give two doses together, and to call the healthcare prescriber or pharmacist if they have questions about dosing.
- Encourage selection of medications that can be given in the fewest number of doses per day to decrease potential of missed doses.
- Instruct the family to contact the healthcare provider if
  - Child develops rash or fever
  - Intravenous access site becomes hard and reddened
  - Unable to flush intravenous access
  - Swelling, redness, pain, or leaking of fluid occurs at intravenous access site during administration of fluids or medications
  - Child has other reactions during therapy

Unexpected Situation

- *Resistance is felt when the saline flush or medication is administered:* Stop the administration and assess the IV site for infiltration or phlebitis. Remove the IV catheter and insert an IV catheter at another site. Proceed with medication administration at the prescribed rate.

Bibliography

Centers for Disease Control and Prevention. (2002). Guidelines for the prevention of intravascular catheter-related infections. *MMWR. Morbidity and Mortality Weekly Report, 51*(No. RR-10), 1–34. Retrieved August 21, 2006, from http://www.cdc.gov/ncidod/hip/iv/iv.htm

Ford, N. A., Drott, H. R., & Cierplinski-Robertson, J. A. (2003). Administration of IV medications via soluset. *Pediatric Nursing, 29*, 283–286, 319.

Gardner, G., Gardner, A., Morley, G., & Watson, A. R. (2003). Managing intervenous medications in the non-hospital setting: An ethnographic investigation. *Journal of Infusion Nursing, 26*, 227–233.

Infusion Nurses Society. (2006). Infusion nursing: Standards of practice. *Journal of Infusion Nursing, 29*(1S), S1–S92.

McCullen, K. L., & Pieper, B. (2006). A retrospective chart review of risk factors for extravasation among neonates receiving peripheral intravascular fluids. *Journal of Wound, Ostomy, and Continence Nursing, 33*, 133–139.

Mirtallo, J. M. (2004). Complications associated with drug and nutrient interactions. *Journal of Infusion Nursing, 27*, 19–24.

Poole, S. M., Nowobilski-Vasilios, A., & Free, F. (1999). Intravenous push medications in the home. *Journal of Intravenous Nursing, 2*, 209–215.

Rothschild, J. M., Keohane, C. A., Cook, E. F., et al. (2005). A controlled trial of smart infusion pumps to improve medication safety in critically ill patients. *Critical Care Medicine, 33*, 533–540.

Taketomo, C. K., Hodding, J. H., & Kraus, D. M. (2004). *Pediatric dosage handbook* (11th ed.). Hudson, OH: Lexi-Comp Inc.

Vesely, T. M., Stranz, M., Masoorli, S., & Hadaway, L. C. (2002). The diverse and conflicting standards and practices in infusion therapy. *Journal of Vascular Access Devices, 7*(3), 9–25.

Wedekind, C. A., & Fidler, B. D. (2001). Compatibility of commonly used intravenous infusions in a pediatric intensive care unit. *Critical Care Nurse, 21*(4), 45–51.

Zenk, K. E., Stills, J. H., & Koeppel, R. M. (2003). *Neonatal medications and nutrition, a comprehensive guide* (3rd ed.). Santa Rosa, CA: NICU Ink Book Publishers.

CHAPTER

67

Medication Administration: Intravenous Cardiovascular

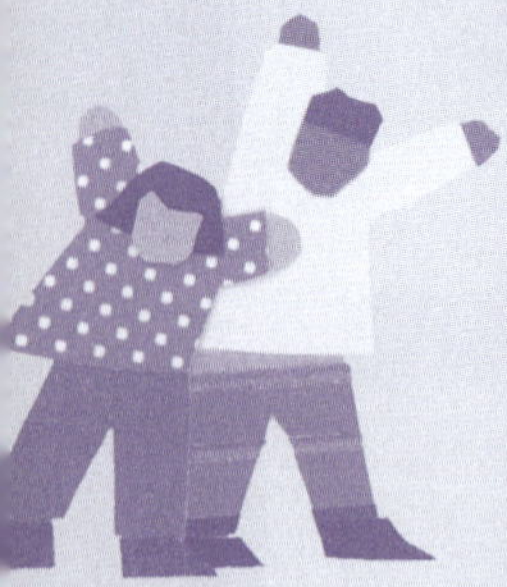

Clinical Guidelines

- A healthcare prescriber orders medications and parameters for titration.
- Medications are administered by a registered nurse (RN) or healthcare prescriber that is knowledgeable about the medication and techniques of administering intravenous cardiovascular medications to a child.
- The RN managing the care of the critically ill child receiving intravenous cardiovascular medications exhibits the following competencies:
  - Education and training in pediatric critical care nursing, including developmental anatomy and physiology, pathophysiology, advanced clinical assessment, and principles of hemodynamic monitoring
  - Comprehensive knowledge regarding the administration, dosing, and monitoring of pharmacologic agents to children, including drug-specific information related to
    - Drug actions and indications for use
    - Pharmacodynamics (onset and duration of action)
    - Pharmacokinetics (absorption, distribution, metabolism, excretion, and half-life)
    - Appropriate dosage and dosage range for age, size, and condition of child
    - Precautions
    - Adverse reactions
    - Side effects
    - Interactions
    - Certification in Pediatric Advanced Life Support (PALS) through the American Heart Association

caREminder

Emergency drugs and equipment appropriate for pediatric resuscitation must be available for immediate use in the event of adverse drug reactions, potential complications, or emergency situations that require advanced life support. Protocols for emergency resuscitation and management are in accordance with those in published references, such as PALS and Advanced Pediatric Life Support (APLS) textbooks.

- Principles of pharmacologic management (see Chapter 6) are followed.
- Intravenous cardiovascular medications are administered to acutely ill children to achieve and maintain hemodynamic stability. Hemodynamic regulation is achieved through pharmaco-

logic intervention aimed at optimizing heart rate and rhythm, blood pressure, tissue perfusion, and measures of preload, afterload, and contractility.

- All continuously infused cardiovascular medications are infused through a volumetric IV-controlled infusion device.
- The child receiving intravenous cardiovascular medications, either by intravenous push (IVP) injection or by continuous infusion administration, must be continuously monitored in a critical care setting. Monitoring of vital signs and hemodynamic responses to cardiovascular pharmacologic therapy requires facilities, equipment, and resources to perform the following procedures before and during drug administration:
  - Continuous electrocardiogram (ECG) monitoring of heart rate and rhythm
  - Continuous oxygen saturation (SaO_2) monitoring by pulse oximetry
  - Continuous intraarterial blood pressure (ABP) monitoring when indicated
  - Continuous central venous pressure (CVP) or right atrial pressure (RAP) monitoring when indicated
  - Continuous pulmonary artery pressure (PAP), pulmonary artery wedge pressure (PAWP), or left atrial pressure (LAP) monitoring when indicated
  - Monitoring of hemodynamic parameters, such as cardiac output (CO) and cardiac index (CI), systemic vascular resistance (SVR), and pulmonary vascular resistance (PVR), when indicated
  - Intermittent monitoring of temperature

EQUIPMENT

- Central venous line access
- Volumetric IV-controlled infusion device that provides consistent continuous flow rate
- Cardiovascular and hemodynamic monitoring equipment as indicated
- APLS drugs and equipment
- Pharmaceutical manufacturer's drug-specific information
- Related institutional guidelines and procedures

CHILD AND FAMILY ASSESSMENT AND PREPARATION

- Establish a baseline assessment of the child; include health history, age, height, weight, review of systems, physical examination, and baseline laboratory values.
- Observe child for signs and symptoms of gradual or acute hypotension or hypertension, dysrhythmias, circulatory collapse, cardiac arrest, hemorrhage, hypoxemia, metabolic acidosis or alkalosis, fluid imbalance, diminished mental status, or laboratory abnormalities.
- Assess child's and parents' understanding of need for the IV medications that will be administered.
- Prepare the child, as appropriate to cognitive level, and parents before medication administration. Explain the medication's actions and side effects.
- Utilize therapeutic play, as indicated, to allow the child to work through his or her fears and master control of the situation (see Chapter 4).
- Assess for drug and latex allergies; if present, implement latex precautions (see Chapter 60) and notify healthcare prescriber of drug allergy. Label child's record and apply identification band indicating allergies.
- Assess existing vascular access for patency and signs of complications with line (e.g., redness, swelling, fluid leaking from site indicating phlebitis or infiltration). If line is not patent or signs of complications exist, ensure a new vascular access is established by the healthcare prescriber prior to administering medication.

PROCEDURE **Preparation, Administration, and Titration of Intravenous Cardiovascular Medications**

Steps	Rationale/Points of Emphasis
1. Record the child's weight in kilograms (kg) in an easily accessible location on the medical record before administration of cardiovascular medications and daily thereafter.	Most cardiovascular drug dosages are administered in milligrams per kilogram per minute (mg/kg/min) or micrograms per kilogram per hour (μg/kg/hr). Quick access to body weight (kg) reduces delay in dosage calculation. **caREminder** *In collaboration with the healthcare prescriber/pharmacist, dosages should be recalculated daily to reflect changes in body weight. Rapid fluctuations in weight can occur in critically ill children as a result of alterations in fluid status.*

Continued

Steps	Rationale/Points of Emphasis
2. Perform hand hygiene.	Reduces transmission of microorganisms.
3. Ensure central venous line access.	Central venous access ensures drug delivery and bioavailability to the systemic circulation.
3a. Administer infusions of cardiovascular drugs that support heart rate, blood pressure, or cardiac output through a central vein.	Central venous administration provides rapid steady drug delivery.
3b. Infusions of vasoconstricting drugs should only be administered through a central vein.	Potent vasoconstricting effects of these drugs can cause tissue ischemia and necrosis if interstitial infusion (infiltration) occurs; central line administration reduces this risk.
3c. Administer highly acidic or alkaline drugs through a central vein.	Extreme deviations in drug pH are not adequately diluted in a peripheral vein and could produce vessel erosion; central line administration reduces this risk.
4. Obtain a volumetric IV-controlled infusion device or utilize "smart pumps" with built-in software to monitor medication administration.	A volumetric IV-controlled infusion device is used to ensure safe accurate delivery and titration of cardioactive or vasoactive medications. "Smart pump" software technology can reduce medication errors by creating safety guardrails for medication administration; however, the devices do not calculate the amount of medication that should be given per weight to each child. This calculation must be completed by the nurse and verified by another nurse or healthcare prescriber. **Alert!** ***The pump must provide a constant continuous flow rate, not intermittent boluses of fluid.***
5. Verify infusion orders. Orders must include a. Concentration—amount of drug per volume of solution b. Type of IV solution that the drug is to be added to c. Dosage to be delivered, calculated in • Units of delivery (e.g., µg/kg/min) and • Corresponding infusion rate in milliliters per hour (mL/hr)	Orders for drug dosages, concentration, and IV solutions or admixtures are verified for accuracy and correct dosing, preparation, and administration instructions. Consult with the clinical pharmacist when necessary with questions regarding individual considerations and drug preparation or administration to ensure safe delivery.
6. Verify orders for titration.	Orders for titration are based on desired effect or therapeutic end point. Orders should specify the goal of therapy and clinical parameters for drug titration (e.g., to keep blood pressure greater than 90 mm Hg).
6a. Orders must include starting dosage to be delivered, calculated in • Units of delivery (e.g., µg/kg/min) and • Corresponding infusion rate in mL/hr	Dosages are titrated within a prescribed dosage range that includes starting dosage and maximum dosage. Generally, the drug is started at the lowest dose and is then titrated upward to achieve the desired effect.
6b. Orders must include maximum dosage drug can be titrated up to, calculated in • Units of delivery (e.g., µg/kg/min) and • Corresponding infusion rate in mL/hr	Orders must clearly specify the clinical parameters for dose titration. Parameters may include heart rate, rhythm, blood pressure, indicators of tissue perfusion, and measures of preload, afterload, and contractility.
7. Calculate dosage (see Chapter 6 for calculation procedures):	
a. For IVP administration, determine duration of administration (e.g., IVP over 3–5 minutes). Refer to pharmaceutical manufacturer's instructions and institutional protocols for appropriate administration time.	Central venous IVP injection times must be strictly followed to prevent untoward reactions.
b. For continuous infusion administration, determine number of mL/hr to deliver desired dose. Preestablished infusion rate tables can be consulted and placed at the bedside for easy reference when titrating dosages.	Reference to preestablished infusion rate tables (available from pharmaceutical manufacturers, pharmacology textbooks, and as software programs) for individual drugs reduces delay in initial dose/rate calculation and in recalculation of rates when titrating dosages.

Steps	Rationale/Points of Emphasis
8. Before administration, verify a. Compatibility with other drugs or IV solutions. b. Time requirement for solution change (e.g., every 24 hours). c. Requirements for protection from heat or light. d. Integrity of IV solution (check expiration date; inspect for turbidity, discoloration, or particulate matter). Expired or potentially contaminated solutions must be discarded and reported to pharmacy. e. Other specific requirements for administration or drug monitoring. **caREminder** *Refer to pharmaceutical manufacturer's instructions, institutional standards and protocols, and compatibility charts for specific preparation and administration requirements.*	Admixture specifications and compatibility requirements must be strictly followed for safe preparation and administration. Many medications become less stable after 24 hours. Some medications must be protected from heat or light to prevent degradation.
9. Verify all dosage calculations with another nurse or pharmacist before the initiation of therapy or drug titration.	Cochecking reduces the risk for dosage errors.
10. Label bottle/bag clearly with drug name. Include date/time hung, and specify date/time to be changed.	Clear labeling reduces the risk of errors. Changing solutions when specified maintains drug effectiveness and reduces the potential for bacterial growth.
11. Flag tubing with name of drug.	Tubings can become intertwined when multiple IV lines are in place. Clear labeling of each tubing reduces the risk for infusion errors.
12. Ensure that all central line connections are securely connected with locking devices (e.g., Luer-Lok connectors).	Secure connection of all central line tubing ensures drug delivery to the intended location and reduces the risk for air embolization, hemorrhage, and bacterial contamination. **caREminder** *Routinely check all IV lines for secure connections throughout the course of therapy.*
13. Use only central venous ports intended for drug administration. Appropriate sites include the introducer line or other central venous ports labeled for infusion access. Intracardiac catheters with PAP or LAP ports are intended for hemodynamic monitoring only and are not to be used for drug administration.	Hemodynamic monitoring cannot be interrupted. An inadvertent bolus injection of medication could be administered if a monitoring line is flushed. Most intracardiac catheters for hemodynamic monitoring have central venous infusion port access specifically intended for IV solution or medication administration. Refer to manufacturer's instructions for medication port access specifications.
14. Verify the medication with the electronic medication record or take the medication record and syringe with bottle/bag of medication and any other IV equipment needed to the child to administer. Verify the child's identity by comparing name on medication (if verified electronically) or on medication record with child's identification band and any other patient identifier required by the institution.	Ensures proper identification of the child utilizing two different patient identifiers (see Chapter 85).
15. Administer medication at ordered dosage/rate. Closely monitor child for expected response, adverse effects, or untoward reactions (refer to Assessment and Monitoring of the Child Receiving Intravenous Cardiovascular Medications). Notify the healthcare prescriber when unexpected responses occur.	Knowledge of expected responses and adverse effects is essential to evaluate the drug's effectiveness and provide safe care.

Continued

Steps	Rationale/Points of Emphasis
16. Titrate dosage per order to achieve desired therapeutic response. Closely monitor child for responses to dosage change with titration (refer to Assessment and Monitoring of the Child Receiving Intravenous Cardiovascular Medications). Notify the healthcare prescriber if the desired therapeutic response does not occur within the ordered titration dosage range.	Titration requires frequent close monitoring of clinical parameters to evaluate drug effectiveness and achieve the desired goals of therapy.
17. Continuously monitor the child's clinical status throughout the course of therapy (refer to Assessment and Monitoring of the Child Receiving Intravenous Cardiovascular Medications).	Clinical changes in the child may require dosage readjustment or weaning during the course of therapy. Discontinuation of a drug may be necessary if unexpected or adverse reactions occur or when a therapeutic response is not achieved.

PROCEDURE Assessment and Monitoring of the Child Receiving Intravenous Cardiovascular Medications

Steps	Rationale/Points of Emphasis
1. Review baseline assessment of the child.	Knowledge of baseline assessment aids in evaluating the child's response to therapy.
2. Evaluate the child's response to therapy. Consider drug pharmacodynamics, pharmacokinetics, therapeutic goals, and potential adverse effects.	Dosage titration is based on the child's clinical response to therapy. Individual responses may require dosage adjustments to achieve therapeutic goals or if adverse reactions occur.
3. Continuously monitor heart rate and rhythm: • Select best electrocardiogram (ECG) lead for continuous monitoring. • Document rate, rhythm, PR interval, QRS width, and QT interval; compare with baseline ECG and expected response to medication. • Obtain 12-lead ECG as indicated. • Ensure availability of PALS drugs and equipment. **caREminder** *A pediatric crash cart must be immediately available.* • Set monitor alarms as appropriate and ensure that they are on at all times. • Notify healthcare prescriber of significant changes.	Continuous cardiac monitoring is required during the administration of cardioactive or vasoactive medications to detect dysrhythmias and evaluate response to therapy. Many cardiovascular drugs can precipitate dysrhythmias, which may require discontinuation of the drug or additional therapies to treat the dysrhythmias. Alarms must be kept on at all times to ensure prompt response to changes in child's status.
4. Monitor systolic, diastolic, and mean arterial blood pressure at frequent regular intervals throughout the course of therapy: • Compare with expected values for age and with the child's baseline. Note widening or narrowing of the pulse pressure. • Monitor blood pressure every 1 to 5 minutes during titration of vasoactive drugs and during IVP administration of antiarrhythmic agents. • Every 8 hours, use cuff blood pressures to validate findings from arterial line pressures. • Notify healthcare prescriber of significant deviations or unexpected changes.	Frequent regular blood pressure monitoring is required with the administration of vasodilators, vasopressors, and antidysrhythmics. Intraarterial blood pressure monitoring is preferred when titrating vasopressors or vasodilators to monitor minute-to-minute changes in response to dosage adjustments.
5. Monitor hemodynamic parameters (CVP, PAP, PAWP, CO/CI, SVR/PVR) as indicated. Notify healthcare prescriber of significant deviations or unexpected changes.	Hemodynamic values are used to make clinical decisions in drug selection, dosing, and titration. Values and trends assist in clinical decision-making aimed at optimizing hemodynamic status.

Steps	Rationale/Points of Emphasis
6. Monitor signs of tissue perfusion, including capillary refill, peripheral pulses, temperature, and color of extremities. Notify the healthcare prescriber of signs of poor tissue perfusion or failure to respond to agents intended to improve cardiac output and tissue perfusion.	Decreased tissue perfusion may occur as a result of hypotension, dysrhythmias, volume depletion, poor myocardial contractility, or high doses of vasopressors. Early detection of signs of altered tissue perfusion is essential to maintaining hemodynamic stability. High doses of vasopressors can compromise tissue perfusion due to the ischemic effects of vasoconstriction.
7. Monitor input and output, urine output (UOP), and daily weight:	
a. Closely regulate fluids; use a volumetric IV-controlled infusion device for all infused fluids.	Fluids must be closely regulated to avoid dehydration or overhydration.
b. Measure urine output hourly (normal UOP is 1 to 2 mL/kg/hr). Compare with expected response to drug.	Urine output is an indicator of renal perfusion and fluid volume status.
c. Weigh child daily.	Weight fluctuations and changes in total body water can rapidly occur in acutely ill children. Individual dosing parameters in children require frequent reassessment of weight and amount of total body water. **caREminder** *Recalculate dosages daily or per institutional policy to reflect changes in body weight.*
d. Assess for signs of volume depletion (i.e., decreased UOP, specific gravity > 1.025, poor skin turgor, hypotension, tachycardia, depressed fontanels, dry mucous membranes, decreased CVP, decreased PAP or PAWP).	Failure of blood pressure to respond to vasopressors may indicate intravascular volume depletion and the need for additional IV fluids. Volume expanders or an increase in IV rate may be ordered.
e. Assess for signs of fluid overload (i.e., fluid intake greater than output, weight gain, pulmonary congestion, dependent edema, bulging fontanels, increased CVP, increased PAP or PAWP).	Diuretics may be ordered to correct fluid overload states. Signs of hypovolemia or hypervolemia require change in therapy to achieve euvolemic status.
f. Notify healthcare prescriber when urine output is abnormal and for signs and symptoms of dehydration or overhydration.	
8. Monitor respiratory status at frequent regular intervals: • Evaluate oxygen saturation and arterial blood gases for hypoxemia or hypercapnia. • Assess for signs of hypoxemia (i.e., restlessness, confusion, tachypnea, decreased or adventitious breath sounds, peripheral or circumoral cyanosis, sternal retraction, nasal flaring). • Notify healthcare prescriber of changes in respiratory status, oxygenation, and acid-base balance.	Adequate oxygenation and maintenance of acid-base balance are critical to achieving hemodynamic stability. Nursing and medical interventions are aimed at correcting O_2 deficiencies and acid-base imbalances.
9. Monitor electrolyte values, especially sodium, potassium, calcium, and magnesium. Notify healthcare prescriber of abnormalities.	Abnormal electrolyte values increase the risk for dysrhythmias and may decrease myocardial contractility. Nursing and medical interventions are aimed at normalizing electrolyte values.
10. Monitor renal function, including blood urea nitrogen (BUN), creatinine, and creatinine clearance, when indicated. Notify healthcare prescriber of abnormalities.	Drug dosage adjustments may be required when renal function is impaired, especially with drugs that are metabolized by the kidneys. Nursing and medical interventions are aimed at optimizing renal perfusion.
11. Monitor hepatic function, including aspartate aminotransferase (AST), alanine aminotransferase (ALT), gamma-glutamyl transpeptidase (GGT), and lactate dehydrogenase (LDH). Notify healthcare prescriber of abnormalities.	Drug dosage adjustments may be required when hepatic function is impaired, especially with drugs that are metabolized by the liver.
12. Reduce myocardial oxygen consumption (e.g., minimize environmental stressors, reduce anxiety, control pain, control fever).	Factors that increase myocardial oxygen consumption impair myocardial performance and affect hemodynamic stability.
13. Monitor serum drug levels (e.g., digoxin, lidocaine, procainamide) when indicated. Notify healthcare prescriber of subtherapeutic or potentially toxic levels.	Serum drug levels should be within the specified therapeutic range for age and size of child.

Continued

Steps	Rationale/Points of Emphasis
14. Assess the central line access site at frequent regular intervals for complications (e.g., signs/symptoms of infection, phlebitis, infiltration, or catheter-related complications). Notify the healthcare prescriber of abnormal findings.	Astute monitoring allows for early detection and treatment of complications.
15. Follow institutional guidelines and procedures for catheter insertion, site care, and dressing change regimens.	Strict adherence to aseptic technique and infection control measures reduces the risk for intravascular catheter-related infections.

CHILD AND FAMILY EVALUATION AND DOCUMENTATION

- Evaluate child's response to the medication(s) for potential side effects or adverse reactions.
- Evaluate the child's and family's understanding of medication and therapy. Determine whether the child or family have additional areas of concern to discuss.
- Document the following:
  - Medication name
  - Route given
  - Drug concentration and intravenous (IV) solution or diluent
  - Dosage
  - Date and time of administration, dosage delivery time if IVP, and corresponding infusion rate in milliliters per hour if continuous infusion or titration
  - Clinical parameters for titration
  - Appearance of central venous access site
  - Child's response to therapy
  - Presence or absence of adverse effects and notification of healthcare prescriber of such
  - Teaching and information given to child and parent

COMMUNITY CARE

- Encourage family members' involvement in child's care while they are still in the hospital so they are better prepared to assume child's care at home.
- Teach family about medications child will likely be taking at home, including dosage, administration procedures, expected responses, potential side effects, and guidelines for missed doses.
- Inform family of expected healing of the central venous access site.
- Initiate appropriate referrals for follow-up care, if needed.
- Instruct the family to contact the healthcare provider if
  - IV insertion site is red, inflamed, or draining.
  - Child has unexpected reactions during therapy.
  - Questions occur regarding dosage, administration, missed dose guidelines, or other concerns.

Unexpected Situation

- *During assessment of the child on intravenous cardiovascular medications, you note a sudden drop in the child's arterial blood pressure:* Complete a rapid assessment of child to determine whether other critical parameters (i.e., heart rate and respirations, skin color, perfusion) have changed. If indicated, initiate CPR. Troubleshoot the arterial blood pressure monitoring system and the intravenous infusion system to ensure equipment is functioning properly, intravenous lines are intact, and medication delivery has been continuing in an uninterrupted fashion. If the systems are intact and infusing properly and the child's blood pressure continues to decrease, titrate the cardiovascular medication per healthcare prescriber's order to maintain the child's blood pressure within acceptable parameters.

Bibliography

American Heart Association. (2000). Guidelines 2000 for cardiopulmonary resuscitation and emergency cardiovascular care. *CURRENTS, 11*(3), 3–27.

Brown, K. & Bocock, J. (2002). Update in pediatric resuscitation. *Emergency Medicine Clinics of North America, 20*(1), 1–20.

Centers for Disease Control and Prevention. (2002). Guidelines for the prevention of intravascular catheter-related infections. *MMWR. Morbidity and Mortality Weekly Report, 51*, (No. RR-10), 1–34. Retrieved August 21, 2006, from http://www.cdc.gov/ncidod/hip/iv/htm

Hazinski, M. F., Zaritsky, A. L., Nadkarni, V. M., et al. (2002). *PALS provider manual.* Dallas, TX: American Heart Association.

Juarez, P. (2005). Safe administration of IV infusions: Part 1. Vasopressors: Pressors in the ICU—the do's and the don'ts. *American Journal of Nursing, 105*(9), 72AA–72FF.

Miller-Hoover, S. R. (2003). Pediatric and neonatal cardiovascular pharmacology. *Pediatric Nursing, 29*(2), 105–114.

Potts, A. L., Barr, F. E., Gregory, D. F., Wright, L., & Patel, N. R. (2004). Computerized physician order entry and medication errors in a pediatric intensive care unit. *Pediatrics, 113*(1), 59–63.

Wiswell, T. (2003). Neonatal resuscitation. *Respiratory Care, 48*(3), 288–295.

CHAPTER
68

Medication Administration: Nasal

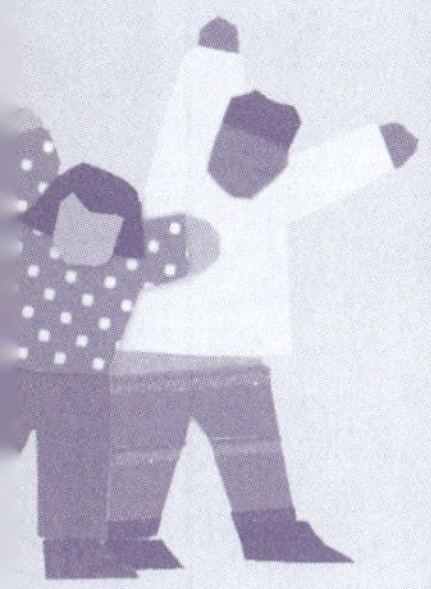

Clinical Guidelines

- A healthcare prescriber orders medications.
- Medications are administered by a registered nurse (RN), licensed practical nurse (LPN), physician, or parent who is knowledgeable about the medication and techniques of administering nasal medications to a child.
- Medications are administered within 1 hour of prescribed time.
- Principles of pharmacologic management (see Chapter 6) are followed.

Equipment

- Nonsterile gloves
- Tissue
- Bulb syringe (if needed)
- Correct medication
- Dropper (if medication bottle does not have one)

Child and Family Assessment and Preparation

- Assess child's previous experiences with receiving nasal medications.
- Assess child's and parents' understanding of need for nasal medication that will be administered.
- Prepare the child, as appropriate to cognitive level, and parents before administration (see Chapter 4). Provide therapeutic play as indicated, or involve a child life specialist, to allow the child to work through his or her fears and master control of the situation.
- Assess for allergies. If latex allergies are present, implement latex precautions (see Chapter 60). Notify healthcare provider ordering medications of drug allergy. Label child's record and apply identification band indicating allergies.

PROCEDURE Administering Nasal Medication

Steps	Rationale/Points of Emphasis
1. Verify the order with the child's medical record and check for allergy to drug; if present, do not administer drug and notify prescriber.	Verifies correct drug, dose, route, time, and patient. Allergic reactions to medications may be life threatening.
2. Perform hand hygiene and don gloves.	Reduces transmission of organisms.
3a. Obtain medication and read the label to verify with the order. Check for expiration date; if expired, do not administer. Identify the correct nostril in which to administer the medication.	To decrease chance of medication error, patient, route, dose, frequency, and time to be administered must be verified each time a medication is administered.
3b. Bring medication to room temperature before administration. Warm the solution by gently rotating the bottle in your hands before administration.	Cold medication increases discomfort when medication is administered nasally. **caREminder** *Nasal medication must be water based and not oil based. This prevents the possibility of aspiration pneumonia and facilitates absorption through nasal mucosa.*
4. Verify medication with the electronic record or take medication record and medication to the child to administer. Verify child's identity by comparing name on medication (if verified electronically) or on medication record with child's identification bracelet band and any other patient identifier required by the institution.	Ensures proper identification of the child.
5. Have the child blow his or her nose before administration. If the child is not old enough to cooperate, use a bulb syringe.	Clears the nose to allow for proper absorption of the medication.
6. Nose drops:	
a. Position the child in the supine position with the head tilted back or place a rolled towel or pillow under the child's neck and shoulder. An older child can extend the head over the side of the bed so that it is lower than the trunk.	Allows medication to coat nasal mucosa.
b. Aim the tip of the dropper toward the nasal passage and instill the ordered number of drops into each nostril, being careful not to touch the sides of the nostril (Figure 68-1).	Deposits the drug within the nose rather than in the throat and ensures administering the correct dose. Prevents contamination of the dropper or bottle.
c. Have the child remain in that position for several minutes, if possible.	Gives time for absorption of the medication.

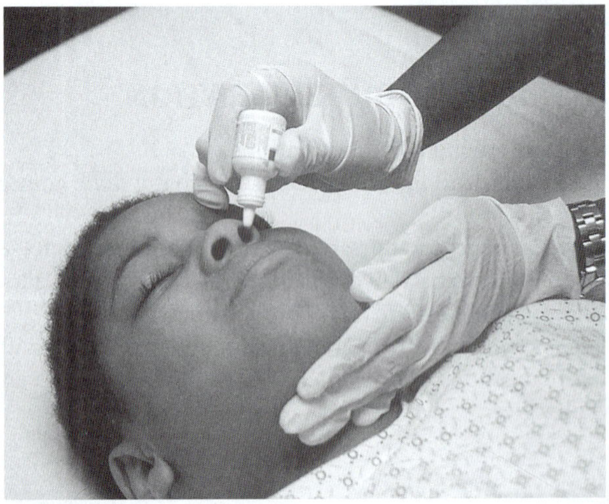

FIGURE 68-1
Position the child in the supine position with the head tilted back. Instill the ordered number of drops into each nostril, being careful not to touch the sides of the nostrils.

Steps	Rationale/Points of Emphasis
7. Nasal spray:	
a. Position the child in a semi-Fowler position with the head tilted slightly back.	Allows medication to coat nasal mucosa.
b. Instill the spray by holding (or having the child hold) one nostril closed while the medication is sprayed into the other nostril. Direct the spray to the side away from the septum and toward the top of the ear on that side.	Allows for full administration of the spray into the nostril.
c. Have the child take a deep breath through the nostril while the medication is being administered.	Facilitates absorption of the medication.
d. If indicated, repeat the procedure on the other nostril.	
8. Remove gloves and perform hand hygiene. Recap the medication. Return medication to appropriate storage area.	Reduces transmission of microorganisms. Provides safe storage of medication.

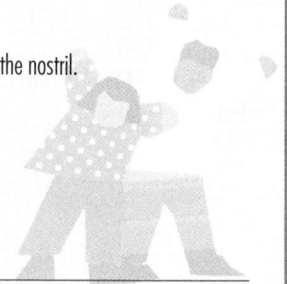

CHILD AND FAMILY EVALUATION AND DOCUMENTATION

- Observe the child after medication administration for any potential side effects. Evaluate the child for change in vital signs, hemodynamic status, and other signs as appropriate after medication administration to assess the effects of the medication.
- Evaluate child's response to the procedure and comfort as needed.
- Evaluate child's and family's understanding of medication. Determine whether the child and family have additional areas of concern to discuss.
- Document the following:
  - Date and time administered
  - Type of medication
  - Dose
  - Route given and site (one or both nares)
  - Presence or absence of adverse effects and notification of prescriber of such
  - Child's response to and tolerance of procedure
  - Teaching and information given to child and parents

COMMUNITY CARE

- If nasal medications are to be given in the home, teach the family the following:
  - Technique to administer medication
  - Signs of adverse reaction
  - Storage of medication
  - Safe storage of supplies
- If nasal medications are to be given in the home, ensure family has
  - Refrigeration (if needed to store medication)
  - Prescriber consent if child is to be given medication at school
- Identify problems that may prevent the parents from obtaining the medications (e.g., inability to pay for medications, lack of transportation to pick them up) and involve social services or support groups as necessary.
- Ensure that all medications have childproof caps and are kept beyond reach of children.
- Advise family members of guidelines regarding when they can still give medication if they forget to give a dose, to not give two doses together, and to call the prescriber or pharmacist if they have questions about dosing.
- Encourage prescriber to select medications that can be given in the fewest number of doses per day to decrease potential of missed doses.
- Instruct the family to contact the healthcare provider if
  - Child develops nasal irritation from medication
  - Medication is not controlling the symptoms for which it was intended

Unexpected Situations

- *The child's nasal passages are blocked by mucus:* Remove the excess mucus by gently suctioning with a bulb syringe before medication administration. Saline nose drops can be used first to loosen the mucus.
- *Child gags and starts to vomit after instillation of medication:* Turn child on his or her side or sit the child up to reduce chance of aspiration.

Bibliography

American Academy of Pediatrics, Committee on Drugs. (1997). Alternative routes of drug administration: Advantages and disadvantages (subject review). *Pediatrics, 100,* 143–152.

Benninger, M. S., Hadley, J. A., Osguthorpe, J. D., et al. (2004). Techniques of intranasal steroid use. *Otolaryngology—Head and Neck Surgery, 130,* 5–24.

Karagama, Y. G., Lancaster, J. L., Karkanevatos, A., & O'Sullivan, G. (2001). Delivery of nasal drops to the middle meatus: Which is the best head position? *Rhinology, 39,* 226–229.

Kayarkar, R., Clifton, N. J., & Woolford, T. J. (2002). An evaluation of the best head position for instillation of steroid nose drops. *Clinical Otolaryngology and Allied Sciences, 27,* 18–21.

Kubba, H., Spinou, E., & Robertson, A. (2000). The effect of head position on the distribution of drops within the nose. *American Journal of Rhinology, 14,* 83–86.

Turker, S., Onur, E., & Ozer, Y. (2004). Nasal route and drug delivery systems. *Pharmacy and World Science, 26,* 137–142.

Wolfe, T. R., & Bernstone, T. (2004). Intranasal drug delivery: An alternative to intravenous administration in selected emergency cases. *Journal of Emergency Nursing, 30,* 141–147.

CHAPTER

69

Medication Administration: Ophthalmic

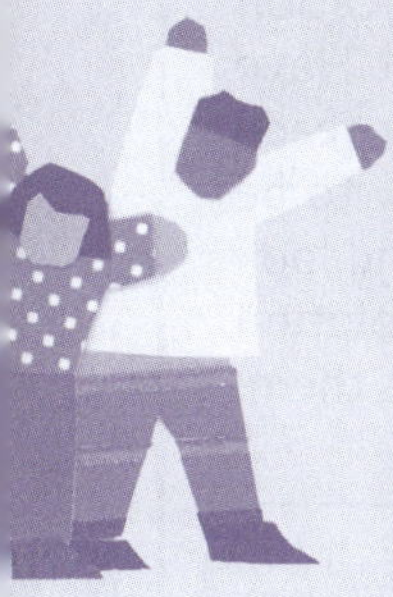

Clinical Guidelines

- Ophthalmic medications are administered by a registered nurse (RN), licensed practical nurse (LPN), physician, or parent who is knowledgeable about the medication and techniques of administering ophthalmic medications to a child.
- A healthcare prescriber orders medications.
- Medications are administered within 1 hour of prescribed time.
- Principles of pharmacologic management (see Chapter 6) are followed.

Equipment

- Correct medication
- Eyedropper
- Cotton ball/2 × 2 gauze
- Tissues
- Nonsterile gloves

Child and Family Assessment and Preparation

- Assess child's previous experiences with receiving ophthalmic medications.
- Assess child's and parents' understanding of need for ophthalmic medications that will be administered.
- Prepare the child, as appropriate to cognitive level, and parents for medication administration.
- Use therapeutic play, as indicated to allow the child to work through his or her fears and master control of the situation (see Chapter 4).
- Assess for drug and latex allergies. If present, implement latex precautions (see Chapter 60). Notify healthcare prescriber of drug allergy. Label child's record and apply identification band indicating allergies.

PROCEDURE Administering Ophthalmic Medications

Steps	Rationale/Points of Emphasis
1. Verify the order with the child's medical record and check for allergy to drug; if present, do not administer drug and notify prescriber.	Verifies correct drug, dose, route, time, and patient. Allergic reactions to medications may be life threatening.
2. Perform hand hygiene.	Reduces transmission of microorganisms.
3. Obtain medication and read the label to verify with the order; verify if the medication is to be administered into both eyes or only one and into which eye if only one. Check for expiration date; if expired, do not administer.	To decrease the chance of medication error, the patient, route, dose, frequency, and time to be administered must be verified each time a medication is administered. **caREminder** *Bring medication to room temperature before administration. If it is not, warm eye drops by holding the vial between the hands until warm because cold medication increases discomfort during oral administration.*
4. Verify medication with the electronic record or take medication record and medication to the child to administer. Verify child's identity by comparing name on medication (if verified electronically) or on medication record with child's identification band and any other patient identifier required by the institution.	Ensures proper identification of the child.
5. Don gloves.	Standard precaution to reduce transmission of microorganisms.
6. Cleanse the eye with cotton ball or gauze soaked with normal saline if necessary. Move from the inner canthus of the eyelid to the outer canthus. Use a new cotton ball each time you sweep the eye.	Old medication or discharge from the eye may mat around the eye. Using a new cotton ball or gauze for each sweep of the eye prevents contamination.
7. Position the child supine in bed, or other flat surface, looking up. Restrain the uncooperative child for administration; obtain another person to assist the child to lie still if needed.	Facilitates safe rapid administration.
8. Rest your dominant hand against the child's forehead. With the other hand, pull down the lower eyelid to expose the conjunctival sac.	Stabilizes hand, prevents poking the child in the eye with the dropper or medication tube, and allows for correct placement of the medication. **KidKare** Instillation of ophthalmic medication may be frightening and intrusive to the child. Have the child keep his or her eyes closed until you are ready to administer. When the medication is ready to be administered, have the child open the eyes and look up. Immediately instill the correct drops of solution or ointment into the eyes when the child opens them.
9. Administer the medication.	
a. Eye drops: If using a dropper, instill the correct amount of drops into the conjunctival sac, being careful not to touch the dropper to the eye (Figure 69-1). An alternate method of administration is to have the child close his or her eyes and tip the head backward. Place the medication drop(s) on the inner canthus and instruct the child to open eyes.	Noncontact prevents contamination of the dropper or bottle. Promotes a more comfortable administration and allows for correct placement of the medication in a more controlled manner.
b. Ointment: If using ointment, twist the ointment tube at the end to dislodge the ointment from the tube and place a thin ribbon of ointment along the entire conjunctival sac from the inner canthus to the outer canthus or as prescribed (e.g., ¼-inch ribbon). Have the child keep his or her eyes closed for up to 1 minute after administration (Figure 69-2).	Allows correct placement of the medication and allows time for the medication to disperse over the eye.

Steps	Rationale/Points of Emphasis

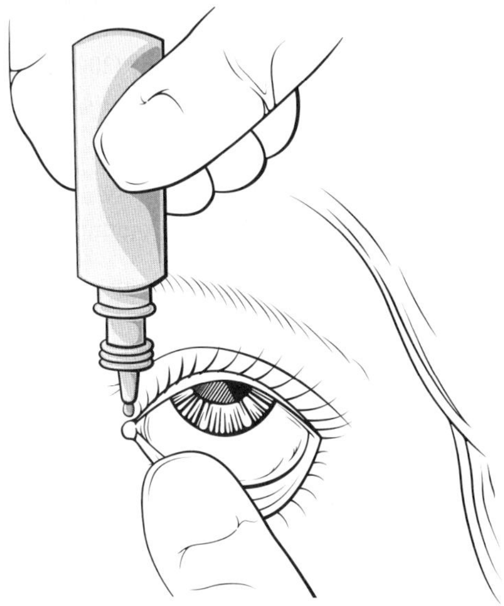

FIGURE 69-1
Instill the correct amount of eye drops into the conjunctival sac, being careful not to touch the dropper to the eye.

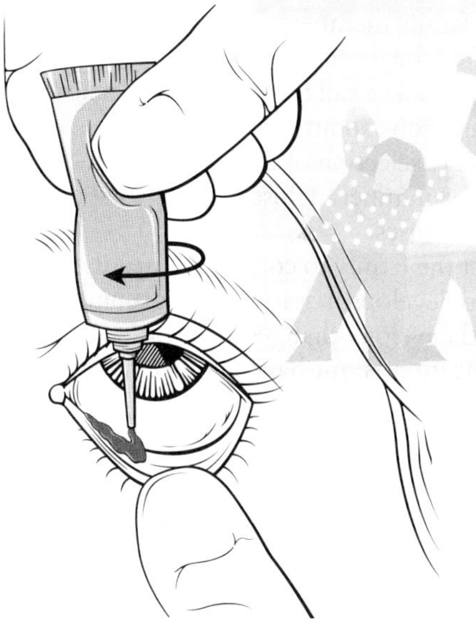

FIGURE 69-2
If using ointment, place a thin ribbon along the entire conjunctival sac from the inner canthus to the outer canthus.

Steps	Rationale/Points of Emphasis
10. Wipe excess medication off with a cotton ball or tissue.	Prevents irritation of medication to the skin surrounding eyes.
11. Remove gloves and perform hand hygiene.	Reduces transmission of microorganisms.
12. Return medication to appropriate storage area.	Provides safe storage of medication.

CHILD AND FAMILY EVALUATION AND DOCUMENTATION

- Observe the child after medication administration for any potential side effects. Side effects from ophthalmic medications may be either local (redness or edema around eyes) or systemic. Evaluate child's response to the procedure and comfort as needed.
- Evaluate child and family's understanding of medication. Determine whether the child and family have additional areas of concern to discuss.
- Document the following:
  - Date and time administered
  - Type of medication
  - Dose
  - Route and site given (right eye, left eye, or both); do not use abbreviations because they are frequently misinterpreted and result in medication errors.
  - Presence or absence of adverse effects and notification of healthcare prescriber of such
  - Child's response to and tolerance of procedure
  - Teaching and information given to child and parents

COMMUNITY CARE

- If ophthalmic medications are to be given in the home, teach the family the following:
  - Technique to administer medication; if the child is uncooperative, teach positioning to administer the medication: sit on the floor with legs extended, lay the child supine between your legs with his or her head positioned between your upper thighs, place your legs over the child's arms and legs to secure them, leaving both your hands free to administer the medication
  - Signs of adverse reaction
  - Storage of medication
  - Safe storage of supplies

caREminder

Ophthalmic medication should not be shared. Teach families that each family member must have his or her own medication to prevent cross-contamination.

- If ophthalmic medications are to be given in the home, ensure that family has
  - Refrigeration (if needed to store medication)
  - Physician consent if child is to be given medication at school
- Identify problems that may prevent the parents from obtaining the medications (e.g., inability to pay for medications, lack of transportation to pick them up) and involve social services or support groups as necessary.

- Ensure that all medications have childproof caps and are kept beyond reach of children.
- Advise family members of guidelines regarding what to do if they forget to give a dose, to not give two doses together, and to call the physician or pharmacist if they have questions about dosing.
- Encourage selection of medications that can be given in the fewest number of doses per day to decrease potential of missed doses.
- Instruct the family to contact the healthcare provider if
  - Child develops irritation in or around the eye
  - Child develops changes in vision
  - Medication is not having desired effect within indicated period of time

Unexpected Situations

- *Infant or child begins to cry:* Quickly console the child to prevent expulsion of the medication with tears.
- *Otic medication is inadvertently administered into the eyes instead of the ophthalmic medication:* Immediately flush eyes with lukewarm water or sterile saline for 10 minutes to reduce potential toxicity and notify the healthcare prescriber.

Bibliography

Coulter, R. A. (2004). Pediatric use of topical ophthalmic drugs. *Optometry, 75*, 419–429.

Institute for Safe Medication Practices. (2005). *ISMP's list of error-prone abbreviations, symbols, and dose designations.* Retrieved December 28, 2005, from www.ismp.org

Luc Van Santvliet, L. V., & Ludwig, A. (2004). Determinants of eye drop size. *Survey of Ophthalmology, 49*, 197–213.

McConnell, E. (1999). Instilling eye ointment. *Nursing1999, 29*, 14.

Ritch, R., Jamal, K. N., Gürses-Özden, R. & Liebmann, J. M. (2003). An improved technique of eye drop self-administration for patients with limited vision. *American Journal of Ophthalmology, 135*, 530–533.

Smith, S. E. (1997). Eyedrop instillation for reluctant children. *British Journal of Ophthalmology, 75*, 480–481.

C H A P T E R

70

Medication Administration: Oral

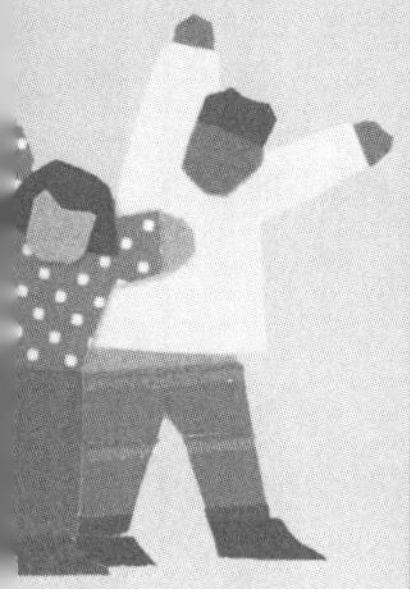

Clinical Guidelines

- Medications are administered by a registered nurse (RN), licensed practical nurse (LPN), physician, or parent who is knowledgeable about the medication and techniques of administering oral medications to a child.
- A healthcare prescriber orders medications.
- Principles of pharmacologic management (see Chapter 6) are followed.
- Use the oral route whenever possible because it is the least invasive method and less traumatic than intramuscular (IM) and intravenous (IV) routes. The gastrointestinal (GI) tract provides a vast absorptive area for medications. This absorption from the GI tract, as well as distribution, metabolism, and elimination, differs with maturation. Factors such as gastric pH, gastric emptying time, motility, absorptive area, enzyme activity, and dietary factors affect GI absorption.
- Medications are administered within 1 hour of prescribed time.
- When using syringes to measure and administer oral medications, use oral syringes (has a smooth versus Luer-Lok tip). Do not use Luer-Lok syringes to help prevent inadvertent IV or IM administration of medication because needles cannot be attached to oral syringes.
- Administer oral medications in a manner consistent with the child's age and developmental abilities. The following are guidelines for administration by age:
  - Infant
    - Up to 3 to 4 months of age: Liquid medication may be put in a nipple or oral syringe. The rooting-and-suck reflex stimulates the infant to suck the medication from the syringe and swallow it.
    - 5 to 12 months of age: Put liquid medication in an oral syringe and administer in small amounts toward the side of the mouth, not toward the throat. Place the syringe across the tongue to keep an older infant from spitting out the medication. Lightly stroking the throat in a downward motion may stimulate the infant to swallow.
    - Oral medicine can be placed on a spoon in a small amount of sweet-tasting food and fed to infant. Do not place medication in large amounts of fluid (e.g., a feeding) because the child may not ingest it all.

Alert! ***Never give honey to an infant because of risk for botulism.***

- Toddler
  - Explain in simple terms the reason for the medication. The same techniques used with the infant, excluding the nipple, can be used. Offer choices of technique when possible, e.g., "Do you want to suck from the syringe or drink from the medicine cup?" Include parents in medication administration. Permit the expression of anger and spend time comforting and praising the child afterward.
- Preschooler
  - Offer choices on technique and fluids to drink afterward. Enlist the child's cooperation.
- School-aged child
  - Give concrete explanations of the purpose of the medications. Offer choices as often as possible concerning administration (e.g., liquid, chewable tablet, or pill). School-aged children are collectors, so offer option of collecting washed-out medication cups or medication labels. Allows independence from parents in the process if the child gets to choose.
- Adolescent
  - Depending on maturity, more abstract rationales for the medication may be given to the adolescent. Use approaches suggested for the school-aged child.

EQUIPMENT

- Nonsterile gloves
- Correct medication
- Oral syringe or medicine cup
- Water or juice to drink or Popsicle
- Flavored syrup, such as cherry or grape (optional)
- Nipple (optional)
- Applesauce (optional)

CHILD AND FAMILY ASSESSMENT AND PREPARATION

- Assess the child's previous experience with oral medications. Parents are a good source of information about their child; ask them how the child best takes oral medications.
- Prepare the child, as appropriate to cognitive level, and parents before administration
- Provide therapeutic play as indicated, or involve a child life specialist, to allow the child to work through his or her fears and master control of the situation (see Chapter 4).
- Explain the medication's actions and side effects.
- Teach parents how to administer oral medications to the child if they have not done so in the past.
- Assess for drug and latex allergies. If latex allergies present, implement latex precautions (see Chapter 60). Notify healthcare prescriber of drug allergy. Label child's record and apply identification band indicating allergies.

PROCEDURE **Administering Oral Medication**

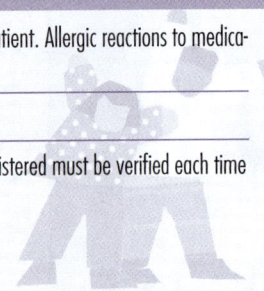

Steps	Rationale/Points of Emphasis
1. Verify the order with the child's medical record and check for allergy to drug; if present, do not administer drug and notify prescriber.	Verifies correct drug, dose, route, time, and patient. Allergic reactions to medications may be life threatening.
2. Perform hand hygiene and don gloves.	Reduces transmission of microorganisms.
3. Obtain medication and read the label to verify with the order. Check for expiration date; if expired, do not administer. ***Alert!*** *Some institutions automatically discontinue oral medications after surgery. Check policy.*	Route, dose, frequency, and time to be administered must be verified each time a medication is given.
4. Check medication form dispensed to ensure that it is appropriate for the child.	Many children are unable to swallow pills or capsules, and the medication may need to be modified. Contact pharmacy for alternate forms of the medication. Solid medications that are not sustained-release preparations may be crushed and mixed with a small amount of nonessential food, such as applesauce or pudding. Check with pharmacy before crushing tablets to ensure it is not contraindicated.
5. Prepare medication for administration. Measure all liquid medications using an oral syringe or medicine cup.	For amounts less than 1 mL or drops, use a tuberculin syringe. Household spoons are inaccurate. Medications must be measured accurately because a small error in amount could be dangerous for the child.

Steps	Rationale/Points of Emphasis
	caREminder *If mixing the medication with food or a liquid, use a small amount so that the child will finish all the medication.*
6. Verify the medication with the electronic record or take medication record and medication to child to administer. Verify the child's identity by comparing name on medication (if verified electronically) or on medication record with child's identification band and any other patient identifier required by the institution.	Ensures proper identification of the child.
7. Elevate the child's head or pick up and hold an infant or small child before administering medication, unless such positioning is contraindicated (Figure 70-1). 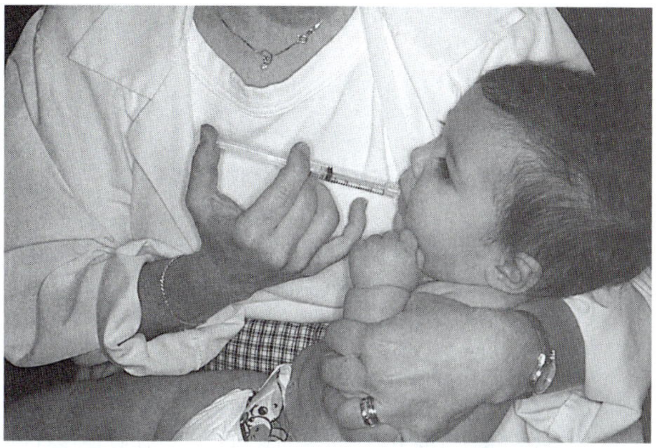 **FIGURE 70-1** When giving oral medication, position the child upright with the head elevated.	An upright position aids swallowing and helps prevent choking and aspiration. **KidKare** Never call medicine candy or a treat to reduce the chance that the child will think it is a treat and then seek out and ingest large amounts. If the medication is mixed in food or liquid, tell the child that the food or liquid contains medication to promote trust between child and care provider.
8. Administer the medication. Deliver liquids in small amounts, placing the syringe to the side of the mouth and allow the child to swallow between amounts.	Administration of 0.2 to 0.5 mL at a time helps prevent choking. Aiming the syringe to the side of the mouth helps prevent gagging and choking on the medication. **KidKare** If the medication is distasteful, offer a Popsicle or iced fluid after swallowing to disguise the taste.
9. Stay with the child until the medication is taken. Never leave medication at the bedside.	Nurse is responsible to ensure the child has received the medication. If left at the bedside, if could be forgotten or taken by another child. **caREminder** *Have parents administer the medication, if they are willing, under nursing supervision to optimize teaching opportunities and to evaluate parental technique.*
10. Dispose of medicine cup, syringe, and other objects in appropriate receptacle.	Ensures equipment is not reused or used for other procedures (e.g., feeding).
11. Remove gloves and perform hand hygiene.	Reduces transmission of microorganisms.

CHILD AND FAMILY EVALUATION AND DOCUMENTATION

- Evaluate child's response to the procedure and comfort as needed.
- Evaluate child and family's understanding of medication. Determine whether the child and family have additional areas of concern to discuss.

> **Alert!** *If the child vomits, assess approximate amount, note time since administration, and contact healthcare prescriber for orders.*

- Document the following:
  - Date and time administered
  - Type of medication
  - Dose
  - Route (oral) and method given (e.g., mixed with juice)
  - Presence or absence of adverse effects and notification of physician of such
  - Child's response to and tolerance of procedure
  - Teaching and information given to child and parents

COMMUNITY CARE

- If oral medications are to be given in the home, teach the family the following:
  - Methods to give oral medications
  - Method to draw up medication from larger container to smaller measuring device
  - Signs of adverse reaction
  - Storage of medication
  - Safe storage of supplies
  - Safe disposal or methods of cleaning for reuse of equipment
- If oral medications are to be given in the home, ensure that family has
  - Equipment to measure doses of liquid medications
  - Refrigeration (if needed to store medication)
  - Healthcare prescriber consent if child is to be given medication at school
- Identify problems that may prevent the child from obtaining the medications (e.g., inability to pay for medications). Assist family to resolve identified problems or refer to social services (e.g., apply for public health insurance [Medicaid]).
- Ensure that all medications have childproof caps and are kept beyond reach of children and pets.
- Advise family members of guidelines regarding when they can still give medication if child vomits immediately after medication administration or if they forget to give a dose. Inform them to not give two doses together and to call the healthcare prescriber or pharmacist with any questions about dosing.
- Encourage selection of medications that can be given in the fewest number of doses per day to decrease potential of missed doses.
- Instruct the family to contact the healthcare provider if
  - Child repeatedly vomits when given medication
  - Child develops a rash or fever
  - Symptoms of condition medication is being given for do not abate

Unexpected Situations

- *The infant or child begins to choke:* Sit the infant or child upright and allow him or her to recover. Continue to administer the medication slowly in small amounts, placing the medication syringe or medicine dropper alongside of the infant or child's tongue.
- *The infant allows the medication to dribble out of the mouth:* Retrieve medication from the lips and chin and refeed the medication, slowly placing the medication syringe or medicine dropper alongside the infant's tongue. Elicit the infant's normal rooting and sucking reflexes.

Bibliography

Bell, E. A. (2004). Improving tastes of liquid antibiotics. *Infectious Diseases in Children, 17*(10), 10–11.

Feldstein, T. J. (1996). Carbohydrate and alcohol content of 200 oral liquid medications for use in patients receiving ketogenic diets. *Pediatrics, 97*, 506–511.

Kraus, D., Stohlmeyer, L., Hannon, P., & Freels, S. (2001). Effectiveness and infant acceptance of the Rx medibottle versus oral syringe. *Pharmacotherapy, 21*, 416–423.

Mennella, J. A., Pepino, M. Y., & Beauchamp, G. K. (2003). Modification of bitter taste in children. *Developmental Psychobiology, 43*, 120–127.

CHAPTER

71

Medication Administration: Otic

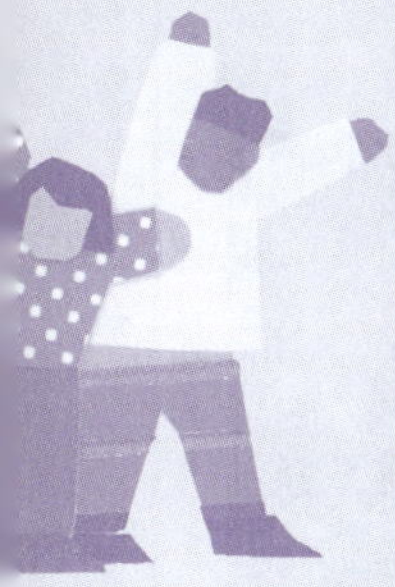

Clinical Guidelines

- A healthcare prescriber orders medications.
- Otic medications are administered by a registered nurse (RN), licensed practical nurse (LPN), physician, or parent who is knowledgeable about the medication and techniques of administering otic medication to a child.
- Principles of pharmacologic management (see Chapter 6) are followed.
- Medications are administered within 1 hour of prescribed time.

Equipment

- Nonsterile gloves
- Otic medication
- Dropper (if needed)
- Cotton ball

Child and Family Assessment and Preparation

- Assess child's previous experiences with receiving otic medications.
- Assess child's and parents' understanding of need for otic medication that will be administered.
- Prepare the child, as appropriate to cognitive level, and parents for medication administration (see Chapter 4). Use therapeutic play to allow the child to work through his or her fears and master control of the situation. Explain that the medication may make the ear tickle.
- Assess for allergies. If latex allergies present, implement latex precautions (see Chapter 60). Notify healthcare provider ordering medications of drug allergy. Label child's record and apply identification band indicating allergies.

PROCEDURE Administering Otic Medication

Steps	Rationale/Points of Emphasis
1. Verify the order with the child's medical record. Check for allergy to drug; if present, do not administer drug, and notify prescriber.	Verifies correct drug, dose, route, time, and patient. Allergic reactions to medications may be life threatening.
2. Perform hand hygiene and don gloves.	Standard precaution to reduce transmission of microorganisms.
3. Obtain medication and read the label to verify with the order. Check for expiration date; if expired, do not administer. Verify in which ear medication is to be administered.	To decrease chance of medication error, patient, route, dose, frequency, and time to be administered must be verified each time a medication is administered.

Alert! *Do not administer otic medication if it is cold. If kept in the refrigerator, allow the medication to come to room temperature before administration. Warm the solution by gently rotating the bottle in your hands before administration. Cold medication may cause discomfort and produce vomiting or vertigo in the child.*

Steps	Rationale/Points of Emphasis
4. Verify the medication with the electronic record or take medication record and bottle of medication to child to administer. Verify the child's identity by comparing name on medication (if verified electronically) or on medication record with child's identification band and any other patient identifier required by the institution.	Ensures proper identification of the child.
5. Have the child lie in a supine position with his or her head turned to the appropriate side; the child can also lie across parent's lap. Turn on cartoons to distract child. Soothe child afterward to keep him or her quiet while the medication is instilling.	Allows entry of the eardrops into the ear canal. **caREminder** *Talk to children, sing to them, or turn on videos to distract them, to facilitate instillation of medication.*
6. Pull the earlobe down and back for children younger than 3 years of age (Figure 71-1A). For older children, pull the pinna up and back (Figure 71-1B).	Straightens the ear canal and facilitates entry of the eardrops into the ear canal.

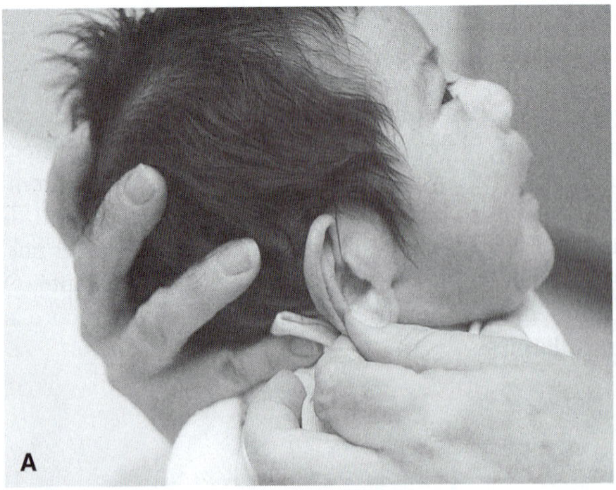

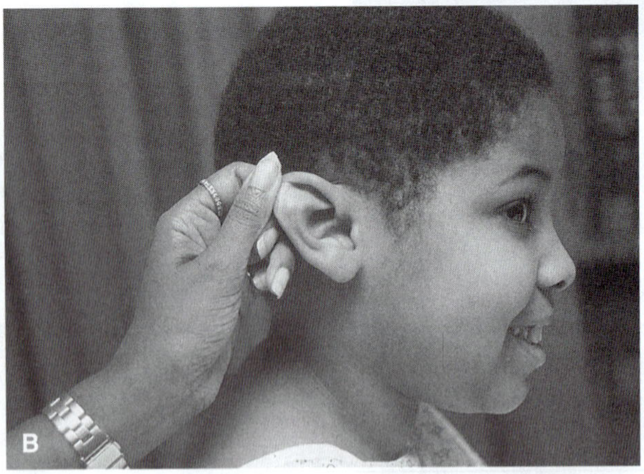

FIGURE 71-1
(**A**) Pull the ear down and back for children under 3 years of age. (**B**) For older children, pull the ear up and back.

Steps	Rationale/Points of Emphasis
7. Administer the ordered amount of drops into the ear canal, holding the dropper ½ inch above the ear canal and being careful not to contaminate the ear dropper.	Reduces transmission of microorganisms onto the dropper.
8. Gently massage the tragus (area anterior to the ear canal) unless contraindicated due to pain.	Facilitates entry of the medication into the ear canal.
9. Have the child remain in the supine position with the head turned for 2 to 3 minutes.	Gives time for the medication to enter the ear canal.
10. Insert a small cotton ball into the entry to the ear canal.	Prevents the medication from leaking out into the external ear. **caREminder** *Moistening the cotton ball with warm water or the otic medication prevents the cotton ball from absorbing the medication in the ear canal.*
11. Repeat with other ear if prescribed.	
12. Remove gloves and perform hand hygiene. Return medication to appropriate storage area.	Reduces transmission of microorganisms. Provides safe storage of medication.

CHILD AND FAMILY EVALUATION AND DOCUMENTATION

- Observe the child after medication administration for any potential side effects, such as dizziness. Evaluate child's response to the procedure and comfort as needed.
- Evaluate child's and family's understanding of medication. Determine whether the child and family have additional areas of concern to discuss.
- Document the following:
  - Date and time administered
  - Type of medication
  - Dose
  - Route and site given (right ear, left ear, or both)
  - Presence or absence of adverse effects and notification of healthcare prescriber of such
  - Child's response to and tolerance of procedure
  - Teaching and information given to child and parents

COMMUNITY CARE

- If otic medications are to be given in the home, teach the family the following:
  - Technique to administer medication
  - Signs of adverse reaction
  - Storage of medication
  - Safe storage of supplies
- If otic medications are to be given in the home, ensure that the family has
  - Refrigeration (if needed to store medication)
  - Prescriber consent if child is also to be given medication at school
- Identify problems that may prevent the parents from obtaining the medications (e.g., inability to pay for medications, lack of transportation to pick them up) and involve social services or support groups as necessary.
- Encourage the prescriber to select medications that can be given in the fewest number of doses per day to decrease potential of missed doses.
- Ensure that all medications have childproof caps and are kept beyond reach of children.
- Advise family members of guidelines regarding when they can still give medication if they forget to give a dose, to not give two doses together, and to call the prescriber or pharmacist with questions about dosing.
- Instruct the family to contact the healthcare provider if
  - Child develops otic irritation from medication
  - Medication is not having desired effect within indicated period of time

Unexpected Situation

- *Child complains of dizziness and starts to fall when standing up after medication administration:* Have child sit down or help him or her to a sitting position; ensure that child is away from sharp edges if he or she should fall. Reinforce that medication should be room temperature when administered and teach child to sit for a few minutes after medication administration.

Bibliography

Goldenberg, D., Golz, A., Netzer, A., & Joachims, H. Z. (2002). The use of otic powder in the treatment of acute external otitis. *American Journal of Otolaryngology, 23*, 142–147.

Hebert, R. L., Vick, M. L., King, G. E., & Bent, J. P. (2000). Tympanostomy tubes and otic suspensions: Do they reach the middle ear space? *Otolaryngology Head and Neck Surgery, 122*, 330–333.

Sood, S., Strachan, D. R., Tsikoudas, A., & Stables, G. I. (2002). Allergic otitis externa. *Clinical Otolaryngology and Allied Sciences, 27*, 233–236.

CHAPTER

72

Medication Administration: Rectal

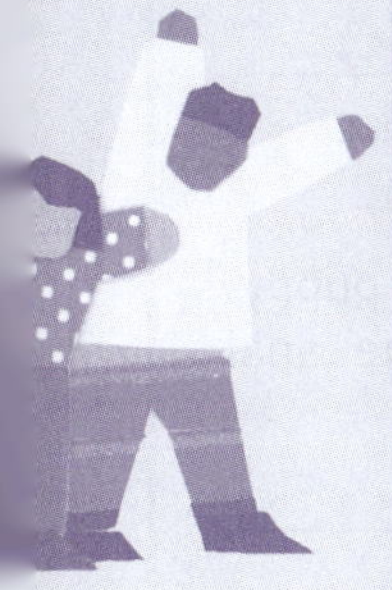

Clinical Guidelines

- Rectal medications are administered by a registered nurse (RN), licensed practical nurse (LPN), physician, or parent who is knowledgeable about the medication and techniques of administering rectal medication to a child.
- A healthcare prescriber orders medications.
- Principles of pharmacologic management (see Chapter 6) are followed.
- The rectal route is not the preferred route because of potential emotional trauma to the child and unpredictable absorption from the colon. Absorption can be further affected by the presence of stool in the colon and rectum. The rectal route may be the best choice for a child who cannot tolerate oral medication and in whom a parenteral route is not available.
- Medications are administered within 1 hour of prescribed time.

Equipment

- Nonsterile gloves
- Water-soluble lubricant
- Medication

Child and Family Assessment and Preparation

- Assess child's previous experiences with receiving rectal medications.
- Assess child's and parents' understanding of need for rectal medication that will be administered.
- Prepare the child, as appropriate to cognitive level, and parents for medication administration.
- Use therapeutic play to allow the child to work through his or her fears and master control of the situation (see Chapter 4).
- Assess for drug and latex allergies; if present, implement latex precautions (see Chapter 60) and notify healthcare prescriber of drug allergy. Label child's record and apply identification band indicating allergies.
- Ask the child if he or she is able to defecate (using terms the child is familiar with) before administration of the suppository. Stool in the colon can affect absorption of medication.

PROCEDURE Administering Rectal Medication

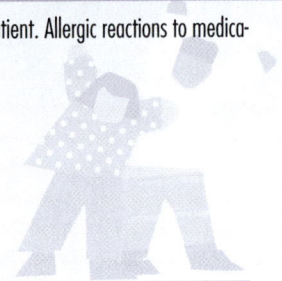

Steps	Rationale/Points of Emphasis
1. Verify the order with the medical record and check for allergy to drug; if present, do not administer drug and notify prescriber. ***Alert!*** *Rectal medication administration is contraindicated in children who are immunosuppressed or thrombocytopenic because of the risk of infection or bleeding.*	Verifies correct drug, dose, route, time, and patient. Allergic reactions to medications may be life threatening.
2. Perform hand hygiene.	Reduces transmission of microorganisms.
3. Obtain medication and read the label to verify with the order. Check for expiration date; if expired, do not administer.	To decrease chance of medication error, patient, route, dose, frequency, and time to be administered must be verified each time a medication is administered.
4. Check medication form dispensed to ensure that it is appropriate for the child.	Suppositories are the most frequent form of rectal administration, although occasionally medication may be administered in an enema form (see Chapter 37). Children are very susceptible to fluid and electrolyte imbalances.
5. Prepare medication for administration. Avoid cutting if possible. If the suppository must be cut to obtain the ordered dose, then it must be cut lengthwise.	Cutting a suppository lengthwise helps absorption at the required rate. The drug may not be dispersed evenly within the suppository.
6. Verify the medication with the electronic record or take medication record and medication to child to administer. Verify the child's identity by comparing name on medication (if verified electronically) or on medication record with child's identification band and any other patient identifier required by the institution.	Ensures proper identification of the child.
7. Don gloves.	Protects the administrator from fecal material, thus reducing transmission of microorganisms.
8. Position the child in a left lateral position with the right leg flexed or in the knee–chest position.	Either of these positions exposes the anus and helps relax the external sphincter for ease of insertion.
9. Remove the suppository packaging and lubricate the suppository with a water-soluble lubricating jelly.	Reduces friction against mucosal surfaces.
10. Gently insert the apex (pointed end) of the suppository past the internal anal sphincter, placing the medication against the rectal wall. In an infant or toddler, insert the suppository with the little finger. The index finger can be used for older children.	The suppository must be past the internal sphincter to prevent expulsion. **KidKare** Instruct the child to pant like a puppy. This provides distraction and relaxes the anal sphincter.
11. Hold the child's buttocks together until the child relaxes or loses the urge to push. If the child has a stool within 30 minutes, examine the stool for the presence of the suppository.	Prevents expulsion of medication. **KidKare** Distraction of the child with games or other activities can help avoid expulsion.
12. Remove gloves. Dispose of gloves in appropriate receptacle. Perform hand hygiene.	Reduces transmission of microorganisms. Standard precautions.

CHILD AND FAMILY EVALUATION AND DOCUMENTATION

- Observe the child after medication administration for any potential side effects. Evaluate the child for change in vital signs, hemodynamic status, and other signs as appropriate after medication administration to assess the effects of the medication.
- Evaluate child's response to the procedure and comfort as needed.
- Evaluate child and family's understanding of medication. Determine whether the child and family have additional areas of concern to discuss.
- Document the following:
  - Date and time administered
  - Type of medication
  - Dose
  - Route given
  - Presence or absence of adverse effects and notification of healthcare prescriber of such
  - Child's response to and tolerance of procedure
  - Teaching and information given to child and parents

COMMUNITY CARE

- If rectal medications are to be given in the home, teach the family the following:
  - Technique to administer medication
  - Signs of adverse reaction
  - Storage of medication in refrigerator
  - Removal of foil from medication before administering
  - Safe storage of supplies
- If rectal medications are to be given in the home, ensure that the family has
  - Nonsterile gloves
  - Refrigeration (if needed to store medication)
  - Healthcare prescriber consent if child is to be given medication at school
  - Identify problems that may prevent the parents from obtaining the medications (e.g., inability to pay for medications, lack of transportation to pick them up) and involve social services or support groups as necessary.
- Ensure that all medications are kept beyond reach of children.
- Advise family members of guidelines of when they can still give medication if they forget to give a dose, to not give two doses together, and to call the physician or pharmacist with questions about dosing.
- Encourage selection of medications that can be given in the least number of doses per day to decrease potential of missed doses.
- Instruct the family to contact the healthcare provider if
  - Child is unable to retain doses of the medication
  - Medication is not controlling the symptoms it was intended for
  - Child develops adverse effects
  - Child has rectal bleeding

Unexpected Situation

- *The infant's or child's rectum is full of stool:* Do not administer and notify the healthcare prescriber; the presence of feces affects absorption of the medication.

Bibliography

American Academy of Pediatrics, Committee on Drugs. (1997). Alternative routes of drug administration: Advantages and disadvantages [subject review]. *Pediatrics, 100,* 143–152.

Kannan, S., & Derrick, G. (2001). Packaging of codeine phosphate suppositories. *Paediatric Anaesthesia, 11,* 124.

Kim, T., Rognerud, C., & Ou, C.-N. (2005). Accuracy in the alteration of acetaminophen suppositories. *Anesthesia & Analgesia, 100,* 1303–1305.

Warren, D. E. (1996), Practical use of rectal medications in palliative care. *Journal of Pain and Symptom Management, 11,* 378–387.

CHAPTER

73

Medication Administration: Subcutaneous

Clinical Guidelines

- A healthcare prescriber orders medications.
- Medications are administered by a registered nurse (RN), licensed practical nurse (LPN), physician, child, or parent who is knowledgeable about the medication and techniques of administering a subcutaneous injection to a child.
- Principles of pharmacologic management (see Chapter 6) are followed.
- Medications are given subcutaneously (SC) when a slower rate of absorption is desired because fatty tissue has fewer blood vessels than muscle. This site can only be used for medications that do not cause tissue irritation.
- Medications are administered within 1 hour of prescribed time.

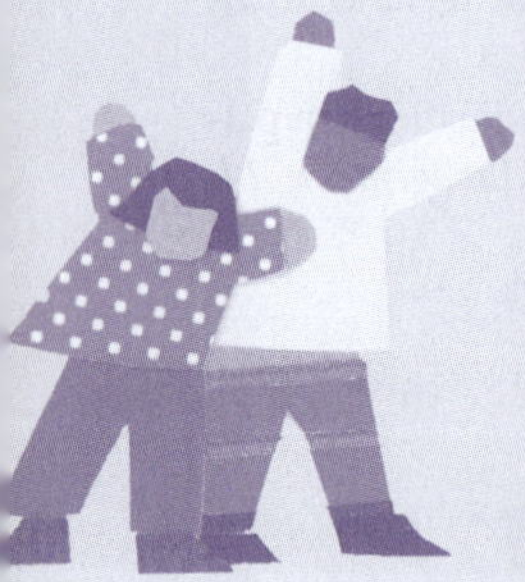

Equipment

- Correct medication
- Syringe, appropriate size
- Needle, appropriate size and length (Table 73-1)
- Antiseptic swab or pledget (alcohol, 2% chlorhexidine, or 10% povidone-iodine)
- Cotton ball
- Nonsterile gloves
- Adhesive bandage

Child and Family Assessment and Preparation

- Assess the child's previous experience with injections.
- Prepare the child, as appropriate to cognitive level, and parents for the injection before administration.

TABLE 73-1

Needle Length and Size Recommendations for Subcutaneous Injection

	Length	Gauge	Amount of Infusion
Adolescent or adult	½ to ⅝ inch	25–27	0.5–1 mL
Obese person	⅞ inch	25–27	0.5–1 mL
Infant or child	⅜ inch	25	No more than 0.1 mL for intradermal No more than 0.5 mL for subcutaneous to small child or 1 mL to preschool-aged or school-aged child

KidKare Enlist the child's cooperation by having the child hold the bandage. Tell the child that it is okay to yell or cry and that his or her job is to stay as still as possible.

- Provide therapeutic play as indicated, or involve a child life specialist, to allow the child to work through his or her fears and master control of the situation (see Chapter 4).
- Assess for drug and latex allergies; if present, implement latex precautions (see Chapter 60) and notify healthcare prescriber of drug allergy. Label child's record and apply identification band indicating allergies.
- Use a topical anesthetic (e.g., EMLA, LMX4, vapo-coolant) if injection is painful and when time allows to reduce pain and trauma of injection (see Chapter 7).

PROCEDURE Administering Subcutaneous Injections

Steps	Rationale/Points of Emphasis
1. Verify the order with the child's medical record and check for allergy to drug; if present, do not administer drug, and notify prescriber.	Verifies correct drug, dose, route, time, and patient. Allergic reactions to medications may be life threatening.
2. Perform hand hygiene.	Reduces transmission of microorganisms.
3. Obtain medication and read the label to verify with the order. Check for expiration date; if expired, do not administer.	To decrease chance of medication error, patient, route, dose, frequency, and time to be administered must be verified each time a medication is administered. **caREminder** *Medication should be at room temperature before administration; cold medication increases discomfort of the injection.*
4. Check the amount of medication to be administered to determine syringe size and appropriateness for the child (see Table 73-1). Limit volume according to the age of the child and the amount of adipose tissue.	Large volumes of medication injected into the subcutaneous tissue can result in tissue injury. The subcutaneous route is occasionally used to administer continuous infusions (e.g., chemotherapy, iron chelation).
5. Choose appropriate needle gauge and length for the medication, child size, and site (see Table 73-1). Do not use a needle longer than ⅝ inch.	Viscous medication requires a larger gauge needle. Use the needle with the smallest bore (large gauge = 25 or 27 gauge) possible. A longer needle may result in intramuscular instead of subcutaneous administration.
6. Draw up correct amount of medication into syringe. If there is a large volume of medication, more than one injection may be needed.	Medications must be measured accurately because a small error in amount may cause serious dosage errors. **KidKare** Draw up the medication in the medication room. The sight of the needle can increase the child's anxiety. **Alert!** *Do not draw up additional air into the syringe. Clearing the needle of medication can affect dose administered.*

Continued

Steps	Rationale/Points of Emphasis
7. Verify medication with electronic record or take medication record and syringe with medication to the child to administer. Verify the child's identity by comparing name on medication (if verified electronically) or on medication record with child's identification band and any other patient identifier required by the institution.	Ensures proper identification of the child.
8. Don gloves.	Standard precaution to reduce transmission of microorganisms.
9. Evaluate the child's subcutaneous tissue; choose the most appropriate site considering the adequacy and condition of subcutaneous tissue and duration of therapy (Figure 73-1). 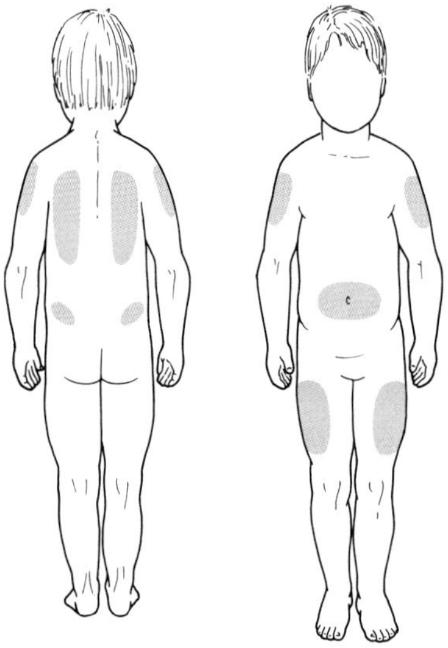 **FIGURE 73-1** Sites for subcutaneous injections.	Subcutaneous injection sites include abdomen, lateral upper arms, and thighs. Wide variations in the amount of subcutaneous fat in children exist. This may necessitate choosing an alternative site in the child. ***Alert!*** ***Do not give in operative site or an extremity that has a pathologic process. Complications associated with giving subcutaneous injections are often the result of inappropriate sites.***
10. Evaluate the use of nonpharmacologic interventions: distraction (storytelling, blowing bubbles), cold therapy, and other methods (see Chapter 7).	May decrease perception of pain sensation. **KidKare** Give the child choices, as appropriate (e.g., which leg or side), which gives the child some control of the situation.
11. Restrain the child securely. Assess the need for additional help holding the child, and obtain help as indicated. Parents should not be responsible for securing the child but may remain to give support, such as holding the child's hand.	Decreases chance of injury from movement because even cooperative children have a tendency to move during injections.
12a. Cleanse the site with antiseptic and allow to dry. 12b. Insulin injections do not require skin preparation. The small-gauge needle used for injection of insulin cannot carry sufficient number of bacteria to cause infection.	Allowing the antiseptic to dry allows antimicrobial action of antiseptic and minimizes pain at the site of injection.
13a. Grasp the site and elevate the tissue. Insert the needle quickly at a 45- to 90-degree angle. Insert at 45 degrees if there is little subcutaneous tissue or at 90 degrees if subcutaneous tissue is abundant.	Elevating the site separates the subcutaneous skin from the muscle.

Steps	Rationale/Points of Emphasis
13b. Aspirate to check for blood. If blood is in the syringe, remove the needle.	Thought to prevent intravenous or intra-arterial administration; no clinical studies confirm or negate this. Do not aspirate when administering insulin or heparin.
13c. If blood is not present, slowly inject the medication.	Slow injection may reduce local damage and pain.
14. Withdraw the needle quickly at the same angle at which it was inserted and apply pressure over the site with a dry cotton ball. **Alert!** *Do not recap the needle, to reduce chance of needle-stick injury.*	Alcohol over an injection site may sting and prolong bleeding.
15. Place adhesive bandage over site.	Young children may believe their insides will leak out the injection site if a bandage is not used. **KidKare** Use character or colorful bandages to comfort the child.
16. Dispose of needle, syringe, and waste in appropriate receptacle. Remove gloves and perform hand hygiene.	Prevents needle-stick injuries. Reduces transmission of microorganisms.
17. Comfort the child and have the parent comfort the child after the injection.	Promotes positive relationship and decreases long-term negative effects of painful procedures. **KidKare** Giving the child a sticker or other reward can help promote comfort and provide positive feelings.
18. Return to the room a short time later for positive interaction with the child.	Playing or other activities will help the child not associate the nurse with only painful procedures. Gives opportunity to further evaluate the child's response to procedure.

CHILD AND FAMILY EVALUATION AND DOCUMENTATION

- Healthcare provider must monitor child for 15 minutes after SC injection of drugs that may potentially cause a reaction for side effects or allergic reactions, such as respiratory distress. Evaluate the child for change in vital signs, hemodynamic status, and other signs as appropriate after medication administration to assess the effects of the medication.
- Evaluate child's response to the procedure and comfort as needed.
- Evaluate child and family's understanding of medication. Determine whether the child and family have additional areas of concern to discuss.
- Document the following:
  - Date and time administered
  - Type of medication
  - Dose
  - Route and site given
  - Presence or absence of adverse effects and notification of healthcare prescriber of such
  - Child's response to and tolerance of procedure
  - Teaching and information given to child and parents

COMMUNITY CARE

- Provide parents instructions regarding expected response to SC medication administration.
- If subcutaneous medications are to be given in the home, teach the family the following:
  - Sites for subcutaneous administration
  - Method to draw up medication
  - Technique to administer medication
  - Signs of adverse reaction
  - Storage of medication
  - Safe storage of supplies (including putting needles and syringes out of reach of small children)
  - Safe disposal of needles and syringes
- If subcutaneous medications are to be given in the home, ensure that the family has
  - Name of medical supply vendor to obtain necessary equipment
  - Needle disposal container

- Refrigeration (if needed to store medication)
- Healthcare prescriber consent if child is to be given medication at school

- Identify problems that may prevent the child from obtaining the medications (e.g., inability to pay for medications or lack of transportation to pick up medications). Assist family to resolve identified problems or refer to social services (e.g., apply for public health insurance such as Medicaid and identify vendors who deliver).
- Ensure that all medications have childproof caps and are kept beyond reach of children.
- Advise family members of guidelines of when they can still give medication if they forget to give a dose, to not give two doses together, and to call the healthcare prescriber or pharmacist with questions about dosing.
- Encourage selection of medications that can be given in the fewest number of doses per day to decrease potential of missed doses.
- Instruct the family to contact the healthcare provider if
  - Child develops rash over body or injection site
  - Child develops a fever
  - Injection site becomes hard and reddened
  - Medication is not causing desired effects or child is experiencing side effects from the medication

Unexpected Situation

- *When you are aspirating for blood return before injecting the medication, the needle pulls out of the skin:* If insulin injection, reattempt injection avoiding previous insertion site. For all other medications, remove and appropriately discard needle. Attach a new needle to syringe and administer injection.

Bibliography

American Diabetes Association. (2004). Position statement: Insulin administration. *Diabetes Care, 27,* S106–S107.

Annersten, M., & Willman, A. (2005). Performing subcutaneous injections: A literature review. *Worldviews on Evidence-based Nursing, 2,* 122–130.

Fleming, D. R. (1999). Challenging traditional insulin injection practices. *American Journal of Nursing, 99*(2), 72–74.

Halperin, S. A., McGrath, P., Smith, B., & Houston, T. (2000). Lidocaine-prilocaine patch decreases the pain associated with the subcutaneous administration of measles-mumps-rubella vaccine but does not adversely affect the antibody response. *Journal of Pediatrics, 136,* 789–794.

Martin, S., Jones, J. S., & Wynn, B. N. (1996). Does warming local anesthetic reduce the pain of subcutaneous injection? *American Journal of Emergency Medicine, 14,* 10–12.

Peragallo-Dittko, V. (1995). Aspiration of the subcutaneous insulin injection: Clinical evaluation of needle size and amount of subcutaneous fat. *Diabetes Educator, 21,* 291–296.

Tubiana-Rufi, N., Kakou, B., Belarbi, N., et al. (1999). Short needles (8 mm) reduce the risk of intramuscular injections in children with type 1 diabetes. *Diabetes Care, 22,* 1621–1625.

Uzun, S., Inanc, N., & Azal, O. (2001). Determining optimal needle length for subcutaneous injection. *Journal of Diabetes Nursing, 5*(3), 83–87.

C H A P T E R

74

Medication Administration: Sublingual and Buccal

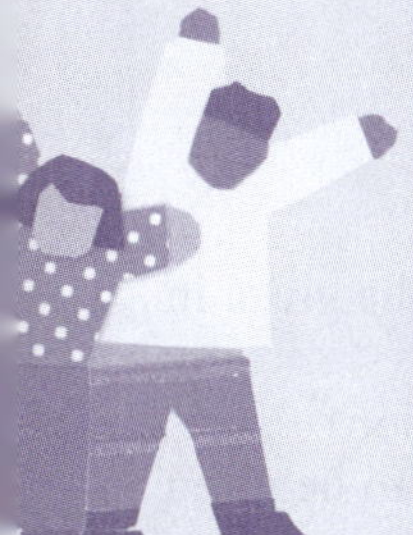

Clinical Guidelines

- A healthcare prescriber orders medications.
- Sublingual (under the tongue) and buccal (between the cheek and gum) medications are administered by a registered nurse (RN), licensed practical nurse (LPN), physician, child, or parent who is knowledgeable about the techniques of administering transmucosal medication to a child as well as the particular medication being used and its possible effects on the child.
- Principles of pharmacologic management (see Chapter 6) are followed.
- Sublingual and buccal medications are absorbed by the oral mucosa, which has a rich vascular supply and lacks a stratum corneum epidermidis; therefore, absorption by this route is rapid. Medications given this way can be detected in the blood within 1 minute, and peak levels are generally achieved within 10 to 15 minutes.
- Medications are administered within 1 hour of prescribed time.

Equipment

- Correct medication
- Nonsterile gloves

Child and Family Assessment and Preparation

- Assess sublingual/buccal mucosa for redness and/or disrupted integrity, and notify prescriber if disruption in mucosal integrity is present.
- Assess child's previous experiences with receiving sublingual or buccal medications.
- Assess child's and parents' understanding of need for sublingual or buccal medication that will be administered.
- Prepare the child, as appropriate to cognitive level, and parents for medication administration (see Chapter 4). Use therapeutic play to allow the child to work through his or her fears and master control of the situation.
- Assess for drug and latex allergies; if present, implement latex precautions (see Chapter 60) and notify healthcare prescriber of drug allergy. Label child's record and apply identification band indicating allergies.

PROCEDURE Administering Sublingual and Buccal Medication

Steps	Rationale/Points of Emphasis
1. Verify the order with the child's medical record and check for allergy to drug; if present, do not administer drug and notify prescriber.	Verifies correct drug, dose, route, time, and patient. Allergic reactions to medications may be life threatening.
2. Perform hand hygiene and don gloves.	Reduces transmission of microorganisms.
3. Obtain medication and read the label to verify that it is the same medication as prescribed in the order. Check for expiration date; if expired, do not administer.	Ensures that correct medication is being given. **caREminder** *Use caution not to get the medication wet or to place it against the skin, because sublingual and buccal medications degrade and are absorbed very rapidly.*
4. Verify the medication with the electronic medication record or take the medication record and medication to the child to administer. Verify the child's identity by comparing name on medication (if verified electronically) or on medication record with child's identification band and any other patient identifier required by the institution.	Ensures proper identification of the child.
5. Place the medication either under the child's tongue (sublingual) or between the cheek and the gum (buccal). If repeated doses are to be administered, alternate sides of the mouth for subsequent doses. The child should not eat, drink, or smoke while the medication is in his or her mouth.	These locations aid in quick absorption of medication. Eating, drinking, and smoking interfere with absorption of the medication. **KidKare** If the child has trouble raising his or her tongue, place one end of a straw in the sublingual pocket and drop the tablet in via the other end. Tell the child not to swallow the medication but to let it be absorbed in the mouth.
6a. Remove gloves and perform hand hygiene. 6b. Return medication to appropriate storage area.	Reduces transmission of microorganisms. Maintains organization and provides safe storage of medication.

CHILD AND FAMILY EVALUATION AND DOCUMENTATION

- Evaluate child's response to the procedure and comfort child as needed. Monitor for desired and untoward side effects of the medication.
- Document the following:
  - Type of medication
  - Dose
  - Site given (sublingual or buccal)
  - Time administered
  - Presence or absence of adverse effects, including signs of mucosal irritation
  - Child's response to and tolerance of procedure
  - Teaching and information given to child and parents

COMMUNITY CARE

- If sublingual or buccal medications are to be given in the home, teach the family the following:
  - To assess sublingual/buccal mucosa for irritation or disrupted integrity
  - Technique to administer medication
  - Signs of adverse reactions
  - Storage of medication and supplies
- If sublingual or buccal medications are to be given in the home, ensure that family has
  - Refrigeration (if needed to store medication)
  - Healthcare prescriber consent if child is to be given medication at school
- Identify problems that may prevent the parents from obtaining the medications (e.g., inability to pay for medications, lack of transportation to pick them up) and involve social services or support groups as necessary.
- Ensure that all medications have childproof caps and are kept beyond the reach of all the children.
- Advise family members of guidelines regarding when they can still give medication if they forget to give a dose, and explain that they should not give two doses together. Advise family members to call the prescriber or pharmacist with questions about dosing.

- Encourage selection of medications that can be given in the fewest number of doses per day to decrease potential of missed doses.
- Instruct the family to contact the healthcare provider if
  - Child develops irritation of the oral mucosa from medication
  - Medication is not causing desired effects
  - Child is experiencing side effects from the medication

Unexpected Situation

- *The child tells you that she wants the medicine because she likes the funny feeling when the medicine is in her mouth:* The fizzing action of many sublingual and buccal medications mimics some types of candy. Caution children and parents that this is a medication, not candy.

Bibliography

American Academy of Pediatrics, Committee on Drugs. (1997). Alternative routes of drug administration: Advantages and disadvantages [subject review]. *Pediatrics, 100,* 143–152.

Springhouse. (2002). *Medication administration made incredibly easy!* Philadelphia: Lippincott Williams & Wilkins.

C H A P T E R

75

Medication Administration: Topical

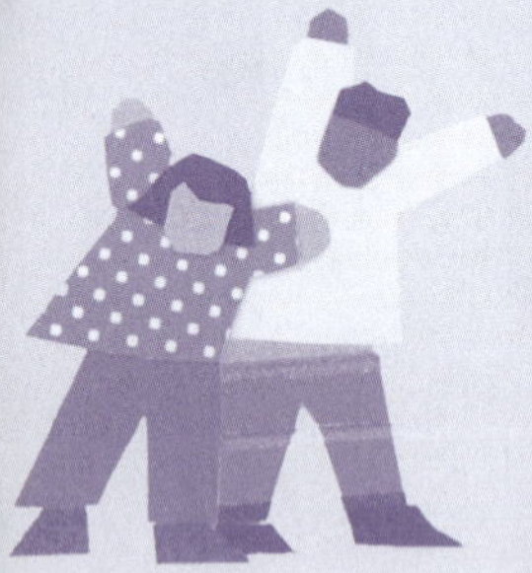

Clinical Guidelines

- A healthcare prescriber orders medications.
- Medications are administered by a registered nurse (RN), licensed practical nurse (LPN), physician, child, or parent who is knowledgeable about the medication and techniques of administering topical medication to a child.
- Principles of pharmacologic management (see Chapter 6) are followed.
- Medications are given topically through the skin (transdermally) and absorbed because of the skin's relatively rich blood supply. Because skin thickness and blood flow to the skin vary with age, the potential for toxic effects of the drug must be considered. Children have a larger body surface area and a thinner layer of cutaneous and subcutaneous tissue than adults, so there is an increased risk for systemic absorption and effects through topical application.
- Do not apply topical medication to skin with open lesions unless ordered.
- Medications are administered within 1 hour of prescribed time.

Equipment

- Topical medication
- Nonsterile gloves
- Washcloth
- Basin of warm water
- Gauze (if needed)
- Appropriate applicator (cotton swab, tongue depressor, or other)
- Sterile dressing (if needed)

Child and Family Assessment and Preparation

- Assess the child's skin integrity before administration of topical medication. Observe for cleanliness and clean off dirt and excess lotions as needed.
- Assess the condition of the child's skin, noting areas of healing, excoriation, edema, rashes, or increased redness.
- Assess the child's previous experience with topical medications.
- Prepare the child, as appropriate to cognitive level, and parents before administration.
- Provide therapeutic play as indicated, or involve a child life specialist, to allow the child to work through his or her fears and master control of the situation (see Chapter 4).

- Teach the child and parents about the medication's actions and side effects, how the medication is to be applied, and the reason for its use.

KidKare Remind the child not to rub or scratch where the medication is to be applied. Scratching or rubbing the area may remove some of the medication, interfere with absorption, and damage the skin or underlying tissue.

- Assess for drug and latex allergies; if present, implement latex precautions (see Chapter 60), and notify healthcare prescriber of drug allergy. Label child's record and apply identification band indicating allergies.

PROCEDURE **Administering Topical Medication**

Steps	Rationale/Points of Emphasis
1. Verify the order with the medical record and check for allergy to drug; if present, do not administer drug and notify prescriber.	Verifies correct drug, dose, route, time, and patient. Allergic reactions to medications may be life threatening.
2. Obtain the ordered topical medication and read the label to verify with the order. Check for expiration date; if expired, do not administer. Use topical medication at room temperature unless otherwise specified.	Room temperature medication may be more comfortable and easier to apply.
3. Perform hand hygiene and don gloves.	Reduces transmission of microorganisms.
4. Verify the medication with the electronic medication record or take the medication record and medication to the child to administer. Verify the child's identity by comparing name on medication (if verified electronically) or on medication record with child's identification band and any other patient identifier required by the institution.	Ensures proper identification of child.
5. Cleanse the skin, as ordered or per reference manual recommendations, before application of the medication. Use a basin of warm water and a washcloth only. If an open wound is present, use gauze instead of a washcloth. Dry skin well after washing.	Some medications require cleansing all old medication off the skin before the application of new medication. Other medications require applying new sterile medication over the old medication without cleansing the area.
6a. Apply topical medication to the site. Use the correct amount as ordered and administration technique for the type of topical medication.	An excessive amount of medication may result in irritation of the skin and adverse systemic effects. Unintentional absorption through mucous membranes can result in systemic toxicity.
6b. Administer gels, ointments, and pastes using cotton swabs or tongue blades.	
6c. Administer lotions and creams using cotton swabs, tongue blades, or the nurse's gloved hands.	Gloves help to reduce transmission of microorganisms and protect the caregiver from absorbing the medication through his or her hands. **caREminder** *Do not apply moisturizers or lubricants to an infant or toddler's diaper area. These products may enhance the incidence of skin breakdown by causing the skin to become overhydrated and act as a friction between the diaper and the child's skin.*
6d. If a powder is ordered, sprinkle it over the site. Ensure that the child's head is turned away to avoid inhalation of the powder (see Chapter 34). If a spray is ordered, check with reference source or manufacturer's recommendations; most sprays must be shaken before administration. Spray over the site and ensure that the child's head is turned away to reduce potential of inhalation.	Powders and sprays are easily inhaled, which may cause lung tissue damage or increase absorption through the respiratory system.
6e. Emulsions are often mixed with water (water temperature should be between 98.6° and 113°F[37° and 45°C]) and the area submerged in the liquid for a specific period of time, usually 15 to 20 minutes. Follow time recommendations closely.	Water temperature that is too hot can cause vasodilation and heat injury. Water that is too cold can cause discomfort and chilling. Prolonged exposure can cause vasodilation of the skin or increased absorption of the medication.

Continued

Steps	Rationale/Points of Emphasis
Alert! *Avoid using products with alcohol, perfumes, or dyes in neonates. The newborn's skin is drier than that of an adult but becomes gradually more hydrated as the eccrine glands mature during the first year of life. Routine use of emollients, such as Aquaphor ointment, can prevent excessive dryness, skin cracking, and fissures in premature and full-term infants. However, perfumes and dyes in these substances can be absorbed and are potential contact irritants.*	
6f. Apply transdermal and topical systemic medication patches to a flat area of the skin; they are self-adhesive. Rotate application sites.	Flat areas help the medication remain in contact with the skin, promoting even absorption. Rotation reduces skin irritation. ***Alert!*** *Do not cut medication patches to fit area because this alters the dose administered. Also, do not cut to reduce dose because the medication may not be distributed evenly on the patch, and there is no way to know the amount of medication left on patch.*
7. Apply a dressing over the site if indicated.	A covering prevents the medication from being rubbed off, protecting clothing and site. ***Alert!*** *Occlusive dressings may increase absorption of the medication and should not be used with topical steroids.* **KidKare** Fluffy toys or other objects may stick to the medication site. Toys should either be kept away or the site covered, whichever is appropriate.
8. Remove gloves and perform hand hygiene. Return medication to appropriate storage area.	Reduces transmission of microorganisms. Provides safe storage of medication.

CHILD AND FAMILY EVALUATION AND DOCUMENTATION

- Evaluate child's tolerance of medication, potential side effects, and changes in the skin condition. If there is any worsening in the skin condition or signs of an allergic reaction, notify the primary care provider.
- Monitor young children so that they do not put the medication in their mouth.
- Evaluate child and family's understanding of medication's effects.
- Document the following:
  - Type of medication
  - Dose
  - Site given (location on skin)
  - Date and time given
  - Condition of the skin
  - Presence and absence of adverse effects
  - Child's response to and tolerance of procedure
  - Teaching and information given to child and parent

COMMUNITY CARE

- If topical medications are to be given in the home, teach the family the following:
  - Technique to administer medication
  - Signs of adverse reaction
  - Storage of medication
  - Disposal of used medication, particularly patches that should be folded over so that adhesive seals together and contains any unused medication.
- If topical medications are to be given in the home, ensure that family has
  - Nonsterile gloves
  - Refrigeration (if needed to store medication)
  - Healthcare prescriber consent if child is also to be given medication at school

- Identify problems that may prevent the child from obtaining the medications (e.g., inability to pay for medications). Assist family to resolve identified problems or refer to social services (e.g., apply for public health insurance [Medicaid]).
- Ensure that all medications have childproof caps and are kept beyond reach of children and pets.
- Advise family members of guidelines regarding when they can still give medication if they forget to give a dose, to not give two doses together, and to call the physician or pharmacist if they have questions about dosing.
- Encourage selection of medications that can be given in the fewest number of doses per day to decrease potential of missed doses.
- Instruct the family to contact the healthcare provider if
  - Child's skin condition does not show improvement
  - Child develops denuded areas, secondary rash, or other irritation from medication
  - Child shows signs of systemic illness

Unexpected Situations

- *The child is found sucking on the area where medication was applied:* Manually remove any medication present and rinse the child's mouth out with water. Notify healthcare prescriber immediately. If the child is in a community setting, instruct parents or caregiver to call Poison Control.
- *The child's skin under a transdermal patch is noted to be swollen and erythematous when the patch is removed:* Wash skin with soap and water and reassess child's history for latex or adhesive allergies. Notify the healthcare prescriber before applying new patch.

Bibliography

American Academy of Pediatrics, Committee on Drugs. (1997). Alternative routes of drug administration: Advantages and disadvantages [subject review]. *Pediatrics, 100,* 143–152.

Howard, R. (2001). The appropriate use of topical antimicrobials and antiseptics in children. *Pediatric Annals, 30,* 219–224.

Lund, C., Kuller, J., Lane, A., Lott, J., & Raines, D. (1999). Neonatal skin care: The scientific basis for practice. *Journal of Obstetric, Gynecologic, and Neonatal Nursing, 28,* 241–254.

Orchard, D., & Weston, W. L. (2001). The importance of vehicle in pediatric topical therapy. *Pediatric Annals, 30,* 208–210.

Rudy, S. J., & Parham-Vetter, P. C. (2003). Percutaneous absorption of topically applied medication. *Dermatology Nursing, 15,* 145–152.

Yosipovitch, G., Maayan-Metzger, A., Merlob, P., & Sirota, L. (2000). Skin barrier properties in different body areas in neonates. *Pediatrics, 106,* 105–108.

CHAPTER

76

Nasotracheal Suctioning

CLINICAL GUIDELINES

- A registered nurse (RN), licensed practical nurse (LPN), or respiratory therapist may perform nasotracheal suctioning.

Alert! *Delegation of the skill of nasotracheal suctioning by the RN to the LPN may not be permissible according to the particular state's scope of nursing practice due to the assessment component required to initiate this procedure.*

- Nasotracheal suctioning is implemented to remove secretions obstructing the trachea and nasopharyngeal airway that cannot be removed by the child's spontaneous cough or less invasive procedures, to obtain secretions for diagnostic purposes, or to prevent infection that can occur from accumulated secretions.
- The care provider uses valid assessment findings (dyspnea, poor skin color, decreased SaO_2 levels, visible or audible secretions, restlessness) to determine the need for nasotracheal suctioning. The care provider is familiar with the potential risks associated with nasotracheal suctioning (Chart 76-1).
- Although the upper airways (oropharynx and nasopharynx) are not a sterile environment, it is recommended to use sterile technique for all suctioning to avoid introducing pathogens into the airways.
- The appropriate subatmospheric pressures to use when suctioning are
  - Neonates: 60–80 mm Hg
  - Infants: 80–100 mm Hg
  - Children: 100–120 mm Hg
  - Adults: 100–150 mm Hg

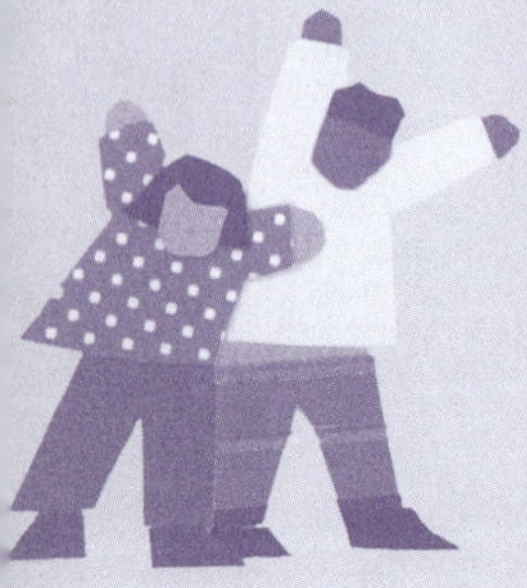

EQUIPMENT

- Portable or wall suction machine with tubing and collection container
- Receiving blanket
- Towel or disposable waterproof pad
- Appropriate-sized sterile suction catheter (the catheter diameter should not exceed half the diameter of the airway)

Age	Catheter Size
Neonate to 18 months	5 to 8 French
18 months to 7 years	8 to 10 French
7 to 10 years	10 to 14 French
11 years to adult	12 to 16 French

- Sterile container for sterile fluids used to lubricate and clear catheter
- Water-soluble lubricant and/or normal saline
- Sterile gloves
- Eye shields/goggles as indicated
- Sterile water

CHART 76-1 COMPLICATIONS OF NASOTRACHEAL SUCTIONING

Trauma to the mucosa
Cardiac dysrhythmias
Changes in heart rate (bradycardia, tachycardia)
Changes in blood pressure (increase or decrease)
Respiratory distress (hypoxia, hypoxemia, respiratory arrest)
Uncontrolled coughing
Gagging/vomiting
Discomfort and pain
Increased intracranial pressure
Nosocomial infection

CHILD AND FAMILY ASSESSMENT AND PREPARATION

- Assess the child's respiratory status. Determine the need for suctioning based on clinical findings:
  - Breath sounds
  - Skin color
  - Breathing pattern and rate
  - Pulse rate, dysrhythmias
  - Color, consistency, and volume of secretions
  - Presence of bleeding or evidence of physical trauma
  - Cough
  - Oxygenation (pulse oximetry)
  - Arterial blood gas (if available)
  - Laryngospasm
- Assess the child or family's readiness to learn.
- Determine whether the child or family understands the procedure and its significance. Explain in age-appropriate terms to the child that suctioning will relieve breathing difficulty but that it will be uncomfortable and might cause him or her to cough, gag, or sneeze.
- Use a doll and a suction catheter in therapeutic play to demonstrate suctioning to the toddler, preschool-aged, or school-aged child to facilitate his or her understanding. A child life specialist can be used to assist in this therapeutic play.

KidKare Encourage a parent to stay with child during the procedure to minimize the child's stress. If no parent is available, elicit assistance from another staff member.

PROCEDURE Nasotracheal Suctioning

Steps	Rationale/Points of Emphasis
1. Gather the necessary supplies and equipment and check for proper functioning.	Promotes efficient time management and provides an organized approach to the procedure. Properly functioning equipment and supplies are needed for beneficial results.
2. Place the supplies on a bedside table, turn on the portable or wall suction apparatus, and set the pressure gauge to the appropriate range.	Appropriate suction pressure decreases the chance of mucosal irritation and damage, hypoxemia, and atelectasis.
3. Perform hand hygiene and don personal protective gear.	Reduces the transmission of microorganisms and maintains standard precautions. **Alert!** *Contact and airborne precautions must be used for children with respiratory illnesses such as respiratory syncytial virus (RSV).*

Continued

Steps	Rationale/Points of Emphasis
4a. Assist the conscious child to assume a semi-Fowler's position. For an infant, place a folded receiving blanket or roll under the shoulders. Place the head in the midline position. Place the unconscious child in the lateral position, facing the person performing the suctioning.	These positions facilitate coughing and the insertion of the catheter in the conscious child. For the unconscious child, the lateral position facilitates drainage of secretions from the pharynx. It also helps to prevent aspiration. **KidKare** An infant may be swaddled with slightly flexed extremities to provide comfort and assist in the procedure. If remaining present for procedure, position parent at head of bed to keep them within immediate eyesight of their child.
4b. Plan method to keep child from touching sterile catheter, such as distraction, swaddling, or obtaining assistance from parent or other staff.	Maintains sterility and prevents introduction of microorganisms.
5. Place a towel or disposable waterproof pad on the child's chest.	Protects the child's clothing.
6a. Aseptically open sterile suction kit or equipment, using the inside of the wrapping as a sterile field. 6b. Set up the sterile cup or container, touching only the outside, and pour sterile water or saline into it, making sure the top of the bottle does not touch the inside of the container. 6c. Open lubricant and squeeze onto the sterile field.	Maintains sterility. The inside of the container is considered to be sterile, and your hands are contaminated. The water is used to clear the catheter of secretions. The lubricant is used to lubricate the catheter, allowing for easier passage, causing less trauma to the nasal mucosa.
7. Don sterile gloves. The dominant hand must remain sterile, and the nondominant hand is considered clean rather than sterile.	The sterile gloved hand maintains sterility of the catheter, and the unsterile hand maintains standard precautions.
8. With the sterile gloved (dominant) hand, pick up suction catheter, being careful to avoid touching nonsterile surfaces. With the clean (nondominant) glove, pick up the connecting tubing and secure it to the catheter.	Maintains catheter sterility. The nondominant hand controls all nonsterile equipment.
9. Check equipment for proper functioning by placing the catheter in the container of solution while holding a sterile gloved finger or thumb over the port of suction catheter to create suction.	Ensures equipment function. Checks for catheter patency.
10. Make an approximate measure of the depth for the insertion of the catheter by measuring the distance from the tragus of the child's ear to tip of the nose. Mark the position on the tube by placing the sterile gloved forefinger and thumb at that point on the catheter.	Ensures proper length of catheter to be inserted for nasotracheal suctioning to prevent airway trauma or vagal stimulation.
11. Reassure the child before initiating the procedure. If possible, encourage the child to cough.	Decreases stress. Coughing helps to pool secretions.
12. Dip the catheter tip into the lubricant.	Reduces friction and facilitates insertion of the catheter.
13. Holding the tip of the catheter between the index finger and thumb of the sterile gloved hand, wrap the rest of the catheter around the sterile hand.	Decreases the potential for contamination of the catheter.
14. Without applying suction, gently insert the premeasured catheter into either naris along the nasal septum and advance caudally along the floor of the nasal cavity (Figure 76-1).	Applying suction during catheter passage can cause hypoxia and tissue damage. Advancing the catheter along the floor of the nasal cavity avoids the nasal turbinates, which are easily ruptured and bleed.

Steps	Rationale/Points of Emphasis

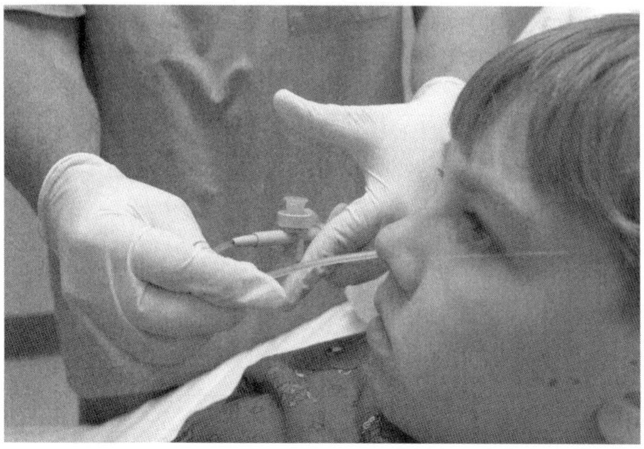

FIGURE 76-1
Suction is not applied while the catheter is gently being inserted into the nares.

Alert! *Use gentle touch because bradycardia may occur as a result of vagal stimulation at the posterior oropharynx with vigorous suctioning.*

caREminder

Never force the catheter if resistance is met; simply remove the catheter and attempt passage through the other naris.

Steps	Rationale/Points of Emphasis
15. Apply suction intermittently by occluding the suction control port with the sterile gloved thumb, removing thumb intermittently, and gently rotating the catheter as it is being withdrawn from the naris. Duration of suctioning should be limited to no more than 15 seconds (Figure 76-2).	Removes secretions. Gentle rotation of the catheter and applying intermittent suction ensures that all surfaces are being reached, avoids tissue trauma to any one area, and prevents hypoxia.

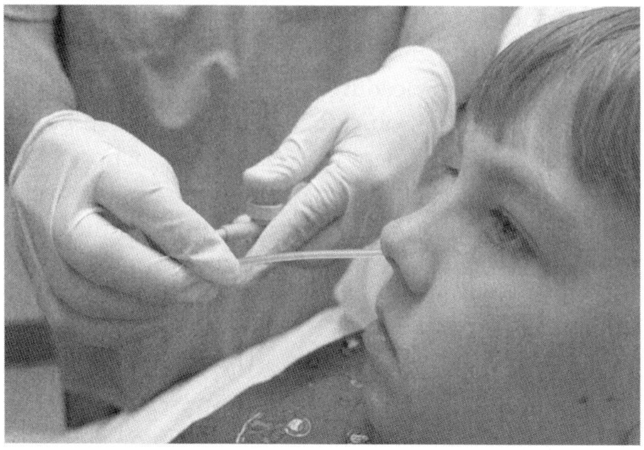

FIGURE 76-2
During the suctioning process, suction is applied intermittently. The duration of suctioning should be limited to no more than 15 seconds.

Steps	Rationale/Points of Emphasis
16. Irrigate the catheter with the sterile water or saline after each suction pass.	Cleans the catheter of occluding secretions.
17. Relubricate the catheter and repeat suctioning as needed or as tolerated by the child, allowing a 20- to 30-second interval between each suctioning. The nares should be alternated if possible when repeated suctioning is required.	Applying suction for prolonged periods can cause secretions to increase and can decrease the oxygen supply. Alternating the nares can help reduce tissue trauma.
18. Assess the child for color, respiratory rate and effort, and Sao_2 levels (if monitored) during suctioning.	Determines adequacy of oxygenation.
19. Gently clean around the child's nares once all suctioning has been completed.	Mucus accumulated around the nares is irritating to the mucous membranes and unpleasant for the child.

Continued

Steps	Rationale/Points of Emphasis
20. When suctioning is completed, remove gloves inside out. Dispose of gloves, suction catheter, and solution container in proper receptacle. Perform hand hygiene.	Standard precautions. Reduces transmission of microorganisms.
21. Praise child for assistance in procedure and provide comfort. **KidKare** Further praise and encouragement to the child for his or her cooperation during this procedure can be implemented by using a reward chart, stickers, or prizes from a treasure box.	Minimizes stress. Provides child with positive feedback.
22. Auscultate child's breath sounds; assess color, secretions, Sao_2 level, dyspnea, and level of anxiety.	Evaluates effectiveness of suctioning.

CHILD AND FAMILY EVALUATION AND DOCUMENTATION

- Evaluate the child's or parents' response to the procedure and reaffirm the reason why the procedure was necessary.

caREminder

Improved blood gas data or pulse oximetry can be used to evaluate the effectiveness of the procedure.

- Document the following
  - Presuctioning assessment findings, including the clinical indicators assessed validating the need for nasotracheal suctioning.
  - Completion of the procedure to include
    - The amount, color, consistency, and odor of secretions obtained
    - Size of catheter used
    - Number of passes of the suction catheter
    - Any difficulties during suctioning, including difficulty passing the catheter in either of the nares
    - Condition of the nares and surrounding skin
    - Nursing interventions used if difficulties in procedure were encountered
    - Tolerance of the suctioning procedure, including any unexpected outcomes during or after the procedure with the appropriate nursing interventions implemented
  - Postsuctioning assessment findings to summarize effectiveness of the procedure.

COMMUNITY CARE

- If a child needs nasotracheal suctioning in the home setting, the parent must be instructed and evaluated for proficiency in performing the procedure before the child's discharge. Home care instructions must also include
  - Basic oxygenation assessment skills
  - Handwashing techniques
  - Storage of materials
  - Contacts of vendors to obtain supplies
- Suctioning in the home setting is considered a clean, not a sterile, procedure.
- A 60-mL irrigation catheter-tip syringe can be used if suctioning equipment is unavailable to suction the nares. The syringe can be carried at all times by the parent in a plastic bag for emergency use outside of the home.
- Instruct parents to keep the suction machine readily available in the home so that it can be quickly reached and connected.
- Instruct the family to contact the healthcare provider if
  - Child experiences bleeding from the nares that cannot be easily stopped after suctioning
  - Child experiences apnea or any degree of cyanosis during the procedure

Alert! *It is a medical emergency if child experiences severe apnea or cyanosis during the procedure and does not quickly return to baseline color, with good respiratory effort present. If the child is in respiratory or cardiac distress, emergency services should be contacted immediately.*

Unexpected Situations

Nasotracheal suctioning should be considered a blind high-risk procedure with at times unpredictable outcomes. Potential complications that must be assessed for during the procedure include

- *Bradycardia; dysrhythmias with possible hypotension:* Nasotracheal suctioning can produce a vagal stimulus, causing the heart rate to drop precipitously. The vagal response in children is stronger than that found in adults. Anxiety to the child can result in brief episodes of tachycardia during the procedure.

- *Hypoxia; bronchospasm; laryngospasm; mechanical trauma to airway; risk for infection:* Suctioning passes that are too long in duration could cause hypoxia, irritation to the airway and to the child, and may cause upper or lower airway to spasm. The suction catheter is a foreign body, and introduction of any foreign body into the airway carries a risk for infection as well as mechanical trauma to friable mucosa lining the airway.
- *Increased blood pressure; vomiting; increased intracranial pressure and emotional distress:* If increasing intracranial pressure is a concern, nasotracheal suctioning should only be undertaken if the airway is at risk for obstruction. Suctioning in itself causes increasing blood pressure and increasing intracranial pressure. Vomiting can be induced by the catheter stimulating the gag reflex, further increasing intracranial pressure and presenting a risk for aspiration.

Bibliography

American Association of Respiratory Care. (2004). Nasotracheal suctioning. *Respiratory Care, 49*(9), 1080–1084.

Czarnecki, M. L., & Kaucic, C. L. (1999). Infant nasal-pharyngeal suctioning: Is it beneficial? *Pediatric Nursing, 25*(2), 193–196, 218.

Vain, N. E., Szyld, E. G., Prudent, L. M., et al. (2004). Oropharyngeal and nasotracheal suctioning of meconium-stained neonates before delivery of their shoulders: Multicentre, randomized controlled trial. *The Lancet, 364*, 597–602.

CHAPTER 77

Neurologic Assessment

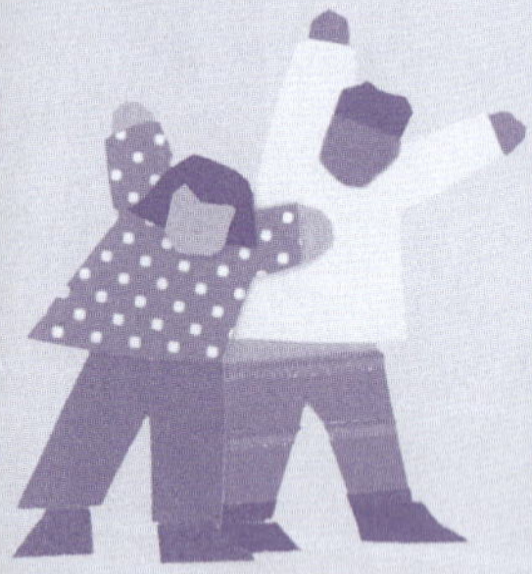

Clinical Guidelines

- The physician, registered nurse (RN), or licensed practical nurse (LPN) performs the neurologic assessment.
- Neurologic status is assessed on admission of all children to an acute care setting as part of the initial physical assessment. The thoroughness of the examination is determined by the child's diagnosis, acuity level, and ability to participate in the examination.
- Neurologic assessments are included in all well-child examinations.
- A comprehensive neurologic examination is presented below. An acute neurologic check should be performed at regularly scheduled intervals for children with known or suspected brain injury, intracranial bleeding, intracranial tumors, or neurologic condition (e.g., meningitis, encephalitis) or after the child has had cranial surgery. Components of an acute neurologic check include level of consciousness (orientation and cognition), pupillary signs (size, reactivity to light, equality of reaction), and motor tone and strength (hand grasps, pronator drift, leg movement, motor strength of extremities).

Equipment

- Measuring tape
- Penlight
- Reflex hammer
- Blunt-tip needle
- Cotton swab
- Children's play materials (e.g., crayons, paper, blocks, colorful pictures, books, ball, Play-Doh)
- Common scents (e.g., peanut butter, peppermint, orange, vanilla)
- Vision chart
- Flavors (salt, sugar, lemon)
- Tongue blade
- O-shaped cereal

Child and Family Assessment and Preparation

- Assess child's previous neurologic, general health, nutritional, and developmental history.
- Assess child's and family's understanding of current health status.
- Explain the procedure and purpose of the neurologic examination to the child and family.
- Review results of child's last neurologic assessment to provide baseline data.
- Review child's medical diagnosis, health history, and developmental history to determine whether any neurologic changes may be consistent with current health problems or medical history.

PROCEDURE Comprehensive Neurologic Assessment

Steps	Rationale/Points of Emphasis
1. Perform hand hygiene	Reduces transmission of microorganisms.
2. Observe child at rest, noting behavior, mood, response to surroundings, and movements.	Initial baseline data of assessment can be gathered through observing child in usual state of play or rest.
3. Assess level of consciousness, noting stimulus needed to elicit arousal, quality of response to stimuli (e.g., eye opening, appropriate verbalization, lack of verbalization), and length of response time (Tables 77-1 and 77-2).	Determines child's current state of responsiveness. **caREminder** *Use of the modified Glasgow coma scale assists in age-specific detailed notation of level of consciousness (see Tables 77-1 and 77-2).*
4. Measure and graph head circumference (see Chapter 44).	Notes child's head growth compared with standardized norms and, most importantly, tracks child's own growth trajectory over time.
5. Inspect child's cranial shape for symmetry and palpate fontanels to assess whether they are open; note if sunken or bulging.	Detects outward signs of neurologic abnormalities. The child's cranial shape should be symmetric, without areas of bogginess or edema. The anterior fontanel is normally closed by 2 years of age. Normally, an open fontanel is slightly depressed, with minimal arterial pulsations detected.
6. Inspect child's skin, noting neurocutaneous findings such as café-au-lait spots, hemangiomas, nonpigmented areas, hairy patches, sacral dimples, or spine curvature.	Neurocutaneous findings may provide clues to neurologic abnormalities.

TABLE 77-1
Pediatric Coma Scale

	Score	Older Than 1 Year of Age	Younger Than 1 Year of Age
Eyes opening	4	Spontaneously	Spontaneously
	3	To verbal command	To verbal stimuli
	2	To pain	To pain
	1	No response	No response
Best motor response	6	Obeys	Localizes pain
	5	Localizes pain	Flexion withdrawal
	4	Flexion withdrawal (decorticate rigidity)	Flexion—abnormal (decorticate rigidity)
	2	Extension (decerebrate rigidity)	Extension (decerebrate rigidity)
	1	No response	No response
	Score	**Older Than 5 Years of Age**	**2–5 Years of Age**
Best verbal response	5	Oriented and converses	Appropriate word phrases
	4	Disoriented and talks	Inappropriate words
	3	Inappropriate words	Cries and/or screams
	2	Incomprehensible sounds	Grunts
	1	No response	No response
Total	3–15		

TABLE 77-2

Glasgow Coma Scale: Verbal Responses of Infants

Score Given	Response
1 month	None
1	
2	
3	
4	
5	
2 months	
1	None
2	Crying to stimuli
3	Shuts eyes to light
4	Smiles when caressed
5	Babbles single-vowel sounds
3 months	
1	None
2	Crying to stimuli (moans)
3	Stares at response and looks at environment
4	Smiles to sound stimulation
5	Chuckles vowels in prolonged manner
4 months	
1	None
2	Crying to stimuli (moans)
3	Turns head to sound
4	Smiles spontaneously or laughs when socially stimulated
5	Modulating voice and perfect vocalization of vowels
5 and 6 months	
1	None
2	Crying to stimuli (moans)
3	Localizes general direction of sound
4	Discrimination of family members
5	Babbles to people, toys
7 and 8 months	
1	None
2	Crying to stimuli (moans)
3	Recognizes familiar voices and family
4	Babbles
5	"Ba," "Ma," "Da"
9 and 10 months	
1	None
2	Crying to stimuli
3	Recognizes (smiles or laughs)
4	Babbles
5	"Mama" and "Dada"
10 months to 1 year	
1	None
2	Crying to stimuli
3	Recognizes (smiles)
4	Babbles
5	Words (especially "Mama" and "Dada")

Courtesy of Dr. Kenneth Shapiro.
From Zimmerman, S. S., & Gildea, J. H. (1985). *Critical care pediatrics.* Philadelphia: W. B. Saunders. Used with permission.

PROCEDURE Cranial Nerve Assessment

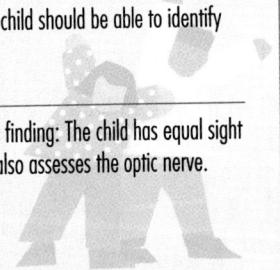

Steps	Rationale/Points of Emphasis
1. Have child close eyes and then smell and identify various common scents (e.g., peanut butter, peppermint, orange, vanilla), if available, with one nostril at a time.	Assesses cranial nerve I (olfactory nerve). The child should be able to identify common scents.
2. Stand in front of the child with your face at the same level as child's face. Ask child to look at your nose while you move your hands around the peripheral vision visual fields. Wiggle one finger at a time and ask child to point to the hand that had the wiggling finger while continuing to look at examiner's nose. To test visual fields in a younger child, have child sit on the parent's lap with attention drawn to an object in front of child. Move another object from behind the child to side of child's head and note when the child's attention is drawn to the new object.	Assesses cranial nerve II (optic nerve). Normal finding: The child has equal sight in peripheral fields. Funduscopic examination also assesses the optic nerve.
3. Test visual acuity if a vision chart is available (see Chapter 128). Ask the child to look at colorful pictures and identify objects or read words from a favorite book. Note whether infant tracks and observes faces and reaches for toys.	Assesses cranial nerve II (optic nerve). At birth, infants see best at a distance of 8 to 12 inches. Toddlers are far-sighted, normally reaching 20/20 acuity by 4 years of age.

Steps	Rationale/Points of Emphasis
4. Using a penlight, check pupil size, noting reactivity to light and symmetry. There should be prompt constriction of the pupils after application of a bright light stimulus. Note response as nonreactive, brisk, or sluggish.	Assesses cranial nerve III (oculomotor nerve).
5. Using a bright object or light, ask the child to follow with eyes only, moving object in front of face past outer border of each eye, past outer corner of each brow, over forehead, over chin, in front of each ear, and in toward the tip of child's nose.	Assesses cranial nerves III, IV, and VI (oculomotor, trochlear, and abducens nerves). Child should have full and symmetric eye movements without nystagmus to six cardinal positions of gaze.
6. Ask the child to bite down hard on tongue blade and then open jaw while the examiner palpates jaw and temporal muscles for strength and symmetry.	Assesses cranial nerve V (trigeminal nerve) motor function. Equal muscle symmetry should be noted bilaterally.
7. Ask the child to close eyes and then touch the child's cheeks and chin with a cotton swab. Ask child to tell you where he or she feels the cotton swab.	Assesses cranial nerve V (trigeminal nerve) sensory function. Child should be able to detect light touch in mandibular and maxillary regions.
8. Ask the child to smile showing teeth, puff out cheeks, shut eyes tightly and open, and raise eyebrows. For an infant, observe for facial symmetry when crying.	Assesses cranial nerve VII (facial nerve) motor function. Normal finding: The face at rest and with expression is symmetric.
9. Ask the child to identify common tastes (e.g., sugar, salt, and lemon), if available, by placing them with an applicator on various locations of the tongue.	Assesses cranial nerves VII and IX (glossopharyngeal) sensory function. Tastes on the anterior two thirds of the tongue evaluate the facial nerve; tastes on the posterior tongue evaluate the glossopharyngeal nerve. The child should be able to identify common tastes.
10. Clap hands from behind infant (not next to ear so air movement is felt) and observe reaction or whisper without older child able to see your lips moving. Ask child to repeat a whispered number or letter.	Assesses cranial nerve VII (auditory or vestibular nerve). Very young infant should startle or respond to sudden noise and, as older, turn toward noise. Older children should respond to whispered request.
11. Assess the child's ability to swallow.	Assesses cranial nerve IX (glossopharyngeal) motor function. Child should demonstrate effective swallow. Child should not choke on solids, liquids, or saliva.
12. Ask the child to open mouth and say "ahhh," noting elevation of uvula and soft palate.	Assesses cranial nerve X (vagus nerve). Uvula and tongue should lay midline. The soft palate normally elevates when the child says "ahhh."
13. Elicit gag reflex by placing tongue blade on posterior palate.	Assesses cranial nerve X (vagus nerve). Gag reflex should be elicited with tongue blade placed at posterior portion of tongue.
14. Ask the child to shrug shoulders while you place hand pressure on shoulders, noting strength and symmetry of movement.	Assesses cranial nerve XI (spinal accessory nerve). Child should be able to equally raise shoulders.
15. Ask the child to turn head side to side while you place your hand alongside child's face to resist this movement.	Assesses cranial nerve XI (spinal accessory nerve). Child should exhibit equal bilateral effort to turn head side to side.
16. Ask the child to stick out tongue and move it in all directions. Place a tongue blade against the side of the child's tongue and ask the child to move it away.	Assesses cranial nerve XII (hypoglossal nerve). Tongue protrusion should be midline, without deviation, and child should be able to move tongue easily from side to side.

PROCEDURE Motor Assessment

Steps	Rationale/Points of Emphasis
1. In infants, note spontaneous movements.	Infants should demonstrate spontaneous and equal movements of extremities.
2. Assess infant reflexes (Table 77-3).	Assesses infant motor and sensory function.

Continued

TABLE 77-3

Assessment of Infant Reflexes

Reflex	How to Test	Usual Response	Abnormal Findings
Newborn reflexes			
Babinski's sign	Stroke sole of foot along lateral edge from heel upward.	Toes fan, dorsiflexion of big toe.	Persistence beyond age 24 months
Crawling	Place infant on abdomen.	Crawling movements with arms and legs.	Asymmetric movements
Dance or stepping	Hold infant with feet lightly touching firm surface.	Feet move up and down.	Persistence beyond age 4–8 weeks
Extrusion	Touch tip of infant's tongue.	Tongue extends out.	Persistence beyond age 4 months
Galant's	Stroke lateral side of spine from shoulder to buttocks.	Back moves to side being stroked.	Persistence beyond age 4–8 weeks
Moro's	Place infant in semiupright position; let head fall backward with immediate resupport with the examiner's hands.	Symmetric abduction and extension of arms, flexion of thumb, followed by flexion and adduction of upper limbs.	Persistence beyond age 4 months; asymmetric or absent response
Palmar grasp	Place finger or object in infant's open palm.	Infant's fingers curve around finger or object and resist its removal.	Absence, or persistence beyond age 10 months
Rooting	Stroke corner of infant's mouth.	Infant opens mouth and turns head to side being stroked.	Absence or depressed; disappears by age 3–4 months when awake
Startle	Clap hands loudly.	Infant extends and flexes arms quickly.	Absence, or persistence beyond age 4 months
Sucking	Place nipple 3–4 cm into the infant's mouth.	Infant begins sucking.	Absence or depressed; disappears at age 3–4 months when awake
Later reflexes			
Parachute	Suspend the infant by the trunk and suddenly flex body forward.	Infant spontaneously extends arms, hands, and fingers.	Normally appears by 6–8 months; remains throughout life
Tonic neck	Turn infant's head quickly to one side when supine.	Extension of arm and leg on side that head turned with flexion in opposite limbs	If locked in the "fencer's position," normal from age 2–6 months

Steps	Rationale/Points of Emphasis
3. Ask child to squeeze your fingers or ask child to mold Play-Doh.	Assesses grip strength. Individual muscle strength (grip, biceps, triceps, quadriceps, gastrocnemius, and tibial-radialis) assessment findings are generally graded from 0 to 5: *0—No movement (no muscle contraction)* *1—Flicker or trace of muscle contraction* *2—Active movement with gravity eliminated (i.e., movement with examiner supporting the body part being assessed)* *3—Active movement against gravity* *4—Active movement against gravity plus resistance* *5—Normal power of movement* **caREminder** *All testing of muscle strength should be conducted bilaterally, noting symmetry.*

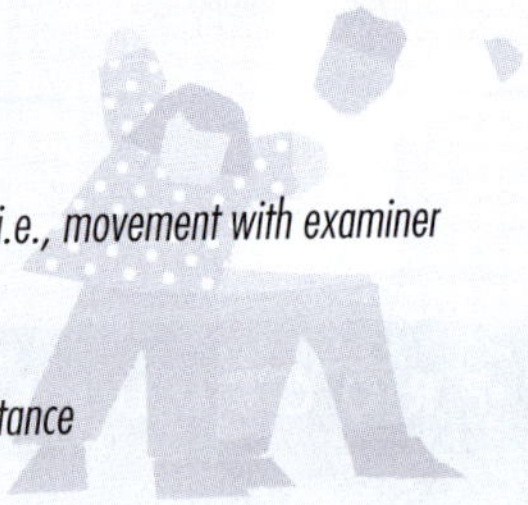

Steps	Rationale/Points of Emphasis
4. Ask the child to "make muscles" by bending arms at elbows with palms of hands facing body and resist your attempt to straighten arm.	Assesses biceps strength.
5. Ask the child to extend arms straight out in front of body and resist your attempt to bend arm.	Assesses triceps strength.
6. While child is seated with legs dangling over edge of bed or table, ask the child to extend each leg straight and resist your attempt to bend leg.	Assesses quadriceps strength.
7. Ask the child to press sole of foot against your hand, to "step on the gas."	Assesses gastrocnemius strength.
8. Ask the child to bend toes up toward his or her face while you place your hand on top of foot.	Assesses tibial-radialis strength.
9. Passively move the child's extremities, noting tone and ease of movement.	Detects spasticity. Movement should be smooth and joints flexible.
10. Lift smaller child under armpits and note child's ability to lock shoulders and prevent slip-through.	Assesses proximal strength. Child should exhibit equal bilateral shoulder strength, preventing slip-through from examiner's hands.
11. Ask the child to lie supine on floor and then rise quickly to standing position.	Assesses proximal strength. Child should be able to rise easily without pushing off from furniture, floor, or self.
12. Ask the child to sit on stool or chair and rise to standing position, keeping arms crossed in front of chest.	Assesses proximal strength. Child should be able to stand without use of arms to push against furniture, floor, or self.
13. Ask the child to draw a picture and build a tower of blocks.	Assesses fine motor dexterity. Child should demonstrate age-appropriate accuracy of fine motor movements: for example, building a tower of blocks (tower of three to four blocks by age 18 months; tower of six to seven blocks by age 24 months; tower of eight blocks or more by age 30 months) and drawing pictures (scribbles spontaneously by age 15 months; imitates circular stroke and vertical line by age 24 months; copies circle and imitates cross by end of age 36 months).
14. Ask the child to pick up a small object, such as a piece of cereal (e.g., Cheerios) or a raisin, observing finger and hand movements bilaterally.	Assesses fine motor dexterity. Children older than the age of about 9 months should demonstrate a pincer grasp using the thumb and pointer finger.
15. With arm lifted away from body, ask the child to quickly press thumb and pointer finger together and apart repeatedly and then have the child use thumb to alternately touch each finger on same hand. Observe movements of one hand and then the other.	Assesses fine motor coordination. Child should exhibit manual dexterity by age 3 years and equal coordination bilaterally.

PROCEDURE Cerebellar Assessment

Steps	Rationale/Points of Emphasis
1. Ask the child to walk, run, hop, skip, and walk heel-to-toe. Techniques to elicit actions include rolling a ball along the floor and asking a young child to go get it or having a child run to try and catch his or her parent.	Assesses balance and coordination. Child should demonstrate age-appropriate gross motor skills that are well balanced.
2. Ask the child to use pointer finger to touch his or her nose, alternately touching your pointer finger in various locations near child's body, noting tremor or past-pointing.	Assesses coordination and sense of body in space. Tremor noted as the child's finger approaches the target may indicate cerebellar dysfunction.
3. To assess Romberg's sign, ask the child to stand with feet together, arms at sides and eyes closed, "like a soldier."	Assesses balance. Child should not lean or fall over.

PROCEDURE Sensory Assessment

Steps	Rationale/Points of Emphasis
1. Follow steps 1, 3, 7, 9, and 10 of the procedure for Cranial Nerve Assessment, above.	Assesses central sensory pathways.
2. Ask an older child to close eyes and identify whether touches are sharp or soft when you use a blunt-tip needle or cotton swab to gently touch various locations on all four extremities.	Assesses pain sensations (anterior and lateral spinothalamic tracts) and light touch sensation (anterior and lateral spinothalamic tracts and posterior columns). Child should be able to discriminate between sharp and soft touches to extremities. Sensation should be equal bilaterally.

PROCEDURE Reflex Assessment

Steps	Rationale/Points of Emphasis
1. Flex the child's forearm, place your thumb over child's antecubital space, and tap with reflex hammer. Deep tendon reflex response is typically graded using a four point scale: *0—No response* *1—Diminished response* *2—Average response* *3—Brisker than average response* *4—Hyperactive (very brisk)*	Assesses biceps tendon reflex. There should be slight flexion of the arm when the tendon is tapped.
2. Abduct the child's arm and support forearm with your hand (forearm hangs free), or hold child's wrist over his or her chest to flex arm at elbow. Tap directly above elbow.	Assesses triceps reflex. There should be partial extension of the forearm when tendon is tapped.
3. Place the child's arm and hand in relaxed position with arm flexed and palm down. Tap the radius about 1 inch (2.5 cm) above wrist.	Assesses brachioradialis tendon reflex. There should be flexion of the forearm and upward turn of the palm when the tendon is tapped.
4. With the child sitting on edge of table or bed with legs dangling, use reflex hammer to tap front outer aspect of child's knee, midline, just below the patella (Figure 77-1).	Assesses quadriceps (patellar) reflex. There should be partial extension of the lower leg when the tendon is tapped.

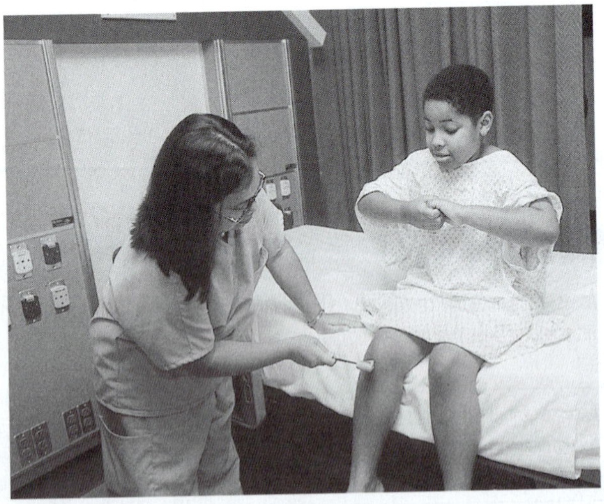

FIGURE 77-1
Use the reflex hammer to tap the front outer aspect of the child's knee just below the kneecap to elicit the reflex.

KidKare To facilitate evaluation of deep tendon reflexes in a child's lower extremities, distract the child by having him or her lock fingers together and then try to pull his or her hands apart.

Steps	Rationale/Points of Emphasis
5. Assist the child to a seated position on the edge of a table or bed. The child's legs should dangle freely over the edge. Support child's foot at a 90-degree angle and use reflex hammer to tap back of child's heel. If child is in supine position, flex one leg at knee and hip, supporting the lower portion of that leg on the opposite shin. Lightly support foot in your hand in dorsiflexion and tap Achilles' tendon.	Assesses Achilles' tendon reflex. Plantar flexion of the foot should occur when the tendon is tapped.
6. Stroke the outer sole of the child's foot from heel to toes with the handle of reflex hammer and note movement of toes. In children older than 2 years of age, the toes should flex downward. Upward movement of the big toe with other toes fanning outward is called Babinski's sign.	A positive Babinski's sign in children older than 2 years of age may indicate upper motor neuron abnormality.
7. With the child lying supine, lift child's leg with flexion of knee and hip. Note any pain or resistance (Kernig's sign).	Pain may be indicative of spinal abnormality.
8. With child lying supine, flex child's neck. Note pain or involuntary flexion of the child's knees or hips (Brudzinski's sign).	Pain may be indicative of meningeal irritation.
9. With the child lying supine, stroke abdominal skin in all four quadrants by moving handle of reflex hammer from the side toward the midline.	Assesses superficial abdominal reflex. The umbilicus should move toward the stroking in children older than 6 months of age.
10. Don gloves. With examiner's gloved index finger, gently stroke inner aspect of a male child's thigh.	Reduces transmission of microorganisms. Assesses cremasteric muscle. The testis on the side of the thigh that is stroked should retract into the inguinal canal.
11. With examiner's gloved index finger or cotton swab, gently stroke perianal skin.	Assesses anal reflex. An "anal wink," or brisk contracture of the anal sphincter, should be noted.
12. Remove gloves and perform hand hygiene. Dispose of equipment and waste in appropriate receptacle.	Reduces transmission of microorganisms. Standard precautions.

Child and Family Evaluation and Documentation

- Document all findings of the neurologic assessment in the child's medical record.
- Refer to physician/nurse practitioner if neurologic assessment elicits abnormalities or if there is deterioration/alteration in findings from previous assessment.
- Explain findings and changes in findings to child and parents.
- Evaluate child and family understanding of current health condition and neurologic findings and answer questions.

Community Care

- Assess discharge needs and modifications that may need to be made in the home environment due to any new neurologic deficit or increased risk for injury. Instruct the family to contact the healthcare provider if
  - Child has increased complaints of headaches
  - Change in child's gait is noticed
  - Child experiences blurred vision
  - Child experiences a trauma to the head

Unexpected Situation

- *Child loses balance during motor evaluation tests:* Protect child from falling. Ensure that the examination area is unobstructed. Ensure appropriate height of examination table.

Bibliography

Hadders-Algra, M., Mavinkurve-Groothuis, A. M., Groen, S. E., et al. (2004). Quality of general movements and the development of minor neurological dysfunction at toddler and school age. *Clinical Rehabilitation, 18*, 287–299.

Hobdell, E. (2001). Infant neurologic assessment. *Journal of Neuroscience Nursing, 33*, 190–193.

Mercuri, E., Guzzetta, A., Laroche, S., et al. (2003). Neurologic examination of preterm infants at term age: Comparison with term infants. *Journal of Pediatrics, 142*, 647–655.

Orfanelli, L. (2001). Neurologic examination of the toddler: How to assess for increased intracranial pressure following head trauma. *American Journal of Nursing, 101*, 24CC–24FF.

Zafeiriou, D. L. (2004). Primitive reflexes and postural reactions in the neurodevelopmental examination. *Pediatric Neurology, 31*, 1–8.

CHAPTER

78

Newborn Care: Immediate Needs of the Stable Newborn

Clinical Guidelines

- Care of the stable newborn is delivered in the room of the recovering mother or in the newborn nursery by the registered nurse (RN) or licensed practical nurse (LPN).
- Apgar scoring is completed at 1 minute and 5 minutes after birth.
- Apical pulse, respiratory rate, and temperature of the stable newborn are assessed every hour for the first 4 hours of life, then every 4 hours for the next 24 hours, and then as ordered.
- Length, weight, and head and chest circumference of the stable newborn are assessed within 2 hours of delivery.
- Weight of the newborn is assessed every 24 hours.
- The newborn's temperature is maintained between 98.2°F and 99.8°F (36.8°C and 37.28°C) axillary. The preterm infant's temperature is maintained between 97.3°F and 98.9°F (36.3°C and 36.9°C).
- Vitamin K is administered intramuscularly to the newborn within 2 hours of delivery.
- Prophylactic eye care is provided to the newborn within 2 hours of delivery.
- Blood glucose is maintained above 40 mg/dL in the newborn.
- The first feeding of the newborn is initiated within 1 to 4 hours of delivery. Breast-feeding should be initiated within the first hour of life.
- Parents demonstrate safe nurturing care of the newborn.
- Infant's cues for care are responded to promptly to facilitate the development of trust.

Equipment

- Identification bands and other security devices per institutional policy
- Ink pad and footprint identification form
- Radiant warmer
- Blankets
- Stockinet cap for infant's head
- Stethoscope
- Thermometer

- Scale
- Tape measure
- Silver nitrate, erythromycin, or tetracycline drops as per institutional policy
- Blood glucose monitoring supplies (see Chapter 19)
- Vitamin K and intramuscular administration supplies (see Chapter 64)
- Bathing supplies (see Chapter 14)
- Formula or breast milk and feeding supplies (see Chapter 43)

CHILD AND FAMILY ASSESSMENT AND PREPARATION

- Explain to parents the immediate care needs of the newborn and all procedures as they are to be performed.
- Involve mother, father, or other care providers in care to be delivered, including first bath and first feeding.
- Ensure Apgar scoring is completed at 1 and 5 minutes after birth. Scoring includes assessment of heart rate, respiratory rate, muscle tone, reflex irritability, and color.

PROCEDURE Infant Identification and Footprinting

Steps	Rationale/Points of Emphasis
1. Apply identification (ID) bands with mother's name and ID number as well as infant's ID number to infant's ankle and wrist before infant leaves the delivery room. Also apply band with infant's number to the mother's wrist. Placement of a similar wristband on the father or significant other should proceed following institutional guidelines. Apply infant security device to infant's ankle per institutional policy, and explain the purpose of the device to parents (see Chapters 85 and 129).	Identifies infant and associates infant with correct mother and father for later ID. Infant security device will stay on the infant's ankle at all times until the nurse takes it off at the time of discharge. The infant security will track the location of the infant for abduction purposes.
2. Once infant is stable, gather footprinting supplies.	Footprinting should be delayed until after infant is stabilized.
3. Press infant's foot firmly to ink pad and then transfer footprint to ID form with firm gentle pressure. The footprints are given to the parents upon discharge.	Provides another means of infant ID.
4. Always check mother's ID band against infant's ID band when bringing infant to mother.	Ensures that correct infant is given to mother. It is unrealistic to expect a newly delivered mother to recognize her newborn.
5. If the newborn must remain hospitalized after maternal discharge, ask the mother to continue to wear her ID band and an ID band matching that of her infant after discharge to ensure that proper identification strategies may be used when she visits her infant.	Allows for accurate mother and infant identification at each visit.

PROCEDURE Thermoregulation

Steps	Rationale/Points of Emphasis
1. Warm the delivery room or nursery. Warm items that will be used in direct infant care, such as blankets, stethoscope, and isolette. **Alert!** *Premature infants are especially vulnerable to hypothermia because of the lack of brown fat stores.*	Prevents newborn hypothermia that may result in increased metabolic needs, apnea, and bradycardia.
2. Perform hand hygiene. Don gloves.	Reduces transmission of microorganisms. Standard precautions.
3. Dry infant immediately after birth.	Prevents unnecessary evaporative heat loss.
4. If possible, keep infant close to mother's body with skin-to-skin contact.	Uses mother's body temperature to warm infant and fosters early maternal–child bonding.

Continued

Steps	Rationale/Points of Emphasis
5. Bundle infant in warmed baby blanket.	Decreases exposure of infant's skin to cooler room temperatures.
6. Cover infant's head with stockinet cap.	Decreases loss of heat through infant's head.
7. Remove gloves and perform hand hygiene.	Reduces transmission of microorganisms.
8. Transport infant in an isolette.	Prevents infant exposure to drafts.
9. If infant's temperature remains unstable, evaluate for possible causes (e.g., hypoglycemia) and keep infant in controlled-temperature environment (isolette) while appropriate actions are taken and until infant's temperature is stable (see Chapters 79 and 135 for further guidelines regarding thermoregulation).	If found, causes of temperature instability should be treated immediately. Infant should be kept in a warm environment. **caREminder** *Instruct others to avoid opening the isolette unnecessarily.*
10. If infant is being warmed using an overhead warmer or isolette, assess infant's temperature every 30 minutes. Once infant's temperature is stable and being maintained in isolette, assess temperature every 1–2 hours.	Ensures that infant's temperature stabilizes without excessive overheating and provides ongoing assessment of temperature stability.

PROCEDURE Monitoring Newborn Vital Signs

Steps	Rationale/Points of Emphasis
1. Monitor infant's color. **Alert!** *Central cyanosis is abnormal and may indicate a respiratory or cardiac problem. Notify healthcare prescriber. Peripheral cyanosis of the hands and feet may normally be present.*	Infant's skin color should be pink and nonmottled. A yellowish color may be indicative of hyperbilirubinemia.
2. Monitor infant's quality of breathing and respiratory rate, counting respirations for a full minute. Use bulb syringe to gently suction airway and remove secretions, if needed. Monitor for signs of respiratory distress.	Infant should have a clear airway with spontaneous respirations. Respirations should be unlabored and without tachypnea, nasal flaring, grunting, retractions, rales, or rhonchi. The normal rate of respiration in the newborn is 30 to 60 breaths/min.
3. Place stethoscope on infant's chest at point of maximum impulse and count infant's heart rate for a full minute, noting irregularities of rhythm and any murmurs.	Infant should have a strong regular heart rate, without murmurs. Many infants have "innocent murmurs"; that is, murmurs with no implication of a pathologic condition or process. All murmurs should be reported to the healthcare prescriber and further assessed to validate the characteristics of the murmur and the degree of further evaluation warranted. The normal heart rate of the newborn is 120 to 160 beats/min.
4. Assess vital signs, including axillary temperature, apical pulse rate, and respirations hourly for the first 4 hours, then once every 4 hours for the next 24 hours, and then as ordered (see Chapters 131, 133, and 134). See Appendix A, Table 2, for normal temperature ranges.	Assesses stability of the infant through adjustment to the extrauterine environment. **caREminder** *Axillary temperature should be obtained in the newborn to avoid possible damage to the rectal mucosa.*

PROCEDURE Assessing Growth Parameters

Steps	Rationale/Points of Emphasis
1. Obtain length, weight, and head and chest circumference of the newborn within 2 hours of birth, after stabilization of temperature (see Chapter 44).	Assesses birth weight, length, and head circumference.
2. Assess infant's weight daily during initial hospital stay.	Assesses weight stability. **caREminder** *An initial weight loss of 5% to 10% during the first few days of life is normal. The infant should be at or above birth weight by the 2-week well-child visit. If initial weight loss is greater than 10%, infant's nutritional and hydration status must be reassessed.*

PROCEDURE Determining Gestational Age of the Newborn

Steps	Rationale/Points of Emphasis
1. Once temperature is stabilized, conduct physical examination, comparing infant findings against the Ballard scale of neuromuscular and physical maturity (Figure 78-1).	The Ballard scale assesses neuromuscular and physical characteristics of the neonate and estimates week of gestational maturity.
2. Once gestational age has been determined, plot the infant's weight, length, and head circumference.	Plotting the infant's size helps determine whether the infant is appropriate for gestational age (AGA), large for gestational age (LGA), or small for gestational age (SGA).

PROCEDURE Prophylactic Eye Care of the Newborn

Steps	Rationale/Points of Emphasis
1. Administer eye care prophylaxis (see Chapter 69) after initial early bonding period between parents and infant.	Eye prophylaxis is delayed until after initial bonding to allow as much initial eye-to-eye interaction between parents and infant as possible. **caREminder** *Eye prophylaxis using silver nitrate drops (one drop of 1% solution to each eye) to prevent gonorrhea ophthalmia or antibiotic drops, such as erythromycin or tetracycline, to prevent chlamydia will be determined by your institution.*
2. Once prophylaxis is administered, monitor infant's eyes for redness, drainage, or crustiness.	Monitors for the presence of infection.

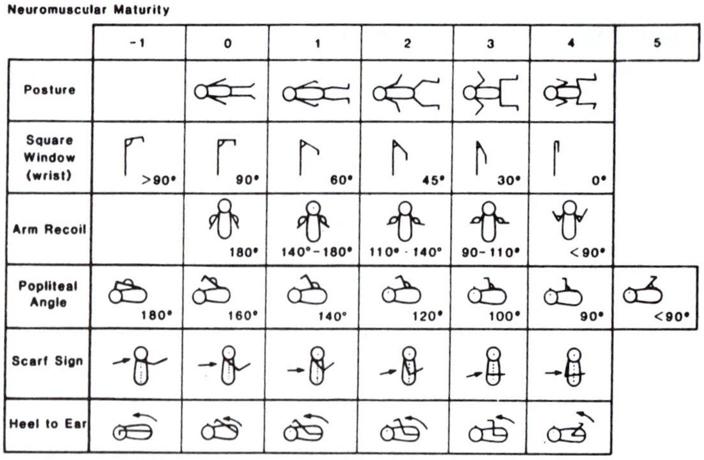
Neuromuscular Maturity
-1
0
1
2
3
4
5
Posture
Square Window (wrist)
>90°
90°
60°
45°
30°
0°
Arm Recoil
180°
140°-180°
110°-140°
90-110°
<90°
Popliteal Angle
180°
160°
140°
120°
100°
90°
<90°
Scarf Sign
Heel to Ear

Physical Maturity

	-1	0	1	2	3	4	5
Skin	sticky friable transparent	gelatinous red, translucent	smooth pink, visible veins	superficial peeling &/or rash. few veins	cracking pale areas rare veins	parchment deep cracking no vessels	leathery cracked wrinkled
Lanugo	none	sparse	abundant	thinning	bald areas	mostly bald	
Plantar Surface	heel-toe 40-50 mm: -1 <40 mm: -2	>50mm no crease	faint red marks	anterior transverse crease only	creases ant. 2/3	creases over entire sole	
Breast	imperceptible	barely perceptible	flat areola no bud	stippled areola 1-2mm bud	raised areola 3-4mm bud	full areola 5-10mm bud	
Eye/Ear	lids fused loosely:-1 tightly:-2	lids open pinna flat stays folded	sl. curved pinna; soft; slow recoil	well-curved pinna; soft but ready recoil	formed &firm instant recoil	thick cartilage ear stiff	
Genitals male	scrotum flat, smooth	scrotum empty faint rugae	testes in upper canal rare rugae	testes descending few rugae	testes down good rugae	testes pendulous deep rugae	
Genitals female	clitoris prominent labia flat	prominent clitoris small labia minora	prominent clitoris enlarging minora	majora & minora equally prominent	majora large minora small	majora cover clitoris & minora	

Maturity Rating

score	weeks
-10	20
-5	22
0	24
5	26
10	28
15	30
20	32
25	34
30	36
35	38
40	40
45	42
50	44

FIGURE 78-1
Ballard scoring system for determining gestational age in weeks. The Neuromuscular maturity criteria are depicted in the top half of the figure. The scores for each criterion are indicated at the top of the vertical columns. Asphyxiated neonates or neonates obtunded by anesthetic agents or drugs will score lower on neuromuscular maturity criteria. In such instances, scoring should be repeated at 24 to 48 hours of age. The physical maturity criteria are shown in the bottom half of the figure and are self-explanatory. The scores for each criterion are again the numbers at the top of the columns. The sum of the scores for all of the neuromuscular and physical maturity items provides an estimate of gestational age in weeks, using the maturity rating scale at the lower right portion of the figure. (From Ballard, J. L., Khoury, J., Wedig, K. et al. (1991). Now Ballard scores expanded to include extremely premature infants. *Journal of Pediatrics, 19*[3], 417–423.)

PROCEDURE Initiating Cord Care

Steps	Rationale/Points of Emphasis
1. Perform hand hygiene and don gloves.	Reduces transmission of microorganisms.
2. Assess vessels of the umbilical cord.	Two arteries and one vein should be present. The presence of only one artery may be indicative of congenital anomalies.
3. Hold stump gently away from infant's abdomen and cleanse site with soap and water. Use a damp cloth or cotton-tipped swabs to clean from base of stump to 1-inch diameter circle of infant's abdomen around base of stump.	A mild soap and water can provide initial cleaning of the cord stump.

Steps	Rationale/Points of Emphasis
4. Subsequently, allow the cord to dry naturally.	Research evidence does not support continued use of alcohol for newborn cord care. Shorter cord separation time has been noted with natural drying of the cord. Alcohol may also destroy normal flora present around the umbilical cord, thus delaying separation time and increasing the risk of infection. Alcohol use is also noted to be more costly than natural drying.
5. Do not submerge cord area in water until stump has fallen off.	Avoids infection of umbilical cord area.
6. Remove clamp from umbilical cord stump when discharging infant to home or after 24 hours of age and dry umbilical cord is observed.	By 24 hours of age, the arteries and vein present in the stump have closed, and there is less risk for hemorrhage.

PROCEDURE Administering Vitamin K

Steps	Rationale/Points of Emphasis
1. Administer vitamin K by intramuscular injection (see Chapter 64).	There is a decrease in vitamin K–dependent factors in neonates between 48 and 72 hours of age due to lack of vitamin K production by the sterile gut of the newborn infant.

caREminder

Infants weighing more than 1,500 g receive 1 mg. Low-birth-weight infants receive 0.5 mg. Vitamin K for oral administration is available and may be used per institutional policy.

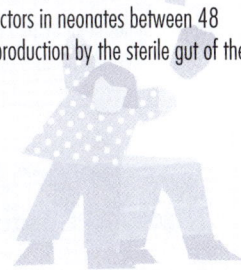

PROCEDURE Assessing Genitourinary and Gastrointestinal Function

Steps	Rationale/Points of Emphasis
1. For the male infant, feel the scrotum on each testicle, and note for descended or undescended testicles.	Both testicles should be in their sacks; if not noted, inform healthcare prescriber.
2. For all infants, note frequency, color, and concentration of urine. **Alert!** *Dark urine with a strong odor may indicate dehydration in the infant.*	Assesses renal functioning of the newborn. Urine of the newborn is usually colorless or pale yellow and without a strong odor. Most infants (more than 90%) void within 24 hours of delivery. Failure to void within 48 hours suggests renal abnormality.
3. Assess bowel sounds.	Bowel sounds are usually present within the first several hours after birth.
4. Document passage of meconium.	Meconium is the first bowel movement that an infant passes after birth. It is a sticky, thick, greenish-black, tarry stool that appears in the first 24 hours and may persist for up to 3 days. Meconium may be passed in utero with postconceptual-age fetuses and infants with a history of fetal distress.
5. After the passage of meconium, document the presence of stools.	The newborn generally has a bowel movement after each feeding, but each infant will establish his or her own bowel habits. Stools of breast-fed infants are usually yellow with a consistency that is soft or resembling thick liquid. Stools of bottle-fed infants may vary from pale yellow-brown thick liquid to pasty greenish-brown stool.

PROCEDURE Monitoring Blood Glucose

Steps	Rationale/Points of Emphasis
1. Assess blood glucose of infants at risk for hypoglycemia by heel-stick method within 1 hour of delivery and hourly for at least 6 hours or per healthcare prescriber's orders (see Chapter 19). **Alert!** *Infants at risk for hypoglycemia include infants of a diabetic mother; small-for-gestational-age infants; premature infants; infants with endocrine disorders, congenital heart disease, or sepsis; and infants who have had an exchange transfusion.*	Assesses newborn's metabolic stability.
2. If newborn is hypoglycemic (blood glucose of 30 mg/dL in term infant and of 20 mg/dL in preterm infant), initiate treatment as ordered.	Signs and symptoms of hypoglycemia include irritability, lethargy, cyanosis, high-pitched cry, tremulousness, apnea, respiratory distress, hyponatremia, pallor, and seizures. Symptomatic hypoglycemia requires immediate treatment with intravenous infusion.
3. If an infant has been treated for hypoglycemia, blood glucose should be assessed every 30 minutes until stable and then every hour for 3 hours.	Determines continued metabolic stability of the infant.

PROCEDURE Initiating Feeding

Steps	Rationale/Points of Emphasis
1. If infant is to be formula fed, initiate first feeding after assessment of gastrointestinal functioning; because of the chance of aspiration of formula, infant should start with 5–10 mL of water (see Chapter 43).	Initial start of formula feeding with water decreases the swallowing difficulty or an unrecognized congenital anomaly, such as esophageal atresia.
2. Assess infant for cyanosis, respiratory distress, or choking with feeding. Assess neonate's ability to suck.	Determines ability of infant to tolerate oral feedings.
3. If mother intends to breast-feed, the infant should be offered the breast within the first hour of life. Thereafter, the infant should be nursed on demand, at least eight times per day.	Encourages maternal–infant bonding while initiating feeding. Frequent nursing leads to development of efficient let-down reflex, decreases infant bilirubin, and prevents breast engorgement.
4. Regardless of type of nutrition, feedings should take place in a relaxed, unhurried, pleasant, and supportive environment.	Fosters parent–infant bonding while meeting infant nutritional needs.

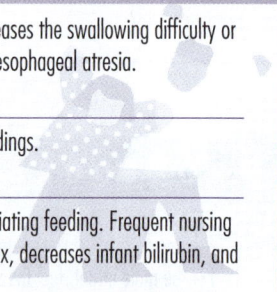

PROCEDURE Parent–Infant Bonding

Steps	Rationale/Points of Emphasis
1. Discuss principles of infant nurturing: • Responding to infant's cry and picking infant up as soon as possible • Holding infant in secure manner • Talking to infant in face-to-face position • Infant's ability to see and hear • Expected course of infant developmental gains • Provision of age-appropriate activities and infant stimulation	Provides information about infant's nurturing needs and appropriate expectations for infant developmental gains.
2. Encourage parent involvement in all care provision.	Provides supervised practice environment for parenting.
3. Verbally praise parent for appropriate nurturing behaviors, such as cuddling and talking to infant and safe handling of infant.	Provides reinforcement of parenting skills.

PROCEDURE Positioning the Infant

Steps	Rationale/Points of Emphasis
1. Infant should be positioned on back position for sleep.	Current research has found that back-to-sleep positioning decreases the incidence of sudden infant death syndrome (SIDS).
2. Elevate infant's head while burping.	Allows for proper burping and decreases chances of aspiration.
3. Elevate head of mattress of bassinet or isolette.	Assists respiratory function.

PROCEDURE Bath and Skin Care

Steps	Rationale/Points of Emphasis
1. Bathe infant with a mild moisturizing soap after the infant's temperature has stabilized in the normal range (98.2–99.8°F or 36.8–37.28°C axillary) and when appropriate care is taken to support thermal stability. Ensure that all areas of infant that are not immediately being bathed are covered (see Chapter 14).	Cleanses infant of birth residue while ensuring regulation of stable infant temperature.
2. Reassess axillary temperature 1 hour after bathing.	Assesses infant temperature stability.
3. After initial bath, infant should be bathed with water alone and a mild moisturizing soap to the perineal area if needed.	Decreases chance of skin irritation or drying.

PROCEDURE Hepatitis B Prophylaxis

Steps	Rationale/Points of Emphasis
1. Assess mother's hepatitis B surface antigen result. If result is positive or unknown, administer hepatitis B immune globulin (0.5 mL) and either Recombivax HB (5 mg) or Energix-B (10 mg) intramuscularly to infant within 12 hours of birth. If result is negative, administer Recombivax HB (5 mg) or Energix-B (10 mg) intramuscularly.	Ensures timely initiation of hepatitis B vaccine series to prevent transmission of disease to infant. Consent from parents is required.

CHILD AND FAMILY EVALUATION AND DOCUMENTATION

- Evaluate parent–newborn interactions.
- Evaluate neonate's ability to suck and ability to complete first feeding.
- Provide parents with documentation of infant's birth weight and length.
- Document the following:
  - Apgar scores
  - Temperature and interventions required to maintain a stable body temperature
  - Vital signs
  - Length, weight, and head and chest circumference
  - Assessment parameters of gestational age
  - Administration of silver nitrate or antibiotic prophylaxis and assessment of infant's eyes after administration, noting any redness and drainage
  - Presence of three vessels in umbilical cord
  - Cleansing of umbilical cord and stump and presence of any redness, drainage, or odor
  - Administration of vitamin K, noting amount given and location of intramuscular administration
  - Genitourinary and gastrointestinal functioning, including accurate intake and output, color of urine, presence of meconium, bowel sounds, and tolerance of feedings
  - Blood glucose determination and treatment of hypoglycemia
  - Parent participation in infant care and assessment of parent–infant bonding

- Maternal hepatitis B surface antigen status and administration of hepatitis B vaccine, if appropriate

COMMUNITY CARE

- Assess home availability of needed supplies.
- Assess infant's home environment for safety (i.e., appropriate-sized crib with rails no greater than $2\frac{3}{8}$ inches apart, needed supplies for infant feeding, blankets and clothing, safe location for infant bath).
- Reinforce importance of provision of a secure, nurturing, loving environment for infant.
- Parent teaching:
  - Bottle-feed infant 1 to 2 ounces every 2 to 3 hours on demand, or breast-feed infant on demand at least eight times per day.
  - Infant may lose several ounces of weight in first week after delivery but should then gain weight consistently. Infant should return to birth weight by the 2-week well-child visit.
- Instruct the family to contact the healthcare provider if
  - Infant has crusty drainage from eyes
  - Odor or discharge is coming from umbilical cord
  - Infant's temperature is more than 100.8°F or 38.8°C
  - Infant displays unusual irritability or lethargy
  - Infant refuses to eat or has persistent vomiting or regurgitation
  - Decrease in number of wet diapers (less than six to eight per day)
  - No passage of stool for more than 1 day, if this is unusual for infant

Unexpected Situation

- *The parent is concerned that there is no "purple dye" on child's umbilical cord, stating, "All of my other children had that on their cord, why did they forget to apply it?":* Explain that the purple dye was from a formula called "triple dye" and that research evidence now indicates the solution does not assist in drying of the cord. Furthermore, the dye may increase the incidence of infection of the cord. Evidence now indicates that natural drying of the cord is the most beneficial method to manage the cord separation.

Bibliography

American Academy of Pediatrics. (1992). Positioning and SIDS. *Pediatrics, 89*(6), 1120–1126.

American Academy of Pediatrics. (1995). Hospital stay for healthy term newborns. *Pediatrics, 96*(4), 788–790.

American Academy of Pediatrics. (1996). Positioning and sudden infant death syndrome (SIDS): Update. *Pediatrics, 98*(6), 1216–1218.

Behring, A., Vezeau, T. M., & Fink, R. (2003). Timing of the newborn first bath: A replication. *Neonatal Network, 22*(1), 39–46.

Dore, S., Buchan, D., Coulas, S., et al. (1998). Alcohol versus natural drying for newborn cord care. *Journal of Obstetric, Gynecologic, and Neonatal Nursing, 27*, 621–627.

Fuloria, M., & Kreiter, S. (2002a). The newborn examination: Part I. *American Family Physician, 65*(1), 61–68.

Fuloria, M., & Kreiter, S. (2002b). The newborn examination: Part II. *American Family Physician, 65*(2), 265–270.

Hackman, P. (2001). Recognizing and understanding the cold-stressed term infant. *Neonatal Network, 20*(8), 35–41.

Lund, C., Kuller, J., Lane, A., Lott, J., Raines, D., & Thomas, K. (2001). Neonatal skin care: Evidence-based clinical practice guidelines. *Journal of Obstetric, Gynecologic, and Neonatal Nursing, 30*(1), 30–40.

Medves, J., & O'Brien, B. (1997). Cleaning solutions and bacterial colonization in promoting healing and early separation of the umbilical cord in healthy newborns. *Revue Canadienne de Sante Publique, 88*(6), 380–382.

Medves, J., & O'Brien, B. (2004). The effect of bather and location of first bath on maintaining thermal stability in newborns. *Journal of Obstetric, Gynecologic, and Neonatal Nursing, 33*, 175–182.

Zupan, J., Garner, P., & Omari, A. (2004). Topical umbilical cord care at birth. *The Cochrane Database of Systematic Reviews*, (3), No. CD001057.

CHAPTER

79

Newborn Care: Maintaining a Thermal Neutral Environment

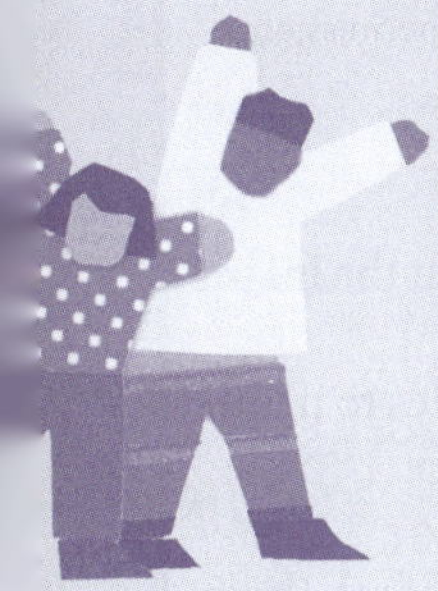

Clinical Guidelines

- Use of selected warming devices to maintain a thermal neutral environment is implemented by the registered nurse (RN) or licensed practical nurse (LPN) with an order from a health-care prescriber. Follow institutional protocols.
- The infant's temperature is maintained within a specific environmental range, called the *thermal neutral zone* (TNZ), in which the rates of oxygen consumption and metabolism are minimal and internal body temperature is maintained because of thermal balance. Specific ranges for ambient environmental temperature vary based on the age and weight of the infant (Table 79-1).
- All newborns have their temperature assessed hourly and as needed for the first 4 hours of life.
- All infants and children have their temperature assessed as per their acuity level and standard of the unit or institution (see Chapter 134).

Equipment

- Temperature measurement device (see Chapter 134 for types of temperature measurement devices)
- Blankets
- Head covers
- Booties

For radiant warmer:
- Radiant warmer
- Servo temperature probe

For isolette:
- Double-walled isolette (Use of porthole sleeves, when available, decreases the amount of ambient heat loss.)
- Servo temperature probe

For chemically heated mattress:
- Chemically heated mattress
- Linen to cover mattress

TABLE 79-1
Thermal Neutral Environmental Temperatures*

Age and Weight	Range of Temperature [°C]
0–6 Hours	
Less than 1200 g	34.0–35.4
1200–1500 g	33.9–34.4
1501–2500 g	32.8–33.8
More than 2500 g (and >36 weeks)	32.0–33.8
6–12 Hours	
Less than 1200 g	34.0–35.4
1200–1500 g	33.5–34.4
1501–2500 g	32.2–33.8
More than 2500 g (and >36 weeks)	31.4–33.8
12–24 Hours	
Less than 1200 g	34.0–35.4
1200–1500 g	33.3–34.3
1501–2500 g	31.8–33.8
More than 2500 g (and >36 weeks)	31.0–33.7
24–36 Hours	
Less than 1200 g	34.0–35.0
1200–1500 g	33.1–34.2
1501–2500 g	31.6–33.6
More than 2500 g (and >36 weeks)	30.7–33.5
36–48 Hours	
Less than 1200 g	34.0–35.0
1200–1500 g	33.0–34.1
1501–2500 g	31.4–33.5
More than 2500 g (and >36 weeks)	30.1–33.2
72–96 Hours	
Less than 1200 g	34.0–35.0
1200–1500 g	33.0–34.0
1501–2500 g	31.1–33.2
More than 2500 g (and >36 weeks)	29.8–32.6
4–12 Days	
Less than 1500 g	33.0–34.0
1501–2500 g	31.0–33.2
More than 2500 g (and >36 weeks)	29.0–32.6
4–5 days	29.5–32.6
5–6 days	29.4–32.3
6–8 days	29.0–32.2
8–10 days	29.0–31.8
10–12 days	29.0–31.4
12–14 Days	
Less than 1500 g	32.6–34.0
1500–2500 g	31.0–33.2
More than 2500 g (and >36 weeks)	29.0–30.8
2–3 Weeks	
Less than 1500 g	32.2–34.0
1500–2500 g	30.5–33.0
3–4 Weeks	
Less than 1500 g	31.6–33.6
1500–2500 g	30.0–32.7
4–5 Weeks	
Less than 1500 g	31.2–33.0
1500–2500 g	29.5–32.2
5–6 Weeks	
Less than 1500 g	30.6–32.3
1500–2500 g	29.0–31.8

*Generally, the smaller infants in each weight group will require a temperature in the higher portion of the temperature range. Within each time range, the younger the infant, the higher the temperature required.

From Klaus, M. H., & Fanaroff, A. A. (1986). *Care of the high-risk neonate* (3rd ed., p. 103). Philadelphia: W. B. Saunders. Used with permission.

For heat lamp:
- Heat lamp
- Yardstick or tape measure

For heat shields or plastic wrap devices:
- Plexiglas heat shield, plastic wrap

For warmed inspired air:
- Oxygen tubing
- Oxygen flowmeter
- Humidification device

CHILD AND FAMILY ASSESSMENT AND PREPARATION

- Educate the parents of the importance of maintaining the infant's body temperature.
- Discuss measures that will be used to maintain the infant in a thermal neutral environment:
  - Explanation of how infant loses heat and tries to maintain heat (Chart 79-1)
  - Measures used to prevent heat loss
  - Measures used to provide heat to the infant (heat production)
  - Manner in which the parents can assist with the infant's care while maintaining the infant's temperature
  - Explanation of all equipment to be used to assist in warming the infant
  - Measures to be used to monitor the infant's temperature
  - How to provide skin-to-skin contact (kangaroo care) to the infant
- Prewarm isolette or warmer in anticipation for admission of the infant.

CHART 79-1 TEMPERATURE REGULATION TERMS

Conduction—heat transfer from one object to another by direct contact (e.g., x-ray plate, scale, mattress).

Convection—heat loss or increase due to air motion (e.g., cool or warm breezes).

Evaporation—heat loss due to moisture vaporizing from the skin surface (e.g., wet infant at birth or due to bath).

Radiation—heat transfer between objects that are not in direct contact with each other (e.g., incubator placed in direct sunlight).

Thermal neutral zone—an environmental range in which the rates of oxygen consumption and metabolism are minimal for the infant and internal body temperature is maintained because of thermal balance.

Thermogenesis—physiologic mechanisms that increase heat production in the newborn. These include increased basal metabolic rate, muscular activity, and chemical thermogenesis (also called *nonshivering thermogenesis*).

PROCEDURE Maintaining a Thermal Neutral Environment

Steps	Rationale/Points of Emphasis
1. Perform hand hygiene; don protective apparel (gown and gloves) for care of infant immediately after delivery. Perform hand hygiene after each contact with the infant and before initiating new contact with infant (see Chapter 52).	Reduces transmission of microorganisms. Protects healthcare provider from exposure to blood and body fluids.
2. Place infant under warming source (on prewarmed warmer or isolette) after birth. Dry infant and remove wet linens. Provide warmed blankets and hat for warmth.	Decreases evaporative heat loss and decreases loss from the head, which is an infant's largest heat-losing body surface.
3. Determine newborn's temperature while under warming source. a. Place servo-control skin probe over abdominal area, avoiding bony areas, using foil protective cover; do not place probe where infant will lie on the sensor. b. Correlate probe readout with infant's temperature when recording vital signs.	The probe must be in good contact with the skin so that it does not cause false high or low temperatures, thus causing the heating element to react and adversely affect the infant's temperature. Ensures correct patient data are being observed and collected. **caREminder** *Do not place probe over stomach area if infant is being fed enterally because the probe will sense the feeding temperature and therefore fluctuate the environment accordingly.*
4. Assess temperature hourly for the first 4 hours of life and then as indicated by infant's acuity level and institutional policy; see Appendix A: Reference Ranges for Vital Sign Measurements for normal ranges. Refer to Chapter 134 for methods to assess temperature.	Ensures that deviation from normal is detected promptly.
5. Offer parents the option of skin-to-skin contact, if infant is stable.	Skin-to-skin contact encourages warmth from convection with parent's body temperature.
6. Give first bath after the infant's temperature has stabilized in the normal range (98.2–99.8°F or 36.8–37.28°C axillary) and when appropriate care is taken to support thermal stability (see Chapter 14).	Prevents hypothermia that can increase oxygen consumption and respiratory distress.

Continued

Steps	Rationale/Points of Emphasis
7a. Assess infant. If stable, clothe infant, put on head covering, bundle in blanket, and move infant to open crib for ongoing observations or transfer to mother or father to hold.	Stability is determined by normal vital signs and no signs of respiratory distress. Easy visualization of infant's chest will aid in prompt detection of increasing respiratory distress. Early transfer to the mother or father promotes parent–infant bonding. **caREminder** *Typically, healthy infants who weigh more than 2,300 g can maintain their temperature when covered, as above, in an open crib.*
7b. Continue to monitor temperature per institutional policy. To prevent exposure and chilling, keep neonate wrapped in a lightweight blanket and accomplish care quickly in a draft-free, warm environment.	Prevents further exposure to cold environment.
8. Provide ongoing warming measures as needed (Figure 79-1).	Prevents hypothermia, which can increase oxygen consumption and respiratory distress. Warming measures are selected based on infant's temperature, age (premature versus term), diagnosis, and the resources available.
a. If unable to maintain temperature within normal range and if signs of respiratory distress or other signs need to be closely observed, keep infant under radiant warmer or move to prewarmed incubator or isolette.	If infant's axillary temperature is below 97.2°F (36.2°C), rewarming should be initiated. The process should be gradual to prevent the possibility of hyperthermia. Servo-control mode is required for slow rewarming of infant. When the new skin temperature is reached, the air temperature is increased in hourly increments of 1.0°C until the desired skin temperature is reached and infant's temperature is stable.

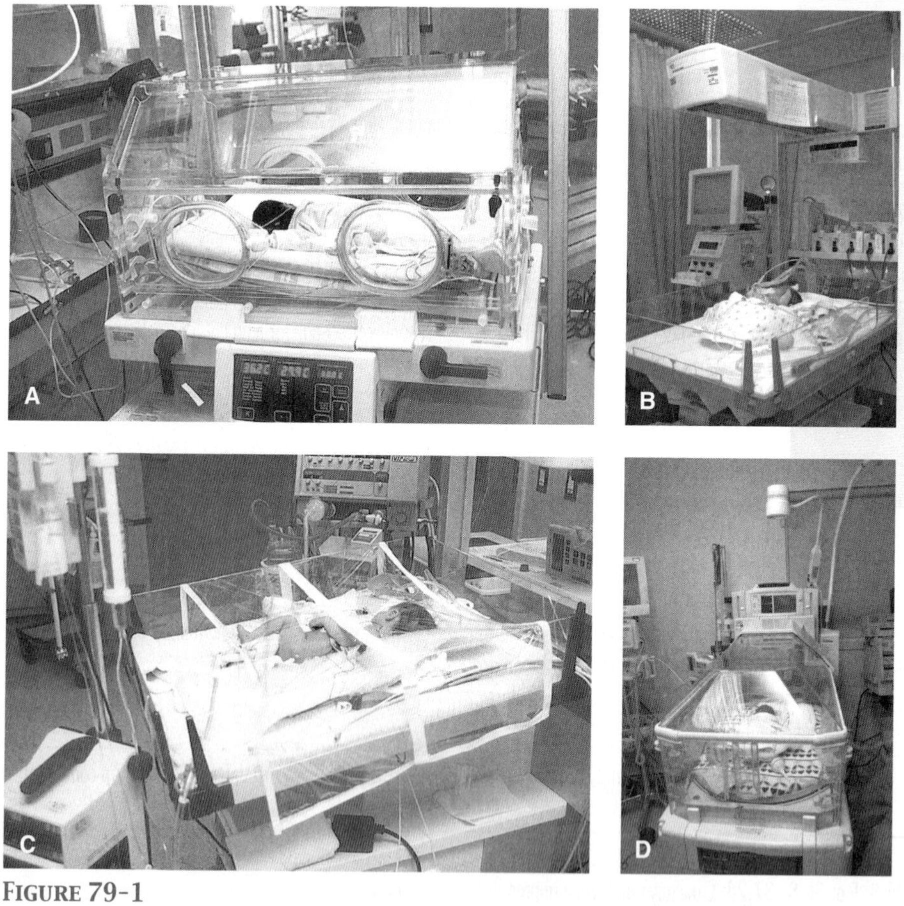

FIGURE 79-1
Various methods help newborns maintain thermoregulation: (**A**) isolette, (**B**) radiant warmer, (**C**) plastic wrap, or (**D**) combination unit, radiant warmer and isolette.

Steps	Rationale/Points of Emphasis
b. Follow procedures in Chapter 135 for use of the following warming devices: • Radiant warmer and isolette • Chemically heated mattress • Heat lamp Place warming device and infant in a draft-free environment, out of direct sunlight, to decrease temperature fluctuations due to convection and radiation.	Ensures that environmental temperature is individualized as appropriate for the infant. Ensures that deviations from normal are detected promptly.
c. For use of plastic wrap as a warming device: • Stretch wrap over the infant across the plastic sides of radiant warmer. • Do not place wrap directly on infant's skin.	Provides barrier to decrease heat loss by convection or evaporation. Contact with infant's skin may cause maceration or burning.
d. For use of Plexiglas heat shield as a warming device: • Place heat shield over infant in incubator or isolette. Do not use when infant is under radiant warmer.	Decreases radiant heat loss. Under the radiant warmer, the heat shield blocks the infrared heat from reaching the infant.
e. For use of warmed inspired air to aid in thermoregulation: • Follow procedure for oxygen administration (see Chapter 83) to provide warm, humidified, inspired air if infant requires supplemental oxygen.	Provides additional measures to decreases evaporative heat loss and insensible heat loss.
9. Continue to monitor temperature per institutional policy. Continue warming measures as needed.	Provides ongoing assessment and reevaluation of interventions.

CHILD AND FAMILY EVALUATION AND DOCUMENTATION

- Compare infant's temperature with previous readings.
- Evaluate infant's response to interventions.
- Evaluate parents' understanding of methods used to monitor and maintain infant's temperature.
- Notify healthcare prescriber if the infant's temperature does not maintain stability in response to the measures used.
- Document the following:
  - Temperature, route obtained, and device used; include manual readings and readings from warming devices (i.e., servo-control on radiant warmer)
  - Interventions implemented to maintain temperature
  - Infant's response to interventions
  - The set point of radiant warmer temperature, incubator, or isolette temperature
  - Education provided to the family
  - Family's participation in infant's care

COMMUNITY CARE

- Instruct parents to clothe infant for the weather; remind parents that an infant loses a large percentage of heat through the head.
- Instruct parents to contact the healthcare provider if
  - Infant's temperature remains outside normal parameters despite appropriate environmental management (e.g., adding or removing layers of clothing, altering room temperature)
  - The infant's extremities are cold to touch and blue in color

Unexpected Situation

- *Newborn has been placed under a radiant warmer to maintain body temperature within normal ranges. After 1 hour, you note that newborn is listless and the skin appears dry and pale. Newborn has a weak cry when stimulated:* Heat and water losses have been noted to be higher in infants under radiant warmers than in incubators. The infant may be hypoglycemic and in need of hydration. Assess all vital signs, complete blood glucose testing, and assess voiding patterns. Report findings to healthcare prescriber. Nutritional/fluid interventions may need to be implemented.

Bibliography

Behring, A., Vezaeu, T., & Fink, R. (2003). Timing of the newborn first bath: A replication. *The Journal of Neonatal Nursing, 22*(1), 39–46.

Blackburn, S., DePaul, D., Loan, L., et al. (2001). Neonatal thermal care. III. The effect of infant position and temperature probe placement. *Neonatal Network, 20*(3), 25–30.

Flenady, V. J., & Woodgate, P. G. (2005). Radiant warmers versus incubators for regulating body temperature in newborn infants. *The Cochrane Database of Systematic Reviews,* (1), No. CD000435.

Hackman, P. S. (2001). Recognizing and understanding the cold-stressed term infant. *Neonatal Network, 20*(8), 35–41.

Horns, K. M. (2002). Comparison of two microenvironments and nurse caregiving on thermal stability of ELBW infants. *Advances in Neonatal Care, 2,* 149–160.

Laroia, N., & Phelps, D. (2003). Double wall vs. single wall incubator for reducing heat loss in very low birth weight infants in incubators. *The Cochrane Database of Systematic Reviews,* (2), No. CD004215.

New, K., Flenady, V., & Davies, M. W. (2004). Transfer of preterm infants from incubator to open cot at lower versus higher body weight. *The Cochrane Database of Systematic Reviews,* (2), No. CD004214.

Sinclair, J. C. (2002). Servo-control for maintaining abdominal skin temperature at 36°C in low birth weight infants. *The Cochrane Database of Systematic Reviews,* (1), No. CD001074.

Varda, K., & Behnke, R. (2000). The effect of timing of initial bath on newborn's temperature. *Journal of Obstetric, Gynecologic, and Neonatal Nursing, 29*(1), 27–32.

CHAPTER 80

Newborn Care: Newborn Screening

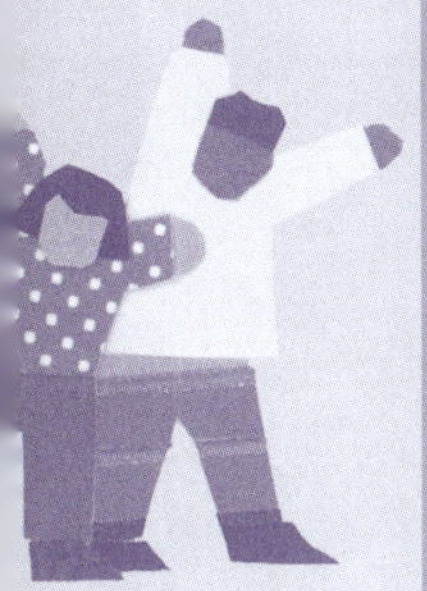

Clinical Guidelines

- A registered nurse (RN) or licensed practical nurse (LPN) may perform newborn screening.
- All newborns are screened for phenylketonuria and hypothyroidism and undergo other state-specific mandated studies, preferably between 24 and 72 hours of age, before hospital discharge, and in no case later than 7 days of life.
- Screening of premature or sick infants is completed as close as possible to the time of discharge from the nursery or at or near the seventh day of age regardless of feeding status.
- If the initial specimen for newborn screening is collected before 12 hours of age, a second specimen should be collected at 1 to 2 weeks of age.
- It is best to complete screening prior to transfusion or dialysis if the child's condition permits. If the infant requires a blood transfusion or dialysis before the specimen is collected, complete newborn screening 24 hours after completion of the blood transfusion/dialysis.
- If the newborn is transferred to another facility for continuing care on or before the seventh day of age, the receiving hospital will obtain the specimen. A "Hospital Report of Newborn Specimen Not Obtained" form must be completed and sent immediately to the Department of Health Services, Genetic Disease Branch.
- Newborn screening is repeated as soon as possible if the initial sample was inadequate.
- Parents/legal guardians may refuse the test on the basis of religious beliefs or practices. A "Newborn Screening Test Refusal" form must be signed and copies sent as directed on the form.
- Newborn screening results are forwarded to the infant's primary healthcare provider.
- The parent is provided with results of newborn screening.
- Abnormalities found through newborn screening are referred to the appropriate provider for follow-up and treatment.

Equipment

- Nonsterile gloves
- Supplies needed for heel-stick blood draw (see Chapter 16)
- Newborn screening blood collection form per state regulation
- Parental information materials about newborn screening tests

CHILD AND FAMILY ASSESSMENT AND PREPARATION

- Instruct parent about procedure and reason for screening.
- Provide family printed information about the screening tests that will be completed.

Alert! *Some states require informed consent from parents to perform newborn screening. Check with the state laws to verify regulations before performing this procedure. In almost all states, required testing can be overridden by invoking a religious exception.*

PROCEDURE Newborn Screening

Steps	Rationale/Points of Emphasis
1. Identify infant and write infant and maternal biographic data on newborn screening blood collection form.	Ensures correct patient for procedure and correct results will be documented for the correct patient.
2. Write hospital data and infant's primary healthcare provider information, including physician license number on newborn screening blood collection form.	Ensures that newborn screening results are forwarded to appropriate primary healthcare provider.
3. Perform hand hygiene and don gloves.	Reduces transmission of microorganisms.
4. Perform heel stick (see Chapter 16).	Obtains blood sample for screening. **caREminder** *A warming device may need to be placed on the area 5 to 10 minutes before puncture to increase blood flow and reduce hemolysis and bruising (see Chapter 16).*
5. Wipe away first drop of blood from heel-stick area with sterile gauze.	Ensures that sample will not be contaminated with alcohol used to clean heel-stick site or serous drainage from heel stick.
6. Allow second large drop of blood to form at site of heel stick and gently apply filter paper to drop of blood, allowing blood to soak into paper, completely filling preprinted circle on newborn screening blood collection form (Figure 80-1).	Collects adequate blood sample.

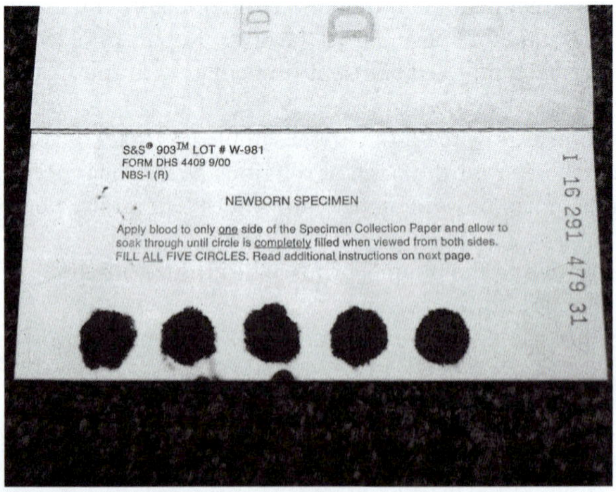

FIGURE 80-1
When collecting blood samples for newborn screening, completely cover the preprinted circles on the form with blood.

Steps	Rationale/Points of Emphasis
7. Repeat procedure, filling each circle completely with an individual drop of blood.	Collects adequate blood sample.
8. Dispose of heel lancet in needle receptacle. Remove gloves and dispose of gloves in appropriate receptacle. Perform hand hygiene.	Promotes needle safety. Reduces transmission of microorganisms.
9. Allow blood-soaked circles to air-dry thoroughly for at least 4 hours.	Drying of blood samples collected on filter paper preserves sample to allow for proper processing.
10. Forward copies of newborn screening blood collection form to appropriate locations, per state protocol. One copy will go to the infant's parents, one copy will go into the infant's medical record, and the remaining copies will be retained with the blood sample.	Provides appropriate notification and documentation that sample has been obtained.
11. Place collected sample on completed newborn screening blood collection form in biohazard bag and forward to testing laboratory.	Prevents healthcare personnel exposure to blood and body fluids and routes sample to appropriate location for processing.

Child and Family Evaluation and Documentation

- Document the following:
  - Completion of newborn screening in infant's medical record. Attach chart copy of newborn screening blood collection form to medical record.
  - Infant's response to procedure in medical record.

Community Care

- Schedule 2-week follow-up well-child appointment with infant's primary healthcare provider before infant's discharge to home after delivery.
- At infant's well-child appointments, assess for signs and symptoms of possible abnormalities on newborn screen (lack of weight gain, persistence of open fontanel, unusual odor of infant, irritability).
- Almost all newborns screened have residual blood samples retained by the state for various lengths of time, some up to 21 years. With parental permission, these samples may be used for population-based epidemiology data on disease prevalence, for research purposes, or for future clinical or forensic testing
- Instruct the family to contact the healthcare provider if
  - Family changes place of residence before getting the results of the newborn screening to ensure adequate follow-up on screening results
  - No communication is received within 1 month of discharge regarding the results of the screening procedures
  - Child develops atypical-smelling urine, listlessness, diminished appetite, or changes in the level of alertness or responsiveness to stimuli
  - Child has seizure activity

Unexpected Situations

- *Parents have stated that they do not want newborn screening testing completed on their child:* Further assessment is needed to determine reason for parent's refusal of newborn screening. Further parent education may be needed. Parents may refuse testing based on religious exception. After further discussion and sharing of information with parents, if they maintain refusal of newborn screening, a "Newborn Screening Test Refusal" form must be completed and signed by the parents. Copies of these forms are filed in the child's medical record at the hospital, given to the parents, and submitted to the state Department of Health Services.
- *Specimen is collected when child is less than 24 hours old:* If the initial specimen is obtained before 24 hours of age, then a second specimen should be obtained at 1 to 2 weeks of age to decrease the probability that PKU and other disorders with metabolite accumulation will be missed as a consequence of testing before adequate protein intake.

Bibliography

American Academy of Pediatrics. (1997). Newborn screening fact sheets. *Pediatrics, 98*, 473–501.

American Academy of Pediatrics. (2000a). Serving the family from birth to the medical home. *Pediatrics, 106*(Suppl. 2), 389–422.

American Academy of Pediatrics. (2000b). Newborn screening: A blueprint for the future executive summary. *Pediatrics, 106*(Suppl. 2), 386–388.

American Academy of Pediatrics. (2000c). *Newborn screening by states and jurisdictions.* Retrieved September 18, 2006, from http://www.aap.org/policy/01565t1.htm

American Academy of Pediatrics. (2002). *A compendium of resources on newborn screening policy and system development.* Washington, DC: U.S. Department of Health and Human Services Administration, Maternal Child Bureau.

Dhanda, R., & Reilly, P. (2003). Legal and ethical issues of newborn screening. *Pediatric Annals, 32*(8), 540–546.

Fearing, M., & Marsden, D. (2003). Expanded newborn screening. *Pediatric Annals, 32*(8), 509–515.

Kerruisch, N., & Robertson, S. (2005). Newborn screening: New developments, new dilemmas. *Journal of Medical Ethics, 31*, 393–398.

McCartney, P. (2003). Newborn identification, screening and DNA. *MCN, 28*(2), 124.

National Newborn Screening and Genetics Resource Center. (2005). *National newborn screening status report.* Updated 6/15/05. Retrieved July 1, 2005, from http://genes-r-us.uthscsa.edu/resources/newborn/newborn_menu.htm

Task Force on Newborn Screening. (2000). Serving the family from birth to the medical home. *Pediatrics, 106*(2 Suppl.), 389–422.

CHAPTER 81

Oral Care

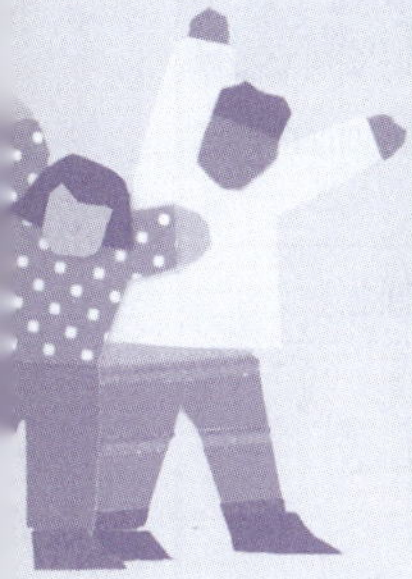

Clinical Guidelines

- Oral care of infants and young children may be performed by a registered nurse (RN), licensed practical nurse (LPN), or an appropriately trained caregiver.
- Oral hygiene should be introduced at an early age, before the eruption of the first tooth, and independence should be encouraged to promote good habits. The caregiver must monitor that the child does not swallow toothpaste. Also monitor brushing and flossing until the child has manual dexterity and the practice is firmly established, often until the child is 8 or 9 years of age.
- Preventative dental care should include the following:
  - Children should receive their first dental checkup when the first tooth appears or no later than the first birthday to determine risk factors and evaluate fluoride needs before the child's permanent teeth come in. Then, depending on oral hygiene, the child should receive a follow-up visit 6 months to 1 year later.
  - At 3 years of age, children should have their first dental cleaning with a checkup. Subsequent dental visits should occur every 6 months thereafter.
  - Infants should never have a propped bottle and should never be put to bed with a bottle to avoid baby-bottle tooth decay and other potential adverse sequelae such as otitis media.
- Perform oral assessments on a daily basis for children receiving chemotherapy treatments or radiation of the head or neck regions or if child has undergone a bone marrow transplantation.
- Perform oral hygiene two to three times a day and more often if needed for children with cancer.
- Pediatric oncology patients with dentition should be referred to a pediatric dentist for evaluation before initiation of chemotherapy, bone marrow transplantation, or radiation.

Equipment

For oral care of infants:

- Soft washcloth or gauze pad
- Clear warm water
- Nonsterile gloves

For oral care of toddlers:

- Soft bristle brush
- Toothpaste with fluoride (if recommended by dentist)
- Dental floss

- Clear water
- Nonsterile gloves

For oral care of children 3 years of age and older:

- Soft bristle brush
- Toothpaste with fluoride
- Dental floss
- Clear water
- Nonsterile gloves

For oncology patients:

- Soft-bristle brush, soft toothettes, or gauze (choice dependent on absolute neutrophil count [ANC] and platelet count)
- Toothpaste with fluoride
- Dental floss
- Clear water
- Nonalcohol 0.1% chlorhexidine mouthwash rinse, saline, sterile water, or sodium bicarbonate
- Nystatin (if ordered)
- Petroleum jelly or topical lubricating anesthetic as needed
- Pain medication as ordered and if needed for severe mucositis
- Nonsterile gloves

CHILD AND FAMILY ASSESSMENT AND PREPARATION

- Assess current dental care practices. If possible, observe the older child performing dental self-care.
- Assess feeding practices (e.g., breast, bottle, cup), sucking practices (pacifier versus thumb), dietary intake (what is consumed, amount of fruits, vegetables, foods with high sugar content), and oral hygiene practices.
- Assess oral cavity for
  - Integrity and color of the lips, tongue, gingivae, and mucous membranes
  - Irritations, potential infections, trauma, or other disease processes
  - Impending tooth eruptions and placement of present teeth
  - Child's ability to salivate, swallow, and eat

caREminder

Children with some medical conditions, such as Down syndrome, have atypical tooth eruption patterns. Children with Down syndrome usually have delayed tooth eruption and an unusual order of eruption.

- Assess for any pain associated with oral cavity.
- Assess caregiver knowledge base regarding tooth eruption and physical side effects (sore red gums, profuse salivation, slight temperature elevation, mild diarrhea, skin eruptions, fussiness).
- Review child's record for any current medical treatments that may impact oral health (e.g., chemotherapy, radiation, bone marrow transplantation).

PROCEDURE Providing Oral Care

Steps	Rationale/Points of Emphasis
1. Perform hand hygiene and gather all necessary supplies.	Reduces transmission of microorganisms. Promotes efficient time management and provides an organized approach to the procedure.
2. Professional caregivers should don gloves before performing procedure.	Maintains standard precautions to protect against contact with body fluids.
Infants	
1. Position infant on lap or in infant seat. Caregiver should have access to mouth. A second person may be necessary for support or restraint.	Maintains child's comfort.
2. Reassure infant; make this a gentle, nonaggressive routine.	Reduces infant crying and fear. If teeth are erupting, gums may be sore, and these procedures will soothe the irritated gums.
3. Clean gums and teeth:	
a. After each feeding, wrap a soft cloth or gauze dampened with warm water around your finger and wipe or massage the gums.	Regular cleansing of the gums soothes the discomfort due to eruptions of new teeth and removes excess plaque and bacteria.
b. As teeth erupt, a dab of fluoride toothpaste (the size of a rice grain) may be added to the cloth and used to wipe teeth.	Eliminates chance of swallowing fluoride-containing toothpaste, resulting in fluorosis (brown discoloration with white specks on teeth). The flavor of adult toothpaste may be too intense, causing an aversion to the procedure, and the toothpaste may contain too much fluoride, leading to chronic excessive fluoride intake.

Steps	Rationale/Points of Emphasis
c. When most of the teeth are in, a soft bristle brush and a dab of fluoride toothpaste may be used to cleanse the teeth twice daily. Adult brands of toothpaste are not recommended for young children.	At about 6 months of age, parental use of toothbrush on the infant's teeth should be promoted. Select a fluoridated toothpaste that is specifically recommended for young children.
d. Clean the gums and the gingival tissue adjacent to any teeth to remove plaque.	Promotes optimal oral cleansing.
e. Excess toothpaste should be spit out, but rinsing should be discouraged.	Residual toothpaste on the teeth increases the caries-prevention effects.
Toddlers	
1. Engage the toddler in the activity of tooth brushing if developmentally appropriate and if the child is medically stable enough to engage in self-care activities. Allow the child to brush his or her teeth, followed by the caregiver brushing the child's teeth until the child can achieve the manual dexterity necessary to complete the task successfully.	Promotes the child's cooperation. The procedure should be routine and not be a reward or punishment. Be cautious in the amount of toothpaste used with children younger than 2 years of age. They are not able to spit the toothpaste out after brushing and tend to swallow it. Too much fluoride taken internally between ages 2 and 4 years can lead to enamel fluorosis, or discoloration of the teeth.
2. Clean teeth and gums:	
a. Choose a toothbrush labeled "very soft" or "soft" and with thin bristles with a short trim height and a small enough head to allow maneuverability within the child-sized oral cavity.	Promotes child's comfort. Prevents plaque buildup and deters dental caries formation.
b. Brush the child's teeth gently, using a pea-sized amount of fluoride toothpaste only if the child is capable of spitting out the toothpaste. If the child is unable to spit out the toothpaste, use warm water for cleansing the teeth.	When toothpaste is used, it is imperative that the child not swallow large amounts of the dentifrice to prevent dental fluorosis.
c. Gently brush the gums.	Removes bacteria from gums.
d. Floss the teeth once it is noted that two of the child's teeth have begun to touch.	
e. Brush teeth at least twice per day; if the child eats highly sweetened foods, then an extra brushing after the snack should occur.	Promotes routine, decreasing child's resistance.
Children Aged 3 Years and Older	
1. Explain the procedure to the child; engage the child in the activity.	Encourages good dental hygiene as a lifelong habit. **KidKare** Use of a timer may be introduced to encourage adequate brushing time.
2. Clean teeth:	
a. Gently brush all the teeth using a soft-bristle brush and a pea-sized amount of toothpaste.	Prevents plaque buildup.
b. Brush all sides and edges of the gums.	
c. Supervision is necessary until the child is at least 8 years old. Toothbrushes with an interdental brush with a small cone shape are helpful in brushing between braces and fixtures.	By 8 years of age, the child should possess the manual dexterity necessary to perform the procedure.
d. Ensure that flossing is completed. Floss at least once per day; a floss holder may facilitate the process.	Prevents plaque from forming. Children have much more space between their teeth initially, and flossing should be easy. Waxed floss may be easier for the child or caregiver to manipulate. Floss holders are plastic forklike devices that hold the floss for you, making it easier to floss in hard-to-reach places.
Oncology Patients	
1. Review health records or discuss with family to determine types of medical interventions that may be affecting oral mucosa (e.g., chemotherapy, radiation).	Rapidly dividing mucosal epithelial cells lining the oral cavity and the gastrointestinal tract are easily damaged by chemotherapeutic agents, with mucosal changes appearing within 2–3 days after chemotherapy administration.

Continued

Steps	Rationale/Points of Emphasis
	Changes in the oral mucosa can also be a result of anorexia, radiation to the oral cavity, and poor oral care. Oral complications of cancer treatment include mucositis, stomatitis, salivary gland dysfunction and xerostomia, infection, tooth demineralization, altered taste perception, nutritional compromise, abnormal tooth and craniofacial development, neurotoxicity, bleeding, radiation caries, trismus and tissue fibrosis, and osteoradionecrosis (Figure 81-1). 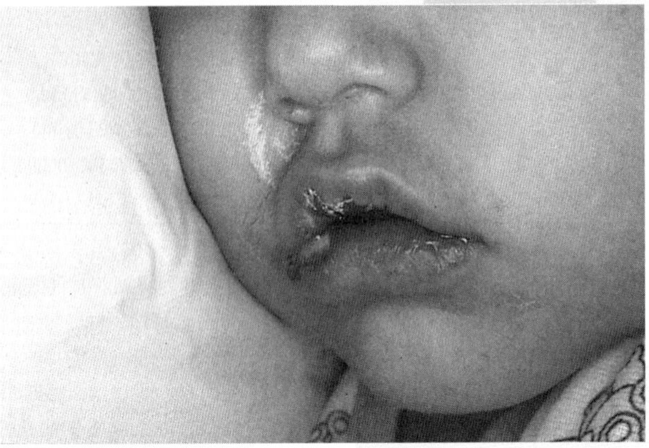 **FIGURE 81-1** The child with stomatitis or mucositis may require specific measures to reduce pain during oral hygiene procedures.
2. In consultation with the oncologist, initiate referral to pediatric dentistry services.	The eradication of active and potential sites for infection before the initiation of chemotherapy, bone marrow transplantation, or radiation is optimal. Ideally, oral assessment by a dentist should occur 7 to 10 days before initiation of chemotherapy or radiation. This may not be possible because of the medical status of the child. The American Academy of Pediatric Dentistry (AAPD) has specific guidelines for the management of pediatric dental patients receiving chemotherapy, bone marrow transplantation, or radiation (AAPD, 2000).
3. Assess child's oral cavity.	The child who is immunosuppressed is at risk for septicemia due to oral infections.
4. Assist child as needed to perform oral hygiene.	Early identification and prompt treatment can decrease the incidence of oral complications.
a. Brush with soft toothettes.	Using toothettes prevents bleeding of the gums that might be caused by harder bristle toothbrushes. The toothettes act to loosen the debris on the oral mucosa and teeth.
b. Use floss when there are no mouth sores or bleeding.	Prevents food particles from remaining between teeth and making the teeth at risk for cavities.
c. Rinse (swish) and spit with 0.1% chlorhexidine mouthwash, saline, water, sodium bicarbonate, or nystatin, as ordered. **Alert!** *These solutions should not be swallowed to prevent them from killing the normal flora of the gastrointestinal tract.*	These solutions assist to keep the oral mucosa clean and free of debris. Research indicates no significant difference between incidence of stomatitis, days to onset of stomatitis, or severity of stomatitis with use of chlorhexidine versus a sterile water mouthwash. Use of sterile water has been found to be as effective as chlorhexidine and more cost effective. **KidKare** For children who are younger than 6 years of age and may not be able to swish and spit, cleansing can be done by dipping the toothette in the solution and using this to clean the mucosa and teeth.
d. Oral intake should be restricted for 30 minutes afterward.	Waiting to eat or drink promotes absorption of the medication into the mucosa.

Steps	Rationale/Points of Emphasis
5. Apply petroleum jelly or lip balm to the lips.	Prevents cracking of the lips. Sore lips can make it difficult for the child to drink or chew.
6. For the child with stomatitis or mucositis: a. Assess for oral pain. Use oral analgesic agents that contain an antacid, diphenhydramine (Benadryl), and a topical anesthetic (viscous lidocaine) for mild discomfort. This agent can be applied directly to sore areas of the mouth or swished and spit. Physician's orders should be obtained for these oral agents.	Pain is highly associated with stomatitis. **Alert!** *Instruct the child not to swallow a solution containing this agent. The dosage should not exceed 15 mL every 3 hours.*
b. When moderate to severe stomatitis or mucositis is present: • Continue meticulous oral hygiene. Oral rinses can be used to clean the teeth, with a toothette used to remove debris loosened by the rinse. • Moderate to severe mucositis pain may be controlled with IV opioids (e.g., morphine or fentanyl). • When severe mucositis is present, premedication (i.e., using viscous lidocaine) to manage pain control may be necessary before oral care can be completed.	Promotes comfort in the presence of stomatitis or mucositis. The side effects of viscous lidocaine include a decreased gag reflex, tingling, and seizures. **Alert!** *If the child is unable to eat or swallow, supplemental intravenous fluids and nutrition must be administered.*
7. When oral care is completed, dispose of equipment and waste in appropriate receptacle. Store reusable supplies (e.g., toothbrush) in secure location away from easy reach of young children. Remove gloves and perform hand hygiene.	Standard precautions. Reduces transmission of microorganisms.

CHILD AND FAMILY EVALUATION AND DOCUMENTATION

- Evaluate caregiver understanding of schedule of eruption of teeth and discuss concerns regarding systemic consequences.
- Evaluate need for referral to appropriate pediatric dental professional.
- Evaluate child or caregiver's ability to perform appropriate oral care.
- Encourage preventative interventions, such as not running with lollipops, toothbrushes, and other items in mouth and the use of a mouth guard while engaging in sports activities.
- Evaluate caregiver understanding of good dietary habits and how they support good oral hygiene.
- Document the following:
  - Child and family assessment of oral health needs
  - Home care practices and teaching provided
  - Status of child's lips and oral cavity
  - Oral hygiene performed, including cleansing solutions used
  - Child's ability to participate in self-care activities

COMMUNITY CARE

- Instruct child and family regarding age-appropriate oral care; provide written instructions.
- Refer family to resources to obtain appropriate pediatric dental care (if needed).
- Initiate referral to dietitian (if needed) to ensure appropriate nutrition.
- Refer to appropriate social agencies if family lacks adequate resources for medical, dental, and nutritional care.
- Dental sealants (thin plastic coatings applied to the chewing surfaces of the molars) may be recommended to prevent tooth decay. Permanent molars are most likely to benefit, and it is best if the sealant is applied soon after the molars erupt (about 6 years of age for first molars and 12 years of age for second molars).
- For children who regularly drink bottled water, well water, or unfluoridated tap water, dietary fluoride supplements are recommended for the child aged 6 months to 16 years. The correct dosage is based on
  - Fluoride level in the local drinking water (if unknown, testing should be completed) (Table 81-1).
  - A complete fluoride history that includes all sources of the child's fluoride intake (e.g., water sources, fluoridated toothpaste).
- For oncology patients, oral hygiene should be completed by the child three or four times a day and as needed whether the child is hospitalized, at home, or participating in activities away from home. To promote healthy oral mucosa, the child needs to
  - Brush with soft-bristle brush, soft toothettes, or gauze (choice dependent on ANC and platelet counts)

TABLE 81-1
Dietary Fluoride Supplement Schedule

	Fluoride Ion Level in Drinking Water (ppm)*		
Age	<0.3 ppm	0.3–0.6 ppm	>0.6 ppm
Birth–6 mo	None	None	None
6 mo–3 yr	0.25 mg/day†	None	None
3–6 yr	0.50 mg/day	0.25 mg/day	None
6–16 yr	1.0 mg/day	0.50 mg/day	None

*0.1 Part per million (ppm) = 1 milligram per liter (mg/L).
†2.2 mg sodium fluoride contains 1 mg fluoride ion.
From National Center for Chronic Disease Prevention and Health Promotion. Available at www.cdc.gov/nccdphp/oh/child-flsupp.htm. Used with permission.

- Use floss when there are no mouth sores or bleeding
- Rinse and spit with 0.1% chlorhexidine mouthwash, saline, or sodium bicarbonate
- Swish and swallow with nystatin, as ordered
- Avoid hard foods that can cause abrasions to the gum line
- Avoid acidic foods, which can irritate tender or sore areas in the mouth
- Maintain a good fluid intake to keep mucous membranes moist
- Keep the lips lubricated with petroleum jelly or some type of lip balm
- Participate in regular dental checkups

- Identify and treat existing oral infections and dental problems.
- Participate in prophylactic antibiotic coverage if the child has an ANC of less than 500/mm or a white blood cell count of less than 2,000/mm, if the child has a central venous catheter, or if the child is taking long-term immunosuppressive drugs (e.g., cyclosporine, prednisone)
- Instruct the family to notify the healthcare provider if
  - Child develops sores/lesions in the oral cavity
  - Child complains of tooth pain or sensitivity of the teeth to hot or cold substances
  - Child has ongoing and persistent halitosis
  - Child is unable to swallow or eat due to lesions in the oral cavity

Unexpected Situations

- *While cleaning the teeth, the child notices there is blood coming from her mouth:* The blood is most likely from the gum line, and bleeding in this area in children most likely indicates gum irritation because they have not been properly brushing this area on a daily basis. Allow the child to gently rinse the mouth with water and spit into the sink or emesis basin. Assist the child to brush the gums in a gentle fashion, demonstrating how to perform this cleansing on a daily basis.
- *The child has braces on the teeth:* Braces collect food particles and need to be brushed extra thoroughly. The orthodontist can provide the child with special toothbrushes that are cone shaped and allow easier access underneath brace wires.
- *The child receiving chemotherapy complains of oral pain:* Assess the child's mouth for signs of mucositis. Implement institution-specific protocols for mucositis prevention and management.

Bibliography

American Academy of Pediatric Dentistry. (2000). *Guidelines for the management of pediatric dental patients receiving chemotherapy, bone marrow transplantation, and/or radiation.* Retrieved August 21, 2006, from www.aapd.org

Clarkson, J. E., Worthington, H. V., & Eden, O. B. (2003). Interventions for preventing oral mucositis for patients with cancer receiving treatment. *The Cochrane Database of Systematic Reviews, 3,* No. CD000978.

Dodd, M., Dibble, S. L., Miaskowski, C., et al. (2000). Randomized clinical trial of the effectiveness of 3 commonly used mouthwashes to treat chemotherapy-induced mucositis. *Oral Surgery, Oral Medicine, Oral Pathology, Oral Radiology, and Endodontology, 90,* 39–47.

Dodd, M., Larson, P., Dibble, S., et al. (1996). Randomized clinical trial of chlorhexidine versus placebo for prevention of oral mucositis in patients receiving chemotherapy. *Oncology Nursing Forum, 23*(6), 921–927.

Douglass, J., Douglass, A., & Silk, H. (2004). A practical guide to infant oral health. *American Family Physician, 70,* 2113–2120, 2121–2122.

Ferretti, G. A., Raybould, T. R., Brown, A. T., et al. (1990). Chlorhexidine prophylaxis for chemotherapy- and radiotherapy-induced stomatitis: A randomized double-blind trial. *Oral Surgery, Oral Medicine, Oral Pathology, Oral Radiology, and Endodontology, 69,* 331–338.

Fulton, J., Middleton, G., & McPhail, J. (2002). Management of oral complications. *Seminars in Oncology Nursing, 18*(1), 28–35.

Green, M., & Palfry, J. (Eds.). (2002). *Bright futures: Guidelines for health supervision of infants, children, and adolescents* (2nd ed., rev.). Arlington, VA: National Center for Education in Maternal and Child Health.

Harris, D., & Knobf, M. (2004). Assessing and managing chemotherapy-induced mucositis pain. *Clinical Journal of Oncology Nursing, 8*(6), 622–628.

McGraw, W. T., & Belch, A. (1985). Oral complications of acute leukemia: Prophylactic impact of a chlorhexidine mouth rinse regimen. *Oral Surgery, Oral Medicine, Oral Pathology, Oral Radiology, and Endodontology, 60,* 275–280.

McGuire, D., Rubenstein, E., & Peterson, D. (2004). Evidence-based guidelines for managing mucositis. *Seminars in Oncology Nursing, 20*(1), 59–66.

National Center for Chronic Disease Prevention and Health Promotion. (2002a). *Children's oral health: Dental sealants.*

Retrieved August 21, 2006, from www.cdc.gov/nccdphp/oh/child-sealants.htm

National Center for Chronic Disease Prevention and Health Promotion. (2002b). *Dietary fluoride supplement schedule.* Retrieved August 21, 2006, from www.cdc.gov/nccdphp/oh/child-flsupp.htm

Sanchez, O. M. & Childers, N. (2000). Anticipatory guidance in infant oral health: Rationale and recommendations. *American Family Physicians, 61*(1), 115–120, 123–124.

U.S. Preventive Services Task Force. (2004). Prevention of dental caries in preschool children: Recommendations and rationale statement. *The American Journal for Nurse Practitioners, 8*(11), 29–35.

Weisdorf, D. J., Bostrom, B., Raether, D., et al. (1989). Oropharyngeal mucositis complicating bone marrow transplantation: Prognostic factors and the effect of chlorhexidine mouth rinse. *Bone Marrow Transplantation, 4*, 89–95.

C H A P T E R

82

Ostomy Care

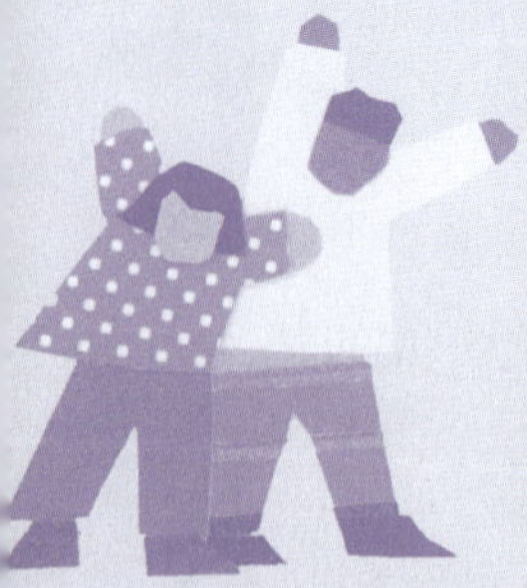

Clinical Guidelines

- Application of the ostomy pouch system and irrigation of the stoma are performed by a registered nurse (RN) or licensed practical nurse (LPN).
- Emptying and cleaning of pouch can be done by older child, parent, or care assistant.
- All school-aged children and adolescents should have the stoma site marked by a wound ostomy certified nurse (WOCN) if surgery is not done as an emergency.
- All fecal stomas (ileostomies and colostomies) should be pouched. A protective barrier is necessary for these stomas.
- Wear time for pouches for infants and children is generally 2 to 4 days.
- Older children and families need to be taught ostomy care skills before discharge.
- Successful stoma management can be measured by the maintenance of skin and stoma integrity.

Equipment

For stoma care immediate postoperative period:

- Nonsterile gloves
- Nonsterile gauze pads
- Vaseline gauze or petroleum jelly

For pouch application:

- Basin with warm water
- Nonsterile gloves (not necessary for parent or other family caregiver)
- Wash cloth, 4 × 4 nonsterile gauze, or soft paper towels
- Paper towel or transparent film
- Scissors
- Ostomy pouch
- Skin barrier (ostomy) paste
- Skin barrier (ostomy) powder
- Skin preparation (no-sting) optional

For emptying and cleaning pouch:

- Basin (with ability to measure output if necessary) or toilet facility
- Nonsterile gloves
- Washcloths, diaper wipes, tissues, or paper towels

CHILD AND FAMILY ASSESSMENT AND PREPARATION

- Assess child and family to determine current knowledge of ostomy care needs and current ability to perform ostomy care.
- Assess chart to determine presence of any allergies, including those to latex, alcohol, and any skincare products.
- Prepare child and family by describing the procedure and, if appropriate, demonstrating on a doll.
- Encourage parents of infants and young children to participate in care at first opportunity. If child is school age or older, encourage child to assist with procedure.

KidKare Shadow Buddies (Hollister, Inc., 1-800-323-4060) are dolls with an ostomy that can be given to children who have ostomies. These dolls can be used for demonstration of care procedures.

PROCEDURE Stoma Care Without Appliance: Immediate Postoperative Period

Steps	Rationale/Points of Emphasis
1. Gather the necessary supplies.	Promotes efficient time management and provides an organized approach to the procedure.
2. Perform hand hygiene. Don gloves.	Standard precautions to reduce transmission of microorganisms.
3. Cover the stoma site with Vaseline gauze or petroleum jelly and gauze until output begins. Check with surgical team as to timing of pouch application.	Keeps the stoma moist, protecting it from friction damage and allowing for ease of observation.
4. Remove gloves and perform hand hygiene.	Reduces transmission of microorganisms.

PROCEDURE Stoma Care: Routine

Steps	Rationale/Points of Emphasis
1. Gather the necessary supplies. Perform hand hygiene.	Promotes efficient time management and provides an organized approach to the procedure. Reduces transmission of microorganisms.
2. Prepare pouch barrier for application:	
a. Measure the stoma with the guide provided with the pouches (Figure 82-1). You may have to start the hole off-center to avoid the umbilicus or other abdominal landmarks. If the stoma is oval or double barreled, make a custom pattern by tracing shape on paper towel or transparent film. Pouch opening should be about 2 mm larger than the base of the stoma. Save pattern to use as a guide in the future.	If new ostomy, need to check stoma size each time pouch is applied. The stoma will decrease in size after surgery as the edema resolves. The guides assist in getting a proper fit around the stoma. The stoma may also change secondary to peristalsis.

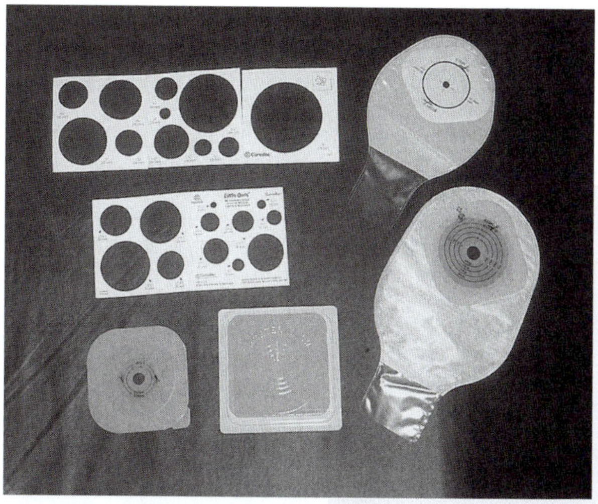

FIGURE 82-1
The measuring guide is used to determine the size of the hole in stomahesive wafer. Templates may need to be customized to fit the child.

Continued

Steps	Rationale/Points of Emphasis
b. Trace the selected circle on the release paper on the back of the wafer or the pouch if one-piece system.	Provides a guide to follow for cutting.
c. Before cutting pouch opening, pull the front of pouch away from wafer or place fingers inside pouch to separate panels and prevent puncturing pouch. Using small scissors (preferably with a rounded tip), cut the barrier on the marked circle.	Provides a guide to follow for cutting. Prevents pouch from being cut. If pouch is accidentally cut, use a new pouch and prepare as above.
d. Smooth the cut edge by running a finger around the circle.	Not all barriers can be smoothed.
e. Some barriers may benefit from being warmed to make them more moldable by placing between your hands or by placing under infant or child while preparing the skin. **caREminder** *Do not warm with heat lamp, heel warmer, or other warming devices that will melt the barrier.*	Assists with the adhesion of the pouch to child's skin contours, especially if barrier is somewhat stiff.
3. Position infant and young child in a supine position, restraining as necessary. Older children and adolescents may sit or stand, depending on which position is more comfortable.	Promotes ease of access to site. Allows child or teen to see stoma site so that he or she can participate actively. Child's privacy must be protected. **caREminder** *Perform the procedure in the bathroom or at bedside based on child and family preference when hospitalized. If working with premature newborns whose temperature is unstable, work through portholes in isolette. You may want to warm infants after procedure with warmed blankets. Excessive exposure of the child during this procedure can cause hypothermia.*
4. Don gloves.	Standard precaution to reduce transmission of microorganisms.
5. Remove old appliance or dressing; cleanse peristomal skin using warm water.	Clean skin allows for better adhesion of pouch. It generally is not necessary to use soap. Soap can leave a film on the skin that interferes with pouch adherence. **caREminder** *Adhesive removers and solvents should not be used on premature infants and rarely on infants or toddlers. Premature infants and young children do not metabolize and excrete chemicals as efficiently as adults and their surface area to body weight is much greater. Therefore it is important to minimize exposure to unnecessary chemicals. A soft cloth dampened with warm water can be used to loosen barrier adhesive.*
6. Dry skin thoroughly. Apply skin preparations only if necessary and allow to dry completely.	Alcohol-free preparations should be used generally on infants and toddlers if used at all. Skin preparations should be used if the pouch being applied has a taped border. Skin preparations can help with adherence. **caREminder** *There is limited safety information on the use of this product with premature infants and infants less than 30 days of age.*

Steps	Rationale/Points of Emphasis
7a. Inspect the child's skin.	Provides early detection of complications from poor pouch adherence. Stoma should be pink to red in color and moist.
7b. Inspect the stoma for color and condition, peristomal hernia, prolapse, retraction, and infection around stoma or incision.	Infants with ileostomies tend to have higher incidence of hernias. If outward telescoping of bowel is present, notify surgeon. Stoma is below skin surface. Pouch opening needs to be slightly larger to keep a good seal. Protect any exposed skin with skin barrier (ostomy) powder and seal with no-sting preparations. Swelling or firm abdomen, redness, tenderness to touch, and/or a fungal rash may all indicate signs of infection.
8. If infant, child, or teen has reddened or denuded skin, a barrier powder should be used on this skin. Apply a small amount of powder to cleansed skin. Gently brush away excess powder with gauze, being careful not to brush toward face. Seal powder with alcohol-free skin prep (3M or Smith and Nephew). Allow to dry completely.	Powder can assist with healing of peristomal skin. Applying powder to moist skin before drying sometimes makes this application easier. For very young infants, use a moistened finger to seal powder in place of skin preparations. Use alcohol-free preparation only to decrease the amount of discomfort with application. When sealing powder, pat (do not wipe) the preparation to trap powder in place. Skin preparations also help seal around the stoma at any irregular areas.
9. If paste is necessary to fill gaps or increase wear time, apply to back of the skin barrier on the pouch after removing the release paper. A thin layer should be applied near the stoma opening only. Use a small syringe to assist in applying a thin line of paste to pouch.	Paste helps to caulk around the stoma and protect the skin. It may also increase wear time of the barrier. **caREminder** *Newborn skin is fragile and is easily traumatized. Using as few products as possible to obtain adequate seal is encouraged. Do not use paste on skin that is not intact because it will cause discomfort.*
10a. Remove paper backing and apply prepared pouch over stoma. Press pouch with fingertips, especially around base of stoma.	
10b. Hold your hand gently over the pouch for 1 to 2 minutes.	Improves adhesion of the pouch.
10c. For infants, it often is easier to place pouch to the side.	Allows for ease of emptying pouch.
11. Close bottom of pouch with tail closure or clamp provided. The tail closure on the infant and pediatric pouch needs to be rolled at least three times before folding ties in. When using a clamp to close the pouch, make sure that the end of the pouch is folded over just one time and clamp is closed.	Keeps drainage in pouch. With infants and toddlers, it is easier to apply the tail closure before applying the pouch. Be careful not to pull on the pouch seal when applying tail closure. If clamp is not closed properly, it may come open and leak from the weight of stool. **KidKare** Do not use small clips or rubber bands with young children because these are choking hazards.
12. Remove gloves and perform hand hygiene. Dispose of waste in appropriate receptacle. Return equipment to secure area.	Reduces transmission of microorganisms. Equipment should be easily located for next use.
13. If a pattern has not been made, save the paper backing to provide a pattern for the next pouch change. Date pattern.	Assists others in preparation of future pouches.

PROCEDURE Emptying/Cleaning Pouch

Steps	Rationale/Points of Emphasis
1. Gather the necessary supplies.	Promotes efficient time management and provides an organized approach to the procedure.
2. Perform hand hygiene. Don gloves.	Standard precautions to reduce transmission of microorganisms.
3a. Position infant or child supine or on side. Position container under end of pouch.	Allows for ease of emptying pouch.
3b. Older children or teens may go into bathroom and sit on toilet or sit on the edge of their bed.	Allows child or teen to develop routine when he or she is at home or school.
4. For younger children, unwind tail closure and empty contents into container or diaper. For older children, using a clamp can open and turn bottom of pouch up to cuff.	Open system for drainage. Maintains a clean system when finished.
5. Empty contents into container or toilet.	Removes feces.
6. For infants and toddlers, cleanse bottom of pouch up to the tail closure both inside and out with paper toilet tissue or diaper wipes. For older children and teens, cleanse bottom of pouch cuff with tissue or paper towel before uncuffing and closing pouch.	Provides clean pouch bottom and decreases odor.
7. Close pouch with tail closure or clamp.	Keeps drainage in pouch.
8. Discard contents of container after measuring, if ordered.	Generally important to know output of infants and young children.
9. Remove gloves and perform hand hygiene. Dispose of waste in appropriate receptacle.	Reduces transmission of microorganisms. Standard precautions.

CHILD AND FAMILY EVALUATION AND DOCUMENTATION

- Evaluate the child or family's ability to perform ostomy care.
- Document the following:
  - Date and time of interaction
  - Assessment of stoma
  - Condition of the skin around the stoma
  - Type of output
  - Application of specific pouch
  - Child's tolerance of procedure
  - Child's and family's involvement and teaching of procedures to child or family

COMMUNITY CARE

- Review stoma and skin care and pouch application, emptying, and cleaning.
- Review the medical condition for which stoma was necessary with child and family.
- Demonstrate procedure to family and observe return demonstration.
- Include in teaching:
  - Odor can be controlled with commercial deodorants, if desired.
  - Baths can be given with or without the pouch in place, although showering is preferred.
  - One-piece garments will discourage a younger child from pulling on the appliance; loose-waist outfits decrease pressure on the area.
  - If the child is ambulatory, position the bottom of the pouch toward the child's thigh. If the child is on bed rest, position the pouch to the side to facilitate draining.
  - Signs and symptoms of diarrhea or dehydration, especially for infants and young children.
- Ensure that family has access to a vendor who can provide needed supplies.
- Ensure that the family has the name of a contact person and knows how to contact that person.
- Instruct the family to notify the healthcare provider if
  - Any changes are noted in the stoma or output, such as skin breakdown, ribbon-like stools, diarrhea, bleeding, no stool or flatus, or prolapse of the stoma.

Unexpected Situations

- *The ostomy bag continually comes loose and falls off:* Cleanse the skin thoroughly with warm water. Use a skin preparation to promote better adhesion of the pouch to the skin.
- *Skin around the stoma is excoriated or irritated:* The appliance may be cut too large, exposing skin inside of the ostomy appliance. Apply additional skin protection under ostomy appliance until skin is healed, and ensure appliance is cut to the correct size so that skin is not exposed.

Bibliography

Harrison, B., & Boarini, J. (2004). Pediatric ostomies: Pathophysiology and management. In J. Colwell, M. Goldberg, & J. Carmel (Eds.), *Fecal & urinary diversions management principles*. St. Louis: Mosby.

Rogers, V. (2003). Managing preemie stomas: More than just the pouch. *Journal of Wound, Ostomy & Continence Nursing, 30*(2), 100–110.

CHAPTER

83

Oxygen Administration

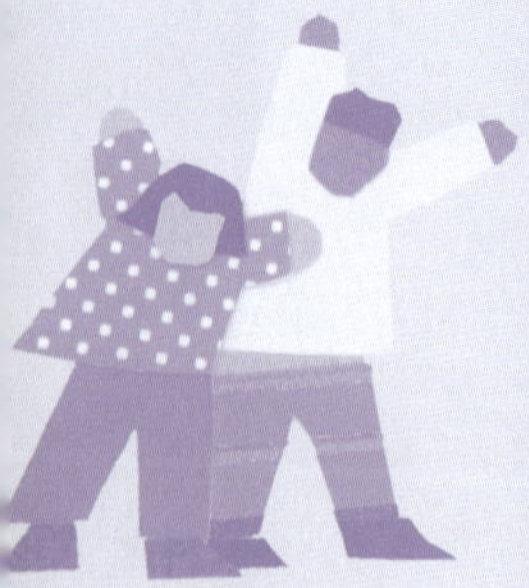

Clinical Guidelines

- Oxygen therapy may be administered by a respiratory therapist, registered nurse (RN), licensed practical nurse (LPN), or appropriately trained parent.
- Oxygen may be administered by use of a nasal cannula, nasopharyngeal catheter, mask, or hood when the oxygen level is below normal or the demand is increased (Table 83-1).
- Nasal cannulas and nasopharyngeal catheters are contraindicated in children with nasal obstruction (e.g., nasal polyps and choanal atresia).
- Nasopharyngeal catheters are contraindicated in those who have sustained a maxillofacial trauma, children in whom a basal skull fracture is present or suspected, and in children with coagulations problems.
- Nasopharyngeal catheters are not appropriate for oxygen administration in the neonatal population.
- Partial rebreathers or non-rebreather masks are not appropriate for use in the neonatal population.
- Restrict use of ignition sources in child's room (e.g., sparking toys, cigarettes, candles) when oxygen is in use.
- Secure cylinders of oxygen in upright position.
- During oxygen administration, the child should not wear clothing made of synthetic fabric that can build up static electricity.
- Oils and oil-based petroleum products should not be used on the child when oxygen is in use. These products are known to ignite spontaneously when used around oxygen (e.g., petroleum jelly should not be used around the child's face).
- The need for oxygen, the type of delivery system, and the amount of oxygen administered are determined by the physician.

Equipment

- Nasal cannula, nasopharyngeal catheter, or masks
- "No smoking" sign
- Oxygen flowmeter
- Oxygen tubing
- Oxygen hood
- Paper tape
- Water-soluble lubricant (for catheter insertion)
- Disposable gloves
- Goggles (if needed)
- Humidification attachment (if ordered)
- Waterproof pad

TABLE 83-1

Modes of Oxygen Delivery

Method of Delivery	Percentage of O_2 Delivered	Liter Flow	Nursing Care Considerations
Nasal cannula	21% O_2 plus 3% per liter	0.5–6 L/min	Dries mucosa; give with humidification. Provides limited O_2 delivery. Easy to use and well tolerated. Child can eat and talk without altering FiO_2. Contraindicated in children with nasal obstruction
Nasopharyngeal catheter	FiO_2 varies with the child's inspiratory flow	<3 L/min	Improper insertion can cause gagging and nasal or pharyngeal trauma. Contraindicated in children with nasal obstruction and in presence of maxillofacial trauma. Not appropriate for the neonatal population
Venturi mask	24–50% FiO_2	3–15 L/min	Adjustable to control percentage of oxygen delivered. Eating disrupts oxygen delivery. Air containment ports can become occluded.
Simple face mask	<40% FiO_2	4–8 L/min	Not a stable delivery system of FiO_2 >40%; good for short-term use (e.g., during procedures, for transport, in emergency situations). Eating disrupts oxygen delivery.
Partial rebreathing mask	50–60% FiO_2	6–10 L/min	Allows greater concentration of O_2 to be delivered. Eating disrupts oxygen delivery. Not appropriate for the neonatal population
Non-rebreathing mask	90–95% FiO_2	6–10 L/min	Allows greater concentration of O_2 to be delivered. Eating disrupts oxygen delivery. Child inhales only from gases in the bag; thus, kinks in the tubing may cause hypoxia. Not appropriate for the neonatal population
Bag-valve mask	65–95% FiO_2	10–15 L/min	Excellent method for assisted ventilation. Mask is selected to fit over the child's mouth and nose.
Air-entrainment mask (AEM) and nebulizers	24–60% FiO_2	3–15 L/min	FiO_2s are changed by selecting or changing the jet adapter or entrainment holes. Humidification of O_2 not required with mask use. Air-entrainment nebulizers share most features of AEMs but provide additional humidification and heat control and produce high noise levels in enclosed environments (e.g., hoods, incubators). Monitor child's temperature if heated nebulizer is used.
O_2-powered device	—	—	Never use in children.
O_2 hood	Can deliver FiO_2 up to 100%	2–3 L/kg/min	Easy visibility and access to child. Need to remove infant for feeding and care. Need oxygen analyzer to gauge percentage of oxygen delivered. Temperature in hood needs to be monitored. High gas flows may produce harmful noise levels.

- Extra baby blankets or bath blankets
- Warm sleepwear and hat for child
- Humidifier and sterile water
- Stimulating pictures to place on outside of hood (optional)

CHILD AND FAMILY ASSESSMENT AND PREPARATION

- Assess child's history to determine rationale for oxygen administration (e.g., chronic or acute pathologies).
- Determine whether there are any contraindications or concerns related to a particular method of oxygen delivery or level of oxygen concentration; inappropriate oxygen flow can result in hypoxemia or hyperoxemia.

Alert! *The role of oxygen in the development of retinopathy of prematurity is controversial. Care should be taken when oxygen is provided to preterm infants (those born before 37 weeks' gestation). Oxygen supplementation should not result in a PaO_2 of more than 80 mm Hg.*

- Use the parents to demonstrate how the equipment is placed on the child's face.
- Explain the procedure to the child/family. Use developmentally appropriate language (e.g., "This is to help you breathe better"). If access to the child is limited because of hood use, discuss with the family alternative methods to provide stimulation to the child and to engage in physical contact with the child.

PROCEDURE Nasal Cannula, Nasopharyngeal Catheter, or Mask

Steps	Rationale/Points of Emphasis
1. Perform hand hygiene. Gather all necessary supplies.	Reduces transmission of microorganisms. Promotes efficient time management and provides an organized approach to the procedure.
2. Select proper size of cannula, catheter, or mask.	Improper sizing of the equipment can lead to nasal obstruction.
3. Remove all friction toys or open flames from the area and display "no smoking" signs.	Sparks or static electricity will ignite the oxygen.
4. Connect the flowmeter to either the oxygen wall unit or the freestanding tank.	Allows for the oxygen to flow from source at the prescribed rate.
5. Connect the humidifier to the oxygen setup.	Provides for moisture in the system. Humidified air is less drying to the nares and to the lungs.
6. Following instructions for the particular oxygen setup, fill reservoir with sterile water.	Use of sterile water decreases the incidence of bacterial growth and mineral buildup within the system.
7a. Attach tubing to the oxygen source. 7b. Check all electrical equipment in area to ensure that it is grounded. 7c. Connect the distal end of oxygen tubing to the delivery device (cannula, catheter, or mask).	Allows oxygen to flow from source to child. Decreases chance of electrical sparks igniting the oxygen. Completes the cycle of supplying oxygen from the source to the patient.
8. Turn on the flowmeter to the prescribed amount and check to see whether you feel oxygen flowing through the system. Flow rates should be as follows: • Nasal cannula: In newborns and infants, flows should be limited to a maximum of 2 L/min. Older children and adolescents can be maintained up to 6 L/min. • Nasopharyngeal catheter: 0.5 L/min through and 8F catheter in infants with pneumonia and 1 L/min in infants up to 12 months of age. • Masks: Flow rates can vary from 5 to 10 L/min. Rebreathing of CO_2 may occur if total O_2 flow is inadequate.	Ensures the child actually receives the amount of oxygen the physician deemed necessary.
9. Don disposable gloves. If child is coughing or has copious secretions, a mask and goggles may also be worn.	Gloves and safety equipment protect against transfer of pathogens.
10. Place child in supine semi-Fowler's position. The neonate's and infant's head should be placed in a midline "sniffing position."	Raising the head of the bed helps protect the airway if the child should vomit during airway placement. Maintains proper alignment of the mouth, pharynx, and trachea.

For nasal cannula:

11. Place the nasal prongs just inside the external meatus of the nares. Either loop the head attachment around the child's ears and tighten it under the chin or loop it around and behind the child's head and tighten (Figure 83-1). Paper tape or other adhesive materials may be used sparingly to secure the tubing to the child's face.	Allows the oxygen to flow in closest proximity to the respiratory system of the child. The means of securing the nasal cannula in place vary based on manufacturer. The result should be the same: a secure nasal cannula. The restless child can easily dislodge the nasal cannula. Displacement can lead to loss of oxygen delivery. Care should be taken to keep cannula tubing and straps away from the neck to prevent airway obstruction in infants.

Alert! *Whatever type of attachment is used, take care to avoid undue pressure on the nasal tissue from tightening the attachment too much. Advise parents to watch for redness and irritation at any pressure points. Pressure on an area of skin can lead to tissue breakdown. Pressure in the nares can cause discomfort and erosion of the mucous membranes of the nares. Skin irritation can also occur from local allergic reaction to the polyvinyl chloride content of cannula.*

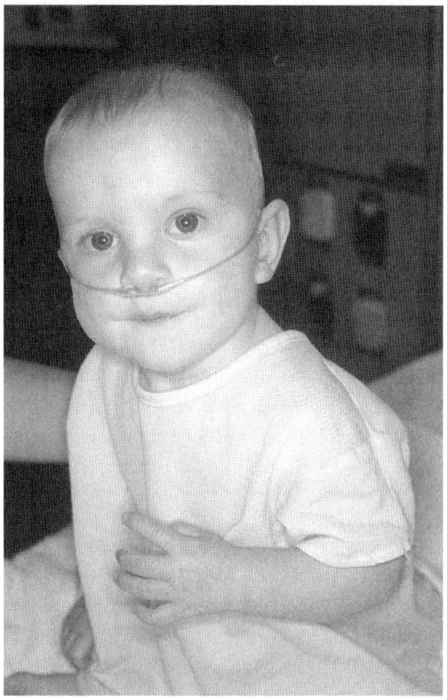

FIGURE 83-1
Nasal prongs are placed inside the external meatus of the nares, and the cannula tubing is secured.

Steps	Rationale/Points of Emphasis
12. Instruct child to breathe through his or her nose.	Provides the prescribed oxygen.
For nasopharyngeal catheter:	
13. Lubricate the tip of the catheter with water-soluble lubricant.	Protects the mucosa as the catheter is glided in place. **caREminder** *During insertion, keep air flow off to prevent irritation to the child as the catheter is being manipulated near the child's face. Begin air flow once the tube is secured in place.*
14. Gently insert the properly sized catheter to a depth equal to the distance from the side of the nose to the front of the ear, so that the tip of the catheter is just visible in the pharynx below the soft palate when the mouth of the infant is open. In infants, this distance is about 7 cm. ***Alert!*** ***Do not use force to place the catheter. If resistance in placement is met, do not proceed.***	Improper insertion can cause gagging and nasal or pharyngeal trauma. Improper sizing can lead to nasal obstruction and irritation. Catheter sizes less than 8F are less effective in oxygen delivery and may easily obstruct with mucus. Use may be limited by excessive mucous drainage, mucosal edema, or the presence of a deviated septum.
15. Secure the tubing to the child's face using paper tape or other adhesive material.	Prevents dislodgement of the catheter when the child moves.
16. Turn on flowmeter, providing humidified oxygen to the child.	Oxygen given with this method is bypassing the humidifying and warming properties of the nose, thus requiring humidification to avoid drying of the pharyngeal mucosa and to reduce the likelihood of producing thick, dry secretions.

Continued

Steps	Rationale/Points of Emphasis
17. Place nasogastric tube through nares not being used. See Chapter 39 for insertion instructions.	The nasopharyngeal catheter can become displaced downward into the esophagus and cause gastric distention. Passage of the nasogastric tube permits rapid decompression of the stomach.
18. Alternate the site of the catheter between nares every 8–12 hours and change the tube daily.	Prevents occlusion of distal holes in catheter. Accumulation of mucus in the catheter can cause upper airway obstruction.

For mask:

19. With the elastic straps very loose, place oxygen mask over the head of the child so that the oxygen tubing travels downward and away from the child's head (Figure 83-2).	This position ensures that the mask is not placed upside down.

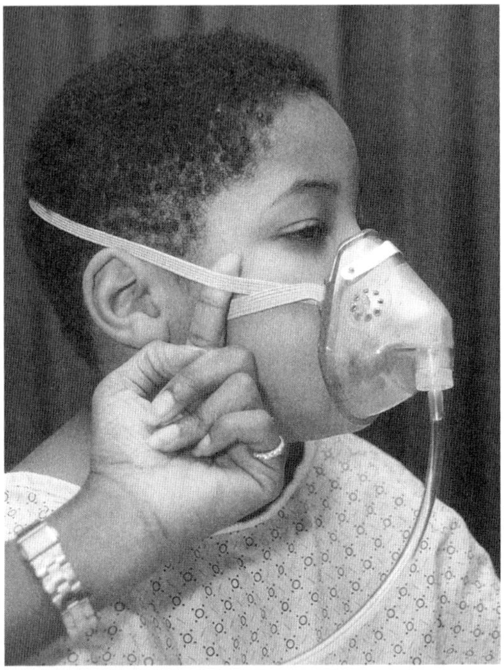

FIGURE 83-2
The oxygen mask is placed over the mouth and nose such that the nurse can easily fit one finger between the strap and the child's face.

20. Tighten the straps attached to the mask until you can easily fit one finger between the strap and the face of the child.	A properly secured mask allows the prescribed amount of oxygen to flow into the respiratory system. Irritation may result from tight application.

Alert! ***Aspiration of vomitus may be more likely when a mask is in place.***

PROCEDURE Oxygen Hood

Steps	Rationale/Points of Emphasis
1. Perform hand hygiene. Gather all necessary supplies	Reduces transmission of microorganisms. Promotes efficient time management and provides an organized approach to the procedure.
2. Remove all friction toys or open flames from the area and display "no smoking" signs.	Sparks or static electricity will ignite the oxygen. **KidKare** Dress child in warm sleepwear and hat because cool, moist oxygen can decrease body temperature enough to cause hypothermia.
3. Line area that the hood covers on the bed with a waterproof pad. Cover the same area with layers of bath or baby blankets.	Humidity from the oxygen delivery system will cause the sheets and mattress to become damp with moisture in a very short time. Having a layered area that can be easily changed will help keep the child from having to lie on damp sheets. **caREminder** *In the preterm neonate population, heated humidifiers rather than nebulizers should be used with the hood. Humidifiers reduce the noise level and minimize cross-contamination. Heated humidifiers are recommended to maintain thermoneutral environments. Temperatures within enclosures should be monitored to reduce the potential for overheating the neonate, resulting in cold stress or apnea.*
4. Connect the humidifying unit to the hood.	Moistened oxygen is less drying to the respiratory system. If unheated, O_2 from nebulizer may induce cold stress in neonates. Temperatures within the hood should be closely monitored to reduce potential for cold stress or apnea.
5. Following the manufacturer's instructions, fill the reservoir with sterile water.	Sterile water is less likely to grow bacteria and clog the system with minerals.
6. Connect the unit to the oxygen source.	This allows the oxygen to move from the source to the child.
7. Place the hood on the crib or bed so that the child's head is inside the unit. The hood should not rest on the child's neck, and the child should be able to turn his or her head side to side easily (Figure 83-3).	Prevents obstruction of the airway. An improperly sized hood can result in irritation to the infant's skin.

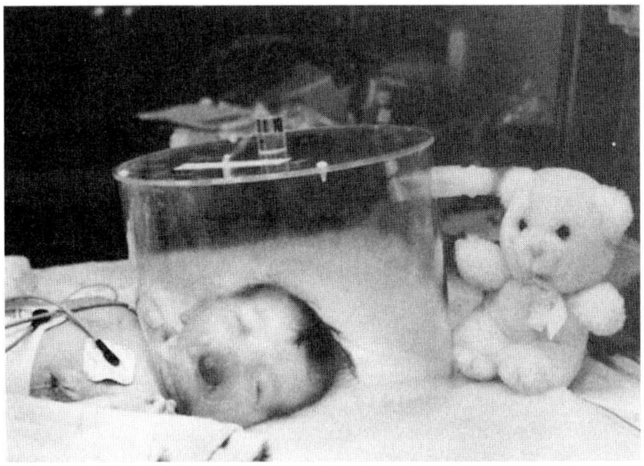

FIGURE 83-3
The child's entire head should be inside the oxygen hood with enough free space to ensure that the hood does not rest on the child's neck.

Continued

Steps	Rationale/Points of Emphasis
8. Turn on the oxygen and humidifying unit to the prescribed setting. Measure oxygen concentration close to the child's nose and mouth. Adjust oxygen to ordered concentration.	Ensures that the ordered oxygen concentration level is available.
9. Encourage family and other staff to limit the amount of time the child is outside of the hood. Removable lids and ports should be used to access the infant. Encourage family to freely touch and stroke the child and to provide auditory and visual stimulation. Nasal O_2 may need to be supplied during feeding and nursing care of the child in a hood.	Limiting the time that the unit is open will maximize the quality of the oxygen therapy. Each time the unit is opened or the infant is removed from the hood, the oxygen level administered to the infant is decreased. **KidKare** Small visually stimulating pictures can be placed on the outside of the hood, facing the infant, to provide infant stimulation. Pictures should not obstruct clear view of infant by healthcare providers.

CHILD AND FAMILY EVALUATION AND DOCUMENTATION

- Evaluate the child/family's level of understanding of how and why oxygen therapy is being used.
- Discuss safety concerns with the family, giving special attention to avoidance of smoking, open flames, and electrical or friction toys.
- Evaluate and document the respiratory status of the child.
- Document the following:
  - Type of oxygen delivery system that is in use (i.e., cannula, mask, or hood)
  - Time that oxygen therapy was initiated
  - Setting of the oxygen flowmeter and the frequency and length of time that the hood is open or the oxygen device is not in place
  - Skin status for redness or irritation at pressure points of straps or cannula

COMMUNITY CARE

- If oxygen therapy is to be continued after discharge, verify with the family which home care companies are covered by their insurance.
- Contact chosen home care company as early as possible to make arrangements for home oxygen administration equipment.
- Arrange for home care nurse to speak with the family.
- Review safety considerations with the family:
  - A minimum of 10 feet must separate oxygen apparatus and open flames.
  - Restrict use of ignition sources (e.g., sparking toys, cigarettes).
  - Secure cigarettes, matches, and lighters in a location away from the area where oxygen therapy is being used.
  - Assess that cylinders of oxygen are secured in an upright position.
  - All electrical equipment and oxygen equipment should be intact, in proper working order, and not emitting sparks. Extension cords should not be used.
  - Avoid the use of synthetic materials around oxygen equipment.
  - Avoid the use of oils and oil-based or petroleum products in the area of oxygen therapy.
- Instruct the family to contact the healthcare provider if
  - Child's respiratory condition worsens
  - Family remains unclear how to operate home care equipment

Unexpected Situations

- *While receiving oxygen via nasal prongs, the child turns blue and desaturates to 80% FiO_2 as measured by pulse oximetry:* Stimulate the child. Quickly assess to ensure the child is breathing and has circulation. Increase the flow rate of oxygen provided until he recovers from cyanotic episode and FiO_2 reading is above 95. Ensure that the oxygen tubing is connected to the flowmeter and that there is nothing obstructing the air flow through the tubing. Once the child has recovered from this cyanotic episode, report episode to physician or advanced practice nurse to determine whether flow rate needs to be maintained at a higher rate or decreased back to previous setting.
- *Child is receiving oxygen via face mask and vomits while wearing mask:* Remove mask immediately. With the assistance of another person, provide oxygen by placing an oxygen catheter near the nose while another person assists in cleaning up the child. Once the child is cleaned up, consider changing oxygen delivery system to nasal prongs.

Bibliography

ARRC Clinical Practice Guidelines. (2002). Selection of an oxygen delivery system for neonatal and pediatric patients. *Journal of the American Association for Respiratory Care, 47*(6), 707–716.

Davies, P., Cheng, D., Fox, A., & Lee, L. (2002). The efficacy of noncontact oxygen delivery methods. *Pediatrics, 110*(5), 964–967.

Frey, B., & Shann, F. (2002). Oxygen administration in infants. *Archives of Diseases in Childhood: Fetal and Neonatal Edition, 88*, F84–F88.

Mishoe, S., Brooks, C., Dennison, F., Hill, K., & Frye, T. (1996). Octave waveband analysis to determine sound frequencies and intensities produced by nebulizers and humidifiers used with hoods. *Neonatal Intensive Care, 9*(2), 20, 23–25, 53–54.

Pruitt, W., & Jacobs, M. (2003). Basics of oxygen therapy. *Nursing2003, 33*(10), 43–45.

C H A P T E R

84

Parenteral Nutrition and Intravenous Fat Emulsion Infusion

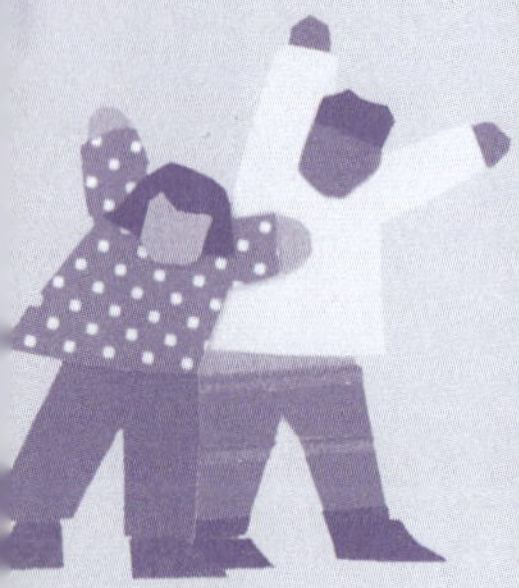

Clinical Guidelines

- Parenteral nutrition (PN) and intravenous fat emulsion (IVFE) are administered by a registered nurse (RN) under order of a healthcare prescriber.
- PN and IVFE are delivered to the neonate, infant, or child through a central or peripheral catheter. Line selection is dependent on the composition of the solution: Peripherally delivered fluids may have no greater than a 10% concentration of dextrose or no greater than 5% concentration of protein. Concentrations above these amounts are delivered though central infusion. Also, if the solution has a pH of <5 or >9, or osmolality >600 mOsm/L, it should be administered through central infusion.
- Central catheter tip location is confirmed by radiography before infusion therapy.
- The infusion line is dedicated to infusion of parenteral nutrition; no other medication or infusion, except intralipids, is infused through this line, except in an emergency.
- PN and IVFE are delivered through an electronic infusion device.

Equipment

- Appropriate venous device in place
- Electronic infusion device
- Tubing for the infusion device
- In-line filter
- For non–lipid-containing solution: 0.2-micron filter containing a membrane that is bacteria and particulate and air eliminating
- For lipid infusions or total nutrient admixtures that require filtration: 1.2-micron filter containing a membrane that is particulate retentive and air eliminating
- Nutrient solution, usually consisting of amino acids, glucose, and electrolytes and/or IVFE solution
- Flush solution (saline or heparin) appropriate to size and weight of child (see Chapters 49 and 104)
- Additives as ordered by the healthcare prescriber
- Disinfectant solution
- Antiseptic swab or pad

CHILD AND FAMILY ASSESSMENT AND PREPARATION

- Assess knowledge base of family and child regarding what parenteral nutrition is and why the child is receiving it.
- Determine family's knowledge level regarding the child's underlying condition.
- Determine child's baseline laboratory values, hydration status, nutritional status, weight, and height.
- Assess catheter site for appropriateness (peripheral versus central, depending on concentration of dextrose and protein), patency, and signs of infection.
- Assess the child for signs and symptoms of septicemia.
- Remove PN or IVFE solutions from refrigerator at least 1 hour before administration to warm to room temperature.

> ***Alert!*** *Child should be weighed daily or per institutional policy to ensure the correct amount of fluid and nutrients are being administered based on child's current weight.*

PROCEDURE **Parenteral Nutrition**

Steps	Rationale/Points of Emphasis
1. Gather the necessary supplies and prepare work surface by cleansing with disinfectant solution. Perform hand hygiene.	Promotes efficient time management and provides an organized approach to the procedure. Reduces transmission of microorganisms.
2. Place solution bag on clean work surface. Solution should be at room temperature. ***Alert!*** *Never warm solution in a microwave; use warm water bath if necessary. Microwaving may cause the solution to heat unevenly and may cause deterioration of components within the solution.*	Infusing a cold solution may cause hypothermia.
3a. Inspect solution. Verify label against healthcare prescriber orders for match. Check expiration date. Examine solution and container for clarity, signs of contamination, or particles. Do not infuse if solution has expired, is cloudy, has crystals, or has leaks.	Reduces chance of child receiving incorrect or contaminated solution.
3b. Identify the child utilizing two different patient identifiers. Match identification with label on the solution bag.	Reduces incidence of solution being administered to the wrong child.
4. Examine infusion device and site for type, placement, patency, and signs of infection. Any signs or symptoms of infection should be immediately reported to the healthcare prescriber and the infusion delayed.	Decreases chance of complications.
5. Maintain aseptic conditions and add additives (many pharmacies send the solution complete with additives, so this step may be eliminated) per following steps: a. Draw up ordered additives. b. Cleanse port with appropriate antiseptic. c. Inject additives into solution; once infusion is started, no other medications may be added. d. Gently agitate solution—do not shake.	Reduces transmission of pathogens into solution. Vigorous shaking causes foaming and delays administration.
6. Set up tubing and pump: a. Add 0.2-micron filter to tubing. b. Spike solution bag. c. Prime tubing according to manufacturer's directions. d. Attach to IV-controlled infusion device according to manufacturer's directions.	Prepares line for infusion.

Continued

Steps	Rationale/Points of Emphasis
Alert! *Change administration sets, using aseptic technique, every 72 hours and immediately upon suspected contamination or when the integrity of the product or system has been compromised to help reduce chance of bacterial growth. Administration sets that have been used for PN and have a piggybacked IVFE must be changed every 24 hours.*	
7. Connect tubing to catheter:	
a. Cleanse catheter port with appropriate antiseptic.	Decreases potential of introducing pathogens because there is a greater potential for pathogen growth and contamination as a result of the dextrose and protein content of the solution.
b. Flush infusion device with normal saline (0.9% NS).	Flushing ensures patency of the line and clears any medication from the line.
c. Secure tubing to device as appropriate or recommended by manufacturer. All administration sets shall be of Luer-Lok design, including all add-on devices and tubing junctions.	
d. Ensure that all connections are secure.	
8. Initiate infusion by setting IV-controlled infusion device to ordered flow rate. Start pump.	Ensures accurate delivery of solution.
9a. Infuse over allocated time period; infusions may be started over a longer time (16–18 hours) and decreased down to 8–10 hours.	Allows body to adapt to metabolizing increasing amounts of dextrose. **KidKare** Administer parenteral nutrition during the night whenever possible so that the child will be free of the tubing and pump during the day. This enables child to more readily engage in developmentally appropriate activities and lead a more normal lifestyle.
9b. Gradually increase flow rate at initiation of high concentrations of dextrose and protein (Figure 84-1).	Prevents hyperglycemia. **caREminder** *Many newer IV-controlled infusion devices have this as a built-in feature.*

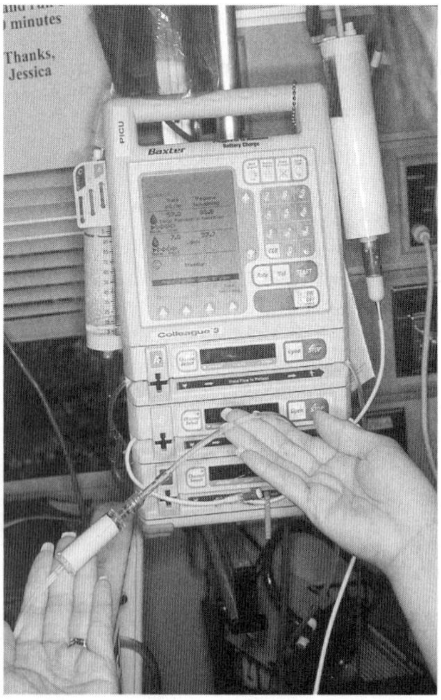

FIGURE 84-1
Parenteral nutrition is administered with an electronic IV-controlled infusion device, using tubing that includes a micron filter.

Steps	Rationale/Points of Emphasis
10a. Monitor child regularly during infusion at least every hour in inpatient facilities and as specified by healthcare prescriber at home for • Metabolic complications: hypoglycemia, hyperglycemia, electrolyte imbalances, azotemia, carbon dioxide retention • Catheter-related problems: breakage, dislodgment, occlusion • Infectious complications: localized site infection, sepsis • Monitor vital signs every 4 hours or as needed.	Enables prompt detection of complications.
10b. Monitor blood glucose every 6 hours initially or if signs of hypoglycemia or hyperglycemia are present. Contact healthcare prescriber if blood glucose is abnormal.	The body adapts to high dextrose concentrations by producing increasing amounts of insulin; when the administration of the high dextrose concentration is suddenly interrupted, the child could experience hypoglycemic episodes because it takes time for the body to react to the change. ***Alert!*** ***If high glucose infusion is suddenly interrupted, be prepared to administer a 5% to 10% dextrose solution to the child until the high glucose solution infusion can resume.***
11. Decrease infusion rate gradually at end of infusion, as ordered.	Enables body to adjust to decreasing dextrose levels; prevents hypoglycemia.
12a. Once infusion is complete, turn off pump.	
12b. Disconnect and discard tubing.	
12c. Cleanse catheter port with appropriate antiseptic.	Reduces the risk for transmission of pathogens into the line.
12d. Flush catheter with normal saline, amount dependent on child and catheter size.	Clears line of dextrose solution, which could potentially cause occlusion or be a growth medium for bacteria.
13. Dispose of equipment and waste in appropriate receptacle. Perform hand hygiene.	Standard precautions. Reduces transmission of microorganisms.

PROCEDURE Intravenous Fat Emulsion

Steps	Rationale/Points of Emphasis
Use the same procedure as in parenteral nutrition, with the following variances:	
1a. When examining solution for contamination and/or decay: lipids appear opaque; inspect for uniformity and no oily separation.	Detects contaminated and decayed solutions. Fat molecules are larger than protein and dextrose molecules and will occlude a finer filter.
1b. IVFEs are usually infused along with the parenteral nutrition through a port below the 0.2-micron filter.	
1c. Change tubing every 24 hours; consecutive units of IVFE may be administered through the same tubing if within 24 hours, and intermittent units of IVFE are administered using a new sterile administration set for each new container. Change add-on devices (e.g., extension tubing, needles) at same time as the tubing.	Prevents potential for pathogen growth.
2. In addition to catheter and infectious complications, monitor triglyceride levels, initially weekly and then as prescribed by the healthcare prescriber.	Provides prompt detection of detrimental effects of IVFE infusion.

Child and Family Evaluation and Documentation

- Evaluate child and family understanding of reason for use of parenteral nutrition, lipids, and treatment plan.
- Evaluate family capabilities if home care is planned.
- Evaluate family understanding of catheter care.
- Document the following:
  - Exact solutions administered, additives, amount, and duration, with time and date infusion started, completed, and by whom
  - Observations of line
  - Any complications that occurred, any side effects, and when healthcare prescriber was notified

Community Care

- If the child will be receiving parenteral nutrition or IVFE at home:
  - Contact the home care agency to coordinate teaching of IV-controlled infusion device to be used at home.
  - Initiate teaching of line care.
  - Initiate teaching regarding symptoms of hypoglycemia and hyperglycemia, other electrolyte imbalances, dehydration, overhydration, infection, and septicemia.
- Instruct family to contact healthcare provider if
  - Signs of infection are seen at infusion insertion site
  - Child has changes in mental status or level of consciousness
  - Child is not voiding
  - Child complains of pain at catheter site

Unexpected Situation

- *During infusion of parenteral nutrition, the young child is playing and disconnects his infusion tubing that is connected to his central line. Blood is now back flowing from the central line to the floor:* Immediately clamp the central line closest to the point of origin. Using aseptic technique, clean the access line and slowly infuse a heparin flush (see Chapter 49), evaluating for clotting. Once patency of the line has been reestablished, administer a 5% to 10% dextrose solution to the child until the high glucose solution infusion can resume. The tubing to the parental solution will need to be changed before being reconnected to the central line. Observe the child for hypoglycemia.

Bibliography

Ainsworth, S., Clerihew, L., & McGuire, W. (2005). Percutaneous central venous catheters versus peripheral cannulae for delivery of parenteral nutrition in neonates. *The Cochrane Database of Systematic Reviews, 2,* No. CD004219.pub2.

American Gastroenterological Association. (2001). American Gastroenterological Association medical position statement: Parenteral nutrition. *Gastroenterology, 121*(4), 966–969.

American Society for Parenteral and Enteral Nutrition. (2002a). Administration of specialized nutrition support. *Journal of Parenteral and Enteral Nutrition, 26*(Suppl. 1), 18SA–21SA.

American Society for Parenteral and Enteral Nutrition. (2002b). Administration of specialized nutrition support—Issues unique to pediatrics. *Journal of Parenteral and Enteral Nutrition, 26*(Suppl. 1), 97SA–110SA.

Duggan, C., Rizzo, C., Cooper, A., et al. (2002). Effectiveness of a clinical practice guideline for parenteral nutrition: A 5 year follow-up study in a pediatric teaching hospital. *Journal of Parenteral and Enteral Nutrition, 26*(6), 377–381.

Infusion Nurses Society. (2006). Infusion nursing: Standards of practice. *Journal of Infusion Nursing, 29*(1S), S1–S92.

Kanfelz, D., Gambarara, M., Diamanti, A., et al. (2003). Complications of home parenteral nutrition support in a large pediatric series. *Transplant Proceedings, 35*(8), 3050–3051.

Kleinman, R., Barness, L., & Finberg, L. (2003). History of pediatric nutrition and fluid therapy. *Pediatric Research, 54*(5), 762–772.

Phillips, S. (2004). Pediatric parenteral nutrition: Differences in practice from adult care. *Journal of Infusion Nursing, 27*(3), 166–170.

Schwenk, W. (2003). Specialized nutrition support: The pediatric perspective. *Journal of Parenteral and Enteral Nutrition, 27*(3), 160–167.

CHAPTER
85

Patient Identification

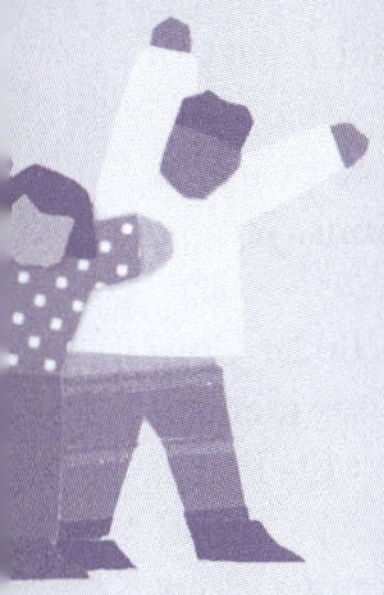

Clinical Guidelines

- All personnel providing care to pediatric patients must properly identify the child utilizing two different patient identifiers.
- Acceptable forms of identification include the child's
  - Name, as provided by the child/parent
  - Hospital identification (ID) number
  - Telephone number
  - Birth date
  - Address
  - Social Security number
  - Government issue or hospital issue photograph identification
  - Bar coding on the hospital ID name band
- Sources of patient identifiers include parent, guardian, and other family members. A child may not serve as the sole verbal source for patient identification about either himself or herself or a family member.

KidKare Have the parent/guardian confirm the child's name band information by saying the child's name and birth date, and ask for agreement from the child.

- In cases where children require emergency care and are unable to identify themselves and/or there is an absence of a parent who can provide identifying information, treatment is administered before identification if this care is necessary to stabilize the child.

On admission:

- All pediatric patients will have an ID name band affixed to an extremity upon admission.
- The parent or legal guardian of the admitted child receives a corresponding ID name band to affix on the wrist at the time of admission.

caREminder

The two-identifier requirement begins at the time of admission whereby the patient identifiers are reliably obtained. The ID name band is attached to the child (e.g., as an armband) and can be used to identify the child and matched to the procedure (medication, blood, sample).

During the child's stay:

- The registered nurse (RN) or licensed practical nurse (LPN) is responsible for assessing the integrity and placement of the ID name band daily.
- The child and parent are expected to wear their ID name bands during the entire course of their stay at the institution.

- If the ID name band is missing or removed for therapeutic purposes, after appropriate identification of the child or parent, a new ID name band will be placed on the child or parent.
- The child's and parent's ID name bands are compared at initial and subsequent visits.
- The child's identification is verified before receiving medications, obtaining specimens, or receiving treatments, procedures, or surgery.

caREminder

The ID name band should rotate freely on the extremity. Care should be taken that the extremity does not become edematous.

When transferring a child to another facility or receiving a child from another facility:

- The parent's ID name band and the child's ID name band are compared and matched by two RNs. Documentation reflects this match.
- Both the staff handing off and the staff receiving the child are responsible for patient identification at the time of transfer.
- Child must be wearing referring facility ID name band at time of transport.

When discharging the child:

- The child's and parent's ID name bands are compared and matched by two RNs.

EQUIPMENT

- Patient ID name bands for child and parent
- Chart with information providing secondary identification information about the child.

CHILD AND FAMILY ASSESSMENT AND PREPARATION

- Provide the child and family members with information regarding patient identification measures and procedures.
- Before affixing ID name bands on the child and parent, verify correct identification and match name band with child's medical record.

KidKare Help the child feel more at ease wearing an ID band by placing a blank ID band on the child's favorite stuffed animal.

CHILD AND FAMILY EVALUATION AND DOCUMENTATION

- Document the following:
  - Presence of correct ID name band on the child at the beginning of each shift
  - Match of parent's ID name band and child's ID name band any time child is transported to or from another institution or to or from another unit within an institution and upon discharge
  - Match of parent's ID name band and child's ID name band at initial and subsequent visits

COMMUNITY CARE

- During preadmission tours and activities, provide the child with a "play" ID name band to assist in the child's familiarity with this safety device. Explain institutional policies regarding patient identification.

Unexpected Situations

- *The child has lost her ID name band:* The child is identified using an acceptable form of identification, which may include the child's name as provided by the child/parent, hospital ID number or bar coding that matches parent's ID name band, telephone number, birth date, address, Social Security number, government issue or hospital issue photograph identification.
- *Patient transport has arrived to take the child to radiology. The child is alone in the room and speaks Spanish only:* Ensure an ID name band is on the child. Verify the child's identification by examination of the ID name band that is affixed to the child. The two-identifier method of patient identification is used without the child or parent having to recite back identifiers.

Bibliography

Beyea, S. C. (2002). Systems that reduce the potential for patient identification errors. *AORN Journal, 76*(3), 504–506.

Beyea, S. C. (2003). Patient identification: A crucial aspect of patient safety. *AORN Journal, 16*(3), 478–482.

Hottinger, J., Carlson, K., Salavec, L., Flade, R. G., & Beard, B. (2005). Managers forum. Two patient identifications. *Journal of Emergency Nursing, 31*(2), 191–192.

Howanitz, P. J., Renner, S. W., & Walsh, M. K. (2002). Continuous wristband monitoring over 2 years decreases identification errors: A College of American Pathologists Q-Tracks Study. *Arch Pathol Lab Medicine, 126*(7), 809–815.

Joint Commission on Accreditation of Healthcare Organizations. (2005). *National patient safety goals.* Retrieved November 1, 2004, from http://www.jcaho.org/acredited-organizations/patient+safety/05_npsg_guidilines_2pdf

Murphy, M. F., & Kay, J. D. (2004). Patient identification: Problems and potential solutions. *Vox Sang, 87*(Suppl. 2), S197–S202.

O'Neill, K. A., Shinn, D., Starr, K. T., & Kelley, J. (2004). Patient misidentification in a pediatric emergency department: Patient safety and legal perspectives. *Pediatric Emergency Care, 20*(7), 487–492.

Parisi, L. L. (2003). Patient identification: The foundation for a culture of patient safety. *Journal of Nursing Care Quality, 18*(1), 73–79.

C H A P T E R

86

Peak Flowmeters and Spacers, Use and Care of

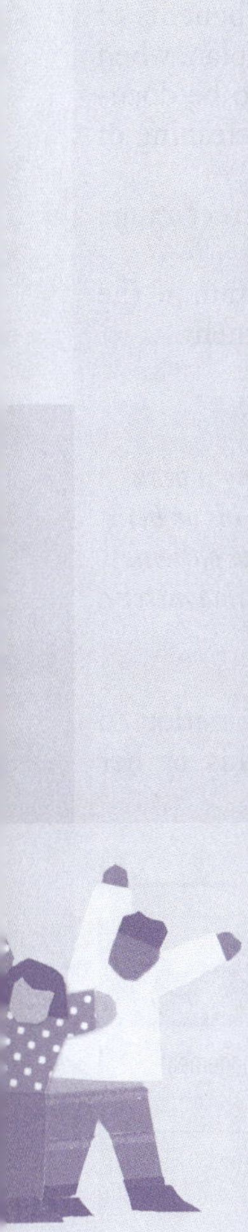

Clinical Guidelines

Peak Flowmeters

- Use of a peak flowmeter is ordered by a healthcare prescriber.
- Assessment of a child's peak flow may be performed by any healthcare provider, family care provider, or child (patient) who is educated about the technique.
- Peak flowmeters measure the greatest flow velocity that can be obtained during a forced expiration; peak flow measures the degree of obstructed airflow and patient's response to medication and can indicate a pattern of improvement or decline over time.
- Peak expiratory flow (PEF) varies with age, height, and sex.
- Peak flow measurements are effort dependent; poor effort results in poor measurements.
- Peak flowmeters are used in the initial, chronic, and long-term management of children with asthma.
- Measurement should not be performed immediately after a meal; this may result in triggering the child to gag or vomit.

Spacers

- Use of a spacer/holding chamber with the delivery of an inhaled medication (as ordered by the healthcare prescriber) may be performed by a registered nurse (RN), licensed practical nurse (LPN), family caregiver, or child (patient) who is educated about the delivery technique.
- Spacers/holding chambers are delivery devices used with a metered dose inhaler (MDI) to assist in the delivery of inhaled medication. In the case of children between 2 and 6 years old, you should use a spacer with a face mask attached or to which one can be attached.

caREminder

Assessment of children, regardless of age, may indicate that a mask is more effective in the delivery of the medication than the mouthpiece, for example, in children who are mouth-breathers, uncooperative, and so on.

- Spacers/holding chambers have a one-way valve that decreases the need for coordinated inhalation with the trigger of the puff of medication. They reduce the delivery of medication to the oropharyngeal region and potentially reduce side effects of inhaled steroids.

EQUIPMENT

For peak flow:

- Child's peak flowmeter (the same meter should be used consistently)
- PEF diary or flow sheet and pen to record

For spacer/holding chamber:

- Child's prescribed medication (MDI) and medication order
- Spacer/holding chamber
- Face mask if used by the child and separate from the spacer/holding chamber

CHILD AND FAMILY ASSESSMENT AND PREPARATION

- Determine whether the child/family routinely assesses PEF with the use of a peak flowmeter.
- For the chronic asthmatic child, engage the family in a discussion of the current home asthma management and the child's baseline "personal best" PEF as documented on his or her flow sheet.
- Review with family the child's green, yellow, and red zones (Chart 86-1) as identified by his or her healthcare provider and documented on his or her personal flow sheet. Have the child and family demonstrate their technique for using the peak flowmeter.

CHART 86-1 PEAK FLOW ZONE READINGS

Green zone = **Good control**—greater than 80% of the child's personal best.

Yellow zone = **Caution**—between 50% and 80% of the child's personal best.

Red zone = **Medical alert**—less than 50% of the child's personal best.

- For the child who is using a peak flowmeter for the first time, explain the procedure in an age-appropriate manner to the child and family, including the benefits of use, correlation between use and treatment plan, when to use the meter, information that needs to be documented with each use, and proper use and cleaning of equipment.
- Check to make sure the child has the correct range flowmeter.
- Provide the child with the opportunity to examine the meter and handle it before the actual assessment.

caREminder

In an outpatient office setting, the child may be using a peak flowmeter with disposable mouthpieces rather than his or her personal meter. Part of the educational plan for new patients may be to advise them to bring their personal peak flowmeter with them to each follow-up visit.

- Evaluate records and medical history information to determine the child's baseline PEF and his or her ranges for green, yellow, and red zones.

PROCEDURE Peak Flowmeter

Steps	Rationale/Points of Emphasis
1. Perform hand hygiene and gather the necessary supplies.	Reduces transmission of microorganisms. Promotes efficient time management and provides organized approach to the procedure.
2. Have child stand if able; otherwise, have child sit up straight with shoulders back. Have child empty the mouth of any solids or liquids	Provides for full expansion of the lungs for an accurate assessment.
3. Put the gauge on the meter to zero or at the bottom of the scale (Figure 86-1).	Provides for an accurate assessment on the gauge/meter.
4a. Have the child blow out to clear the airways.	Clears the airways to allow for a complete/full breath in. **KidKare** Have the child role-play huff cough, huff cough onto a mirror or blowing out candles on an imaginary cake. Demonstrate to the child the process and then have him or her return the demonstration so that when you are ready to perform the test, the child can clear the airways appropriately.

Steps	Rationale/Points of Emphasis

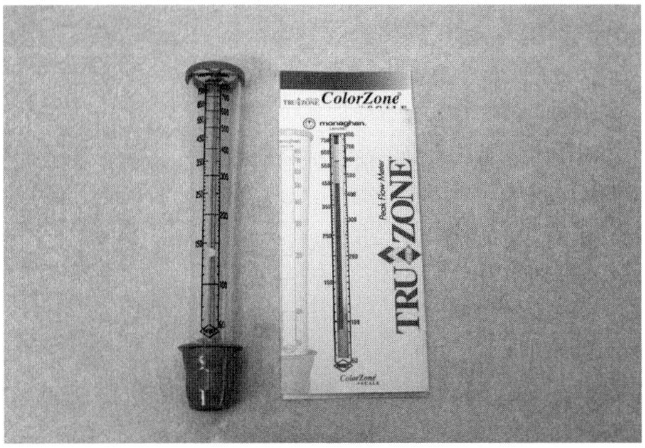

FIGURE 86-1
Peak flowmeter.

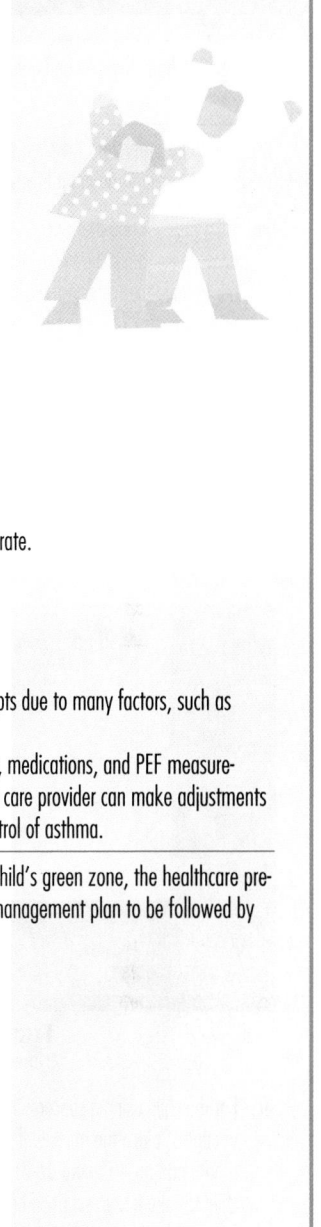

Steps	Rationale/Points of Emphasis
4b. Have the child take a deep breath in and then place the mouthpiece into child's mouth (lips around the mouthpiece), keeping the tongue away from the mouthpiece. Have the child blow out as hard and fast as he or she can. (Be sure your fingers are not in the way of the slide/gauge of the peak flowmeter.) Document the number.	This ensures that the measurement is accurate.
4c. Repeat steps 4a and 4b a minimum of two more times and record.	Some children may need additional attempts due to many factors, such as learning curve, fatigue, and cooperation.
4d. Select the best of three readings and document this in your charting and in the child's peak flow zone diary/log/worksheet. Also make notations regarding any current symptoms, activities, and/or medications.	By keeping a diary that reflects symptoms, medications, and PEF measurements across a period of time, the asthma care provider can make adjustments to your management plan to optimize control of asthma.
5. Compare the value obtained for the PEF with the orders/parameters. Where does it fall with regard to the child's personal best percentage? Initiate preestablished management plan to administer medication if child's results are in yellow or red zone (see procedure for Spacers, below). Obtain feedback from parent about child's past performance efforts as compared with current effort and progress.	For anything less than a value within the child's green zone, the healthcare prescriber will have previously established a management plan to be followed by the child.

caREminder

Factors that may influence the child's "personal best" include child's degree of effort, prior experience, ability to cooperate (regardless of age), and fatigue. Peak flow measurements are one tool used in the evaluation process.

Steps	Rationale/Points of Emphasis
6. Clean peak flowmeter per manufacturer's recommendations.	Standard precaution to reduce transmission of microorganisms.
7. Perform hand hygiene. Return equipment to secure area.	Reduces transmission of microorganisms. Equipment should be easily located for next use.

PROCEDURE Spacers

Steps	Rationale/Points of Emphasis
1. Perform hand hygiene and gather necessary supplies.	Reduces transmission of microorganisms. Provides efficient time management and provides organized approach to the procedure.
2. Verify the order with the child's medical record and check for allergy to drug; if present, do not administer drug and notify prescriber.	Verifies correct drug, dose, route, time, and patient. Allergic reactions to medications may be life threatening.
3a. Take the MDI and the spacer/holding chamber to the child and family and allow them to put the two together if developmentally appropriate. Remember to have them shake the inhaler before attaching the inhaler to the back of the spacer.	Shaking the inhaler is a recommended part of delivery of medication to ensure medication is thoroughly mixed.
3b. Have the child breathe out fully and place the spacer with inhaler attached into his or her mouth (Figure 86-2). For controlling medications (those used to prevent an asthma exacerbation), have the child or parent press down on the inhaler and have the child breathe in slowly and as deeply as possible. Have the child hold breath for a count of 8–10 seconds and then remove the spacer and breathe out slowly. Repeat the procedure to deliver a second puff. Remove spacer from mouth.	Breathing in slowly allows the proper delivery of medication and holding the breath at the end facilitates the delivery of medication to the lungs rather than being expelled.

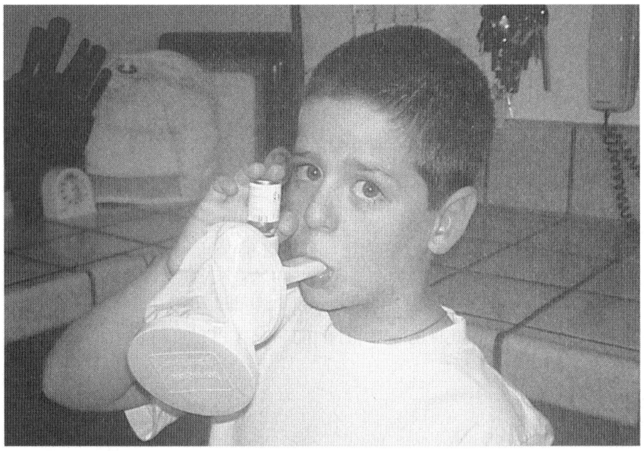

FIGURE 86-2
Use of a metered dose inhaler.

Steps	Rationale/Points of Emphasis
3c. For the child using a spacer with a mask attached (usually ages 6 and younger), place the mask with spacer and inhaler attached over his or her mouth and nose (Figure 86-3). Press down on the inhaler and instruct the child to take five to six good breaths to clear the chamber. Refer to manufacturer's instructions for number of breaths to clear spacer with mask attached. Immediately repeat the procedure to deliver the second puff. Remove spacer with mask from mouth.	Most spacer devices require five to six breaths to clear chamber when a mask is attached.

KidKare Allow younger children who are using a spacer with mask to play with the spacer, with adult supervision, so that damage to the device is avoided, to reduce anxiety at medication time. Use dramatic medical play with a doll and the spacer with mask. Older children can also practice with the spacer and slow breathing. Follow the manufacturer's recommendations about the use of the spacer, because some may have a one-way valve or a built-in flow signal. Because of the one-way valve in the spacer, if a child is breathing too fast or too deeply, the valve will whistle; children can practice so that this does not occur. For example, the AeroChamber MAX with mask has a flow signal to monitor the breaths but does not have an audible whistle.

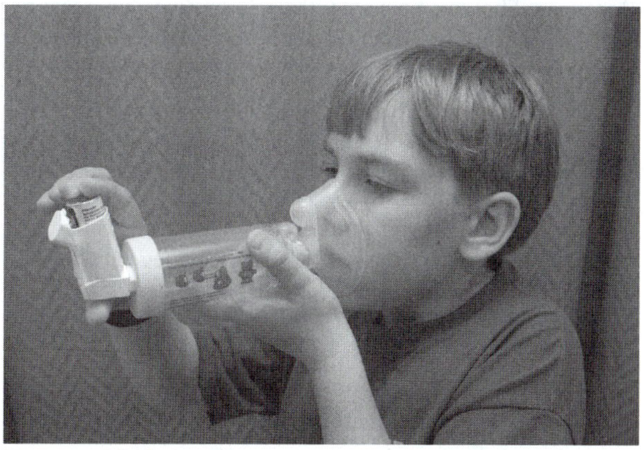

FIGURE 86-3
Spacer with a mask attached; the mask covers both the mouth and nose.

Steps	Rationale/Points of Emphasis
4. Clean spacer per the manufacturer's instruction. Generally, this is before the first use and weekly thereafter. When used with inhaled steroids, the spacer should be cleaned after each use. To clean the spacer, remove the back piece (do not remove the valved end) and soak both parts in lukewarm water with liquid detergent. Before removal, agitate gently. Rinse in clean water, shake excess water from the chamber, and allow to dry in a vertical position. Replace the back piece when the chamber is dry and ready for use.	The spacer chamber will have molecules of medication and propellant attached to the sides of it; these need to be removed on a regular basis, based on manufacturer's recommendations.
5. Clean the inhaler as needed. Look at the hole where the medication sprays from the inhaler to the spacer. If there is "powder" in or around the hole, it is time to clean the inhaler. Remove the metal canister from the L-shaped plastic mouthpiece. Place the mouthpiece and cap in warm water and agitate gently. Rinse and allow to dry overnight. Do not place the metal canister (medication canister) in water.	Standard precaution to reduce transmission of microorganisms.
6. Perform hand hygiene. Return equipment to secure area.	Reduces transmission of microorganisms. Equipment should be easily located for next use.

CHILD AND FAMILY EVALUATION AND DOCUMENTATION

- Evaluate previous assessments from the documentation record. Assess the child's current respiratory rate and effort.
- Inform healthcare prescriber of any significant changes in the PEF (a change from green to yellow or red zone).
- Document the following:
  - The best out of three attempts unless there are medical orders to the contrary. Include additional notes such as more attempts needed based on assessed effort, cooperation, and key interventions that may facilitate the child to effectively perform.
  - Administration of inhaled medication.
  - Child's respiratory status, including respiratory rate, characteristics of breathing, and any signs of respiratory distress.
  - Teaching provided.

COMMUNITY CARE

- If family members are using the peak flowmeter, instruct them to
  - Have the child stand for PEF assessment
  - Make sure the gauge on the meter is at zero or the bottom when starting the assessment
  - Record the best of three assessments
  - Keep peak flow zone chart/guidelines from the healthcare prescriber available at all times and make sure this information is included in the child's health file at school

- Perform an assessment each morning (before taking any medication) and in the evening. You also need to perform an assessment anytime there are symptoms or an attack, and approximately 15 minutes after taking medications for an attack. Assess at any other times as recommended by your physician or nurse practitioner.
- If family members are using the spacer/holding chambers, instruct them to
  - Use the spacer with each dose of medication from the MDI
  - With their school nurse and the healthcare prescriber, complete the appropriate paperwork to have the spacer and MDI at school and, if age appropriate, for young adolescents or school-aged children to carry their rescue medication and spacer with them while at school
- Remind the child and family to not share the MDI/spacers.
- Instruct the family to contact the healthcare provider if
  - PEF drops into the yellow zone or red zone (see Chart 86-1)
  - Child is having difficulty breathing and unable to obtain a PEF
  - Inhaled medication is administered per healthcare prescriber's parameters and child continues to have respiratory distress (e.g., stridor, nasal flaring, retractions)

Unexpected Situation

- *The child completes peak flow measurement and the reading is noted to be in the "yellow zone" (50–80% of personal best):* Review child's management plan to determine what treatment should be initiated at this time. Assist in administration of inhaled medication as prescribed. Reevaluate child's status after implementation of management plan.

Bibliography

American Thoracic Society. (2004). Guidelines for assessing and managing asthma risk at work, school and recreation. *American Journal of Respiratory Critical Care Medicine, 169*(7), 873–881.

Burkhart, P. V., Rayens M. K., & Bowman R. K. (2005). An evaluation of children's metered-dose inhaler technique for asthma medications. *Nursing Clinics of North America, 40*(1), 167–182.

Dolovich, M., Ahrens, R. C., Hess, D. R., et al. (2005). Device selection and outcomes of aerosol therapy: Evidence-based guidelines (Special Report). American College of Chest Physicians/American College of Asthma, Allergy, and Immunology. *Chest 127*(1), 335–371.

National Asthma Education and Prevention Program. (2002). Guidelines for the diagnosis and management of asthma update on selected topics. Expert panel report. *Journal of Allergy and Clinical Immunology, 110*(Suppl 5), S141–S219.

National Heart Lung and Blood Institute. (1997) *Practical guide for the diagnosis and management of asthma.* NIH Publication No. 97-4503. Washington, DC: National Institutes of Health.

Pruitt, W. C. (2005). Teaching your patient to use a peak flow meter. *Nursing2005, 35*(3), 54–55.

Williams, S., Schmidt, D., Redd, S., & Storms, W. (2003). Key clinical activities for quality asthma care: Recommendations of the National Asthma Education and Prevention Program. *MMWR Recommendations Report, 28*(RR-6), 1–8.

CHAPTER

87

Pediculosis and Scabies Management

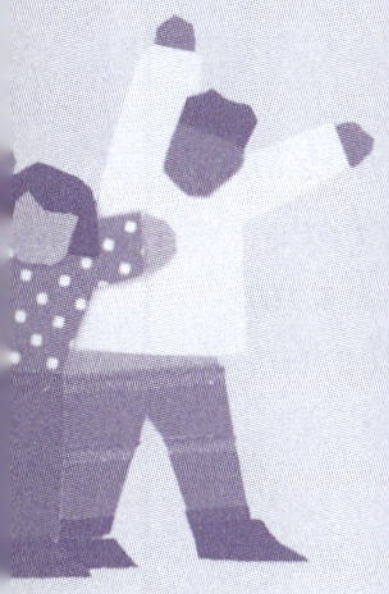

Clinical Guidelines

- A registered nurse (RN), licensed practical nurse (LPN), or unlicensed assistive personnel (UAP) may perform interventions to alleviate pediculosis.
- Implement standard precautions with the child with suspected or known pediculosis infestation.
- Treat sexual contacts of the child or adolescent when the presence of pubic lice or scabies is discovered. Referral may be needed if sexual abuse is suspected.
- Upon detection of pediculi, it may be advised to simultaneously treat the child, the family, and any other close contacts per healthcare prescriber's order.
- Upon detection of scabies, the child and all other members of the household and any other close contacts will be treated simultaneously per healthcare prescriber's order.

Equipment

For screening:

- Nonsterile gloves
- Patient gown or other nonsterile gown
- Nit comb
- Magnifying glass (if needed)

For treatment:

- Nonsterile gloves
- Patient gown or other nonsterile gown
- Plastic bag and secure fastener
- Prescribed medication or shampoo
- Soap
- Nonmedicated shampoo
- Clean, dry towels
- Clean clothes for the child
- Regular comb
- Nit comb
- White vinegar (if needed)

CHILD AND FAMILY ASSESSMENT AND PREPARATION

- Assess the parent's knowledge of pediculosis infestation and etiology of child's current exposure.
- Determine by child's history, secondary reporting, or direct examination of child whether or not child is at risk for pediculosis infestation and requires further evaluation and treatment.
- Teach the parent about pediculosis transmission and the importance of treatment.

caREminder

Parents may request information about alternative nontoxic remedies for head lice infestation such as putting mayonnaise, petroleum jelly, or tea tree oil on the child's hair. None of these methods has any proven effectiveness and may even be harmful to the child.

- Assess the child's home environment and the parent's access to needed supplies.

caREminder

Emphasize to the family that the child should be treated in a nonjudgmental manner and should not be ostracized because of lice or scabies.

- If infestation is suspected, determine child's recent contacts and discuss the need to have these contacts referred for assessment of lice or scabies.

PROCEDURE Screening for Pediculosis and Scabies

Steps	Rationale/Points of Emphasis
1. Interview child and parent about potential or known exposure to lice or scabies. Determine symptoms, length of time of infestation, possible exposure route, and treatment already initiated.	Pediculosis is transmitted through close contact with individuals already infested. Pubic lice or scabies may be associated with sexually transmitted diseases. Pubic lice or scabies infestation in the young child should raise suspicion of sexual activity and abuse. **caREminder** *Pruritus is the primary symptom in children affected by head lice, pubic lice, or scabies.*
2. Perform hand hygiene. Don nonsterile gloves. Don gown (as needed).	Reduces transmission of microorganisms and potential contact with pediculi.
3a. Assessing for lice or nits: Separate the hair into sections and carefully inspect the scalp and hair for the presence of lice or nits. A nit comb may be used to assist with hair separation and inspection. A magnifying glass may be used to assist in visualization of the nits.	Determines whether or not lice or nits are present. Keeping yourself positioned away from the child will prevent your body and clothing from coming into contact with lice or nits. **caREminder** *Nits appear as yellowish or white oval-shaped eggs stuck on the hair shaft. Head lice are clear in color after they have hatched. They may change in color to reddish or black with feeding. Pubic lice are brown or black colored after they are hatched, and their body appears more rounded.*
3b. Assessing for scabies: Examine the child's skin at locations of pruritus as well as skin areas where scabies are most commonly found, such as web areas between fingers and toes and inner aspect of elbows, axilla, wrist, groin, and waistband area.	Determines whether or not scabies are present. Scabies are attracted to warm areas of the body. **caREminder** *Scabies mites are too small to be seen without magnification. The mites cause small, itchy bumps and blisters due to how they burrow into the top layer of human skin to lay their eggs. The burrows sometimes appear as short, wavy, reddish, or darkened lines on the skin's surface, especially around the wrists and between the fingers. A child who has contracted scabies can also develop a bumpy red rash. Burrows are difficult to detect in areas of excoriation of simultaneous infection, such as impetigo.*

Steps	Rationale/Points of Emphasis
4. Remove gloves, and perform hand hygiene.	Reduces transmission of microorganisms or pediculosis.
5. Review findings of examination with child and parent and answer questions. Advise about treatment, if necessary.	Imparts information about child's condition and provides opportunity for teaching.

PROCEDURE Treating Lice

Steps	Rationale/Points of Emphasis
1. Perform hand hygiene. Don nonsterile gloves and gown.	Reduces transmission of microorganisms and potential contact with pediculi.
2. Undress child and place clothes in secured plastic bag. Give bag to the parent and provide instructions for cleaning the clothes (see Community Care).	Reduces transmission of lice.
3a. Bathe child with soap and water. Shampoo hair and pubic area with regular shampoo.	Cleanses body and hair of superficial dirt in preparation for the application of pediculocide. **caREminder** *Do not use conditioner or combination shampoo/conditioner, because the oils in conditioners may enhance absorption of chemicals.*
3b. Towel-dry child's hair with clean towel.	Removes excess water.
4. Place used towels in appropriate receptacle.	Reduces risk of transmission of lice to others.
5a. Apply antilice shampoo or treatment per package instructions or per order of a healthcare prescriber. Massage product into the base of the hair shafts where live lice and nits occur.	Kills lice. The majority of head lice die of starvation unless they have access to a human blood meal at least every 48 hours. Head lice are host specific; they do not live on live pets and do not jump or fly. **KidKare** While applying treatment, avoid contact with child' eyes and mucous membranes by protecting the child's eyes with a towel or washcloth.
5b. Never leave product in child's hair longer than directed. Do not use shower cap. Do not mix products or follow one treatment with another.	Leaving antilice treatments in a child's hair longer than directed prevents unnecessary exposure to toxins. Misuse or overuse of some antilice products has been reported to cause neurotoxic effects. Caution must be used, especially in treatment in children younger than the age of 2 years. Because of the risk of neurotoxic effects, antilice products are not often used on small children. Instead, use of a nit comb can remove nits and lice from the fine hair of young children. **Alert!** *Lindane (Kwell) is no longer recommended as a pediculocide by the Food and Drug Administration and has been banned from use in many countries and certain states. Lindane has a tendency to accumulate in lipid tissue and has a propensity for the lipid matter of the brain, thus leading to neurotoxicity manifested as generalized seizures and bone marrow suppression.*
6. Rinse hair thoroughly until water runs clear.	Removes all chemical products from child's skin to limit unnecessary exposure to chemicals.
7a. Remove child from bath, and dry child's body and hair with clean, dry towels. Place used towels in appropriate receptacle.	Reduces risk of transmission of lice to others.
7b. Dress child in freshly laundered clothing.	Provides for child's comfort and helps prevent reinfestation.

Continued

Steps	Rationale/Points of Emphasis
8. Comb tangles out of child's hair with regular comb.	Later use of nit comb will be easier in untangled hair.
9. Part the child's hair into small, easy-to-handle sections. Using the nit comb, comb each section of hair to remove nits, starting at the scalp and working down in a meticulous fashion and with special attention to the nape of the neck and behind the ears, rinsing comb frequently in water.	Some antilice treatments do not kill the eggs, so removal of the nits helps prevent reinfestation. Small, close teeth in a nit comb allow more effective removal of nits and nit shells.
10. Remove gloves and gown and perform hand hygiene.	Reduces transmission of microorganisms or pediculosis.

PROCEDURE **Treating Scabies**

Steps	Rationale/Points of Emphasis
1. Perform hand hygiene. Don nonsterile gloves and gown.	Reduces transmission of microorganisms and potential contact with pediculi.
2. Undress child and place clothing in a secured plastic bag. Give bag to parent and provide instructions for cleaning the clothes (see Community Care).	Reduces the transmission of scabies. Scabies mites can survive up to 4 days off the host. During that time reinfestation is possible. The female mite burrows under the skin and lays 10 to 25 eggs before dying. Three days later, the eggs hatch. The larvae move to the skin surface and mature into adults after 14 to 17 days.
3. Apply antiscabies cream or lotion to child's entire body from the neck down per package instructions or per order of a physician or healthcare prescriber. Be sure to apply cream to the navel area, between fingers and toes, and in body folds and creases. Leave some cream/lotion under child's fingernails. Avoid contact with mucous membranes.	Correct application of the antiscabies cream or lotion will rid the child of infestation. Misuse of some antiscabies products has been reported to cause neurotoxic effects. Caution must be used, especially in the treatment of premature infants less than 2 months and in children with a preexisting seizure disorder. The areas of the body most commonly affected by scabies are the hands and feet (especially the webs of skin between the fingers and toes), the inner part of the wrists, and the folds under the arms. It may also affect other areas of the body, particularly the elbows and the areas around the breasts, genitals, navel, and buttocks. **KidKare** Applying cream is best done before bedtime because the cream must remain on for 8 to 12 hours before it can be washed off.
4. Dress child in freshly laundered clothing.	Provides child's comfort and helps prevent reinfestation.
5. Wait 8–14 hours (consult package instructions for specific time) and then bathe the child to remove the cream or lotion.	Removes all chemical products from the child's skin to limit unnecessary exposure.
6a. Remove child from bath, and dry child's body and hair with clean, dry towels. Dispose of towels in appropriate receptacle. 6b. Dress child in freshly laundered clothing.	Reduces risk of transmission of lice to others. Standard precautions. Provides for child's comfort and helps prevent reinfestation.
7. Remove gloves and gown and perform hand hygiene.	Reduces transmission of microorganisms or pediculosis.

CHILD AND FAMILY EVALUATION AND DOCUMENTATION

- Evaluate parent's understanding of pediculosis transmission, correct use of prescribed medications, and the necessary actions to rid the family environment of pediculosis infestation. Treatment failure may be related to misunderstanding of instructions, insufficient dose time, frequency or quantity of product applied, or failure to remove live eggs.

CHART 87-1 HOME CARE OF PEDICULOSIS AND SCABIES

Treatment	• Repeat the application of antipediculosis treatment in 7–10 days if indicated in package directions. • For head lice: check the heads of everyone in the home and treat anyone with crawling lice or nits within ½ inch of the scalp with antilice shampoo or cream. • For scabies: everyone living in the house should be treated preventively simultaneously with an application of scabies medicine. Close contacts of the affected child should also be treated. • Notify the child's school or day care facility of the diagnosis, and examine close contacts and treat prophylactically. • Notify sexual partner of the diagnosis.
Managing the Home Environment	• Wash the child's bed linens, pajamas, underwear, recently worn clothing, washable stuffed animals, hats, scarves, hooded jackets, and so forth in a washing machine with hot water and laundry detergent. Dry items on the hot setting for at least 20 minutes. • Dry clean unwashable bed linens or other unwashable items in the child's environment or place items in a sealed plastic bag for 2–3 weeks for scabies and 48 hours for lice. • Vacuum all floors, carpets, and furniture in child's play and sleep areas. Do not use sprays or have the house fumigated. Pesticide sprays add toxins to the child's environment. If the family leaves the home for 48 hours they can expect to return to a head-lice free environment because the lice die of starvation unless they have access to a human blood meal at least every 48 hours. • Soak family combs and brushes in hot water (above 130.8°F [54.9°C) for 1 hour. Add pediculocide or a disinfectant to the water. • Wash or vacuum the child's stroller, car seat, and any sports helmets.
Managing the School or Day Care Environment	• Children can return to school after 1 treatment with shampoo or medicine. • Children infested with lice should not attend school or day care until treated. Children who have nits do not need to be excluded, but should have repeated examinations to detect the presence of crawling lice. • Teach children not to share combs, brushes, clothing or headgear. • Hang each child's coat separately with the respective hat and scarf tucked into the sleeve. • Label sleeping mats individually, store in separate cubbies, and wash frequently. • Vacuum carpeted areas frequently.

- Document the following
  - Intervention measures that were implemented.
  - Instructions given to family regarding ongoing care.

COMMUNITY CARE

- Provide written instructions regarding home/community care to include the following (Chart 87-1):
  - Treatment
  - Managing the home environment
  - Managing the school or day care environment
- Instruct the family to contact the healthcare provider if
  - Itching interferes with sleep (advise the parent that the rash or itch may continue for 2–3 weeks after treatment)
  - Rash clears, then returns
  - Rash or sores begin to look reddened, are warm to touch, or are oozing secretions
  - Child develops a fever
  - New nits or burrows appear

Unexpected Situation

- *While getting a haircut, the hairdresser notes that you have head lice. You recall that you cared for a child 3 days previously with pediculosis:* You need to be treated for head lice following instructions for home care of lice and scabies (see Chart 87-1). You may return to work after one antilice shampoo has been completed.

Bibliography

Burkhart, C. (2004). Relationship of treatment-resistant head lice to the safety and efficacy of pediculicides. *Mayo Clinical Practice*, *79*, 661–666.

Centers for Disease Control and Prevention. (1999). *Parasitic disease information fact sheet.* Retrieved August 21, 2006, from http://www.cdc.gov/az.do

Centers for Disease Control and Prevention. (2000). *Pubic lice fact sheet.* Retrieved August 21, 2006, from http://www.cdc.gov/az.do

Centers for Disease Control and Prevention. (2001). *Treating head lice fact sheet.* Retrieved August 21, 2006, from http://www.cdc.gov/az.do

Centers for Disease Control and Prevention. (2003). *Head lice infestation fact sheet.* Retrieved August 21, 2006, from http://www.cdc.gov/az.do

Flinders, D., & De Schweinitz, P. (2004). Pediculosis and scabies. *American Family Physician, 69*(2), 341–348.

Koch, T, Brown, M., Selim, P., & Isam, C. (2001). Towards eradication of head lice: Literature review and research agenda. *Journal of Clinical Nursing, 10*, 364–367.

LaFuente, C. (2003). Is it scabies? How to tell. *The Nurse Practitioner, 28*(6), 57–59.

Monsen, K., & Keller, L. (2002). A population-based approach to pediculosis management. *Public Health Nursing, 19*(3), 201–208.

Scott, P., Gilmer, M., & Johannessen, W. (2004). The nit rating scale. *Journal of School Health, 74*(3), 108–110.

Venna, S., Fleisher, A. B., & Feldman, S. R. (2001). Scabies and lice: Review of the clinical features and management principles. *Dermatology Nursing, 13*(4), 257–262.

Williams, L. K., Reichert, A., MacKenzie, W. R., Hightower, A. W., & Blake, P. A. (2001). Lice, nits, and school policy. *Pediatrics, 107*, 1011–1015.

Zepe, B. Treatment of head lice: Therapeutic options. *American Family Physician, 69*(3), 655.

C H A P T E R

88

Pet Therapy

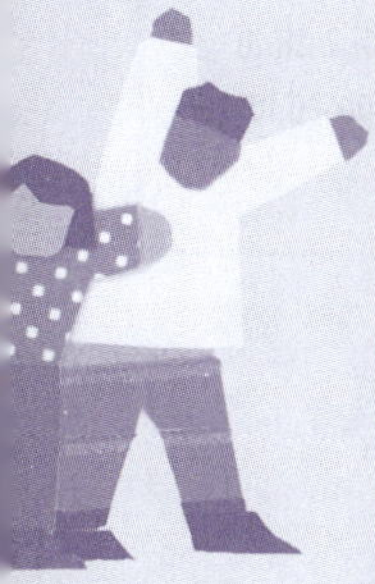

Clinical Guidelines

- Pet therapy or visitation is an intervention involving the use of animals to promote beneficial responses from the patient. These responses include but are not limited to promoting attachment, bonding, pain management, stress management, motivation, support, communication, improved body image, physiologic stability, coping, and comfort.
- Pet therapy animals are trained to participate in pet therapy visitation programs by certified organizations. This ensures the animals used are of good temperament, receive adequate health maintenance, and are up to date with vaccinations.
- Child/family consent for pet therapy is attained before the therapy.
- Pet therapy animals are bathed by caretaker within 24 hours before the pet therapy visit. The animals should be free from ticks, fleas, and obvious signs of illness.
- Provisions and arrangements for animal excrement, nutrition, and water needs are predetermined by the institution, the pet therapy organization, and the caretaker before the pet therapy visitation.
- The facility establishes guidelines for transport of animal and caretaker to area where pet therapy will be administered. Generally, animals are escorted by caretaker on a leash. The animal usually wears a T-shirt to control dander while being escorted through the hospital.
- Contraindications for pet therapy in the pediatric patient include allergies to animals or pet dander, the presence of an open draining wound, and fear of animals.
- Immunocompromised children do not need to be excluded from interaction with animals, according to the Centers for Disease Control and Prevention (CDC), as long as certain guidelines are adhered to. The participation of an immunocompromised child in pet therapy should be cleared by the attending healthcare professional in conjunction with the parents.
- The following animals are not suitable for pet therapy in a healthcare facility due to the high risk of infectious zoonosis: reptiles, birds, rodents, and exotic nondomestic animals.
- Pet therapy animals are kept from food preparation, linen, supply, and sterile areas.
- If assistance is required for sanitation of animal excrement, use universal precautions and contact facility's environmental services for a more thorough cleaning.

Equipment

- Certified therapy animal
- Animal caretaker or handler
- Clean towel/sheet if child is to hold the animal
- Disinfectant hand gel or soap and sink

Child and Family Assessment and Preparation

- Assess child for contraindications to pet therapy, and obtain attending healthcare professional clearance for pet therapy if child is immunocompromised. This ensures that pet therapy will not be administered inappropriately and put the child at undue risk for infection, allergies, or fear.
- Explain the procedure, purpose of the procedure, and possible benefits of the procedure to the child (in an age-appropriate manner) and family. This allows the child and family time to prepare and/or decline the intervention. Documented benefits include decreased blood pressure, decreased vital sign fluctuations, decreased muscle tension, and decreased risk for cardiovascular disease.

PROCEDURE Providing Pet Therapy

Steps	Rationale/Points of Emphasis
1. Identify area for pet therapy. If pet therapy is to take place at child's bedside, obtain permission from child's roommate; otherwise, an alternative area for pet therapy must be designated.	Children and their families who do not wish to participate or cannot participate in pet therapy must not be unduly exposed to pet therapy animals.
2. Check identification of animal and caretaker according to facility guidelines.	Ensures identity of pet therapy caretaker and animal and provides security.
3. Escort animal and caretaker to designated therapy area.	Prevents unnecessary exposure of animal to the healthcare facility.
4. Perform hand hygiene and instruct and observe child and any other staff to perform hand hygiene before contact with the therapy animal.	Reduces transmission of microorganisms.
5. If child will be holding animal in lap, cover the child's lap with a towel or clean sheet. If animal is placed on child's bed, cover the bed with a towel or clean sheet.	Contains pet dander in healthcare facility and prevents shedding onto child's clothes and bedding.
6. Observe child during pet therapy. During the therapy period, the child is permitted to touch and gently handle the animal. The child may also choose to sit quietly and enjoy having the pet in his or her presence without initiating physical contact with the pet. The length of therapy is based on tolerance of the pet and child and other variables that might impact the child's schedule (e.g., mealtime).	Evaluates tolerance to procedure.
7. At completion of therapy, remove linen upon which the animal had been placed and place in appropriate receptacle. Perform hand hygiene and instruct child and any other staff to perform hand hygiene after contact with pet therapy animal.	Reduces transmission of microorganisms.
8. Escort animal and caretaker from the child's room, ensuring that contact with other children is not made unless otherwise prearranged.	Ensures safe removal of animal. Children and their families who do not wish to participate or cannot participate in pet therapy must not be unduly exposed to pet therapy animals.

Child and Family Evaluation and Documentation

- Document child's tolerance to the procedure and any noted changes in affect, mood participation, or pain level.
- If child is being monitored, document any changes in vital signs or pain level.

Community Care

- If immunocompromised child is going home to an environment with animals, instruct the child in an age-appropriate manner and family on guidelines to reduce risk of infection.

Unexpected Situation

- *During the therapy session the child becomes agitated and starts crying:* Remove the pet from the child's lap or bed, ensuring that this is done in a calm and gentle manner so as not to further agitate the child or the pet. Provide distance between the child and pet. Determine source of child's agitation. Based on this information, pet therapy sessions may be discontinued at this time.

Bibliography

Brodie, S. J., & Biley, F. C. (1999). An exploration of the potential benefits of pet-facilitated therapy. *Journal of Clinical Nursing, 8*, 329–337.

Brodie, S. J., Biley, J., & Shewring, M. (2002). An exploration of the potential risks associated with using pet therapy in healthcare settings. *Journal of Clinical Nursing, 11*, 444–456.

Centers for Disease Control and Prevention. (1999). *Preventing infections from pets: A guide for people with HIV.* Retrieved August 21, 2006, from http://www.cdc.gov/hiv/pubs/brochure/oi_pets.htm

Centers for Disease Control and Prevention. (2004). *Healthy pets, healthy people.* Retrieved August 21, 2006, from http://www.cdc.gov/healthypets.

Freeman, L., Stewart, P., & Hooker, S. D. (2002). Pet therapy research: A historical review. *Holistic Nursing Practice, 17*(1), 17–23.

Giuliano, K. K., Bloniasz, E., & Bell, J. (1999). Implementation of a pet visitation program in critical care. *Critical Care Nursing, 19*(3), 43–50.

Kaminski, M., Pellino, T., & Wish, J. (2002). Play and pets: The physical and emotional impact of child-life and pet therapy on hospitalized children. *Children's Healthcare, 31*(4), 321–335.

National Association of State Public Health Veterinarians. (2003). Compendium of measures to prevent disease and injury associated with animals in public settings. Retrieved August 21, 2006, from http://www.avma.org/pubhlth/comp_animals_public_settings.asp

Schulster, L. M., Chinn, R. Y. W., Arduino, M. J., et al. (2004). *Recommendations of the CDC and Healthcare Infection Control Practices Advisory Committee. Guidelines for environmental infection control in healthcare facilities.* Chicago, IL: American Society for Healthcare Engineering/American Hospital Association.

Wu, A. S., Niedra, R., Pendergast, L., & McCrindle, B. W. (2002). Acceptability and impact of pet visitation on a pediatric cardiology inpatient unit. *Journal of Pediatric Nursing, 17*(5), 354–362.

CHAPTER

89

pH Study

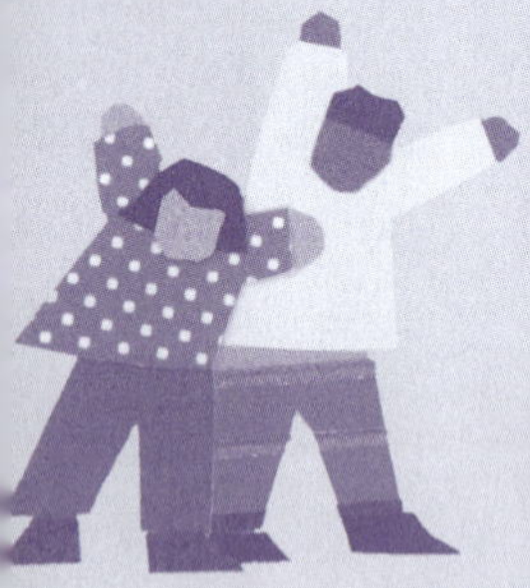

Clinical Guidelines

- The pH probe is inserted and removed by a physician or by an appropriately trained registered nurse (RN) or technician.
- An unlicensed assistive personnel (UAP) may act as an assistant during probe placement and may record observed events on the pH study log.
- Initiation and discontinuation of continuous pH monitoring require an order from a physician or advanced practice nurse (APN).
- A physician's or APN's order is required if restraints are to be used during the continuous pH monitoring.

Equipment

- pH probe
- Batteries
- pH monitor
- Buffer solution(s)
- Water-soluble lubricant
- Nonsterile gloves
- Tape measure (in centimeters)
- Tape or transparent dressing
- Lead wire with electrode, if applicable
- Electrode gel, if applicable
- Emesis basin
- Tissues
- pH study flow sheet

Child and Family Assessment and Preparation

- Assess the child's and family's understanding of the test's purpose, the basic procedure, and when to expect test results. Explain procedure as age appropriate.
- Explain parent's role in maintaining probe placement and documenting events during the test.

- Ensure that the parent or legal guardian has signed a consent form for pH monitoring before initiating the procedure.
- Assess for past history of symptoms, such as frequent coughing, choking or vomiting, irritability, poor eating, failure to thrive, apnea, bronchiolitis, pneumonia, asthma, hoarseness, stridor, and croup, which are often associated with gastroesophageal reflux (GER).
- Assess usual dietary habits, time of last feeding or meal, and any medications that child has taken in the previous 7 days.
- Assess need for sedation for probe insertion, if indicated. Allow adequate time for sedation to take effect.

PROCEDURE **pH Monitoring**

Steps	Rationale/Points of Emphasis
1. Ensure that the child has had nothing by mouth for 2 to 4 hours before probe placement.	Inserting the probe in the immediate postprandial period increases the risk for bronchial aspiration.
2. Notify the physician or APN if the child has taken any of the following within the time frames noted: • Histamine receptor antagonists (e.g., Tagamet, Zantac, Pepcid) within 72 hours of testing • Proton pump inhibitors (e.g., Prilosec, Prevacid, Nexium) within 7 days of testing • Prokinetics (e.g., Reglan) within 72 hours of testing • Antacids within 6 hours of testing	These medications tend to decrease the frequency or severity of acid reflux, producing inaccurate test results. However, the physician or APN may choose to do the study while the child is on medication.
3. Assemble equipment, perform hand hygiene, and don gloves.	Facilitates initiating the test with minimal delays and institutes standard precautions.
4. Attach the pH probe to the monitor, turn it on, and calibrate and record per the pH system manufacturer's instructions.	Proper calibration is necessary for accurate test results.
5. Estimate the position of the lower esophageal sphincter (LES) using the following formula: (length from nares to LES $= 5 + 0.252 \times$ height [cm]).	This is a commonly used formula to estimate position of tube, developed by Strobel and colleagues (Little et al., 1997).
6. Multiply the above value by 0.87 (87%). Mark the pH probe at this number.	The probe tip is placed at a distance 13% above the LES.
7. With an assistant's help, position the child supine with chin flexed to chest (place a pillow or towel roll under head to aid positioning). Older children may sit up with head forward. Secure both hands away from the face. Have emesis basin and tissues readily available.	Proper head placement decreases risk for inserting probe in the trachea and restraining hands decreases the risk of the child pulling out the probe. Sitting upright may increase the child's sense of control and decrease fear. Emesis basin is ready if child gags or vomits; tissues if slight bleeding from nose occurs.
8. Apply water-soluble lubricant to probe tip. Topical analgesic spray may be used at the back of the throat, analgesic gel may be used on the probe, or sedation may be used, as needed, with a physician's or APN's order.	Although tube placement is uncomfortable rather than painful, evaluate the needs and perceptions of the child on an individual basis. **KidKare** The child may suck on a bottle or sip water, depending on preference of person inserting probe; peristalsis with swallowing may help pass the probe. Do not use this technique in conjunction with analgesic sprays or sedation.
9. If a nasogastric tube is in place, pass through the same naris. Insert the probe through the child's naris and into the esophagus. Slowly advance the probe to the stomach (the pH will drop to less than 4). Then pull back until the premeasured mark is at the naris opening.	Oral placement is contraindicated in children with teeth. Occlusion of both nostrils is prevented when a nasogastric tube is in place. Advancing the probe to the stomach further confirms it is not in the airway.
10. Secure the probe to the cheek area beside the nares with tape or transparent dressing, making sure there is no pressure on the nares. Loop the probe tube over the top of the nearest ear and tape to the child's neck and back.	Secures the probe to maintain consistent placement during the pH study.

Continued

Steps	Rationale/Points of Emphasis
11. Dispose of equipment and waste in appropriate receptacle. Remove gloves and perform hand hygiene.	Standard precautions. Reduces transmission of microorganisms.
12. Obtain a single-view anteroposterior chest x-ray and assist with positioning, as needed. If necessary, per recommendation of the radiologist, physician, or APN, adjust the tube as directed.	Proper tube placement must be confirmed by x-ray to ensure safety and accuracy of test results.
13. If the pH monitor requires an electrode, once probe placement is confirmed, place a well-gelled electrode over the area of the spine.	Serves as a ground wire.
14. If a pH study flow sheet is being used, record the following information on a pH study flow sheet, noting exact times each event occurs, along with pH reading on the monitor: feeding, positioning changes, sleep–wake cycles, and any observed symptoms (e.g., coughing, vomiting, or gasping). If event recording is done using the monitor, refer to manufacturer's instructions.	Factors that precipitate GER can be identified by the physician or APN when the log, with exact times, is compared with the pH study recording strip. Food ingestion and physical activity often provoke GER. Normal pH range is 4.0 to 9.0. **caREminder** *When apnea monitoring or pulse oximetry is being used, note those readings in conjunction with the above-mentioned events to assist in providing a clear clinical picture of the child during the pH study.*
15. Teach all caregivers who will be with the child for the 24-hour test period to participate in recording the pH study log or event recording using the monitor.	Reduces chance of nonrecording of events. Test may run a minimum of 16–18 hours, including a sleep–wake cycle, but normally runs for 24 hours.
16. Encourage parents to constantly monitor the child and use techniques such as touching, hugging, and distraction to keep the child from removing the probe.	Ensures that the test will not be disrupted because of accidental probe removal. **caREminder** *It may be necessary to place mittens over the hands of infants and young children or use armboards, especially while child is sleeping, to help prevent inadvertent pH probe removal or dislodging of the probe.*
17. Allow the child to resume eating, per physician or APN order.	Allows evaluation of the child under typical conditions.
18. During the pH study, notify the physician or APN if any the following occur: • Child experiences significant distress or change in clinical status • pH readings change significantly during study • Equipment malfunction or probe displacement is suspected	Ensures patient safety and allows for early correction of any possible test malfunctions. **caREminder** *If child vomits, assess breath sounds and check for respiratory distress. Also, check probe because displacement of the pH probe may occur during vomiting.*
19a. Upon completion of the study, turn off the monitor following the manufacturer's instructions. With clean gloved hands, remove the ground wire from the child's back, if used, and discard the electrode. Loosen the tape, holding the tube in position. Adhesive removal pads may be used. Ask the child to swallow as the tube is removed. Discard the pH probe.	Peristalsis with swallowing may ease removal of the probe.
19b. Remove gloves and perform hand hygiene.	Reduces transmission of microorganisms.

Steps	Rationale/Points of Emphasis
20. Forward the monitor and log if applicable to the appropriate department or follow manufacturer's instructions for extracting information from the monitor.	Recorded information must be analyzed to obtain results.
21. The child may continue with his or her prestudy diet and routine, unless otherwise ordered by the physician or APN.	Allows the child to resume what is comfortable and familiar to him or her.

CHILD AND FAMILY EVALUATION AND DOCUMENTATION

- At time of insertion of pH probe, document the following:
  - Time pH probe was inserted
  - Time study was initiated
  - Time study was discontinued
  - How the child tolerated the procedure
  - Probe placement in centimeters
  - Family instruction provided
  - If restraints applied
- During the study, document the following:
  - Child's clinical status and any changes
  - Exact times each event occurs along with the pH reading on the monitor
  - Times and duration of feedings
  - Positioning changes
  - Sleep–wake cycles
  - Any observed symptoms (i.e., coughing, vomiting, or gasping)
  - Probe and wires (if used) are intact and note the pH reading at least every 2 hours.

COMMUNITY CARE

- If the test is to be completed in the home setting, ensure that parents understand how to properly record events, signs to watch for and report, and whom to call if problems or questions arise.
- Instruct family to return with the child the following day, at the specified time, for the test to be discontinued or inform the family of when to expect a professional to be at the home to discontinue the test there.
- Reinforce teaching regarding test results, diagnosis, care, and treatment, including medication administration, as appropriate.
- Instruct family to contact healthcare provider if
  - Child experiences significant distress or change in clinical status
  - pH readings change significantly during study
  - Equipment malfunction or probe displacement is suspected

Unexpected Situation

- *After the pH probe is placed and taped securely, the child has increased coughing and is not comfortable, and he states he is having trouble breathing:* Remove the tube and ensure that the coughing and difficulty breathing resolve (administer blow-by oxygen if the child is unable to stabilize). The probe was most likely placed in the airway instead of the esophagus. Call physician or APN if breathing difficulty continues.

Bibliography

Bagucka, B., Badriul, H., Vandemaele, K., Troch, E., & Vandenplas, Y. (2000). Normal ranges of continuous pH monitoring in the proximal esophagus. *Journal of Pediatric Gastroenterology and Nutrition, 31*, 244–247.

Hassall, E. (2005). Decisions in diagnosing and managing chronic gastroesophageal reflux disease in children. *Journal of Pediatrics, 146*(3 Suppl), S3–S12.

Little, J. P., Matthews, B. L., Glock, M. S., et al. (1997). Extraesophageal pediatric reflux: 24-hour double probe pH monitoring of 222 children. *Annals of Otology, Rhinology, & Laryngology, 169*(Suppl), 1–16.

Patwari, A. K., Bajaj, P., Kashyp, R., et al. (2002). Diagnostic modalities for gastroesophageal reflux. *Indian Journal of Pediatrics, 69*, 133–136.

Society of Gastroenterology Nurses and Associates, Inc. (2004). *Manual of gastrointestinal procedures* (5th ed.). Chicago, IL: Author.

Wenzl, T. G. (2003). Evaluation of gastroesophageal reflux events in children using multichannel intraluminal electrical impedance. *American Journal of Medicine, 18*(Suppl 3A), 161S–165S.

CHAPTER

90

Phototherapy

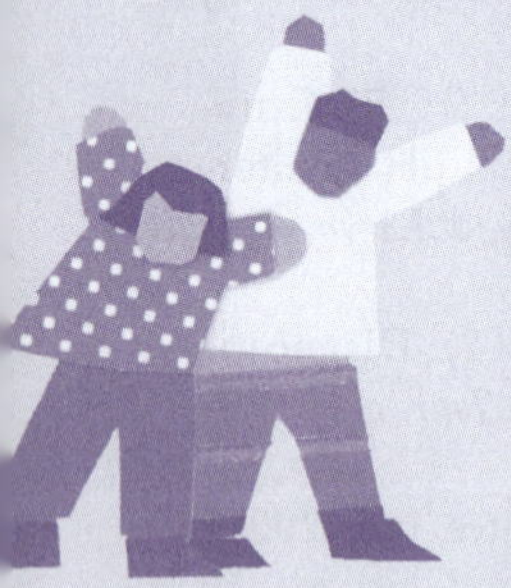

Clinical Guidelines

- A healthcare prescriber orders phototherapy.
- The registered nurse (RN), licensed practical nurse (LPN), and parent are involved with the delivery of care during the phototherapy treatment. The RN or LPN is responsible for verifying the intensity of phototherapy lights.
- Phototherapy is recommended for term neonates if total serum bilirubin (TSB) levels rise above 5 mg/dL in the first day of life. TSB greater than 8 mg/dL in the first 24 hours of life is considered "pathologic" and should be evaluated for hemolytic disease or other disorders.
- Phototherapy is generally initiated sooner and at lower levels in premature neonates and infants with risk factors (e.g., cephalohematoma, hemolytic disease of the newborn, polycythemia, sepsis).
- After the first 24 hours of life, phototherapy is recommended to treat serum bilirubin levels greater than 15 to 22 mg/dL based on age (in hours), risk factors, and clinical assessment of the infant.
- Intensity of the phototherapy lights is checked daily.
- Serum bilirubin levels are checked as ordered or per protocol.
- Infants receiving phototherapy treatment are weighed daily.

Equipment

For phototherapy lights:

- Overhead phototherapy lights
- Isolette
- Eye shields or surgical mask (for smaller infants)
- Disposable diapers
- Towel or disposable waterproof pad
- Bilirubin light meter
- Isolette temperature monitor
- Baby scale
- Thermometer
- Documentation sheets for intake and output

For fiberoptic phototherapy pads or blankets:

- Fiberoptic blanket or pad with light source box
- Surge-protected power strip
- Disposable sheath for covering pad or blanket

- Extra bulb
- Baby scale
- Documentation sheets for intake and output
- Thermometer

CHILD AND FAMILY ASSESSMENT AND PREPARATION

- Assess child's history to determine risk factors for hyperbilirubinemia (e.g., Rh or ABO incompatibility, polycythemia, sepsis, prematurity, malpresentation).
- Check available blood values (e.g., infant's hematocrit, blood type, mother's blood type, Coombs test).
- Before initiating phototherapy, assess the infant for the following:
  - Respirations, pulse, and temperature to establish baseline parameters
  - Weight
  - Level of hydration
  - Level of consciousness
  - Signs of cephalohematoma, ecchymosis, and abrasions. Any suggestion of traumatic delivery may indicate extravascular hemolysis that adds to the bilirubin production.
  - Signs of jaundice
  - Presence of petechiae, which may be indicative of congenital infection, overwhelming sepsis, or severe hemolytic disease
  - Presence of hepatosplenomegaly, which may be indicative of chronic intrauterine infection and hemolytic anemia
- Explain to family members the following information:
  - Reason for phototherapy treatment
  - Reason for covering child's eyes whenever phototherapy lights are turned on
  - Reason for the child's loose stools and methods to treat skin irritation
  - The importance of checking the child's diaper every hour and of maintaining good skin care

caREminder

It is important to provide support and encouragement to the parents because they experience a major disruption in their ability to bond with their newborn child. Plan activities such as feeding or bathing the infant so that family members may fully participate in the child's care and enjoy what access they have to their child while phototherapy is in progress.

PROCEDURE Use of Phototherapy Lights

Steps	Rationale/Points of Emphasis
1. Gather the necessary supplies. Perform hand hygiene.	Promotes efficient time management and provides an organized approach to the procedure. Reduces transmission of microorganisms.
2. Determine whether the infant will be able to maintain his or her temperature and can be nursed in an open bassinet. If so, set up bassinet. If not, set up an isolette following the manufacturer's instructions.	Neonates have limited ability to regulate or maintain body temperature and must be protected against hypothermia and hyperthermia. Relatively healthy term neonates should be able to maintain their temperature; preterm or sick neonates often cannot maintain adequate temperature and thus must be placed in an environment where temperature can be regulated for them.
3. Set up the fluorescent overlights, following manufacturer recommendations, as close to the infant as possible: in an open bassinet, about 4 inches (10 cm) from the infant; in an isolette, about 15 to 18 inches (38 to 46 cm) from the infant.	Bilirubin absorbs visible light in the range of 400 to 500 nm. The distance of the light source from the infant affects how well the light penetrates skin and is absorbed by bilirubin (this effect is most significant when special blue tubes are used). **Alert!** *Halogen lamps emit more heat than fluorescent bulbs and therefore increase the risk of a burn; do not position close to infant. Follow manufacturer's instructions for distance when using halogen lights.*
4. Turn the light unit on. Using a light meter, verify that the level of irradiance is appropriate to the manufacturer's recommendations for the system in use, approximately 12 to 15 μW/cm²/nm for low intensity (conventional or single phototherapy) or 30 to 35 μW/cm²/nm for high intensity (intensive or double phototherapy) (Figure 90-1).	Intensity of lights may decrease over time. Lights of less intensity may be ineffective or may require longer lengths of exposure to the infant to achieve the desired therapeutic effect.

Continued

Steps	Rationale/Points of Emphasis

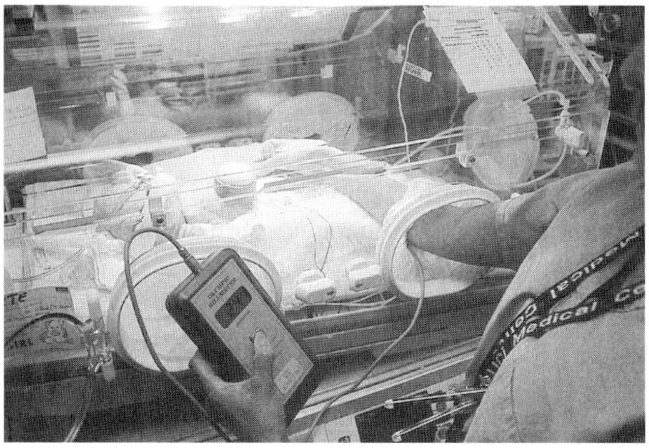

FIGURE 90-1
A light meter is used to verify the light of irradiance, ensuring the minimum of 10 to 12 μW/cm²/nm.

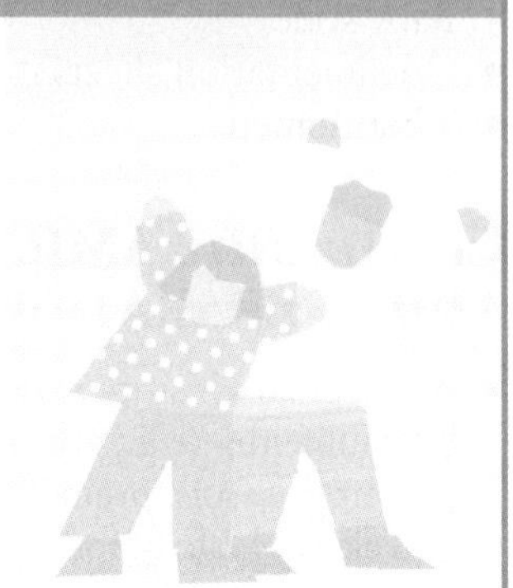

Steps	Rationale/Points of Emphasis
5. Perform hand hygiene.	Reduces transmission of microorganisms.
6. Undress the infant, leaving a diaper in place to cover the genitals. Use a surgical mask for a diaper if diapers cover too much skin area of a small infant.	Undressing the infant increases the amount of skin surface area exposed. The diaper protects the gonads against chromatic radiant damage from the phototherapy light exposure.
7. Ensuring that the infant's eyelids are closed, carefully cover the eyes completely with protective shields, making sure not to obstruct the nares. Remove eye patches a minimum of every 4 hours.	The infant's eyes are closed to prevent corneal excoriation. The infant's eyes are covered by protective eye shields at all times during use of overhead phototherapy to protect them against retinal damage.

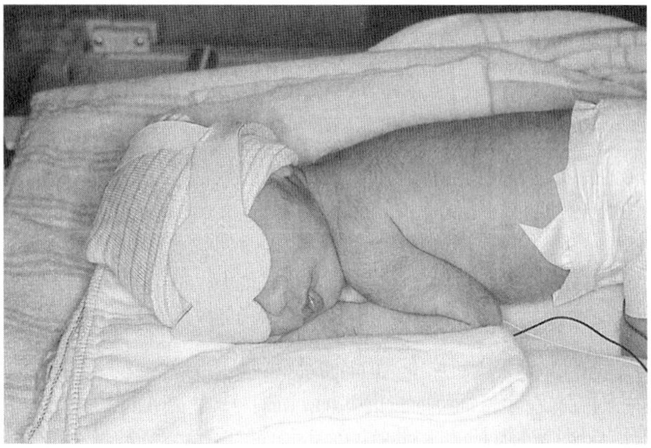

FIGURE 90-2
Properly positioned patches do not put pressure over the bridge of the nose, which could cause airway compromise.

caREminder

Check the position of the eye patches every hour. Infants often wiggle enough to push the eye patches either above or below the eyes, leaving them exposed. If the eye shields have slipped during treatment, damage can be done to the eyes. Also, the edges of the patches can dig into the eyes or compress the nose and can therefore interfere with the infant's breathing (Figure 90-2). If adhesive is used to fasten the eye patches, check for skin irritation. Remove the eye shields and inspect for purulent drainage and abrasion each time the lights are turned off for feedings, parental contact, or diaper-area care. If eye discharge is present, cleanse with wet warm gauze or cotton ball from the inner to the outer eye.

Steps	Rationale/Points of Emphasis
8. Place the infant in the bassinet or isolette. Ensure that the position of the lights is maintained about 4 inches (10 cm) from the infant in a bassinet or about 15 to 18 inches (38 to 46 cm) from the infant in an isolette.	For the overhead lights to be safe and effective, an exact distance from the lights must be maintained throughout the treatment.
9. Turn the infant every 2 hours, assessing skin integrity, hydration, temperature, and neurologic status.	Ongoing skin surveillance can detect problems early and prevent dehydration or damage to the infant's skin integrity.

Steps	Rationale/Points of Emphasis
	caREminder *Turn the lights off when changing the infant's diapers or when collecting blood specimens for bilirubin levels.*
10. Monitor the infant's temperature in an open bassinet every 30 minutes for the first hour and then every 2 hours and as needed after that. If in an isolette, monitor the infant's temperature every 2 to 3 hours.	Verifies that the naked infant in an open bassinet can maintain his or her temperature in a safe range and to detect alterations promptly. Although the isolette has a servocontrol, the thermal homeostasis of the infant can be compromised. A neutral thermal environment needs to be maintained.
11. Remain vigilant in keeping the diaper area as clean as possible.	Excretion of bilirubin and exposure to phototherapy cause the infant's skin to be at greater risk for compromise.
12. Provide both breast-fed and formula-fed infants with nutrition every 2 to 3 hours. Water supplements are not recommended.	Provides the caloric support for hepatic processing of bilirubin and stimulates peristalsis, which allows the bilirubin-rich meconium stool to be excreted. **caREminder** *Because of increased insensible stool water losses, encourage increased fluid intake. Bilirubin binds with protein; because there is no protein in water, it allows for limited flushing of the bilirubin. Water also supplies no nutrients, but it will fill the newborn's stomach, and the infant will then feed less frequently.*
13. Ensure that bilirubin blood monitoring is completed as ordered by the physician.	Evaluation of bilirubin levels provides data needed to determine when phototherapy can be discontinued.
14. Discontinue therapy when ordered by the physician/advanced practice nurse.	Therapy can be discontinued when bilirubin levels fall into normal range for the infant.

PROCEDURE Use of the Fiberoptic Phototherapy Pads and Blanket

Steps	Rationale/Points of Emphasis
1. Perform hand hygiene. Gather fiberoptic blanket/pad and light source box.	Handling equipment with clean hands decreases the chances of pathogens being transferred to the cleaned equipment.
2. Place light source box on a noncarpeted surface.	A noncarpeted surface, such as a piece of plywood or a tile floor, does not absorb heat as quickly as carpet and thus helps to keep the unit from overheating.
3a. Verify that the unit is at least 6 feet away from radiators or air vents. 3b. Verify that the unit is within 4 feet from where the child will be sleeping or will be held.	Heat from radiators or air ducts may lead to overheating of the illuminator. The fiberoptic cable that is used to transfer the light from the illuminator to the child stretches for a distance of about 4 feet.
4. Connect the fiberoptic cable to the light source box.	The light source box is an illuminator that contains a 150-watt quartz halogen bulb and a fan. The fiberoptic cable contains a bundle of plastic fibers that transmit light but no heat. At the distal end of the cable, the fibers fan out to create a flat flexible blanket or pad that contains the bands of light that wrap around the child.
5. Plug in the entire unit and verify that light actually travels through the cable.	Verifying that the unit is in good working order before beginning phototherapy decreases the anxiety of the family and sets the stage for your teaching.
6. When it is not in use, turn off the fiberoptic unit.	The life of a halogen bulb is limited and therefore should be conserved while the unit is not actually in use.

Continued

Steps	Rationale/Points of Emphasis
7. Insert fiberoptic blanket into disposable panel cover.	Protects infant from direct contact with light panel, thus providing a more comfortable contact between the device and the infant's skin.
8. With infant dressed only in diaper, wrap the covered panel under the infant's arms. The lower part of the panel will be on the outside of the diaper (Figure 90-3). Be sure that the diaper is folded down below the infant's navel in front and as far down as possible in the back.	The effectiveness of phototherapy is dependent on the amount of circulating blood that is exposed to ultraviolet light. **caREminder** *After securing the fiberoptic blanket, check to make sure that you can easily slip your fingers between the blanket and under the infant's arms. If the blanket still rubs under the infant's arms, try lining the immediate area with a soft cotton cloth or with a foam edge protector. A blanket applied too tightly or too closely under the arms causes tissue breakdown.*

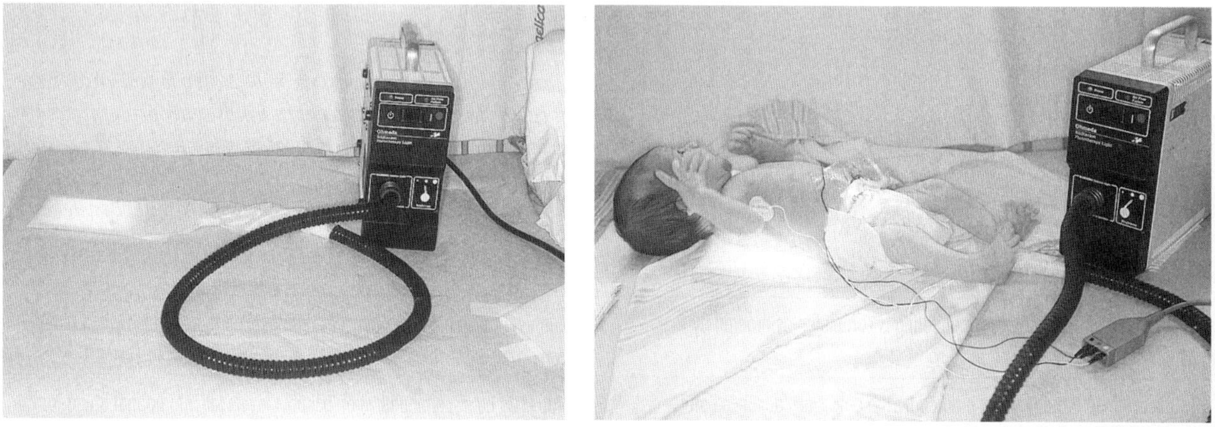

FIGURE 90-3
The fiberoptic blanket is positioned to cover the infant from the nipple line down. Ensure that the blanket does not rub under the infant's arm.

Steps	Rationale/Points of Emphasis
9. Fasten the panel in place with tape tabs.	Allows for quick and easy release of the fiberoptics.
10. If a pad is being used instead of wrapping a blanket, a pad may be placed under the infant. No tabs are used.	Flat pads do not require securing.
11. Redress the infant in a kimono or a sleeper that covers both the infant and the blanket.	Thermal instability in neonates may lead to hypothermia unless the infant is covered. The fiberoptic blanket does not transfer any heat from the halogen light.
12. Turn on the illuminator. The infant's abdomen will appear to glow through the infant's clothes.	Light is reflected through the fiberoptics onto the light panel to produce the therapeutic effect to the child.
13. Instruct the family that the infant may be held, may be fed, or may sleep while the phototherapy is taking place. Care must be taken to hold the infant securely and not to allow the fiberoptic cord to pull on the infant's chest.	The fiberoptic unit is attached to the infant and does not require that the infant be confined to an isolette. This form of phototherapy provides greater support for maintaining and promoting parent–child bonding practices. ***Alert!*** *Turn off and remove the fiberoptic blanket when bathing the infant. There is no electricity flowing through the blanket or pad; however, bathing gives the skin under the unit a chance to breathe and gives the caregiver an opportunity to assess the infant's skin for any changes.*
14. Discontinue therapy when ordered by the physician/advanced practice nurse.	Therapy can be discontinued when bilirubin levels fall into normal range for the infant.

CHILD AND FAMILY EVALUATION AND DOCUMENTATION

- Evaluate the family's understanding of hyperbilirubinemia and phototherapy.
- Determine the amount of involvement the family is willing to undertake in the care of the infant receiving phototherapy.
- Document the following:
  - Date and time bilirubin levels obtained
  - Intake and output during the entire course of treatment
  - Level of alertness
  - Skin integrity
  - Temperature of the infant and of the isolette, if in use
  - Level of hydration
  - Placement of the eye patches
- If overhead lights are being used:
  - Evaluate the infant's temperature every 2 to 3 hours or as indicated
  - Verify and document the intensity of the lights every 24 hours
  - If the infant is in an isolette, verify the temperature in the isolette every 8 hours

COMMUNITY CARE

- If the mother is breast-feeding, provide mother with information about lactation resources available in her community. Early and frequent breast-feeding decreases hyperbilirubinemia through stimulation of gut motility and prevention of bilirubin reabsorption.
- If phototherapy is administered in the home, teach parents use of phototherapy (fiberoptic pad or blanket or lights), following previously presented procedure; ensure home health referral is completed. Provide instructions regarding follow-up with healthcare provider and laboratory screening of bilirubin levels. The home health nurse will evaluate infant and mother, intensity of the light (if overhead lights in use), and parental understanding of infant care needs.
- Instruct the family to contact the healthcare provider if
  - Infant's skin becomes reddened or excoriated
  - Infant experiences decreased intake
  - Infant experiences change in activity level (e.g., lethargy, little movement or vigor)
  - Infant's skin remains yellow toned
  - Infant arches back or neck
  - Infant develops a screeching or high-pitched cry

Unexpected Situation

- *The infant's serum bilirubin continues to increase despite use of phototherapy:* Verify the light intensity of the equipment is at least 10 to 12 μW/cm²/nm. Ensure an adequate amount of infant skin is exposed to the phototherapy. Determine whether or not the infant is adequately hydrated.

Bibliography

American Academy of Pediatrics. (2004). Management of hyperbilirubinemia in the newborn infant 35 or more weeks of gestation. *Pediatrics, 114*, 297–316.

Frank, C. G., Cooper, S. C., & Merenstein, G. B. (2002). Jaundice. In G. B. Merenstein & S. L. Gardner (Eds.), *Handbook of neonatal intensive care* (5th ed., pp. 443–461). St. Louis: Mosby.

Gracey, K., & Stokowski, L. A. (2002). Family teaching toolbox: Newborn jaundice. *Advances in Neonatal Care, 2*, 115–116.

Maisels, M. J., & Watchko, J. F. (2003). Treatment of jaundice in low birthweight infants. *Archives of Disease in Childhood Fetal and Neonatal Edition, 88*, F459–F463.

Palmer, R. H., Clanton, M., Ezhuthachan, S., et al. (2003). Applying the "10 simple rules" of the Institute of Medicine to management of hyperbilirubinemia in newborns. *Pediatrics, 112*, 1388–1393.

Ross, G. (2003). Hyperbilirubinemia in the 2000s: What should we do next? *American Journal of Perinatology, 20*, 415–424.

Stokowski, L. A. (2002). Early recognition of neonatal jaundice and kernicterus. *Advances in Neonatal Care, 2*, 101–114.

Watson, R. L. (2004). Gastrointestinal disorders. In M. T. Verklan & M. Walden (Eds.), *Core curriculum for neonatal intensive care nursing* (3rd ed., pp. 685–697). St. Louis: Elsevier.

CHAPTER

91

Pneumogram: Two- or Four-Channel

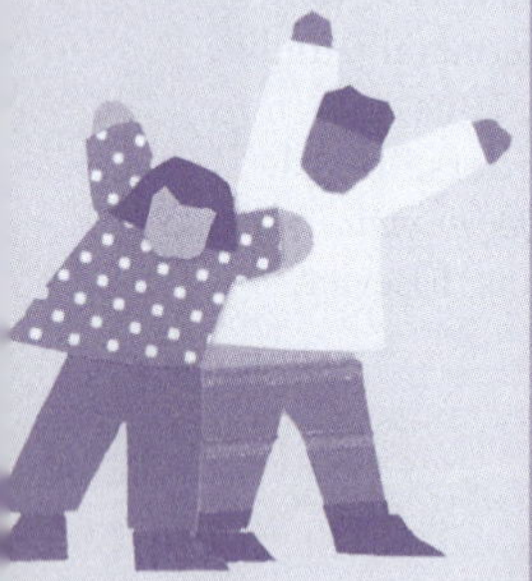

Clinical Guidelines

- A physician's order is required before initiating a two- or four-channel pneumogram.
- A registered nurse (RN), respiratory therapist, or electrodiagnostic technician who has completed the appropriate training and demonstrated competency may administer a pneumogram or polysomnogram.
- A properly trained electrodiagnostic technician completes computer analysis of the test results.

Equipment

For a two-channel pneumogram:

- Pneumogram computerized recorder with interface cable
- Apnea monitor with patient cable, lead wires, and electrodes
- Pneumogram log
- Computer printer with software to download data once pneumogram is complete
- Blank formatted disk, if needed per manufacturer's instructions

For a four-channel pneumogram:

- Apnea monitor with patient cable, charger cable, lead wires, and electrodes
- Digital recorder with multisensor cable assembly, locking charger cable, oximeter probe, monitor interface cable, and airflow sensor
- Pneumogram log

Child and Family Assessment and Preparation

- Assess the child's and family's understanding of the test's purpose, the basic procedure, and when to expect test results.
- Assess child's medical history, including prematurity, recent history of respiratory infections, current medications, reports of blue spells, breath holding, or gasping for air, which may be associated with apnea.

PROCEDURE Measuring Heart Rate and Respiratory Impedance With a Two-Channel Pneumogram

Steps	Rationale/Points of Emphasis
1. Review the explanation of the procedure, including the parent's role in documenting events during the test.	Helps to relieve anxiety and gains family cooperation with the procedure.
2. Start the test in the evening and discontinue it in the morning after at least 12 hours of monitoring.	Allows an adequate test period during the infant's sleep cycle.
3. Perform hand hygiene.	Reduces transmission of microorganisms.
4. Gather the necessary supplies. If recorder parameters and demographics have not been preset (and per manufacturer's instructions): a. Attach recorder to computer with interface cable and plug into an electrical outlet. b. Switch from off to stand-by to initiate a memory test. c. When the main menu appears, select pneumogram and enter. d. Enter the appropriate information for each prompt. e. When complete, switch recorder from stand-by to save data and follow prompts. f. When complete, switch to save data.	Promotes efficient time management and provides an organized approach to the procedure. Prepares the recorder to accept data, based on the child's gestational age, medication history, and appropriate limits for apnea delay, bradycardia, and tachycardia.
5. Apply apnea monitor to the infant, ensuring that settings are correct and appropriate for gestational age.	Prepares for testing.
6. Attach the recorder to the monitor with an interface cable, switch the recorder to stand-by until only the green charger light and red stand-by lights are on, and then switch to record and wait for the red record light to illuminate.	Initiates the test by starting data recording.
7. Note time the test was initiated and record the following information on the pneumogram log with each monitor alarm: a. Time of occurrence b. Type of alarm c. Lowest or highest heart rate noted d. Presence of cyanosis e. Interventions used to terminate the episode	Offers valuable information to the physician and technician interpreting the pneumogram by providing corresponding clinical data.
8. Teach those who will be with the infant during the test to participate in noting and recording clinical information on the log.	Decreases the chance that significant details of apneic and bradycardiac events will be missed and go unrecorded.
9. To discontinue the pneumogram after 12 hours of recording, switch the recorder to save data, note the time, disconnect from the apnea monitor, and unplug from the electrical outlet.	This concludes the test and is essential in ensuring that the data will not be lost. **caREminder** *Instruct parents to notify staff if they notice that the "memory full" light is illuminated, so that the test can be discontinued without loss of data. The recorder will store up to 12 hours of data or 400 events, whichever comes first. When one of the limits is reached, the "memory full" light will illuminate.*
10. Return the recorder to the appropriate department for computer analysis.	This allows preparation of the data for interpretation by the physician.

PROCEDURE Measuring Heart Rate, Respiratory Impedance, Airflow, and Oxygen Saturation With a Four-Channel Pneumogram

Steps	Rationale/Points of Emphasis
1. Review the explanation of the procedure, including the parent's role in documenting events during the test.	Helps relieve anxiety and gains family cooperation with the procedure.
2. Start the test in the evening and discontinue it in the morning after at least 12 hours of monitoring.	Allows an adequate test period during the infant's sleep cycle to evaluate respiratory cycle during sleep.
3. Perform hand hygiene.	Reduces transmission of microorganisms.
4. Apply apnea monitor to the infant, ensuring that settings are correct and appropriate for gestational age.	Prepares for testing; monitors for apnea and bradycardia.
5. Attach the pulse oximeter probe to the infant and ensure that it is attached to the recorder cable.	Prepares for testing; monitors oxygen saturation.
6. Apply the airflow sensor by positioning the prongs directly under the nares; tape securely above the lip to the patient's cheek.	Proper placement is critical to obtaining accurate airflow measurements.
7. Set up recorder as follows (and per manufacturer's instructions): a. Turn recorder on and to the setup mode. b. Enter the appropriate information for each prompt. c. When signals have been checked, advance to the ready mode. d. Recording will begin, and a message such as, "Recording data, sensors OK" will be visible.	Prepares the recorder to record the four channels being monitored. If a sensor is not properly connected, that sensor will be indicated on the screen until the connection has been properly established.
8. Note time the test was initiated and record the following information on the pneumogram log with each monitor alarm: a. Time of occurrence b. Type of alarm c. Lowest or highest heart rate noted d. Presence of cyanosis e. Interventions used to terminate the episode	Offers valuable information to the physician and technician interpreting the pneumogram by providing corresponding clinical data.
9. Teach those who will be with the infant during the test to participate in noting and recording clinical information on the log.	Decreases the chance that significant details of apneic and bradycardic events will be missed and go unrecorded.
10. To discontinue the recording, turn the recorder off and detach the sensors from the patient and the cables from the recorder.	This concludes the test. **caREminder** *Instruct parents that the recording will automatically end when any of the following occurs: the memory becomes full, all cables are detached from the recorder, the power supply becomes disconnected, or the recorder is turned off. Education of parents reduces the risk for inadvertent or premature discontinuance of the pneumogram.*
11. Return the recorder to the appropriate department for computer analysis.	Allows preparation of the data for interpretation by the physician.

CHILD AND FAMILY EVALUATION AND DOCUMENTATION

- Record time study was initiated and discontinued.
- During the study, note clinical status and any significant changes.
- Document that the recorder is on and functioning at least every 2 hours.

COMMUNITY CARE

- If the test is to be completed in the home setting, ensure that parents understand
  - How to properly document on the pneumogram log
  - Signs to watch for and report
  - How to save data if the recorder memory is full
  - Whom to call if problems or questions arise
- Inform family members regarding when they can expect a professional to be at their home to discontinue the test and when test result can be expected.
- Instruct the family to contact the healthcare provider if
  - Equipment appears to be malfunctioning
  - Child's clinical status deteriorates

Unexpected Situation

- *The child experiences clinical status changes evidenced by activated alarms on monitoring equipment (low heart rate; low respiratory rate; low oxygen saturation, if using pulse oximetry monitoring):* Assess child's status to differentiate between actual clinical changes and artifact readings on monitoring equipment. If actual physiologic compromise is clinically evident, initiate appropriate rescue or emergency actions. Teach parents signs and symptoms of respiratory distress and physiologic changes, as well as appropriate interventions. Parents should be trained in CPR before managing child's monitoring at home.

Bibliography

American Academy of Pediatrics (AAP). (2002). Clinical practice guideline: Diagnosis and management of childhood obstructive sleep apnea syndrome. *Pediatrics, 109*, 704–712.

Kirk, V. G., Bohn, S. G., Flemons, W. W., et al. (2003). Comparison of home oximetry monitoring with laboratory polysomnography in children. *Chest, 124*, 1702–1708.

Ohayon, M. M., Carskadon, M. A., Guilleminault, C., & Vitiello, M. V. (2004). Meta-analysis of quantitative sleep parameters from childhood to old age in healthy individuals: Developing normative sleep values across the human lifespan. *Sleep, 27*, 1255–1273.

CHAPTER 92

Poison Management

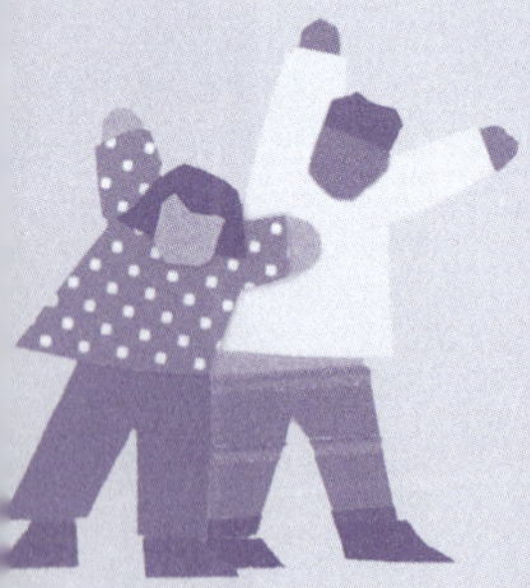

Clinical Guidelines

- A registered nurse (RN), licensed practical nurse (LPN), or unlicensed assistive personnel (UAP) may obtain vital signs. When obtained by the UAP, any variance from baseline or deviance from previous measurement is reported to the licensed caregiver.
- Medications and treatments are administered by an RN, LPN, or physician within their scope of practice.
- Laboratory tests and treatments are performed upon order of a physician or advanced practice nurse.
- In children, treat the symptoms, not the toxin.
- Contact your regional Poison Control Center for additional management of specific exposures. The National Poison Control number is 800-222-1222.

Equipment

- Antidotes/reversal agents for common toxins and drug overdose
- Rectal thermometer
- Stethoscope
- Electrocardiogram (ECG) monitor, electrodes
- Sphygmomanometer and cuff
- Pulse oximeter
- Length-based resuscitation tape (if needed)
- Percussion hammer
- Penlight
- Tongue depressor
- Ophthalmoscope
- Orogastric/nasogastric tube, largest size appropriate for child

Child and Family Assessment and Preparation

- Explain each procedure before performance if time allows. If emergent, provide explanation as procedure is performed.
- Assess child's and family's understanding of necessity for procedures and what will happen.

PROCEDURE Assessing Airway, Breathing, Circulation (ABCs), and Mental Status

Steps	Rationale/Points of Emphasis
1. Determine whether the child is breathing and has a pulse. Be prepared to assist with intubation. Assess mental status.	Compromised airway/respiratory depression and altered mental status are common with certain exposures.
2. Obtain intravenous access, if necessary.	Enables immediate administration of fluids and necessary medication.
3. Have appropriate antidote or reversal agent ready to administer on physician's order. Examples include • Naloxone (Narcan) to children with respiratory depression • Thiamine to malnourished children • Glucose to any child with an altered mental status	Have available to treat or reverse effects of the poison. Naloxone is an opioid antagonist. Thiamine helps control energy metabolism and a deficiency may impair glucose utilization. Administration of glucose excludes hypoglycemia as the cause of altered mental status.
4. Look for evidence of pill fragments, poison plant matter, or smell of toxin in or near mouth. Inspect clothing for presence of possible toxin.	May aid in verification of toxin, which will aid in delivery of appropriate treatment.

PROCEDURE Assessing History

Steps	Rationale/Points of Emphasis
1. Obtain patient demographic information: • Weight • Age • Sex	The ability to metabolize a drug changes with age and dose; toxicity often relates to the size of the child. Information on gender is obtained for epidemiologic tracking.
2. Obtain exposure information: • Name of the product • Amount of product to which the patient was exposed (if known) • Route of exposure • Time of exposure • Reason for exposure (intentional or unintentional)	There are many types of medications on the market with varying ingredients and amounts; the route and time of exposure may predict level of toxicity and outcome. Intentional overdoses often involve large amounts and multiple ingestions. Amount of product can predict the effects. Many poisonings and medication overdoses involve more than one agent, resulting in a compounding of effects.
3. Obtain symptom history: • Onset • Duration • Progression	Determining whether the symptoms have started, continued, lessened, or worsened helps to determine outcome. Sustained-release or extended-release products have the potential to create prolonged or delayed clinical effects.
4. Obtain medical/medication history: • Medications patient is currently taking • Medications available in the household	Helps to form a more complete differential diagnosis.

PROCEDURE Assessing Vital Signs

Steps	Rationale/Points of Emphasis
1. Perform hand hygiene.	Reduces transmission of microorganisms.
2. Determine respiratory rate. Note the depth, pattern, and effort. Place pulse oximeter for continuous readings.	Changes in respiratory rate are affected by direct effects on the respiratory center, either suppression or stimulation; increased metabolic requirements; or acid-base disorders. Tachypnea is seen with aspirin, cocaine, and amphetamines, among other substances. Bradypnea is associated with agents that cause overall depressed central nervous system effects (e.g., barbiturates, clonidine, opioids, and ethanol).

Continued

Steps	Rationale/Points of Emphasis
3. Obtain pulse rate, and provide continuous electrocardiogram monitoring.	Many toxins and drugs cause a change in heart rate and conduction. Bradycardia is seen with antidysrhythmics, clonidine, and opioids. Prolongation of the QRS complex can be seen with tricyclic antidepressants and selective serotonin reuptake inhibitors. Agents such as cocaine, theophylline, amphetamines, and organophosphates may cause tachycardia. Respiratory depression may result in hypoxia, causing dysrhythmias.
4. Obtain blood pressure.	Hypotension is noted in β-blockers, calcium channel blockers, methanol, and tricyclic antidepressants, among others. The most common reason hypotension develops in poisoned patients is intravascular volume depletion. Hypertension may develop because of increased release of norepinephrine. Some agents that may cause this effect include epinephrine, phenylephrine (Neo-Synephrine), and ergotamines (agents that are often contained in OTC cold preparations and diet pills).
5. If weight is unknown, weigh child or use length-based resuscitation tape to estimate weight.	The length-based resuscitation tape is a rapid noninvasive method that converts the child's length into a probable weight range.
6. Obtain rectal temperature.	Slight variations in temperature are noteworthy in poison exposures. Rectal temperature is the preferred method because it reflects the core temperature.

PROCEDURE Performing Specific Systems Assessments

Steps	Rationale/Points of Emphasis
1. Assess neurologic status:	
a. Evaluate the child's level of consciousness (orientation to people, place, and time) as age appropriate.	Level of consciousness changes can range from lethargy to coma. Agents that produce this effect include benzodiazepines, phenothiazine, sedative-hypnotics, and certain household products.
b. If the child is comatose, determine whether the child responds to painful stimuli.	Indicates depth of coma.
c. Determine pupil size and reactivity to light. Note any variation in symmetry, color, or movement of pupils, iris, or sclera.	Mydriasis occurs with tricyclic antidepressants, cocaine, and drug withdrawal, whereas miosis occurs with organophosphates, nicotine, opioids, and sedating agents. Nystagmus is seen with phencyclidine (PCP), carbamazepine, and other drugs.
d. Observe for signs of visual or auditory hallucinations and seizures. If seizures occur, determine type of seizure. Maintain seizure precautions.	Reduces chance of injury if seizure occurs.
2. Perform abdominal assessment specific for distention and bowel sounds.	Hyperactive bowel sounds are associated with cholinergic crisis, as with organophosphates (dermal and oral exposures), and diminished bowel sounds are associated with anticholinergic effects. Drugs that cause a decrease in gastrointestinal motility include diphenhydramine and tricyclic antidepressants. **Alert!** *Determining the presence of bowel sounds is essential before the administration of activated charcoal. If the bowel is not active, activated charcoal will not have the intended effect and may cause further problems if it accumulates.*
3. Evaluate skin for moisture, turgor, and edema.	Anticholinergic agents such as tricyclic antidepressants and diphenhydramine cause the skin to become warm, red, and dry. Organophosphates produce a cholinergic crisis, which manifests with diaphoresis.

PROCEDURE Obtaining Laboratory Tests, as Ordered

Steps	Rationale/Points of Emphasis
1. Obtain electrocardiogram (ECG); serial ECGs may be warranted.	ECG changes are associated with overdoses, such as a widening QRS complex (noted with tricyclic antidepressants), heart block, and dysrhythmias. Digoxin may cause first-degree heart block. Sympathomimetics, cocaine, calcium channel blockers and other cardiac medications, chloral hydrate, and phenothiazine can cause a variety of altered rhythms.
2. Obtain blood electrolyte levels and determine whether an anion gap is present.	An elevation in the patient's anion gap is associated with certain toxins. The mnemonic MUDPILES is used to identify toxins/conditions that produce an anion gap. They include methanol, uremia, diabetes mellitus, phenformin, iron, isoniazid, lactic acidosis, ethylene glycol, and salicylates.
3. Obtain chest x-ray.	Some medications, such as iron tablets and chloral hydrate, are radiopaque and can be seen on x-ray. When a hydrocarbon or a toxin that causes respiratory symptomology is ingested, an x-ray is indicated.
4. Obtain acetaminophen levels in all patients suspected of overdose. Obtain other pertinent levels, such as lithium, phenobarbital, and methanol, when history or symptoms indicate.	Studies indicate that acetaminophen is a common coingestant in many overdoses. A 4-hour postexposure acetaminophen level is predictive of toxicity. Studies have shown that many patients presenting to a healthcare facility for an intentional overdose have a toxic acetaminophen level. **caREminder** *Severe symptoms of acetaminophen overdose are not present until hepatic failure begins to develop.*
5. Obtain arterial blood gas when the risk of respiratory or metabolic instability is present and evaluate values.	Indicates acid-base and oxygenation status.
6. Determine whether patient's presenting findings are consistent with common toxidromes.	A constellation of symptoms is associated with specific toxins, such as the toxidrome for opioids, which includes miosis and hyperpnea. The toxidrome for organophosphates includes SLUDGE (salivation, lacrimation, urination, defecation, gastrointestinal distress, and emesis).

PROCEDURE Continuing Care

Steps	Rationale/Points of Emphasis
1. Continuously reassess ABCs, vital signs, neurologic status, and significant symptoms.	Some poisons worsen or vary their effect over time. Some treatment interventions may have a shorter effect than the agents they treat (e.g., naloxone has a shorter half-life than the opioids) and may require repeated administration.
2. Perform hand hygiene before and after physical interventions.	Reduces transmission of microorganisms.

PROCEDURE Gastrointestinal Decontamination

Steps	Rationale/Points of Emphasis
1a. Activated charcoal—single dose: • Children up to 1 year of age: 1 g/kg • Children 1–12 years of age: 25–50 g • Adolescents and adults: 25–100 g • Administer orally or through orogastric tube	Activated charcoal absorbs the toxin from the gastrointestinal tract, thereby decreasing the risk for systemic toxicity. Some ingestants, such as lithium, iron, caustics, and alcohol, are not bound to charcoal; therefore, charcoal is not indicated.

Alert! *Do not use with an unprotected airway and when there is a risk for aspiration (decreased level of consciousness, decreased gag reflex). When administering through a nasogastric tube, ascertain that the tube is in the stomach. Assess the child's respiratory status and skin color.*

Steps	Rationale/Points of Emphasis
1b. Activated charcoal—multiple dosing: • Administer 0.25 to 2 g/kg every 1–6 hours, depending on the toxin	Multiple dosing of activated charcoal is useful with drugs that slow gastrointestinal motility (e.g., phenothiazine), drugs that form concretions (e.g., aspirin), and sustained-release preparations; in these cases, a single dose of charcoal is insufficient to bind to the toxin. Multiple dosing is also indicated for drugs that go through enterohepatic circulation (e.g., theophylline, diphenhydramine). Vomiting sometimes occurs after the administration of activated charcoal. This has been associated with route of administration, prior vomiting, and the effects of the poisoning. The administration of an antiemetic (e.g., Zofran) before the administration of charcoal is sometimes warranted. **KidKare** To mask the sight of the charcoal and make it more palatable, put cover on cup and offer through straw when administering orally.
2. Orogastric lavage: a. Evaluate child's level of consciousness and mechanism of injury before lavage. b. Intubate with endotracheal tube before lavage if the child has absent or depressed gag reflex.	Injury to the oral cavity or esophagus would contraindicate orogastric lavage. Children with altered LOC are at increased risk for aspiration.

Alert! *Lavage should be performed only if a life-threatening ingestion has occurred or within 1 hour of exposure. Lavage is contraindicated in a child who has a depressed mental status if the airway is unprotected because this increases the risk of aspiration; in the child who has ingested a product that is easily aspirated, such as a hydrocarbon, or has ingested a corrosive substance; or in the child who has a surgical or medical condition that increases the risk for hemorrhage or gastrointestinal perforation.*

Steps	Rationale/Points of Emphasis
c. Place nasogastric tube; use a 24–28 French gauge tube in children and a 36–40 French gauge in adolescents; verify tube placement (refer to Chapter 39).	Large-bore tubes should be used so they are bigger than the pill fragments or poison to be extracted.
d. Position child in the left lateral decubitus position or in a supine position with the head elevated, depending on age and clinical condition of the child.	Gastroesophageal reflux is more common in the right than in the left lateral position. Elevation of head discourages aspiration of gastric contents by using gravity to keep fluid down when lavaging.

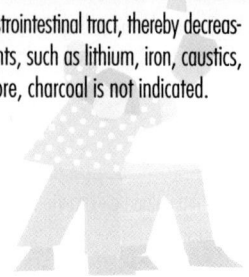

Steps	Rationale/Points of Emphasis
e. Instill 10 mL/kg of lavage solution for children younger than 5 years and 150–200 mL in children older than 5 years. In young children, because of the risk of hypothermia, only warmed normal saline is recommended; water is not used in children because of the risk for developing hyponatremia and water intoxication. In adolescents, normal saline is used.	Warmed fluids help to minimize development of hypothermia. To avoid electrolyte imbalance, the volume of lavage return should equal the amount of fluids given.
f. Instill fluid at consecutive intervals until the fluid aspirate is clear.	Clear aspirate indicates that particulate matter has been removed.
3. Whole bowel irrigation: • Irrigate with polyethylene glycol electrolyte solution: ▪ In children younger than 12 years of age, use 500 mL/hr. ▪ In children older than 12 years of age, use 2 L/hr. • Administer the solution orally or by nasogastric tube. • End point is when the rectal effluent is clear.	In cases in which activated charcoal is not useful, such as with lithium and iron, as well as when a sustained-release product has been ingested, whole bowel irrigation works by cleansing the bowel and decontaminating the entire gastrointestinal tract.

PROCEDURE Treatment Measures

Steps	Rationale/Points of Emphasis
1. Urine alkalinization: • Administer sodium bicarbonate, 1–2 mEq/kg IV bolus, followed by three ampules of sodium bicarbonate, 44 mEq Na^{++} in 1 liter D_5W infused at two times maintenance fluid to maintain blood pH between 7.45 and 7.55. • Do not give $NaHCO_3$ bolus if blood pH is above 7.45. • Maintain urine pH higher than 7.0. • Monitor for hypokalemia; correct as needed.	Useful for salicylates and phenobarbital overdoses because it increases the urinary pH of the urine, thereby enhancing the elimination of these drugs.
2. Serum alkalinization: • Administer sodium bicarbonate, 1–2 mEq/kg IV bolus, followed by a solution of three ampules of 44 mEq Na^{++} in 1 liter of D_5W at a rate of 1.5–2 times maintenance. • Monitor arterial blood gases to a pH of 7.45–7.55. • Repeat bolus as needed, but do not let pH rise above 7.55. • Monitor child's cardiovascular and pulmonary status.	Indicated for tricyclic antidepressant overdose if the QRS is more than 100 msec; continuous cardiac monitoring assists with accurate evaluation of the effects of the bicarbonate solution. A QRS complex wider than 100 msec is associated with seizure activity.
3. Extracorporeal filtration: • Hemodialysis or hemoperfusion	Hemodialysis is indicated for ingestants that have a low volume of distribution and low protein binding, such as toxic alcohols, salicylates, and lithium. Hemoperfusion is sometimes useful for drugs such as theophylline.
4. Eye irrigation: • In the home setting, instruct parent to take child into the shower and irrigate eyes for 15–20 minutes with copious amounts of tepid water. • In a healthcare facility, irrigate eyes for 15–20 minutes with water or normal saline. • Lid retraction and eversion are necessary for complete irrigation. • Assist with ophthalmology examination, including slit-lamp examination, as needed.	Irrigation dilutes the toxin in the eye, removes the toxin from the eye, removes the particles from the eye, and normalizes the pH of the eye.
5. Skin decontamination: • Wash exposed areas with copious amounts of water or flush with normal saline. • Evaluate the skin for signs of burns, irritation, or allergic reaction.	Washing helps to minimize absorption and, therefore, systemic toxicity.

Continued

Steps	Rationale/Points of Emphasis
6. Antidotes: • Use based on symptoms and toxins, in conjunction with gastrointestinal decontamination and supportive care. • Flumazenil is used to reverse the effects of benzodiazepines. **Alert!** *Flumazenil should be used cautiously when there is a possibility that a tricyclic antidepressant was ingested or it is unknown what the child ingested. The use of flumazenil and tricyclic antidepressants together has been known to precipitate seizures and ventricular dysrhythmias.* • Naloxone reverses the effects of opioids. • Mucomyst (*N*-acetylcysteine) is used for acetaminophen toxicity. • Vitamin B_6 is used for isoniazid toxicity. • Ethanol and fomepizole are used for ethylene glycol and methanol exposures.	Antidotes reverse the effects of the toxin.

Child and Family Evaluation and Documentation

- Evaluate the child's and parents' understanding of the dangers of poisons.
- Provide written poison prevention information; include the National Poison Control number (1-800-222-1222).
- Refer child to appropriate psychiatric or referral agents if this was an intentional abuse or misuse of a drug.
- Document all procedures performed, child and family response to procedures, teaching, and follow-up.

Community Care

- Provide child and family with poison prevention teaching before discharge from the healthcare facility after being treated for a poison exposure.
- Include poison prevention information in parenting classes:
  - Never call medicine "candy."
  - Lock all medications out of a child's reach and use child-resistant caps.
  - Never put poisons in empty food containers.
  - Wash out all bottles and cans in the recycling bin and keep the recycling bin out of a child's reach.
  - Never dispose of topical medication patches within the reach of children (e.g., nitroglycerin, opioids).
- Provide poison prevention information to preschool-aged and young school-aged children:
  - Never eat or drink anything without first checking with a grown-up.
  - Never eat berries, mushrooms, or plants growing outside.
  - Never take medication, including vitamins, on your own.
- Teach school-aged children about the dangers of "huffing" and using inhalants as well as the dangers of drug abuse. Include information on the toxicity of over-the-counter drugs, herbal medications, and drugs of abuse.
- Teach children never to share their medication.
- Teach senior citizens that when they have small children visiting, they need to child-proof their house. All medications should be labeled and out of reach. Avoid mixing pills in the same container.
- Instruct the family to contact the healthcare provider or nearest Poison Control Center if
  - It is known or suspected that the child has ingested or been exposed to a poisonous substance.
  - Symptoms return or worsen
  - The child demonstrates atypical behaviors
  - Further exposure occurs

Unexpected Situation

- *A 2-year-old presents with symptoms of bradycardia and lethargy. Mother gives history of child being out of her sight for an unknown period of time previous to symptom onset. The only medications in the home are an unopened bottle of acetaminophen and antacids. All household products are in a locked cabinet in the garage:* Ask specifically about the presence of herbal remedies in the home. These are typically viewed as natural agents and not mentioned unless specifically queried.

Bibliography

American Academy of Pediatrics. (2003). Poison treatment in the home. *Pediatrics, 112,* 1182–1185.

American Association of Poison Control Centers. Retrieved September 23, 2006, from www.aapcc.org

Bryant, S., & Singer, J. (2003). Management of toxic exposure in children. *Emergency Medicine Clinics of North America, 21,* 101–119.

Demorest, R. A., Posner, J. C., Osterhoudt, K. C., & Henretig, F. M. (2004). Poisoning prevention education during emergency department visits for childhood poisoning. *Pediatric Emergency Care, 20,* 281–284.

Dorrington, C. L., Johnson, D. W., Brant, R., & Multiple Dose Activated Charcoal Complication Study Group. (2003). The frequency of complications associated with the use of multiple-dose activated charcoal. *Annals of Emergency Medicine, 41,* 370–377.

Goldfrank, L. R., Flomenbaum, N. E., Lewin, N. A., Weisman, R., Howland, M. A., & Hoffman, R. S. (1998). *Goldfrank's toxicologic emergencies* (5th ed.). Norwalk, CT: Appleton-Lange.

Kao, L. W., Kirk, M. A., Furbee, R. B., Mehta, N. H., Skinner, J. R., & Briwnsinw, E. J. (2003). What is the rate of adverse events after oral N-acetylcysteine administered by the intravenous route to patients with suspected acetaminophen poisoning? *Annals of Emergency Medicine, 42,* 741–750.

Krenzelok, E. P., Mcguigan, M., & Lheur, P. (1997). American Board of Applied Toxicology and the Canadian Association of Poison Control Centers position papers on gastrointestinal decontamination. *Clinical Toxicology, 35,* 695–762.

Osterhoudt, K. C., Alpern, E. R., Durbin, D., Nadel, F., & Henretig, F. M. (2004). Activated charcoal administration in a pediatric emergency department. *Pediatric Emergency Care, 20,* 493–498.

Osterhoudt, K. C., Durbin, D., Alpern, E. R., & Henretig, F. M. (2004). Risk factors for emesis after therapeutic use of activated charcoal in acutely poisoned children. *Pediatrics, 113,* 806–810.

Shannon, M. (2000). Ingestion of toxic substances by children. *The New England Journal of Medicine, 342,* 186–192.

CHAPTER

93

Postanesthesia Care

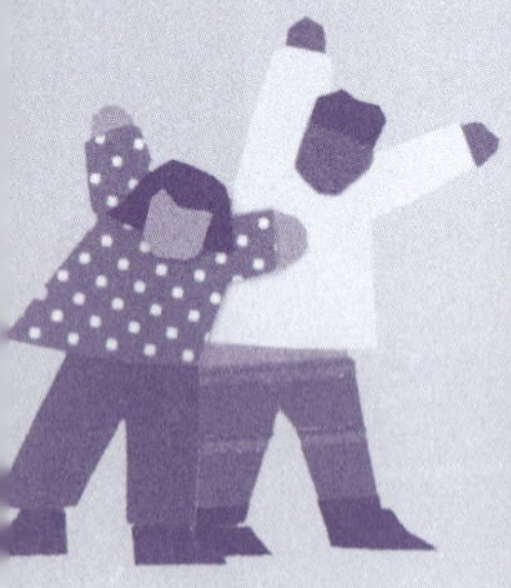

Clinical Guidelines

- A registered nurse (RN) or licensed practical nurse (LPN) performs postanesthesia care.
- Age-appropriate resuscitation equipment is available in the postanesthesia area.
- Safety of the child during the postanesthesia period is maintained: Use of sedation or restraints to restrict movement and to keep intravenous (IV) lines or tubes in place may be needed and implemented following a physician's order (see Chapter 102).
- Parents or other trusted caregivers are allowed in the postanesthesia recovery area to provide support to the child and to reduce the child's sense of isolation and separation anxiety.

Equipment

- Nonsterile gloves
- Stethoscope
- Thermometer (see Chapter 134)
- Blood pressure monitor (see Chapter 130)
- Fluids and nutrition for child (as ordered)
- Bedpan or urinal
- Blankets and warming devices (see Chapter 135)
- Incentive spirometer (see Chapter 51)
- Pillow for splinting
- Pain medications (as ordered)
- Resuscitation and intubation equipment (see Chapters 24 and 59)
- Oxygen and oxygen delivery system (see Chapter 83)
- Cardiopulmonary monitoring equipment (see Chapter 23)
- Pulse oximetry monitoring equipment (see Chapter 100)
- Ventilation device (available if needed)

Child and Family Assessment and Preparation

- Assess child for developmental stage and level of cognitive functioning.
- Assess operative and recovery room course and records for type of anesthesia, medications, vital signs, blood loss, fluid and blood replacement, procedural information, and complications.
- Determine whether family members would like to visit. Respect the child's feelings. Explore the visiting family members' understanding and provide age-appropriate information before

they come to see the child. If possible, utilize child life specialists to provide information to siblings before they visit the child.

KidKare Visual aids, such as picture books, photographs, and drawings, can familiarize children with what they will see.

PROCEDURE Immediate Postanesthesia Recovery Period

Steps	Rationale/Point of Emphasis
1. Perform hand hygiene. Don gloves if assessing wounds, drains, or tubes.	Reduces transmission of microorganisms.
2a. Assess airway; level of consciousness; breath sounds; bowel sounds; neurologic and neurovascular status; bladder functioning or distention; and status of drains, tubes, IV lines, monitoring devices, appliances, incision, dressing, skin integrity, pain status, positioning, and alignment (Table 93-1). The frequency of these assessments should be based on the child's condition.	Initial findings of the nurse become the baseline for comparing postoperative changes.
2b. Assess vital signs per institutional standard for frequency.	Vital signs are evaluated in terms of side effects from anesthesia and signs of impending shock or respiratory compromise.
2c. Compare data to preoperative baseline.	Postoperative condition can change rapidly.
3. Assess child and parents for fear, anxiety, and questions.	Review the child's knowledge to clarify misconceptions. Encouraging expression of feelings will facilitate coping. Research indicates that children who were anxious during the induction of anesthesia have an increased likelihood of developing postoperative negative behavioral changes (e.g., nightmares, separation anxiety, and aggression toward authority). Parents' emotional states are important indicators of children's emotional states and subsequently their pain experience. Involving the family and helping parents to reduce their own anxiety will affect emotional responses of the child.
4. Assess for knowledge of postanesthesia self-care measures (i.e., use of bedpan/urinal, mobility, deep breathing/incentive spirometer, coughing, splinting incision site with pillow), as indicated.	The nurse can support or correct perceptions and procedures to assist the child in achieving mastery of the skill.
5. Maintain adequate ventilation: • Assess breath sounds; document location of adventitious breath sounds. • Assess oxygenation, pulse oximetry, and blood gases, as applicable. • Facilitate coughing and deep breathing using splinting technique, as indicated. • Facilitate use of incentive spirometer; advise child to use 10 times every hour while awake or as ordered.	Anesthesia agents may depress respiratory function because lungs may not be fully inflated during surgery, cough reflex is suppressed, and mucus collects in airway passages.
6. Maintain neurologic and neurovascular status: • Monitor neurologic status: level of consciousness, protective reflexes (i.e., gag reflex, swallowing, pupil checks). • Monitor extremities for color, skin temperature, capillary refill, sensation, and motion. • Reposition frequently; turn every 2 hours as indicated. • Monitor pain because it is a possible indicator of complications. • Maintain patency and integrity of drainage systems. • Maintain antiembolytic device as indicated. Do not restart antiembolytic device if the device has been off for an hour or longer.	Medications, electrolyte and metabolic changes, pain, and emotional factors can influence the level of consciousness. Recent research shows that removing antiembolytic devices and then restarting them after 1 hour or longer increases the changes of emboli.
7. Maintain adequate intake, output, and electrolyte balance: • Maintain IV or IV access lock, as indicated. • Monitor electrolyte laboratory results, as indicated. • Offer fluids, as indicated. Increase diet as ordered from sips of clear fluids to full liquids, as indicated.	Ensures maintenance of the vital functions, provides nutrition, and prevents dehydration and electrolyte imbalances. Advancement of fluids from clear liquids to full liquids may occur after discharge to the home or to another healthcare setting.

Continued

TABLE 93-1

Postanesthesia Concerns in Children

Reasons for Concerns	Interventions
Laryngospasm after extubation	Position the child to maintain airway—head midline, may need to displace mandible anteriorly, open mouth. Administer 100% oxygen by positive-pressure ventilation if laryngospasm occurs. Anesthesia care practitioner may administer a dose of succinylcholine. Assist with reintubation, if needed.
Postintubation croup	Provide humidified mist to child. Give racemic epinephrine treatment through aerosol nebulizer, as ordered. Give corticosteroids before extubation, if ordered. If croup persists longer than 2 to 4 hours, expect to hospitalize the child overnight for observation.
Apnea	Use a cardiac monitor, apnea monitor, and pulse oximeter to monitor the child's status. Provide assisted ventilation as necessary. Keep appropriate pediatric resuscitative equipment available at the bedside.
Airway complications caused by bleeding after nasopharyngeal surgery	Assess the oral and nasal cavities for bright red blood. Observe for excessive swallowing. Monitor for changes in vital signs. Provide fluid resuscitation. Elevate the head of the bed. Apply an ice pack to neck or nose. Keep the child as quiet as possible. Do not remove clots. Administer pain medications as needed.
Aspiration	Suction the mouth, pharynx, and trachea if vomiting or excessive accumulation of secretions occurs. Administer oxygen. Position the patient prone or on the side.
Delayed return to consciousness	Before extubation, assess child's muscular strength, respiratory effort, airway protection, and eye opening. Identify any residual effects of drugs.
Preexisting volume depletion due to illness	Closely monitor intake and output. Urine output should average 1 mL/kg/hr.
NPO status before surgery	Establish and protect venous access.
Child's body surface area is greater than adults; during illness, trauma, or stress, the child's extracellular fluid is easily depleted.	Administer maintenance fluids that are hypotonic and contain glucose.
Although children have relatively greater fluid demands than adults, the actual amount of fluids required is small.	Prevent fluid overload by administering all fluids, blood, and blood products with a volumetric infusion pump.
Accelerated hypoglycemic reactions due to fluid loss and stress of illness and surgery	Monitor for symptoms of hypoglycemia; check blood glucose if symptoms are present.
External loss of fluid from vomiting, diarrhea, and nasogastric suctioning	Administer isotonic replacement fluids.
Postoperative hemorrhage due to bleeding of an open vessel, continuous third-spacing fluid shift, or coagulopathy.	Monitor circulatory status by assessing vital signs, urine output, central venous pressure, and pulmonary artery pressure. Give blood or blood products as needed.

TABLE 93-1

Postanesthesia Concerns in Children (continued)

Reasons for Concerns	Interventions
Risk factors, including previous history of seizures; intracranial injury, hemorrhage, or tumor; increased intracranial pressure; or metabolic or nutritional disorders that may result in electrolyte imbalances, such as hypoglycemia, hypocalcemia, and hyponatremia	Assess the child for predisposing factors that increase risk for seizures. Treat seizures promptly with diazepam or lorazepam, as ordered. Ensure the child's airway is maintained. Provide additional respiratory support after any drug therapy begins. Keep resuscitative equipment immediately available. Prepare the child for a complete diagnostic work-up as needed to determine the cause of the seizure.
Children have a high ratio of body surface area to body mass and a large head in relation to body size and thus lose heat readily. Hypothermia with increased risk for apnea, hypoventilation, hypotension, hypoglycemia, and metabolic acidosis (in neonates) Cool operating room Postoperative shivering, which can increase oxygen requirements by 400%–500% Hypothermia causes slowed recovery from anesthetic agents and may delay elimination of muscle relaxants. Heat loss by vasodilation, lack of muscle tone, and inhibition of temperature regulation caused by general anesthesia and neuromuscular block	Use warming lights and heating blankets to keep the child warm. Wrap the child's head to preserve body heat. Give the child supplemental oxygen. Use pulse oximetry to monitor the adequacy of oxygen therapy. Treat shivering with small dose of IV meperidine, or place heat on the child's skin.
Increased prevalence of agitation in children and young adults May be exacerbated by hypoxia, nausea, dizziness, inability to move, pain, fear, anxiety, full bladder, hypotension, gastric distension, and pharmacologic agents or postoperative medications	Involve the parents in recovery by having them hold, reassure, and comfort the child. Immediately rule out hypoxia as the cause. Give narcotics to treat pain. Catheterize the bladder, if warranted. Use a soft, soothing voice and light touch to calm the child. Protect the child from self-injury by padding the bed or crib rails. Relax physical restraints if they cause the child to fight harder. Secure all venous access devices, tubes, drains, and dressings.
Emergency equipment too large for the child Immediate need for pediatric dosages of resuscitation medications	Always use equipment specifically designed for pediatric patients. Organize resuscitation equipment for pediatric patients on a cart, including defibrillator paddles, intraosseous and IV needles, and oxygen equipment. Ensure that the staff is competent in using pediatric equipment. Keep essential resuscitation medications immediately available in pediatric dosages. Ensure that the child's age and weight are easily retrieved from the chart. Keep pediatric emergency drug dosage calculation cards handy.

Data from Meyer-Pahoulis, E., Williams, S. L., Davidson, S. I., McVey, J. R., & Mazurek, A. (1993). The pediatric patient in the post anesthesia care unit. *Nursing Clinics of North America, 28*, 519–530.

Steps	Rationale/Points of Emphasis
• Monitor for signs and symptoms of fluid and electrolyte imbalance. • Monitor output of tubes, drains, and body fluids.	
8. Maintain urinary output: • Check voiding. Monitor intake and output every 8 hours; notify physician if output is less than 1–2 mL/kg per hr. • Assess for retention or incontinence. • Catheterize as ordered or indicated. • Provide perineal care and catheter care, as indicated.	Anesthetic agents may temporarily depress bladder tone and response. Accurate recording of intake and output helps to assess renal and circulatory function.
9. Maintain normal bowel elimination: • Assess normal and baseline bowel pattern. • Assess bowel sounds: note signs and symptoms of distension, nausea and vomiting, abdominal pain, and flatus. • Monitor bowel movements.	Anesthetic agents may depress peristalsis and normal gastrointestinal function.
10. Prevent infection: • Assess and maintain surgical site dressing integrity; consult with physician regarding first surgical dressing change. • Use sterile dressings and technique in postoperative period. • Assess for signs and symptoms of drainage: odor, increased pain, redness, swelling, and constriction of circulation. • Maintain patency and integrity of drainage systems, as indicated.	The goal is to minimize the risk for infection and early detection of the infection.
11. Promote comfort and pain reduction: • Provide warming measures to reduce postoperative shivering and hypothermia. • Use a developmentally appropriate pain assessment method and teach the child to use it (follow practices initiated in preoperative area; see Chapter 7). Determine the level of pain above which adjustment of analgesia or other interventions will be considered. • Provide the child with education and information about pain control, including training in nonpharmacologic options such as relaxation and distraction. **KidKare** Explain to child that it is easier to prevent pain than to reduce it once it has become established and that communication of unrelieved pain is essential to its relief. Emphasize the importance of a factual report of pain, avoiding stoicism or exaggeration. • Assess the child's perception of pain along with behavioral and physiologic responses (remember that observations of behavior and vital signs should not be used instead of a self-report unless the child is unable to communicate). • Assess and reassess pain frequently during the immediate postanesthesia period. Determine the frequency of assessment based on the operation performed and the severity of the pain; for example, pain should be assessed every 2 hours during the first postoperative day after major surgery. • Increase the frequency of assessment and reassessment if the pain is poorly controlled or if interventions are changing.	Promoting comfort and minimizing pain will allow the child to rest comfortably and participate cooperatively in postoperative procedures.

PROCEDURE During Ongoing Recovery Period on Nursing Unit or in Postanesthesia Unit Before Discharge

Steps	Rationale/Points of Emphasis
1. Continue assessments as outlined above.	
2. Maintain adequate nutritional intake: • Increase diet as ordered from clear liquids to full liquids to solids. Avoid greasy, spicy, or rich foods the first 24 hours. Avoid large amounts of carbonated beverages. • Assess ability for self-feeding; assist as needed. • Encourage intake of appropriate foods to promote healing. • Initiate dietary supplements or parenteral nutrition as ordered and indicated.	Alteration in nutritional, circulatory, and metabolic states may predispose patients to infection and delayed healing. Do not press intake of solid food; let the child eat what he or she feels like eating. Push intake only if no intravenous fluids are being administered.
3. Promote mobility and self-care: • Assess restrictions as indicated; encourage activity as tolerated by the child. • Plan methods of self-care with the child. • Assist the child with mobilization as indicated; use mobilization assistance devices as needed.	Gives the child some control when participating in his or her care and promotes independence.
4. Provide sensory input: • Orient the child to time, place, environment, and circumstances. • Using age-appropriate language, explain all procedures and instructions. • Utilize an interpreter and written, visual, or auditory communication, as indicated.	Provides cognitive stimulation to the child.
5. Provide psychosocial support: • Assess the child's understanding of diagnosis, treatment, and procedures. • Encourage the child to verbalize his or her needs, concerns, and questions. • Involve the child and parents in the child's care. • Encourage diversional activities for the child.	Provides mechanisms to increase child's degree of comfort in unfamiliar situation and promotes trust with parents.

PROCEDURE Discharge Criteria for Same-Day Surgery

Steps	Rationale/Points of Emphasis
1. Child's vital signs are stable, similar to preoperative baseline vital signs, with no signs of respiratory distress.	Return to baseline indicates lack of respiratory distress, pain, fever, and fluid depletion.
2. Child has no complications related to anesthesia or specific type of operation (e.g., no excessive bleeding from wound; minimal nausea, vomiting, and dizziness).	See Table 93-1. Complications such as airway complications, fluid volume depletion, hypothermia, and seizures must be treated immediately to maintain safety and overall welfare of the child.
3. Child's pain is well controlled.	Minimizing pain will allow the child to rest comfortably and participate cooperatively in home care procedures.
4. Child has regained preoperative cognitive functioning.	Failure to return to baseline may indicate that hypoxic episode has occurred or that sedative agents continue to impact child's level of arousal. **caREminder** *The child may still be sleepy or need assistance with motor functions.*

Continued

Steps	Rationale/Points of Emphasis
5. Child ingests and retains fluid if he or she chooses to drink.	The approach to minimizing nausea and vomiting in the postoperative period is multifactorial and includes proper preoperative preparation, use of intraoperative antiemetic prophylaxis, choice of appropriate anesthetic agents and techniques, and appropriate plan of care in the postoperative period (e.g., advancement of diet, hydration status, use of antiemetics). **caREminder** *Letting the child choose to drink or not reduces the immediate postoperative incidence of vomiting.*
6. Child has voided.	Ensures that renal system is functioning and child is not dehydrated.
7. Child's parents understand the postoperative care needs and signs of complications and when to contact the healthcare provider. Written instructions and prescriptions have been provided to the family.	Ensures that child's home care needs will be met by parents who are fully informed of child's healthcare issues.

CHILD AND FAMILY EVALUATION AND DOCUMENTATION

- Evaluate child's and parent's understanding of surgical event and postanesthesia care and needs.
- Evaluate child's health status, including vital signs, respiratory and neurologic status, and integrity of all drains, tubes, appliances, and dressings.
- Document the following:
  - Vital signs
  - Input and output
  - Status of drains, tubes, appliances, and dressings
  - Respiratory assessment and interventions
  - Neurologic assessment
  - Postanesthesia complications and subsequent interventions
  - Pain assessment findings and pain management interventions
  - Teaching provided to child and parent

COMMUNITY CARE

- Initiate referrals as indicated (e.g., social services/home health, physical/occupational therapist, dietitian, respiratory therapist).
- After same-day surgery, instruct the parent and provide written instructions concerning the following:
  - Activity restrictions—usually restrict to quiet activities for 24 hours because of effects of anesthesia; no unsupervised activities for 24 hours that require coordination, such as stair climbing and sports, and then as appropriate to the procedure, for example, when myringotomy tubes are placed, child must wear earplugs when in water (e.g., baths, swimming)
  - Intake—clear liquids and then increase as tolerated or as specific to procedure (e.g., soft foods post-tonsillectomy); how to tell if the child is drinking enough (if voiding once every 8 hours, the child probably has sufficient intake); tips to promote fluid intake (offer Popsicles, serve fluid in small cups, encourage a few sips with every television commercial); avoid large amounts of carbonated beverages
  - Incision and wound care—if appropriate, whether to change dressing or not; amount and type of drainage expected; any special site care (e.g., elevation, ice, cleansing)
  - Pain management—how to assess as developmentally and child appropriate; pharmacologic and nonpharmacologic management strategies with potential side effects of drugs and actions to minimize these (e.g., child should drink plenty of fluids if taking codeine to counter constipating effects)
  - Proper use of any equipment, such as crutch walking
  - Signs of complications pertinent to procedure: excessive bleeding; acute onset, excessive, or poorly controlled pain; unable to tolerate oral fluids; insufficient urine output; altered motor or cognitive functioning; lethargy
- For the child being discharged several days after surgery, instruct the parent concerning the following:
  - Activity restrictions
  - Dietary restrictions (if any)
  - Incision and wound care
  - Pain management—review with the child and parent pain interventions used and their efficacy and provide specific discharge instructions regarding pain and its management
  - Proper use of equipment
  - Signs of complications
- Instruct the family to contact the healthcare provider if
  - Child begins to vomit or complain of ongoing nausea
  - Child develops a fever

- Child complains of pain that is not alleviated by prescribed pain medications and nonpharmacologic interventions
- Child has difficulty breathing
- Child refuses to eat or drink and has poor urinary output
- Child becomes unresponsive

Unexpected Situations

- *Heart rate is increased from baseline in the absence of fever:* This may be a sign of blood loss. Assess incision/dressing for bleeding; reinforce dressing if needed, but do not remove original dressing. Internal bleeding may be present. Notify physician.
- *Child reports or has signs of pain, unrelieved by ordered medications and nonpharmacologic methods:* Perform complete pain assessment (location, description, intensity, causal and alleviating factors) and notify healthcare prescriber.

Bibliography

Association of Operating Room Nurses. (1989). *Standards of perioperative nurse practice.* Denver: Author.

Collett, L., & D'Errico, C. (2000). Suggestions on meeting ASPAN standards in a pediatric setting. *Journal of Perianesthesia Nursing, 15,* 386–391.

Cropper, J., Hutchison, L., & Llewellyn, N. (2003). Postoperative retention of urine in children. *Paediatric Nursing, 15*(7), 15–18.

Hung, L., & Lam, B. (2004). Management of postoperative urinary retention: A randomized trial of in-out versus overnight catheterization. *Australian and New Zealand Journal of Surgery, 74,* 658–661.

Kain, Z. N., Mayes, L. C., Caldwell-Andrews, A. A., et al. (2002). Sleeping characteristics of children undergoing outpatient elective surgery. *Anesthesiology, 97,* 1093–1101.

Koomen, E., Janssen, S., & Anderson, B. J. (2002). Use of ultrasound bladder monitoring in children after caudal anaesthesia. *Paediatric Anaesthesia, 12,* 738–741.

LaMontagne, L., Hepworth, J., & Salisbury, M. (2001). Anxiety and postoperative pain in children who undergo major orthopedic surgery. *Applied Nursing Research, 14,* 119–124.

Manworren, R. C. B., Paulos, C. L., & Pop, R. (2004). Treating children for acute agitation in the PACU: Differentiating pain and emergence delirium. *Journal of Perianesthesia Nursing, 19,* 183–193.

Munro, H. (2000). Postoperative nausea and vomiting in children. *Journal of Perianesthesia Nursing, 15*(6), 401–407.

Pölkki, T., Pietilä, A., & Vehviläinen-Julkunen, K. (2003). Hospitalized children's descriptions of their experiences with postsurgical pain relieving methods. *International Journal of Nursing Studies, 40*(1), 33–44.

Ringdal, M., Borg, B., & Hellström, A. (2004). A survey on incidence and factors that may influence first postoperative urination. *Urologic Nursing, 23,* 341–346, 354.

Schreiner, M. (1994). Preoperative and postoperative fasting in children. *Pediatric Clinics of North America, 41,* 111–120.

Tripi, P. A., Palermo, T. M., Thomas, S., Goldfinger, M. M., & Florentino-Pineda, I. (2004). Assessment of risk factors for emergence distress and postoperative behavioural changes in children following general anaesthesia. *Paediatric Anaesthesia, 14,* 235–240.

CHAPTER

94

Postmortem Care

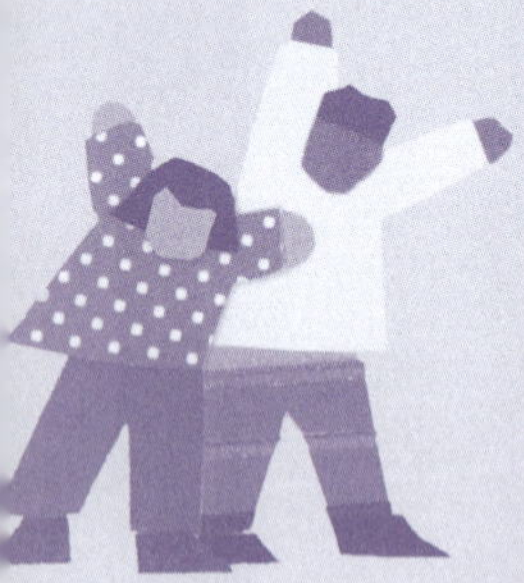

Clinical Guidelines

- A registered nurse (RN) or licensed practical nurse (LPN) is responsible for ensuring that all aspects of postmortem care are completed.
- Family members may participate in activities (e.g., bathing) to complete end-of-life care needs.
- Religious practices, cultural rituals, and any other requests are taken into consideration and implemented as possible during this period.
- All deceased children are treated with respect while being provided end-of-life care.

Equipment

- Towels, washcloths
- Bath basin with warm water
- Toiletry articles (e.g., soap, brush)
- Nonsterile gloves
- Clean linens, clothes
- Shroud pack with tags
- Death certificate
- Family support materials (e.g., list of local support groups, list of local mortuaries, reading materials about loss and grief)
- Keepsake kit, to include Polaroid camera, stamp pad and paper, scissors, small plastic bags or envelopes for hair locks
- Organ procurement consent (if needed)
- Autopsy or genetic workup consent (if needed)

Child and Family Assessment and Preparation

- Verify that all necessary parties involved have been notified of child's death (e.g., primary medical staff, coroner, grief counselor or bereavement team, religious cleric).
- Determine whether family needs assistance with funeral arrangements or legal issues.
- In collaboration with social services, assess any special requests that the family may have with regard to religion, culture, and end-of-life care needs.

- Verify that all forms have been reviewed with family and signed (e.g., tissue/organ donation, autopsy request, release of remains).
- If organ donation is to be implemented, initiate institutional procedures for procurement. In some states, it is mandated that the organ procurement agency be notified about every death and within a certain time frame, and it is requested that only agency members initiate family contact. Be sure to review the statutes before the death of the child.
- Check criteria for death to be reported to the coroner because this will modify the procedure to follow. Ascertain whether tubes and lines should be left in or removed when speaking to the coroner.
- Ensure that the child's medical record is ready to be sent to medical records.

PROCEDURE Providing Postmortem Care

Steps	Rationale/Points of Emphasis
1a. After the physician has pronounced the child's time of death, provide psychosocial support to family. If family is not present, confirm with physician that he or she will notify them. 1b. Provide privacy (e.g., pull curtains, close doors).	The loss of a child is a devastating experience for families; the nurse can help the family find needed privacy and can help facilitate communication among family members and members of the healthcare team. Allows family and significant others to begin the grieving process and to have some special time with the deceased child.
2. Ask family members if they would like to assist with cleaning and changing of the child.	Gives the family a sense of control in being part of the care of the deceased child. Respects and acknowledges cultural and religious beliefs.
3. Perform hand hygiene.	Reduces transmission of microorganisms.
4. Gather the necessary supplies and basin of warm water.	Promotes efficient time management and provides an organized approach to the procedure during postmortem care.
5. Don gloves. If the deceased child had been in isolation for any reason, the same isolation practices need to be followed after death; label the body accordingly.	Standard precaution to reduce transmission of microorganisms.
6. Cleanse the body. If an autopsy is to be performed, initiate procedural paperwork for autopsy.	Conveys respect and prepares the body for parents' viewing, if not already present. Many coroners and pathologists no longer require that lines and tubes be left in for autopsy cases. **Alert!** *If child has a pacemaker, place tape across chest with the word "pacemaker" written across to alert mortician.*
7. Prepare the child and the room for the family's visit, if not already present: • Provide clean bed linens as needed. • Dress the child in clothes brought from home or provided by the hospital. • Position the child in a pose of comfort; close child's eyes, if open. • Turn off and push equipment to side. • Deodorize room, if needed.	Familiar clothing reinforces the unique and special characteristics of this child to the family. Comfortable appearance of child and calm room may comfort the family. **caREminder** *It may be beneficial to leave much of the resuscitation equipment in the room to reinforce the fact that efforts were taken to save the child.*
8. Use "keepsake kit" to take photos of the child in an aesthetically pleasing manner. Make hand and/or footprints. Collect a lock of the child's hair and place in a plastic bag. Collect the clothes the child was wearing, if appropriate, and place in a sealable plastic bag. Offer these mementos to the family, or place them with the medical record to be given to the family at a later date.	Mementos give the family reminders of the child. Sealing the plastic bag may help preserve the child's scent on the clothes. The family may not be ready for the photos and other mementos at this time in their grieving process; however, many families often change their minds and want these items at later dates.

Continued

Steps	Rationale/Points of Emphasis
9a. If family members have not assisted up until this point, accompany them to the bedside and allow for privacy with the deceased child. If the family has been assisting, allow them time with the deceased child alone.	Many families experience a sense of comfort when allowed private time with a deceased child.
9b. Without forcing, encourage family members to spend as much time as they wish with the child.	The length of the final visit should be determined by the needs of the individual family.
9c. Support the family as necessary. Offer the family the opportunity to hold the child, and assist as needed. If siblings of a deceased child are present, discuss with the parents allowing siblings to see the child. Use child life specialists, if available, to assist in preparing the siblings to see the child.	Viewing or holding the deceased child reinforces the reality of death and may help in saying farewell to child. **KidKare** Inform siblings of what happened and give them an opportunity to express their questions and fears and to see their brother or sister if requested.
9d. Provide support for the completion of any requested religious practices, such as baptizing or blessing the child.	Demonstrates respect for cultural and spiritual needs and practices associated with the child's death.
10. Inventory the child's personal belongings and give them to the child's parents. If family is not present, turn personal belongings over to security. Have the parents sign the appropriate documents (e.g., donor papers, autopsy).	Ensures that the family obtains the child's belongings, which can help the family in the grieving process.
11. Before the family has departed, ensure that the child has on the correct armband. If armband is not in place, apply one.	The family provides positive identification of the child.
12. After the family leaves, fill out the labels of the shroud pack with the appropriate information.	Ensures correct identification of child among medical team, mortician, and organ procurement agency or coroner, if involved.
13. With assistance if needed, roll deceased child onto plastic sheet in shroud kit.	Keeps body fluids that may be released because of relaxed sphincters from contaminating any surface that the body may be moved to.
14a. Attach one of the labels to either the great toe or ankle. 14b. Loosely tape wrists or ankles to maintain alignment of body if necessary; do not use cording or other ties.	Ensures proper identification of child. The ties may cause damage to the skin and tissues of the deceased child.
15. Fold plastic sheet around body, securing ends and closing with tape.	Maintains body fluids in that space.
16. Remove gloves and perform hand hygiene.	Reduces transmission of microorganisms.
17. Attach second label securely with tape to top portion of covered body.	Ensures proper identification of child.
18. Obtain stretcher for transporting deceased child to morgue, and place deceased child onto stretcher.	Provides easier transportation than moving the entire bed.
19. Notify security or other personnel as required by institution for escorting the deceased child to the morgue.	Facilitates transport into the morgue.
20a. Escort deceased child to morgue with second person. 20b. Verify identity of child and accuracy of accompanying records upon arrival at morgue. Complete documentation and dispense the medical record per institution policy.	Provides emotional support for unit personnel after a death and safe and discreet physical transport. Reduces chance of identity errors. Provides permanent record of care.
21. Enter the necessary information into the morgue log book, and fill out other unit documents as appropriate.	Ensures proper identification of deceased child for anyone working with body.
22. Upon return to the child's room, don gloves.	Reduces transmission of microorganisms.
23. Clean room of linen and equipment; dispose of equipment and waste in appropriate receptacle.	Prepares room for terminal cleaning. Standard precautions.
24. Remove gloves and perform hand hygiene.	Reduces transmission of microorganisms.

CHILD AND FAMILY EVALUATION AND DOCUMENTATION

- Evaluate family's needs for support.
- Notify any family or support people if necessary.
- Allow family time to ask questions and share concerns.
- Determine that all consents have been signed and appropriately distributed.
- Complete narrative notes with time of death, name of physician who pronounced the child, follow-up care given, disposition of remains and personal effects, support of family, and referrals given to family.
- Document child's death in unit log book and discharge from hospital bed.

COMMUNITY CARE

- Determine if hospice services were used; these services are available in most communities to support families of infants and children who are terminally ill or have died. Contact social services or use the telephone book as a source of further information.
- Provide follow-up care to the family as appropriate (e.g., cards, letters, and phone calls from healthcare personnel or grief counselors).
- Provide follow-up debriefing to the hospital staff as needed utilizing chaplains, pastoral care, social workers, or grief counselors.

Unexpected Situation

- *After a child's death, the family insists on someone staying with their child because their religious beliefs dictate that the body not be left alone:* Make every attempt to accommodate the family's wishes. Arrange for the mortuary to pick up the body directly from the unit instead of sending the child to the morgue. If this is too disruptive for the unit, arrange for the child to be transported to the morgue after the mortuary staff arrives.

Bibliography

American Academy of Pediatrics and the American College of Emergency Physicians. (2002). Death of a child in the emergency department: Joint statement. *Pediatrics, 110,* 839–840.

American Association of Colleges of Nursing & City of Hope. (2004). *End-of-life nursing education consortium pediatric palliative care* (ELNEC PPC). Washington, DC: Author.

Cook, P., White, D. K., & Ross-Russell, R. I. (2004). Bereavement support following sudden and unexpected death: Guidelines for care. *Archives of Diseases in Childhood, 87,* 36–38.

Davies, R. (2004). New understandings of parental grief: Literature review. *Journal of Advanced Nursing, 46,* 506–513.

King, P. (2003). Listen to the children and honor their pain. *Oncology Nursing Forum, 30,* 779–780.

Meert, K. L., Thurston, C. S., & Thomas, R. (2001). Parental coping and bereavement outcome after the death of a child in the pediatric intensive care unit. *Pediatric Critical Care Medicine, 2,* 324–328.

Murphy, S. A., Johnson, L. C., Wu, L., Fan, J. J., & Lohan, J. (2003). Bereaved parents' outcomes 4 to 60 months after their children's deaths by accident, suicide, or homicide: A comparative study demonstrating differences. *Death Studies, 27,* 39–61.

Riely, M. (2003). Facilitating children's grief. *Journal of School Nursing, 19,* 212–218.

Servaty-Seib, H. L., Peterson, J., & Spang, D. (2003). Notifying individual students of a death loss: Practical recommendations for schools and school counselors. *Death Studies, 27,* 167–186.

CHAPTER

95

Postural Screening

Clinical Guidelines

- Physicians and registered nurses (RNs), with the proper training, may perform postural screening. Some states mandate screening for scoliosis and spinal abnormalities. In this case, most screenings are performed by the school nurse and educational staff who are properly trained by clinicians, depending on district policy.
- Screenings may be performed at any age but are usually performed during adolescence when the body is going through rapid physical growth. During mass screening, boys and girls must be screened separately and individually.

Equipment

- Scoliometer
- A secluded area with adequate lighting
- Pen
- Record sheet

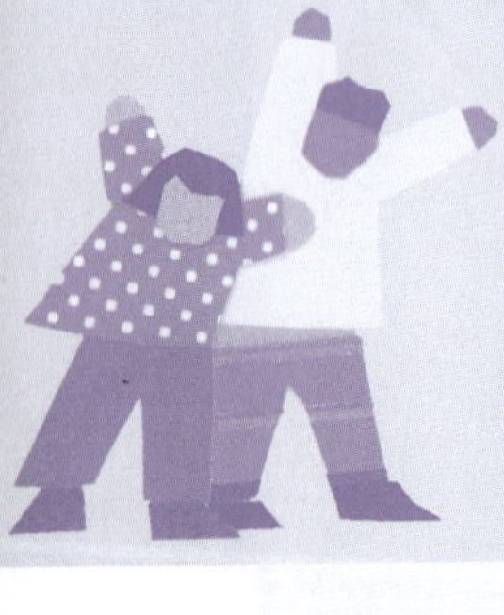

Child and Family Assessment and Preparation

- Obtain history of back pain and family history of spinal curvatures.
- Advise the child/adolescent that the shirt and shoes must be removed during screening; girls may keep their bra on.
- Children and adolescents are often embarrassed by the screening procedure. Teach them that the entire procedure takes 1 to 2 minutes and should effectively detect or rule out early signs of spine curvature. Early identification allows for prompt evaluation and treatment, avoiding possible cosmetic concerns and functional impairment.

PROCEDURE Conducting Postural Screening

Steps	Rationale/Points of Emphasis
1. Perform hand hygiene.	Reduces transmission of microorganisms.
2. Ask the child to remove shirt and shoes. Girls may keep their bra on if not wearing a gown.	The bare back must be viewed to properly see the curves of the spine. The feet must be flat on the floor to avoid any false curvature caused by improper stance or shoes. **KidKare** When mass screening is performed (e.g., at school) have girls wear or bring a bathing suit top to wear on the day of scoliosis testing; sports bras may cover the scapula and obscure visualization and therefore are not optimal. It may facilitate testing if a placement marker (e.g., an object or tape line) is placed to guide the child where to stand.
3. Ask the child to stand erect, arms hanging relaxed at his or her sides.	Allows the body to assume a relaxed position.
4. Stand in front and then behind the child, assessing for obvious abnormalities: • Visualize the back and assess the position of the spine for curvature. • Compare the shoulder and hip level for equality or if one side is higher than the other. • Compare the shoulder blades; evaluate if one side is more prominent than the other. • Look at the space between the arms and the body for equal distances between the arms and the flank. • Observe waist crease, if present; evaluate if the creases or skin folds at the waist are equal on both sides. • Compare leg lengths for equality. This is done by comparing hip symmetry while feet are flat on the floor in a standing position.	Shoulders, shoulder blades, and hips should be level, spine straight, and arms should have equal distances from the body. Leg length and waist creases, if present, should be equal on both sides. Possible scoliosis if inequality is present. **caREminder** *If hips are not symmetric while standing, have the child sit on the edge of a chair or bench and assess the hip and shoulder symmetry. If the hips and shoulders are symmetric while sitting, then the legs are not equal.*
5. Instruct the child to assume the forward bend position (Adams test), observing from the front, side, and back: • Feet 4 inches apart • Knees straight • Bend at the waist at 90 degrees • Arms hanging, relaxed • Palms of the hand facing each other, like diving into a pool • Head down, chin to chest	Position allows observation of the spine while it is curved. Asymmetry in upper or lower back, rib cage, and hip level or lateral curvature of the spine suggest scoliosis. Excessive prominence of the thoracic spine suggests kyphosis, and excessive sway back suggests lordosis.
6. If any asymmetry or prominence is noted, measure the angle of truncal rotation (ATR) by placing the scoliometer at the top of the thoracic spine, with the 0 (zero) mark over the spinous process, and slowly move the scoliometer down the spine noting the degree of truncal rotation by reading the number where the ball moves in line, either to the left or the right of the zero mark. This is the degree of rotation.	Determines degree of curvature. **caREminder** *If asymmetry is present in both the upper and lower back, obtain two scoliometer readings. In this instance the curves typically go in the opposite direction because of compensatory mechanisms.*
7. Ask the child to put his or her shirt and shoes back on and commend for a job well done.	Positive reinforcement allows the child to walk away from the screening feeling proud and alleviates the initial feelings of embarrassment and anxiety.
8. Perform hand hygiene.	Reduces transmission of microorganisms.

CHILD AND FAMILY EVALUATION AND DOCUMENTATION

- If screening results are positive, furnish a letter of referral to the primary care provider indicating the positive findings. Criteria for referral include
  - Any child with an obvious deformity
  - Lordosis or kyphosis
  - Curvature of the spine: 5 degrees or more ATR on the scoliometer
  - Two or more of these signs: shoulder or scapula asymmetry of at least 1 inch, hip asymmetry of at least ½ inch, larger space between arm and flank on one side, uneven waist creases, and leg length difference of at least ½ inch
- Record screening results on appropriate form.

COMMUNITY CARE

- Advise the parent of the results of screening, emphasizing referral and follow-up for children with positive findings.
- Teach children proper body mechanics while carrying their backpacks, sitting in class, using a computer, and performing other activities of daily living.
- Instruct the family to contact the healthcare provider if
  - Child complains of back pain
  - Parent notices abnormal gait or stance

caREminder

Scoliosis typically does not cause back pain; however, poor posture and weak musculature is related to back pain and pain and scoliosis can coexist.

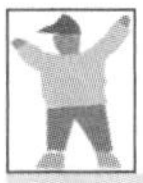

Unexpected Situation

- *When examining the child's back, you observe a rash:* Refer child to primary care provider to determine cause of rash and potential need for treatment.

Bibliography

Burwell, R. G., Aujla, R. K., Cole, A. A., et al. (2002). Back shape assessment in each of three positions in preoperative patients with adolescent idiopathic scoliosis: Evaluation of a 10-level scoliometer method interpolated to 18-levels. *Studies in Health Technology and Informatics, 91*, 119–122.

Huang, S.-C. (1997). Cut-off point of the scoliometer in school scoliosis screening. *Spine, 22*, 1985–1989.

Reamy, B. & Slakey, J. (2001). Adolescent idiopathic scoliosis: Review and current concepts. *American Family Physician, 64*, 111–116.

Ryberg, J. (2004). *Postural screening guidelines for school nurses.* (National Association of School Nurses Publication No. S013). Scarborough, ME: National Association of School Nurses.

United States Department of Health and Human Services. (2001). *Scoliosis in children and adolescents.* (NIH Publication No. 01-4862). Retrieved on November 16, 2004 from http://www.niams.nih.gov/HI/topics/scoliosis/ScoliosisRP.pdf

United States Preventive Services Task Force. (2002). *Guide to clinical preventive services* (pp. 373–382). McLean, VA: International Medical Publishing, Inc.

Yawn, B. P., & Yawn, R. A. (2000). The estimated cost of school scoliosis screening. *Spine, 25*, 2387–2391.

CHAPTER 96

Potassium Infusion, Administration of

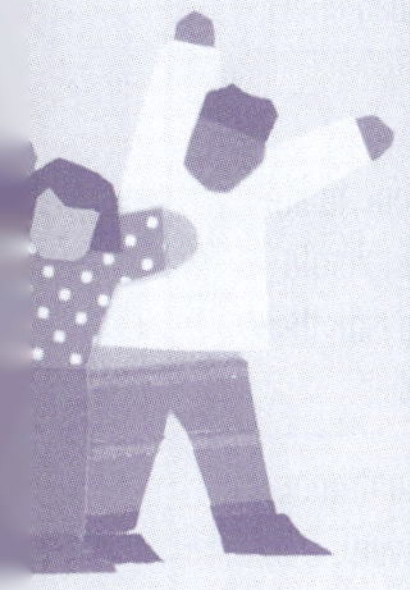

Clinical Guidelines

- A healthcare prescriber orders potassium infusions.
- Potassium infusions are administered by a registered nurse (RN) or healthcare prescriber who is knowledgeable about administering potassium.
- Before administration, the potassium infusion must be verified by two of the above providers to check child's identification, weight, physician order, drug concentration, and rate of infusion.
- Principles of pharmacologic management (see Chapter 6) are followed.
- Intravenous potassium is administered to achieve and maintain electrolyte balance.
- Serum potassium concentrations should always be interpreted using the child's current pH. If the pH is to be corrected, potassium supplementation should be dependent on the results of the pH correction. For example, a low potassium concentration may be adequate if the child is alkalotic and the alkalosis is going to be corrected; therefore, potassium replacement may not be necessary.
- Hypokalemia may be treated orally or parenterally. Nonsymptomatic hypokalemia should be treated, whenever possible, with oral supplementation.
- Hypokalemia-related dysrhythmias should be treated with IV supplementation with the patient continuously monitored in a critical care setting. Because potassium contributes to the resting membrane potential of the cells, this may result in acute and dramatic fluctuations in serum potassium levels that can precipitate life-threatening dysrhythmias.
- Monitoring of vital signs and cardiac response to the potassium acute infusion requires facilities, equipment, and resources to perform the following before, during, and after the potassium infusion:
  - Continuous electrocardiogram (ECG) monitoring of heart rate and rhythm
  - Pediatric advanced life support
  - Treatment of life-threatening dysrhythmias
- The maximum concentration for acute potassium infusions should be no greater than 0.4 mEq/mL for central line infusion and 0.2 mEq/mL for peripheral line infusion.
- The maximum acute infusion rate should be 0.5 mEq/kg per dose or less (infused over an hour or more).
- Emergency drugs and equipment must be available for immediate use in the event of adverse drug reactions, potential complications, or emergency situations that require advanced life support (see Chapters 24 and 67).

EQUIPMENT

- Existing access, central or peripheral (if not present, see Chapters 55 to 58)
- IV-controlled infusion device with appropriate tubing
- Premixed dose of potassium in either a bag or syringe
- Needleless access device
- Alcohol swabs
- Cardiopulmonary monitoring when appropriate

CHILD AND FAMILY ASSESSMENT AND PREPARATION

- Establish a baseline assessment of the child; include health history, age, height, weight, review of systems, physical examination, baseline laboratory values, baseline cardiac rate and rhythm, and child's previous experience with potassium infusions.
- Assess for drug or latex allergies.
- Assess existing vascular access for patency, blood return, redness, pain, or leaking at the site. If necessary, establish new vascular access.
- Assess the child's and parent's understanding for the need for the potassium infusion.
- Prepare the child, as appropriate, and parents before the potassium infusion. Explain the medication's actions and side effects.

PROCEDURE Administering a Potassium Infusion

Steps	Rationale/Points of Emphasis
1. Gather the necessary supplies.	Promotes efficient time management and provides an organized approach to the procedure.
2. Verify the order with the medical record and check for allergy to drug; if present, do not administer drug and notify prescriber. **Alert!** *Acute potassium infusions may cause life-threatening dysrhythmias. The word* bolus *infers a rapid infusion over minutes and therefore should not be used when ordering potassium. Potassium orders should always indicate an acute infusion, meaning an infusion over an hour or more.*	Verifies correct drug, dose, route, time, and patient. Allergic reactions to medications may be life threatening.
3. Obtain the premixed potassium from the pharmacy and read the label to verify with the order. Check for expiration date; if expired, do not administer.	Route, dose, frequency, and time to be administered must be verified each time a medication is administered. Expired medications may not give the intended effect.
4. Perform hand hygiene and don gloves.	Reduces transmission of microorganisms.
5. Place the child on a cardiopulmonary monitor if the patient is symptomatic.	Children who are symptomatic with a low potassium level are more prone to life-threatening dysrhythmias during the infusion. Pediatric patients usually tolerate hypokalemia well, without significant incidence of atrial or ventricular dysrhythmias. One exception to this is the patient with congenital heart anomalies.
6. With a second nurse, verify the medication with the electronic medication record or take the medication record and medication to the child to administer. Verify the child's identity by comparing name on medication (if verified electronically) or on medication record with child's identification band and any other patient identifier required by the institution. In addition, verify child's weight, physician order, drug concentration, and rate of infusion.	Ensures proper identification of child. Orders for potassium dose, concentration, preparation, and rate are verified for accuracy to help ensure safe delivery. Double checking reduces the risk of errors. **KidKare** Lidocaine may be added to the potassium acute infusion to help lessen the amount of discomfort at the IV site. Be sure to indicate on the child's medical record and plan of care that lidocaine was used.
7. Ensure vascular access.	Extravasation of potassium into the tissues may cause necrosis.

Steps	Rationale/Points of Emphasis
8. Spike medication bag with tubing or place tubing on syringe pump containing the medication, prime tubing, and clearly label tubing.	Clear labeling reduces the risk for errors.
9. Obtain a volumetric IV-controlled infusion device or use "smart pumps" with built-in software to monitor medication administration. Set rate. **Alert!** *The pump must provide a constant continuous flow rate, not intermittent boluses of fluid.*	A volumetric IV-controlled infusion device is used to ensure safe accurate delivery and titration of cardioactive or vasoactive medications. "Smart pump" software technology can reduce medication errors by creating safety guardrails for medication administration.
10. Start infusion. Stop acute infusion if the child complains of pain or burning at the IV site. If not previously done, obtain an order for lidocaine, or reduce the concentration of the potassium, or reduce the rate.	Adding lidocaine anesthetizes the area and reduces discomfort. Reducing the concentration or rate also decreases discomfort.
11. Remove gloves and perform hand hygiene.	Reduces transmission of microorganisms.
12. Continuously monitor the child's clinical status throughout the course of therapy.	Clinical changes in the child may require dosage readjustment or weaning during the course of therapy. Discontinuation of a drug may be necessary if unexpected or adverse reactions occur or when a therapeutic response is not achieved.

Child and Family Evaluation and Documentation

- Evaluate the child's response to the potassium infusion.
- Determine whether the child or family have additional questions regarding therapy.
- Document the following:
  - Medication(s) given
  - Route given
  - Drug concentration and diluent
  - Dosage
  - Date and time of administration
  - Child's response to medication
  - ECG rhythm strip (pre- and postinfusion), if applicable
  - Presence or absence of adverse reactions
  - Notification of physician if applicable
  - Teaching and information given to child and parent

Community Care

- Encourage family members' involvement in child's care while he or she is still in the hospital so they are better prepared to assume child's care at home.
- Teach family about medications child will likely be taking at home, including dosage, administration procedures, expected responses, potential side effects, and guidelines for missed doses.
- Initiate appropriate referrals for follow-up care, if needed.
- Instruct the family to contact the healthcare provider if
  - IV insertion site is red, inflamed, or draining
  - Child has unexpected reactions during therapy
  - Questions occur regarding dosage, administration, missed dose guidelines, or other concerns

Unexpected Situations

- *Child complains of pain at the IV site:* Stop infusion and consider the following:
  - Need for new vascular access
  - If access is patent, then consider adding lidocaine
  - Or reduce the concentration of the drug
  - Or reduce the rate of the infusion
- *Infusion causes extravasation into the tissues:* Stop the infusion. Warm compresses will help the medication absorb into the tissues.
- *Child develops a dysrhythmia during the infusion:* Stop infusion and call the physician. Monitor patient for continued dysrhythmias. If possible, move to critical care unit for continued observation. For life-threatening dysrhythmias that are symptomatic, initiate CPR immediately.

Bibliography

American Association of Critical Care Nurses. (2006). *Core curriculum for pediatric critical care nursing.* Philadelphia: W. B. Saunders.

Gunn, V. L., Nechyba, C., & Barone, M. A. (Eds.). (2003). *The Harriet Lane handbook: A manual for pediatric house officers* (16th ed.). St. Louis: Mosby.

Slonirn, A., Pollack, M. M., Bell, M. J., et al. (2006). *Pediatric critical care medicine.* Philadelphia: Lippincott, Williams & Wilkins.

Taketomo, C. K., Hodding, J. H., & Kraus, D. M. (2005). *Pediatric dosage handbook* (12th ed.). Hudson, OH: Lexi-Comp Inc.

CHAPTER

97

Preoperative Care

CLINICAL GUIDELINES

- Preoperative preparation is provided to the child and parent by the child life specialist, registered nurse (RN), or licensed practical nurse (LPN).
- An RN or LPN completes the preoperative checklist before transportation of the child to surgery.
- A signed surgical consent form is present in the front of the child's medical record. The site and laterality (right, left, midline, or bilateral) of all procedures is spelled out in its entirety on the consent form.
- Parents accompany the child to surgical waiting area.

EQUIPMENT

- Identification band for child
- Surgical clothing for child
- Stethoscope
- Thermometer
- Blood pressure monitor
- Pulse oximetry monitor
- Scale
- Preoperative checklist
- Razor (if needed)
- Preoperative medications (if prescribed)

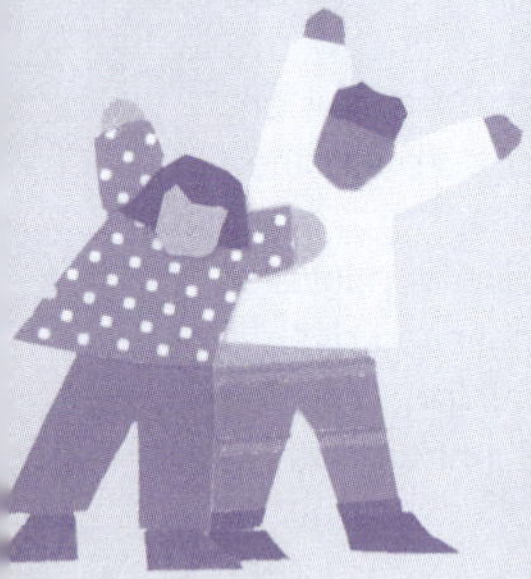

CHILD AND FAMILY ASSESSMENT AND PREPARATION

- Verify identification of the child with two identifiers (e.g., name, date of birth, medical record number). Verify that child's identification band matches identification number on medical record.
- Assess child for developmental stage and level of cognitive functioning
- Ensure consent form is completed, signed, and placed in front of the child's chart.
- Verify that the site and laterality of the procedure is completely spelled out on the consent form.
- Verify that the child's chart contains the following:
  - History and physical examination completed by physician or advanced practice nurse, per state and facility protocol
  - Current nursing flow sheet

    - Relevant laboratory values
    - Preoperative checklist
- Verify the site and laterality of the procedure with the parent and child as appropriate, child's chart, preoperative checklist, and consent.
- Check that preoperative laboratory tests were completed and assess values to identify any that lie outside normal ranges.
- Ensure that child's old medical records are available if needed.
- If ordered, determine that blood is available for possible transfusion during surgery.
- Determine the child's preoperative fasting status (Chart 97-1).
- Determine child's isolation status; note any specific precautions on the chart and communicate status with other care providers.
- Determine whether child completed any antimicrobial skin preparation before admission.
- Assist child to don surgical gown.
- Verify that parent knows location of waiting room, anticipated length of surgery, and areas to obtain amenities (e.g., coffee, bathrooms). Give family name and location of a contact person to answer questions or concerns about the surgery.

KidKare Many facilities allow children to wear their pajamas into surgery, changing their clothes after they have received light anesthesia. Allow children to carry a favorite toy or blanket with them into the surgical area. If at all possible, allow parents to be with their child during the initial induction so that the parents are the last thing the child remembers before going to sleep.

PROCEDURE Complete Preoperative Assessment

Steps	Rationale/Points of Emphasis
1. Assess child's history, with special emphasis on experiences with pain and pain management beliefs, risk factors (nutrition, allergies, medications, mobility, gastrointestinal and genitourinary function, skin integrity), and previous operating room procedure and anesthesia (Table 97-1).	When presenting new information, build on the child's previous experiences. **caREminder** *The child with an upper respiratory tract infection does not automatically need to have his or her surgery canceled. Based on the admission assessment of the child and on post-surgical management of the child, perioperative respiratory complications may be easily managed and not associated with any adverse sequelae.*
2. Obtain baseline pertinent physical examination data, including current height and weight.	Establishes normal values for the child and alerts the nurse to possible post-operative complications.

CHART 97-1 PREOPERATIVE FASTING INSTRUCTIONS*

- Normal meals and snacks may be eaten until bedtime on the evening before the day of surgery.
- After bedtime, no foods or fluids should be ingested, except for *clear* fluids such as water, apple juice, cranberry juice, Jell-O, and ginger ale. These clear fluids may be ingested until 2 hours before the child's arrival at the hospital. Fluids that should *not* be ingested include milk, orange juice, and other fluids that contain particulate matter and are not clear.
- Infants who receive formula should finish their last feeding 6 hours before the start of surgery. Like older children, they may drink *clear* fluids up to 2 hours before coming to the hospital.
- Infants who are breast fed may nurse until 3 hours before scheduled to arrive at the hospital.
- The anesthesiologist, taking into account the health status and special considerations of the individual child, may make exceptions to the above rules.
- If the child must take any oral medication, generally it may be taken with a small sip of water. Medications that are important to continue include antibiotics, anticonvulsants, bronchodilators, and other drugs ordered by the surgeon or anesthesiologist. The health care team should be informed of these and any other medications that the child is currently taking.

*This is an example of information the nurse may provide to the patient and family before surgery. Specific instructions may vary. Check your facility's protocol.

TABLE 97-1

Pediatric Presurgical Check

Aspect of Care	Nursing Action	Rationale
Identification verification	Verify that identification band corroborates with patient and family statement and chart documentation.	The identification band functions as a safety measure so that the proper patient receives the correct surgery.
Preoperative workup within hospital parameters (often 72 hours)	Check that laboratory values are in the chart. Assess laboratory values for relationship to normalcy and identify any values that lie outside normal ranges. Physician should be notified of outliers.	Special attention should be paid to potentially significant outliers that may indicate change in patient status or electrolyte imbalance.
Consents completed: General consent Surgical consent	Confirm that all required consent forms are completed, with dates, proper procedure identified, and witness.	Lack of properly signed consents can result in litigation and refusal of reimbursement to the institution.
Surgical attire	Dress child per facility's policy regarding perioperative attire.	Some facilities allow the children to wear underwear to the operating room (OR) in order to reduce anxiety.
Family notification	Verify that the family/guardian is informed regarding location of surgical waiting room, anticipated length of surgery, and areas to obtain amenities such as coffee and refreshments.	Concerned family members generally want to remain nearby when possible, in order to be notified as to the ongoing status or outcome of surgery as soon as possible.
Allergy status	Prominently note known or suspected allergies in the chart. If available, place allergy wristband on child.	Patient or family members should be asked about any allergies, including episodes of hives and food or medication allergy.
Familial history of problems with anesthesia	Elicit family history of reaction to anesthesia.	Intolerance or adverse reactions to anesthesia can be life threatening and may be hereditary.
Vital signs	Chart current vital signs; identify any unusual trends or values outside the norm.	Unusual patterns or change in vital signs may indicate change in patient status.
Body weight and height	Document current height and weight.	Height and weight are the primary parameters used to determine drug dosages, blood volume, and fluid requirements.
Elimination: urine	Encourage child to void before surgery, and document; note any changes or unusual appearance in urine.	The opportunity to void in the OR may be limited, and the child will receive generous amounts of IV fluids intraoperatively.
NPO status	Keep the child NPO as ordered; inform family of underlying rationale.	Stomach contents may be aspirated during intubation. Anesthesia may reduce gastric motility as well as cause nausea and vomiting.
Removal of foreign objects or personal belongings	Check for and ask the child about the possible presence of hair pins, jewelry, and so forth. Remove these before transport to the OR. If items (such as a ring) are not removable, the OR nurse should be notified of their presence so that any hazard that these may produce can be minimized.	Metal or other materials may be a risk factor for burns from the cautery used in surgery or form pressure sores during prolonged surgery. Check even infants for earrings; older children may have other body areas pierced, such as umbilicus.
Removal of prostheses	Remove contact lenses, eyeglasses, and orthodontic appliances before transport to the OR. Note any exceptions.	Items such as contact lenses and orthodontic appliances are commonly encountered in the pre-adolescent and adolescent population.

TABLE 97-1

Pediatric Presurgical Check (continued)

Aspect of Care	Nursing Action	Rationale
Nail bed assessment	Remove any nail polish from fingers and toes before transportation to the OR.	Nail polish can obscure the ability to accurately assess for oxygenation and capillary refill.
Dentition	Examine the mouth, and inquire about potentially loose teeth. If identified, note and report to the OR nurse or anesthetist.	Children intermittently loosen their "baby teeth," which can pose a hazard should the patient be intubated.
Preoperative medication	Administer any prescribed medications before transport to OR. If IM medications are ordered, check with anesthesia care practitioner to give by a different route.	Light sedation is often desirable to allay anxiety associated with surgery. Medication should be administered with enough time to achieve desired effect, and the patient is monitored or observed for any adverse reactions.
Operative site preparation	Comply with facility standards for skin preparation for cleansing or shaving of operative skin.	The skin at the operative site should be as free of oil and debris as possible, to reduce risk for infection.

PROCEDURE Complete Preoperative Teaching

Steps	Rationale/Points of Emphasis
1. Assess child for knowledge of perioperative procedures. Determine what role the parents have played in preparing the child for surgery. Activate and use the child life specialist, if available, early in the preoperative preparation period.	The nurse may need to reinforce information given by the parents. The child life specialist plays a key role in the psychological preparation of children and their families. **KidKare** Because of the wide range of developmental variances in the pediatric population, one type of preparation may not benefit all children equally; a variety of strategies may need to be tried. Communicate and document effective strategies to all members of the healthcare team.
2. Assess child for fear and anxiety. Determine the coping mechanisms used by the child: • Encourage child to verbalize fears and anxieties. • Ask parents to assist in interpreting child's behaviors (e.g., does silence mean the child has no questions or does it indicate fear?). • Orient the child to the environment. • Explain all procedures to the child. • Use anxiety-reducing techniques (e.g., relaxation, imagery, diversional activities).	Children often develop fantasies or distorted ideas when they do not have accurate knowledge. Preoperative teaching reduces anxiety and fear, promotes cooperation, supports coping skills, and may facilitate a feeling of mastery over a potentially stressful event. A sense of security and comfort is important in the child. Parents' emotional states are important indicators of children's emotional states and subsequently their pain experience. Involving the family and helping parents to reduce their anxiety will affect emotional responses of the child.
3. Assess child and parent knowledge of postoperative self-care measures.	Involving child helps gain his or her cooperation. Parents relate their fears and anxieties to their children verbally and nonverbally. Therefore, parents need assurance that their child is receiving adequate medical treatment, they need information to allow them to understand their child's medical status, and they need to know how they can be involved in their child's care.

Continued

Steps	Rationale/Points of Emphasis
KidKare Siblings can be a source of support and strength for the child. Therefore it is desirable to involve them in the preparation process.	
4. Provide explanation of preoperative and postoperative activities and expectations.	Research indicates that all children can benefit from preoperative preparation. Children need an explanation for anything that involves them. Ensure that explanation is short, simple, and appropriate to child's level of understanding.
5. Describe typical sensory experiences (e.g., discomfort or pain, position, temperature) that the child may expect to encounter during the operative experience.	Provision of sensory-procedural information and helping the child develop coping skills are effective preparations for painful procedures.
6. Instruct the child in coughing and deep-breathing mobility and other self-care measures.	Rehearsing the events will familiarize the child with medical procedures and decrease anxiety and better prepare the child to participate in his or her care.
7. Instruct the child and parent regarding anticipated postoperative tubes and drains.	Children who are prepared may experience less anxiety.
8. Instruct the child and parent regarding postoperative pain management: • Provide age-appropriate information about pain management therapies that are available and the rationale underlying their use. • With the child and parent, develop a plan for pain assessment and management. • Determine a pain assessment method, and teach the child and parent to use it. Determine the level of pain above which adjustment of analgesia or other interventions will be considered. • Provide the child and parent with education and information about pain control, including demonstration of nonpharmacologic measures (see Chapter 7). • Inform the child and parent that it is easier to prevent pain than to try to reduce it once it has become established and that communication of unrelieved pain is essential to its relief. Emphasize the importance of the factual report of pain, avoiding either stoicism or exaggeration.	Provides a baseline assessment for pain. Introduces the child, while awake and alert, to the pain assessment tool that will be used throughout the child's surgical stay.

PROCEDURE Provide Ongoing Care Until Time of Surgery

Steps	Rationale/Points of Emphasis
1. Maintain nutritional and fluid balance: • Initiate intravascular access if needed to provide nutritional and fluid support in cases of extensive NPO or multiple traumas.	The surgical patient is vulnerable to fluid and electrolyte imbalances. **KidKare** IV access is often not initiated until after the child has received some light anesthesia to reduce the trauma associated with IV starts.
2. Maintain skin integrity: • Anticipate the need for pressure prevention device or specialty bed. • Provide skin preparation as ordered.	The skin contains multiple microorganisms that grow and multiply when the integrity is damaged. Some facilities aspire to achieve such a progressive reduction of bacteria that children are instructed to begin antimicrobial skin preparation at home before admission. Skin cleansing before surgery assists in removing microbes, flakes of dead skin cells, oils, and other debris that foster growth of bacteria.

Steps	Rationale/Points of Emphasis
KidKare Hair removal is rarely deemed necessary in prepubescent children because they have scant amounts of body hair. Hair removal, if necessary, should be completed after the child is anesthetized to reduce anxiety in the child and to minimize scratches and nicks associated with sudden movements made by an alert child. Place hair from the child's head that is removed as a result of surgery in a plastic bag and offer to the parents.	
3. Administer preoperative medications, as ordered. Intervene to keep the child as calm as possible.	Sedatives (e.g., midazolam) and antibiotic therapy may be ordered to be given before entering the operating room. A mild sedative may reduce anxiety and assist the child to relax. Children who are anxious during the induction of anesthesia have an increased likelihood of developing postoperative negative behavioral changes (e.g., nightmares, separation anxiety, and aggression toward authority).

CHILD AND FAMILY EVALUATION AND DOCUMENTATION

- Evaluate child's and parent's understanding of surgical event and preoperative and postanesthesia care.
- Evaluate child's health status, including vital signs, respiratory and neurologic status, mobility, and self-care capabilities.
- Complete the institutional preoperative checklist.
- Document the following:
  - Vital signs
  - Body weight and height
  - NPO status
  - Allergy status
  - Family history
  - Physical assessment findings
  - Dentition
  - Removal of foreign objects or personal belongings
  - Preoperative medications
  - Operative site preparations (ensure the site is marked by the surgeon or designee before entering the surgical suite)
  - Pain assessment findings
  - Child and family teaching provided

COMMUNITY CARE

- Encourage parents to complete laboratory work before the date of the surgery.
- Provide child with opportunity for preoperative hospital tour (see Chapter 4).
- Refer family to educational resources (e.g., television educational channel, pamphlets, and visual aids).
- Instruct the family to contact the healthcare provider if
  - Child develops a cold or fever before scheduled surgery

Unexpected Situations

- *Child's preoperative laboratory values are abnormal:* Notify the physician because some abnormalities may postpone the surgery.
- *Child or parent reports that child ingested fluids shortly before scheduled surgery time:* Notify physician; depending on amount and type of fluid and child's risk factors, surgery may be postponed to reduce aspiration risk.

Bibliography

American Academy of Pediatrics Policy Statement. (1996). *Evaluation and preparation of pediatric patients undergoing anesthesia (RE9633).* Retrieved January 3, 2005, from www.aap.org

American Academy of Pediatrics Policy Statement. (1999). *Guidelines for pediatric perioperative anesthesia environment (RE9820).* Retrieved January 3, 2005, from www.aap.org

American Society of Anesthesiologists. (n.d.) *Practice guidelines for preoperative fasting and the use of pharmacologic agents to reduce the risk of pulmonary aspiration: Application to healthy patients undergoing elective procedures.* Retrieved January 3, 2005, from http://www.asahq.org/publicationsAndServices/NPO.pdf

Association of periOperative Registered Nurses (AORN). (2003). *Guidelines to eliminate wrong site surgery.* Retrieved January 3, 2005, from http://www.aorn.org/about/positions/pdf/Wrong-site% 20Surgery.pdf

Bellew, M., Atkinson, K. R., Dixon, G., & Yates, A. (2002). The introduction of a paediatric anaesthesia information leaflet: An audit of its impact on parental anxiety and satisfaction. *Paediatric Anaesthesia, 12,* 124–130.

Chan, C. S., & Molassiotis, A. (2002). The effects of an educational programme on the anxiety and satisfaction level of parents having parent present induction and visitation in a postanaesthesia care unit. *Paediatric Anaesthesia, 12,* 131–139.

Collett, L., & D'Errico, C. (2000). Suggestions on meeting ASPAN standards in a pediatric setting. *Journal of Perianesthesia Nursing, 15*, 386–391.

Cook-Sather, S. D., Harris, K. A., Chiavacci, R., Gallagher, P. R., & Schreiner, M. S. (2003). A liberalized fasting guideline for formula-fed infants does not increase average gastric fluid volume before elective surgery. *Anesthesia & Analgesia, 96*, 965–969.

Friesen, R. H., Wurl, J. L., & Friesen, R. M. (2002). Duration of preoperative fast correlates with arterial blood pressure response to halothane in infants. *Anesthesia & Analgesia, 95*, 1572–1576.

Garcia-Miguel, F. J., Serrano-Aguilar, P. G., & López-Bastida, J. (2003). Preoperative assessment. *The Lancet, 362*, 1749–1757.

Leelanukrom, R., Somboonviboon, W., & Sriprachittichai, P. (2002). Parental presence during induction of anesthesia in children: A study on parental attitudes and children's cooperation. *Medical Journal of the Medical Association of Thailand, 85*, S186–S192.

Li, H. C. W., & Lam, H. Y. A. (2003). Paediatric day surgery: Impact on Hong Kong Chinese children and their parents. *Journal of Clinical Nursing, 12*, 882–887.

Maxwell, L. G. (2004). Age-associated issues in preoperative evaluation, testing, and planning: Pediatrics. *Anesthesiology Clinics of North America, 22*, 27–43.

Messeri, A., Caprilli, S., & Busoni, P. (2004). Anaesthesia induction in children: A psychological evaluation of the efficiency of parents' presence. *Paediatric Anaesthesia, 14*, 551–556.

O'Connor, S. (2000). Preparing children for surgery: An integrative research review. *AORN Journal, 71*, 334–343.

Oshodi, T. O. (2004). Clinical skills: An evidence-based approach to preoperative fasting. *British Journal of Nursing, 13*, 958–962.

Tait, A., Voepel-Lewis, T., & Malviya, S. (2000). Perioperative consideration for the child with an upper respiratory tract infection. *Journal of Perianesthesia Nursing, 15*, 392–396.

Wang, S. M., Maranets, I., Weinberg, M. E., Caldwell-Andrews, A. A., & Kain, Z. N. (2004). Parental auricular acupuncture as an adjunct for parental presence during induction of anesthesia. *Anesthesiology, 100*, 1399–1404.

Wisselo, T. L., Stuart, C., & Muris, P. (2004). Providing parents with information before anaesthesia: What do they really want to know? *Paediatric Anaesthesia, 14*, 299–307.

CHAPTER

98

Procedures: General Guidelines

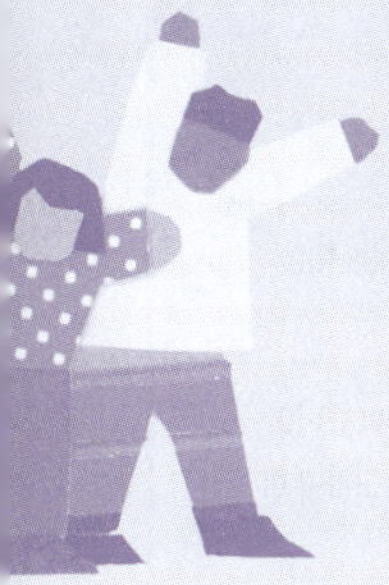

Clinical Guidelines

- Procedures are performed within the scope of practice of the healthcare provider.
- If a procedure is painful or involves tissue trauma, pain is managed as appropriate to degree of anticipated tissue trauma (e.g., sedation, local anesthesia, topical anesthetic, opioids) (see Chapter 7).
- The child is transported to the site where the procedure will be completed in a safe and age-appropriate manner (see Chapter 115).
- Family members will be permitted in the patient care area during invasive procedures.

Equipment

- As indicated for the procedure

Child and Family Assessment and Preparation

- Assess severity of child's illness and determine whether there is adequate time for explanation and use of topical anesthesia. If emergent, explain procedure as it is being performed.
- Assess child and family for prior adverse experiences during a procedure.
- Assess child for any allergies (including allergies to medication, adhesive tape, and topical solutions [e.g., chlorhexidine]) and for latex sensitivity; if present, initiate appropriate precautions (see Chapter 60).
- Assess child and parent's understanding of the procedure.
- Provide developmentally appropriate teaching before procedure to the child and family (see Chapter 3).
- Inform child and parent what is expected of child during the procedure as developmentally appropriate (e.g., hold still, take a deep breath).
- Explain normal and abnormal sensation that child might experience during the procedure (e.g., the cleaning medicine will feel cold, or some children say it feels like someone is pushing on them).
- Give parents and child an approximate length of time to complete the procedure.
- Discuss any restraint that might be used during procedure (e.g., "I'm going to help you keep your hand still.") (see Chapter 102).
- Inform parents that they may choose to stay with their child during the procedure and that it is okay to leave while the procedure is being performed. If parents choose to stay with

the child during the procedure, it should be explained to them that their role is to be supportive to the child. Give the parents concrete things that they can do to provide support (e.g., read a pop-up book, hold the child's hand, sing songs, advocate for child if he or she needs a break, tell child how much longer). Instruct parent to inform nurse if he or she feels uncomfortable, lightheaded, dizzy, or ill. Provide seating for parent during the procedure if possible.

- Child may be NPO (nothing by mouth) before procedure, depending on the risk for aspiration.
- Assess the young child for self-comforting behaviors, or ask the family. Ask the older child, using developmentally appropriate terminology, what comforts him or her (e.g., "If you are scared, what helps you to not be scared?" "What helps you to calm down/feel less stressed?"). Encourage the family to promote the use of self-comforting behaviors. Provide the child and family with information about other nonpharmacologic pain relief measures, incorporating these measures during and after procedure (see Chapters 7 and 132).
- Discuss pharmacologic pain relief measures with healthcare prescriber (e.g., topical anesthetics, local anesthetics, conscious sedation) and prepare needed equipment.
- Check laboratory values before procedure, if ordered, and notify healthcare prescriber of results.
- Obtain consent if indicated (see Chapter 53).
- Ensure that all equipment, including emergency equipment, is the appropriate size and is functioning properly.
- Ensure appropriate place for procedure other than child's room whenever possible (e.g., treatment room) and that child is transported to this location in a safe and age-appropriate manner.
- Follow the Universal Protocol for Preventing Wrong Site, Wrong Procedure, and Wrong Person Surgery:
  - Use verification procedures, especially when the patient has different parents, before sedation if possible, and before going to surgery or the procedure room. A preoperative checklist helps ensure patient safety by providing complete information. Prevents surgery on wrong patient.
  - Check to see whether operative site has been marked with permanent marker. Prevents surgery on wrong site.

> **Alert!** *Although protocol calls for using a permanent marker to mark the correct operative site, do not follow this protocol for premature infants. Differences in skin structure make premature infants more vulnerable to toxic effects of the marker.*

  - Using a checklist, take "time out" before beginning the procedure where the whole team verifies that the patient, procedure, site, and implants/equipment are correct. Prevents surgery on wrong patient, wrong site, or with the wrong equipment.

PROCEDURE General Guidelines for Performing a Procedure

Steps	Rationale/Points of Emphasis
1. Perform hand hygiene. Don gloves as indicated (sterile/nonsterile) for the specific procedure.	Reduces transmission of microorganisms.
2. Premedicate as ordered.	Managing pain or discomfort in the child helps to decrease fear and aids the child in maintaining control.
3. Gather the necessary supplies. Obtain extra set of supplies if appropriate (e.g., extra needles, gloves, catheters).	Promotes efficient time management and provides an organized approach to the procedure. Avoids increasing child's and family's anxiety due to waiting or seeing equipment. Having an extra set avoids prolonging procedure.
4a. Escort family members to waiting area or have family members accompany child and healthcare personnel to location that where the procedure will be completed.	Family presence during invasive procedures has been demonstrated to be beneficial to the child and the participating family members. Families perceive themselves as active participants, caring for the child with the staff. Family presence has been viewed by families as a right, obligation, and natural event.
4b. When possible, assign a family facilitator to the family members.	The facilitator plays a role to initiate interventions to assist the family and provide emotional and psychosocial support.

Steps	Rationale/Points of Emphasis
5. Whenever possible, move child to treatment room to perform painful procedures.	If painful or traumatic procedures are performed in the child's room, he or she might be fearful during the entire hospital stay that people entering his or her room are there to perform a painful procedure. In the outpatient setting, procedures should be performed in a provided area, away from general viewing by other children and their families. Young children may be traumatized witnessing other children receive painful procedures.
6. Monitor child's status as indicated.	Some procedures or medications may have an adverse effect on the child's hemodynamic status.
7. Assist with or perform the procedure.	Completes required task.
8. Return child to room, as appropriate.	Provides child with a feeling of safety.
9. Discard biohazards and trash in appropriate containers.	Prevents injury or biohazard exposure to staff or others.
10. Remove gloves and perform hand hygiene.	Reduces transmission of microorganisms.
11. Monitor child's vital signs and condition as appropriate for procedure and child's status.	Ensures prompt detection of adverse effects resulting from procedure or medication, if administered.
12. Provide period of debriefing for family members both present and not present during the procedure. Address family's concerns, provide comfort measures, and address other psychosocial needs identified during the intervention.	Provides consistent and ongoing support to the family members.

CHILD AND FAMILY EVALUATION AND DOCUMENTATION

- Evaluate child's status as appropriate to procedure.
- Evaluate child's tolerance of procedure and child's and family's response to and coping with procedure.
- Document in medical record:
  - Time of procedure
  - Name of person performing procedure
  - Medication administered
  - Number of attempts at procedure
  - Type and size of supplies used
  - Presence of parents during procedure
  - Method of transportation, if transported
  - Hemodynamic monitoring, if performed
  - Child's response to and tolerance of procedure

COMMUNITY CARE

- Upon discharge, educate child and family regarding
  - Adverse symptoms that indicate complications associated with procedure (e.g., pain, bleeding, limited range of motion) or sedation (e.g., vomiting, changes in level of consciousness), if used
  - Activity limitations and length of time to limit activity
  - Use and dosage of medications, if ordered
  - Equipment, supplies, wound care as appropriate
- Instruct family to contact the healthcare provider if
  - Signs of complications appear
  - Child's pain cannot be managed

Unexpected Situation

- *The nurse from the pediatric intensive care unit has come to transport the adolescent to the unit to perform an intravenous cutdown procedure. Upon reviewing the chart, it is noted that there is no signed informed consent form present. The parents are not at the bedside. The adolescent is upset and states he or she did not know anything about this procedure being done:* Unless this is an emergency situation, the procedure may not proceed without parental informed consent and assent from the adolescent. Parents need to be contacted and asked to return to the hospital to discuss the procedure with the healthcare prescriber and the adolescent. The procedure cannot be completed until family preparation and informed consent has been completed.

Bibliography

Joint Commission on Accreditation of Healthcare Organizations (JCAHO). (2003). *The universal protocol for preventing wrong site, wrong procedure, and wrong person surgery*™. Retrieved October 1, 2006, from http://www.jointcommission.org/NR/rdonlyres/E3C600EB-043B-4E86-B04E-CA4A89AD5433/0/universal_protocol.pdf

Malviya, S., Voepel-Lewis, T., Tait, A. R., & Merkel, S. (2000). Sedation/analgesia for diagnostic and therapeutic procedures in children. *Journal of Perianesthesia Nursing, 15*, 415–422.

Meyers, T., Eichhorn, D., Guzzetta, C., et al. (2004). Family presence during invasive procedures and resuscitation. *Topics in Emergency Medicine, 26*(1), 61–73.

Ng, E., Taddio, A., & Ohlsson, A. (2003). Intravenous midazolam infusion for sedation of infants in the neonatal intensive care unit. *The Cochrane Database of Systematic Reviews*, (1), No. CD002052.

Stephens, B. K., Barkey, M. E., & Hall, H. R. (1999). Techniques to comfort children during stressful procedures. *Advances in Mind-Body Medicine*, *15*, 49–60.

Weisman, S. J., Bernstein, B., & Schechter, N. L. (1998). Consequences of inadequate analgesia during painful procedures in children. *Archives of Pediatrics & Adolescent Medicine*, *152*, 147–149.

C H A P T E R

99

Prostheses and Orthoses

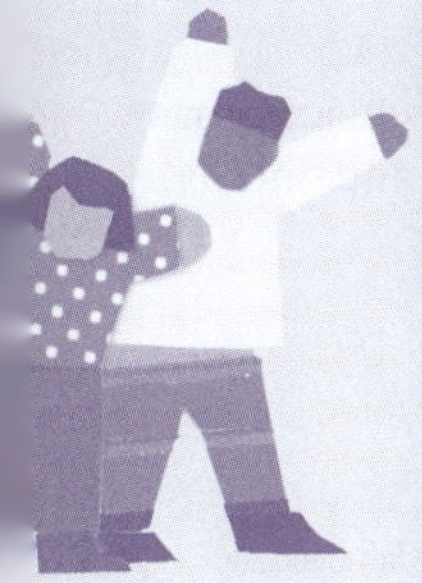

Clinical Guidelines

Prostheses

- Prosthesis is Greek for "an addition," such as an artificial limb or artificial eye.
- Management of the prosthesis while in the hospital should be completed by the registered nurse (RN) or licensed practical nurse (LPN) within the framework of orders by the healthcare prescriber. If the prosthesis is new, the physical therapy team will also be involved in the management of the prosthesis and establishing the break-in period procedure.
- The prosthesis is not worn at all times but needs to be available to the child at all times. Storage of the device should be in close proximity to the child to promote age-appropriate independence.
- All prostheses should have routine care and maintenance programs to ensure the proper function and long-term use of the device. A maintenance program includes the orthotist/prosthetist, the patient, and the family as well as the treating healthcare provider. The maintenance program includes
  - Daily care of devices such as cleaning and inspection
  - Weekly inspection for any defects, loose screws, weakened rivets, or nicks and scratches
  - Regular adjustment and service of devices that have mechanical components/moving parts or are subjected to load (such as an artificial knee and lower leg) to prevent damage and loss of use
- Routine care includes cleaning the plastic parts with antibacterial soap, rinsing thoroughly with cold water, and drying. The prosthesis should be air-dried because the plastics can be damaged by heat (i.e., do not dry with blow dryer).

Orthoses

- An orthotic or orthosis is a brace or a device that provides correction or support for weak or imbalanced muscles. The words *brace*, *splint*, and *orthotic* tend to be used interchangeably. Examples include leg braces, arm braces, spine braces, shoe inserts, shoe lifts, cranial molding helmets, and several other devices. These are typically used for a prolonged period of time. A splint, however, usually refers to a supportive device that is used for a shorter period of time, after injury or surgery.
- The uses of orthotics include stabilizing unstable joints, counteracting the force of a spastic muscle, protecting fragile bones, preventing progression of a deformity, and replacing the function of damaged or defective limb or anatomic structure. The orthosis cannot be used to correct a rigid-type deformity, such as a clubfoot.

- Orthoses are defined or described by the area of the body that they are treating. A common one used in children would be the ankle-foot orthosis (AFO).
- Management of the orthosis while in the hospital should be completed by the RN within the framework of orders by the healthcare prescriber. If the orthosis is new, the physical therapy or occupational therapy team will also be involved in the management of the orthotic and establishing the break-in period procedure.
- Orthoses as a rule are custom designed and custom fit for the child. Most orthoses/braces must be adjusted or revised every 6 months based on growth.
- All orthoses should have routine care and maintenance programs to ensure the proper function and long-term use of the device. A maintenance program includes the orthotist, the patient, and the family as well as the treating healthcare provider. The maintenance program includes
  - Daily care of the devices such as cleaning and inspection
  - Weekly inspection for any defects, loose screws, weakened rivets, or nicks and scratches
  - Regular adjustment and service of devices that have mechanical components/moving parts or are subjected to load (such as a leg brace) to prevent damage and loss of use
- Routine care includes cleaning the plastic parts with antibacterial soap, rinsing thoroughly with cold water, and drying. The orthotic device should be air-dried because the plastics can be damaged by heat (i.e., do not dry with blow dryer).

Equipment

- Prosthesis or orthosis
- Any special liners or skin protection garment

Child and Family Assessment and Preparation

- Evaluate child's and family's knowledge and understanding of the use of the orthosis or prosthesis if he or she is admitted with the device.
- Clarify with child and family when the child does not use the device and how they prefer to store the device. Identify a location that is safe and easily accessible for the storage of device during admission. This will ensure that the device does not become lost or damaged when not in use.
- If newly fitted with device, confirm that the family has a wearing/break-in schedule for the device. This will minimize problems with skin intolerance and avert such problems as excessive redness, chafing, and blisters.

Child and Family Evaluation and Documentation

- Document the following:
  - Type of orthotic/prosthetic device (e.g., bilateral AFO, Milwaukee brace, Boston brace, lumbar-sacral orthosis [LSO], wrist-hand orthosis [WHO], knee-ankle foot orthosis [KAFO], or Aspen cervical orthosis [neck orthosis])
  - Note if the device is solid, articulating, or dynamic
  - Location of the device, such as the extremity, back, neck, or, in the case of a prosthesis, the limb or organ that is the prosthetic device

Community Care

- Upon discharge, educate child and family regarding:
  - Skin care and monitoring for skin breakdown
  - Care of the orthosis or prosthetic should be done in accordance with manufacturer guidelines or clinical protocol; include contact name and number of orthotist or prosthetist for questions and concerns regarding malfunctions
- Assist the family in preparing the child's peers, teacher, and school in what to anticipate with the child's return to school with an orthosis or prosthesis if it is obvious. This may include a 504 accommodation from the school to make modifications to the school environment to allow the child to participate fully in his or her school program.
- Instruct the family to call the healthcare provider if
  - Child develops area of skin breakdown as evidenced by redness, sores, or blisters
  - Child loses appliance and it needs to be replaced; in most cases a new set of measurements and molds need to be taken to ensure correct fitting

Unexpected Situation

- *When assisting child to remove his or her prosthetic device, the skin under the device is noted to be red and has areas where blisters have developed:* Assess the skin for breakdown. Document findings and notify the healthcare prescriber. The extent of the skin break-down will determine skin care to be provided. Extensive skin breakdown may require consultation of a skin care specialist and a period of time in which the prosthetic device is not applied. Complete normal cleaning and storage of the prosthetic device, with special attention given to the area of the device in contact with the skin to decrease transmission of microorganisms from the area of the skin breakdown.

Bibliography

Armstrong, P. F. (2002). Orthotics, braces, and splints. In L. T. Staheli (Ed.), *Pediatric orthopaedic secrets* (2nd ed., pp. 75–79). Philadelphia: Hanley & Belfus, Inc.

Lusardi, M., & Nielsen, C. (2000). *Orthotics and prosthetics in rehabilitation.* Boston, MA: Butterworth-Heinemann.

Patel, D. R., & Greydanus, D. E. (2002). The pediatric athlete with disabilities. *Pediatric Clinics of North America, 49,* 803–827.

Wenger, D. R., & Mercer, R. (1993). *The art and practice of children's orthopaedics.* New York: Raven Press.

CHAPTER 100

Pulse Oximetry

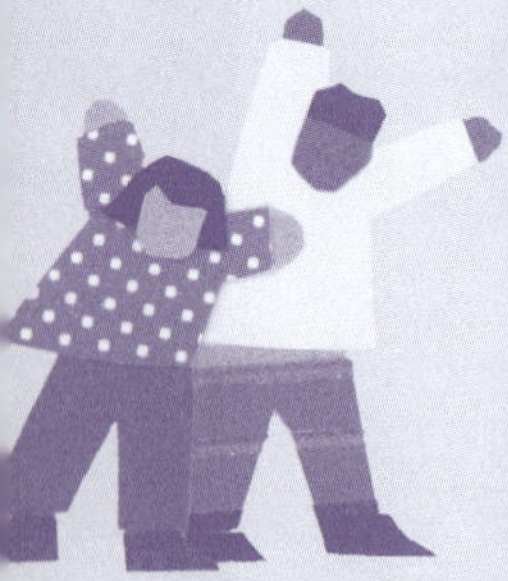

Clinical Guidelines

- Pulse oximetry may be performed by a respiratory therapist (RT) or registered nurse (RN) per healthcare prescriber's orders or as an acute emergent evaluation of child's status without a direct healthcare prescriber's order. A pulse oximetry sensor may be placed on the child by a licensed practical nurse (LPN) or unlicensed assistant personnel (UAP) with the data given to the licensed personnel for assessment.
- Child receives pulse oximetry monitoring as per healthcare prescriber's order, which specifies frequency (continuous or spot check). Orders may be written as guidelines to adjust oxygen administration based on pulse oximetry saturation level.
- Acceptable ranges for the child's saturation levels are prescribed by the healthcare provider or per unit protocol. Parameters are based on the child's underlying clinical condition and past medical history. Normal saturation levels for healthy children are considered to range between 97% and 99%.
- All patients receiving continuous pulse oximetry are assessed by an RT or RN every 2 hours or more frequently as indicated by the child's status. Assessment should include respiratory status, pulse oximetry reading, skin integrity at the site, circulation distal to the sensor site, and knowledge of the child's baseline diagnosis and status.
- All pulse oximetry spot checks are performed and evaluated by an RT or an RN.
- Pulse oximetry is used when a child is undergoing a procedure that requires sedation and when observation may be difficult.
- All children on pulse oximetry will have appropriately sized oxygen delivery devices readily available (e.g., bag-mask, oxygen tubing, oxygen source).

Equipment

- Pulse oximeter saturation monitor
- Pulse oximeter probe, either disposable or nondisposable, and age and size appropriate
- Tape
- Bedside oxygen delivery equipment, including oxygen source, flowmeter and bag-mask (size appropriate)

Child and Family Assessment and Preparation

- Identify the child and explain the purpose of the equipment to the child and parent based on the child's developmental level of understanding. Explain the child's and parents' role in assisting maintenance of proper placement of the sensor.

CHART 100-1 VARIABLES IMPACTING PULSE OXIMETRY READINGS

No Readings or False Readings Too Low

Sensor not secured properly to skin

Poor positioning

Motion artifact

Sensor pulse rate and apical pulse rate that do not correspond

Incorrect positioning of the sensor (not at level of the heart)

Nail polish

False nails

Recent use of intravenous dyes

Bright overhead lights (e.g., those used during surgery or during a procedure)

Shivering

Hyperbilirubinemia

Peripheral vasoconstriction

Diaphoresis

Underperfusion and cardiac arrest, which can cause hypovolemia, hypotension, and hypothermia

False Readings Too High

Child exposed to smoke inhalation or carbon monoxide poisoning

Anemia

- Assess pertinent history, focusing on events that may have precipitated respiratory distress. Also assess for recent intravascular use of lipids or dyes, which could interfere with the accuracy of pulse oximetry readings.
- Assess physical findings, including respiratory rate and effort, use of accessory muscles, shape of chest, position of child (i.e., sitting, standing), breath sounds, perfusion, vital signs, and presence and degree of restlessness and anxiety. Also check for an elevated bilirubin level, if available, which may falsely lower oxygen saturation readings.
- Ensure that child's fingernail beds are clean and free of nail polish to decrease interference in providing accurate oximetry readings (Chart 100-1).

PROCEDURE Performing Pulse Oximetry

Steps	Rationale/Points of Emphasis
1. Perform hand hygiene.	Reduces transmission of microorganisms.
2. Gather the necessary equipment and supplies. Plug pulse oximeter into wall outlet.	Promotes efficient time management and provides an organized approach to the procedure. Facilitates initiating the monitoring with minimal delays.
3. Select the appropriate sensor and attach the cable to the pulse oximeter unit.	Base sensor selection on child's age, size, and preferred site to be used.
4. Attach sensor to the selected site with the light source on one side of the tissue pad and the sensor on the other side, facing each other. For optimal performance, keep the sensor site at the level of the heart. ***Alert!*** *Research has indicated that during neonatal resuscitation efforts, applying the sensor to the infant before connecting to the oximeter resulted in quickest acquisition of accurate heart rate.*	Allows measurement of the light transmitted through a pulsating arterial vascular bed to calculate the percentage of hemoglobin saturated with oxygen (Sao_2). Avoid placing the sensor over thick skin, nail polish, false nails, extremities that are moved excessively by the child, and areas where perfusion is known to be poor (see Chart 100-1). These sites are least restrictive and easiest to maintain in infants. • In neonates, suggested sites include ▪ Sole of the foot below the toes, with the cable extending toward the heel ▪ Palm of the hand ▪ Wrist ▪ Forehead • In infants, suggested sites include ▪ Great toe, with the cable extending toward the heel (Figure 100-1) ▪ Ball of foot below the toes

Continued

Steps	Rationale/Points of Emphasis

- Palm of the hand
- Wrist
- Forehead (Figure 100-2)

- In children, suggested sites include
  - Index finger (preferred location), with the light source centered on the fingertip (Figure 100-3)
  - Forehead

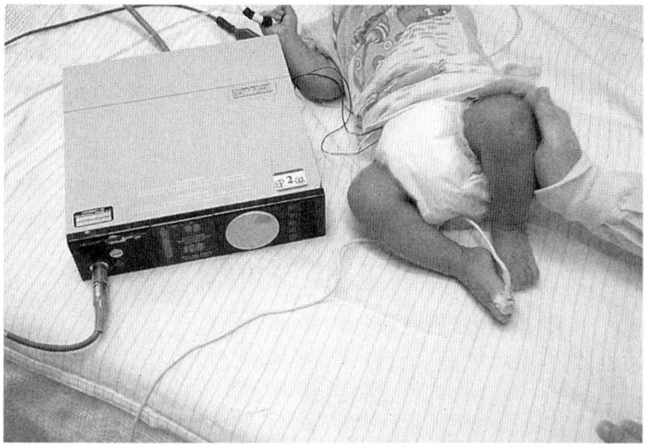

FIGURE 100-1
Position the sensor on the great toe with the light source on one side and the sensor on the other side, facing each other. The cable should extend toward the heel.

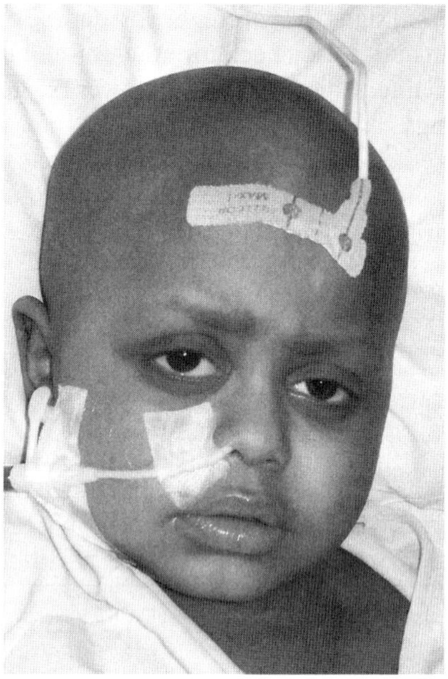

FIGURE 100-2
Placement of the sensor on the forehead is effective because blood supply to the forehead precludes minimal vasoactivity.

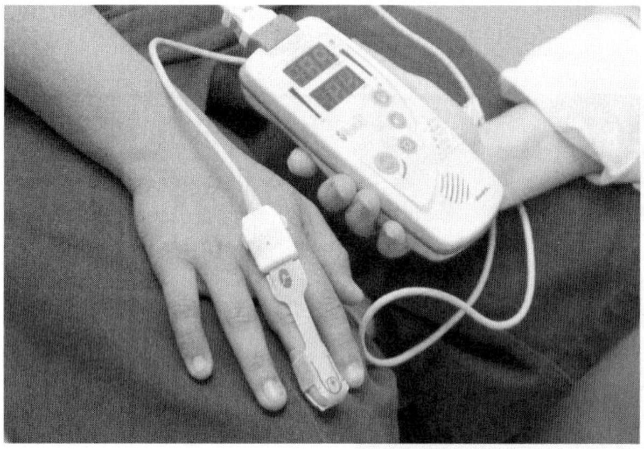

FIGURE 100-3
When using the finger, position the sensor with the light source centered on the fingertip.

Steps	Rationale/Points of Emphasis
5. Tape sensor in place, loosely but securely.	Failure to position and to secure properly may cause motion artifact and thus incorrect Sa_{O_2} measurement. Taping too tightly may impede circulation, causing an incorrect reading and potential damage to the child's fragile skin.
6. Cover sensor site with an opaque material.	Excessive light, such as from phototherapy, direct sunlight, or excessive ambient lighting, can interfere with the sensor's ability to produce an accurate reading.
7. Turn pulse oximeter on and verify that child's apical pulse rate corresponds to the pulse rate shown on the monitor. If machine has a visual waveform display or other bar graph indicator to indicate that an accurate signal is being received, ensure that the reading is present at the highest level and that the waveform shows a good trace.	Lack of correlation between child's actual pulse rate and pulse rate shown on the monitor indicates the unreliability of the Sa_{O_2} findings. The reliability of the Sa_{O_2} findings will be greater if the waveform display is reading at a high, as opposed to a low, level.

Steps	Rationale/Points of Emphasis
8a. Alarm limits should be determined in conjunction with the healthcare prescriber and take into consideration the child's age, underlying condition, and past history of normal parameters for that child.	When alarms are set correctly, the oximeter can detect hypoxemia before the child becomes cyanotic and the nurse can be alerted to a downward trend and deterioration in the child's status. Although oxygen saturation of 95% and 96% are adequate (i.e., not requiring acute oxygen therapy), these values are associated with higher rates of airway pulmonary or cardiovascular system involvement and should be considered potentially abnormal. Oxygen saturation of 97% is on the border of normal. Normal saturations can occur with airway pulmonary or cardiovascular system involvement or respiratory infectious conditions, but saturation less than 97% is associated with a higher risk of an airway pulmonary or cardiovascular system involvement or respiratory infectious conditions in children (Mau, Yamasato, & Yamamoto, 2005).
8b. Set alarm limits as follows and refer to manufacturer's instructions. **Alert!** *Once alarm limits are set, these will default to the manufacturer's settings for the monitor when the monitor is switched off and then on again. Each time the monitor is turned on, the alarm limits must be rechecked.*	
8c. Set sensitivity by pushing high-rate and low-rate buttons simultaneously. Turn wheel while depressing buttons to set desired sensitivity. 8d. Set low-saturation limit and low-pulse alarm by simultaneously pushing each button and turning the wheel to the predetermined numeric value as defined by healthcare prescriber or hospital policy.	Possible settings are 1, 2, and 3, with 3 being the least sensitive to artifact and nonsensitive to pulse. Set low-saturation alarm at 92% in most cases. This allows for early intervention and treatment if oxygen is to be delivered once a 90% saturation level is observed. Low-pulse alarms are often set as follows, based on child's age: • <1 month—80 beats/min • 1–3 months—70 beats/min • >3 months—60 beats/min **caREminder** *The pitch of the audible pulse signal falls with reducing values of saturation.*
9. Determine with the healthcare prescriber when oxygen should be administered or increased based on Sao_2 values and the child's clinical presentation.	Oxygen should be given if the Sao_2 values are 90% or below. This may vary depending on the child's underlying medical condition (e.g., cardiac anomaly). **Alert!** *Pulse oximetry saturation for newborns is lower at higher altitudes than at sea level.*
10. Dispose of equipment and waste in appropriate receptacle. Perform hand hygiene.	Standard precautions. Reduces transmission of microorganisms.
11. When responding to alarms, assess for the following: • Respiratory distress, failure, or insufficiency (note child's color, respiratory effort, and rate) • Pulse rate on the oximeter corresponds with child's pulse rate monitor or apical heart rate • Oxygen equipment is functioning properly • Good adhesion of the sensor to the skin site • Light source on the probe is functioning, and oximetry cables are properly connected • Opaque cover is in place over the sensor • Limb being used is not being moved excessively • Sensor is at the level of the heart • Hypothermia • Hypotension • Vasoconstriction • Diaphoresis	Pulse oximetry is used as an early detector of hypoxemia in children. Children have lower pulmonary reserves than adults and can decompensate more quickly if oxygen levels are not stabilized. All the assessments indicated here, with the exception of respiratory failure or insufficiency (which warrants immediate intervention by, and notification of, the healthcare prescriber), can produce inaccurate readings and false alarms and need to be corrected once discovered. **caREminder** *Readings from the oximeter should always be interpreted in association with the child's clinical condition. Strong lighting such as phototherapy lights will interfere with accurate readings.*
12. Rotate the sensor site a minimum of once every 2 hours or as unit-specific criteria specifies.	Decreases the risk for tissue breakdown.

CHILD AND FAMILY EVALUATION AND DOCUMENTATION

- Falling percentiles in oximetry readings should be brought to the attention of the healthcare prescriber as soon as possible.
- Document the following:
  - Respiratory status
  - Pulse oximeter reading
  - Skin integrity at the site
  - Circulation distal to the sensor site
- If alarm sounds, document the reason for the alarm and the intervention required to alleviate the problem. Note the condition of the child both at the time of the alarm and after any interventions to stabilize the child's status.

COMMUNITY CARE

- If pulse oximetry is to continue at home, instruct the family on
  - Use of the equipment
  - How to troubleshoot problems
  - Signs of problems with oxygenation or complications to monitor and report
- Instruct the family to contact the healthcare provider if
  - Child develops signs of fever or respiratory distress
  - Child's oxygen saturation levels consistently fall below designated parameters
  - Equipment malfunctions

Unexpected Situation

- *Infant's pulse oximeter alarms frequently:* First assess child to determine whether there is a change in the respiratory status. If none is noted, this could be an equipment malfunction. Rotate the site of the sensor. A new sensor may be needed. Check that alarm limits are set correctly. If the assessment verifies there is a change in child's respiratory status (e.g., apneic, irregular respirations, change in skin color), observe child to note whether regular respirations resume and oxygen saturation levels increase. If child remains apneic, stimulate the child and administer oxygen via face mask. Implement emergency resuscitation procedures as needed. Notify healthcare prescriber of child's altered respiratory status.

Bibliography

Bakr, A., & Habib, H. (2005). Normal values of pulse oximetry in newborns at high altitude. *Journal of Tropical Pediatrics, 51*(3), 170–173.

Cardiopulmonary Diagnostics Guidelines Committee. (1991). AARC clinical practice guideline: Pulse oximetry. *Respiratory Care, 36*, 1406–1409.

Considine, J. (2005). The reliability of clinical indicators of oxygenation: A literature review. *Contemporary Nurse: A Journal for the Australian Nursing Profession, 18*(3), 258–267.

Mau, M., Yamasato, K., & Yamamoto, L. (2005). Normal oxygen saturation values in pediatric patients. *Hawaii Medical Journal, 64*(2), 42, 44–45.

O'Donnell, C., Kamlin, C., Davis, P., & Morley, C. (2005). Obtaining pulse oximetry data in neonates: A randomized crossover study of sensor application techniques. *Archives of Disease in Childhood, 90*(1), F84–F85.

Pulse Oximetry Forum, Child Health Corporation of America. (2002). Recommendations on best practices in pediatric pulse oximetry. *AARC Times, 24*(4), 36–44.

Salyer, J. (2003). Neonatal and pediatric pulse oximetry. *Respiratory Care, 48*(4), 386–398.

Tanen, D., & Trocinski, D. (2002). The use of pulse oximetry to exclude pneumonia in children. *American Journal of Emergency Medicine, 20*, 521–523.

Urguhart, C., & Bell, G. (2005). Ear probe pulse oximeters and neonates. *Anaesthesia, 60*(3), 294.

CHAPTER

101

Range-of-Motion Exercises

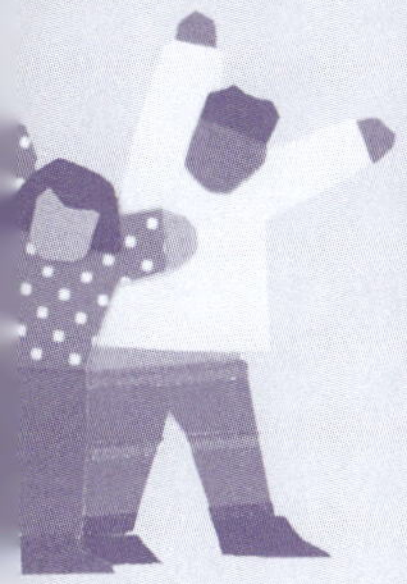

Clinical Guidelines

- A registered nurse (RN), licensed practical nurse (LPN), physical therapist (PT), or physical therapy technician may complete range-of-motion (ROM) exercises.
- ROM exercises are used when all or some of the normal physical activities are not able to be completed due to the physical condition of the child. Attention is given to the joint not being used through provision of active or passive ROM exercises. Active ROM exercises are those that the patient does for himself or herself. Passive ROM exercises are those performed by the family member or the healthcare provider without participation by the child.
- ROM exercises are completed twice a day, with three to five repetitions of each movement unless otherwise prescribed by the physical therapist.
- ROM exercises are completed as appropriate to the child's physical condition (Table 101-1 and Figures 101-1 to 101-11).

Equipment

- Nonsterile gloves
- Bed with firm mattress or padded table
- Blanket for privacy

Child and Family Assessment and Preparation

- Review the child's history for contraindications to ROM exercises, determining limitations of joint movement and impact on function. In cases of joint inflammation, dislocation, or fracture, ROM exercises may be contraindicated.
- Review child's chart to determine whether a specific ROM exercise plan has been provided in the interdisciplinary patient orders.
- Explain to the child and family the purpose and the plan of ROM exercises.
- Initiate pain control measures if needed 30 minutes before beginning ROM exercises.
- Provide antispasmodic medications, if ordered, 30 minutes before beginning ROM exercises.

caREminder

Children with conditions such as cerebral palsy or hemiplegia will be more comfortable during ROM activities when given muscle relaxants before the procedure.

TABLE 101-1

Range of Motion Terminology

Movement	Definition	Use
Circumduction	Movement of the joint in a full circle	Used in movement of the shoulder
Hyperextension	Movement of the joint in the direction of extension beyond a straight line	Used in movement of the arms, legs, hands, and wrists
Flexion	The bending of the joint in which the two adjacent parts move toward each other, thus reducing the angle of the joint between two parts. Decreasing the angle between two bones	Used in the shoulder, elbow, knee, and finger joints
Extension	Movement increasing angle between two adjoining bones	Used in the shoulder, elbow, knee, and finger joints
Internal rotation	Turning away from the midline	Used in movement of the head from side to side
Abduction	Movement away from the midline of the body	Used in movement of the legs, arms, and fingers
Adduction	Movement toward the midline of the body	Used in movement of extremities; legs, arms, and fingers
Pronation	Turning the forearm so that the palmar surface of the hand is facing downward	Used in movement of the hand and wrist
Supination	Turning the forearm so that the palmar surface of the hand is facing upward	Used in movement of the hand and wrist
Deviation	Abduction or adduction of the wrist	Used in movement of the wrist
Opposition	Placement of the palmar surface of the thumb so that it touches the base of the fingers	Used in movement of the hand

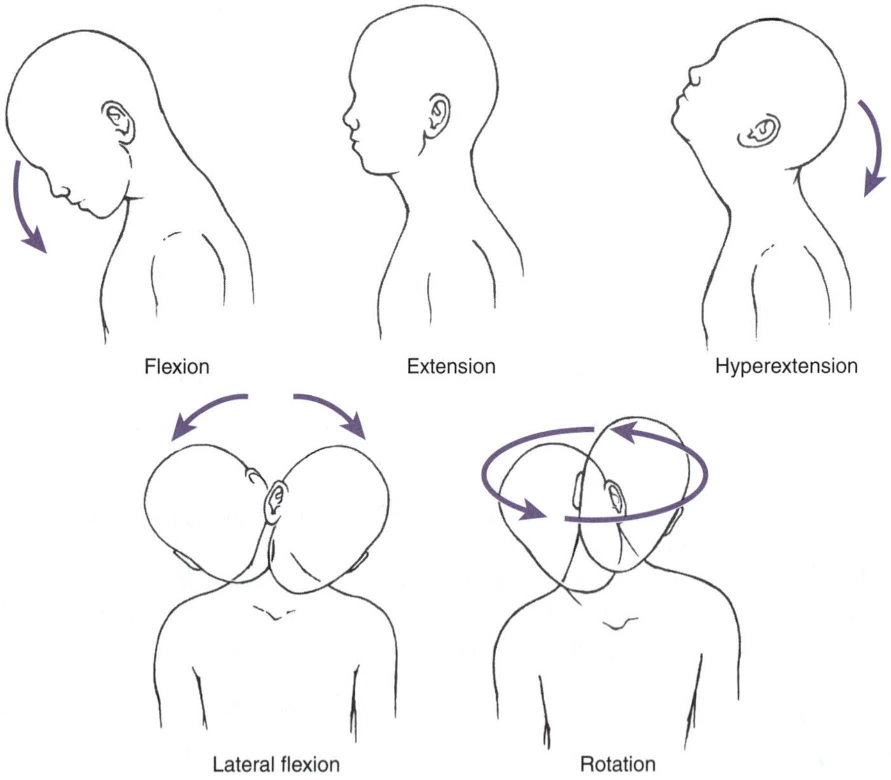

FIGURE 101-1
During neck range-of-motion exercises, support the child's head while tilting the head up and down and moving the head from side to side.

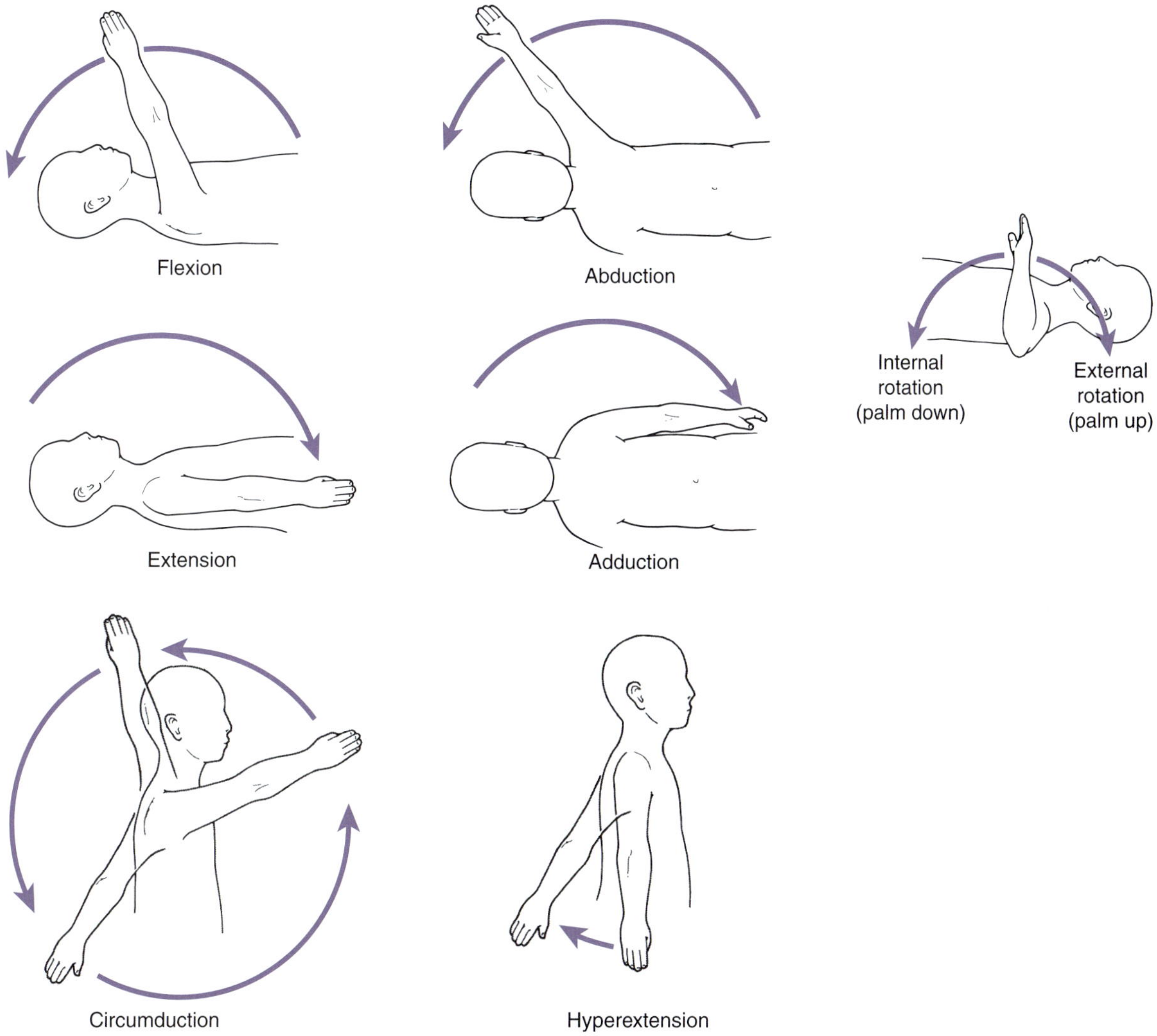

FIGURE 101-2
During shoulder range-of-motion exercises, grasp child's arm at the elbow and use your other hand to support the patient's shoulder.

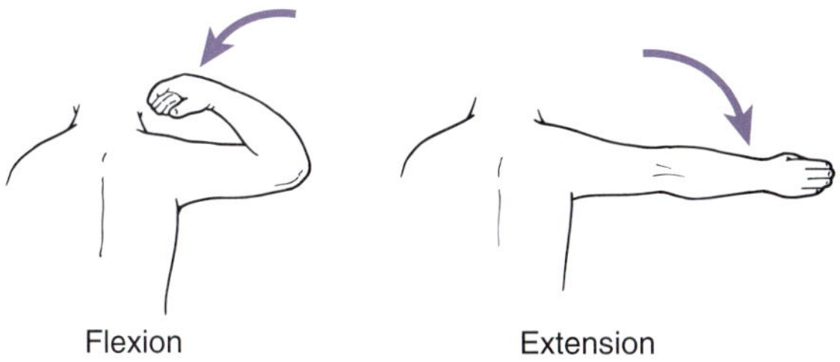

FIGURE 101-3
During elbow ROM exercises, grasp child's arm at the elbow and use your other hand to support the patient's wrist and hand.

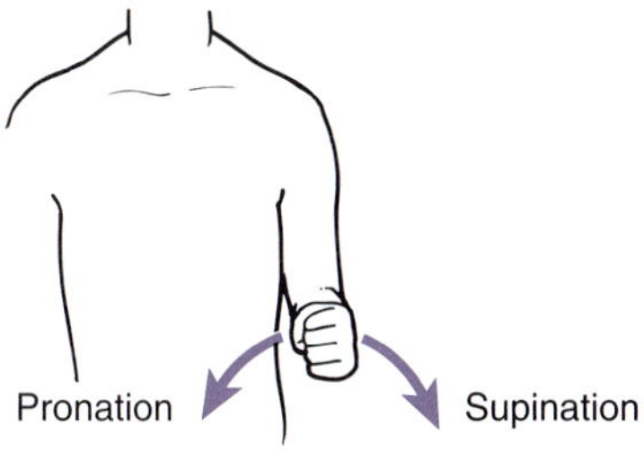

FIGURE 101-4
During forearm ROM exercises, grasp the child at elbow with one hand and grasp child's hand with your other hand.

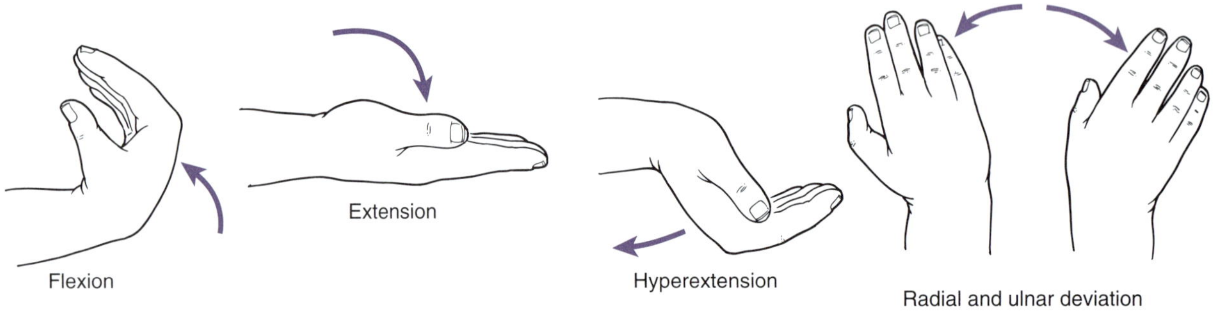

FIGURE 101-5
During wrist ROM exercises, grasp the child's forearm just above the wrist with one hand and use the other hand to grasp child's hand.

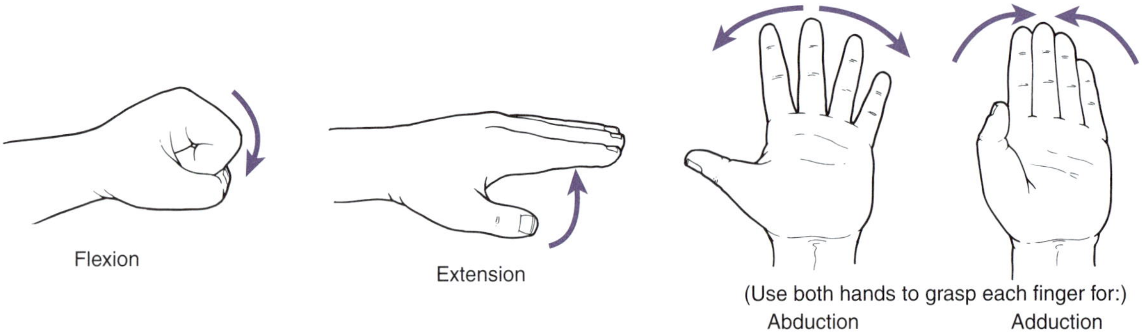

FIGURE 101-6
During finger ROM exercises, support the child's wrist with one hand and use the fingers of your other hand. Flex fingers with wrist extended and extend fingers with wrist flexed.

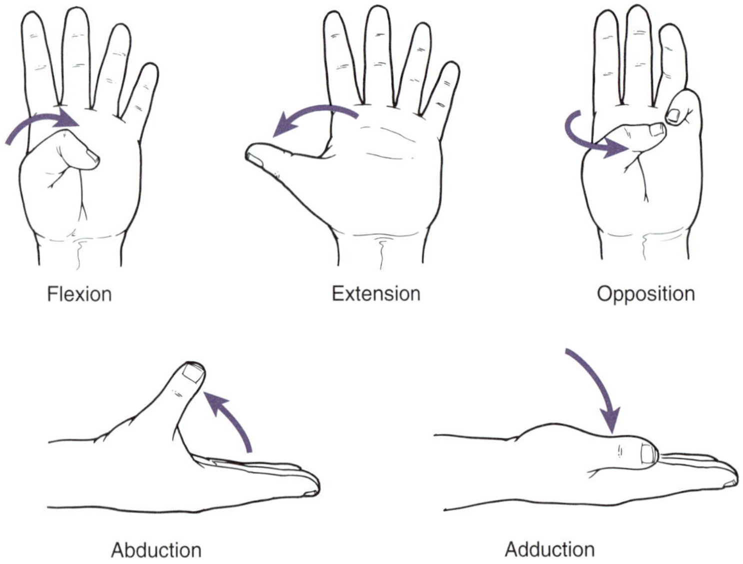

FIGURE 101-7
During thumb ROM exercises, support child's hand and fingers with one hand and grasp his or her thumb with the other hand.

- Provide for privacy.
- Schedule ROM activities to coincide with routine care. An ideal time to do the exercise is during morning care or bath time. Include child and family in planning for ROM activities (e.g., when and where to perform).
- Dress child in nonrestrictive loose-fitting clothing.
- Assess vital signs to provide a baseline for comparison if changes occur.
- Determine the baseline activity and condition for the child.
- Observe the equality of movement of each joint. The movement of the joints should be equal bilaterally.
- Note the condition of the joint. The joint should be free of pain, spastic movement, deformity, and crepitation. There should be no limitation of movement.

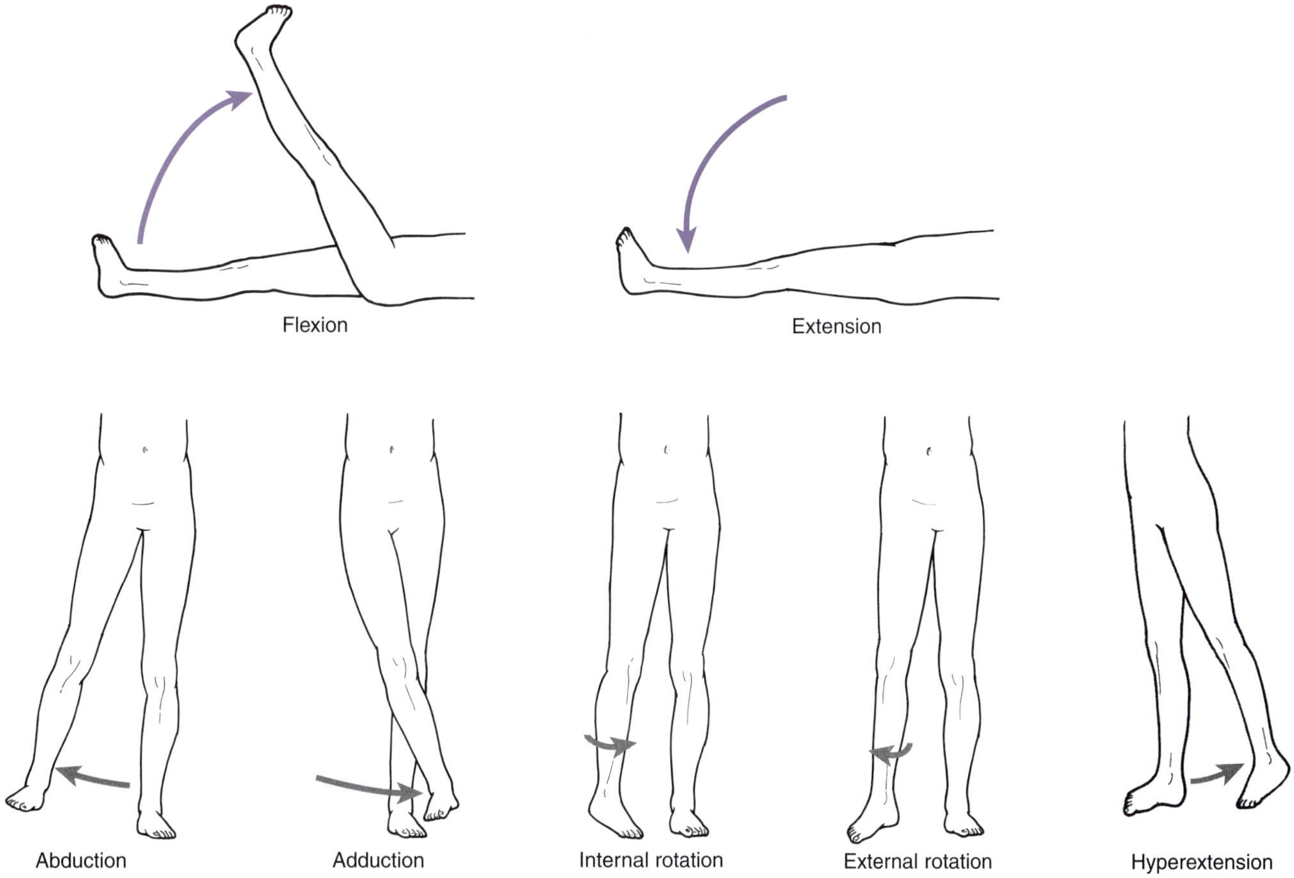

FIGURE 101-8
During hip ROM exercises, support child's leg by placing his or her ankle in one hand and holding his or her knee in extension with your other hand.

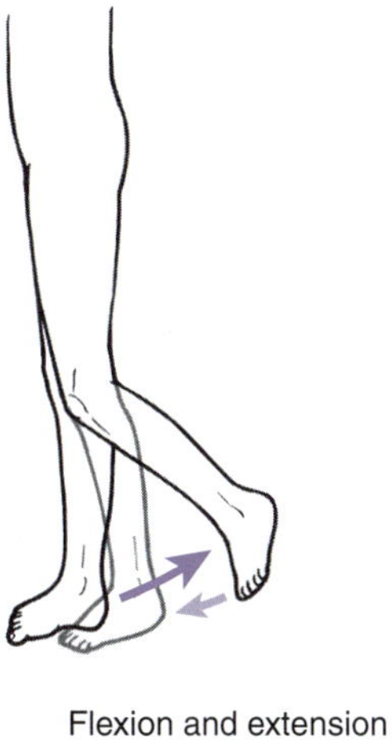

FIGURE 101-9
During knee ROM exercises, flex child's hip approximately 90 degrees and support his or her leg by placing one hand just above the knee and grasping the ankle with the other hand.

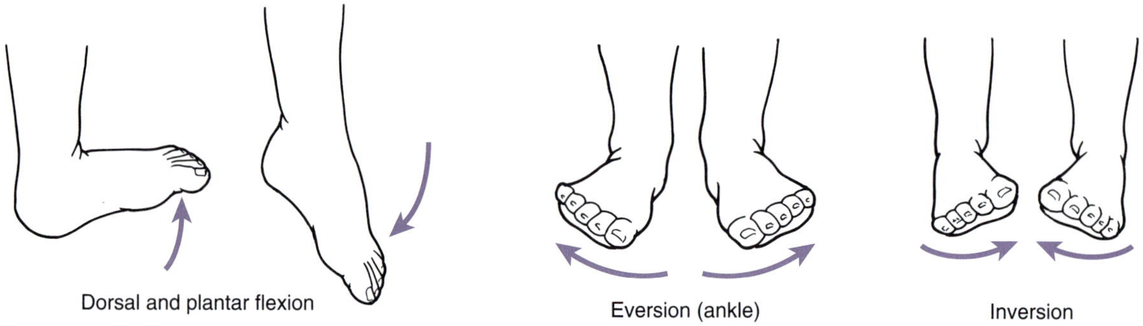

FIGURE 101-10
During ankle ROM exercises, with child's leg resting on the bed, place one hand on his or her knee to keep it from flexing. Grasp the heel in the palm of your other hand with the sole of his or her foot resting against your forearm.

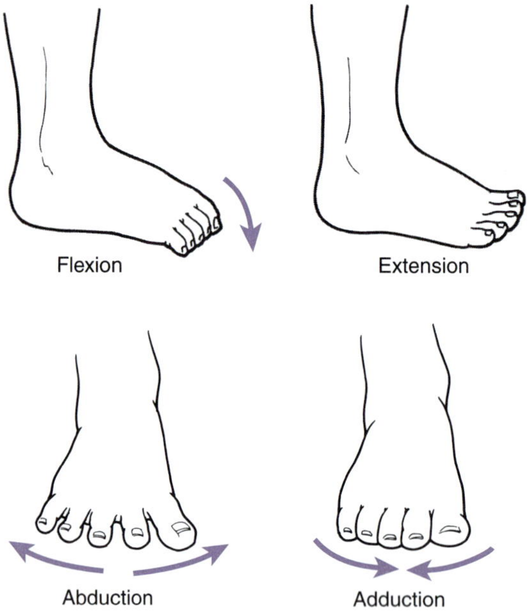

FIGURE 101-11
During toe ROM exercises, hold patient's foot with one hand and use the other hand.

PROCEDURE Performing Range-of-Motion Exercises

Steps	Rationale/Points of Emphasis
1. Raise bed or padded table to a comfortable working level for the practitioner.	Promotes proper body mechanics.
2. Perform hand hygiene, and don sterile gloves if contact with body fluids is possible.	Reduces transmission of microorganisms and prevents direct contact with body fluids.
3. Position child in a supine position on bed or padded table.	Allows for proper range of motion of body parts.
4. Cover the child with a blanket, exposing only the extremity involved in each specific exercise.	Promotes privacy. Keeps the child warm.
5a. Conduct appropriate exercises along the cephalocaudal axis, first on one side of the body and then on the other side (see Figures 101-1 to 101-11).	Promotes efficient use of energy.

Steps	Rationale/Points of Emphasis
5b. Each exercise should be performed three to five times in a slow, smooth, even movement.	Muscle contractions need to be held for 6 to 10 seconds and to be repeated three to five times to be effective.
5c. Support the dependent extremity while putting an immobilized joint through ROM exercises.	Provides for optimal comfort while performing the exercise.
6. If muscle spasm occurs, decrease the pressure slightly and keep the joint in a functional position until spasm eases.	If the joint is moved past the point of resistance, injury may occur.
7. If the child exhibits pain or discomfort, discontinue exercise.	Moving the joint to a point of pain or discomfort may cause injury to the joint.
8. Observe the child for respiratory or cardiac distress during the procedure.	ROM exercises increase energy use of the body and may cause stress on other systems.
9. Provide child with positive reinforcement for performing ROM exercises.	Positive reinforcement encourages willingness of the child to participate in these ongoing activities. Younger child may benefit from the use of a sticker or star chart.
10. Return bed or padded table to low position. If child was moved from own bed, assist child back to his or her room and return the child to a comfortable and safe position in his or her bed.	Promotes safety of child.
11. Remove gloves, if donned, and perform hand hygiene.	Reduces transmission of microorganisms.

CHILD AND FAMILY EVALUATION AND DOCUMENTATION

- Evaluate child's response to ROM activities, noting any complaints of pain during the activities.
- Document the following:
  - Vital signs before the procedure
  - Pain control measures initiated before, during, or after the procedure
  - ROM exercises performed
  - Assessment of joint mobility before and after activities performed, noting if movements were bilaterally equal and able to move to full extent
  - Child's response to ROM activities
  - Presence of pain or spasms during ROM activities
  - Parent teaching about completing ROM activities
  - Competency of parent or family member in providing ROM exercises

COMMUNITY CARE

- Refer to physical therapy services as indicated.
- Provide parents with instruction regarding how to provide passive-assisted or active ROM exercises at home if warranted.
- Assist family to develop a schedule for active ROM exercises.
- Instruct the family to contact the healthcare provider if
  - Child complains of acute pain during exercises
  - Child's physical limitations worsen

Unexpected Situations

- *While performing ROM exercises on the child's arm, child complains of sharp pain in that extremity:* Stop the ROM exercises. Further evaluate the pain. ROM exercises should not be painful. Joints are moved until there is resistance; however, sharp pain should not be present. Notify the healthcare prescriber of the child's pain to further determine whether the exercise plan should be revised.
- *During ROM exercises, child falls asleep:* Stop the exercises and allow child to rest. Reschedule the activity for a time when child is more alert.

Bibliography

Cadenhead, S., McEwen, I., & Thompson, D. (2002). Effect of passive range of motion exercises on lower-extremity goniometric measurements of adults with cerebral palsy: A single-subject design. *Physical Therapy, 82*(7), 658–669.

Dawe, D., & Curran-Smith, J. (1994). Going through the motions: Range of motion exercises. *Canadian Nurse, 90*(1), 31–33.

Oagley, C. (1992). Basic ROM exercises for forearm and wrist. *Patient Care, 26*(4), 104.

Pelland, L., Brosseau, L., Wells, G., et al. (2004). Efficacy of strengthening exercises for osteoarthritis (part I): A meta-analysis. *Physical Therapy Reviews, 9*(2), 77–108.

Sullivan, P., & Markos, P. (1993). *Clinical procedures in therapeutic exercise.* Norwalk, CT: Appleton & Lange.

CHAPTER

102

Restraint and Seclusion

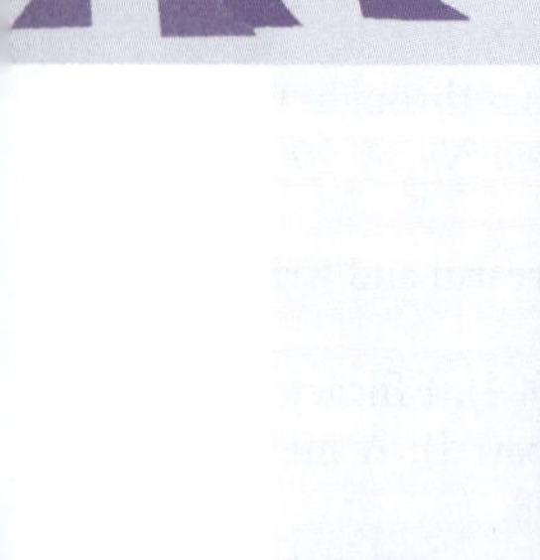

Clinical Guidelines

- A restraint or seclusion is only applied under the provision of a healthcare prescriber (physician or licensed independent practitioner [LIP]). The order includes reason for restraint, type of restraint to be used, and length of time the restraint may be in place.
- If the child's behavior presents a clear threat to self or others, the child may be placed in restraint at the discretion of the registered nurse (RN). As soon as possible but no longer than 1 hour after initiation of restraint or seclusion, the healthcare prescriber must be notified, and a verbal or written order must be obtained (Table 102-1). See Chapter 103 for guidelines regarding safety measures.
- Licensed practical nurses (LPNs) and unlicensed assistive personnel (UAP) may apply restraints and monitor patients who are restrained under the direction of the RN. Personnel using restraints have been instructed and demonstrate competence in using alternatives to restraints, correct application of the restraints, monitoring of the child while restrained, and recognizing when emergent healthcare prescriber referral is needed.
- A restraint is defined as any physical or chemical mechanism used to restrict a child's movement or physical activity. Restraint is used to maximize patient safety and prevent potential injury. The only indications for the use of restraint and seclusion are to prevent dangerous behavior to self/others or to prevent complete disruption of the child's treatment program.
- Physical restraints include, but are not limited to, elbow restraints, jacket restraints, and limb restraints such as No-No arm wraps.
- Chemical restraints include, but are not limited to, psychotropic medications, tranquilizers, and hypnotics.
- Children with any of the following contraindications should not normally be sedated with chemical restraints:
  - Abnormal airway (including large tonsils and anatomic abnormalities of upper or lower airway)
  - Raised intracranial pressure
  - Depressed conscious level
  - History of sleep apnea
  - Respiratory failure
  - Cardiac failure
  - Neuromuscular disease
  - Bowel obstruction
  - Active respiratory tract infection
  - Known allergy to sedative drug/previous adverse reaction
  - Child too distressed despite adequate preparation
  - Older children with severe behavioral problems
  - Informed refusal by the parent/guardian/child

TABLE 102-1

Restraint Orders

	Type of Restraint	Justification [Based on Child's Behavior]	Time Limits for Restraint Order	Licensed Independent Practitioner Evaluation
Medical-surgical restraint	Mummy restraint Elbow restraint Arm boards Protection of surgical and treatment sites Jacket restraint Orthopedic appliances Tabletop chairs Helmets Postural support devices	Limitation of mobility related to medical, diagnostic, or surgical procedures and related postprocedures care practices Adaptive support based on patient need Use of side rails and safety belts as routine protective care, not restraint	No PRNs Not to exceed 24 hours	In person, every 24 hours
Behavioral restraint	Elbow restraint Jacket restraint Leather restraint Seclusion	Climbing out of bed Pulling at tubes or lines Combative Aggressive/assaultive behavior resulting in danger to self or others	No PRNs Not to exceed • 4 hours: 18 years of age and older • 2 hours, 9–17 years of age • 1 hour, younger than 9 years of age	In person, within 1 hour of restraint initiation Ongoing evaluation in person • Every 8 hours, 18 years of age and older • Every 4 hours, 17 years of age and younger

- Seclusion is defined as the involuntary confinement of a person in a room or an area where he or she is physically prevented from leaving.
- Restraint and seclusion standards do not apply to limitation of mobility related to medical, diagnostic, or surgical procedures and related postprocedure care practices (e.g., positioning during procedures, intravenous [IV] armboards, protection of surgical and treatment sites) and adaptive support based on patient need (e.g., orthopedic appliances, tabletop chairs).
- Restraints and seclusion should not be used as punishment or for the convenience of the program.
- Children should never be left alone while in behavioral restraint or while secluded.
- The use of side rails, safety belts, tabletop extensions, protective nets, helmets, and postural support devices used to promote good body alignment are not restraints.
- The standard for restraints and seclusion does not apply when a staff member physically redirects or holds a child, without the child's permission, for 30 minutes or less.
- Verbal and written orders for restraint and seclusion are limited to
  - 4 hours for patients 18 years of age and older
  - 2 hours for children 9 to 17 years of age
  - 1 hour for children younger than 9 years of age
- Healthcare prescriber orders and assessments are required to continue restraint beyond 24 hours.
- Seclusion or restraints should not be ordered on a PRN basis.
- Reevaluation of the need for restraints or seclusion of the child takes place every
  - 4 hours for patients 18 years of age and older
  - 2 hours for children 9 to 17 years of age
  - 1 hour for children younger than 9 years of age
- All pediatric patients in seclusion or restraints must be monitored continuously.
- The healthcare prescriber conducts an in-person reevaluation of the child at least every 8 hours for youth 18 years of age and older and every 4 hours for children 17 years of age and younger.
- Chemical or physical restraints are used only after all other alternatives are exhausted.
- The child is assessed at the initiation of restraint or seclusion and every 15 minutes thereafter. This assessment includes, as appropriate to the type of restraint or seclusion used
  - Signs of injury associated with application of restraint or seclusion
  - Nutrition and hydration
  - Circulation and range of motion of extremities
  - Vital signs

- Hygiene and elimination
- Physical and psychological status and comfort
- Readiness for discontinuation of restraint or seclusion
- Immobilizing restraints are released and range-of-motion exercises are performed every 2 hours.
- Restraints are placed on the patient according to manufacturer's instructions.
- Restraints are fastened to the bed frame or structure of vehicle, never to the side rails or moving parts of the frame.
- Clinical leadership is immediately notified when a child remains in restraint or seclusion for more than 12 hours or experiences two or more separate episodes of restraint or seclusion of any duration within 12 hours. Thereafter, the leadership is notified every 12 hours if either of the above conditions continues.
- Child's well-being, dignity, and rights are protected at all times.
- Child's family is notified promptly of the initiation of restraints or seclusion.
- As early as possible, make the child aware of the rationale for restraint or seclusion, and present the behavioral criteria for discontinuation.
- Restraints are released when essential medical devices are no longer in place or the child is no longer a danger to self or to others. If restraints are released and the child manifests the same behavior that required restraint, the original order can be reapplied if not expired and alternatives to restraint are ineffective.
- The child or family and staff participate in a debriefing about the restraints or seclusion episode. Debriefing includes a review of the events that triggered the seclusion or restraints, alternatives to avoid similar incidents, and, if appropriate, the child making amends if anyone was injured.

EQUIPMENT

For a mummy restraint:

- Receiving blanket, blanket, or sheet
- Tape

For a jacket restraint:

- Jacket or vest of appropriate size

For an elbow device:

- Commercial cuff
- Tongue depressors
- Tape

CHILD AND FAMILY ASSESSMENT AND PREPARATION

- Assess the child for
  - Preexisting medical condition or physical disability and limitations that would place the child at greater risk during restraint or seclusion
  - History of sexual or physical abuse that would place the child at greater psychological risk during restraint or seclusion
- Attempt to find an alternative to using restraints. Some options are
  - Increased supervision of child by hospital personnel or parents
  - Modification of the environment
  - Redirection of the child
  - Diversionary activities such as television or radio
  - Preparing the child for a procedure with a simple explanation if developmentally appropriate
  - Using protective cover devices or camouflage over IV sites
  - Removing lines (e.g., IV, urinary catheter) as soon as possible
- Explain to parents the need for restraint, alternatives to restraint, the positive and negative aspects of restraint, and the consequences of not using restraints. Use the parents' assistance to obtain the child's cooperation.
- Actively listen to the child as to why the child is uncooperative; address this when possible.
- Explain to the child why the restraint is necessary.
- Obtain an order from the healthcare prescriber. Clarify institution's policy for order renewal. Use the least amount of restriction as possible.

PROCEDURE Using a Mummy Restraint

Steps	Rationale/Points of Emphasis
1. Place blanket on bed or examination table on a diagonal. Fold down one corner.	Used to immobilize infants/young children during procedure.
2. Place child on the blanket with shoulders in line with the fold. Use firm gentle motions. Continually speak soothingly to child.	Reassures child.

Steps	Rationale/Points of Emphasis
3. Firmly pull one corner of the blanket over the infant's body and tuck under the opposite shoulder. Pull the opposite side over and tuck it under the infant's back. Pull the bottom up and secure ends of the blanket with tape to keep in place (Figure 102-1).	Positions child securely and restrains safely.

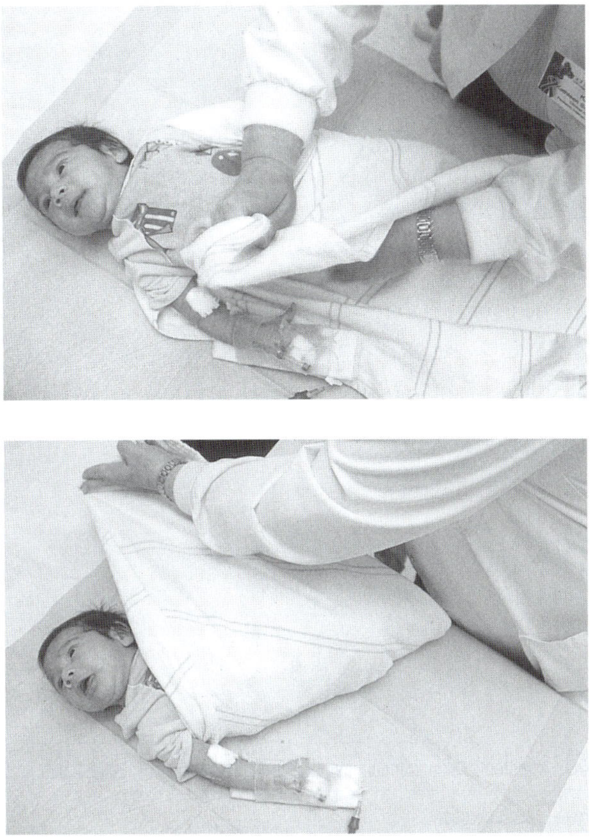

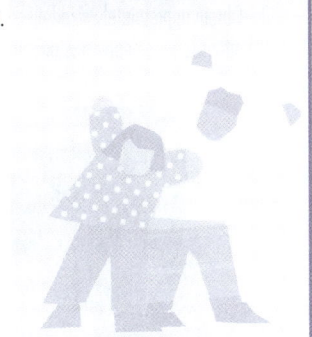

FIGURE 102-1
Mummy restraint.

Steps	Rationale/Points of Emphasis
4. Do not cover child's face. Ensure that wrapping is not obstructing the child's airway or circulation. Monitor airway and circulation throughout restraint.	Prevents and ensures prompt detection of complications.
5. Modify wrap to give access to chest and groin: Instead of wrapping the blanket corner over chest, promptly wrap blanket around the infant's arms and under back. Roll the edges around the legs and secure with tape. Ensure that the wrap does not obstruct circulation of the limbs.	Secures child safely. Prevents/detects complications.

PROCEDURE Using an Elbow Restraint

Steps	Rationale/Points of Emphasis
1. Obtain a healthcare prescriber's order. Explain to the child and parents what is going to occur and why.	Healthcare prescriber's orders are needed to apply continuous restraints. Explanation helps reduce fear and feeling of being disobedient.
2. Examine skin and document condition before applying restraint. Do not apply over open wounds or over restrictive clothing.	Provides baseline for evaluation. Restrictive clothing may impair circulation.

Continued

Steps	Rationale/Points of Emphasis
3. Obtain appropriately sized elbow restraints that keep arms straight with either tongue depressors or commercial plastic devices (Figure 102-2).	Too small a restraint can break or be ineffective; too large a restraint may slip.

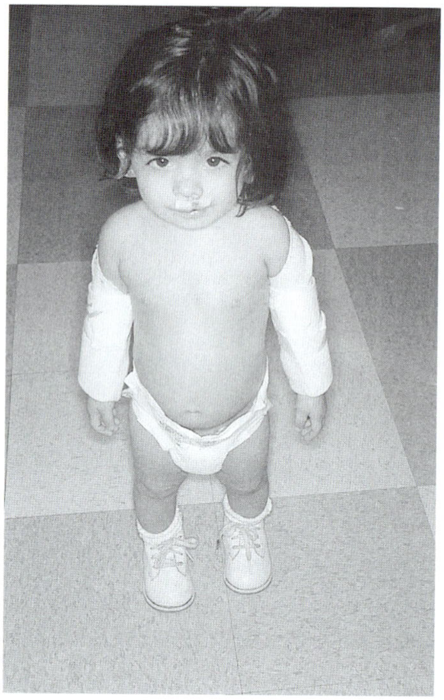

FIGURE 102-2
Elbow restraints.

Steps	Rationale/Points of Emphasis
4. Pad child's skin under restraint with towel or gauze padding.	Reduces potential skin irritation and increases effectiveness of the restraint.
5. Secure restraint using ties. Ensure that there is adequate circulation to limb.	Prevents complications.
6. Remove restraints and check skin condition at least every 2 hours. Provide range of motion. Document.	Provides early detection of compromised skin integrity. Prevents stiffness and encourages circulation.

PROCEDURE Using a Jacket Restraint

Steps	Rationale/Points of Emphasis
1. Obtain a healthcare prescriber's order.	Healthcare prescriber's orders are needed to apply continuous restraints.
2. Explain to child and parents what is going to be done and why.	Developmentally appropriate explanation to the child may elicit the child's cooperation. Parents will be more willing to assist and cooperate if they are prepared.
3. Obtain a jacket of the appropriate size.	Improves effectiveness and decreases chance of injury in either too small or too large a jacket.

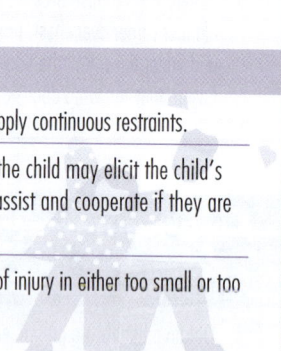

Steps	Rationale/Points of Emphasis
4. Place child's arms through the armholes. Secure jacket on child—most jackets have ties in the back or wrap the ties across the back and loop through the side (Figure 102-3).	Positions jacket to avoid child slipping down in jacket and causing airway obstruction.

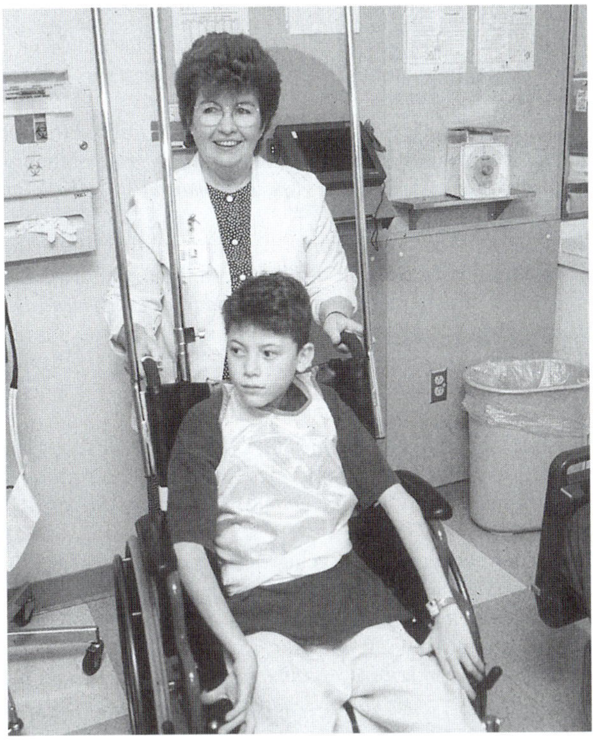

FIGURE 102-3
Jacket restraint.

Steps	Rationale/Points of Emphasis
5. Secure ties of jacket to a nonmovable part of the bed frame (not side rails) or wheelchair. Use a knot that can be quickly released.	Reduces chance of injury and airway occlusion caused by pulling on restraint with equipment movement. In case of an emergency, the child can be readily removed from restraint.
6. Reposition the child, release immobilizing restraints, and perform range of motion every 1 to 2 hours.	Prevents stiffness and promotes comfort.

CHILD AND FAMILY EVALUATION AND DOCUMENTATION

- Healthcare prescriber performs a face-to-face evaluation of the child within 1 hour of initiation of restraints.
- Nurse performs an assessment of the child every 15 minutes to include
  - Signs of injury associated with the application of restraint or seclusion
  - Nutrition and hydration
  - Circulation and range of motion of the extremities
  - Vital signs
  - Hygiene and elimination
  - Physical and psychological status and comfort
  - Readiness for discontinuation of restraint
- The RN evaluates the continuing need for restraint and documents this every
  - 4 hours for youths 18 years of age and older, up to a maximum of 24 hours of restraint
  - 2 hours for children 9 to 17 years of age, up to a maximum of 24 hours of restraint
  - 1 hour for children younger than 9 years of age, up to a maximum of 24 hours of restraint
- Periodically evaluate use of alternative methods to remove need for restraints; document child's response.
- Healthcare prescriber performs a face-to-face evaluation of the continuing need for restraint every 8 hours for youths 18 years of age and older and every 4 hours for children 17 years of age and younger.

- Document the following:
  - Reason for restraint or seclusion
  - Child's condition when restraints applied
  - Alternative measures used to avoid restraint use
  - Rationale for the type of physical intervention selected
  - Notification of the child's family
  - Child and parent teaching
  - Behavioral criteria for discontinuation
  - Notification of healthcare prescriber
  - Each in-person healthcare prescriber evaluation and reevaluation of the child
  - Assistance provided to the child to help him or her meet behavior criteria for discontinuation of restraint or seclusion
  - Findings from every-15-minute assessments
  - Child's condition after restraints removed
  - Debriefing with the staff
  - Notification of clinical leadership of restraint use (see Clinical Guidelines)

COMMUNITY CARE

- Teach parents alternatives to restraint and appropriate methods of restraint, including potential complications of each.

caREminder

The use of restraints in the home is not recommended but may be necessary in some cases, such as the neurologically impaired child who is seated in a wheelchair.

- Assess the potential for neglect and abuse in the implementation of some methods of restraint, including chemical restraints and seclusion. Report suspected abuse to appropriate authorities.
- Instruct the family to contact the healthcare provider if
  - Complications occur associated with restraint use (e.g., skin breakdown)
  - An increasing need for home use of restraint occurs

Unexpected Situations

- *Elbow restraints are causing skin breakdown:* Ensure that the restraints are removed routinely for at least 30 minutes and complete a skin assessment. Use padded dressing to prevent further friction between the reddened area and the restraint.
- *Child in jacket restraint slides down in wheelchair and neck is caught in the restraint:* Immediately release the restraint. Determine whether size of restraint was too large. Put on smaller restraint or select another method for restraining.

Bibliography

American Academy of Child and Adolescent Psychiatry. (2001). Practice parameter for the prevention and management of aggressive behavior in child and adolescent psychiatric institutions with special reference to seclusion and restraint. *Journal of the American Academy of Child and Adolescent Psychiatry, 41*(2 Suppl.), 4S–25S.

American Academy of Pediatrics. (1997). The use of physical restraint interventions for children and adolescents in the acute care setting. *Pediatrics, 99*(3), 497–498.

Day, D. (2002). Examining the therapeutic utility of restraints and seclusion with children and youth: The role of theory and research in practice. *The American Journal of Orthopsychiatry, 72*(2), 266–278.

Delaney, K. (2006). Evidence base for practice: Reduction of restraint and seclusion use during child and adolescent psychiatric inpatient treatment. *Worldviews on Evidenced-Based Nursing, 3*(1), 19–30.

Dorfman, D., & Kastner, B. (2004). The use of restraint for pediatric psychiatric patients in emergency departments. *Pediatric Emergency Care, 20*(3), 151–156.

Fenton, M., Bowers, L., Jones, J., Lakeman, R., & Morrison, E. (2000). Containment strategies for those with serious mental illness. *The Cochrane Database of Systematic Reviews,* (2), No. CD002084.

International Society of Psychiatric Nursing. (2001). ISPN position statement on the use of restraint and seclusion. *Journal of Child and Adolescent Psychiatric Nursing, 14*(3), 100–101.

Joint Commission on Healthcare Organizations (JCAHO). (2006). *Comprehensive accreditation manual for hospitals: Behavioral healthcare restraint and seclusion standard.* Oakbrook Terrace, IL: Author.

Ofoegbu, B., & Playfor, S. (2005). The use of physical restraints on paediatric intensive care units. *Paediatric Anesthesia, 15*(5), 407–411.

Sailas, E., & Fenton, M. (2000). Seclusion and restraint for people with serious mental illnesses. *The Cochrane Database of Systematic Reviews,* (1), No. CD001163.

Scottish Intercollegiate Guidelines Network–National Government Agency. (2004). *Safe sedation of children undergoing diagnostic and therapeutic procedures. A national clinical guideline.* Scottish Intercollegiate Guidelines Network (SIGN). Retrieved October 1, 2006, from www.sign.ac.UK/guidelines/fulltext/58/index.html

Selekman, J., & Snyder, B. (1995). Nursing perceptions of using physical restraints on children, *Pediatric Nursing, 21,* 460–464.

Selekman, J., & Snyder, B. (1996). Uses and alternatives to restraints in pediatric settings. *AACN Clinical Issues, 7,* 603–610.

Selekman, J., & Snyder, B. (1997). Institutional policies on the use of physical restraints on children. *Pediatric Nursing, 23,* 531–537.

Snyder, B. (2004). Preventing treatment interference: Nurses' and parents' intervention strategies. *Pediatric Nursing, 30,* 31–40.

Sorrentino, A. (2004). Chemical restraints for the agitated, violent, or psychotic pediatric patient in the emergency department: Controversies and recommendations. *Current Opinion in Pediatrics, 16*(2), 201–205.

Swauger, K., & Tomlin, C. (2000). Moving toward restraint-free patient care. *Journal of Nursing Administration, 30*(6), 325–329.

CHAPTER

103

Safety Measures

Clinical Guidelines

- All healthcare team members incorporate safety factors into care of the child and his or her family.
- To use safety measures, the guidelines from these chapters must be followed:
    - Chapter 15: Bed and Crib Choices
    - Chapter 43: Feeding, Infant: Breast-Feeding and Formula-Feeding
    - Chapter 85: Patient Identification
    - Chapter 102: Restraint and Seclusion
    - Chapter 110: Toys: Distribution, Cleaning, and Storage
    - Chapter 115: Transition Management: Discharging and Transferring the Child
    - Chapter 129: Visitor Identification and Management
- Child and family are provided information regarding safety measures in the healthcare institution.
- Child and family are provided anticipatory guidance regarding child safety issues.
- All healthcare providers are responsible for implementing measures to ensure the safety of the child and family while in the healthcare setting.

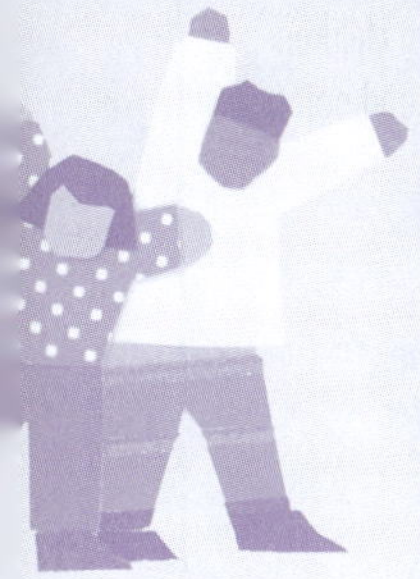

Equipment

- Age-appropriate bed
- Developmentally appropriate toys and equipment
- Shoes or slippers for child
- Age-appropriate clothes
- Restraints (if ordered)
- Child and parent identification bands

Child and Family Assessment and Preparation

- Evaluate child's and family's knowledge and understanding of safety needs of child on admission or initial contact with the healthcare provider or healthcare system.
- Assess the current history of child to determine type of safety measures used in the home and presence of accident-prone behaviors (e.g., risk-taking activities, multiple trips to emergency room).
- Assess for physical signs on the child's body that may indicate a history of accidents (scars, bruises, cuts).
- Assess developmental age of child.
- Determine child's and family's willingness to learn about child safety issues.

PROCEDURE Assessing Environmental Factors for Safety

Steps	Rationale/Points of Emphasis
1. Clear floors of fluid and other objects.	Decreases risk for falls.
2. Confirm that showers and tubs have nonskid surfaces.	Provides traction to decrease risk for falls.
3. Ensure that electrical equipment is maintained in good working order with no broken plugs or exposed wires. All electrical outlets should have child safety covers.	Prevents injury from electrical shock.
4. Follow facility policy for use of personal electronic devices (radio, hairdryer, etc.).	Use of personal electronic devices may produce a safety hazard.
5. Monitor use of personal devices such as compact disc (CD) or MP3 players.	Excessive noise levels can damage hearing and can be disturbing to other patients. Cords from headphones may present a strangulation hazard.
6. Ensure that patient care instruments, supplies, and solutions are kept out of reach of the child and on shelves where ambulatory children and child visitors cannot access them.	Children may mistake solutions for food or candy. Prevents accidental injury.
7. Do not store medications in the child's room.	Children may mistake medications for food or candy and may ingest them.

PROCEDURE Assessing Beds and Cribs for Safety (see also Chapter 15: Bed and Crib Choices)

Steps	Rationale/Points of Emphasis
1. Ensure that the catches on the crib are in good working condition. Place the wheel of crib or bed in a locked position.	Latches in good working order prevent side rails from falling down when child leans on them or pulls up from a sitting to standing position using the rail. Wheels locked in place prevent rolling of the bed.
2. Keep crib and bedside rails up when the child is in the bed.	Prevents falls from the crib or bed.
3. Use bumper pads as necessary around cribs of small infants and children who are at risk for injury if they hit the side rails of the crib or bed. Bumper pads may also be used in beds for children with a history of seizures and for the agitated child (e.g., post–head injury).	Prevents child from getting caught between the mattress and the crib or bed side and from hitting a part of his or her body on the rails. Prevents injury if child has a seizure while in bed. Bumper pads should not be used with children who can stand on their own because they can then stand on the pad and potentially climb out of the crib. **Alert!** *Bumper pads should not be used at home. These products may actually place the child at greater risk for suffocation and death.*
4. Crib side rails must be less than $2\frac{3}{8}$ inches apart.	Prevents child from getting his or her head caught between rails.
5. Add net or bubble tops to the crib as needed.	Prevents child from crawling out over top of side rails.
6. "Hi-lo" beds should remain in the low position.	Allows toilet-trained children to easily and safely climb out of bed to use bathroom.

PROCEDURE Assessing Toys and Other Equipment for Safety (see also Chapter 110: Toys: Distribution, Cleaning, and Storage)

Steps	Rationale/Points of Emphasis
1. Use toys that are developmentally appropriate, allergy free, washable, unbreakable, and have no removable parts.	The young child can easily aspirate small parts.
2. Do not use friction toys under an oxygen tent.	Sparks in any high-oxygen environment can cause spontaneous combustion.
3. Avoid toys with strings.	Prevents accidental strangulation.
4. Select age-appropriate toys.	Children under age 3 years should not have toys with removable parts that are smaller than $1\frac{1}{4}$ inches in diameter and less than $2\frac{1}{4}$ inches long.
5. Balloons are hazardous at any age but may not be given to children under the age of 8.	Broken, uninflated, or underinflated balloons can be aspirated and cause suffocation. Balloons may also contain latex, which may compromise a latex-free environment.
6. Clean toys after use by a child and before distribution to another child.	Reduces transmission of microorganisms.
7. Do not use infant walkers in the healthcare setting; instruct parents not to use at home.	Data indicate a considerable risk for major and minor injury and even death from the use of infant walkers. Data indicate no clear benefit from walker use. The American Academy of Pediatrics recommends a ban on the manufacture and sale of mobile infant walkers.
8. Select clothing for the child that fits properly.	Clothing that is too small is uncomfortable. Clothing that is too large may cause injury as the child moves.
9. Children should wear foot covering with a hard sole when out of bed.	Prevents child from stepping on items that can injure the foot and from slipping easily on the floor.

PROCEDURE Managing Transition for Safety (see also Chapter 115: Transition Management: Transferring and Discharging the Child)

Steps	Rationale/Points of Emphasis
1. Infants may be transported to other areas in their cribs or bassinets or using strollers with a seat belt.	An infant or child should not be carried because the nurse may fall and injure the child.
2. Transport children who are able to sit up without support by a gurney, their bed, a wheelchair, or a wagon.	Provides safe transportation of child.
3. Transport infants and children unable to sit without support in their bed or crib or in a wheelchair with a seat belt.	Provides safe transportation of child. Protects the child from falling over during transportation.
4. Parents are highly encouraged to accompany the child whenever transported.	Parental presence provides support for the child.
5a. All newborns who are to be discharged home in a car shall be transported in a car seat that meets federal safety requirements. Infants and older children shall be discharged and transported home in a car seat following federal guidelines according to age, weight, and medical condition of the child. Older children should be discharged and transported home in car with the child restrained using a seat belt.	Recommendations are supported by the American Academy of Pediatrics and include the standard that the healthcare facility should make available an appropriate car safety seat by sale, short-term loan, or donation to parents before discharge if the parents are unable to provide their own.
5b. Provision of information and training for parents and guardians should be presented before discharge on the generic issues related to correct use of car safety seats. Hands-on teaching, including "return demonstration," should be a part of this instruction.	Ensures parents fully understand safe use of a car seat and regulations regarding forward versus rear facing and car seat versus booster seat based on age and weight of child.
5c. The installation of a specific car seat in a specific car is the responsibility of the parent.	Ensures liability of safe installation of the car seat is the responsibility of the parent and not the healthcare facility.

PROCEDURE Patient and Visitor Identification (see also Chapter 85: Patient Identification and Chapter 129: Visitor Identification and Management)

Steps	Rationale/Points of Emphasis
1. Identify all children and their parents using identification name bands.	Protects security of the child. Prevents inaccurate identification of child and parents, especially during medication administration and for procedures.
2. Ensure visitors have been identified per institutional policies, including identification of visitors by use of temporary name badges.	Protects child and family from unwanted visitors and from possible abduction by unidentified personnel in the area.
3. Provide comfortable and safe areas for visitors to wait.	Prevents visitors obstructing hallways and waiting in areas that need to be highly accessed by healthcare personnel.

PROCEDURE Food Management (see Chapter 43: Feeding, Infant: Breast-Feeding and Formula-Feeding)

Steps	Rationale/Points of Emphasis
1. Do not prop bottles for infant feeding.	Propping bottles can cause aspiration and discourages parent–child interactions.
2. Treat expressed breast milk as a bodily fluid and follow universal precautions for handling of bodily fluids.	Reduces spread of viruses. Use of breast milk is advocated as providing the best nutrition for infants before the age of 6 months.
3. Monitor infants and toddlers placed in high chairs for meals during the meal and as long as they remain in the high chair.	Protects child from injury while in high chair. Young children can easily choke on food and therefore should be monitored while eating.
4. Disinfect high chair trays, arms, seats, and other soiled areas after each use.	Reduces spread of microorganisms.
5. Verify the child has no food allergies.	Prevents allergic/anaphylactic reaction.
6. Serve commercially prepared infant food from dish rather than from the original jar or package.	Allows examination of food before serving for spoilage or contaminants.
7. Avoid foods that can be aspirated (e.g., peanuts, popcorn, raisins, and hot dogs).	Small foods given to infants and toddlers can lead to aspiration.
8. Children may keep food in their room when cleared with the healthcare provider and if kept in sealed containers.	Food that is not appropriately contained can attract bugs, rodents, and microorganisms. Food kept in the room should be monitored to ensure that it is consistent with child's current diet.

PROCEDURE Restraints (see also Chapter 102: Restraint and Seclusion)

Steps	Rationale/Points of Emphasis
1. Apply restraints as needed to protect child from injury to self or others. A physician's order must be obtained to use restraints.	Restraints may be needed to prevent child from pulling out IV lines or other tubes. Alternative measures to avoid use of restraints should be used first (e.g., added supervision of the child, distraction activities).
2. Monitor restrained child at least every 15 minutes or following facility policy.	Prevents injury or death; assesses for comfort. Assess for possible discontinuation of restraints.

CHILD AND FAMILY EVALUATION AND DOCUMENTATION

- Evaluate child's and family's knowledge and understanding of safety rules and precautions while in the healthcare setting.
- Evaluate child's and family's knowledge and understanding of developmentally and age-appropriate safety measures for the child.
- Document the following:
  - Verbal teaching provided to the child and family regarding safety issues
  - Distribution and use of child safety multimedia materials used with the child and family
  - Measures used by the healthcare provider to ensure child safety (e.g., side rails up, child accompanied to events off the unit, slippers worn while out of unit bed)
  - Inconsistent or gross failure of family to provide and implement safety precautions on behalf of the child while under management of the healthcare services

COMMUNITY CARE

- Present family with teaching materials and resources (e.g., websites) to provide family counseling for anticipatory guidance of safety issues in the home and school.
- Advise family to access reputable websites such as the Consumer Product Safety Commission (www.cpsc.org) and the American Association of Pediatrics (www.aap.org) for updated childcare information and recalls.

Unexpected Situations

- *When you walk into child's room, you notice the crib side rails are down on one side and the 2-year-old is asleep in the crib. The mother was watching television in the room, but she has stepped out to get a drink:* Raise the side rail on the bed, and make sure the bubble top or net is also in place. The 2-year-old can awaken at any time and get out of the crib or could easily roll over in his or her sleep and fall out of the bed. When the mother returns, review with her that crib side rails must remain up whenever child is in the bed, unless a parent or other caregiver is at the immediate bedside with the child.
- *While walking by a room, you notice a 4-year-old child digging through the trash in her room. The father has fallen asleep in a chair near the bed:* This is a good reminder that you should never throw any medical equipment discharge or biohazardous waste in the trashcan of the room of a young, curious child. Children need to be supervised if they can get out of bed in the room. Wake the father and explain to him the need to supervise child. Determine whether child can go to the playroom. It may be necessary to place the trashcan out of sight in the bathroom.

Bibliography

American Academy of Pediatrics. (n.d.). *Toy safety.* Retrieved October 4, 2006, from http://www.aap.org/pressroom/toymatrelease.pdf

American Academy of Pediatrics. (1999). Safe transportation of newborns at hospital discharge. *Pediatrics, 104*(4), 986–987.

American Academy of Pediatrics. (2001). Injuries associated with infant walkers. *Pediatrics, 108*(3), 790–792.

American Academy of Pediatrics. (2003). *Holiday safety tips.* Retrieved October 4, 2006, from http://www.aap.org/advocacy/archives/dectips.htm

American Academy of Pediatrics. (2004a). *Healthy Child Care America Back to Sleep campaign speaker materials: Reducing the risk of SIDS in child care.* Retrieved September 4, 2004, from http://healthychildcare.org/section_SIDS.cfm

Gielen, A., Wilson, M., McDonald, E., et al. (2001). Randomized trail of enhanced anticipatory guidance for injury prevention. *Archives of Pediatrics and Adolescent Medicine, 155*(1), 42–49.

Irving, M. (2000). Approaches to child safety and accident prevention. *Community Nurse, 6*(7), 23–24.

McDonald, J., Rutherford, G., & Kennedy, J. (2001). Keeping children safe. *Consumer Product Safety Review, 5*(3), 1–3.

Ricci, F. (2000). Strategies for teaching safety education to children with special needs. *International Journal of Trauma Nursing, 6*(4), 129–132.

Stower, S. (2000). Keeping the hospital environment safe for children. *Paediatric Nursing, 12*(6), 37–43.

Thain, J. (2000). Protecting children: The challenge for all primary care practitioners. *Primary Health Care, 10*(4), 18, 20–21.

CHAPTER

104

Saline Lock/Flush

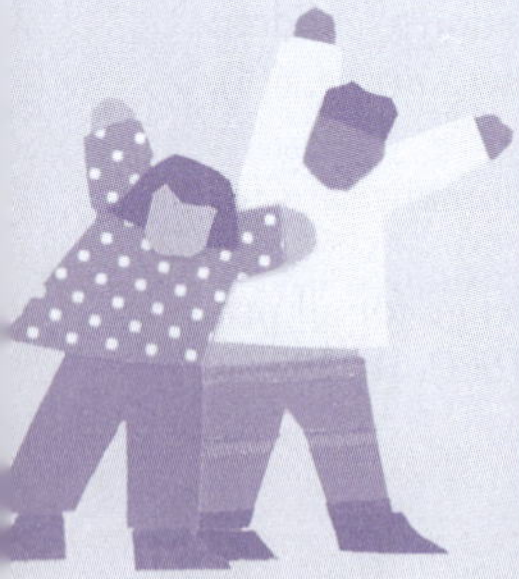

Clinical Guidelines

- A healthcare prescriber must order saline locks and flushes.
- A physician, registered nurse (RN), or licensed practical nurse (LPN) may administer saline flushes per state practice acts.
- Children who do not require continuous intravenous (IV) infusion but who may still require IV access for intermittent intravascular medication administration are considered candidates for a saline lock.
- The efficacy of saline flushes to maintain the patency of an intermittent IV access site has been demonstrated to be safe for children of all ages, including neonates, using catheters 24 gauge and larger.
- Saline flushes and assessment of the IV site must be administered every 6 to 8 hours as ordered for optimal catheter maintenance.
- Flush peripheral catheters with saline using the following:
  - Children and infants—preservative-free normal saline
  - Neonates—weight 800 to 1500 g, preservative-free normal saline; less than 800 g, 5% dextrose solution
- See Chapters 56, 57, and 58 for recommendations regarding heparin flushing of other types of infusion access devices.

Equipment

- Nonsterile gloves
- Alcohol swabs
- Vial of sterile saline solution 0.9%
- Needleless male adapter (injection cap) (if converting an IV continuous infusion to a lock)

Child and Family Assessment and Preparation

- Assess the cognitive level, readiness, and ability to process information of the child and family. The readiness to learn and process information may be impaired as a result of age, stress, or anxiety.
- Reinforce the need and identify and discuss the risks and benefits of saline lock placement, as appropriate, to both the child and family. Explain the signs and symptoms that may indicate the need for IV catheter site change should the saline lock become infiltrated or clotted. This enables the child or family to recognize when the IV is not functioning properly and when to notify the nurse.
- Explain the procedure, as appropriate, to both the child and family. Use therapeutic play as indicated. Be honest; never say "it won't hurt."
- Assess the IV site for signs of infiltration, irritation, or phlebitis.

PROCEDURE Administering a Saline Lock/Flush

Steps	Rationale/Points of Emphasis
1. Check healthcare prescriber's orders and medication records for time intervals for administration.	Flushing of the IV cannula with saline at prescribed intervals improves the duration of catheter patency. Studies indicate that catheters flushed every 6 to 8 hours remain patent significantly longer than catheters flushed at 4-hour intervals.
2. Perform hand hygiene and gather the necessary equipment and supplies.	Reduces transmission of microorganisms. Promotes efficient time management and provides organized approach to the procedure.
3. Use a commercially available prefilled syringe of normal saline or draw up 1 to 3 mL of normal saline and label with child's name and name of solution.	Using a commercially available prefilled syringe reduces medication error. Labeling syringe provides for safe administration of right drug to right patient. The amount of flush delivered is based on child's age, fluid restrictions, and length of tubing to be flushed.
4. Identify the child using two different patient identifiers.	Reduces incidence of treatment being administered to wrong child.
5. Don gloves.	Standard precautions to reduce transmission of microorganisms.
6. Assess IV site.	The IV site should be free from signs of infection or infiltration before heparin is administered.
7. To convert a primary continuous infusion to a saline lock: • Clamp T-connector tubing closest to catheter hub. • Remove the IV administration set tubing from the T-connector tubing or from the hub on the catheter cannula (if no T-connector tubing is present). • Attach a needleless male adapter (injection cap) to the end of the T-connector tubing or to the hub on the catheter cannula.	This is done to keep the IV line available in case it is needed later or to keep the line open for administration of IV medication. With a pediatric patient, it may be hospital policy to keep the IV site patent until the child is discharged.
8. Flush lock with saline solution.	
a. Cleanse needleless male adapter (injection cap) with alcohol pad for at least 3 seconds or per institutional policy.	Reduces presence of microorganisms.
b. Insert needleless syringe with saline solution into injection cap. Unclamp white side clamp on T-connector tubing if necessary.	All connections must be unclamped to allow flow of saline from syringe into catheter.
c. Gently pull back to check for blood flow.	Lack of blood flow is not an accurate determination of cannula placement because a fibrin shield may have formed at the tip of the cannula.
d. Gently inject saline solution into the catheter while assessing for resistance. If resistance is felt, never continue to apply force. Stop and evaluate cause.	The volume of the flush should be equal to the volume capacity of the cannula and add-on device times two. Resistance may mean the catheter is blocked or otherwise not functioning properly.
e. Inject last 0.1 mL while removing the syringe tip or closing white side clamp on T-connector (positive fluid displacement).	Provides positive pressure as syringe tip is being removed. Prevents blood from accumulating at IV catheter tip.
f. Close the clamp.	Positive fluid displacement must be maintained within the cannula lumen during and after a flush to prevent reflux of blood into the lumen.
9. To convert a saline lock to a primary continuous infusion:	
a. Cleanse injection cap with alcohol.	Reduces presence of microorganisms.
b. Insert needleless syringe with saline solution into injection cap. Unclamp T-connector if necessary. Gently inject 1 mL of saline while assessing for resistance or signs of swelling.	Ensures patency of access site before starting a continuous infusion of fluids. If resistance is felt, never continue to apply force. Stop and evaluate cause. If swelling occurs, stop flush because this indicates an infiltration.
c. Attach an IV administration set tubing to the injection cap.	IV administration set provides mechanism to administer fluids over a continuous period of time.
d. Start infusion. Monitor for infiltration.	Signs of infiltration include immediate swelling at the insertion site or fluid leaking from the insertion site.
10. Assess IV site after manipulation of the catheter.	Checks for infiltration at the cannula site of insertion.
11. Dispose of the syringe in appropriate needle receptacle. Remove gloves and perform hand hygiene.	Promotes safety. Reduces transmission of microorganisms.

Child and Family Evaluation and Documentation

- Document the following:
  - Date, time, concentration, and amount of flush solution used
  - Presence or absence of blood return and any resistance to flushing
  - Site appearance (presence or absence of redness, swelling, drainage, tenderness, or streaking)
  - Steps taken to intervene if complications are present (see Table 56-1 in Chapter 56).
  - Evaluate the IV site every 8 hours for complications and discontinue the catheter as necessary.
- Change the IV access site dressing per type of catheter (e.g., tunneled, PICC, peripheral) requirements and if dressing becomes damp, loosened, soiled, or when inspection of the catheter site is necessary. Use aseptic technique while observing proper wound site care. Label the dressing with the time, date, and initials when reapplied to ensure proper change times.
- Determine whether the child and family have other areas of concern to discuss.

Community Care

- If the child is to be discharged home with a saline lock and orders for intermittent IV infusions and medications, discharge planning with a home health nurse should begin as early as possible.
- Communication with the home care provider should include type of catheter, including manufacturer and size if known; date of insertion; dressing change and flush protocol taught in healthcare setting; and notification of any complications after placement.
- Parents should be instructed in performing hand hygiene; dressing changes; flushing the IV line; medication administration and syringe pump use, as applicable; disposal techniques for syringes; and developmentally and age-appropriate methods to maintain the saline lock.
- Before discharge, have the family repeat what they've learned about the most common complications of IV therapy (i.e., sepsis and accidental removal), what to look for, and actions to take in the event of complications to ensure they understand the information.
- Instruct the family to contact the healthcare provider if
  - IV insertion site is reddened or oozes fluid or blood
  - IV becomes dislodged
  - Child develops a fever

Unexpected Situations

- *When administering the saline flush, fluid is seen leaking from the infusion site and resistance is noted:* Stop administering the saline flush. The catheter is infiltrated and needs to be removed from the extremity. Restart the IV in a different location.
- *During the saline flush process, the tip of the saline syringe touches the child's hand:* Discard the syringe of saline. Prepare a new saline flush for administration.

Bibliography

Beecroft, P., Bossert, E., Chung, K., et al. (1997). Intravenous lock patency in children: Dilute heparin versus saline. *Journal of Pediatric Pharmacology Practice, 2*(4), 211–223.

Campbell, S., Trojaniwski, J., & Ackroyd-Stolarz, S. (2005). How often should peripheral intravenous catheters in ambulatory patients be flushed? *Journal of Healthcare Nursing, 28*(6), 399–404.

Crews, B. E., Gnann, K. K., Rice, M. H., & Kee, C. C. (1997). Effects of varying intervals between heparin flushes on pediatric catheter longevity. *Pediatric Nursing, 23*(1), 87–91.

Gyr, R., Smith, K., Pontious, S., et al. (1995). Double blind comparison of heparin and saline flush solutions in maintenance of peripheral infusion devices. *Pediatric Nursing, 21*(4), 366, 383–389.

Hanrahan, K., Kleiber, C., & Berends, S. (2000). Saline for peripheral intravenous locks in neonates: Evaluating a change in practice. *Neonatal Network, 19*(2), 19–24.

Heilskov, J., Kleiber, C., Johnson, K., et al. (1998). A randomized trial of heparin and saline for maintaining intravenous locks in neonates. *Journal of the Society of Pediatric Nurses, 3*(3), 111–116.

Infusion Nurses Society. (2006). Infusion nursing: Standards of practice. *Journal of Infusion Nursing, 29*(1S), S1–S92.

Knue, M., Doellman, D., & Jacobs, B. (2006). Peripherally inserted central catheters in children: A survey of practice patterns. *Journal of Infusion Nursing, 29*(1), 28–33.

Kyle, L., & Yurner, B. (1999). Efficacy of saline versus heparin in maintaining 24-gauge intermittent intravenous catheters in a rabbit model. *Neonatal Network, 18*(6), 49–54.

LeDuc, K. (1997). Efficacy of normal saline solution versus heparin solution for maintaining patency of peripheral intravenous catheters in children. *Journal of Emergency Nursing, 23*(4), 306–309.

Mudge, B., Forcier, D., & Slattery, M. (1998). Patency of 24-gauge peripheral intermittent infusion devices: A comparison of heparin and saline solutions. *Pediatric Nursing, 24*(2), 142–146.

O'Grady, N. P., Alexander, M., Dellinger, E. P., et al. (2002). Guidelines for the prevention of intravascular catheter-related infections. *MMWR Morbidity and Mortality Weekly Report, 51*(RR-10), 1–29.

Shah, P., Ng, E., & Sinha, A. (2002). Heparin for prolonging peripheral intravenous catheter use in neonates. *Cochrane Database System Reviews*, (4), No. CD002774.

CHAPTER

105

Sedation

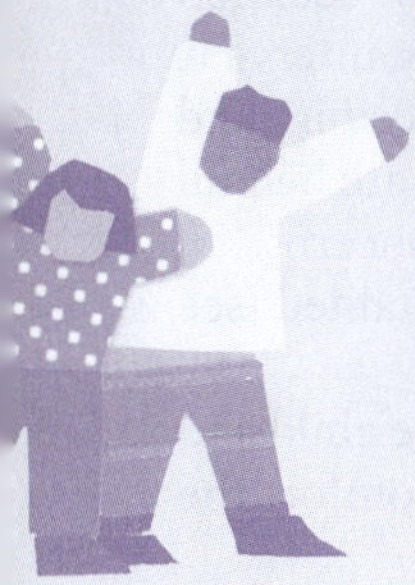

Clinical Guidelines

- Sedation is ordered by a healthcare prescriber. Medications to achieve sedation are selected based on type of procedure, length of the procedure, medical condition of the child, age and weight or body surface area (BSA) of the child, expected painfulness, and the need for amnesia.
- The healthcare prescriber, registered nurse (RN), or licensed practical nurse (LPN) may administer sedation medications, as within their scope of practice. Practitioners who care for children receiving moderate sedation have received competency-based education regarding medication administration and assessment of the child before, during, and after sedation. Practitioners possess the skills to manage a compromised airway and provide adequate oxygenation and ventilation, should these become necessary.
- Moderate sedation is used for diagnostic and therapeutic procedures that are painful or for which the child must remain immobile. Moderate sedation is a drug-induced depression of consciousness; the child can still respond purposefully, maintaining a patent airway and adequate spontaneous ventilation. A key consideration is that sedation to anesthesia is a continuum. Individuals react differently to medications, and healthcare practitioners must be competent to manage a child who enters a deeper than intended level of sedation.
- At least one individual capable of establishing a patent airway and positive-pressure ventilation, other than the practitioner performing the procedure, is present to monitor the child during sedation procedures. This individual's primary responsibility is to monitor the child, but the person may perform interruptible tasks in the room (e.g., charting) after the child's vital signs and level of sedation-analgesia have stabilized, when adequate monitoring of the child's level of sedation and response is maintained.
- The person monitoring the child possesses the requisite knowledge and skills to assess, diagnose, and intervene in the event of complications or undesired outcomes and to institute nursing interventions in compliance with orders (including standing orders) or institutional protocols or guidelines. This individual meets institutional requirements for clinical competency related to monitoring the child receiving sedation. Competencies include pediatric basic life support and knowledge of the following:
  - The anatomy, physiology, pharmacology, and ability to recognize cardiac arrhythmia and complications related to IV sedation and medications
  - Total patient care requirements during IV sedation and recovery. Physiologic measurements should include respiratory rate, oxygen saturation, blood pressure, cardiac rate and rhythm, and patient's level of consciousness.
  - The role of reversal agents for narcotics and benzodiazepines
  - The signs, treatment, and interventions associated with clinical complications
  - The principles of oxygen delivery, respiratory physiology, transport and uptake, and the ability to use oxygen delivery equipment

  - The use of emergency equipment, including airway management resuscitation
- Personnel who are expert in airway management, emergency intubation, and pediatric advanced life support (PALS) are immediately available (within 5 minutes) if complications arise.
- Emergency equipment is present and ready to use in case the child experiences complications. Airway management and breathing equipment are checked for appropriate function before each sedation.
- Oral intake before scheduled procedures is limited as follows (or as otherwise ordered):
  - All children are NPO for 2 hours before procedure.
  - Clear liquids may be consumed up to 2 hours before the procedure.
  - Breast milk may be consumed up to 4 hours before the procedure.
  - Infant formula, nonhuman milk, and light foods (no fried or fatty foods or meat) may be consumed up to 6 hours before the procedure.
- Children at risk for pulmonary aspiration of gastric contents (e.g., history of gastroesophageal reflux, esophageal dysfunction, and extreme obesity) are evaluated for necessity of pharmacologic treatment to reduce gastric volume and increase gastric pH.
- In an emergency when the child has had recent oral intake, the increased risks of sedation are evaluated against its potential benefit, and the need to protect the airway is evaluated before sedation.
- Oxygen saturation level, heart rate, and ventilatory function are monitored continuously during the procedure and documented every 5 minutes. Level of consciousness, response to verbal commands, respiratory rate, and blood pressure are monitored and documented every 5 minutes during the procedure, unless it would interfere with the procedure (e.g., a child undergoing magnetic resonance imaging). In children with a history of cardiovascular disease or anticipated arrhythmia problems, a cardiac monitor is recommended. Oxygen delivery, suctioning, and/or repositioning may be necessary to support ventilatory function.
- Monitoring continues after the procedure until the child is in a state in which safe discharge or transfer to a less acute unit is possible. If the child is transported from the procedure area to a recovery area, the practitioner or RN must remain with the child and continuously monitor by direct observation and pulse oximetry during transport.
- When a reversal agent has been given, the child is monitored for at least 1 hour after the last dose.
- Verbal and written discharge instructions are given to the family before discharge.

EQUIPMENT

- Sedation documentation record
- Pulse oximeter
- Positive-pressure oxygen delivery system, capable of administering greater than 90% oxygen for at least 60 minutes
- Supplemental oxygen
- Functional suction apparatus with appropriate suction catheters
- Sphygmomanometer and blood pressure cuff
- Automated blood pressure monitoring device that uses oscillometric or Doppler technique
- Stethoscope
- Cardiac monitoring equipment
- Emergency cart or kit with age-appropriate drugs and appropriately sized equipment to establish and maintain an airway, and supplies for vascular access
- Medications: sedation-analgesia and appropriate reversal agents (e.g., naloxone, flumazenil)

CHILD AND FAMILY ASSESSMENT AND PREPARATION

- Determine whether the patient's status fits the criteria for American Society of Anesthesiologists class I (normal healthy patient) or class II (patient with mild systemic disease) candidate, frequently considered appropriate candidates for moderate or deep sedation. Children who are class III or IV require additional consideration.
- Assess child's and family's understanding of sedation and the subsequent procedure. Preparatory interventions such as careful explanation of the procedure and the effects of sedatives before the procedure are helpful in alleviating child's distress and parental concerns.
- Ensure that informed consent has been obtained (see Chapter 53).
- If appropriate, invite parents to stay with the child and instruct them on their role to soothe and comfort the child.
- Complete pain assessment with child and family. As needed, review age-appropriate pain assessment scale with child and family to assist in postprocedural pain evaluations.

PROCEDURE Preprocedure Evaluation

Steps	Rationale/Points of Emphasis
1. Document the last time the child consumed food or liquids.	An empty stomach reduces potential aspiration of stomach contents.
2. Ensure that a history has been taken that includes the following: • Preexisting medical conditions • Previous experiences with anesthesia and sedation, including medications given • History of alcohol or substance use • Current medications • Allergies • Presence of gastric reflux	Previous analgesia/sedation experiences and medications taken before the procedure can influence the action of medications given during the procedure and child's response, and they alert the healthcare provider to potential complications and risk factors.
3. Ensure that the physical examination findings are on the chart, including: • Evaluation of the airway • Cardiac assessment • Respiratory assessment	Provides information about the child's preprocedure status to anticipate potential adverse responses.
4. Document recent height and weight.	Height and weight are used to calculate drug dosage.
5. Check condition of tongue, teeth, and ability to open mouth.	Alerts to variances in the event that emergency intubation is needed.
6. Ensure that room is prepared for completing sedation and that all equipment is in proper working condition. Equipment to gather includes pulse oximeter, cardiac monitoring equipment, positive-pressure oxygen delivery system, supplemental oxygen, functional suction apparatus with appropriate suction catheters, vital signs monitoring equipment, emergency cart, and medications for the procedure.	Promotes efficient time management and provides an organized approach to the procedure. Ensures patient safety when all emergency equipment (i.e., oxygen delivery system) is in working order.

PROCEDURE Presedation

Steps	Rationale/Points of Emphasis
1. Perform hand hygiene.	Reduces transmission of microorganisms.
2. Immediately before sedation, record vital signs, level of consciousness, skin color, respiratory status, and oxygenation.	Baseline assessment serves as a guideline for assessing variances during and after the procedure.
3. Apply pulse oximeter probe; turn on machine.	Alerts to reduced blood oxygen saturation levels.
4. Ensure that a patent IV is in place or that a person skilled in establishing IV access in a child is immediately available.	Vascular access is essential in pediatric advanced life support for administration of fluids and medications.
5. Ensure that medication dosages are calculated correctly based on the child's weight or body surface area.	Prevents medication errors.

PROCEDURE Intraprocedure

Steps	Rationale/Points of Emphasis
1. Continuously monitor: • Oxygen saturation • Heart rate • Airway patency • Adequacy of ventilation	To anticipate and recognize potential complications of level of sedation in relation to the type of medication being administered.

Continued

Steps	Rationale/Points of Emphasis
2. Monitor the following at least every 5 minutes (unless it would interfere with procedure):	Alerts to deviance from baseline so that interventions can be implemented promptly to avoid complications.
• Respiratory rate	Ensures airway patency.
• Blood pressure	Evaluates adequacy of ventilation and circulation.
• Head position	Evaluates level of sedation—in a state of moderate sedation, the child should be able to respond to physical stimulation or to a verbal command, such as, "Open your eyes."
• Adequacy of restraining device and circulation of hand/foot that is restrained	Evaluates adequacy of ventilation and circulation.
• Adequacy of chest expansion	
• Level of consciousness	
3. Monitor for complications, and provide interventions as indicated (Chart 105-1).	Ensures safety of the child.

CHART 105-1 NURSING INTERVENTIONS FOR THE COMPLICATIONS OF SEDATION

Complication	Nursing Interventions	Rationale
Airway obstruction or respiratory depression	• Reposition head. • Suction. • Insert oral airway. • Tell child to take a deep breath. • Stimulate child by rubbing arms or legs. • Administer oxygen. • Manually ventilate with a bag-valve-mask device.	Opens airway; assists oxygenation.
Oversedation	• Maintain airway, breathing, and circulation. • Have drugs to reverse sedation immediately available and administer, as ordered, if child is too deeply sedated (e.g., naloxone for opiates, flumazenil for benzodiazepines). • Monitor respiratory status until stable.	Treatment depends on which drug is used for sedation.
Cardiac arrhythmias	• Note baseline heart rate and rhythm. • Obtain apical pulse for 1 full minute. • Examine electrocardiogram patterns if indicated. • Ensure that child has patent airway. • Monitor oxygen saturation levels. • Administer oxygen. • Administer fluids and antiarrhythmic drugs as ordered.	The two most common cardiac arrhythmias that occur during conscious sedation are bradycardia and tachycardia. Bradycardia may be due to hypoxemia or vagal stimulation from the procedure. Tachycardia may be due to pain, anxiety, hypoxemia, or hypovolemia.
Hypotension	• Investigate possible causes. • Support respiratory status. • Administer fluids and vasopressors as ordered.	During conscious sedation, the blood pressure may fluctuate up to 10% from baseline. A drop of 20% to 30% below normal pressure sustained for more than a few minutes may indicate a problem.
Hypertension	• Administer additional sedation or analgesia.	Hypertension may be the result of pain or the stress of the procedure.

PROCEDURE Postprocedure

Steps	Rationale/Points of Emphasis
1a. Monitor every 15 minutes for 1 hour or until sedation level is at the presedation assessment level for two consecutive 15-minute assessments and discharge criteria are met: • Heart rate • Respiratory rate • Blood pressure • Oxygen saturation • Level of consciousness	Detects adequate recovery and provides early recognition of complications.
1b. When a reversal agent has been given, monitor the child for at least 1 hour after the last dose.	Ensures that sedation and cardiorespiratory depression do not recur after the effect of the antagonist dissipates.

PROCEDURE Discharge

Steps	Rationale/Points of Emphasis
1. Discharge child when following criteria have been met:	
a. Stable serial vital signs.	Demonstrates stable and satisfactory cardiovascular function and airway patency.
b. Alert and oriented as before sedation. Child can talk, if age appropriate.	Indicates recovery.
c. Exhibits protective reflexes of cough and gag and sucking and swallowing at presedation level.	Reduces the potential for aspiration or airway compromise. Protective reflexes are normal.
d. Child is not experiencing significant pain or nausea.	Severe pain and inability to retain fluids indicate that further intervention is needed.
e. State of hydration is adequate. Child is able to tolerate oral fluids (unless contraindicated).	Avoids complications associated with dehydration.
f. Child is able to ambulate at presedation level. The very young or the handicapped child demonstrates the presedation level of responsiveness.	Indicates recovery from sedation medications.
g. Dressings, if present, without evidence of bleeding.	Ensures prompt detection of bleeding.

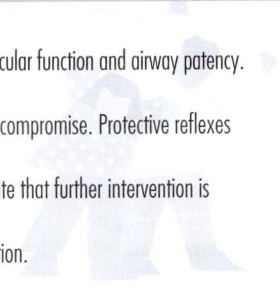

CHILD AND FAMILY EVALUATION AND DOCUMENTATION

- Evaluate child for attainment of discharge criteria and level of comfort.
- Ensure that signed forms are maintained in the child's chart.
- Document the following:
  - Informed consent obtained
  - Instructions and information provided to the responsible person and the person's understanding of such
  - Child's dietary status before sedation
  - Child's age and weight
  - Vital signs at discharge, including temperature
  - Complete institutional sedation record to include
    - Medications given: time, name, route, site, dosage, patient effect of administered drug
    - Monitoring parameters: presedation, intraprocedure, and postprocedure
  - Interventions and child's response
  - Child's status postprocedure and as recovering from sedation
  - That discharge criteria are met and time attained
  - The discharge instructions are given and to whom

COMMUNITY CARE

- Adolescents of driving age may not drive themselves home but must be discharged with a responsible adult who will provide transportation.
- Discharge instructions for the child going home after sedation should include the following:
  - Quiet activities for 24 hours after discharge, no activities requiring coordination (e.g., bicycle riding, playground equipment); other activity restriction specific to procedure
  - Consciousness checks
  - Dietary instructions

    - Medication instructions (e.g., pain medications)
    - Medication resumption
    - Care needs associated with specific procedure completed (e.g., dressing care)
    - Signs of complications and actions to take
    - Phone number of person to contact in emergency
    - Follow-up care needed (e.g., appointments with healthcare provider)
- Instruct family to contact healthcare provider if
    - Child appears lethargic and listless
    - Child has adverse sequelae due to procedure (bleeding, pain, fever)

Unexpected Situation

- *A 9-month-old child has received sedation to complete a bone marrow aspiration procedure. During the procedure, the child becomes tachycardic, oxygen saturation drops to 85%, and capillary refill is diminished:* Complete a respiratory assessment. Open airway and provide oxygen. Reassess child. More sedation may be needed.

Bibliography

American Academy of Pediatrics, Committee on Drugs. (2002). Guidelines for monitoring and management of pediatric patients during and after sedation for diagnostic and therapeutic procedures: Addendum. *Pediatrics, 110*(4), 836–838.

American Nurses Association. (September 6, 1991). *Board of Directors policy/position, endorsement of position statement on the role of the registered nurse (RN) in the management of patients receiving IV conscious sedation for short-term therapeutic, diagnostic, or surgical procedures.* Retrieved July 11, 2006, from www.nursingworld.org/readroom/position/join/jtsedate.htm

American Society of Anesthesiologists. (2005). *Sedation model policy (amended 02/25/2005).* Retrieved [month, date, year] from http://www.asahq.org/practice/sedation/sedation1017.pdf

Cravero, J., & Blike, G. (2004). Review of pediatric sedation. *Anesthesia & Analgesia, 99,* 1355–1364.

Krause, B., & Green, S. M. (2006). Procedural sedation and analgesia in children. *Lancet, 367,* 766–780.

Lahoud, G. (2005). Conscious sedation for children. *Anaesthesia, 60*(2), 199–201.

Leitch, J., Lennox, C., & Robb, N. (2005). Recent advances in conscious sedation. *Dental Update, 32*(4), 199–200, 202–203.

Lightdale, J. (2004). Sedation and analgesia in the pediatric patient. *Gastrointestinal Endoscopy Clinics of North America, 14,* 385–399.

Matharu, L., & Ashley, P. (2005). Sedation of anxious children undergoing dental treatment. *Cochrane Database of Systematic Reviews* (3), No. CD003877.

Overley, C., & Rex, D. (2004). A nursing perspective on sedation and nurse-administered propofol for endoscopy. *Gastrointestinal Endoscopy Clinics of North America, 14,* 325–333.

Pershad, J., & Godambe, S. (2004). Propofol for procedural sedation in the emergency department. *The Journal of Emergency Medicine, 27*(1), 11–14.

Reeves, S., Havidich, J., & Tobin, D. (2004). Conscious sedation of children with propofol is anything but conscious. *Pediatrics, 114,* 74–76.

Roberts, J. (2004). Conscious sedation. *British Dental Journal, 196*(12), 731–733.

CHAPTER 106

Seizure Precautions

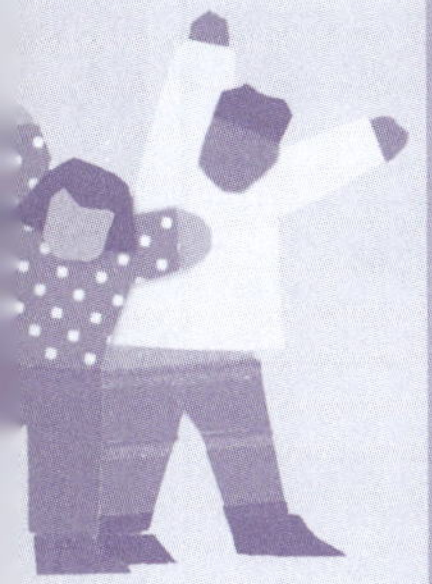

Clinical Guidelines

- A registered nurse (RN), licensed practical nurse (LPN), or unlicensed assistive personnel (UAP) may institute seizure precautions. An RN calculates weight-appropriate dosages for emergency seizure medications.
- Seizure precautions are implemented for children with
  - Known seizure disorder
  - History of seizure in the last 6 months (Chart 106-1)
  - New onset of seizures
  - Known risk for seizures from head trauma, severe electrolyte imbalance, or drug overdose
- Seizure precautions are implemented for the first 24 hours postprocedure or postsurgery on all children with a past history of seizures if the current surgery requires the use of general anesthesia, narcotics, or bowel-cleansing preparations.

Alert! *Most breakthrough seizures occur as a result of missed seizure medications. Therefore, children whose diet status is NPO should have the order written as "NPO, except for seizure medications." If the prescriber prefers nothing to be administered by mouth, then the IV route should be ordered for medications.*

Equipment

- Bed pads
- Bedside oxygen delivery equipment, including oxygen source, flowmeter, and bag-mask (size appropriate)
- Suction apparatus and suction catheters
- Pulse oximeter
- Cardiac/apnea monitor
- Seizure record
- Vital sign equipment (e.g., stethoscope, thermometer, blood pressure cuff) (see Chapters 130, 131, 133, and 134)
- Blood glucose monitor equipment (as ordered) (see Chapter 19)
- Completed emergency medication list

CHART 106-1 Seizure: The Risk of Recurrence

- Highest recurrence risk after the first unprovoked seizure is in the first year at approximately 40%.
- The rate of recurrence decreases dramatically beyond the first seizure-free year after a first unprovoked seizure. The probability for recurrent seizures in children with a first unprovoked seizure plateaus at approximately 60% after 2–3 years.
- The recurrence rate at 2 years varies by neurologic history. Only about one third of those children with previously normal cognition and motor function and no prior neurologic injury will have had a seizure recurrence after 2 years. However, in children with previously abnormal cognition or motor function, it is found that about two thirds of them will have had a seizure recurrence after 2 years.
- Almost 90% of children whose seizures recur do so within 2 years of the initial event.

Child and Family Assessment and Preparation

- Assess child's perinatal development and birth history.
- Assess child's seizure history, including
  - Type of seizures
  - Typical frequency of seizures
  - Description of events
  - Typical length of seizure events
  - Auras the child experiences before seizures

Alert! *The initial assessment and history for a first unprovoked seizure are crucial in determining baseline functioning and the diagnostic modalities selected. Focal onset seizures and seizures associated with new persistent focal deficits are more likely to be caused by intracranial lesions (tumor, stroke, abscess, vascular malformation).*

- Assess child's and family's understanding of seizures.
- Assess child's and family's understanding of current antiepileptic medications, including purpose, side effects, and importance of adherence to medication regimen.
- Explain to child and family why seizure precautions are necessary, using developmentally appropriate language (e.g., "The pad on the railing is soft, so you won't hurt yourself if you bump it.")
- Instruct the child and family to inform the nursing staff if the child senses an aura or exhibits any seizure activity.

PROCEDURE Room Preparation

Steps	Rationale/Points of Emphasis
1. Perform hand hygiene.	Reduces transmission of microorganisms.
2. Follow basic steps of room preparation (see Chapters 9 and 10).	Provides basic safety and comfort measures. Additional safety needs to be taken for the child at risk for seizure activity.
3. Select age-appropriate bed or crib (see Chapter 15).	Proper type and size of bed decreases the likelihood of falls.
4. Pad side rails.	Prevents injury in the event of patient seizure. **KidKare** If available, use colorfully decorated, child-friendly pads to help decrease child's anxiety.
5. Set up suction at bedside, including a Yankauer and appropriately sized suction catheters. Test the equipment to make sure it is working.	During the postictal period of a seizure, suction may be required to prevent aspiration.
6. Place emergency equipment, including an oxygen flowmeter, a partial rebreather, and an Ambu bag at the bedside.	Prevents wasted time locating equipment in the event that emergency measures need to be taken after prolonged seizures or if there are complications/sedation after administration of antiepileptic medications.

Steps	Rationale/Points of Emphasis
7. Keep bed in lowest position with brakes locked and side rails up.	Prevents injury if child falls from bed. Prevents bed from moving.
8. Place seizure record at bedside.	Conveniently located documentation tools allow personnel to accurately document seizure activity, which can aid in diagnosis and treatment by helping to determine what type of seizures the child is experiencing.
9. Calculate weight-appropriate dosage for emergency seizure medication and place list at bedside. List should include • Lorazepam (Ativan) • Diazepam (Valium) • Phenytoin sodium (Dilantin) • Phenobarbital	Antiepileptic medications may be administered for prolonged seizures.
10. Place child on continuous pulse oximetry and cardiac/apnea monitoring while unattended.	Provides mechanism to notify staff if child exhibits changes in heart rate, respiratory rate, or oxygenation, which may indicate seizure activity.

PROCEDURE Nursing Care During a Seizure

Steps	Rationale/Points of Emphasis
1. Protect the child's head. Lower child to the floor, if standing.	Falls to the ground or violent seizure may cause the head to hit hard surfaces.
2. Place child in side-lying position if possible. **Alert!** *If the child may have sustained a head or neck injury due to an unwitnessed fall, implement spine precautions.*	Prevents aspiration.
3. Loosen tight clothing, especially from around the neck.	Assists in maintaining an open airway.
4. Do not restrain child during a seizure.	Restraint of movements could cause injury to child or staff.
5. Do not force anything into child's mouth during a seizure.	Forcing tongue blades or other objects into the child's mouth may cause tooth loss, lacerations, vomiting, or respiratory distress.
6. Stay with the child and call for help.	Allows monitoring of child throughout seizure and arrival of other personnel as appropriate.
7. Draw bedside curtains; close doors as appropriate.	Protects the privacy of the child and the family.
8. Assess the child's airway, breathing, and circulation (ABCs) and provide support as needed.	Most seizures require minimal airway intervention (e.g., positioning to maintain a patent airway), but oxygen administration and/or bag-valve mask ventilation may be required for prolonged seizures.
9. Initiate IV access if there is none or if IV is not patent (see Chapter 56).	A seizure lasting more than 5–10 minutes will likely require administration of antiepileptic medications. Treatment after a first unprovoked seizure appears to decrease the risk of a second seizure, but there are few data from studies involving only children. The decision as to whether or not to treat children and adolescents who have experienced a first unprovoked seizure must be based on a risk–benefit assessment that weighs the risk of having another seizure against the risk of chronic antiepileptic drug (AED) therapy. **Alert!** *Obtain a finger-stick blood glucose level from any child who presents with a seizure and a persistent altered level of consciousness.*

PROCEDURE Nursing Care After a Seizure

Steps	Rationale/Points of Emphasis
1. Place child in side-lying position.	Prevents aspiration during postictal phase.
2. Suction child's mouth and nose as needed.	Prevents aspiration during postictal phase.
3. Monitor the child's vital signs and respiratory status, including breath sounds, respiratory rate, depth, and effectiveness; skin color; and pulse oximetry every few minutes until he or she regains consciousness. Measure the child's blood pressure. A finger-prick blood glucose may be ordered if the child is still seizing or is not fully alert.	Some children may have shallow ineffective breathing or may stop breathing during the postictal phase, requiring positioning to maintain a patent airway, oxygen administration, or bag-mask ventilation. Temperature readings will assist in identifying if the seizure is related to fever (febrile seizure). Children with afebrile seizures often present with systematic hypertension and/or low blood sugar. Data collected will assist in investigation of origin of seizures.
4. Adjust bed to lowest position.	Prevents falls if child is disoriented.
5. Reassure and support child and family. Encourage questions and expression of feelings regarding the event.	Seizures are a frightening experience for both the child and those who witness the event. **KidKare** Explain in simple language, "Johnny had a seizure. It is over now. Everything is okay."
6. Allow child to rest or sleep.	Children are often tired or sleepy after a seizure.
7. Perform hand hygiene.	Reduces transmission of microorganisms.

CHILD AND FAMILY EVALUATION AND DOCUMENTATION

- Evaluate child's and family's understanding of seizure event.
- Document all seizure activity descriptions on bedside seizure record, including
  - Time that seizure started
  - Duration of seizure
  - Description of seizure event
  - Aura before seizure, if present
  - Color change of skin or mucous membranes
  - Presence of incontinence
  - Postictal response
  - Level of consciousness
  - Nursing interventions and patient's response
  - Any injury to the child
- Once the bedside seizure record is full or child is discharged, place it in the medical record.

COMMUNITY CARE

- Assess the immediate environment of a child who is at risk for seizures and institute changes that will maximize safety should a seizure occur.
- Give the child and family information about managing the condition and support in the form of talking to other children with seizures. Refer the child and family to support services, such as the Epilepsy Foundation.
- It is recommended that discussion of the risk of injury be held with parents of a child after a first unprovoked seizure. Children with seizure disorders have been found to be at an elevated risk of injury during play, recreation, and activities of daily living such as bathing.
- Children with seizure disorders have been found to be at significantly elevated risk of drowning and injury. It is recommended that parents never leave children who have confirmed or suspected seizure disorders alone in a bathtub or swimming area.
- Children with seizure disorders should always wear a helmet and other protective gear when riding on bicycles, skateboards, or motorized recreational vehicles.
- Potentially suffocating bedding should be avoided (especially in younger children and infants).
- Febrile seizures are different from epilepsy; they are usually benign and do not require treatment with antiepileptic medications. Antipyretics have neither been shown to prevent nor stop febrile seizures.
- Help family identify precipitating factors such as sleep deprivation, missed medications, illness, and hypoglycemia. Encourage child to get plenty of rest, take

medications as prescribed, see a doctor with any signs of illness, and eat a balanced diet.

- Teach family members, teachers, coaches, and daycare providers about appropriate actions for the care of a child experiencing a seizure:
  - Place the child in a side-lying position during the seizure.
  - Remove any nearby objects that may cause injury.
  - Do not place anything into the child's mouth during the seizure.
  - Do not try to restrain the child.
- Instruct parents to call emergency transport if
  - Seizure does not end within 10 minutes
  - Child is not able to be aroused after a seizure
  - Child stops breathing
- Instruct the family to contact the healthcare provider if
  - Child is injured while having a seizure
  - Child is extremely irritable or has a stiff neck immediately after the seizure ends
  - The frequency, intensity, or duration of the child's seizures changes

Unexpected Situation

- *Most seizures are self-limiting and require minimal intervention. However, your patient has a seizure lasting longer than 5 to 10 minutes and does not regain consciousness:* The child is in status epilepticus. This is a medical emergency that requires immediate intensive monitoring and treatment. Stay with child and call for help. Initiate the emergency response system within your facility and notify the healthcare prescriber immediately. Assess ABCs. Maintain a patent airway and provide suctioning, oxygenation, and bag-mask ventilation as needed until further help arrives. Every few minutes, reassess ABCs. Follow procedure for nursing care during a seizure.

Bibliography

Armon, K., Stephenson, T., MacFaul, R., et al. (2003). Childhood seizure guideline: An evidence and consensus based guideline for the management of a child after a seizure. *Emergency Medicine Journal, 20,* 13–20.

Aytch, L., Hammond, R., & White, C. (2001). Seizures in infants and young children: An exploratory study of family experiences and needs for information and support. *Journal of Neuroscience Nursing, 33*(5), 278–285.

Baumer, J. (2003). Evidence based guideline for post-seizure management in children presenting acutely to secondary care. *Archives of Disease in Childhood, 89,* 278–280.

Cincinnati Children's Hospital Medical Center. (2002). *Evidence based clinical practice guideline for first unprovoked seizure for children 2 to 18 years of age.* Cincinnati, OH: Cincinnati Children's Hospital Medical Center. Retrieved September 18, 2006, from http://www.guidelines.gov

Hirtz, D., Berg, A., Bettis, D., et al. (2003). Practice parameter: Treatment of the child with a first unprovoked seizure. Report of the Quality Standards Subcommittee of the American Academy of Neurology and the Practice Committee of the Child Neurology Society. *Neurology, 60*(2), 166–175.

Marthaler, M. (2004). Critical care: Seizures revisited. *Nursing Management, 35*(4), 71–74.

Warden, C., Zibulewsky, J., Mace, S., et al. (2003). Evaluation and management of febrile seizures in the out-of-hospital and emergency department settings. *Annals of Emergency Medicine, 41,* 215–222.

Wehrle, L. (2003). Epilepsy: Its presentation and nursing management. *Nursing Times, 99*(20), 30–33.

C H A P T E R

107

Skeletal Pin Site Care

Clinical Guidelines

- Pin site care may be performed by a registered nurse (RN), licensed practical nurse (LPN), or healthcare prescriber.
- Pin site should be assessed every shift.
- Pin sites are redressed 24–72 hours after the procedure per healthcare prescriber's orders and as warranted by the amount of drainage.
- After the first 48–72 hours, pin site care is performed daily or weekly for sites with mechanically stable bone–pin interfaces.
- Showering with bacterial soap and drying the pin site with a towel or hair dryer is allowed 5–10 days after insertion.

Equipment

- Sterile gloves
- Sterile applicators
- Sterile container
- Chlorhexidine 2 mg/mL solution or swabs
- Absorbent nonstick dressing
- Sterile water
- Wrap or Ace-type compression bandage (optional)

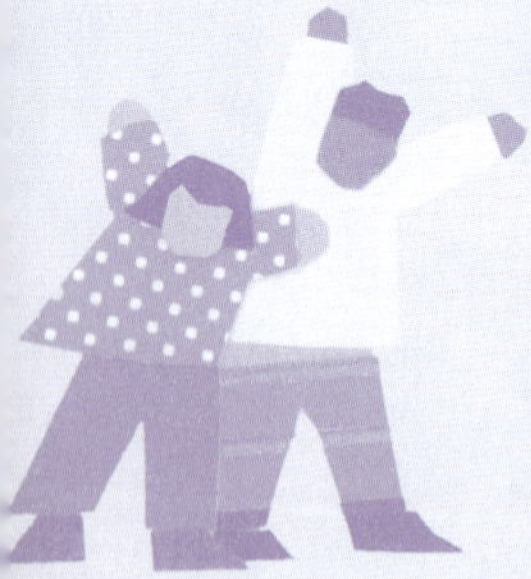

Child and Family Assessment and Preparation

- Explain the procedure you will be completing to the child and family.

KidKare Do not tell the child that he or she has a "hole" in his or her hurt extremity. Rather, use words such as "opening" or "small cut." Emphasize that the cut will heal or the opening will close quickly after the pin is taken out.

- Explain sensations the child may feel; for example, "There may be a feeling of cold when I put the cleansing solution on."
- Follow traction care guidelines (see Chapter 114) in regard to evaluation of the traction apparatus, skin, neurovascular status, and presence of pain.
- Assess for indications of infection (Chart 107-1).

CHART 107-1 THE CHECKETTS-OTTERBURNS GRADING SYSTEM

Grade	Appearance	Treatment
1	Slight redness, little discharge	Improved pin site care
2	Redness of skin, discharge, pain, and tenderness in the soft tissues	Improved pin site care, oral antibiotics
3	Grade 2 but not improved by antibiotic	Affected pin or pins resited and external fixation can be continued
4	Severe soft tissue infection involving several pins, sometimes with associated loosening of the pin	External fixation must be abandoned
5	Grade 4 but also involvement of the bone; also visible on radiographs	External fixation must be abandoned
6	This infection occurs after fixator removal. The pin track heals initially, but will break down and discharge in intervals. Radiograph shows new bone formation and sometimes sequestra.	Curettage of the pin track

From Checketts, R. (2000). Pin track infection and the principles of pin site care. In A. DeBastiani, A. Graham Apley, & D. E. Goldberg (Eds.). *Orthofix external fixation in children: Trauma and orthopaedics* (pp. 97–103). Berlin: Springer.

***Alert!** Studies indicate that pins located in areas not considered soft tissue should be considered at greater risk for infection. Higher rates of infection have been reported in femoral pins compared with tibial pins and in proximal pins when compared with lower and middle pins (Holmes, Brown, & Pin Site Expert Panel, 2005).*

- Medicating for pain is not necessary because skeletal pin site care is generally not painful. For the child who is anxious about the procedure, diversionary measures or relaxation techniques should be used (e.g., listening to selected music, watching a video).
- Allow child to watch the procedure if desired. Use of a hand mirror held by the parent may assist the child to watch the procedure and view the pin site.
- Allow the school-aged child or adolescent who is willing and able to assist in the cleaning and dressing change process. Child's physical skills and location (placement) of the pin must be considered.

PROCEDURE Caring for the Skeletal Pin Site

Steps	Rationale/Points of Emphasis
1. Gather the necessary supplies.	Promotes efficient time management and provides an organized approach to procedure.
2. Perform hand hygiene and don sterile gloves.	Reduces transmission of microorganisms. Sterile technique for the hospitalized child is recommended because the child's natural defenses against infection may be compromised during the acute phase of his or her recovery.
3. Remove the soiled pin site dressing. Place the dressing in proper receptacle.	Standard precautions for disposal of body fluids.
4. Inspect the wound site. Observe for redness, swelling, tenderness, or purulent drainage (see Chart 107–1). Notify healthcare prescriber if these signs occur.	Indicates possible infection.
5. Observe for loosening of pins.	Slippage or movement of the pins may interfere with the effectiveness of the traction. Excessive motion of the pin may result in increased drainage, which creates an environment conducive to bacterial growth and infection formation.

Continued

Steps	Rationale/Points of Emphasis
6. Observe for skin adherence to pin.	Adherence of skin may be painful and cause further tissue damage at the site.
7. Remove gloves and perform hand hygiene.	Reduces transmission of microorganisms.
8. Open sterile packages and containers. Pour cleaning solution into sterile container. Place applicators in solution.	Using sterile technique reduces transmission of microorganisms.
9. Don sterile gloves.	Standard precaution reduces transmission of microorganisms and maintains asepsis.
10. Using applicators and the chlorhexidine cleansing solution, cleanse the area starting at the insertion site and working outward away from the pin site. Use each applicator once. Remove exudates or dried crust or blood. Lightly massage area.	Studies indicate chlorhexidine solution may be more effective in preventing site infection compared with other solutions. Povidone-iodine and hydrogen peroxide at certain concentrations may be cytotoxic to osteoblasts and damaging to healthy tissue. Hydrogen peroxide at 1:10 or 1:5 concentrations may not be bactericidal. Further research is needed to determine the most effective cleansing agent. Removal of crust is recommended to allow exudate to escape from pin site, thereby preventing site contamination and abscess formation. Massage is believed to assist in preventing skin adherence to pin.
11. Leave the wound dry after cleaning.	Moisture encourages colonization of bacteria. Ointments applied to the site appear to block the normal drainage of exudates, thereby increasing the risk for infection.
12. Clean metal of pin using sterile water and sterile applicators or sterile gauze pads.	Removes bacteria and wound exudates.
13. Apply absorbent nonstick dressing to site. Apply wrap or Ace-type compression bandage if site continues to have drainage.	The dressing provides a protective barrier against airborne infection and contamination by parents' or child's hands. A dressing should be used that applies only a small amount of pressure to the site.
14. Dispose of equipment and waste in appropriate receptacle. Return reusable supplies to convenient location. Perform hand hygiene.	Standard precautions. Reduces transmission of microorganisms.
15. Notify healthcare prescriber of any unusual findings.	Communicates concerns that may need additional interventions.

Child and Family Evaluation and Documentation

- Evaluate child's and family's understanding of procedure and ability to provide self-care.
- Document the following:
  - Completion of pin site care
  - Condition of the skin, including color, discharge, tenderness, swelling, and skin adherence
  - Condition of the pin (e.g., slippage, position)
  - Neurovascular status
  - Results of pain assessment and interventions implemented to relieve pain

Community Care

- In cooperation with the family, determine which aspects of home care the parents, the child, or the home care nurse will complete.
- Have the child's home care provider demonstrate pin care before discharge as indicated.
- Provide the child and family with written instructions regarding pin care and signs and symptoms of infection.
- To clean the pin site at home, child should
  - Shower and dry the fixator with a clean towel used only for pin care purposes.
  - Actively clean the pin site only if exudates are present. Clean technique is used.
  - Loosely wrap a gauze dressing on the site after the shower.
- Review activity limitations and suggest diversionary activities for the child.
- Encourage child to eat a well-balanced diet to promote adequate healing and to prevent weight gain during this period of inactivity.
- Instruct the family to contact the healthcare provider if
  - Child has an elevated temperature
  - Pin site shows signs of redness, swelling, tenderness, or oozing secretions
  - Pin site has an odor
  - Child complains of pain at the pin site
  - Pin moves from the original site

Unexpected Situation

- *During pin site care, you note that several of the pins move and slide in the pin tract:* Assess the site for infection, including redness, swelling, tenderness, or purulent drainage. Assess child for fever and pain. Assess the extremity for neurovascular changes such as changes in circulation, temperature, and sensation. Notify healthcare prescriber of the findings.

Bibliography

Bernardo, L. (2001). Evidence-based practice for pin site care in injured children. *Orthopedic Nursing, 20*(5), 29–34.

Checketts, R. (2000). Pin track infection and the principles of pin site care. In A. DeBastiani, A. Graham Apley, & D. E. Goldberg (Eds.), *Orthofix external fixation in children: Trauma and orthopaedics* (pp. 97–103). Berlin: Springer.

Davis, P., Lee-Smith, J., Booth, J., Mann, S., Santy, J., & Kneale, J. (2001). Pin site management: Towards a consensus (Part 2). *Journal of Orthopedic Nursing, 5*(2), 125–130.

Gordon, J., Kelly-Hahn, J., Carpenter, C., & Schoenecker, P. (2000). Pin site care during external fixation in children: Results of a nihilistic approach. *Journal of Pediatric Orthopedics, 20*(2), 163–165.

Holmes, S., Brown, S., & Pin Site Care Expert Panel. (2005). Skeletal pin site care. *Orthopaedic Nursing, 24*(2), 99–107.

Lee-Smith, J., Santy, J., Davis, P., Jester, R., & Kneale, J. (2001). Pin site management: Towards a consensus (Part 1). *Journal of Orthopaedic Nursing, 5*(1), 37–42.

McKenzie, L. (1999). In search of a standard for pin site care. *Orthopedic Nursing, 18*(2), 73–78.

Moroni, A., Vannini, F., Mosca, M., & Giannini, S. (2002). State of the art review: Techniques to avoid pin loosening and infection in external fixation. *Journal of Orthopaedic Trauma, 16*(3), 189–195.

Sims, M., & Saleh, M. (2000). External fixation—the incidence of pin site infection: A prospective audit. *Journal of Orthopaedic Nursing, 4*(2), 59–63.

Sims, M., & Whiting, J. (2000). Pin site care. *Nursing Times, 96*(48), 46.

Temple, J., & Santy, J. (2004). Pin site care for preventing infections associated with external bone fixators and pins. *The Cochrane Database of Systematic Reviews,* (1), No. CD004551.

W-Dahl, A., & Toksvig-Larsen, S. (2003). The difference between daily and weekly pin site care: A randomized study of 50 patients with external fixation. *Acta Orthopaedica Scandinavica, 74*(6), 704–708.

W-Dahl, A., & Toksvig-Larsen, S. (2004). Pin site care in external fixation: Sodium chloride or chlorhexidine solution as a cleansing agent. *Archives of Orthopaedic Trauma Surgery, 124*(8), 555–558

CHAPTER

108

Stool Collection and Analysis

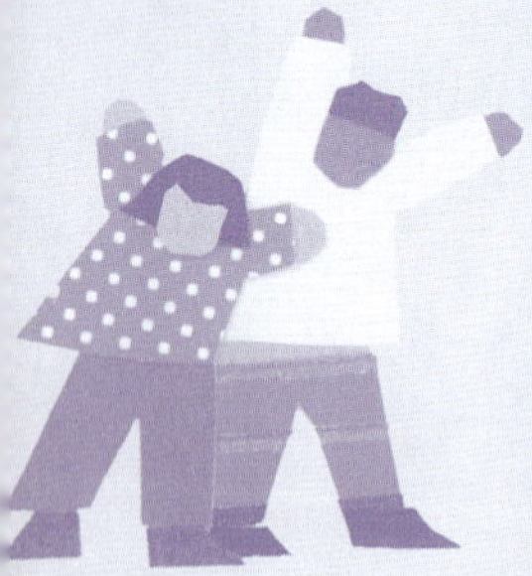

Clinical Guidelines

- A healthcare prescriber's order is required to obtain a stool specimen for bedside testing or laboratory analysis.
- A registered nurse (RN), licensed practical nurse (LPN), or unlicensed assistive personnel (UAP) who has demonstrated competency may obtain a stool specimen for analysis.
- The child should be isolated if an acute infectious gastroenteritis is suspected, although children with similar symptoms may be cohorted, if necessary.

Equipment

If obtaining a laboratory stool specimen:

- Tongue blade
- Nonsterile gloves
- Bedpan or commode specimen container, as appropriate
- Urine bag, if needed
- Specimen container with lid or swab and culture tube for laboratory specimens
- Adhesive label
- Laboratory request form
- Self-sealing plastic biohazard bag

If obtaining a rectal swab, additional equipment:

- Normal saline or broth medium
- Soap, water, and washcloth
- Rectal swab

If obtaining a stool sample by enema, additional equipment:

- Saline solution or tap-water enema

If obtaining a stool specimen for bedside testing:

- Tongue blade or other wood instrument
- Nonsterile gloves
- Diaper (for infants and children who do not have bowel and bladder control)
- Bedpan or commode specimen container (for children who have bowel and bladder control)
- Urine bag, if needed (for children who are diapered)

If testing for fecal occult blood, additional equipment:

- Hematest reagent tablet test kit or Hemoccult fecal blood test kit

If testing stool pH, additional equipment:

- pH paper and color chart

If testing stool for reducing substances, additional equipment:

- Test tube
- Clinitest tablets and color chart

CHILD AND FAMILY ASSESSMENT AND PREPARATION

- Assess pertinent history to include
  - Length of illness
  - Clinical symptoms
  - Contacts with other ill persons, particularly at home, school, or child care
  - Recent travel
  - Recent diet
  - Current medications
  - Normal and current bowel patterns
  - Recent gastrointestinal tests
- Assess the child's (when appropriate for developmental level) and family's knowledge regarding the reason for testing, method used to collect the specimen, and when to expect test results.
- Determine what terms the child and family use to describe relevant body parts and bodily functions.
- Explain the stool collection procedure to the child and family, using terms they can understand. This helps to relieve anxiety, gains patient and family cooperation with the collection procedure, and helps to avoid inadvertent disposal of stool specimen.
- Provide privacy for the child, regardless of age, during procedure and handle specimen discretely.

PROCEDURE **Obtaining a Voided Stool Specimen**

Steps	Rationale/Points of Emphasis
1. Gather the necessary supplies and perform hand hygiene.	Promotes efficient time management and provides an organized approach to the procedure. Reduces transmission of microorganisms.
2. Prelabel specimen container with the following information: patient's name, date of birth, room or patient ID number, date and time of collection, and initials of person collecting sample.	Ensures that correct test is done on the correct patient.
3. Complete a laboratory requisition slip indicating the desired tests; include any relevant patient history.	Providing relevant patient history notifies the laboratory of events or circumstances that could influence or explain test results.
4a. If stool is to be collected from a diaper, check frequently for defecation while wearing gloves.	Ensures collection of a fresh specimen, which will not be distorted by time lapse. **caREminder** *For water-loss stools, use a urine bag to collect either the urine or the stool. This prevents contamination of the stool specimen by urine, which could distort test results.*
4b. Remove soiled diaper, clean perineal area, and apply a clean diaper.	Cleaning the perineal area prevents skin irritation from the stool.
5a. Instruct the child with bowel and bladder control to notify you when having the urge to defecate and then have the child defecate in a clean dry bedpan or commode specimen container.	Ensures collection of a fresh specimen, which will not be distorted by time lapse. **KidKare** Tell child to urinate in the commode before defecating into collection container. This prevents contamination of the stool specimen by urine, which could distort test results.
5b. Have child wipe perineal area with toilet paper and wash rectal area and hands thoroughly.	Cleaning the perineal area prevents skin irritation from the stool, and hand washing prevents patient contamination.

Continued

Steps	Rationale/Points of Emphasis
	caREminder *Do not place toilet paper or paper towels in container with stool and do not allow toilet water to come in contact with stool sample. Toilet paper and paper towels contain bismuth, which interferes with test results. Toilet water also interferes with results.*
6. While wearing gloves and before transferring stool to specimen container, assess color, consistency, and odor. Also observe for foreign material, such as blood, mucus, or pus.	Observed abnormalities may give insight into possible pathology.
7. Transfer the most representative stool specimen from the diaper, bedpan, or commode container to the appropriate specimen container using tongue blade and then tightly secure the cap, being careful not to contaminate the outside of the container.	Begins preparation of the specimen for safe transport to the laboratory.
8. Wrap tongue blade in paper towel and dispose of waste in appropriate receptacle. Remove gloves and perform hand hygiene.	Standard precautions. Reduces transmission of microorganisms.
9. Place specimen container in a self-sealing biohazard bag and send, with laboratory slip, immediately to the laboratory.	Delays in stool specimen processing can adversely affect test results.
10. Perform hand hygiene.	Reduces transmission of microorganisms.

PROCEDURE Obtaining a Specimen by Rectal Swab

Steps	Rationale/Points of Emphasis
1. Gather the necessary supplies. Perform hand hygiene and don gloves. ***Alert!*** *Rectal swabbing should not be done in a child with a hematology or oncology diagnosis, immunosuppression, rectal malformation, or pelvic or rectal staged surgical procedure. Immunosuppression increases the potential for infection if the rectal mucosa tears; an area undergoing reconstruction may be damaged by swabbing.*	Promotes efficient time management and provides an organized approach to the procedure. Reduces transmission of microorganisms.
2. Prelabel specimen container with the following information: patient's name, date of birth, room or patient ID number, date and time of collection, and initials of person collecting sample.	Ensures that correct test is completed on the correct patient.
3. Complete a laboratory requisition slip indicating the desired tests; include any relevant patient history.	Providing relevant patient history notifies the laboratory of events or circumstances that could influence or explain test results.
4. Clean area around child's anus using a washcloth with soap and water.	Removes any organisms or residue that could interfere with sample collection.
5. Insert swab, moistened with normal saline or broth medium, through the anus and advance anywhere from 1 cm in infants to 4 cm in larger adolescents.	Allows for safe specimen collection.
6. Move swab side to side and keep in rectum for 30 seconds.	Allows for absorption of organisms.
7. While withdrawing swab, gently rotate against the walls of the lower rectum.	Provides a sample of a large area of the rectal mucosa.

Steps	Rationale/Points of Emphasis
8. Place swab in culture tube and secure the lid. Crush the base to release holding media, if applicable.	Begins preparation of the specimen for safe transport to the laboratory.
9. Dispose of equipment and waste in appropriate receptacle. Remove gloves and perform hand hygiene.	Standard precautions. Reduces transmission of microorganisms.
10. Place specimen container in a self-sealing biohazard bag and send, with laboratory slip, immediately to the laboratory.	Delays in stool specimen processing can adversely affect test results.
11. Perform hand hygiene.	Reduces transmission of microorganisms.

PROCEDURE Specimen Collection for Frequently Used Laboratory Tests

Steps	Rationale/Points of Emphasis
Follow the steps in the previous procedures (Obtaining a Voided Stool Specimen and Obtaining a Specimen by Rectal Swab) for specimen collection, with the following test-specific modifications:	
1. Cultures:	
a. Collect 1–2 g of stool using a sterile tongue blade into a sterile container, or use a sterile swab and place in a sterile culturette for transport.	Decreases the likelihood of contaminating the specimen.
b. Pay particular attention to history of recent travel or antimicrobial therapy.	Some diseases are endemic to particular geographic areas; recent antimicrobial therapy may decrease bacterial growth in a specimen.
c. Use a transport medium or transport the specimen to laboratory promptly.	Failure to handle specimen properly may result in loss of enteric pathogens or overgrowth of nonpathogenic organisms.
2. Rotavirus:	
a. Collect 1 g of stool in a preservative-free sterile tube or vial. If a swab is used, it must be heavily stained with stool.	Ensures an adequate sample without interfering factors.
b. Specimen may be refrigerated for up to 24 hours, if necessary.	Preserves the specimen without damage to the organisms.
3. Ova and parasites:	
a. Collect two or three specimens 1–2 days apart.	Some organisms may only be passed intermittently because of cyclic shedding.
b. Send the entire stool, whenever possible, or 30–50 mL of liquid stool. If a specially prepared kit is used, fill each container to the specified mark and follow package directions carefully.	This increases the likelihood that organisms will be discovered, when present.
c. Note whether any of the following were used within the past 7–10 days: barium, castor or mineral oil, magnesium, bismuth, antacids, anti-diarrheal agents, or antibiotics. Keep stool from coming in contact with urine or toilet water.	These agents can destroy organisms or otherwise interfere with laboratory results.
d. Pay particular attention to recent dietary and travel history as well as use of antiparasitic drugs within 2 weeks of test.	Certain parasites are common to certain countries.
e. Liquid or soft stool specimen must be kept warm and transported to the laboratory within 30 minutes. Formed stool may be placed in preservative and kept at a neutral temperature if immediate transport is not possible.	Some organisms can degrade beyond recognition in as little as 30 minutes. Excessive heat or cold can destroy parasites.
f. Oral laxatives may be used to assist in producing a stool specimen. Collection by enema or rectal swab is not appropriate.	Parasites rarely locate in the distal colon.
4. Pinworms:	
a. Collect specimen early in the morning, before patient bathes or defecates, whenever possible.	Female pinworm usually deposits ova at night.
b. Use manufacturer-made specimen kit, or place a piece of cellophane tape, sticky side out, on the end of a tongue blade and press it firmly on the anal area. Transfer tape, sticky side down, to a slide.	Pinworm ova rarely appear in the feces because the female migrates to the anus and deposits ova there.

Continued

Steps	Rationale/Points of Emphasis
5. Fecal fat:	
a. Expect child to be on a high-fat diet 1–3 days before and throughout testing.	A diet of 100 g of fat per day is recommended to make excretion of fecal lipids (steatorrhea) evident, if present.
b. Pay particular attention to recent drug history.	Certain drugs can interfere with test results.
c. Requires collection of all stools for a 72-hour period.	Consider the first stool passed by the child as the start of the collection period.
d. Do not collect stool in a waxed container.	Wax may become incorporated into the stool and interfere with test results.
e. Send each sample, as obtained, or refrigerate or freeze stool in collection container and send entire specimen to the laboratory at the end of the collection period.	Preserves the specimen without damage to the fecal lipids.
6. Gram stain (for white cells):	
a. Collect a stool specimen or rectal swab and send immediately to the laboratory.	Ensures a proper sample for testing.
b. Pay particular attention to recent history of gastrointestinal tests.	Barium may interfere with test results.
7. α_1-Antitrypsin:	
a. Send 5 g of stool promptly to the laboratory after collection.	Ensures a sufficient quantity of stool for testing.
b. Specimen may be refrigerated or frozen, if necessary.	For this test, cold temperatures do not adversely affect stool contents.
8. *Clostridium difficile* toxin assay:	
a. Send 1–2 g of stool promptly to the laboratory.	Ensures an adequate sample for testing.
9. Group B streptococcus screen:	
a. Obtain a rectal swab and transport to the laboratory in a culturette.	Provides the laboratory with an appropriate specimen.
10. Miscellaneous laboratory stool tests:	
a. Consult the laboratory to obtain information regarding stool sample size, handling requirements, and any special considerations.	Ensures that an adequate sample is obtained and handled properly.

PROCEDURE Bedside Stool Testing

Steps	Rationale/Points of Emphasis
caREminder *When using any test kit, always review package inserts and instructions before performing a test.*	
Begin with steps 1 through 6 from the first procedure (Obtaining a Voided Stool Specimen) and then:	
1. Occult blood (general):	
a. Expect child to be on a meatless high-residue diet, with no turnips or vitamin C supplements for 2–3 days before test. Pay particular attention to recent drug and dietary history.	Ensures testing accuracy by allowing for the possibility of test updates or manufacturer variations. Red meat, iron, iodine, turnips, horseradish, melons, radishes, chlorophyll, and various drugs (such as aspirin or anti-inflammatory drugs) and dyes can cause false-positive reactions. Vitamin C, charcoal, antacids, and some foods can cause false-negative results.

Steps	Rationale/Points of Emphasis
	caREminder *In neonates and newborns, meconium and transitional stools will test positive for occult blood. After birth, newborns shed maternal blood cells swallowed from amniotic fluid. When testing postpubescent girls, wait 3 days after menses has stopped before collecting a stool sample. Testing during menses can produce false-positive test results. If testing cannot be delayed, provide perineal care and then place a gauze pad or tampon (if patient has used one previously) in the vaginal orifice.*
b. Perform test immediately on freshly excreted stool.	Increases test accuracy because hemoglobin is not stable in stool.
c. Test samples from several different portions of the same specimen.	Blood from the upper gastrointestinal (GI) tract may not be evenly disbursed throughout a formed stool. Lower GI bleeding may appear primarily on the outer surface of the stool.
d. To confirm positive test results, repeat the test at least three times while child is on a proper diet and drug regimen.	A single positive test does not necessarily confirm GI bleeding.
2. Hematest reagent tablet test:	
a. After collecting stool sample and while wearing gloves, smear a bit of stool on the kit's filter paper with a tongue blade or swab.	Prepares the specimen for testing.
b. Place one reagent tablet in the center of the stool smear. Remember to close the cap tightly on the reagent tablet bottle immediately after use.	To remain effective, reagent tablets must be protected from moisture, heat, and light.
c. Add one drop of water to the tablet and allow it to soak in for 5–10 seconds. Add a second drop, allowing it to run from the tablet onto the stool specimen and filter paper.	Allows the reagent to react to the presence of occult blood.
d. After 2 minutes, the filter paper will turn blue if the test is positive for occult blood.	Will react positively to blood loss of greater than 5 mL in 24 hours. Do not read the color that appears on the tablet or filter paper after the 2-minute period.
e. Wrap the tongue blade and filter paper in a paper towel and discard. Flush remaining stool sample in commode. Remove and discard gloves. Perform hand hygiene.	Standard precautions. Reduces transmission of microorganisms.
3. Hemoccult fecal occult blood test:	
a. After collecting stool sample and while wearing gloves, open flap on slide packet and apply a thin smear of stool on the exposed filter paper in box A with a tongue blade or swab.	Prepares the specimen for testing.
b. Apply a second smear from another part of the stool specimen to the exposed filter paper in box B and then close the slide packet's cover.	Location of blood within a stool sample can vary with the location or source of the bleed.
c. Open the rear flap on the slide package and place two drops of Hemoccult developing solution on the paper over each stool smear.	Allows the reagent to react to the presence of occult blood.
d. A blue reaction will appear on this side in 30 to 60 seconds if the test is positive.	Reacts positively to blood loss of greater than 5 mL in 24 hours.
e. Wrap the tongue blade and filter paper in a paper towel and discard. Flush remaining stool sample in commode. Remove and discard gloves. Perform hand hygiene.	Standard precautions. Reduces transmission of microorganisms.
4. Stool pH:	
a. Dip one end of a strip of pH paper into freshly excreted liquid stool.	Allows paper to react to stool pH.
b. Immediately compare the resulting color change on the pH paper with the accompanying color chart.	Alkaline stool may reflect a high-protein intake. Acidic stool (pH 6.0) may reflect a high-carbohydrate diet or may be an indicator of malabsorption.
c. Wrap used pH paper in a paper towel and discard. Flush stool sample in commode. Remove and discard gloves. Perform hand hygiene.	Standard precautions. Reduces transmission of microorganisms.

Continued

Steps	Rationale/Points of Emphasis
5. Reducing substances:	
a. Mix 5 drops of freshly excreted liquid stool with 10 drops of tap water in a test tube.	Prepares the sample for testing.
b. Add one Clinitest tablet and wait for boiling to stop completely. Do not shake tube.	Allows the testing agent to react to the stool contents.
c. Once boiling action has stopped, shake the test tube and, within the next 15 seconds, compare the color of the liquid with the Clinitest color chart. Ignore the color of the resulting sediment.	The reaction to the stool's sugar content happens with the liquid, and the visible color becomes inaccurate after 15 seconds. Greater than 0.5% reducing substances indicates malabsorption of sugars.
d. Flush stool sample and material in test tube in commode. Remove and discard gloves. Perform hand hygiene.	Reduces transmission of microorganisms.

CHILD AND FAMILY EVALUATION AND DOCUMENTATION

Document the following:

- Stool color, odor, amount, consistency, and any unusual characteristics.
- For laboratory specimen:
  - Record time and method of sample collection
  - Required storage (if applicable)
  - Time of transport to the laboratory
  - Type of tests requested
- For bedside testing:
  - Record time and method of sample collection and test results
  - Note condition of skin in perineal area and document any treatment
  - Document child's tolerance of the procedure
  - Notify healthcare prescriber of any significant abnormalities found during assessment or testing
  - Resume pretest diet and medications, as appropriate

COMMUNITY CARE

- Reinforce information given by healthcare prescriber regarding test results.
- Explain any monitoring, follow-up appointments, or repeat tests that may be needed.
- Instruct child (as appropriate) and family regarding appropriate perineal skincare based on child's age and skin condition.
- For specimen collection at home, instruct child (as appropriate) and family regarding proper collection method, handling, and transport to the laboratory.
- A piece of plastic wrap can be placed under the commode seat over the commode opening to collect stool as it is being voided.
- If specimen is to be stored in the refrigerator, instruct family to keep specimen container in a paper or plastic bag, stored away from food.
- Instruct the family to contact the healthcare provider if
  - Child's condition worsens
  - Child has not received results of tests after time frame needed to complete specific test

Unexpected Situation

- *Child is menstruating or has discarded toilet paper in the commode with stool:* Contact the laboratory to discuss possible effects of these situations on test results. Not all stool samples are affected by contamination from menses blood or toilet paper.

Bibliography

Dammel, T. (1997). Looking for hidden danger: Fecal occult blood testing. *Nursing, 27*(7), 44–45.

Davis, C. E. (1996). Fresh vs. preserved stool specimens for detection of parasites. *Journal of the American Medical Association, 275*(4), 326–327.

Denno, D., Stapp, J. R., Boster, D. R., et al., (2005). Etiology of diarrhea in pediatric outpatient settings. *Pediatric Infectious Disease Journal, 24*(2), 142–148.

Koontz, F., & Weinstock, J. V. (1996). The approach to stool examination for parasites. *Gastroenterology Clinics of North America, 25*(3), 435–449.

McConnell, E. A. (1995). Testing stool for occult blood. *Nursing, 25*(6), 26.

Meropol, S. B. (1997). Yield from stool testing of pediatric inpatients. *Archives of Pediatrics & Adolescent Medicine, 151*(2), 142–145.

Peredy, T. R., & Powers, R. D. (1997). Bedside diagnostic testing of body fluids. *American Journal of Emergency Medicine, 15*(4), 400–407.

Stokamer, C., Tenner, C., Chaudhun, J., Vazquez, E., & Bini, E. (2005). Randomized controlled trial of the impact of intensive patient education on compliance with fecal occult blood testing. *Journal of General Internal Medicine, 20*(3), 278–282.

Young, G. P., Sinatra, M. A., & St. John, D. J. (1996). Influence of delay in stool sampling on fecal occult blood test sensitivity. *Clinical Chemistry, 42*(7), 1107–1108.

CHAPTER

109

Suture/Staple Removal

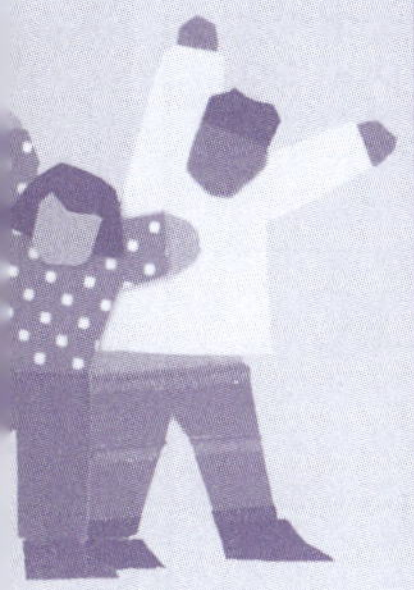

Clinical Guidelines

- The registered nurse (RN) when ordered to do so by the healthcare prescriber may perform suture/staple removal.
- The method of suture removal is determined by the suturing technique used. For instance, a running or continuous suture may need to be removed by gently pulling one end of the suture after the knot is cut. Other sutures are meant to reabsorb over time. If you are unsure of the method of suture removal, ask the physician, nurse practitioner, or physician assistant before attempting suture removal.
- Different parts of the body require suture/staple removal at different times. The general guidelines are as follows:
  - Face: 3–4 days
  - Neck: 5 days
  - Scalp: 6 days
  - Chest or abdomen: 7 days
  - Arms and back of hands: 7 days
  - Legs and top of feet: 10 days
  - Back: 10 days
  - Palms and soles of feet: 14 days
- Suture/staple removal is performed using aseptic technique.

Equipment

- Suture/staple removal kit

OR

- Sterile suture scissors/sterile stitch cutter
- Sterile forceps
- Staple remover
- Nonsterile gloves
- Adhesive strips or bandages
- Sterile saline
- Cotton swabs
- Gauze pads: 2 × 2 or 4 × 4
- Nonsterile drapes
- Adhesive solution (if needed)
- Adhesive remover (if needed)

CHILD AND FAMILY ASSESSMENT AND PREPARATION

- Determine child's and family's knowledge of the procedure.
- Explain the steps of the procedure to the child and family, and encourage questions. Having knowledge of what will occur during the procedure can decrease fear and anxiety.

KidKare Explain to the child that when the sutures are removed he or she will feel a pulling sensation as the sutures/staples are being tugged away from the skin.

- Assess for allergies to acetone if adhesive remover is to be used.
- Assess the need for pain medication, distraction methods, or child life specialist intervention before starting the procedure. Instruct the parent(s) how to provide distraction during the procedure.
- Use child life therapist to provide distraction to the child during the procedure.

KidKare Have the child demonstrate the procedure on a favorite doll or stuffed animal to help become more familiar with equipment and to reduce fear.

PROCEDURE Removing Sutures/Staples

Steps	Rationale/Points of Emphasis
1. Gather the necessary supplies.	Promotes efficient time management and provides an organized approach to the procedure.
2a. Assist the child into a comfortable position for the procedure. Be sure that the child's position does not create tension on the suture line. 2b. Drape the child so that only the suture area is exposed.	Proper positioning should facilitate patient comfort and removal of sutures/staples. Tension on the sutures will cause more pain during removal. Provides for privacy and protects the modesty of the child. **KidKare** Whenever possible, the child should be positioned so that the parent(s) can provide comfort during the procedure. Parents can provide diversionary measures to aid in the child's anxiety/pain relief. The child can be instructed to blow out through pursed lips during the procedure. If the child is extremely anxious, "proximal diversion" can be used. The RN will put pressure with the hand on an area proximal to the suture line (i.e., the upper thigh if sutures are in lower thigh) while pulling the suture out.
3. Perform hand hygiene and don gloves.	Standard precaution to reduce transmission of microorganisms.
4. Remove any dressing that may be covering site. Use adhesive remover as needed to remove old adhesive from skin.	Prepares site for cleaning.
5. Remove gloves, and discard dressing and gloves in appropriate receptacle.	Adheres to standard precautions.
6. Assess the site for redness, heat, swelling, and drainage. Note if the wound margins are well approximated. Share any abnormal findings with the physician, nurse practitioner, or physician assistant.	If the wound is not adequately healed, the sutures/staples may need to remain in place longer. Any evidence of infection may require pharmacologic intervention. **caREminder** *There may be a localized reaction to the suture material that causes some faint erythema. This is normal but must be differentiated from pathologic erythema.*

Steps	Rationale/Points of Emphasis
7. Perform hand hygiene and don gloves.	Standard precaution to reduce transmission of microorganisms.
8. Cleanse incision site with warm saline-soaked gauze. Begin at the edges of the suture site and move around the skin, making increasingly larger circles until the area that was covered by the dressing is clean. Repeat if necessary with new gauze pad.	Removes microorganisms and helps ease suture/staple removal. **caREminder** *Always wipe from clean area to dirty area; innermost area to outermost area.*
9. Remove the suture/staple in succession or skip every other one until you reach the end and then return to the top and remove the rest.	Dehiscence can be detected early, if removing every second stitch is done and then every other suture/staple can be left in place if needed.
For suture removal:	
10a. Hold forceps in nondominant hand, and use them to grasp the suture near the knot. Gently lift the knot up off the skin.	Pulls the suture up and away from the skin, while avoiding tension on the suture line. The exposed part of the suture may harbor pathogens that can trigger infection if pulled under the skin.
10b. Place the curved edge of the scissors under the suture, either directly under or near the knot (Figure 109-1). If using a stitch cutter, place the curved edge of the cutter directly under or near the knot.	Prepares suture to be cut.

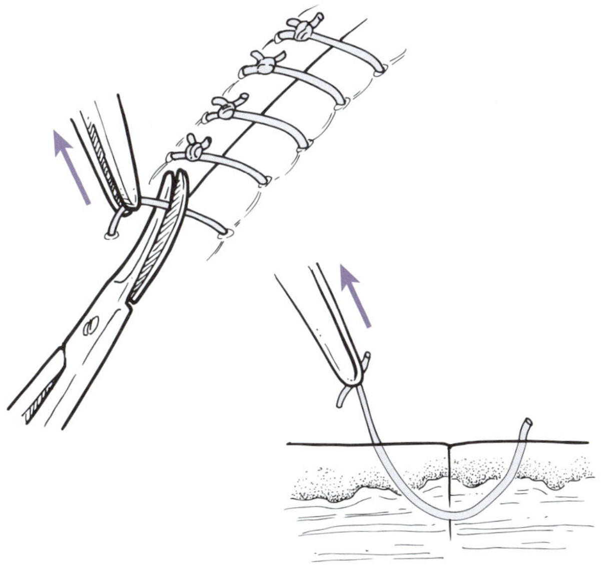

FIGURE 109-1
To begin suture removal, the curved edge of the scissors is placed under the suture, near the knot.

Steps	Rationale/Points of Emphasis
10c. Cut the suture. Pull out the suture in one piece with the forceps, and discard the sutures onto a gauze pad. If using a stitch cutter, use an upward motion away from the child's body to "slice" the stitch.	Removes suture from skin, and adheres to aseptic technique.
For staple removal:	
11a. Place the bottom of the staple remover under the center of the first staple (Figure 109-2).	Prepares staple to be removed. **caREminder** *If the staple is in at an angle, it should be straightened before attempting to remove to minimize damage to underlying tissue during the removal process.*

Continued

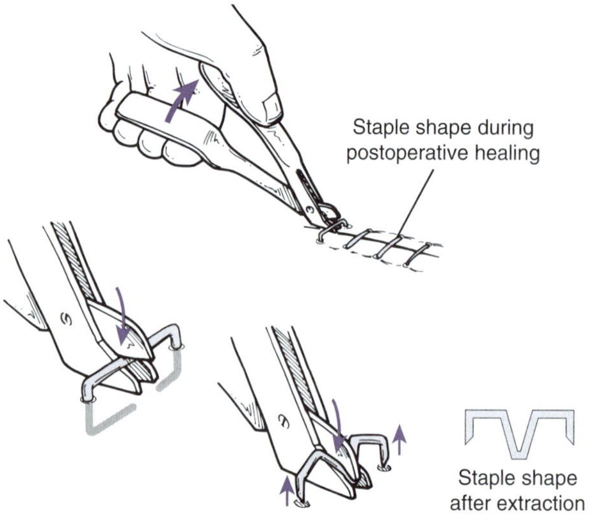

FIGURE 109-2
To begin staple removal, the bottom edge of the staple remover is placed under the center of the first staple.

Steps	Rationale/Points of Emphasis
11b. Keeping the lower jaw of the instrument against the skin, squeeze the handles of the staple remover together to close it. Lift the staple out of the skin in a swift smooth motion (there is less pain associated if the staple is removed quickly), and discard staple onto gauze pad.	Removes staple from tissue, and adheres to aseptic technique.
12. Assess the site for approximation of margins, redness, heat, swelling, and drainage. Report any abnormal findings to healthcare prescriber.	May indicate infection or incomplete healing.
13. Remove all remaining sutures/staples.	All sutures/staples should be removed after the wound is well healed.
14. If needed, cleanse incision site again with warm saline-soaked gauze. Begin at the edges of the suture site and move around the skin, making increasingly larger circles until the area that was covered by the dressing is clean. Repeat if necessary with new gauze pad.	Removes microorganisms and helps ease suture/staple removal.
15. If needed, adhesive strips (i.e., Steri-Strips) may be applied to support the suture line. These should be applied approximately ½ inch apart or closer depending on the size and location of the suture line. Adhesive solution (i.e., Mastisol) may be used to keep adhesive strips in place. Follow manufacturer's instructions for use.	May aid in wound healing. **KidKare** Depending on age, many younger children will want an adhesive bandage covering the site. A corresponding bandage can be placed on a favorite doll or stuffed animal. The child may also want to keep his or her stitches. Stitches can be placed in a sterile container with a lid and given to the child. Inform parents before giving them to the child.
16. Dispose of equipment and waste in appropriate receptacle.	Standard precautions.
17. Remove gloves and perform hand hygiene.	Reduces transmission of microorganisms.

CHILD AND FAMILY EVALUATION AND DOCUMENTATION

- Document assessment of surgical site before and after suture/staple removal including
  - Appearance of surgical site
  - Approximation of margins
  - Redness, heat, swelling, or drainage
- Communicate to the physician, nurse practitioner, or physician assistant any signs of infection (redness, swelling, odor, or exudates).

COMMUNITY CARE

- Clean technique should be used for changing dressings or adhesive bandages at home. The affected area can be washed as normal depending on other nearby accessory dressings.
- Adhesive strips should remain in place until they come off naturally. This may take longer than expected. Loose edges may be trimmed.
- Instruct family to contact healthcare provider if
  - Redness, heat, swelling, or drainage is noted from the site
  - The suture line separates or a suture comes out early
  - Child develops a fever

Unexpected Situation

- *While removing the sutures you note that a small area of the wound has not healed:* Not all stitches must be removed. If a small area remains unhealed, notify the healthcare prescriber. Then if ordered, remove sutures from the healed area only.

Bibliography

Barton, S., & American Academy of Pediatrics. (2004). *Pediatric telephone protocols: Office version 2004 edition.* Philadelphia: Lippincott Williams & Wilkins.

Hrouda, B. (2000). How to remove surgical sutures and staples. *Nursing2000, 30,* 54–55.

Kanegaye, J. T., Vance, C. W., Chan, L., & Schonfeld, N. (1997). Comparison of skin stapling devices and standard sutures for pediatric scalp laceration: A randomized study of cost and time benefits. *Journal of Pediatrics, 130,* 808–813.

Sadovsky, R. (1997). Skin stapling vs. suturing for pediatric scalp laceration. *American Family Physician, 56,* 2114.

CHAPTER

110

Toys: Distribution, Cleaning, and Storage

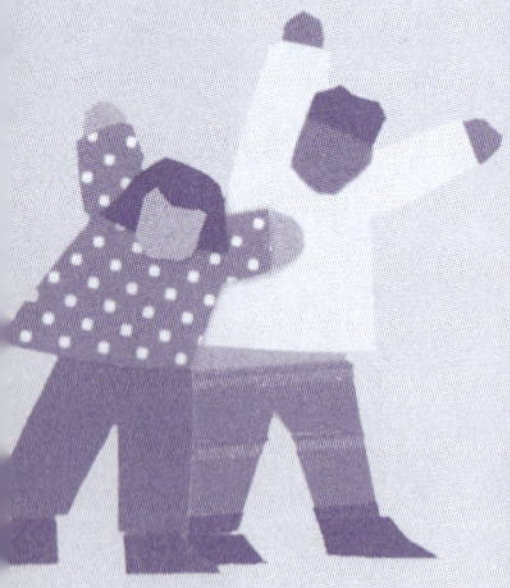

Clinical Guidelines

Distribution

- Developmentally appropriate safe toys are provided to children in the acute care and outpatient settings to be used for play activities and for therapeutic play (Chart 110-1).
- All toys in the clinical facility have property labels. Such labels designate the toy as belonging to a specific child or the property of the clinical facility.
- Infants and toddlers do not share toys because of the risk for sharing germs after toys are put in their mouths.
- Toys selected for children in diapers should be washable.

Cleaning

- Stuffed toys should be used by only a single child and washed after that child's use.
- When an infant or toddler is finished with a toy, remove the toy from the area and place in a bin reserved for dirty toys.
- Wash and disinfect dirty hard plastic toys:
  - Scrub the toy in warm soapy water; use a brush to clean out the crevices.
  - Rinse the toy in clean water.
  - Immerse the toy in a mild bleach solution and allow it to soak for 10 to 20 minutes (1:100 bleach-to-water).
  - Remove the toy from the bleach solution and rinse well in cool water.
  - Air-dry.
- If a dishwasher is available to use, then do not need to use above disinfection treatment.
- Wash stuffed or cloth toys in the hot water cycle of a washing machine; no additional disinfection treatment is needed. Stuffed toys used by a single child should be cleaned in a washing machine every week or more frequently if soiled.

caREminder

Placing stuffed toys in a pillowcase and knotting the ends before placing in the washing machine will cause less damage to the toy.

- Toys and equipment used by older children (and not placed in their mouths) should be cleaned weekly or more frequently if soiled. A soap-and-water wash followed by clear-water rinsing and air-drying is adequate. No disinfection is required unless the child has an infectious process.

CHART 110-1 SELECTING SAFE TOYS FOR ALL AGES

Do not choose

- Toys and objects with easily dislodged parts that fit in an infant's or toddler's mouth
- Toys and objects with parts smaller than 1¼ inches in diameter and 2¼ inches in length
- Toys with sharp points and edges
- Toys with loose string, rope, ribbons, or cords
- Toys that make loud noises or shrilling sounds
- Coins
- Marbles
- Plastic bags or Styrofoam objects
- Rubber balloons
- Safety pins

Do choose toys that are

- Age appropriate
- Made of nontoxic materials
- Washable
- Creative and engaging

Storage

- Store toys in an area that is easily accessible to staff. Toys should not be stored so that they directly contact the floor; rather, use storage baskets and bins to place toys in areas out of reach of children.

EQUIPMENT

- Age-appropriate toys
- Mechanism to place property labels on all toys
- Warm soapy water
- Cleaning brush
- Ten percent bleach solution
- Storage area for toys
- Dishwasher (if possible)
- Washing machine (if possible)

CHILD AND FAMILY ASSESSMENT AND PREPARATION

- Assess child's chronologic age and developmental milestones achieved.
- In discussion with the child and parents, determine the types of toys the child is interested in playing with.
- Ensure that the toys the child brought from home are appropriately labeled with his or her name.
- Review with the child and parents safety issues and use rules associated with toys and equipment to be used by the child (e.g., child may not take the toy home, all pieces of a toy must be returned, child should not place toys in mouth).

CHILD AND FAMILY EVALUATION AND DOCUMENTATION

- Evaluate appropriateness of toy for child.
- Document parental education about toy safety, cleaning, and storage.

COMMUNITY CARE

- Provide parents with recommendations for safe inexpensive toys appropriate for the age and developmental level of the child.
- Encourage thoughtful creative parental selection of toys and discourage the belief that a toy must be trendy or expensive.
- Discourage the purchase of toys for children as bribes and remind parents that their positive attention and interaction are the most effective rewards to encourage good behavior.
- Caution parents about being influenced by the marketing of toys that purport to contribute in a specific manner to the development, especially intellectual or motor development, of infants and young children.
- Provide parents advice as requested regarding safe and unsafe toys.
- Instruct parents to periodically check toys for pieces coming off (eyes) or chipping of plastic or metal parts.
- Provide parents the contact number for the Consumer Product Safety Commission (800-638-2772) and have available current list of recalled toys.
- Emphasize to parents that toys can never substitute for appropriate interactions between the child and parent or caregiver.
- Discuss with parents methods to clean toys.
- Display posters from the American Academy of Pediatrics and the Consumer Product Safety Commission regarding age-appropriate toys and safety recalls.

Unexpected Situation

- *When you enter the room of a 7-month-old, you note he has thrown toys on the floor. The mother has begun to pick them up and place them back in the crib. Meanwhile, the toddler in the next bed space is walking around the room and is also picking up some of the toys off of the floor:* Discuss with the parents of both children the importance of ensuring that each child has his or her own set of toys and that the toys should not be shared with other children to reduce toy-associated spread of infection. Instruct the mother of the infant to wash the toys before placing them back in the crib as it is likely the child will take the "dirty" toys and place them in his mouth, thus also increasing incidence of transmission of microorganisms.

Bibliography

All Family Resources. (1999). *Washing and disinfecting toys.* Retrieved April 25, 2005, from http://www.familymanagement.com/childcare/practices/washing.toys.practices.html

Avila-Aguero, M., German, G., Paris, M., Herrera, J., & the Safe Toys Group. (2004). Toys in a pediatric hospital: Are they a bacterial source? *American Journal of Infection Control, 32*(5), 287–290.

Glassy, D., Romano, J., & the Committee on Early Childhood, Adoption, and Dependent Care. (2003). Selecting appropriate toys for young children: The pediatrician's role. *Pediatrics, 111*(4), 911–913.

Goodson, B., & Bronson, M. (2002). *Which toys for which child: A consumer's guide for selecting suitable toys, ages birth through five.* Washington, DC: Consumer Product Safety Commission. Retrieved April 25, 2005, from http://www.cpsc.gov/cpscpub/pubs/ 285.pdf

Stephenson, M. (2005). Danger in the toy box. *Journal of Pediatric Health Care, 19*, 187–189.

CHAPTER

111

Tracheostomy: Stoma Care and Management

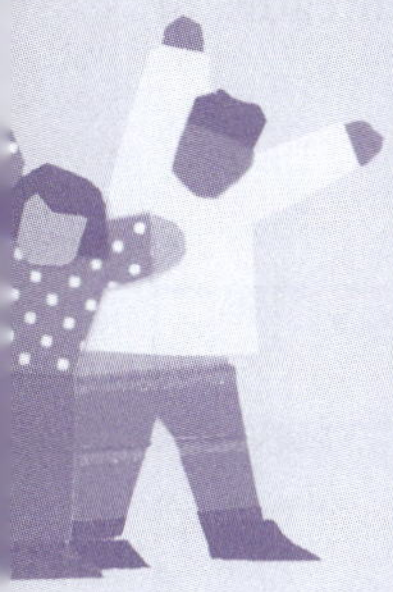

Clinical Guidelines

- The registered nurse (RN), licensed practical nurse (LPN), respiratory therapist, or parent or caregiver performs tracheostomy care, including suctioning, tie change, and stoma care as needed to provide safe effective management of the airway.
- An assistant is always present when tracheostomy care is performed.
- A comprehensive oral hygiene program (per facility policy) is provided daily to the child with a tracheostomy.
- Stoma care is be provided every shift and more frequently based on the clinical assessment and individual characteristics of the child, including:
  - Age
  - Muscular and neurologic status
  - Activity level
  - Ability to generate an effective cough
  - Viscosity and quantity of mucus
  - Maturity of the stoma
- Cleaning of the fresh stoma should be completed every 8 hours or more frequently if indicated by the accumulation of secretions.
- After tracheostomy tube placement, stoma integrity and the area under the tracheostomy ties are assessed every 2 hours for the first 48 hours and then every 8-hour shift.
- The frequency of tracheostomy tie changes varies from child to child based on the particular type of tie (twill tape, Velcro tie, or stainless steel beaded metal chain) and the condition of the tie (e.g., unraveling ends, soiled or wet ties).
- Care and management techniques may vary based on the setting of the child.
  - Sterile technique (sterile catheters, sterile dressings, sterile gloves) or a modified clean technique (sterile catheters, nonsterile gloves and sterile dressings) is used in the acute care and outpatient settings per institutional policies.
  - Clean technique (clean catheters, nonsterile dressings and nonsterile disposable gloves or freshly washed clean hands) is used in the home, school, and other community settings.
- Equipment is available at the bedside at all times for suctioning, ventilatory breaths, and recannulation.
  - The tracheostomy obturator and a tracheostomy tube of the same type and size as being used by the child remain in a visible or readily accessible location at all times.

- Before discharge, two adults, who will be consistent caregivers to the child, are trained in all aspects of the child's care.

EQUIPMENT

For stoma cleaning and outer and inner cannula cleaning:

- Shoulder roll—diapers or small rolled towel
- Gloves (sterile or nonsterile, depending on type of technique used)
- Appropriate protective gear (gown and face shield)
- Gauze or cotton swab applicators
- Towel (sterile or clean, depending on type of technique used)
- Hydrogen peroxide solution (1.5%)
- Sterile or clean cup to soak inner cannula
- Soft sterile brush or sterile pipe cleaners
- Water (sterile or clean, depending on type of technique used)
- Washcloth
- Split gauze dressing (sterile or nonsterile, depending on type of technique used)

For changing tracheostomy ties:

- Scissors
- Split gauze dressing
- Twill tape, Velcro ties, or stainless steel beaded metal chain (rarely used)
- Appropriate protective gear (gown and face shield)
- Stethoscope
- Manual ventilation bag (as needed for ventilatory breaths)
- Suction equipment (as needed) (see Chapter 112)
- Oxygen source (if needed)

For use in emergencies:

- Extra obturator
- Extra tracheostomy tubes of same size as being used by the child and one a size smaller
- Suction equipment (see Chapter 112)
- Manual ventilation bag (as needed for ventilatory breaths)

CHILD AND FAMILY ASSESSMENT AND PREPARATION

- Assess chart for previous history of child's condition, current healthcare status, and for a summary of care needs in relation to tracheostomy.

> **Alert!** *Maintenance of adequate hydration is of utmost importance in a child with a tracheostomy to prevent crusting and secretions around the trachea.*

- Explain the procedure to the child and the family.
- Determine family's ability to perform procedure and, if appropriate, have family perform this procedure.
- Determine the need for distraction measures to be implemented with the child to enhance cooperation during the procedure.
- Assess condition of the stoma for redness, swelling, character of secretions, granulation, presence of purulence, or bleeding.
- Assess the condition of the skin under the tie area.
- Assess neck range of motion.
- Assess child's breath sounds and work of breathing.
- Suction the child before initiating tracheostomy care (see Chapter 112).
- Ensure that equipment is available at the bedside for use if child requires suctioning, ventilatory breaths, or recannulation.

PROCEDURE Preprocedural Care

Steps	Rationale/Points of Emphasis
1. Perform hand hygiene.	Reduces transmission of microorganisms.
2. Gather the necessary supplies. Assemble near child's bed. Select the type of tie material to be used.	Promotes efficient time management and provides an organized approach to the procedure. A potential problem with twill tape is unraveling of the ends of ties or accidental unraveling of the knots used to secure the twill tape. Twill tape may trap moisture and irritate the skin. Velcro ties degrade over time, especially when washed in hot water. One-person tie changes are easier with the Velcro ties than with other materials. Velcro ties are wider than other ties and thus have less tendency to abrade the skin. Velcro ties are easily adjustable. Stainless steel beaded chain does not trap moisture. Tie changes are required less frequently. Because beaded chains hook in the same position every time, they maintain a consistent tension. The chain may not be used with all tracheostomy tubes because it is threaded across the anterior neck between the flanges of the tracheostomy tube.

Steps	Rationale/Points of Emphasis
Alert! *There is concern that young children may pull Velcro ties apart, leading to accidental decannulation. This type of tie may not be indicated for young active children.*	
3. Open sterile supplies (if used).	Healed tissue is less susceptible to infection. **caREminder** *If this is not a new tracheostomy, the procedures may be done using a modified clean procedure as opposed to a sterile procedure.*
4. Position child in supine position with neck slightly extended. Place rolled towel or diaper under child's shoulders.	Straightens airway and optimizes path for removal and placement of tracheostomy. Slightly extends neck for optimal positioning, bringing tracheostomy tube forward.
5. Don appropriate protective gear and gloves.	Face shield should be used if the child is infectious or has copious secretions that may come into contact with the caregiver. Reduces transmission of microorganisms.

PROCEDURE Cleaning the Stoma and Outer Cannula

Steps	Rationale/Points of Emphasis
1. Cleanse the external end of the tracheostomy tube (outer cannula) with peroxide-soaked gauze sponge. Make only one sweep with each gauze pad before discarding.	Removes mucus and crusts on tracheostomy tube.
2. Clean the stoma area with peroxide-soaked gauze sponges. Make only one sweep with each gauze pad before discarding.	Hydrogen peroxide will assist in loosening dry crusts.
3. Utilize sterile cotton swab applicators to loosen and remove crusts from the stoma site.	Assists in loosening and removal of dry crusts.
4. Clean the stoma area with sterile water-soaked gauze sponges. Make only one sweep with each gauze pad before discarding.	Ensures that all hydrogen peroxide is removed.
5. Clean the stoma area with dry gauze sponges. Make only one sweep with each gauze pad before discarding.	Ensures dryness of the area. Wetness will promote infection and skin irritation.
6. Use water-soaked gauze pads or a washcloth to cleanse neck, under the ties.	Maintains cleanliness of skin and helps to prevent skin breakdown.
7. Dry the neck area with dry gauze pads or towel.	Moisture under the ties will increase bacterial growth and cause skin irritation.

PROCEDURE Cleaning the Inner Cannula

Steps	Rationale/Points of Emphasis
1. Remove the inner cannula (Figure 111-1).	Inner cannulas designed for reuse can be removed for cleaning.
2. If the inner cannula is reusable, clean the cannula by soaking and scrubbing it in a sterile or clean cup of half-strength hydrogen peroxide solution. Use a soft sterile brush (for metal cannulas) or sterile pipe cleaners to remove all secretions from the inner cannula.	Cleanses encrusted secretions from the lumen of the cannula. Use of a brush may damage plastic inner cannulas.

Continued

Steps	Rationale/Points of Emphasis

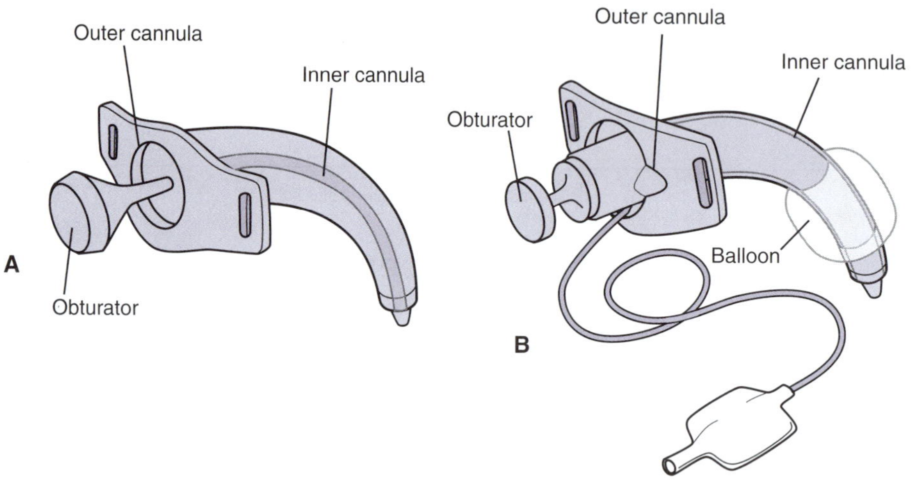

FIGURE 111-1 Parts of the tracheostomy tube. (**A**) Uncuffed. (**B**) Cuffed.

Steps	Rationale/Points of Emphasis
3. Rinse the cannula with sterile water.	Removes remaining debris and hydrogen peroxide solution from cannula.
4. Reinsert the cannula. • Turn the cannula 90 degrees from its usual orientation. Introduce the tip into the stoma, and slowly advance the cannula while rotating it back 90 degrees to its final orientation. • Lock the cannula into place by either pushing it in or twisting or squeezing the clips and clipping the cannula to the tracheostomy per the manufacturer's instructions.	Locking mechanism is used to prevent accidental removal.

PROCEDURE Changing Tracheostomy Ties

Steps	Rationale/Points of Emphasis
1. Cut old ties while holding tracheostomy tube securely in place.	Decreases chance of accidentally dislodging tracheostomy. Minimizes irritation and coughing due to tube manipulation. A second person is recommended to assist by holding the tracheostomy tube.
2. Remove the old ties carefully and replace the tracheostomy ties. • Twill ties ▪ Grasp slit end of clean tape and thread one end through the opening on the side of the tracheostomy tube. ▪ Pull other end of tape securely through the slit end of the tape. ▪ Repeat on the other side. ▪ Tie tapes with a square knot on the side or back of the neck. • Manufactured Velcro ties (Figure 111-2) ▪ Grasp end of Velcro tie and thread through opening on the side of the tracheostomy tube. Use Velcro tab to secure the tie to itself. ▪ Bring the loose end of the tie around the back of the neck. Thread the end of the tie through the opening on the other side of the tracheostomy tube. Use Velcro tab to secure the tie to itself. ▪ Adjust right and left Velcro tabs as needed to ensure that tie is on securely.	Keeping the neck area as clean and dry as possible helps to prevent skin breakdown. Tying the tie too tightly may lead to skin breakdown and vascular obstruction. Tying too loosely may lead to decannulation. **caREminder** *The securing tie should be tight enough for an adult to slip one finger under the tie easily.*

Steps	Rationale/Points of Emphasis
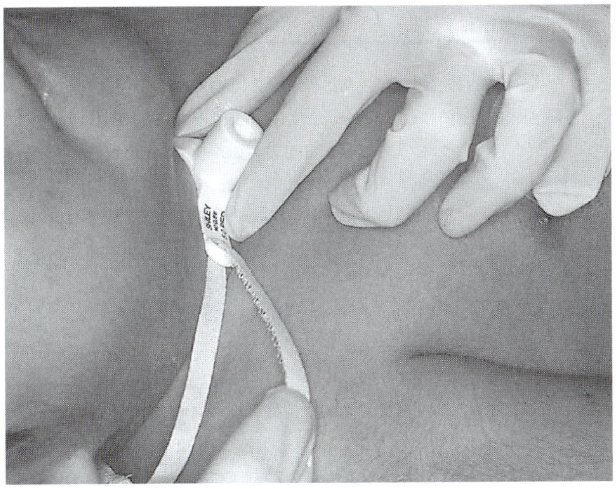 **FIGURE 111-2** Tying the tie too tightly may lead to skin breakdown and vascular obstruction. Tying too loosely may lead to decannulation.	
3. If split gauze dressing is ordered as dressing under outer cannula, secure in place.	A dressing may not be used around the stoma because many clinicians believe that the dressing keeps the area moist and dark, promoting stomal infections. A dressing is recommended if the child has increased secretions or if secretions are draining onto subclavian or neck intravenous sites or other dressings in the neck region. **caREminder** *Use prepackaged split gauze, rather than cutting gauze to split yourself. Cutting gauze to split it may allow threads from the gauze to pull away and become lodged in the trachea.*
4. Dispose of all used equipment, protective gear, and gloves in appropriate disposal receptacles. Perform hand hygiene.	Standard precautions. Reduces transmission of microorganisms.
5. Remove shoulder roll and place child in position of comfort with head elevated 30 degrees.	This position facilitates ease of breathing.

CHILD AND FAMILY EVALUATION AND DOCUMENTATION

- Evaluate child's tolerance of the procedure.
- Document the following:
  - Date and time of procedure
  - Child's tolerance of the procedure
  - Any difficulties encountered while performing care
  - Use of oxygenation during the procedure
  - Quality of breath sounds before and after procedure
  - Appearance of stoma and skin under ties (irritation, redness, edema, subcutaneous air)
  - Character of secretions (color, consistency, odor)
  - Type of tracheostomy tie used
  - Presence of dressing around stoma site
  - Teaching completed with the child and the family and their response to the teaching
  - Involvement of the family in completing the procedure
- Report changes in stoma appearance or secretions to the physician.

COMMUNITY CARE

- Provide the caregivers in the home/school with the knowledge, skills, and equipment to manage care of the child with a tracheostomy tube (Chart 111-1).

CHART 111-1 TRACHEOSTOMY TRAINING FOR CAREGIVERS: KNOWLEDGE, SKILLS, AND EQUIPMENT

The family will be able to demonstrate the following outcomes:

1. Explain the basic anatomy of the trachea and its relationship to adjoining structures.
2. Explain the rationale for tracheostomy and the status of the airway in this child.
3. State elements of respiratory assessment and signs of illness; demonstrate counting of respiratory rate and apical heart rate. Signs of illness may include:
   - Change in amount, color, odor, or consistency of secretions
   - Change in respiratory rate or rhythm
   - Increased respiratory effort
   - Diaphoresis
   - Color change
   - Hemoptysis
   - Fever
4. State actions to be taken in the event of tube obstruction, accidental decannulation, and bleeding. State that tube obstruction is the most common cause of severe respiratory distress in the child with a tracheostomy and must be treated as an emergency; when in doubt: change the tracheostomy tube!
5. Keep an emergency travel kit with the child containing the following supplies:
   - Manual resuscitation bag of appropriate size
   - Suction source
   - Suction catheter
   - Delee suction traps
   - One tracheostomy tube of current size with ties in place
   - One tracheostomy tube that is one size smaller with ties in place
   - Extra ties
   - Shoulder roll
   - A 15-mm adapter for children with metal tracheostomy tubes
   - Suction catheter that can be used if necessary to guide new tube through stoma into tract
   - Scissors
   - Emergency phone numbers
   - Brief description of medical history
   - Description of airway status (i.e., does anatomy preclude oral or nasal intubation and/or ventilation through upper airway?)

   Have contents of the bag checked at least annually by the health care team and updated as needed.
6. Demonstrate cardiopulmonary resuscitation (CPR). Instruction in CPR should include bag-to-tracheostomy ventilation, as well as mouth-to-mouth with stoma occlusion in a child with a patent upper airway.
7. Notify the local emergency services and ascertain their ability to provide services to this child. Verify that telephone services and electricity are available in the home.
8. State the type and size of tracheostomy tube; name the parts of the tube and purpose of each part; demonstrate use of the cuff and state guidelines for its use. If a fenestration is present, understand the emergency implications of this type of tube.
9. State the importance of humidification and method of delivery and demonstrate care of the equipment.
10. Assess the need for suctioning. Demonstrate proper technique for suctioning, cleaning the inner cannula, and cleaning suction equipment. Use premarked catheters and twirl the catheter between the fingertips during suctioning. State indication for lavage and demonstrate lavage technique. The home care suction machine should also operate on a battery source.
11. Assemble supplies and demonstrate a tracheostomy tube change:
    a. Check tube integrity and flexibility; check cuff integrity (if present).
    b. Place obturator in a new tube (if used).
    c. Suction child's tracheostomy tube.
    d. Position child with neck in slight extension, using a small roll under shoulders.
    e. Deflate cuff (if present).
    f. Cut strings or detach ties.
    g. Remove the tube in an upward and outward arc.
    h. Insert a new tube in a downward, inward arc.
    i. Immediately remove the obturator (if used).
    j. Reposition the child in a neutral position by removing the shoulder roll.
    k. Secure ties.
    l. Inflate cuff (if used).
    m. Lock inner cannula in place.

    Ideally, two trained adults should be present for the tube change; special circumstances may exist in a home with a single parent.
12. State the principles of skin care. Prevention is the key to skin care in the tracheostomy patient. State that the primary principles of skin care are to keep the skin clean and dry and to avoid pressure necrosis. Regular daily cleansing is performed with soap and water. A solution, such as 1.5% hydrogen peroxide, can be used to remove encrusted secretions.

CHART 111-1 TRACHEOSTOMY TRAINING FOR CAREGIVERS: KNOWLEDGE, SKILLS, AND EQUIPMENT (CONTINUED)

After its use, the skin is cleansed with water and dried thoroughly. The peristomal area and the neck skin are carefully inspected daily. Children who are mechanically ventilated or infants with short, fat necks are at risk for infection and pressure necrosis and require even more meticulous care. Products such as Duoderm can be used to cushion the skin beneath the tracheostomy ties. Soft tracheostomy ties may be less irritating than strings. The routine use of ointments and creams is avoided. Petroleum-based products are contraindicated. Dressings, if used, should promote the movement of moisture away from the skin. In the early postoperative period, if dressings are used, they should be loose and nonocclusive.

13. Discuss and implement safety measures. Child and parents will attempt to avoid all dust, smoke, lint, pet hair, powder, sprays, and small toys and objects. The child should not be in contact with fuzzy toys, clothes, or bedding. Contact sports and water sports are not permitted. The child may be bathed in 1–2 inches of water with a trained caretaker in attendance. Showers may be permissible for older children.
14. Discuss and implement infection control practices. Care practices include
    - Proper handwashing before and after procedure
    - Cleaning and disinfecting all equipment and supplies:
        a. Clean with detergent and water.
        b. Follow with 60-minute soak in a solution of vinegar and water with an acetic acid content ≥ 1.25% or quaternary ammonium compound or glutaraldehyde.
    - Proper storage of equipment and supplies between use
    - Proper disposal of used supplies and infectious waste
15. Be aware of, and participate in, goals and plans for feeding program, occupational therapy, physical therapy, and speech therapy.
16. Be aware of, and participate in, the plan for return to school/classroom and any out-of-home arrangements, such as day care. Children who are most at risk for a serious episode of tracheostomy obstruction are younger children who do not yet attend school. However, in older, school-aged children who have a critical airway in which the risk for obstruction is high, a trained caregiver should be in attendance throughout transport to and from school and while child is attending school.
17. Be aware of monitoring needs, if prescribed. Be able to operate the monitor correctly and to act on the information it provides.
18. Be aware of projected decannulation plan.
19. Discuss the plan for follow-up care with the parents/caregivers.

Information from American Thoracic Society. (2000). Care of the child with a chronic tracheostomy. *American Journal of Respiratory and Critical Care Medicine, 16*(1), 297–308; and McInturff S., Make B., Robart, P., & Saposnick, A. (1999). AARC clinical practice guidelines: Suctioning of the patient in the home. *Respiratory Care, 44*(1), 99–104.

KidKare A doll or mannequin with a tracheostomy can be used for practice. Role-playing helps to reinforce skills and basic confidence. When possible and appropriate, siblings should participate in the teaching program.

- Ensure home/school caregivers are instructed in cardiopulmonary resuscitation techniques including bag to tracheostomy ventilation and mouth to mouth with stoma occlusion in a child with a patent upper airway.
- Arrange for the caregivers in the home to participate actively in all aspects of the tracheostomy tube suctioning and tie change before discharge from the acute care setting. Provide family with opportunity for a rooming-in period before discharge to ensure that they feel comfortable with the child's care needs. A day pass to the home may also be considered.
- Ensure that all home care equipment, including portable equipment, is used in the hospital before discharge.
- Provide the family with the location of a local vendor or supplier of tracheostomy equipment.
- Instruct the family to contact the healthcare provider if
    - Tracheostomy tube becomes displaced
    - Child develops a fever
    - Child is having an increased amount and frequency of mucus production
    - Mucus is green or dark in color and/or is foul smelling
    - Child develops signs of skin breakdown around tube site or under tracheostomy ties
    - Child has sustained period of increased respirations or decreased respirations
    - Blood is present in the tracheal secretions

Unexpected Situation

- *While changing tracheostomy ties, child starts to kick and move his or her arms. The tracheostomy tube becomes dislodged:* A spare tracheostomy and obturator should be kept at the bedside. The obturator is inserted into the new tracheostomy. Reinsert the tracheostomy into the stoma. Remove obturator. Secure the ties. Assess child's respiratory status, ensuring breath sounds present bilaterally. Notify healthcare prescriber of tube dislodgement and reinsertion of new tracheostomy.

Bibliography

American Thoracic Society. (2000). Care of the child with a chronic tracheostomy. *American Journal of Respiratory and Critical Care Medicine, 16*(1), 297–308.

Pate, M., & St. John, R. (2004). Placement of endotracheal and tracheostomy tubes. *Critical Care Nurse, 24*(3), 13–14.

Russell, C. (2005). Providing the nurse with a guide to tracheostomy care and management. *British Journal of Nursing, 14*(8), 428–433.

Smith, J., Williams, J., & Gibbin, K. (2003). Children with a tracheostomy: Experience of their carers in school. *Child: Care, Health and Development, 29*(4), 291–296.

Sole, M., Byers, J., Ludy, J., & Ostrow, C. (2002). Suctioning techniques and airway management practices: Pilot study and instrument evaluation. *American Journal of Critical Care, 11*(4), 363–368.

Sole, M., Poalillo, F., Byers, J., & Ludy, J. (2002). Bacterial growth in secretions and on suctioning equipment of orally intubated patients: A pilot study. *American Journal of Critical Care, 11*, 141–149.

St. Clair, J. (2005). A new model of tracheostomy care: Closing the research-practice gap. *Advances in patient safety: From research to implementation.* Volume 3, AHRQ Publication Nos. 050021 (1–4). February 2005. Rockville, MD: Agency for Healthcare Research and Quality. Retrieved October 6, 2006, from http://www.ahrq.gov/ qual/advances/

Tablan, O. C., Anderson, L. J., Besser, R., Bridges, C., & Hajjeh, R. (2004). Guidelines for preventing health-care–associated pneumonia, 2003: Recommendations of CDC and the Healthcare Infection Control Practices Advisory Committee. *MMWR Morbidity and Mortality Weekly Report, 53*(RR-3), 1–36.

Tamburri, L. (2000). Care of the patient with a tracheostomy. *Orthopedic Nursing, 19*(2), 49–60.

Wilson, M. (2005). Tracheostomy management. *Paediatric Nursing, 17*(3), 38–43.

C H A P T E R

112

Tracheostomy: Suctioning

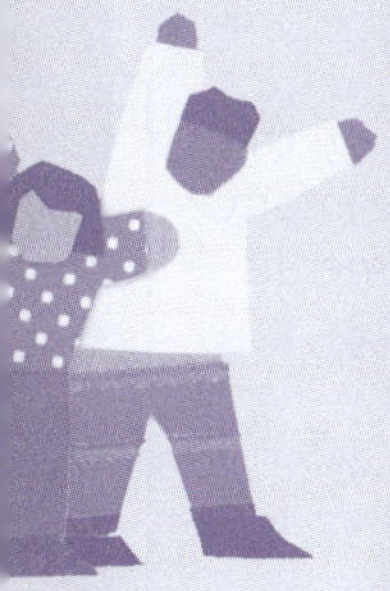

Clinical Guidelines

- The registered nurse (RN), licensed practical nurse (LPN), respiratory therapist (RT), and parent or caregiver may perform tracheostomy care, including suctioning, tie change, and stoma care, as needed to provide safe effective management of the airway (see Figure 111-1).
- Suctioning is performed on the basis of clinical assessment and individual characteristics of the child:
  - Age
  - Muscular and neurologic status
  - Activity level
  - Ability to generate an effective cough
  - Viscosity and quantity of mucus
  - Maturity of the stoma
- Perform suctioning if the child exhibits difficulty in breathing, if there is the sound of mucus in the tracheostomy tube that cannot be removed by coughing, or when there are adventitious breath sounds.
- In children with no evidence of secretions, institute a minimum of suctioning, at morning and bedtime, to check patency of the tube.
- Suctioning techniques may vary based on the setting of the child.
  - Sterile technique (sterile catheters, sterile dressings, sterile gloves) or a modified clean technique (sterile catheters, nonsterile gloves and sterile dressings) is used in the acute care and outpatient settings per institutional policies.
  - Clean technique (clean catheters, nonsterile dressings and nonsterile, disposable gloves or freshly washed clean hands) is used in the home, school, and other community settings.
- Premarked suction catheters are recommended to ensure insertion of the catheter to the proper depth.
- Routine instillation of normal saline in the tracheostomy tube would not be initiated to stimulate cough, to loosen or thin secretions, or to serve as a vehicle to remove mucus.
- Equipment is available at the bedside at all times for suctioning, ventilatory breaths, and recannulation.
  - The tracheostomy obturator and a tracheostomy tube of the same type and size being used by the child remain with the child in a visible or readily accessible location at all times.
- Before discharge, two adults, who will be consistent caregivers to the child, are trained in all aspects of the child's care.

EQUIPMENT

- Shoulder roll—diapers or small rolled towel
- Suction machine
- Suction catheter (sterile or clean, based on type of technique used)
- Collection container for secretions
- Sterile normal saline
- Sterile and clean gloves
- Appropriate protective gear (gown and face shield)
- Water (sterile or clean based on type of technique used)
- Manual ventilation bag (as needed for ventilatory breaths)

CHILD AND FAMILY ASSESSMENT AND PREPARATION

- Assess chart for previous history of child's condition and for a summary of care needs in relation to tracheostomy.
- Assess child's breath sounds and work of breathing.
- Explain the procedure to the child and the family.
- Determine family's ability to perform procedure and, if appropriate, have family perform this procedure in your presence.
- Determine the need for distraction measures to be implemented with the child to enhance cooperation during the procedure.

PROCEDURE Performing Suctioning

Steps	Rationale/Points of Emphasis
1. Verify that the gauge on the suction machine or manometer is set between 80 and 100 mm Hg and that the suction equipment is attached appropriately to the suction machine and the collection container for secretions.	Pressure that is too great may cause a change in the negative pressure of the lungs, leading to pneumothorax.
2. Perform hand hygiene. Gather the necessary supplies.	Reduces transmission of microorganisms. Promotes efficient time management and provides an organized approach to the procedure. **caREminder** *The suction catheter should be one half the internal diameter of the tracheostomy tube. Large-bore tube removes secretions more efficiently than a small-bore catheter. Using the correct size minimizes the chance of creating negative pressure that could lead to atelectasis.*
3. Place infant or child in supine position with neck slightly extended. If child is old enough, have him or her raise head into a "sniffing" position.	Extension of neck enables the suction catheter to more easily follow the natural curve of the trachea. **KidKare** To increase the comfort level of the child, a family member may want to hold the infant or child during the procedure or provide some distraction measures.
4. Open sterile supplies (if used).	Healed tissue is less susceptible to infection. **caREminder** *If this is not a new tracheostomy, the suctioning may be done using a modified clean procedure as opposed to a sterile procedure.*
5. Pour a small amount of sterile normal saline into a disposable container.	Sterile normal saline is used to lubricate the tip of the suction catheter and to cleanse the suction catheter of mucus between passes.
6. Don appropriate protective gear (optional) and gloves.	Face shield should be used if the child is infectious or has copious secretions that may come into contact with the caregiver. Reduces transmission of microorganisms.

Steps	Rationale/Points of Emphasis
7. Determine the length of catheter to be inserted in the tracheostomy tube during suctioning. A tracheostomy tube the same size as the one in the child may be used to measure the exact depth to insert the catheter (Chart 112-1).	Ensures catheter is not inserted too far during suctioning.

CHART 112-1 TYPES OF SUCTIONING

Shallow suctioning describes the insertion of a catheter just into the hub of the tracheostomy tube to remove secretions child has coughed up to the opening of the tracheostomy tube.

Premeasured technique involves inserting a catheter with holes close to the distal end, to a premeasured depth, with the most distal holes just exiting the tip of the tracheostomy tube.

Deep suctioning involves inserting the catheter until resistance is met and withdrawing the catheter slightly before applying suctioning. Special circumstances may necessitate the occasional use of deep suctioning. In general, this method should not be used because this causes epithelial damage.

Steps	Rationale/Points of Emphasis
8. Pick up the sterile suction catheter and attach to the suction tubing. The hand grasping the suction catheter at the point that it connects with the suction tubing is now no longer considered sterile and should not be used to insert the catheter down the tracheostomy tube.	Designating one hand as clean and using only this hand to pass the catheter into the tracheostomy assists in minimizing transmission of organisms.
9. Using the sterile dominant hand, lubricate catheter with normal saline.	Small amount of lubricant eases the passage of the catheter into the tracheostomy tube. **caREminder** *Hyperventilation or hyperoxygenation breaths are not recommended before initiating suctioning. Delivering a manual breath when secretions are bubbling in the tube only serves to force these secretions into the more distal parts of the airway. Stable children with a tracheostomy and no additional respiratory support, such as a ventilator, continuous positive airway pressure, or high levels of supplemental oxygen, typically do not require extra breaths or oxygenation before suctioning.*
10. If the child has a mask applied over the tracheostomy tube to deliver oxygen and humidification, move the mask aside at this time.	Mask must be moved to access entrance to tracheostomy tube.
a. Using the sterile dominant hand, grasp the catheter; insert the catheter by gently twirling or rotating the catheter between the fingers and thumb.	Twirling the catheter reduces friction so that the catheter can be more easily inserted.

Continued

Steps	Rationale/Points of Emphasis
b. Use the premeasured technique to insert the catheter to the exact depth to which the catheter should be inserted.	The premeasured technique ensures that the catheter is not inserted too far.
c. Do not apply suction while the catheter is being inserted.	While the American Thoracic Society (2000) consensus document recommends applying suction while inserting the catheter in the tracheostomy tube, no research could be found to support this action. More evidence is needed to determine the effects on the child's oxygen saturation and blood gas levels.
11. As the catheter is removed, apply intermittent suction as you gently rotate or twirl the catheter between the thumb and forefinger and withdraw the catheter.	Removes secretions. The catheter should not be stirred with the entire hand. Twirling the catheter between the fingers reduces friction so that the catheter is more easily removed. This method also moves the side holes of the catheter in a helix, thereby helping to remove secretions off all areas of the tracheostomy tube wall.
a. Using the premeasured technique, complete suctioning in 5 seconds or less. If deep suctioning is used, complete suctioning in 15 seconds or less.	Prolonging suctioning results in hypoxia and can lead to atelectasis.
b. Do not introduce saline into the tracheostomy tube in an attempt to loosen the mucus.	Studies have shown that instilling saline before suctioning has an adverse effect on oxygen saturation, which may last up to 5 minutes. Also, instilling saline during suctioning dislodges bacteria into the lower airway. Studies do not demonstrate the efficacy of normal saline in thinning mucous secretions.
c. In children with secretions, an initial pass of the catheter should be made first to quickly clear the tube of any visible or audible secretions.	Quickly clears the tube of loose secretions.
12. Rinse the catheter tip in a container of sterile water.	Aids in unclogging tube of mucus.
13. Assess respiratory status and determine need for postsuctioning hyperventilation or hyperoxygenation breaths.	
a. Assess breath sounds after suctioning or assess for other signs of improved respiratory status (e.g., pinker skin color, decreased "gurgling" sounds when child is breathing, no expelling of mucus from the tube during respirations, end-tidal CO_2 measurements, increased oxygen saturation).	Bag ventilation support may be required if the suctioning caused decreased breath sounds. If the child is hypoxic or if heart rate is highly elevated, further suctioning should not be attempted until the child's status is stable.
b. If child was receiving oxygen and humidification by mask before the suctioning, reapplication of the mask between passes may be warranted (Figure 112-1).	Assists child in maintaining adequate levels of oxygenation. Humidification assists in thinning secretions.
c. Provide hyperventilation or hyperoxygenation breaths using bag ventilation if indicated.	The use of postsuctioning breaths varies depending on the child's needs. Children who are prone to atelectasis may need bag hyperinflation after the passes of the catheter.
14. Repeat procedure until breath sounds are relatively clear.	Too many suction attempts can irritate the mucosal lining of the trachea.

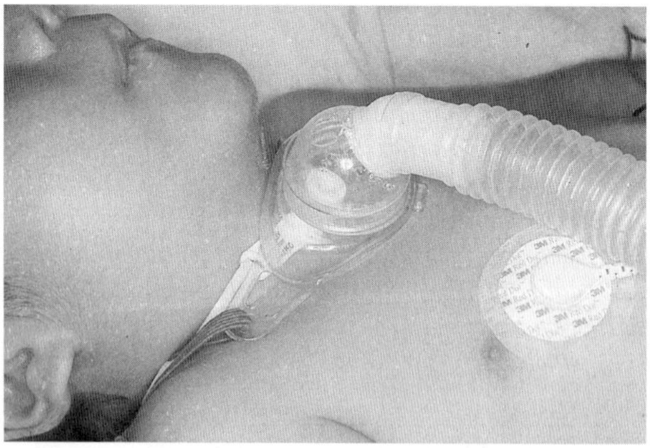

FIGURE 112-1
Providing humidified oxygen/air helps thin secretions.

Steps	Rationale/Points of Emphasis
15. Cleanse the suction catheter and tubing one more time by placing tip in a container of sterile water and applying suction pressure. Detach suction catheter from suction tubing.	Clears suction tubing of mucus and allows mucus to collect in suction collection receptacle. Cleansing the tube helps to prevent contaminates from remaining in the tube.
16. Dispose of suction catheter, water container, mask, and gloves in the appropriate trash receptacle. Turn off suction equipment. Perform hand hygiene.	Reduces transmission of microorganisms. Suction equipment should not remain running when not in use.
17. Remove shoulder roll and place child in position of comfort with head elevated 30 degrees.	This position facilitates ease of breathing.

CHILD AND FAMILY EVALUATION AND DOCUMENTATION

- Evaluate child's tolerance of the procedure.
- Document the following:
  - Color, odor, amount, and consistency of mucus
  - Breath sounds and respiratory effort before and after suctioning
  - Depth used to insert premeasured catheter
  - Use of hyperventilation or hyperoxygenation
  - Time of procedure
  - Child's tolerance of procedure
  - Teaching completed with the child and the family and their response to the teaching
  - Involvement of the family in completing the procedure
- Report changes in stoma appearance or secretions to the physician.

COMMUNITY CARE

- Provide the caregivers in the home with the knowledge, skills, and equipment to manage care of child with a tracheostomy tube (see Table 111-1).

KidKare A doll or mannequin with a tracheostomy can be used for practice. Role-playing helps to reinforce skills and basic confidence. When possible and appropriate, siblings should participate in the teaching program.

- Ensure home/school caregivers are instructed in cardiopulmonary resuscitation techniques including bag to tracheostomy ventilation and mouth to mouth with stoma occlusion in a child with a patent upper airway.
- Arrange for the caregivers in the home to participate actively in all aspects of the tracheostomy tube suctioning and tie change before the child's discharge from the acute care setting. Provide parents with an opportunity for a rooming-in period before discharge to ensure they feel comfortable with child's care needs. A day pass to the home may also be considered.
- Ensure that all home care equipment, including portable equipment, is used in the hospital before discharge to let family see how everything is used.
- Provide the family with the location of a local vendor or supplier of tracheostomy equipment.
- In the home, clean technique can be used to suction the child:
  - Caregivers should wash their hands thoroughly before and after each suctioning procedure. Alcohol or disinfectant foam is an acceptable substitute when soap and water are not available.
  - Preoxygenation or hyperinflation before the suctioning event may not be routinely indicated. When preoxygenation and/or hyperinflation are indicated, a manual resuscitation bag with supplemental oxygen is used.
  - Nonsterile disposable gloves should be worn for the protection of any caregiver who is not a family member or by anyone who is concerned about infection.
  - Individual catheters can be used as long as they remain intact.
  - Instruct the caregivers how to clean suction catheters in the home:
    - Wash and flush the used catheters with hot, soapy water.
    - Disinfect the catheters by soaking them in a vinegar-and-water solution or a commercial disinfectant.
    - Rinse the catheters inside and out with clean water. A hydrogen peroxide flush can be used when particularly adherent secretions are present.
    - Allow catheters to air-dry.
    - Store in a clean, dry container with a lid.
- Instruct the family to contact the healthcare provider if
  - Tracheostomy tube becomes displaced
  - Child develops a fever
  - Child is having an increased amount and frequency of mucus production
  - Mucus is green or dark in color and/or is foul smelling
  - Child develops signs of skin breakdown around tube site or under tracheostomy ties
  - Child has sustained period of increased or decreased respirations
  - Blood is present in the tracheal secretions

Unexpected Situation

- *During suctioning, child becomes cyanotic and bradycardic. Oxygen saturation levels decrease:* Stop suctioning child. Auscultate lung sounds. Manually hyperventilate child if needed to increase oxygen saturation levels. Remain with child until vital signs return to presuctioning state. Document episode in chart. Notify respiratory therapist and healthcare prescriber of incident.

Bibliography

Akgul, S., & Akyolcu, N. (2002). Effects of normal saline on endotracheal suctioning. *Journal of Clinical Nursing, 11*, 826–830.

American Thoracic Society. (2000). Care of the child with a chronic tracheostomy. *American Journal of Respiratory Critical Care Medicine, 161*(1), 297–308.

McInturff, S., Make, B., Robart, P., & Saposnick, A. (1999). Clinical practice guideline: Suctioning the patient in the home. *Respiratory Care, 44*(1), 99–104.

Pate, M., & Zapata, T. (2002). How deeply should I go when I suction an endotracheal (ETT) or tracheostomy tube (TT)? *Critical Care Nurse, 22*(2), 130–131.

Raymond, S. (1995). Normal saline installation before suctioning: Helpful or harmful? A review of the literature. *American Journal of Critical Care, 4*(4), 267–271.

Russell, C. (2005). Providing the nurse with a guide to tracheostomy care and management. *British Journal of Nursing, 14*(8), 428–433.

Sole, M., Byers, J., Ludy, J., & Ostrow, C. (2002). Suctioning techniques and airway management practices: Pilot study and instrument evaluation. *American Journal of Critical Care, 11*(4), 363–368.

Sole, M., Poalillo, F., Byers, J., & Ludy, J. (2002). Bacterial growth in secretions and on suctioning equipment of orally intubated patients: A pilot study. *American Journal of Critical Care, 11*, 141–149.

St. John, R. (2004). Airway management. *Critical Care Nurse, 4*. Retrieved December 18, 2004, from http://findarticles.com/p/articles/mi_m0NUC/is_2_24/ai_n6175383/print

Tamburri, L. (2000). Care of the patient with a tracheostomy. *Orthopedic Nursing, 19*(2), 49–60.

Wilson, M. (2005). Tracheostomy management. *Paediatric Nursing, 17*(3), 38–43.

CHAPTER

113

Tracheostomy: Tube Change

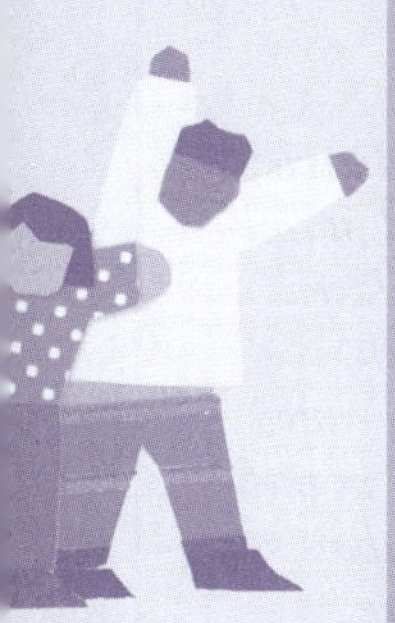

Clinical Guidelines

- The initial tracheostomy tube change is completed by the physician with subsequent changes done by the registered nurse (RN), licensed practical nurse (LPN), respiratory therapist (RT), parent, or caregiver.
- Tracheostomy tube changes are completed to
  - Reduce the incidence of tube occlusion from increased secretions
  - Decrease the possibility of airway infection and airway granulomas
  - Assist the caregiver in maintaining competency in tube changing
- The tracheostomy tube change is usually done about 5 days after the tracheostomy is performed and then weekly or as ordered by the physician. Tube changes should occur 2 to 3 hours after meals. Check manufacturer's recommendation for time frame regarding tube changes.
- Depth of suctioning is reassessed and measured with any change in tracheostomy tube size.
- If accidental decannulation occurs, the tracheostomy tube is replaced with a tube of the same size or one smaller size. If a tracheostomy tube cannot be placed, the child is intubated.
- All tracheostomy tubes have a 15-mm universal adapter to allow bag ventilation in an emergency.
- Equipment is available at the bedside at all times for suctioning, ventilatory breaths, and recannulation.
  - The tracheostomy obturator and a tracheostomy tube of the same type and size being used by the child and one tube a size smaller remain with the child in a visible or readily accessible location at all times.
- Before discharge, two adults, who will be consistent caregivers to the child, are trained in all aspects of the child's care.

Equipment

- Two sterile tracheostomy tubes of appropriate size, with obturator in place (one is left in place at the bedside at all times)
- Water-based lubricant
- Shoulder roll—diapers or small rolled towel
- Nonsterile gloves
- Appropriate protective gear (gown and face shield)

For changing tracheostomy ties (see Chapter 111):

- Scissors
- Twill tape, Velcro ties, or stainless steel beaded metal chain (rarely used)
- Appropriate protective gear (gown and face shield)
- Stethoscope
- Oxygen source (if needed)
- Manual ventilation bag (as needed for ventilatory breaths)
- Suction equipment (as needed) (see Chapter 112)

Child and Family Assessment and Preparation

- Assess chart for previous history of child's condition and for a summary of care needs in relation to tracheostomy.
- Determine date of last tube change.
- Assess child's breath sounds and work of breathing.
- Explain the procedure to the child and the family.
- Determine family's ability to perform procedure and, if appropriate, have family perform this procedure.
- Suction the child before initiating tracheostomy care (see Chapter 112).
- Ensure that equipment is available at the bedside for use if child requires suctioning, ventilatory breaths, or recannulation.
- Determine the need for distraction measures to be implemented with the child to enhance cooperation during the procedure.

PROCEDURE Tube Change

Steps	Rationale/Points of Emphasis
1. Perform hand hygiene.	Reduces transmission of microorganisms.
2a. Gather all necessary supplies. Assemble near the child's bed.	Promotes efficient time management and provides an organized approach to the procedure.
2b. Based on healthcare prescriber's orders, select appropriately sized tracheostomy tube.	Tracheostomy tubes must fit the airway and the functional needs of the child. Tube size is determined based on tracheal size and shape, indications for the tracheostomy, lung mechanics, upper airway resistance, and the needs of the child for speech, ventilation, and airway clearance. Length, curvature, flexibility, and composition of the tube are also considered. Because a stoma may become slightly smaller over time, a second replacement tube at the bedside should be the next smaller size from that of the patient. **caREminder** *The indications for cuffed tracheostomy tubes in pediatrics are limited. Cuffed tracheostomy tubes may be used in children requiring ventilation with high pressures, children requiring only nocturnal ventilation, and those with chronic translaryngeal aspiration. The exact role of cuffed tracheostomy tubes in children has not been defined in the literature. Should a cuffed tube be present, ensure that secretions are cleared from above the tube cuff before deflating the cuff before removal.*
3. Inspect tracheostomy tube for stiffness, cracks, and tears. Damaged tubes or flexible tubes that are becoming stiff should be discarded and replaced with new tubes.	Individual flexible polyvinyl chloride (PVC) tracheostomy tubes may be in intermittent use by the child for 6 months to 1 year before stiffening. With use, these tubes become progressively more rigid and may develop splits or cracks. Silicone tracheostomy tubes do not stiffen after repeated use or after cleaning and disinfection. Metal tracheostomy tubes can be used indefinitely. Metal tubes can occasionally crack at the soldered joint.
4. Attach tie to opening on one end of tracheostomy tube (see Chapter 111). Ensure that the obturator is inserted in the new tube.	Use of obturator gives stability to the tracheostomy.

Steps	Rationale/Points of Emphasis
5. Lubricate the end of the new tracheostomy tube with water-based lubricant. Place back in open package nearby the child.	Lubrication decreases the trauma to tracheal tissue.
6. Position child in supine position with neck slightly extended. Place rolled towel or diaper under child's shoulders.	Straightens airway and optimizes path for removal and placement of tracheostomy. Slightly extends neck for optimal positioning, bringing tracheostomy tube forward. A second person is recommended to assist by holding the child's shoulders to prevent movement.
7. Don appropriate protective gear (optional) and gloves.	Face shield should be used if the child is infectious or has copious secretions that may come into contact with the caregiver. Reduces transmission of microorganisms.
8. Remove old ties. The child, a parent, or another healthcare provider should hold the tracheostomy tube in place.	Velcro ties are easily removed by releasing the Velcro tabs. Care should be taken to prevent cutting the child's skin when removing twill ties.
9. With one hand, remove old tracheostomy tube and tracheostomy set and move it to one side out of the way.	Tracheostomy tubes and sets may be cleaned and reused. Routine tracheostomy tube changes result in fewer complications from infection and formation of granulation tissue requiring surgical intervention.
10. Gently and quickly insert the new tube, pushing back and then down, in an arcing motion.	Back and downward motion follows the natural curve of the trachea. Tube should extend at least 2 cm beyond the stoma and no closer than 1–2 cm to the carina. Curvature should be such that the distal portion of the in situ tracheostomy tube should be concentric and colinear with the trachea.
11. Immediately remove the obturator (Figure 113-1).	Obturator occludes the patency of the tracheostomy.

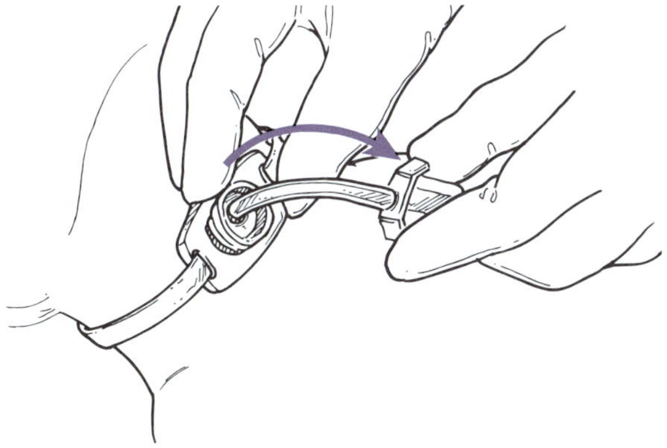

FIGURE 113-1
Once the new tube has been inserted, stabilize the flanges of the outer cannula with the fingers of one hand while immediately withdrawing the obturator with the other hand.

Steps	Rationale/Points of Emphasis
12. Assess for patency of the tube by using stethoscope to listen for air movement.	If there is no air movement, the procedure will need to be repeated. A tracheostomy tube whose distal position is not collinear with the trachea may cause complications, such as esophageal obstruction or partial occlusion of the tracheostomy tube tip by the tracheal wall. Other complications include tracheal wall erosion, trachea–innominate artery fistula, tracheoesophageal fistula, and stomal breakdown.
13. Hold the outer cannula of the tracheostomy tube in place and secure the tracheostomy ties (see Chapter 111).	One person should hold the tube in place, while the assistant secures the ties.
14. If a cuffed tube is used, inflate the cuff to the proper volume using a syringe.	Cuff pressures should be kept as low as possible to protect the airway and prevent leaks. Consult the healthcare prescriber for cuff pressure to be applied. In general, cuff pressures below 20 cm H_2O are well tolerated by children.
15. Provide oxygenation/ventilation breaths as needed using a manual ventilation bag if indicated based on child's respiratory status.	If the child experiences respiratory distress during the procedure, extra breaths will assist in reestablishing the child to his or her baseline respiratory status.

Continued

Steps	Rationale/Points of Emphasis
16. Dispose of used tracheostomy tube, mask, and gloves in the appropriate trash receptacle. Perform hand hygiene. Turn off suction equipment.	Reduces transmission of microorganisms. Suction equipment should not remain running when not in use. **caREminder** *The tracheostomy tube may be cleansed for future use depending on institutional policy. Families should be encouraged to reuse the tubes when performing this procedure at home.*
17. Remove shoulder roll and place child in position of comfort with head elevated 30 degrees.	This position will facilitate ease of breathing.

CHILD AND FAMILY EVALUATION AND DOCUMENTATION

- Document the following:
  - Date and time of procedure
  - Child's tolerance of the procedure
  - Any difficulties encountered while performing care
  - Use of oxygenation during the procedure
  - Quality of breath sounds before and after procedure
  - Appearance of stoma and skin under ties (irritation, redness, edema, subcutaneous air)
  - Character of secretions (color, consistency, odor)
  - Presence of dressing around stoma site
  - Size of tracheostomy used
  - Teaching completed with the child and the family and their response to the teaching
  - Involvement of the family during the procedure.

COMMUNITY CARE

- Provide the caregivers in the home with the knowledge, skills, and equipment to manage care of the child with a tracheostomy tube (see Chart 111-1).

KidKare A doll or mannequin with a tracheostomy can be used for practice. Role-playing helps to reinforce skills and basic confidence. When possible and appropriate, siblings should participate in the teaching program.

- Ensure home/school caregivers are instructed in cardiopulmonary resuscitation techniques including bag to tracheostomy ventilation and mouth to mouth with stoma occlusion in a child with a patent upper airway.
- Arrange for the caregivers in the home to participate actively in all aspects of the tracheostomy tube suctioning and tie change before discharge from the acute care setting.
- Provide family with opportunity for a rooming-in period before discharge to ensure that they feel comfortable with child's care needs. A day pass to the home may also be considered.
- Ensure that all home care equipment, including portable equipment, is used in the hospital before discharge.
- Provide the family with the location of a local vendor or supplier of tracheostomy equipment.
- Instruct the parents and other caregivers how to clean tracheostomy tubes in the home:
  - Wash and flush the used tubes with hot, soapy water.
  - Disinfect the tubes by soaking them in a vinegar-and-water solution or a commercial disinfectant.
  - Rinse the tubes inside and out with clean water. A hydrogen peroxide flush can be used when particularly adherent secretions are present.
  - Allow tubes to air-dry.
  - Assess for stiffness, cracks, or tears. Discard stiff or damaged tubes.
  - Store in a clean, dry container with a lid.
- Instruct the family to contact the healthcare provider if
  - Tracheostomy tube becomes displaced
  - Child develops a fever
  - Child is having an increased amount and frequency of mucus production
  - Mucus is green or dark in color and/or is foul smelling
  - Child develops signs of skin breakdown around tube site or under tracheostomy ties
  - Child has sustained period of increased respirations or decreased respirations
  - Blood is present in the tracheal secretions

Unexpected Situation

- *You have removed the outer cannula for cleaning. While attempting to reinsert the cannula, you are not able to fit it into the opening:* First consider that child may not be in a good position, and thus access to the airway may not be optimal. Reposition the child. The stoma skin may also need to be slightly spread to allow better access. If these interventions do not work, placed at the bedside is a spare tracheostomy tube one size smaller than the tracheostomy tube in place. Use the smaller size cannula to replace in the opening. Notify the healthcare prescriber of the change in cannula size.

Bibliography

American Thoracic Society. (2000). Care of the child with a chronic tracheostomy. *American Journal of Respiratory and Critical Care Medicine, 161*(1), 297–308.

Carr, M., Poje, C., Kingston, L., Kielma, D., & Heard, C. (2001). Complications in pediatric tracheostomies. *The Laryngoscope, 111,* 1925–1928.

Russell, C. (2005). Providing the nurse with a guide to tracheostomy care and management. *British Journal of Nursing, 14*(8), 428–433.

Tamburri, L. (2000). Care of the patient with a tracheostomy. *Orthopedic Nursing, 19*(2), 49–60.

Wilson, M. (2005). Tracheostomy management. *Paediatric Nursing, 17*(3), 38–43.

Yaremchuk, K. (2003). Regular tracheostomy tube changes to prevent formation of granulation tissue. *The Laryngoscope, 113,* 1–10.

CHAPTER

114

Traction Care

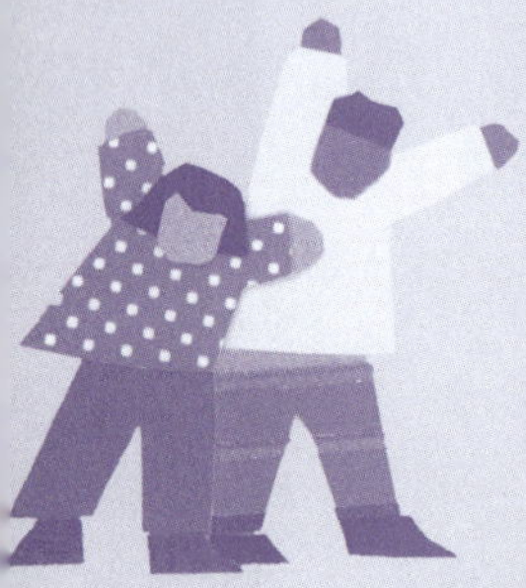

Clinical Guidelines

- The registered nurse (RN), licensed practical nurse (LPN), or orthopedic technician (where applicable) is responsible for daily care needs of the child in traction.
- Weights may not be added or removed without a healthcare prescriber's order.
- Skeletal traction may not be removed without a healthcare prescriber's order.
- Remove skin traction straps every 4 hours or as ordered.
- Remove skin traction boot every 8 hours or as ordered.
- Assess neurovascular status every 4 hours.
- Assess skin integrity before the application of the traction and every 4 hours.
- Assess for pain every 2 to 4 hours during the acute phase and every 4 hours thereafter.
- Evaluate integrity of traction and stabilizing devices every shift.

Equipment

- Skin cleansing supplies
- Skeletal pin site care supplies (see Chapter 107)
- Pillows

Child and Family Assessment and Preparation

- Review chart to determine
  - Diagnosis and type of fracture/surgery the child has sustained
  - Physical condition and integrity of the skeletal system
  - Purpose and type of traction being used (Tables 114-1 and 114-2)
  - Age and weight of child
  - Traction weights ordered by the healthcare prescriber
  - Presence of possible adhesive or latex allergies
- Assess child's vital signs to determine presence of fever, increased respiratory rate, and/or increased heart rate that may indicate presence of infection.
- Assess child for pain and muscle spasms and provide interventions as indicated (see Chapter 7).
- Administer pain medication when indicated, at least 30 minutes before moving or assessing the child.
- Use diversional activities and other nonpharmacologic interventions (e.g., music, stroking of unaffected extremities) to distract the child and assist in pain management during the procedure. Collaborate with child life specialist to provide diversional activities.
- Perform range-of-motion exercises to all extremities, unless contraindicated, every shift.
- Explain to the child and family the care you will be providing.
- Encourage parent and family members to stay with the child during traction care.
- Have the child assist in the examination according to his or her developmental level.

TABLE 114-1

Types of Skin Traction*

Type	Illustration	Uses	Nursing Considerations
Cervical skin	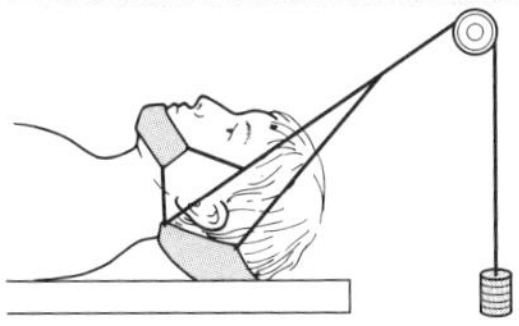	Neck sprains or strains Torticollis Cervical nerve trauma Nerve root compression	There is a 5–7 lb limit of weights. Avoid compressing the throat or ears with the chin strap.
Side-arm 90–90	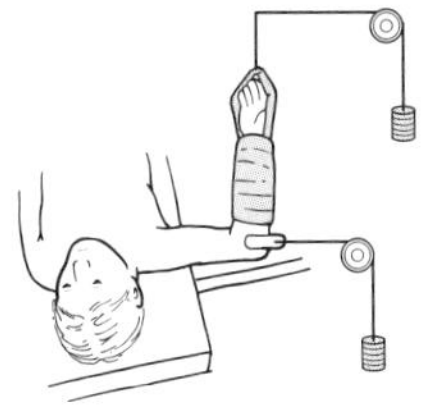	Fractures and dislocations of the upper arm or shoulder	Hand may feel cool because of its elevation. Hand can be covered with sock or mitten if desired.
Dunlop	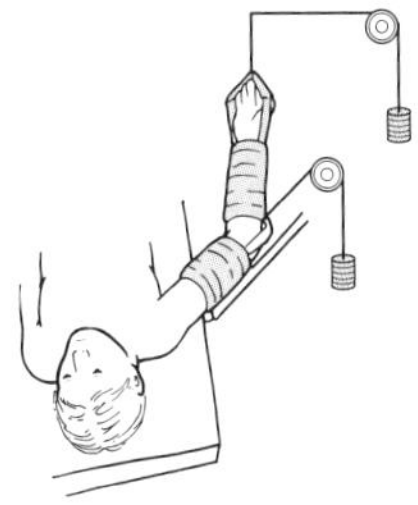	Supracondylar elbow fracture of the humerus	Avoid pressure over bony prominences or nerves.
Pelvis sling	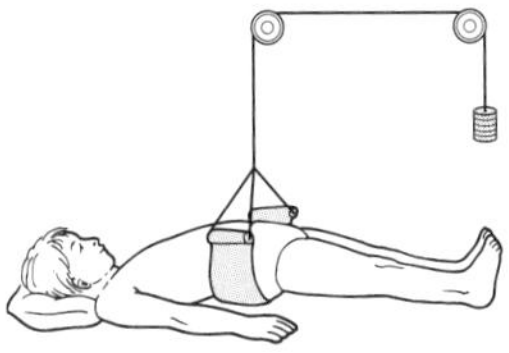	Pelvic fractures	There is a 10–25 lb limit of weights. Ensure proper size of belt and apply it just over iliac crest.
Bryant's traction	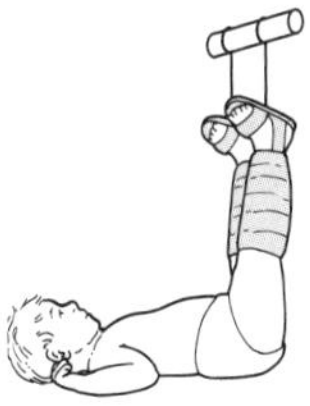	Infant with a femur fracture or developmental dislocated hip	Supply plenty of diversional activities. If child flips over, a sheet or Posey restraint may be used. Avoid pressure over dorsum of foot and heel.
Buck's traction	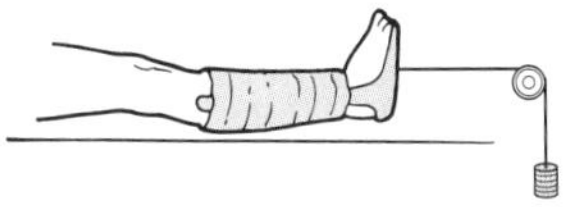	Hip and knee contracture Legg-Calvé-Perthes disease Slipped capital femur epiphysis (SCFE)	Remove boot every 8 hr and assess skin. Leg may be slightly abducted.
Russell's traction	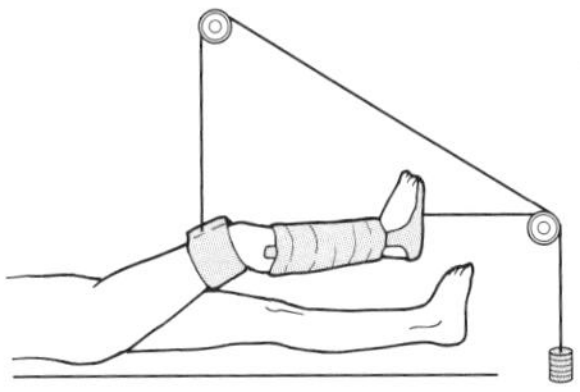	Supracondylar femur fracture Hip and knee contracture	Sling may need to be repositioned often; mark leg to ensure proper placement.
Split Russell's	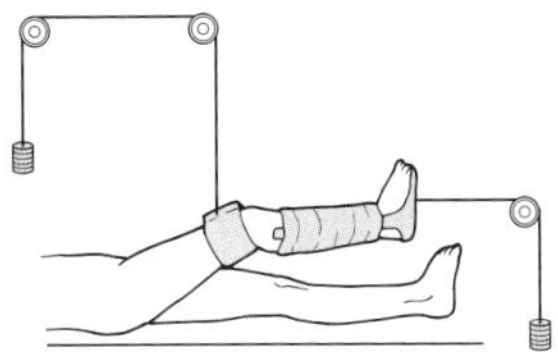	Femur fracture SCFE Legg-Calvé-Perthes disease	Avoid pressure over bony prominences or nerves. Weights are not added or removed without a physician's order.

**Skin traction* refers to any traction apparatus where the pull force is applied to the affected body part via the soft tissue. Traction is applied to the skin by using skin adherents, Ace wraps, commercial traction tapes, or special foam boots. Weights applied to skin traction should not exceed 3.5 kg or 8 lb.

TABLE 114-2
Types of Skeletal Traction*

Type	Illustration	Uses	Nursing Considerations
Cervical skeletal tongs	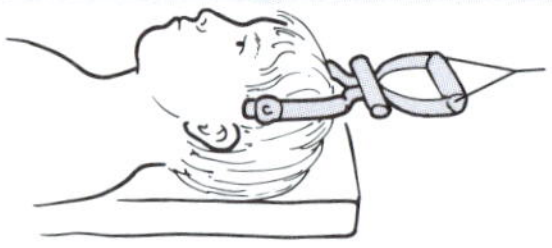	Preoperative spine distraction Fractures or dislocations of cervical or high thoracic vertebrae	A special bed may be used to assist with turning patient. Logroll patient.
Halo cast or vest	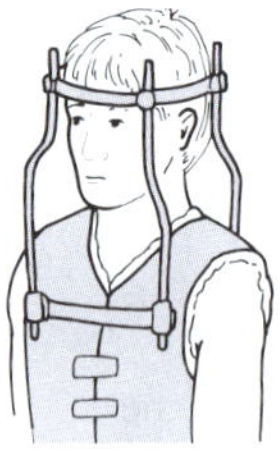	Postoperative immobilization after cervical fusion Fracture or dislocation of cervical or high thoracic vertebrae	A small wrench is taped to the front of the brace to remove front panel in case of emergency. If patient is in halo cast, a cast saw must be with her or him in case of emergency. Balance is altered with a halo cast; patients ambulating need close supervision.
Dunlop's side-arm 00–90	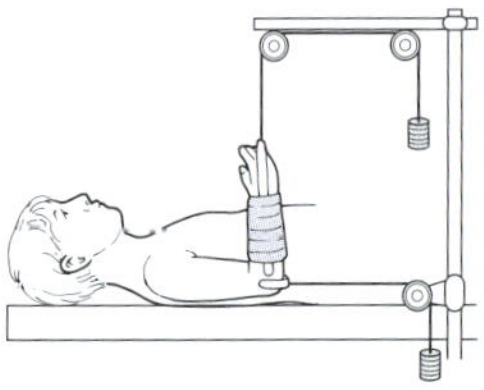	Fractures of upper arm	Turn patient toward the affected side only. Hand may feel cool despite intact neurovascular status; cover hand with mitten or sock if desired.
Knee 90–90	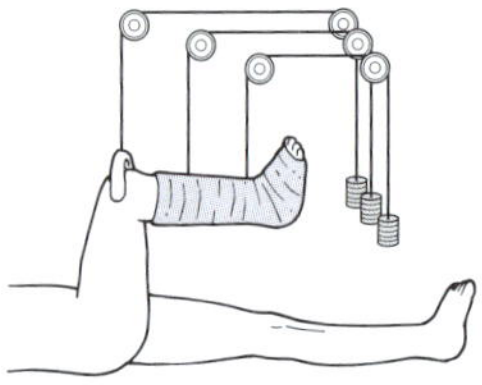	Femur fractures	Encourage child to dorsiflex foot often to prevent foot drop; apply splint if necessary. Ensure weights do not catch on bottom of the bed.
Thomas ring with Pearson attachment (balanced suspension)	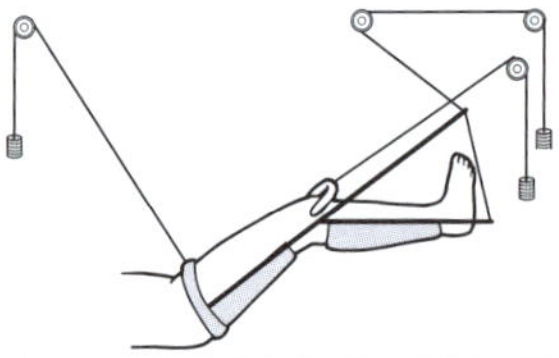	Femur fracture Hip fracture Tibial fracture	Avoid pressure to the area behind the knee, which could cause popliteal nerve injury. If the system is truly balanced, the splint can be placed at any height and it will remain there.

*_Skeletal fracture_ refers to any traction apparatus where the pull force is applied directly to the skeleton via pins, wires, screws, and/or tongs that are inserted into the appropriate area of bone. Weights applied can be 4.5 kg or 10 lb, up to 11.5 kg or 25 lb. Skeletal traction is beneficial for unstable or fragmented fractures that are not amenable to surgical intervention. Skeletal traction would also be used if there were skin damage associated with the fracture.

PROCEDURE Traction Care

Steps	Rationale/Points of Emphasis
1. Perform hand hygiene.	Reduces transmission of microorganisms.
2. Assess child's positioning in bed relative to traction apparatus. a. Reposition the child in supine position with alignment of shoulder, hip, and legs in a midline position. The child's heel should not be digging into the mattress.	Proper alignment prevents pressure on the affected extremity, promotes healing, and ensures good mechanical function of the traction equipment.

Steps	Rationale/Points of Emphasis
Alert! *The side-lying and semi-Fowler positions are contraindicated.*	
b. Elevate head of bed to the angle ordered.	In general, the child should not have the head of the bed elevated more than 20 degrees and should not be allowed to sit up. When the head of the bed is maintained at the proper angle, it provides adequate countertraction. If the force of pull of the traction is greater than the countertraction supplied by the body weight, the child will slide toward the traction force or the traction splint may impinge on the traction pulley.
c. Apply trapeze for convenience in moving in bed (if not contraindicated, as in spinal injuries or bilateral upper extremity injuries).	Children in lower extremity traction can be turned one quarter to the uninvolved side to enable back care or to place a fracture bedpan if they are unable to lift their hips. This turn will not result in misalignment and is important for relieving pressure.
3. Ensure the traction apparatus is properly secured to the bed. Assess the traction setup, including the amount of weights ordered.	
a. Full inspection of traction apparatus verifies alignment of traction cords; integrity of rope, tightness of knots, and securing of tape and bed linen is not interfering with line of traction.	For traction to work effectively, countertraction must be maintained. There must be a reasonable balance between traction forces and countertraction forces to achieve optimal healing and patient comfort. Interruption of the "line of pull" can cause disruption of healing that has occurred in the bones and soft tissue. As movement occurs, inflammation is stimulated. The movement therefore can cause muscle spasm, bleeding, and pain.
b. Ensure weights are hanging free of bed and floor while verifying that the correct amount of weights are used. Reposition weights as needed at a reasonable level from the floor, a considerable distance from the pulley, hanging free of the bed, and always away from the child.	Balanced traction is designed to maintain a constant pull on child, and adequate weight provides countertraction needed to keep bones aligned for optimal healing. Weights should never be removed or added without specific healthcare prescriber orders.
Alert! *Weights should not be removed when lifting or moving a child. Do not release traction unless instructed to do so by the healthcare prescriber.*	
4. Perform neurovascular assessment (see Chapter 77).	Promotes early identification of neurovascular problems and promotes prompt interventions to diminish compromised circulation and oxygenation of tissues.
5. Perform skin assessment.	Promotes early identification of skin problems and promotes prompt interventions to diminish disruptions to skin integrity.
6. Assist child to perform passive and active range of motion of all extremities at least every shift (see Chapter 101).	Helps to maintain muscle tone. Venous thrombosis is a serious complication of immobility; interventions to prevent thrombosis include flexion, extension, and rotation exercises to joints, especially the ankles.
7. Complete interventions to prevent complications of immobility and promote healing (Table 114-3).	Ongoing assessment and implementation of a variety of nursing interventions will assist to prevent skin breakdown, infection, and pain.
8. Notify healthcare prescriber of any abnormal findings.	Early identification of abnormal findings is the key in the prevention and treatment of complications of fractures. Subtle findings will often indicate an impending complication at the earliest stage.

TABLE 114-3

Promoting Healing and Preventing Complications of Immobility

Nursing Diagnosis	Clinical Manifestations	Nursing Interventions	Rationale
Ineffective Breathing Pattern	Slower and more shallow respirations Pooling of secretions Decreased cough reflex	Evaluate respiratory status each shift. Encourage child to cough and deep breathe. Initiate the use of incentive spirometer and chest physiotherapy as needed. Mobilize child as soon as possible.	Immobilization leads to decreased lung expansion, decreased respiratory effort, decreased cough reflex, and pooling of secretions. Baseline assessment provides data for early interventions. Pulmonary status is evaluated to prevent atelectasis. Early interventions reduce respiratory complications.
Ineffective Tissue Perfusion: Cardiopulmonary	Circulatory stasis Venous dilation in dependent parts Decreased thoracic and abdominal pressures Decreased cardiac rate, circulatory volume, and arterial pressure	Turn child every 2 hr. Encourage active/passive range-of-motion activities. Apply elastic stockings to lower extremities. Mobilize child as soon as possible.	Muscular inactivity may lead to vasodilatation and impaired venous return.
Risk for Peripheral Neurovascular Dysfunction	Capillary refill > 3 seconds Pain Pallor of the extremity Decrease pulse or pulselessness of the extremity Diminished sensation in extremity swelling	Assess the child's extremities, comparing both affected and unaffected extremities. Assess for the five P's of vascular impairment: pain, pallor, pulselessness, paresthesia, and paralysis. Assess temperature of extremities. Assess capillary refill by pressing on fingers/toes and observing time for capillary refill. Assess level of swelling in the fingers/toes distal to the fracture site. Monitor motor function and range of motion by having child move fingers/toes.	The unaffected extremity can be used as a baseline for assessment. Starting the exam on the healthy limb may calm the child. Tissue ischemia, nerve damage, tight bandages, and compartment syndrome are serious complications of fractures and need to be identified early. Normal capillary refill is 1–3 seconds. Greater than 3 seconds is indicative of inadequate arterial supply. Swelling peaks within 24–48 hr unless there is extensive tissue damage. Sensation is documented as present, absent, or abnormal. If child's nervous system is intact, sensation should be felt at areas of innervation above and below the injury. Motion distal to the fracture would be normal range of motion, painful, or minimal.
Hyperthermia	Increase in body temperature Flushed skin Increased respiratory rate and heart rate Warm to touch	Monitor child's temperature for fever. Monitor laboratory values for elevated white blood cells or elevated erythrocyte sedimentation rate.	Elevated temperatures may indicate infection. Fever of 101.0°F (38.3°C) or higher should be reported. Elevated white blood cell count and elevated erythrocyte sedimentation rate are indications of infection and/or inflammation.
Impaired Physical Mobility	Decreased muscle mass and strength Decreased bone mass and strength	Encourage active/passive range-of-motion activities. Encourage isometric/isotonic exercises. Mobilize child as soon as possible.	Imbalance between osteoblastic and osteoclastic activity leads to calcium and phosphorus loss, resulting in decreased muscle tone and decreased bone stress.

TABLE 114-3

Promoting Healing and Preventing Complications of Immobility (continued)

Nursing Diagnosis	Clinical Manifestations	Nursing Interventions	Rationale
Imbalanced Nutrition: Less Than Body Requirements	Decreased efficiency in using nutrients Increased potassium and calcium excretion Decreased appetite	Give small, frequent meals. Give increased fiber, protein, vitamin C, and acidifying foods. Limit calcium intake. Mobilize child as soon as possible.	Inactivity will result in decreased basal metabolic rate and oxygen consumption. Nitrogen loss and negative nitrogen balance can occur due to protein loss from loss of muscle mass. Balanced nutritional intake is needed to promote healing.
Impaired Skin Integrity	Increased potential for skin breakdown	Inspect child's skin for rashes, redness, irritation, or pressure sores. Avoid positions that put pressure on bony prominences. Turn child every 2 hr. Keep child's skin clean and dry. Apply lotion to dry skin areas. Apply pressure-equalizing and pressure-reducing devices.	Skin assessment includes looking at the bony prominences and at any area that is in contact with the traction or suspension apparatus, cast, and bedding material. Continuous pressure on any area can compromise skin integrity.
Constipation Impaired Elimination	Constipation Urinary retention Renal calculi Anorexia	Evaluate elimination patterns. Individual has established elimination patterns concerning amount, consistency, and frequency of bowel movement. Encourage fluid intake and roughage. Encourage small, frequent meals. Provide privacy for elimination. Administer stool softeners or suppositories as ordered. Monitor urine output and characteristics of urine every shift. Offer acidic juices such as apple or cranberry.	General muscle weakness and atrophy with inactivity slow peristalsis and cause urinary stasis in renal pelvis. Fluid intake should consist of water and juices; milk intake should be limited. Both are important for maintaining bowel and bladder function, as constipation and renal calculi are both related to immobility. The privacy issue is especially important to children who are school-aged through adolescence. A stool softener or suppository helps facilitate a bowel movement.
Acute Pain	Discomfort Observed evidence of pain Sleep disturbance Guarded behavior Changes in appetite and eating Child's self-report of pain	Assess for cause of pain Use pharmacologic and nonpharmacologic measures for pain management. Position for comfort.	Actual or potential tissue damage can cause pain. Pain may indicate compartment syndrome.
Deficient Diversional Activity	Boredom Irritability Regressive behaviors	Provide a stimulating environment with age-appropriate toys, posters, and music. Provide age-appropriate toys or activities for the child in traction. Encourage a family member to stay with the young child. Allow friends and classmates to visit. Have classmates telephone or write letters to the hospitalized child.	Imposed immobility associated with musculoskeletal conditions and traction can cause disruptions in child's independence, body image, and self-esteem. Stress and changes in role can bring about anxiety and fear. Sensory deprivation can lead to boredom and a sense of being forgotten.

Continued

TABLE 114-3

Promoting Healing and Preventing Complications of Immobility (continued)

Nursing Diagnosis	Clinical Manifestations	Nursing Interventions	Rationale
		Encourage movement by having the child perform appropriate self-care. Enlist child life personnel and physical therapy in providing activities that encourage movement without disrupting traction. A hospital or school tutor can be contacted to continue the school-aged child's schooling. Encourage the child to be an active participant in his or her care. Encourage age-appropriate behavior. Allow for regressive behavior without punishment. Provide methods by which the child can express anger appropriately.	Peer interactions are especially important to school-aged children and adolescents. Move the bed to the playroom daily to change the environment. An immobilized child may regress to an earlier developmental level.

PROCEDURE Specific Interventions for the Child in Skin Traction

Steps	Rationale/Points of Emphasis
1. Remove skin traction straps every 4 hours and boot every 8 hours or per healthcare prescriber's order.	Skin traction is achieved by using a variety of soft materials (moleskin or foam boot), bandages, and wraps that are directly applied to the skin. Skin traction may be removed and reapplied immediately (see Table 114-1). Removing the straps and boot provides access to the extremity to assess for potential complications.
2. Check bony prominences for skin breakdown, abrasions, and pressure areas.	Pressure and friction between the extremity and the tractions and boot may compromise skin integrity.
3. Don gloves.	Reduces transmission of microorganisms.
4. Cleanse, dry, and massage the child's skin beneath the traction areas and dependent areas daily.	Cleanses area and promotes circulation in the affected areas.
5. Replace the traction. Remove gloves and dispose in appropriate receptacle.	Replacing traction is necessary to provide continuing immobilization of the extremity and to promote healing. Standard precautions.
6. Assess position of bandages, wraps, or straps.	Bandages, wraps, and straps should only be applied over intact or protected skin to prevent skin breakdown.

Alert! *Excessive weight, tight bandaging, and incorrectly sized splints and slings in skin traction have the potential to cause the child further harm by creating pressure areas, nerve impingement, or vascular compromise.*

a. Ensure wrapping material is not wrinkled on the skin.	Can lead to skin breakdown.
b. Assess for loosening or slipping of devices.	The devices can slip or loosen with movement.

PROCEDURE **Specific Interventions for the Child in Skeletal Traction**

Steps	Rationale/Points of Emphasis
1. Assess pin site for signs of redness, swelling, or drainage every shift.	Skeletal traction applies force directly to the bone by using ascetically inserted pins, wires, or tongs. Weights are adjusted as necessary to keep the bone in alignment. Skeletal traction may not be removed without a healthcare prescriber's order (see Table 114-2). Children with skeletal pins are at higher risk for osteomyelitis. The organism, often *Staphylococcus aureus* in children, can enter the body through an open fracture or from an upper respiratory infection.
2. Perform pin site care as needed (see Chapter 107).	Prevents pin site infection.
3. Check that pins are secure and not slipping.	Slippage or movement of the pins may interfere with the effectiveness of the traction. The site of a loose pin is at higher risk for infection because of irritation of the bone and surrounding muscle.

CHILD AND FAMILY EVALUATION AND DOCUMENTATION

- Evaluate child's and family's understanding of need to
  - Maintain proper body alignment
  - Report sensations of discomfort and pain
  - Support environment where child is free from injury
- Document the following:
  - Assessment findings, including vital signs, neurovascular, circulation, respiratory, elimination, and skin
  - Position of child and condition and stability of traction apparatus
  - Pain medication administration and child's response to pharmacologic and nonpharmacologic interventions
  - Teaching completed with the family and educational materials provided to child and family

COMMUNITY CARE

- After traction is discontinued the child may be sent home in a cast. See Chapter 25 for community care instructions related to cast care.
- Ensure safe transportation home and address the importance of follow-up appointments.
- Instruct the family to contact the healthcare provider if
  - Child has blue, cold, or very swollen fingers or toes
  - Child has pain that is not relieved by oral analgesics

Unexpected Situation

- *A 1-month-old child has been placed in Bryant's traction for developmental dysplasia of the hip. You note that the feet are cold with diminished pedal pulses:* Remove traction and perform neurovascular and skin assessments. Reposition child in bed as needed. Reapply the traction and reassess neurovascular status in 15 minutes. Notify healthcare prescriber if these symptoms persist.

Bibliography

Draper, P., & Scott, F. (1998). Using traction. *Nursing Times, 94*(12), 31–32.

Hanson, S. T., Jr., & Swiontkowski, M. F. (1993). *Orthopaedic trauma protocols.* New York: Raven Press Ltd.

Harvery, C. (1998). Challenges of traction in critical care: A case study. *Critical Care Nursing Quarterly, 21*(2), 1–13.

McCloskey Docterman, J. & Bulecheck, G. M. (Eds.). (2004). *Nursing interventions classifications (NIC).* St. Louis: Mosby.

Mellett, S. (1998). Care of the orthopedic patient with traction. *Nursing Times, 94*(22), 52–54.

Osmond, T. (1999). Principles of traction. *Australian Nursing Journal, 6*(Suppl. 7), 1–4.

Strycula, L. (1994a). Traction basics (Part I). *Orthopedic Nursing, 13*(2), 71–74.

Strycula, L. (1994b). Traction basics (Part II). Traction equipment. *Orthopedic Nursing, 13*(3), 55–59.

Strycula, L. (1994c). Traction basics (Part III). Types of traction. *Orthopedic Nursing, 13*(4), 34, 38–44.

Strycula, L. (1994d). Traction basics (Part IV). Traction for lower extremities. *Orthopedic Nursing, 13*(5), 59–68.

CHAPTER

115

Transition Management: Discharging and Transferring the Child

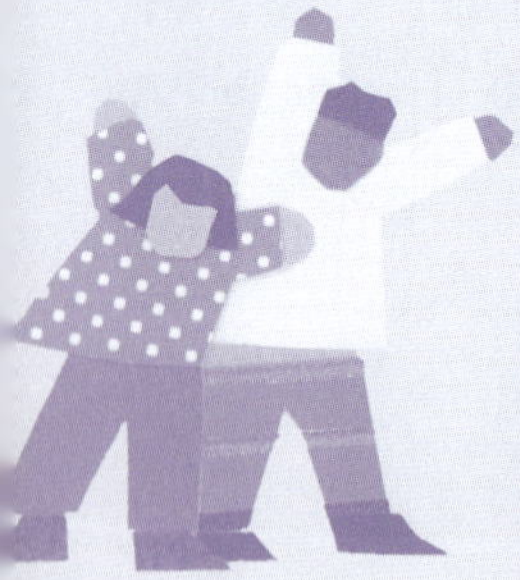

Clinical Guidelines

- A healthcare prescriber's order is required to discharge a child or transfer a child to a different level of care.
- A minor must be discharged to his or her parent or legal guardian, unless other arrangements have been made and are documented in the child's medical record.
- Written parental informed consent should be obtained to transfer the child to another facility.
- Transfer to another facility is treated as a discharge.
- The healthcare prescriber is notified immediately if a parent or legal guardian wishes to take the child from the hospital against medical advice (AMA).
- To ensure the child's safety during transport, use the mode of transport most appropriate to the child's age, developmental level, and condition.
- All written instructions for the family are in a language, reading level, and format that the parent verifies he or she can understand.

Equipment

If discharging a child to parent or legal guardian:

- Medical chart
- Discharge care plan
- Written instructions for home care, including follow-up appointments
- Medications and prescriptions, as appropriate
- Plastic bag for child's personal belongings

If releasing a child to someone other than a parent or legal guardian:

- The above for discharging a child
- Completed Authorization for Release of a Minor form

If transferring a child to another room/unit:

- Medical chart, including care plan or care path
- Medications
- Personal belongings
- Transfer vehicle (wheelchair, bed, gurney)

If transferring a child to another facility:

- The above for discharging a child
- Completed Authorization for Release of a Minor form
- Completed Permission to Release Medical Records form
- Copy of medical records, including radiology files and studies
- Care plan or care path with summary of status in meeting outcomes (goal summary)
- Medications
- Plastic bag for child's personal belongings
- Transfer vehicle

If transferring a critically ill child to another unit or facility, the following additional equipment is needed:

- Blood pressure monitor
- Pulse oximeter
- Cardiac monitor/defibrillator
- Bag-valve mask device
- Oxygen tank and tubing
- Basic resuscitation medications and equipment (for interfacility transports)

If releasing a child against medical advice:

- The above for discharging a child
- AMA form

PROCEDURE **Discharging a Child**

Steps	Rationale/Points of Emphasis
Before the Day of Discharge	
1. Begin discharge planning upon child's admission and continue the process throughout the hospitalization.	Facilitates a smooth transition to home or other facility.
2. Collaborate with the healthcare prescriber, other multidisciplinary team members, and parents in planning for discharge.	Provides the most comprehensive understanding and approach to discharge needs, existing barriers, and available resources.
3. Identify the child's primary caregivers in the home setting.	Allows teaching to be done with the appropriate individuals.
4. Assess the family's knowledge regarding the child's illness, possible complications, and care and treatments to be continued at home.	Understanding the child's healthcare needs improves the likelihood of successful home care.
5. Monitor the parent's readiness and willingness to learn, and provide teaching regularly. For children with complex care needs, evaluate need for parents to assume responsibility for providing total care before discharge, with nursing staff available to assist.	Ongoing teaching assists in knowledge retention and allows repeated opportunities to practice new skills. Family provision of care provides an opportunity to evaluate parent proficiency and reinforce teaching, and it reinforces parent competence and decreases anxiety.
6. Review cares and procedures that will need to be performed at home. Provide demonstrations and written instructions. Evaluate parent understanding and perform return demonstration of proficiency; if unable to perform at a safe level, arrange for alternative providers (e.g., other family members, home healthcare, clinic visits).	Ensures skill proficiency and allows time for questions to be answered. Written materials reinforce in-hospital teaching once the child is at home.
7. Initiate referrals and orders for home care, supportive therapies, equipment, and supplies, as needed, and provide information about available community healthcare resources. Notify Social Services and Case Management of discharge needs.	Aids continuity of care across the healthcare continuum. **caREminder** *To create continuity of care between inpatient and outpatient care, consider a predischarge home evaluation when the child will go home technology dependent. This will help troubleshoot problems in the physical environment that may interfere with setup and care. Contact a home health nursing agency to give report and discuss plan of care (if applicable).*

Continued

Steps	Rationale/Points of Emphasis
8. Assess the family's emotional preparedness for discharge. Arrange predischarge contact with a support person or group, as needed.	Promotes healthy family coping skills. **caREminder** *Arrange respite care for the family of a child with continuous medical needs to provide parents with periodic breaks from complex medical home care responsibilities.*
9. Inform parents of the anticipated date and time of discharge as soon as it is known. Notify Social Services if transportation may be needed.	Allows the family to make necessary arrangements and helps to prevent last-minute delays.
10. Educate parents regarding the laws pertaining to use of a child restraint system in their motor vehicle. Assist in arranging for a special car seat or restraint system, as needed.	Increases safety of transport. Children for whom standard care seats or restraint systems may not be appropriate include • Premature and low-birth-weight infants • Children with tracheostomies or poor head control • Children in a body or hip spica cast • Infants/children requiring prone or supine positioning
On Day of Discharge	
1. Review healthcare prescriber's discharge orders for medications, treatments, equipment, or supplies.	Acts as a safeguard to double-check the accuracy of discharge orders and provides a foundation for final discharge teaching.
2. Confirm arrangements for outpatient and continuing services, home medical care, and equipment with the appropriate vendor or agency.	Ensures that the family will have what they need to provide ongoing care at home.
3. Review the discharge care plan with the child (as appropriate) and his or her family.	Establishes common goals to be met for discharge.
4. Gather prescriptions and any hospital medications that have been relabeled for home use. Review with family the prescribed medications, including the proper dose, route, time schedule, and possible adverse reactions.	Helps to promote proper drug administration. **caREminder** *To promote compliance with the medication regimen, ensure that the child's medication schedule is compatible with the family's normal routine.*
5. Review cares and procedures that will need to be performed at home. Provide demonstrations and written instructions. Evaluate parent understanding and ability to perform cares.	Ensures skill proficiency and allows time for questions to be answered. Written materials reinforce in-hospital teaching once the child is at home.
6. Review dietary or activity restrictions that are applicable and the reason they are necessary. Provide written instructions.	Helps to increase understanding of why adherence to a restriction may promote health.
7. Instruct parent regarding follow-up appointments or outpatient procedures that are needed. Provide written instructions. Assist with scheduling when appropriate.	Promotes continuity of care after discharge.
8. Confirm transportation arrangements with the family. Notify Social Services if last-minute assistance is needed.	Decreases the likelihood of unnecessary discharge delays.
9. Verify the child has been cleared for discharge through the financial and business offices. If not, refer parent to the appropriate office to arrange for clearance.	Ensures that the proper financial arrangements have been made with regard to the hospitalization.
10. Perform a physical assessment of the child. Notify the healthcare prescriber of any abnormal findings.	An abnormal finding may warrant a change in the discharge plan.

Steps	Rationale/Points of Emphasis
11. Gather child's belongings, including hospital hygiene supplies, into a bag. Make every effort to prevent hospital property from being removed with the child's belongings.	Ensures that the child goes home with the appropriate belongings and controls costs for the family and institution.
12. Have parent assist child to dress in street clothing.	Physically prepares the child for transition to home or other facility.
13a. Obtain parents' signatures on discharge instruction sheet and instruct them to bring it to the next follow-up appointment. 13b. Answer any final questions.	Verifies that instructions have been discussed and received and promotes continuity in follow-up care. Ensures parent understanding of home care responsibilities. **caREminder** *Being able to understand the provided instructions at home is necessary for compliance with a therapeutic regimen. All written instructions should be in a language, reading level, and format that the parents can understand. Use pictures or color coding, as necessary. Use an interpreter as necessary. The interpreter should not be anyone under 16 and should not be a family member if possible.*
14. Follow facility policy for checking identification of the parent or legal guardian before releasing the child into their care.	Acts as a security safeguard.
15. Once the child and his or her family have their medications, prescriptions, belongings, and discharge instructions, escort them, either walking or in a wheelchair, to the front lobby for transport home.	Ensures safety while exiting the hospital facility.
16. Remind parents to use appropriate car seat or child restraint system. If the child is going home with equipment, such as an apnea monitor, oxygen, or suction, instruct parents on how to secure it in their motor vehicle.	Promotes safety.
17. Complete discharge summary (see Child and Family Evaluation and Documentation at end of this chapter).	Documents care given and child's condition at discharge.
18. Once the child has left the patient care area, notify housekeeping and arrange for the room to be cleaned.	Facilitates timely preparation of the room for a new patient.

PROCEDURE Releasing a Child to Someone Other Than a Primary Caregiver or Legal Guardian

Steps	Rationale/Points of Emphasis
1. If the child is to be released to a relative (by blood or marriage) or to another healthcare facility, the parent or legal guardian must sign an authorization to release the minor before discharge.	Facilitates a safe and legally appropriate discharge.
2. If the child is younger than 16 years old and is to be released to someone other than a relative (e.g., baby-sitter, neighbor), a report to the State may be required. This report needs to be completed and signed by the parent or legal guardian before discharge.	Ensures that legal requirements are followed where care of a minor is involved. **caREminder** *In certain circumstances, a minor may be released to an agent of a public or law enforcement agency without parent consent. Consult Social Services in this event. A court order can override the usual parent rights. Social Services can assist in making the appropriate arrangements.*

Continued

Steps	Rationale/Points of Emphasis
3. If a child is to be released to someone other than a relative or to an agent of a public or law enforcement agency, the authorized individual's identification needs to be checked, at discharge, and his or her signature obtained on the appropriate form.	Verifies identify of individual and ensures legal parameters of release of a minor are being followed.

PROCEDURE Transferring a Child to Another Room

Steps	Rationale/Points of Emphasis
1. Determine the reason for a room change in collaboration with the charge nurse or unit coordinator. Arrange for an appropriate room, considering child's needs, safety issues, and child and family wishes. Consider age, gender, condition, and isolation requirements when evaluating roommate compatibility.	Allows for the most appropriate placement of the child within the unit.
2. Notify the child (as appropriate) and the family about the room to which the child will be transferred, reason for transfer, and date/time the transfer will occur.	Minimizes child and family anxiety.
3. After verifying that the new room is ready, transfer the child, along with his or her reusable supplies, equipment, and personal belongings.	Avoids loss of articles during transfer, and prevents duplicate patient charges for equipment and supplies.
4. Notify the unit secretary, healthcare prescriber, and Admitting and other departments (e.g., Pharmacy, Dietary) involved in the child's care of the room change.	Ensures that child's medication, meals, and therapies continue to be provided without error or delay. Allows visitors to locate the child.
5. Notify housekeeping when the child's original room has been vacated and arrange for the room to be cleaned.	Facilitates timely preparation of the room for a new patient.

PROCEDURE Transferring a Child to Another Unit

Steps	Rationale/Points of Emphasis
1. Determine the need for transfer in collaboration with the attending healthcare provider, based on changes in the child's condition and the availability of specific cares and resources.	Allows for the most appropriate placement of the child within the facility.
2. Obtain transfer orders that identify the unit to which the child will be transferred and the receiving healthcare prescriber.	Identifies healthcare provider who will be assuming legal responsibility for the child's care.
3. Notify the child (as appropriate) and the family about the unit to which the child will be transferred, reason for transfer, and date/time the transfer will occur.	Minimizes child and family anxiety.
4. Before transporting the child to the new unit, provide verbal report to the nurse who will be assuming care of the child; include the child's current condition and plan of care, necessary therapies, medications and treatments, and special nursing care needs.	Allows receiving nurse to prepare adequately for the child's arrival and promotes continuity of care between units.
5. Ensure that all documentation in the child's chart is complete and accurate.	Allows receiving unit to continue care without error or delay.

Steps	Rationale/Points of Emphasis
6. Gather the following in preparation for transfer: • Reusable supplies • Necessary equipment • Medical record • Medications • Child's personal belongings	Avoids loss of articles during transfer, and prevents duplicate patient charges for medications, equipment, and supplies.
7a. After verifying that the room in the receiving unit is ready, transfer the child along with the items listed in step 6.	Avoids delays upon arrival to receiving unit and loss of articles during transfer.
7b. Obtain assistance, as needed, to transport the child. Additional personnel may be needed based on child's condition and amount of support equipment.	If the transfer is emergent or the child is in critical condition, the receiving nurse from the unit of higher level of care may assist with transport to new unit. It is recommended that a minimum of two people accompany the critically ill patient. The receiving attending healthcare professional should also accompany an unstable child on transport to new unit. Ensure that emergency equipment and airway management and competent staff are present for transport of child (see equipment list).
7c. Report may be delayed for initial stabilization of child. Remain with child to assist receiving nurse and ensure continuity of care in the unit of higher level of care as needed and then proceed with steps 8–10 when appropriate.	Accompanying personnel should have proficient knowledge and skills to deal with rapid changes in the child's condition. Should the child's health status deteriorate rapidly, the priority is to stabilize the child's health condition and place the child on monitoring devices in the new unit as quickly as possible.
8. Notify the receiving unit's nursing station of the child's arrival, and assist in transporting the child to the room. Introduce the child and family to the receiving nurse; provide the nurse with the medical record, equipment, and medications; and answer any questions regarding the child's condition or care.	Allows for a smooth transition and completes the transfer process.
9. Notify Admitting and other departments (e.g., Pharmacy, Dietary) involved in the child's care of the unit transfer.	Ensures that child's medication, meals, and therapies continue to be provided without error or delay. Allows visitors to locate the child.
10. Notify housekeeping when the child's original room has been vacated and arrange for the room to be cleaned.	Facilitates timely preparation of the room for a new patient.

PROCEDURE Transferring a Child to Another Facility

Steps	Rationale/Points of Emphasis
1. Determine the need for transfer in collaboration with the attending healthcare provider and family, based on changes in the child's condition, the availability of needed cares and resources at other facilities, and the family's preference of the available options.	Allows for the most appropriate placement of the child.
2. In collaboration with the receiving agency to which the child will be transported, determine the most appropriate mode of transport based on the child's physical condition. The mode of transport is based on the urgency of the medical condition. • A stable child may be transferred by van or car. • A child requiring more intense physical monitoring must be transported in an ambulance. • A long-distance emergency transfer may require air transport. Ensure that appropriate transportation is arranged in advance.	Ensures appropriate level of monitoring to detect potential complications during transport.
3. Obtain transfer orders that identify the receiving facility and the receiving healthcare prescriber.	Identifies healthcare provider who will be assuming legal responsibility for the child's care.

Continued

Steps	Rationale/Points of Emphasis
4. Explain to the child (as appropriate) and the family the purpose of the transfer, the risks and benefits of the transfer, name and location of the receiving facility, and how and when the transfer will take place. Provide family with map, telephone number, and contact name for new facility.	Minimizes child and family anxiety. Family may wish to meet child at new facility.
5a. Obtain written parent informed consent for the transfer.	Current regulations require that informed consent be given for interhospital transfers. If circumstances do not allow for the informed consent process (e.g., life-threatening emergency), then both the indications for transfer and the reason for not obtaining consent should be documented in the medical record.
5b. Obtain parent or legal guardian signature on the Permission to Release Medical Records form. Forward the form to the Medical Records department, along with the chart to be copied.	The medical record provides the receiving facility with the necessary information to determine needed medications, care, services, and therapies.
6. Document a summary of nursing care and discharge evaluation of achievement of goals for transfer. Give report, by phone, to the receiving nursing unit, if possible.	Facilitates continuity of nursing care and assists in a smooth care transition.
7. Perform a physical assessment of the child; notify healthcare prescriber of any abnormal findings.	An abnormal finding may warrant a change in the transfer plan.
8a. Ensure that all documentation in the child's medical record is complete and accurate.	Allows receiving facility to accurately continue the child's care.
8b. The child's medical records should be sent to the new facility following the original facility's safeguards to protect patient data. Documents may need to be sent before the child's departure to ensure new facility has full understanding of child's health status.	Patient confidentiality and how health information is transferred is regulated by the Health Information Portability and Accountability Act of 1996.
9. Gather child's belongings, including hospital hygiene supplies and any hospital medications that have been relabeled for discharge use, and place them in a bag. Make every effort to prevent hospital property from being removed with the child's belongings.	Ensures that the child is transferred with the appropriate belongings and controls costs for the family and institution.
10. Have parent assist the child to dress in personal pajamas or street clothes, as appropriate.	Physically prepares the child for transfer.
11. When transporter arrives, check identification, complete the Authorization for Release of a Minor form, and obtain transporter's signature.	Facilitates a safe and legally appropriate transfer.
12. When the child has left the patient care area, notify housekeeping and arrange for the room to be cleaned.	Facilitates timely preparation of the room for a new patient.

PROCEDURE Releasing a Child Against Medical Advice (AMA)

Steps	Rationale/Points of Emphasis
1. If a parent expresses a desire to take the child from the hospital before discharge and AMA, notify the attending healthcare prescriber immediately. Implement institution-specific guidelines to safeguard child as healthcare providers discuss situation with the family.	Gives the healthcare prescriber an opportunity to explain the risks of leaving, the advantages of continued hospitalization, and any alternatives to hospitalization, such as transfer to another facility or outpatient treatment. **caREminder** *Medical neglect and child endangerment are reportable, by law. When the decision to take a child from the hospital AMA may cause harm or death, consult Social Services to assist in filing a report with Child Protective Services.*

Steps	Rationale/Points of Emphasis
2a. If the parent persists in the decision to take the child from the hospital, present him or her with an AMA form and ask for his or her signature in the presence of a witness; file the signed form in the medical record.	Ensures documentation for healthcare facility and provides legal verification of parents' informed choice to leave the facility with their child. **caREminder** *Do not detain a parent and his or her child for refusal to sign an AMA form. If they refuse to sign the form, they must still be allowed to leave the facility.*
2b. If the parent refuses to sign an AMA form, note this on the form, along with the date, time, circumstances of refusal, and name of the person who refused, and obtain the signature of a witness. File the form in the medical record.	Ensures proper legal documentation.
3. Complete a Patient Safety Adverse Event form according to institutional policy.	Provides documentation for review by a quality management department.
4. Document, in the child's chart, a summary of the events leading up to and including the incident.	Provides a factual account for the child's permanent medical record. A signed AMA form does not necessarily release the healthcare facility or professionals from legal liability.
5. Complete the discharge procedure (see Discharging a Child, On Day of Discharge Procedure, steps 1–18), as permitted by the parent.	Assists in facilitating a smooth transition to home, as the circumstances allow.

CHILD AND FAMILY EVALUATION AND DOCUMENTATION

Discharge (Planned or AMA)

- Document the following in the child's medical record:
  - Instructions given regarding the child's illness, drug therapy, diet, activity level, treatments, follow-up appointments, possible complications, and which conditions warrant immediate notification of a healthcare prescriber
  - Date and time of discharge and with whom the child was discharged
  - Child's physical condition at discharge (physical assessment)
  - Evaluation of the care plan goals and care path outcomes

Transfer

- For transfer of a child to another room in the same unit, document the following in the child's medical record:
  - Reason for transfer
  - Date, time, and room to which the transfer took place
  - Child's tolerance of the transfer
- For transfer of a child to another unit, document the following in the child's medical record:
  - The transferring nurse documents:
    - Reason for transfer, including changes in child's condition that may have indicated need for transfer
    - The date, time, unit to which child was transferred, and method of transport
    - Child's condition at time of transfer
  - The receiving nurse documents:
    - The date and time of arrival and method of transport
    - Child's condition and tolerance of the transfer
    - Care provided
  - For transfer of a child to another facility, document the following in the child's medical record:
    - Reason for transfer, including changes in child's condition that may have indicated need for transfer
    - Date and time of release to the transport personnel; name of person released to
    - Method of transport to the transport vehicle
    - Child's condition at the time of discharge
    - Notification of primary healthcare prescriber and ancillary departments regarding child's transfer
    - Evaluation of the care plan goals and care path outcomes

COMMUNITY CARE

- Communicate home care needs, as appropriate, to those agencies or individuals who will be following the child in the community setting (e.g., home care agency, equipment vendor, public health nurse, social worker, school nurse).
- Provide anticipatory guidance to the family about child's responses to hospitalization, noting that developmental

regression is not uncommon and that the family should provide support and consistent routine for the child.

- Instruct the family when to call the healthcare provider (varies based on reason for hospitalization), and ensure that the family has the name of provider and contact information.

Unexpected Situations

- *At the time of discharge, the parent who arrives to pick up child is not recognized as the legal guardian of child:* Child may not be released to this parent. The legal guardian should be contacted and informed that child may only be discharged to his or her care. If the parent present becomes agitated, security may need to be called.
- *Child is ready for discharge and is noted to have a fever. The previous vital signs were within normal range:* Retake child's temperature in 30 minutes. If still elevated, notify the healthcare prescriber of child's change in condition. Discharge may be delayed based on child's current condition and previous health status.

Bibliography

American Academy of Pediatrics. (1996). Safe transportation of premature and low birth weight infants. Policy statement (RE9617). *Pediatrics, 97*, 758–760.

American Academy of Pediatrics. (1999a). Care coordination: Integrating health and related systems of care for children with special care needs. *Pediatrics, 104*, 978–981.

American Academy of Pediatrics. (1999b). Guidelines for developing admission and discharge policies for pediatric intensive care unit. *Pediatrics, 103*, 840–842.

American Academy of Pediatrics. (1999c). Safe transportation of newborns at hospital discharge. Policy statement (RE9854). *Pediatrics, 104*, 986–987.

American Academy of Pediatrics. (1999d). Privacy protection of health information: Patient's rights and pediatrician responsibilities. *Pediatrics, 104*, 973–976.

American Academy of Pediatrics. (1999e). Transporting children with special health care needs. Policy statement (RE9852). *Pediatrics, 104*, 988–992.

Bakewell-Sachs, S., & Porth, S. (1995). Discharge planning and home care of the technology-dependent infant. *Journal of Obstetric, Gynecologic, and Neonatal Nursing, 24*(1), 77–83.

Devitt, P. J., Devitt, A. C., & Dewan, M. (2000). Does identifying a discharge as "against medical advice" confer legal protection. *The Journal of Family Practice, 49*(3), 224–226.

Dodds-Azzopardi, S. E., & Chapman, J. S. (1995). Parent's perceptions of stress associated with premature infant transfer among hospital environments. *Journal of Perinatal and Neonatal Nursing, 8*(4), 39–45.

Green, P., Watts, D., Pool, S., & Dhopesh, V. (2004). Why patient's sign out against medical advice: Factors motivating patients to sign out AMA. *The American Journal of Drug and Alcohol Abuse, 30*(2), 489–493.

Heward, Y. (2003). Transfer from ward to PICU: A standard. *Paediatric Nursing, 15*(1), xi–xiii.

Jaimovich, D., & Committee on Hospital Care and Section on Critical Care. (2004). Admission and discharge guidelines for the pediatric patient requiring intermediate care. *Pediatrics, 113*, 1430–1433.

Waisman, Y., Siegal, N., Siegal, G., Amir, L., Cohen, H., & Mimouni, M. (2005). Role of diagnosis-specific information sheets in parents' understanding of emergency department discharge instructions. *European Journal of Emergency Medicine, 12*(4), 159–162.

Warren, J., Fromm, R. E. Jr., Orr, R. A., Rotello, L. C., & Horst, H. M. (2004). Guidelines for the inter- and intrahospital transport of critically ill patients. *Critical Care Medicine, 32*(1), 256–262.

Williams, D. M., Counselman, F. L., & Caggiano, C. D. (1996). Emergency department discharge instructions and patient literacy: A problem of disparity. *American Journal of Emergency Medicine, 14*(1), 19–22.

Worthington, R. C. (1995). Effective transitions for families: Life beyond the hospital. *Pediatric Nursing, 21*(1), 86–87.

CHAPTER 116

Urinary Catheterization: Insertion and Removal of Indwelling Catheter

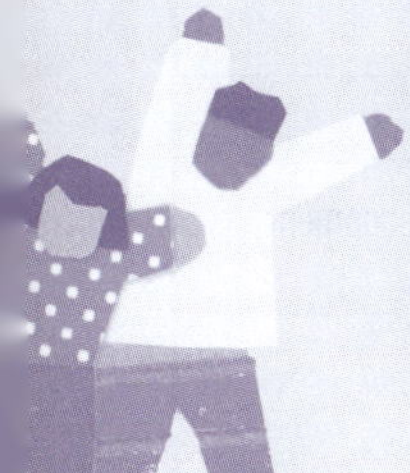

Clinical Guidelines

- A healthcare prescriber's order is required for placement, removal, and replacement of a urinary catheter when it is no longer needed or has become obstructed or requires changing.
- A healthcare prescriber's order is required for use of 2% lidocaine (Xylocaine) water-soluble lubricant in catheterizing a child.
- 2% lidocaine gel has shown effectiveness in reducing discomfort associated with insertion of the catheter. However, because lidocaine gel takes at least 8 minutes for the anesthetic effect to be complete, use of nonanesthetic lubricant with 2% lidocaine gel as lubricant must be considered based on the child's age, level of anxiety, and urgency of the procedure. The use of lidocaine lubricant may be more appropriate with older adolescents because in the younger child it may increase the length of the procedure and, therefore, the child's anxiety. A delay before starting the catheterization maximizes absorption of the anesthetic in the urethra.
- A healthcare prescriber, registered nurse (RN), or licensed practical nurse (LPN) inserts and removes a urinary catheter.

Equipment

- Gloves, gown, and protective eyewear
- Basin with soap and warm water, washcloths, and towels
- Waterproof pad
- Nonallergenic tape
- Prepackaged catheter insertion kit, which includes (obtain the following items if your institution does not supply prepackaged kit)
  - Sterile gloves
  - Sterile povidone-iodine swabs
  - Sterile water-soluble lubricant
  - Sterile towels and drapes
  - Sterile syringe filled with 3 to 5 mL of sterile water
  - Sterile gravity drainage and collection bag
  - Sterile catheter (Table 116-1)

TABLE 116-1

Selection of Urinary Catheter

Age (yr)	Recommended Catheter Size (French)*
0–2	6 F
2–5	6–8 F
5–10	8–10 F
10–16	10–12 F

*Feeding tubes are more prone to knotting and should not be used. Because of its two internal lumens, the balloon catheter must have a larger external diameter than might otherwise be necessary for adequate drainage of urine. In small-sized balloon catheters, the stylet provided for insertion may increase the risk for false passage or bladder perforation. If balloon catheters are used, they should be made of silicone or coated with Teflon to reduce irritation and inflammation of the urethral mucosa.

- Applicator with 2% lidocaine water-soluble lubricant (if ordered)
- Waste receptacle
- Sheet to be used as a drape (may not be necessary for infants and small children)
- Examination light (optional)

CHILD AND FAMILY ASSESSMENT AND PREPARATION

- Assess the cognitive level, readiness, and ability to process information by the child and family. The readiness to learn and process information may be impaired as a result of age, stress, or anxiety.
- Assess the child for signs and symptoms of urinary tract or bladder infection, including fever, inability to void, burning on urination, feeling of fullness, bladder spasms, foul-smelling urine, redness or irritation of urethral opening, urethral discharge, crying without consolation, or discomfort.
- Assess the child for signs and symptoms of a distended bladder or residual urine, for which bladder emptying would be required.
- Identify and discuss the risks and benefits of placing an indwelling catheter. Assure the parents that the catheterization will not harm the child or damage the urethra or hymen.
- Reinforce the need for catheter placement, as appropriate, to both the child and the family.
- Provide the opportunity to ask questions and alleviate fears.
- Explain the procedure, as appropriate, to both the child and the family.

KidKare Reassure the toddler and older child that the catheter is flexible and will feel like a noodle and will produce a feeling of pressure and a desire to urinate.

- Provide instruction on pelvic muscle relaxation whenever possible. To relax pelvic and periurethral muscles, teach the child to blow a pinwheel and to press the hips against the bed or examination table during the catheterization. Next, teach the child to contract and relax the pelvic muscles and to repeat this relaxation procedure during catheter insertion.

PROCEDURE **Insertion of an Indwelling Catheter**

Steps	Rationale/Points of Emphasis
1a. Perform hand hygiene and gather the necessary supplies.	Reduces transmission of microorganisms. Promotes efficient time management and provides an organized approach to the procedure. **caREminder** *Another nurse may be necessary to assist if the child is unable to cooperate for any reason.*
1b. Select catheter appropriate for child (see Table 116–1).	Selection of the catheter is based on the child's age and gender, construction material of the catheter, and the internal and external diameter of the catheter. Small catheter sizes promote comfort and are adequate for specimen collection. Use of shorter-length urinary catheters and basing length on gender and age can reduce incidence of knotting (e.g., for toddlers and younger females, insert 2 inches; for male infants, insert 3 inches; for male toddlers, insert 3 to 4 inches).
1c. Have extra catheters readily accessible during the procedure.	If a catheter becomes contaminated, is inadvertently placed in the vagina, or turns out to be the incorrect size, an extra catheter will be immediately needed to maintain sterility and complete the procedure in a timely manner.

Steps	Rationale/Points of Emphasis
2. Close the door to the child's room or draw the curtains around the child's bed.	Provides privacy during the procedure.
3. Raise the bed to a comfortable working height, or stand on a step stool at crib side.	Reduces the strain placed on your back.
4. Don gloves and protective apparel.	Standard precaution to reduce transmission of microorganisms.
5a. Place a waterproof pad under the child's/infant's buttocks while positioning the child/infant.	Prevents the bed linens from being soiled.
5b. Position females in the supine position with the heels of the feet together and the knees tilted outward (called the frog position). Use rolled blankets, pillow, or towels to support legs in this position.	This position facilitates visualization of the inner labia.
5c. Position males in the supine position with the legs together. Use rolled towels under knees. Raise the penis and scrotal sac to rest on top of the thighs.	This position facilitates visualization of the urethral opening. Bending the knees slightly may be a more comfortable position for the child. **KidKare** Remind the child to keep his or her buttocks on the bed or table and to keep the perineal muscles relaxed. The child will most likely need to be reminded of this several times during the procedure.
6. Place a drape over the child/infant. In females, place the drape in a diamond configuration with one corner at the child's sternum, one corner over each knee, and one corner over the perineum. In males, cover the child's chest and lower extremities with a sheet, leaving only the genital area exposed.	Allows exposure of the child's perineum while covering the rest of the body, allowing for privacy.
7. Wash the child's genital area with warm water and soap. Rinse and dry the area.	Removes secretions and feces.
8. Remove gloves and perform hand hygiene	Reduces transmission of microorganisms.
9. Establish a sterile working area, using a sterile towel spread open.	Establishes a space from which to gather sterile equipment and proceed with catheterization without contamination.
10. Using sterile technique, open the sterile catheter, sterile povidone-iodine, sterile lubricant, swabs, and sterile prefilled syringe of water and drop them on the sterile towel. Open the sterile gravity drainage and collection bag and leave it sitting in the packaging container.	Facilitates ease of access to the equipment. If lidocaine gel is to be used, assemble lidocaine applicator according to the manufacturer's instructions and follow procedure for use of lidocaine lubricant gel.
11. Aseptically place a sterile towel between the female child's legs under the perineal area or on the thighs of a male child.	The pad becomes an extension of the sterile work area.
12. Don sterile gloves.	Reduces introduction of microorganisms into the urinary tract, which is normally sterile.
13. Attach the prefilled syringe of water to the secondary lumen balloon port of the urinary catheter and inflate the balloon with the sterile water and then deflate the balloon, retaining the sterile water in the syringe.	Ensures that the balloon of the retention catheter is working and does not have a leak.
14a. While laying your nondominant arm across the midsection of the lower abdomen, use the thumb and middle finger of your nondominant sterile hand to spread open the female child's labia.	Allows for exposure and visualization of the urethral opening. Swelling of the labia in neonates, due to maternal hormones, may make it difficult to visualize the urethral opening. A flashlight or examination light may be helpful in locating the urethral opening. If locating the urethra in females is difficult, have an assistant, wearing sterile gloves, grasp the labia majora and gently pull forward, forming a cave-like opening and causing the hymen and urethra to drop open.

Continued

Steps	Rationale/Points of Emphasis
14b. For a male child, follow the same procedure and use your nondominant hand to position the child's penis perpendicular to the body. In an uncircumcised male, withdraw the foreskin just far enough to visualize the urethral opening. Do not pull back behind the glans.	Withdrawing the foreskin further will be painful to the child and could cause tears that could lead to potential sites of infection.
15. With your dominant sterile hand, cleanse the area around the urethral opening with the sterile povidone-iodine swabs and discard them in a nearby waste receptacle. In females, using a separate povidone-iodine swab for each stroke, cleanse both the right and left side of the inner labia with one downward stroke. Then clean midline, from the clitoris down to the rectum with one stroke. In males, cleanse the penis in an outgoing circular motion, from the urethral opening to the base of the penis, using a new povidone-iodine swab each time.	Prevents contamination of the catheter by microorganisms on the skin and prevents introduction of open organisms into the patient's urethra and bladder. **caREminder** *The labia should not be allowed to close during the entire procedure because this contaminates the sterile field. If the labia do close, stop the procedure, don new sterile gloves, and start over at this step.*
16. With your sterile dominant hand, lubricate the tip of the sterile catheter with the water-soluble lubricant that has been squirted on the sterile field. The catheter should be lubricated about 2 inches for a female child and about 6 inches for a male child.	Lubricant decreases the friction between the catheter and the urinary tract during catheterization. In males, using lubricant on the tip of the catheter promotes opening of the sphincter mechanism.
17a. Lift the lubricated tip of the catheter with your dominant sterile hand and gently insert it into the child's urethral opening.	Allows for catheterization to obtain sterile urine specimen.
17b. Do not touch the child's perineal hair or skin as the catheter is advanced.	Hair or skin contaminates the catheter.
17c. In males, insert the lubricated catheter tip into the urethra without allowing the intraurethral lubricant (if lidocaine gel was used) to exit the urethral meatus. Because gentle pressure may cause an erection in an adolescent male, hold the penis firmly but not tightly. If held tightly, pressure will collapse the urethra and will prevent advancement of the catheter.	If the adolescent has an erection, stop the procedure until there is a nonerectile state, and then continue with the procedure.
17d. Ask the child to take a deep breath while you insert the catheter.	Taking a deep breath helps to relax the urinary tract. **KidKare** The child may state he or she needs to urinate during catheter insertion. Tell child to go ahead and try to do so; this opens the urethra for passage of the catheter.
18. Insert the catheter until urine begins to flow. If an obstruction is encountered, *do not* force the catheter. If the catheter is inadvertently placed in the vagina, leave it in place and put a second catheter in the other opening (urethra). After second catheter is in place, remove catheter from the vagina. In males, the prepuce is retractable; put it back in the natural position after inserting the catheter. ***Alert!*** ***When the catheter reaches the striated sphincter (proximal urethra in males and midurethra in females), the child may vigorously contract the pelvic muscles, temporarily stopping insertion of the catheter. Hold the catheter in place with steady gentle pressure. Assist the child to press the hips against the bed or examination table and relax the pelvic muscles before gently advancing the catheter into the bladder. Wait for the sphincter to relax before advancing the catheter. If still unable to advance the catheter, discontinue the procedure and notify the healthcare prescriber.***	A rule of thumb for catheter length in males is twice the length of the penis plus 4 cm. Placing the catheter too far into the bladder can cause irritation to the bladder wall and/or knotting of the catheter. Forcing the catheter can cause trauma, bleeding, and possible scar formation, which can lead to strictures and obstruction of the urethra. If lidocaine gel is used it will increase the volume of intraurethral lubricant. Therefore urine return may not be as rapid as when minimal amounts of water-soluble lubricant are used. Avoids possible painful swelling of the glans (paraphimosis).

Steps	Rationale/Points of Emphasis
19. After urinary flow is established, insert the catheter approximately 1–2 cm further and inflate the secondary lumen balloon port of the catheter with sterile water to the amount specified (usually specified on the balloon port itself) and disconnect the syringe.	Prevents the catheter from slipping and from accidental dislodgment. Overinflation of the balloon can cause balloon rupture. Use only the amount specified by the manufacturer. **KidKare** If the child complains of pain or burning, the urinary catheter may not be fully seated in the bladder. Deflate the balloon, advance the catheter further, and reinflate the balloon.
20. Gently tug or pull back slightly on the catheter.	Ensures that the catheter is securely seated in the bladder and not floating.
21. Tightly connect the sterile gravity drainage and collection bag to the urinary catheter; tape the connections and ensure the urine continues to flow out the tubing.	Provides for a closed-system collection of urine output.
22. Attach the bag to the frame of the bed or crib below the level of the bladder, ensuring there are no kinks or obstructions in the tubing.	Positioning the bag below the level of the bladder prevents reflux of urine through the tubing and back into the bladder.
23. Wash and cleanse the child's perineal area and return the foreskin to its natural position after cleansing on the uncircumcised male.	Cleansing promotes the child's comfort and sense of well-being, while removing the povidone-iodine solution from the area. Failure to return the foreskin can lead to swelling of the penis and impairment of circulation.
24. Tape the catheter tubing to the thigh of the older child. For small male infants and neonates not using a balloon catheter, tape the catheter to the lower abdomen or upper perineum, allowing the penis to point upward toward the umbilicus. For small female infants or neonates not using a balloon catheter, tape the catheter at its closest point outside on the left or right labia.	Taping prevents any tension from being placed on the catheter from inside the bladder and avoids dislodgment from accidental pulling or tugging. Movement of the catheter in and out can lead to contamination from microorganisms. **caREminder** *Ensure there are no pressure points or areas of skin breakdown before taping to the thigh, leg, abdomen, or perineum.*
25. Return the child's bed to the lowest position or to a level that is age appropriate.	Reduces potential injury from falls.
26. Dispose of used equipment and waste in appropriate receptacle.	Standard precautions
27. Remove gloves and perform hand hygiene.	Reduces the transmission of microorganisms

PROCEDURE Use of Lidocaine Lubricant Gel

Steps	Rationale/Points of Emphasis
1. Complete steps 1–12 above.	
2. With sterile gloves on, assemble the applicator with 2% lidocaine lubricant gel. Place nickel to quarter size amount of lubricant on a sterile cotton ball.	Facilitates ease of access to the equipment. Standard applicators come with either 5 or 10 mL of 2% lidocaine gel.
3. For males, use forceps to place the gel-covered cotton ball on the meatus; leave in place for at least 2 minutes. For females place a lidocaine-soaked cotton ball on the urethral meatus; leave in place for at least 2 minutes. Place the applicator with the rest of the lubricant in it on the sterile field. Set aside one cotton ball for additional lidocaine gel applications.	The lubricant is used to numb the external meatus and reduce discomfort associated with inserting the catheter. This is the first of four applications of the lubricant gel.

Continued

Steps	Rationale/Points of Emphasis
4. During wait period, continue to set up the catheterization kit. With your sterile dominant hand, lubricate the tip of the sterile catheter with the 2% lidocaine solution or water-soluble lubricant that has been squirted on the sterile field. Lubricate the catheter about 2 inches for a female child and about 6 inches for a male child.	Both lubricants decrease the friction between the catheter and the urinary tract during catheterization. In males, using lubricant on the tip of the catheter promotes opening of the sphincter mechanism.
5. Attach the prefilled syringe of water to the secondary lumen balloon port of the urinary catheter and inflate the balloon with the sterile water, and then deflate the balloon retaining the sterile water in the syringe.	Ensures that the balloon of the retention catheter is working and does not have a leak.
6. After 2 minutes, use forceps to remove and discard the first cotton ball from the meatus of the male or female.	First application of lidocaine has been completed.
a. Continue with the process of sterile cleaning of the perineal area. While laying your nondominant arm across the midsection of the lower abdomen, use the thumb and middle finger of your nondominant sterile hand to spread open the female child's labia.	Allows for exposure and visualization of the urethral opening. Swelling of the labia in neonates, due to maternal hormones, may make it difficult to visualize the urethral opening. A flashlight or examination light may be helpful in locating the urethral opening. If locating the urethra in females is difficult, have an assistant, wearing sterile gloves, grasp the labia majora and gently pull forward, forming a cave-like opening and therefore allowing the hymen and urethra to drop open.
b. For a male child, follow the same procedure and use your nondominant hand to position the child's penis perpendicular to the body. In an uncircumcised male, withdraw the foreskin just far enough to visualize the urethral opening. Do not pull back behind the glans.	Withdrawing the foreskin further will be painful to the child and could cause tears that could lead to potential sites of infection.
7. With your dominant sterile hand, cleanse the area around the urethral opening with the sterile povidone-iodine swabs and discard them in a nearby waste receptacle. In females, using a separate povidone-iodine swab for each stroke, cleanse both the right and left side of the inner labia with one downward stroke. Then clean midline, from the clitoris down to the rectum with one stroke. In males, cleanse the penis in an outgoing circular motion, from the urethral opening to the base of the penis, using a new povidone-iodine swab each time.	Prevents contamination of the catheter by microorganisms on the skin and prevents introduction of open organisms into the patient's urethra and bladder. **caREminder** *The labia should not be allowed to close during the entire procedure because this contaminates the sterile field. If the labia do close, stop the procedure, don new sterile gloves, and start over at this step.*
8. In males, begin installation by gently touching the applicator to the meatus. Slowly instill the lidocaine gel into the meatus (see Table 116-2 for amount of lubricant to be used). Place a cotton ball on the meatus. Hold the lubricant in place by gently squeezing the distal penis (behind the glans penis). Wait 2 minutes. In females, use the applicator to drip lidocaine gel downward from the clitoris onto the urethral opening. Place a second lidocaine gel–soaked cotton ball on the meatus. Wait 2 minutes.	Instilling the lidocaine too quickly causes a burning sensation and irritation of the meatus. The amount of lubricant instilled depends on length and diameter of urethra. Though the female urethra is generally shorter, the amount administered is the same for females and males.

TABLE 116-2

Total Amount of Lidocaine Gel Installed Over Three Installations

Age	Measurement
Infant	½–1½ mL
Toddler	1½–2½ mL
School-aged	2½–5 mL
Adolescent	3–5 mL

Steps	Rationale/Points of Emphasis
9. For males, repeat the numbing and instillation process in step 7 two more times. For females, gently touch the meatus with the applicator and then gently instill a small amount of lubricant into the urethra. Place a cotton ball over the urethra. Wait 2 minutes. Repeat installation of lidocaine one more time and wait 2 minutes.	Repeated applications ensure efficacy of anesthetic.
10. For males, instill extra sterile water-soluble gel into urethra.	Dilates urethra and acts as additional lubricant.
11. Continue with catheterization procedure following steps 16–27 of the procedure for Insertion of an Indwelling Catheter.	Placement of catheter should proceed in atraumatic fashion as a result of lidocaine gel applications.

PROCEDURE Removal of an Indwelling Catheter

Steps	Rationale/Points of Emphasis
1. Collaborate with child, family, and healthcare prescriber regarding time to remove catheter. If routine removal after a procedure, remove the catheter in the late evening.	Ensures child is prepared for the procedure. Studies of midnight versus early morning catheter removal on adult patients reveal that removal at midnight resulted in significantly earlier discharge from the hospital compared with those with morning removal, if discharge was dependent on successful catheter removal.
2. Perform hand hygiene and collect all necessary equipment and supplies for removal.	Reduces transmission of microorganisms. Promotes efficient time management and provides an organized approach to procedure.
3. Close the door to the child's room or draw the curtains around the child's bed.	Provides privacy during the procedure.
4. Raise the bed to a comfortable working height, or stand on a step stool at crib side.	Reduces the strain placed on your back.
5. Don gloves, gown, and protective eyewear.	Standard precautions to reduce transmission of microorganisms.
6. Place a waterproof pad under the child's buttocks while positioning the child/infant. Position the child/infant supine, legs spread apart, with access to the urinary catheter.	Prevents the bed linens from being soiled. Facilitates visualization of the inner labia or the urethral opening.
7. Place a drape over the child/infant.	Allows exposure to the child's perineum while covering the rest of the body, allowing for privacy.
8. Gently remove any tape holding urinary catheter in place.	Provides ease of access to catheter for removal.
9. Attach a syringe to the secondary lumen balloon port of the urinary catheter and deflate the balloon of its entire contents of sterile water (usually the balloon capacity is specified on the balloon port itself).	Allows for atraumatic removal of the retention catheter. **Alert!** *If the catheter is removed without the balloon being fully deflated, bladder or urethral trauma can occur.*
10. Gently remove the urinary catheter by withdrawing slowly and evenly. If resistance is felt, do not pull harder; stop and notify healthcare prescriber.	Reduces trauma and irritation to the urethra. Any resistance to removal may suggest kinking, knotting, the balloon's failure to deflate, or stone formation.
11. Wash the child's genital area with warm water and soap. Rinse and dry the area.	Removes secretions, any urine that may have leaked out, and feces. Drying the area makes the environment less hospitable to microorganisms.
12. Remove the waterproof underpad and re-cover the child as appropriate.	Maintains dry linens for the child and promotes sense of well-being.
13. Return the child's bed to the lowest position or to a level that is age appropriate.	Reduces potential injury from falls.

Continued

Steps	Rationale/Points of Emphasis
14. Dispose of equipment and waste in appropriate receptacle, noting the final amount of urine collected.	Standard precautions.
15. Perform hand hygiene	Reduces the transmission of microorganisms.
16. Monitor child for first void after catheter removal. Note the amount, color, and any sediment of the urine when the child does void.	Decreased bladder function may occur after the catheter is removed. Encourage the child to drink plenty of fluids. Most symptoms of dysuria, enuresis, and hematuria abate after 1 or 2 days. A warm Sitz bath may help children who have voiding difficulties. Urinary tract infections can develop as a result of catheterization.

CHILD AND FAMILY EVALUATION AND DOCUMENTATION

- Evaluate the amount, color, clarity, and odor of the urine and the presence of any sediment at least once per shift (or more often, as indicated by child's condition).
- Evaluate child for signs and symptoms of a urinary tract infection, including fever, tachycardia, foul-smelling urine or perineum, perineal discharge, cloudy or sedimented urine, or urine discoloration.
- Document the following:
  - Completion of the procedure
  - The size of catheter inserted and removed
  - Amount of sterile water inserted and removed from the balloon
  - Amount, color, clarity, and odor of the urine and presence of any sediment
  - Child's response to catheterization and removal
  - Signs and symptoms of urinary tract infection

COMMUNITY CARE

- If the procedure is completed in an outpatient setting, encourage parents to offer fluids to the child on the trip to the office or clinic.
- If the child is discharged with an indwelling catheter, it should be changed at prescribed intervals by a visiting home nurse.
- If the procedure is performed at the child's home, instruct the family to
  - Care for the indwelling catheter, including perineal and catheter hygiene and bag emptying
  - Offer frequent fluids
  - Assess the urinary output
  - Assess for signs and symptoms of urinary tract infection
  - Dispose of excess urine in home lavatory
  - Remove and dispose of catheter (as appropriate)
- Instruct the family to contact the healthcare provider if
  - Urine is cloudy or dark
  - Blood is present in the urine or a change in smell of the urine occurs
  - Child has nausea or vomiting
  - Child has chills or fever
  - Child has flank pain
  - Child is lethargic
  - Child has painful voiding or frequent urgency to void
  - Swelling or redness occurs around the urethral opening

Unexpected Situations

- *When catheterizing a female child, no urine flow is obtained:* Try to visualize whether the catheter is in the vaginal orifice. If this is the case, leave the catheter in place as a landmark. Don fresh gloves. Using a new catheter, attempt to place the tube in the urethral orifice directly above the misplaced catheter.
- *Immediately after the catheter is placed and the balloon is inflated, the child voids a large amount around the balloon:* Ensure that the correct amount of fluid has been injected into the balloon. Do not overinflate the balloon. Leaking around the balloon when the catheter is initially inserted is not uncommon due to the large amount of urine pressure. Place a disposable waterproof pad underneath the child's buttocks and monitor for further leaking. If leaking continues, the child may need a larger catheter inserted.

Bibliography

Bardsley, A. (2005). Use of lubricant gels in urinary catheterization. *Nursing Standard, 20*(8), 41–46.

Bray, L., & Sanders, C. (2006). Nursing management of paediatric urethral catheterization. *Nursing Standard, 20*(24), 51–60, 62, 64.

Bukowski, T., & Freedman, A. (1999). Urethral catheterization: The case for caution. *Contemporary Pediatrics, 16*(4), 100–104.

Carlson, D., & Mowrey, B. (1997). Standards to prevent complications of urinary catheterization in children: Should and should-knots. *Journal of the Society of Pediatric Nurses, 2*, 37–41.

Getliffe, K. (2001). Review of catheter care guidelines. *Nursing Times, 97*(20), 70–71.

Gerard, L., Cooper, C., Duethman, K., et al. (2003). Effectiveness of lidocaine lubricant for discomfort during pediatric urethral catheterization. *Journal of Urology, 170*(2, Part 1), 564–567.

Griffiths, R., & Fernandez, R. (2005). Policies for the removal of short-term indwelling urethral catheters. *The Cochrane Database of Systematic Reviews,* (1), No. CD004011.

Gray, M. (1996). Atraumatic urethral catheterization of children. *Pediatric Nursing, 22,* 306–310.

Niël-Weise, B. S., & van den Broek, P. J. (2005). Urinary catheter policies for long-term bladder drainage. *The Cochrane Database of Systematic Reviews,* (1), No. CD004201.

Siderias, J., Guadio, F., & Singer, A. J. (2004). Comparison of topical anesthetics and lubricants prior to urethral catheterization in males: A randomized controlled trial. *Academic Emergency Medicine, 11,* 703–706.

Simpson, L. (2001). Indwelling urethral catheters: Reducing the risk of potential complications through proactive management. *Primary Health Care, 11*(2), 57–64.

Tanabe, P., Steinmann, R., Anderson, J., et al. (2004). Factors affecting pain scores during female urethral catheterization. *Academic Emergency Medicine, 11,* 699–702.

Turner, T. (2004). Intravesical catheter knotting: An uncommon complication of urinary catheterization. *Pediatric Emergency Care, 20,* 115–117.

Vaughn, M., Paton, E., Bush, A., & Pershad, J. (2005). Does lidocaine gel alleviate the pain of bladder catheterization in young children? A randomized, controlled trial. *Pediatrics, 116,* 917–920.

C H A P T E R

117

Urinary Catheterization: Management of Indwelling Catheter

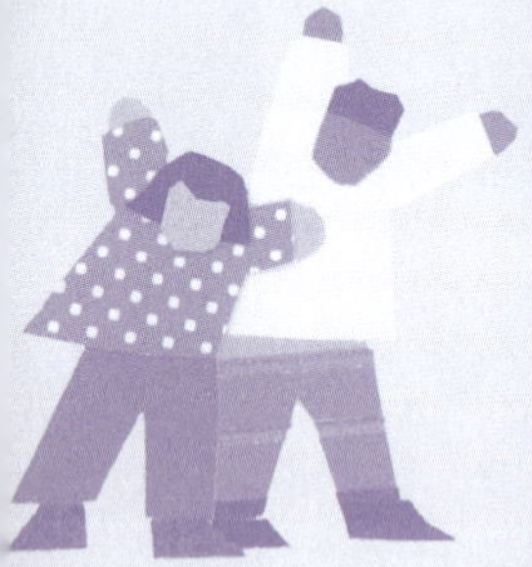

Clinical Guidelines

- A healthcare prescriber's order is required for placement, removal, and replacement of a urinary catheter when it is no longer needed, has become obstructed, or requires changing.
- A registered nurse (RN), licensed practical nurse (LPN), or unlicensed nursing personnel (UAP) performs hygienic care at least twice a day for children with an indwelling catheter.
- Placement of an indwelling or retention catheter is performed for many reasons, including but not limited to
  - Insertion before, for, and after surgery
  - Assisting in urinary elimination of those who are unable to void spontaneously
  - Maintaining an empty bladder
  - Instilling medications
  - Splinting the urethra
  - Precisely measuring urine output
  - Obtaining urine for analysis over an extended period
  - Urinary incontinence and bladder training
- Institutional policy dictates how long the urinary catheter may remain in place without being changed.
- Children with an indwelling urinary catheter are observed for signs and symptoms of urinary tract infection as long as the catheter is in place and for several days after it is removed.

Equipment

- Gloves
- Syringe
- Basin with soap and warm water, washcloths, and towels
- Waterproof pad
- Sheet to be used as a drape (may not be necessary for infants and small children)
- Examination light (optional)

Child and Family Assessment and Preparation

- Assess the cognitive level, readiness, and ability to process information by the child and family. The readiness to learn and process information may be impaired as a result of age, stress, or anxiety.

- Provide the opportunity to ask questions and alleviate fears.
- Explain the procedure, as appropriate, to both the child and the family. Reassure the toddler and older child that the procedure will not hurt and will consist only of a mild cleansing and examination of the perineum.
- Assess the child for pain from the catheter.
- Assess the child for signs and symptoms of urinary tract or bladder infection, including fever, inability to void, burning on urination, feeling of fullness, bladder spasms, foul-smelling urine, redness or irritation of urethral opening, urethral discharge, crying without consolation, or discomfort.
- Assess for signs of lower abdominal distention. Use of certain medications (e.g., opioids, sedatives) may cause urinary retention.
- Assess the child for signs and symptoms of a distended bladder or residual urine, for which bladder emptying would be required.

PROCEDURE **Managing an Indwelling Catheter**

Steps	Rationale/Points of Emphasis
1. Perform hand hygiene and gather the necessary supplies.	Reduces the transmission of microorganisms. Promotes efficient time management and provides an organized approach to the procedure.
2. Close the door to the child's room or draw the curtains around the child's bed.	Provides privacy during the procedure.
3. Raise the bed to a comfortable working height or stand on a step stool at crib side.	Reduces the strain placed on your back.
4. Don gloves.	Standard precaution to reduce transmission of microorganisms.
5. Place a waterproof pad under the child's/infant's buttocks while positioning the child/infant. Girls should be placed in the supine position with their legs spread apart. Boys should be placed in the supine position with their legs straight.	Allows for ease of access. This position facilitates visualization of the inner labia or the urethral opening.
6. Place a drape over the child/infant. For girls, place the drape in a diamond configuration with one corner at the child's sternum, one corner over each knee, and one corner over the perineum. For boys, cover the child's chest and lower extremities with a sheet, leaving only the genital area exposed. A flashlight or examination light may be helpful in locating the urethral opening.	Allows exposure of the child's perineum while covering the rest of the body, allowing for privacy.
7. Attach the syringe to the secondary lumen balloon port of the urinary catheter and then deflate the balloon, retaining the sterile water in the syringe. Note the amount of water and air collected in the syringe and reinflate the balloon.	Ensures patency of balloon of indwelling catheter. Sterile water within the balloon may evaporate or leach out, causing the balloon to deflate and the urinary catheter to slip out of the bladder. Reinflate the balloon with the manufacturer-specified amount of water to ensure patency.
8. Wash the child's genital area with warm water and soap. Cleanse around the urinary meatus and around the catheter itself, being careful not to manipulate the catheter back and forth. Gently retract the foreskin of the uncircumcised boy and cleanse the area. Return the foreskin to its normal position.	Removes secretions, smegma, and fecal matter. Movement of the catheter can introduce organisms into the urinary tract. Failure to return the foreskin can lead to swelling of the penis and impair circulation.
9. Observe for any signs of irritation, trauma, secretions, or incrustations on the catheter. Assess for any foul smells emanating from the urethra.	These signs can indicate a urinary tract infection.
10. Rinse and dry the child's perineum.	Reduces creating a conductive environment for microorganism growth.
11. Assess the drainage tubing for urine flow. Observe that there are no kinks or obstructions in the tubing and make sure that all connections are tightly secured.	Provides for a closed system collection of urine output, with free flow of urine and prevents microorganism introduction into the catheter.
12. Ensure the collection or drainage bag is attached to the frame of the bed or crib below the level of the bladder.	Positioning the bag below the level of the bladder prevents reflux of urine through the tubing and back into the bladder.
13. Ensure that the catheter is taped to the thigh of the older child. For small male infants not using a balloon catheter, tape the catheter to the lower abdomen or upper perineum, allowing the penis to point upward toward the umbilicus. For small female infants not using a balloon catheter, tape the catheter at its closest point outside on the left or right labia.	Taping is done to prevent any tension from being placed on the catheter from inside the bladder and to avoid dislodgment from accidental pulling or tugging. Movement of the catheter in and out can lead to contamination from microorganisms.

Continued

Steps	Rationale/Points of Emphasis
	caREminder *Ensure there are no pressure points or areas of skin breakdown before taping to the thigh, leg, abdomen, or perineum.*
14. Remove the waterproof underpad and re-cover the child as appropriate.	Maintains dry linens for the child and promotes sense of well-being.
15. Return the child's bed to the lowest position or to a level that is age appropriate. Place the child in a position of comfort.	Reduces potential injury from falls.
16. Dispose of used equipment and waste in appropriate waste containers.	Standard precautions
17. Remove gloves and perform hand hygiene.	Reduces transmission of microorganisms.

CHILD AND FAMILY EVALUATION AND DOCUMENTATION

- Evaluate the amount, color, clarity, and odor of the urine and the presence of any sediment.
- Evaluate the child for signs and symptoms of a urinary tract infection, including fever, tachycardia, pain, foul-smelling urine or perineum, perineal discharge, cloudy or sedimented urine, or urine discoloration.
- Evaluate child's response to the procedure.
- Document the following:
  - Completion of hygienic care
  - Catheter size
  - Amount of sterile water taken and reinserted into the balloon
  - Condition of child's skin in and around genital area
  - Color, clarity, and odor of urine
  - Signs and symptoms of urinary tract infection (if present)
  - Child's response to the procedure

COMMUNITY CARE

- If the procedure is done at the child's home, provide the family with instruction regarding
  - Care for the indwelling catheter, including perineal and catheter hygiene and bag emptying at least twice a day for children with indwelling catheters
  - Importance of offering plenty of oral fluids
  - Assessment of urinary output
  - Assessment for signs and symptoms of urinary tract infection
  - Disposal of excess urine in the home lavatory
- Instruct the family to contact the healthcare provider if
  - Catheter becomes dislodged and the child and family do not know how to reinsert the catheter
  - Urine is cloudy or dark
  - Blood is present in the urine or a change in smell of the urine occurs
  - Child has nausea or vomiting
  - Child has chills or fever
  - Child has flank pain
  - Child is lethargic
  - Child has painful voiding or frequent urgency to void
  - Swelling or redness occurs around the urethral opening

Unexpected Situation

- *A 20-month-old child with an indwelling urinary catheter complains of flank pain and has a low-grade fever:* Urinary tract infection should be considered in children younger than age 2 with unexplained fever. Assess the child for dehydration and other signs of urinary tract infection (e.g., foul-smelling urine, nausea, vomiting). Notify the healthcare prescriber and obtain a urine specimen for microbial analysis. If urinalysis suggests UTI, initiate antimicrobial therapy per healthcare prescriber's orders.

Bibliography

Bray, L., & Sanders, C. (2006). Nursing management of paediatric urethral catheterization. *Nursing Standard, 20*, 51–60.

Carlson, D., & Mowrey, B. (1997). Standards to prevent complications of urinary catheterization in children: Should and should-knots. *Journal of the Society of Pediatric Nurses, 2*, 37–41.

Getliffe, K. (2001). Review of catheter care guidelines. *Nursing Times, 97*(20), 70–71.

McConnell, E. (2001). Clinical do's and don'ts. Preventing nosocomial urinary tract infections. *Nursing2001, 31*(5), 17.

Pomfret, I. (2000). Catheter care in the community. *Nursing Standard, 14*, 46–51.

Simpson, L. (2001). Indwelling urethral catheters: Reducing the risk of potential complications through proactive management. *Primary Health Care, 11*(2), 57–64.

CHAPTER
118

Urinary Catheterization: Self-Intermittent Catheterization

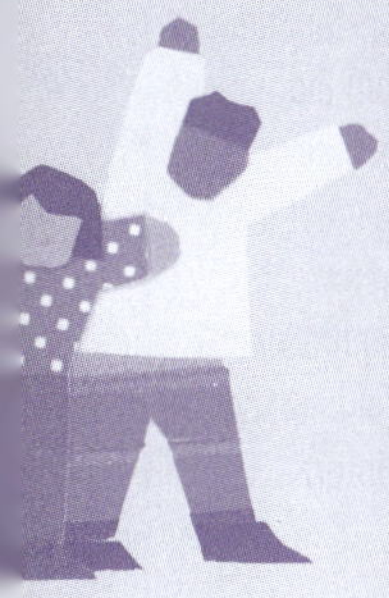

Clinical Guidelines

- Self-intermittent catheterization is ordered by a healthcare prescriber.
- The procedure may be taught to the child/family by the healthcare prescriber, a registered nurse (RN), or a licensed vocational nurse (LVN). The procedure is performed by the child and parent who have received education and training to perform self-catheterization.
- Intermittent self-catheterization may be necessary to implement for any number of reasons, including but not limited to
  - Child has a neurogenic bladder
  - Child has inability to void spontaneously
  - Child has inability to empty the bladder properly
  - Child's bladder leaks urine
  - Child has need for bladder training
- The goal of intermittent self-catheterization is to prevent urinary tract infections while still completely emptying the bladder.
- For most children, intermittent self-catheterization is a clean procedure. The same catheter can be used for weeks at a time. When this procedure is completed in the acute care setting by healthcare staff, it is a sterile procedure and should follow the guidelines in Chapters 116 and 123.
- Clean intermittent self-catheterization is contraindicated whenever the urethra cannot be safely catheterized. False passages or urethral stricture disease must first be managed to allow safe nontraumatic catheterization.

Equipment

- Soap, warm water, washcloth, and towel
- Drainage or collection container and lavatory
- Catheter (Table 118-1)
- Water-soluble lubricant (optional)

TABLE 118-1

Selection of Urinary Catheter for Self-Catheterization

Age (yr)	Recommended Catheter Size* (French or coudé tip)
0–2	6F
2–5	6–8F or coudé tip
5–10	8–10F or coudé tip
10–16	10–12F or coudé tip

*Feeding tubes are more prone to knotting and should be used only for small urethras.

Child and Family Assessment and Preparation

- Assess the cognitive level, readiness, and ability to process information of the child and family. The readiness to learn and process information may be impaired as a result of age, stress, or anxiety. Most children and parents can be taught to perform this procedure. They must learn the basic location of urologic landmarks and have the ability to manipulate the equipment involved. (Those who cannot visualize the urethra may be taught how to feel for the proper location of the urethral meatus.)
- Identify and discuss the risks and benefits of intermittent self-catheterization.
- Assure the parents/child that the catheterization will not harm the child or damage the urethra or hymen.
- Reinforce the need for intermittent self-catheterization, as appropriate, to both the child and the family. The program must be one the child can carry out with the feeling that his or her quality of life is improved or maintained.
- Urodynamic testing may be required before beginning intermittent self-catheterization to ensure there are no urethral strictures, false passages, vesical neck contractures, tumors, or stones that may interfere with catheterization.
- Instruct the child on the times and intervals per day to catheterize. Children should be instructed to catheterize, if it is time to do so, even if soap and water are unavailable.

KidKare Reassure the toddler and older child that the catheter is flexible, will feel like a noodle, and will produce a feeling of pressure and a desire to urinate.

- Instruct the child to try to urinate before self-catheterization, if possible.

PROCEDURE Assisting With Self-Intermittent Catheterization

Steps	Rationale/Points of Emphasis
1. Perform hand hygiene and collect all necessary equipment and supplies for catheterization. Selection of the catheter is based on the child's age and gender, construction material of the catheter, and the internal and external diameter of the catheter (see Table 118-1).	Reduces transmission of microorganisms. Promotes efficient time management and provides an organized approach to the procedure. Actual catheter size is selected after the clinician has assessed the urethral opening. Catheters that are used for clean intermittent self-catheterization are slightly different from the catheters used for indwelling (long-term) catheterization. Self-catheters are straight plastic tubes without the side balloon inflation port and balloon that are used to keep an indwelling catheter in place. They are more rigid than an indwelling catheter, making insertion a little easier. Use of shorter-length urinary catheters and basing length on gender and age can reduce incidence of knotting (e.g., for toddler and younger girls, insert 2 inches; for male infants, insert 3 inches; for male toddlers, insert 3 to 4 inches).
2. Assist, as needed, the child or parent performing the procedure to perform hand hygiene.	Reduces transmission of microorganisms.
3. Assist the child or parent to wash the genital area with warm water and soap. • **For boys:** With your nondominant hand, hold the penis on the sides, perpendicular to the body, while retracting the foreskin. Cleanse the penis and urethral opening and bladder. • **For girls:** Spread the labia open with the fingers of one hand. Cleanse the vulva and urethral opening. Wipe from front to back to prevent contaminating the area with fecal contents. Rinse and dry the area.	Removes secretions and feces. Prevents contamination of the catheter by microorganisms on the skin and prevents introduction of organisms into the child's urethra.

Steps	Rationale/Points of Emphasis
Note: Steps 4–15 are completed by the person performing the self-catheterization.	
4. Lubricate approximately the first 3 inches of the tip of the catheter.	The lubricant is used to reduce discomfort and decreases the friction between the catheter and the urinary tract during catheterization.
5. Hold the catheter as if it were a pencil or a dart, with your dominant hand, about 1 inch from its tip.	Enables manual insertion.
6. Locate the urethral opening. • **For boys:** With your nondominant hand, hold the penis on the sides, perpendicular to the body, while retracting the foreskin. • **For girls:** Spread the labia open with the fingers of the nondominant hand, keeping a finger free to feel for the urinary meatus (located below the clitoris and above the vagina). Some girls may be instructed to perform clean intermittent self-catheterization standing up with one foot on the toilet. This position is also recommended when there is a question about the cleanliness of the toilet, such as in public facilities.	Allows for exposure of the urethral opening during self-catheterization. **KidKare** Because gentle pressure may cause an erection in an adolescent male, the penis should be held firmly but not tightly. If held tightly, pressure collapses the urethra and prevents advancement of the catheter. If the adolescent has an erection, stop the procedure until there is a nonerectile state, and then continue with the procedure.
7. With the dominant hand, begin to gently insert the lubricated catheter into the urethra, in an upward direction toward the umbilicus. Ask the child to take a deep breath while inserting the catheter.	Allows for catheterization to obtain urine. Taking a deep breath helps to relax the urinary tract.
8. Insert the catheter until urine begins to flow. Continue to advance the catheter approximately 1 inch further and hold in place until the urine flow stops and the bladder is empty. Pressing down on the abdominal muscles may be required to assist in emptying the neurogenic bladder.	Allows for bladder emptying of urine. ***Alert!*** *When the catheter reaches the level of the prostate in boys or the striated sphincter (proximal urethra in boys and midurethra in girls), resistance may be met. Instruct the child to relax by deep breathing and continue to advance the catheter. Forcing the catheter can cause trauma, bleeding, and possible scar formation, which can lead to strictures and obstruction of the urethra.*
9. Drain the urine into a waste container or lavatory.	Allows for disposal of expelled urine.
10. Withdraw the catheter in small increments and return the foreskin on the uncircumcised boy to its normal position.	Allows all urine to drain. Failure to return the foreskin can lead to swelling of the penis and impairment of circulation.
11. Wipe off any excess lubricant or urine from the perineal area. Assist child to redress.	Keeps clothing clean and dry. Decreases medium for bacterial growth.
12. Perform hand hygiene.	Reduces transmission of microorganisms.
13. Wash the catheter with soap and water. Rinse the catheter completely and dry the outside of the catheter.	Washing and drying the catheter makes its environment less hospitable to microorganism growth.
14. Store the catheter in a clean, dry, secure location.	Allows for reuse at a later time.
15. Perform hand hygiene.	Reduces transmission of microorganisms.

Child and Family Evaluation and Documentation

- Evaluate the child's response to self-catheterization and determine areas of further teaching needed.
- Document the following:
  - Person who completed the catheterization
  - Amount of urine obtained
  - Time of procedure
  - Competency of care provider and teaching provided

Community Care

- A clean intermittent self-catheter may be reused for 2 to 4 weeks. Teach the child to clean the catheter following instructions and to discard the catheter when it becomes heavily soiled or begins to break down.
- It may be helpful to soak the reused catheter in white vinegar solution once a week to control odor and remove thick mucus deposits.
- Instruct the family to contact the healthcare provider if
  - Urine is cloudy or dark or there is a change in the smell of the urine
  - Blood in the urine
  - Child has nausea or vomiting
  - Child has chills or fever
  - Child has flank pain
  - Child is lethargic
  - Voiding is painful
  - Swelling or redness occurs around the urethral opening

Unexpected Situation

- *Female child is unable to correctly place catheter:* Nurse or parent can use a mirror to assist child to find correct placement position. Child may need to change positions, placing one leg up on toilet seat, to better access urethral opening.

Bibliography

Barton, R. (2000). Intermittent self-catheterization. *Nursing Standard, 15*(9), 54–55.

Carlson, D., & Mowrey, B. (1997). Standards to prevent complications of urinary catheterization in children: Should and should-knots. *Journal of the Society of Pediatric Nurses, 2*, 37–41.

Duffin, H. (2000). Intermittent self-catheterization. *Journal of Community Nursing, 14*(10), 29–30.

Gray, M. (1996). Atraumatic urethral catheterization of children. *Pediatric Nursing, 22*(4), 4, 306–310.

Lemke, J., Kasprowicz, K., & Worral, P. (2005). Using the best evidence to change practice. Intermittent catheterization for patients with neurogenic bladder: Sterile versus clean: Using evidence-based practice at the staff nurse level. *Journal of Nursing Care Quality, 20*, 302–306.

CHAPTER

119

Urine Collection: 24-Hour Specimen

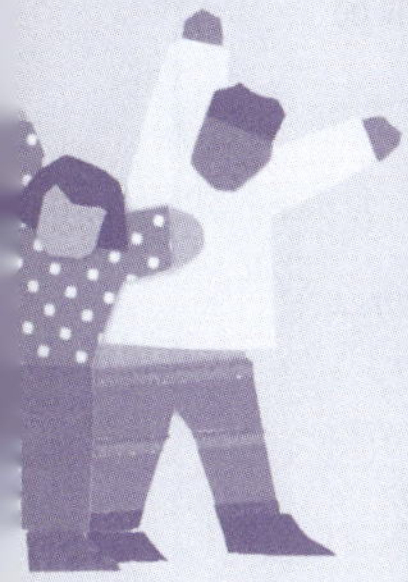

Clinical Guidelines

- Urine collection for diagnostic analysis is ordered by a healthcare prescriber.
- A registered nurse (RN), licensed practical nurse (LPN), or unlicensed assistive personnel (UAP) may collect urine for diagnostic analysis.
- Urine is collected over a 24-hour period to determine the excretion rate of certain hormones, proteins, and electrolytes. The laboratory supplies the container and any necessary preservatives.
- If urine is discarded accidentally after the urine collection has begun, the healthcare prescriber should be notified, and the test should be started again. Any loss of urine invalidates the results of the test.

Equipment

- Large-capped collection container (containing preservative, if necessary)
- Clean bedpan or toilet specimen container, adhesive urine collection bag, or clean urinal, if an indwelling catheter is not in place
- Large basin with ice (freshened with new ice, when the ice melts)
- Adhesive label or marker
- Signs: "24-Hour Urine Collection in Progress"
- Gloves

Child and Family Assessment and Preparation

- Assess the cognitive level, readiness, and ability to process information by the child and family.
- Reinforce the need for the urine specimen collection, as appropriate, to both the child and the family.
- Instruct the child and the family in saving voided urine and notifying nursing personnel of each void.

PROCEDURE 24-Hour Urine Specimen Collection

Steps	Rationale/Points of Emphasis
1. Obtain a collection container from the laboratory to be kept at the bedside. If the child will be voiding using a bedpan or toilet specimen container, instruct the child to place the container toward the perineum or the front of the toilet so that if the child has the urge to defecate, the feces will not mix with the urine in the collection container.	Urine must be kept and stored together in the same collection container over a 24-hour period. **caREminder** *Check with the institution's laboratory manual to determine specific handling and storage procedures. The type of container (some tests require storage in a dark container), type of preservative in the container, and refrigeration or freezing during collection is determined by the type of urine substance being tested.*
2. Post signs on the door to the child's room, above the child's bed, and in the bathroom saying that a 24-hour urine test is in progress.	Reminds all nursing personnel and family members to save the child's urine. A 24-hour collection of urine is needed; if any urine is discarded, test results will be invalid. The total volume of urine collected during the 24-hour period is a factor used to calculate the excretion rate of the substance. Feces and toilet tissue may alter the test results.
3. Don gloves to handle voided specimens.	Standard precautions to reduce transmission of microorganisms.
4. If the child is able, have him or her void to empty the bladder and discard the voided urine. If an indwelling catheter is in place, discard any urine already in the drainage bag.	Because the 24-hour urine is a timed quantitative determination, it is essential to start the test with an empty bladder. **caREminder** *If the child is unable to void on command and does not require an indwelling catheter, place an adhesive urine collection bag over the perineum and discard the first voided urine.*
5. Note the time that the first urine was discarded.	This time is the beginning of the 24-hour collection period.
6. Pour urine from each void into the collection container and keep the collection container on ice. If indwelling catheter or urine collection bag is in place, empty and add to collection container on ice at least every 2 hours. It is not necessary to measure the volume of a voiding unless specifically ordered.	Ice is used for preservation and to control bacterial growth. Results may be altered by urine that is not properly stored. **caREminder** *Remind the child to use toilet paper after the specimen has been transferred into the appropriate container. Toilet paper placed in with the specimen contaminates the specimen and decreases the amount of urine for analysis.*
7. Before the end of the 24-hour collection period, ask the child to void one last specimen. Pour this final specimen into the collection container.	This is necessary for all urine excreted during the 24-hour time period to be collected. The last specimen should be obtained as closely as possible to the stated end time of the test.
8. Label the collection container and send it to the laboratory immediately after the 24-hour period.	Test results depend on an accurate measurement of time and quantitative urine. Test results may be altered because the urine is no longer on ice.
9. Remove gloves and perform hand hygiene after each contact with the urine specimen.	Reduces transmission of microorganisms.

CHILD AND FAMILY EVALUATION AND DOCUMENTATION

- Assess color and clarity of the urine, presence of any sediment, and any unusual odor of the urine.
- Document the following:
  - Time the collection began and time completed
  - Color and clarity of the urine, presence of any sediment, and any unusual odor of the urine.
  - Child's response to the specimen collection process.

COMMUNITY CARE

- If the collection is to be done at the child's home, write specific instructions for the child and family to follow. Ensure family has a collection container with an appropriate preservative.
- If the specimen is to be kept cool, make sure that the family has ice or refrigeration available.
- Make specific arrangements to return for the specimen and transport the specimen in a cooler.
- Instruct the family to contact the healthcare provider if
  - The 24-hour collection is interrupted for some reason
  - Urine is cloudy or dark
  - Blood is present in the urine or a change in smell of the urine occurs
  - Child has nausea or vomiting
  - Child has chills or fever
  - Child has flank pain
  - Child is lethargic
  - Child has painful voiding or frequent urgency to void
  - Swelling or redness occurs around the urethral opening

Unexpected Situations

- *Child or parent forgot to save specimen for collection:* The test must be started again. Unless all urine from the 24-hour period is saved, the test results will not be accurate.
- *An adolescent girl starts her menstrual cycle right before the urine collection period was to begin:* During periods of heavy menstrual flow, the test usually should not be conducted. Cleansing of the perineal area is typically not sufficient to avoid contamination of the specimen. Notify the laboratory personnel and the girl's physician to verify that the test should be postponed.

Bibliography

Burke, N. (1995). Alternative methods for newborn urine sample collection. *Pediatric Nursing, 21*(6), 546–549.

Fischbach, F. (2004). *A manual of laboratory and diagnostic tests* (7th ed.). Philadelphia: Lippincott Williams & Wilkins.

Schultz, C. J., Dalton, R. N., Turner, C., Neil, H. A., & Dunger, D. B. (2000). Freezing method affects the concentration and variability of urine proteins and interpretation of data on microalbuminuria. The Oxford Regional Prospective Study Group. *Diabetic Medicine, 17*(1), 7–14.

CHAPTER

120

Urine Collection: Clean Catch (Midstream)

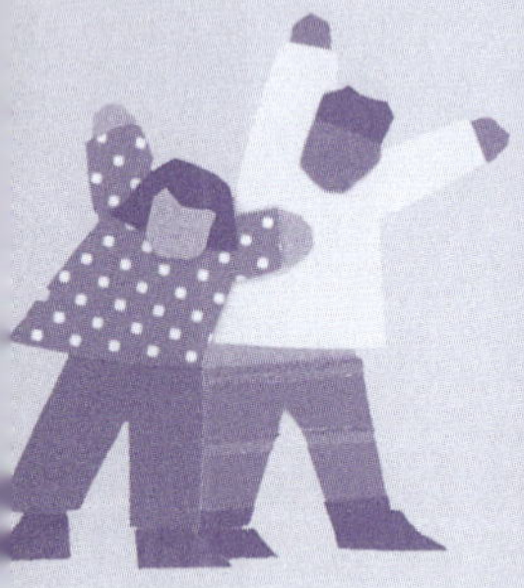

Clinical Guidelines

- Urine collection for diagnostic analysis is ordered by a healthcare prescriber.
- A registered nurse (RN), licensed practical nurse (LPN), or unlicensed assistive personnel (UAP) may collect urine for diagnostic analysis.
- A clean-catch (midstream) urine specimen is collected when a urinary tract infection is suspected and uncontaminated urine is needed for a urine culture and sensitivity. Confirmation of a diagnosis of a urinary tract infection is completed using transurethral bladder catheterization or suprapubic aspiration (see Chapters 123 and 124).

caREminder

The diagnosis of urinary tract infection cannot be established by a culture of urine collected in a bag.

- Specimens needed from infants must be collected using an adhesive urine collection bag or urine collection pad as outlined in Chapter 122.
- If possible, collect the child's first voiding in the morning because bacterial counts are the highest in this voiding.

Equipment

- Gloves
- Basin with soap and warm water, washcloth, and towel
- Sterile specimen container
- Adhesive label or marker
- Antimicrobial perineal wipes, swabs, or sponges
- Biohazard bag for transporting the specimen to the laboratory
- 4 × 4 gauze pads or tampon, if needed, for pubescent girls

Child and Family Assessment and Preparation

- Assess the cognitive level, readiness, and ability to process information by the child and family. The readiness to learn and process information may be impaired as a result of age, stress, or anxiety.

KidKare The child may have difficulty understanding the request. The adolescent may be reluctant to have the test completed or may be unable to void on request. The nurse should use simplistic terms and words the child uses, such as "pee-pee," to make the request. Provide privacy for the older child.

- Assess the present history for toilet training, if age appropriate.
- Before use, assess for allergies to antimicrobial agents.
- Reinforce the need for the urine specimen collection, as appropriate, to both the child and the family.
- Provide the opportunity to ask questions and alleviate fears.
- Explain the procedure, as appropriate, to both the child and the family.

PROCEDURE Clean-Catch (Midstream) Urine Collection

Steps	Rationale/Points of Emphasis
1. Perform hand hygiene. Gather the necessary supplies.	Reduces transmission of microorganisms. Promotes efficient time management and provides an organized approach to the procedure.
2. Close the door to the child's room and draw the curtains around the bed to provide privacy, as appropriate. Assist child to the bathroom.	Provides privacy during the procedure.
3. Don gloves.	Standard precautions to reduce transmission of microorganisms.
4. Remove the lid of the sterile specimen container and place it with the inside of the lid facing up, on a clean surface within easy reach.	Touching the inside of the lid causes contamination.
5. If parent is assisting or child is performing self-care, he or she should perform hand hygiene and don gloves (optional).	Standard precautions to prevent contamination of specimen from microorganisms.
6a. Clean around the child's urethral opening with antimicrobial wipes, swabs, or sponges and discard them in a nearby open waste receptacle. Allow the area to dry.	Prevents contamination of the specimen by microorganisms on the skin.
6b. For girls, using a separate antimicrobial swab for each stroke, open the child's labia and cleanse both the right and left side of the inner labia with one downward stroke. Then clean midline, from the clitoris down to the rectum, with one stroke. The nurse may need to assist the child in keeping the labia open while voiding. If the child is old enough, she may be able to do this herself, although she may then need assistance holding the specimen cup.	Prevents contamination of the sterile field. The labia should not be allowed to close during the entire procedure. If the labia do close, stop the procedure, don new sterile gloves, and start over at this step.
6c. A menstruating girl should place a tampon or a gauze pad in her vaginal orifice after cleansing the perineal area with soap and warm water.	Menses may cause a false-positive result when testing for blood in the urine.
6d. For boys, retract the foreskin (if present). Cleanse the penis in an outgoing circular motion, from the urethral opening to the base of the penis, using a new antimicrobial wipe, swab, or sponge each time.	Removes secretions and smegma and reduces microorganisms.
7. If possible, instruct the child to void a small amount of urine into the toilet or urinal. For infants and young children, use an adhesive urine collection bag or urine collection pad as outlined in Chapter 122 to collect the specimen.	This cleanses the meatus of any remaining bacteria. **KidKare** Run water in the sink to trigger voiding.
8. Have the child urinate 10–20 mL directly into a sterile specimen container; the child can then finish urinating in the toilet or urinal.	Urinating directly into the specimen container decreases the possibility of contaminating the specimen.
9. Place the lid back on the specimen container. Avoid touching the inside of the lid or of the container. Wipe off the outside of the container.	If hands or any other body part or nonsterile object touches the lid or the inside of the container, the specimen is contaminated by outside bacteria.
10. Assist the child with wiping/cleansing the perineal area after voiding is complete, as needed.	Promotes cleanliness.
11. Assist the child to return to bed, or other activity, after disposing of gloves and performing hand hygiene.	Reduces transmission of microorganisms.

Continued

Steps	Rationale/Points of Emphasis
12. Label the specimen, and place it in a biohazard bag.	Standard precautions.
13. Send the specimen to the laboratory immediately.	Urinalysis results may be altered if the specimen is more than 1 hour old. If the specimen is not fresh, bacteria may enter the urine, and other components can break up and disintegrate.
14. Dispose of equipment and waste in appropriate receptacle. Remove gloves. Perform hand hygiene.	Standard precautions. Reduces transmission of microorganisms.

CHILD AND FAMILY EVALUATION AND DOCUMENTATION

- Evaluate child for presence or absence of signs and symptoms of urinary tract or bladder infection, including fever, inability to void, burning on urination, feeling of fullness, bladder spasms, foul-smelling urine, redness or irritation of urethral opening, urethral discharge, and crying without consolation or discomfort.
- Document the following:
  - Amount, color, clarity, and odor of the urine and the presence of any sediment
  - Child's response to the specimen collection
  - Presence or absence of signs and symptoms of a distended bladder or residual urine, for which bladder emptying would be required

COMMUNITY CARE

- If the procedure is performed in a healthcare provider's office or clinic, encourage parents to offer fluids to the child on the trip to the office or clinic.
- If the procedure is done at the child's home, instruct the family to
  - Transport the specimen in a cooler from the home to the laboratory to keep it as fresh as possible
  - Dispose of excess urine in home lavatory
- Instruct the family to contact the healthcare provider if
  - Urine is cloudy or dark
  - Blood is present in the urine or a change in smell of the urine occurs
  - Child has nausea or vomiting
  - Child has chills or fever
  - Child has flank pain
  - Child is lethargic
  - Child has painful voiding or frequent urgency to void
  - Swelling or redness occurs around the urethral opening

Unexpected Situation

- *Child has the urge to defecate while collecting specimen:* Presence of feces will contaminate the specimen. Encourage the child to finish voiding. Assist with transfer of the urine to the collection receptacle while the child proceeds to defecate.

Bibliography

Al-Orifi, F., McGillivray, D., Tange, S., & Kramer, M. S. (2000). Urine culture from bag specimens in young children: Are the risks too high? *Journal of Pediatrics, 13*, 221–226.

American Academy of Pediatrics. (1999). The diagnosis, treatment, and evaluation of the initial urinary tract infection in febrile infants and young children. *Pediatrics, 103*, 843–852.

Farrell, M., Devine, K., Lancaster, G., & Judd, B. (2002). A method comparison study to assess the reliability of urine collection pads as a means of obtaining urine specimens from non-toilet trained children for microbiological examination. *Journal of Advanced Nursing, 37*, 387–393.

Liaw, L., Nayar, D., Pedler, S., & Coulthard, M. (2000). Home collection of urine for culture from infants by three methods: Survey of parents' preferences and bacterial contamination rates. *British Medical Journal, 320*, 1312–1313.

Lifshitz, E., & Kramer, L. (2000). Outpatient urine culture: Does collection technique matter? *Archives of Internal Medicine, 160*(16), 2537–2540.

Loane, V. (2005). Obtaining urine for culture from non-potty trained children. *Paediatric Nursing, 17*(9), 39–42.

McGillivray, D., Mok, E., Mulrooney, E., & Kramer, M. (2005). A head-to-head comparison: "Clean-void" bag versus catheter analysis in the diagnosis of urinary tract infection in young children. *The Journal of Pediatrics, 147*, 451–456.

Ramage, I., Chapman, J., Hollman, A., et al. (1999). Accuracy of clean-catch urine collection in infancy. *Journal of Pediatrics, 135*(6), 765–767.

Rao, S., Bhatt, J., Houghton, C., & Macfarlane, P. (2004). An improved urine collection pad method: A randomized clinical trial. *Archives of Disease in Childhood, 89*, 773–775.

Schroeder, A., Newman, T., Wasserman, R., et al. (2005). Choice of urine collection methods for the diagnosis of urinary tract infection in young, febrile infants. *Archives of Pediatric and Adolescent Medicine, 159*, 915–922.

Thomas, J., Kurien, A., & Philipraj, S. (2006). Methods for collecting urine samples in adults and children with suspected urinary tract infection (Protocol). *The Cochrane Database of Systematic Reviews*, (2), No. CD006025.

Wald, E. (2005). To bag or not to bag. *The Journal of Pediatrics, 147*, 418–420

C H A P T E R

121

Urine Collection: Indwelling Catheter

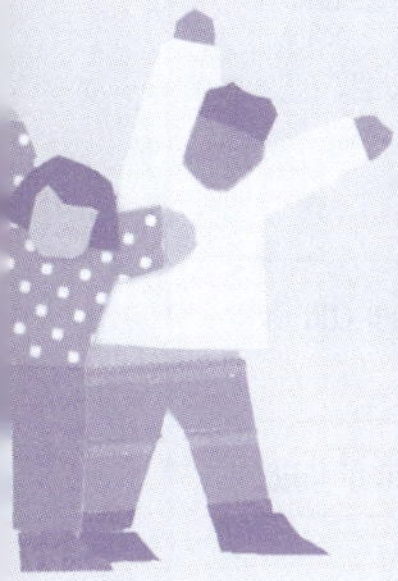

Clinical Guidelines

- Urine collection for diagnostic analysis is ordered by a healthcare prescriber.
- A registered nurse (RN) or licensed practical nurse (LPN) may collect the specimen from the indwelling catheter.
- A urine specimen is collected from an indwelling catheter when a urinary tract infection is suspected and a sterile urine specimen is needed for a urine culture and sensitivity test.
- The specimen must be obtained aseptically so as not to contaminate the closed drainage system or contaminate the specimen.

Equipment

- Clamp
- Gloves
- Sterile alcohol swabs
- Sterile 3- to 10-mL syringe
- Sterile 21- to 25-gauge needle or sterile needleless syringe adaptor
- Clean towel
- Specimen container and label (if the specimen obtained is to be sent to the laboratory for culture and sensitivity, the container for collection must be sterile)
- Biohazard bag for transporting the specimen to the laboratory

Child and Family Assessment and Preparation

- Assess the cognitive level, readiness, and ability to process information of the child and family. The readiness to learn and process information may be impaired as a result of age, stress, or anxiety.
- Reinforce the need for the urine specimen collection, as appropriate, to both the child and the family.
- Provide the opportunity to ask questions and alleviate fears.
- Assess the color and clarity of urine in the catheter drainage tubing.

PROCEDURE Indwelling Catheter Urine Collection

Steps	Rationale/Points of Emphasis
1. Perform hand hygiene. Gather the necessary supplies.	Reduces transmission of microorganisms. Promotes efficient time management and provides an organized approach to the procedure.
2. Close the door to the child's room and draw the curtains around the bed to provide privacy, as appropriate.	Provides privacy during the procedure.
3. Clamp the indwelling catheter just below the aspiration site. Clamps need to remain in place long enough for urine to collect in the drainage tubing.	Allows urine to collect in the drainage tube. Amount of time necessary for urine to collect may vary from child to child.
4. Establish a clean working area, using a clean towel spread open.	Establishes a space from which to gather equipment and proceed with collection without contamination.
5. Using sterile technique, open the sterile alcohol swabs, sterile 3- or 5-mL syringe, sterile 21- to 25-gauge needle, and sterile specimen container and place them on the towel in their packages to maintain the sterility of the supplies.	Facilitates ease of access to the equipment.
6. Don gloves.	Reduces transmission of microorganisms.
7. Wipe the aspiration site of the catheter with friction using sterile alcohol swabs and allow it to air-dry.	Prevents contamination of the aspiration site and specimen by microorganisms and prevents introduction of organisms into the closed catheter system.
8. Withdraw fresh urine from the aspiration site using a needleless adaptor with syringe (preferred) or a 23- or 25-gauge needle.	Allows for specimen to be obtained. Urine should not be collected from the urine collection bag because that urine is contaminated and the components of the urine change when the urine has been sitting at room temperature.

caREminder

Aspirate about 10 mL of urine for a culture or urinalysis. Consult with the institution laboratory manual for all other exact amounts needed for each laboratory test. Many laboratories can complete the tests with very little urine collected.

Steps	Rationale/Points of Emphasis
9. Withdraw the needleless adaptor or needle and syringe and inject the urine directly into the sterile specimen container.	Draining the urine directly into the specimen container decreases the possibility of contaminating the specimen.
10. Put the lid on the container, label the specimen, and place it in a biohazard bag.	Standard precautions.
11. Unclamp the indwelling catheter tubing.	Allows urine to flow into the drainage bag. Stasis of urine in the bladder can cause urinary tract infections.
12. Send the specimen to the laboratory immediately.	Results of the test may be altered if urine is allowed to sit for any length of time.
13. Dispose of used equipment and waste in appropriate receptacle. Perform hand hygiene.	Standard precautions. Reduces transmission of microorganisms.

CHILD AND FAMILY EVALUATION AND DOCUMENTATION

- Evaluate child for presence or absence of signs and symptoms of urinary tract or bladder infection, including fever, feeling of fullness, bladder spasms, foul-smelling urine, redness or irritation of urethral opening, urethral discharge, and crying without consolation or discomfort.
- Document the following:
  - Amount, color, clarity, and odor of the urine and the presence of any sediment
  - Child's response to the specimen collection

- Presence or absence of signs and symptoms of a distended bladder or residual urine, for which bladder emptying would be required

COMMUNITY CARE

- If the procedure is done at the child's home, instruct the family to
  - Transport the specimen in a cooler from the home to the laboratory to keep it as fresh as possible
  - Dispose of used needles and syringes in biohazard sharps container
  - Dispose of used equipment in a sealed plastic bag
- Instruct the family to contact the healthcare provider if
  - Catheter becomes dislodged and the child and family do not know how to reinsert the catheter
  - Urine is cloudy or dark
  - Blood is present in the urine or a change in smell of the urine occurs
  - Child has nausea or vomiting
  - Child has chills or fever
  - Child has flank pain
  - Child is lethargic
  - Child has painful voiding or frequent urgency to void
  - Swelling or redness occurs around the urethral opening

Unexpected Situation

- *Several hours after urine sample is gathered, you note that the urine flow has dwindled from the child's catheter:* Check the tubing for kinks. Make sure you removed the clamp to the catheter tubing applied during the process of obtaining the urine sample. If the child has changed position, the tubing and drainage bag may need to be repositioned to facilitate drainage of the urine.

Bibliography

American Academy of Pediatrics. (1999). The diagnosis, treatment, and evaluation of the initial urinary tract infection in febrile infants and young children. *Pediatrics, 103*, 843–852.

McGillivray, D., Mok, E., Mulrooney, E., & Kramer, M. (2005). A head-to-head comparison: "Clean-void" bag versus catheter analysis in the diagnosis of urinary tract infection in young children. *The Journal of Pediatrics, 147*, 451–456.

Schroeder, A., Newman, T., Wasserman, R., et al. (2005). Choice of urine collection methods for the diagnosis of urinary tract infection in young, febrile infants. *Archives of Pediatric and Adolescent Medicine, 159*, 915–922.

Thomas, J., Kurien, A., & Philipraj, S. (2006). Methods for collecting urine samples in adults and children with suspected urinary tract infection (Protocol). *The Cochrane Database of Systematic Reviews*, (2), No. CD006025.

CHAPTER

122

Urine Collection: Routine Voided Urine Specimen

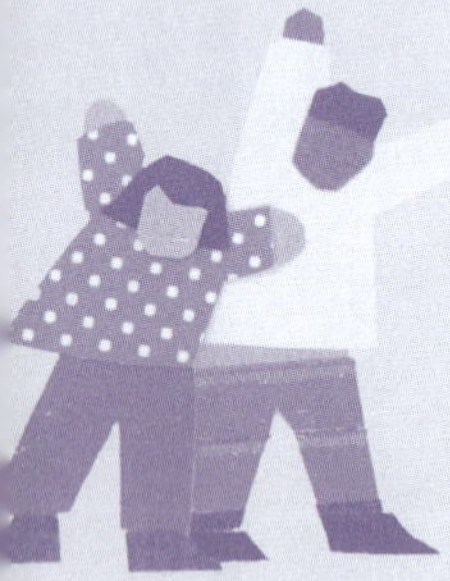

Clinical Guidelines

- Urine collection for diagnostic analysis is ordered by a healthcare prescriber.
- A registered nurse (RN), licensed practical nurse (LPN), or unlicensed assistive personnel (UAP) may collect urine for diagnostic analysis.
- Routine voided specimens are collected for routine urinalysis and can be used to examine the urine for color, specific gravity, pH, protein, glucose, acetone, bilirubin, or the presence of blood.
- A routine voided specimen is usually collected on the child's admission to the hospital, before surgery, or during a visit to the healthcare provider's office for a well-child visit.
- Methods of collection include a clean bedpan, urinal, or toilet specimen container for the toilet-trained child. For the child who is not toilet trained, collect urine using an adhesive urine collection bag, urine collection pad, or cotton balls.
- A routine voided specimen can be used to check for bacteria in the urine; however, it is not used to make a final determination of the presence of bacteria.
- Collect the urine specimen at the child's first void of the morning, if possible. Such a specimen is more likely to reveal abnormalities than a later voiding.

Equipment

- Gloves
- Basin with soap and warm water, washcloth, and towel or perineal wipe
- Waterproof pad
- Age-appropriate urine collection device:
  - Bedpan
  - Urinal
  - Toilet specimen container
  - Sterile foil bowl
  - Adhesive urine collection bag
  - Urine collection pad
  - Cotton balls
- Urine specimen container
- Adhesive label or marker
- Biohazard bag for transporting the specimen to the laboratory
- 4 × 4 gauze pads or tampon, if needed, for pubescent girls during menses

CHILD AND FAMILY ASSESSMENT AND PREPARATION

- Assess the cognitive level, readiness, and ability to process information of the child and family. The readiness to learn and process information may be impaired as a result of age, stress, or anxiety.
- Assess the present history for toilet training, if age appropriate.
- For a young or cognitively delayed child, ask the parents what word the child uses for urine and use that word when talking with the child about the procedure.
- Reinforce the need for the urine specimen collection, as appropriate, to both the child and the family.
- Offer the child something to drink before the procedure to encourage voiding.
- Provide the opportunity to ask questions and alleviate fears.
- Explain the procedure, as appropriate, to both the child and the family.

KidKare The child may have difficulty understanding the request. The adolescent may be reluctant to have the test completed or may be unable to void on request. The nurse should use simplistic terms and words the child uses, such as "pee-pee," to make the request.

- Provide privacy for the child, regardless of age, during procedure and handle specimen discreetly.

PROCEDURE Routine Voided Urine Specimen Collection

Steps	Rationale/Points of Emphasis
1. Perform hand hygiene. Gather the necessary supplies.	Reduces transmission of microorganisms. Promotes efficient time management and provides an organized approach to the procedure.
2. Close the door to the child's room and draw the curtains around the bed to provide privacy, as appropriate. Assist child to bathroom.	Provides privacy during the procedure.
3. Don gloves.	Standard precaution to reduce transmission of microorganisms.
4. As age appropriate, have the child urinate in a clean bedpan, urinal, or toilet specimen container or use a urine collection device to collect urine from the child who is not yet toilet trained.	Adapt the procedure to the child's developmental ability to understand request and to child's physical maturation. Infants and toddlers will be unable to void upon request until myelinization of the spinal cord is complete and potty training practices have been fully mastered. **KidKare** If the child is having difficulty voiding, run water in the sink to trigger voiding.
5. For specimen collected in a bedpan or urinal:	
a. Position the child on the back with the head of the bed slightly elevated.	This position makes it easier to void and allows gravity to aid in elimination.
b. Place a waterproof pad under the child's buttocks.	Prevents the bed linens from being soiled.
c. Wash the child's genital area with warm water and soap. Rinse and dry the area.	Cleanses perineal area. **KidKare** The child and family can be instructed in performing this step themselves.
d. Place the bedpan under the child or place the urinal such that the penis is inserted in the opening.	Having the bedpan or urinal in the proper position prevent spills on the bed.
e. Once the child has voided, remove the bedpan or urinal, offer toilet paper, and assist child to place underwear back on. Assist child to perform hand hygiene.	Cleaning the perineal area prevents odors and irritations to the skin. Hand hygiene prevents transmission of microorganisms.
6. For child using a toilet specimen container:	
a. Explain to the child and family how to clean the genitalia area. Instruct the child not to defecate at the same time and not to contaminate the specimen with toilet paper.	Use age-appropriate terminology. Feces and toilet paper can alter the results of urinalysis.

Continued

Steps	Rationale/Points of Emphasis
b. A menstruating girl should place a tampon or a gauze pad in her vaginal orifice after cleansing the perineal area with warm soap and water.	Menses may cause a false-positive result when testing for blood in the urine.
c. Give the container to the child and explain how to hold the container while voiding.	Proper handling reduces transmission of microorganisms.
d. Ask the child to leave the sample in the bathroom after the specimen is obtained.	Prompt transfer to an appropriate specimen container optimizes accuracy of results.
e. Ask the child to perform hand hygiene after the specimen has been obtained.	Reduces transmission of microorganisms.
f. Once specimen has been obtained, don gloves. Pour the fresh urine in the specimen container and put the lid on the container.	Standard precaution to reduce transmission of microorganisms. Prepares urine for transfer to laboratory.
7. For specimen collected using a urine collection bag:	
a. Position the child on the back with the legs in a frog-like position.	This position exposes the genitalia to facilitate cleansing of the area and proper placement of the collection bag.
b. Remove the diaper and clean the perineum or prepuce of the infant.	Prevents contamination of the urine specimen
c. Apply a chemical adhesive (e.g., tincture of benzoin).	Helps to maintain seal between bag and child's skin.
Alert! *Do not use chemical adhesive on premature infants or neonates because this will cause transdermal tearing.*	
d. Attach a urine collection bag to the infant by removing the protective backing from the adhesive. Make sure bag does not cover anus. • For boys, insert penis and scrotum into bag opening; adhesive adheres to perineum and symphysis (Figure 122-1). • For girls, position lower half of adhesive on bag on perineum first and then press on adhesive up toward symphysis (Figure 122-2).	Proper placement of the bag avoids having to repeat the procedure.
e. Cut a hole in the diaper, pulling the urine bag through the opening.	When the child voids, it is easily visible, and the urine bag can be removed immediately.
f. Replace diaper and wait for child to void.	Child may not void immediately.
g. Remove gloves and perform hand hygiene.	Reduces transmission of microorganisms.
h. After child has voided, don gloves and remove bag from infant. Transfer urine to specimen container by holding urine bag over open specimen container; remove tab over opening in lower bag or cut off tip of bottom corner of bag.	Prepares specimen for submission to laboratory.
i. Remove gloves and perform hand hygiene.	Reduces transmission of microorganisms.

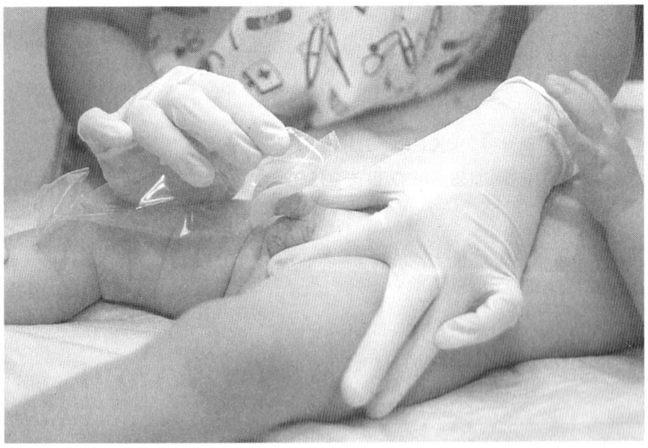

FIGURE 122-1
For males, insert penis and scrotum into bag opening; adhesive adheres to perineum and symphysis.

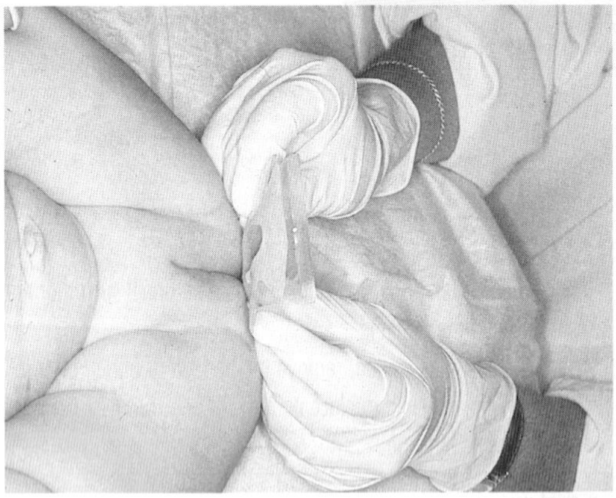

FIGURE 122-2
For females, position lower half of the bag on the perineum first and then press adhesive up toward symphysis.

Steps	Rationale/Points of Emphasis
8. For specimen collected using a urine collection pad:	
a. Remove the diaper and clean the perineum or prepuce of the infant.	Prevents contamination of the urine specimen.
b. Place urine collection pad across urethra or penis in lengthwise fashion.	Urine collection pads have been found to be an effective method to retrieve urine for analysis. This method is more cost effective than urine collection bags and is ideal as a means to rule out urinary tract infection in children in whom this is unlikely to be the focus of infection and where initiation of antibiotic therapy is not urgent. The diagnosis of urinary tract infection is best confirmed by transurethral bladder catheterization or suprapubic aspiration.
c. Remove adhesive backing from pad and replace diaper, ensuring the adhesive strip secures to the inside of the diaper.	Diaper assists to hold adhesive pad in place.
d. Once infant has voided, don gloves and remove the diaper with the absorbent pad in it from the infant.	Urine-saturated pad must be retrieved to obtain specimen.
e. Place clean diaper on infant.	Prevents infant from voiding on bed linen.
f. With gloved hands, squeeze out urine from the absorbent pad into appropriate urine container or onto urine testing strips.	Prepares specimen for submission to laboratory.
g. Dispose of absorbent pad and diaper in appropriate receptacle.	Standard precautions.
h. Remove gloves and perform hand hygiene.	Reduces transmission of microorganisms.
9. For specimen collected using foil bowl:	
a. Remove the diaper and clean the perineum or prepuce of the infant.	Prevents contamination of the urine specimen.
b. Have a nurse or parent sit down with a waterproof pad placed across the lap.	Protects parent's lap and clothes from getting soiled.
c. Place the child on the lap of the parent. The parent holds a sterile foil bowl underneath the child's genitalia.	This method has been compared with suprapubic aspirations and has been found to yield a good association between the results found from using the two methods. Thus, this method is considered less invasive, less costly, and reliable in assessing for microorganisms in the urine. Although the method appears to be time consuming, most specimens can be collected in less than 1 hour.
d. Offer the child oral fluids and await urine collection.	Additional fluids may enhance potential for voiding.
e. Once a specimen is collected, don gloves, replace a diaper on the child, and proceed with preparing the specimen for the laboratory.	Standard precautions to reduce transmission of microorganisms. Diaper contains child's excretions. Prepares specimen for submission to laboratory.
10. For specimen collected using cotton balls:	
a. Remove the diaper and clean the perineum or prepuce of the infant.	Prevents contamination of the urine specimen.
b. Place cotton balls near the urethra.	Use 100% cotton balls. Cotton ball aspiration is a safe valid way to collect urine for pH, specific gravity, and latex-particle agglutination. Urine should not be aspirated from the diaper for specimen collection for testing of specific gravity, pH, or protein. Disposable diapers with absorbent gel are difficult to aspirate from and yield inaccurate results.
c. Replace diaper.	Diaper assists to hold cotton balls in place.
d. Once infant has voided, don gloves and remove the diaper with the cotton balls in it from the infant.	Urine-saturated cotton balls must be retrieved to obtain specimen.
e. Place clean diaper on infant.	Prevents infant from voiding on bed linen.
f. With gloved hands, squeeze out urine from the cotton balls into appropriate urine container or onto urine testing strips.	Prepares specimen for submission to laboratory.
g. Dispose of cotton balls and diaper in appropriate receptacle.	Standard precautions.
h. Remove gloves and perform hand hygiene.	Reduces transmission of microorganisms.
11. Label the specimen, and place it in a biohazard bag.	Standard precautions.
12. Send the specimen to the laboratory immediately.	Urinalysis results may be altered if the specimen is more than 1 hour old. If the specimen is not fresh, bacteria may enter the urine, and other components can break up and disintegrate.
13. Dispose of equipment and waste in appropriate receptacle. Remove gloves. Perform hand hygiene.	Standard precautions. Reduces transmission of microorganisms.

CHILD AND FAMILY EVALUATION AND DOCUMENTATION

- Evaluate child for presence or absence of signs and symptoms of urinary tract or bladder infection, including fever, inability to void, burning upon urination, feeling of fullness, bladder spasms, foul-smelling urine, redness or irritation of urethral opening, urethral discharge, and crying without consolation or discomfort.
- Document the following:
  - Amount, color, clarity, and odor of the urine and the presence of any sediment
  - Child's response to the specimen collection
  - Presence or absence of signs and symptoms of a distended bladder or residual urine, for which bladder emptying would be required

COMMUNITY CARE

- If the procedure is performed in a healthcare provider's office or clinic, encourage parents to offer fluids to the child on the trip to the office or clinic.
- If the procedure is done at the child's home, instruct the family to
  - Transport the specimen from the home to the laboratory in a cooler with ice packs to keep it as fresh as possible
  - Dispose of excess urine in home lavatory
- Instruct the family to contact the healthcare provider if
  - Urine is cloudy or dark
  - Blood is present in the urine or a change in smell of the urine occurs
  - Child has nausea or vomiting
  - Child has chills or fever
  - Child has flank pain
  - Child is lethargic
  - Child has painful voiding or frequent urgency to void
  - Swelling or redness occurs around the urethral opening

Unexpected Situation

- *While checking the infant's diaper, you note that the urine collection bag has become detached and the child has voided into the diaper:* Remove the bag. Perform perineal care. Apply a chemical adhesive (e.g., tincture of benzoin) and then apply a new collection bag.

Bibliography

Al-Orifi, F., McGillivray, D., Tange, S., & Kramer, M. S. (2000). Urine culture from bag specimens in young children: Are the risks too high? *Journal of Pediatrics, 13*, 221–226.

American Academy of Pediatrics. (1999). The diagnosis, treatment, and evaluation of the initial urinary tract infection in febrile infants and young children. *Pediatrics, 103*, 843–852.

Farrell, M., Devine, K., Lancaster, G., & Judd, B. (2002). A method comparison study to assess the reliability of urine collection pads as a means of obtaining urine specimens from non-toilet trained children for microbiological examination. *Journal of Advanced Nursing, 37*, 387–393.

Kirkpatrick, J., Alexander, J., & Cain, R. (1997). Recovering urine from diapers: Are test results accurate? *MCN: American Journal of Maternal Child Nursing, 22*, 96–102.

Liaw, L., Nayar, D., Pedler, S., & Coulthard, M. (2000). Home collection of urine for culture from infants by three methods: Survey of parents' preferences and bacterial contamination rates. *British Medical Journal, 320*, 1312–1313.

Lifshitz, E., & Kramer, L. (2000). Outpatient urine culture: Does collection technique matter? *Archives of Internal Medicine, 160*(16), 2537–2540.

Loane, V. (2005). Obtaining urine for culture from non-potty trained children. *Paediatric Nursing, 17*(9), 39–42.

McGillivray, D., Mok, E., Mulrooney, E., & Kramer, M. (2005). A head-to-head comparison: "Clean-void" bag versus catheter analysis in the diagnosis of urinary tract infection in young children. *The Journal of Pediatrics, 147*, 451–456.

Ramage, I., Chapman, J., Hollman, A., et al. (1999). Accuracy of clean-catch urine collection in infancy. *Journal of Pediatrics, 135*(6), 765–767.

Rao, S., Bhatt, J., Houghton, C., & Macfarlane, P. (2004). An improved urine collection pad method: A randomized clinical trial. *Archives of Disease in Childhood, 89*, 773–775.

Thomas, J., Kurien, A., & Philipraj, S. (2006). Methods for collecting urine samples in adults and children with suspected urinary tract infection (Protocol). *The Cochrane Database of Systematic Reviews*, (2), No. CD006025.

Wald, E. (2005). To bag or not to bag. *The Journal of Pediatrics, 147*, 418–420.

CHAPTER

123

Urine Collection: Straight Catheter

Clinical Guidelines

- A healthcare prescriber's order is required for one-time catheter placement to collect a urine specimen.
- A healthcare prescriber's order is required for use of 2% lidocaine (Xylocaine) water-soluble lubricant in catheterizing a child.
- 2% lidocaine gel has shown effectiveness in reducing discomfort associated with insertion of the catheter. However, because lidocaine gel takes at least 8 minutes for the anesthetic effect to be complete, use of nonanesthetic lubricant with 2% lidocaine gel as lubricant must be carefully considered based on the child's age, level of anxiety, and urgency of the procedure. The use of lidocaine lubricant may be more appropriate with older adolescents because in the younger child it may increase the length of the procedure and therefore the child's anxiety. A delay before starting the catheterization maximizes absorption of the anesthetic in the urethra.
- A healthcare prescriber, registered nurse (RN), or licensed practical nurse (LPN) inserts and removes a urinary catheter.

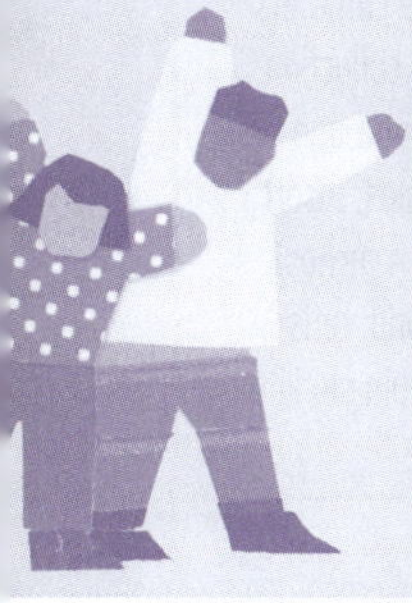

Equipment

- Examination light (optional)
- Gloves, gown, and protective eyewear
- Basin with soap and warm water, washcloth, and towel
- Waterproof pad
- Prepackaged straight catheter kit, which includes (obtain the following items if your institution does not supply prepackaged kit):
  - Sterile gloves
  - Water-soluble lubricant
  - Sterile povidone-iodine swabs
  - Sterile towels and drapes
  - Sterile straight catheter (see Table 116-1)
- Applicator with 2% lidocaine lubricant (if ordered)
- Sterile specimen container and label (if the specimen obtained is to be sent to the laboratory for culture and sensitivity)
- Biohazard bag for transporting the specimen to the laboratory
- Urine receptacle
- Waste receptacle
- Sheet to be used as a drape (may not be necessary for infants and small children)

CHILD AND FAMILY ASSESSMENT AND PREPARATION

- Assess the cognitive level, readiness, and ability to process information of the child and family. The readiness to learn and process information may be impaired as a result of age, stress, or anxiety.
- Identify and discuss the risks and benefits of placing an "in-and-out" catheter. Ensure the parents that the catheterization will not harm the child or damage the urethra or hymen.
- Assess the child for signs and symptoms of urinary tract or bladder infection, including fever, inability to void, burning on urination, feeling of fullness, bladder spasms, foul-smelling urine, redness or irritation of urethral opening, urethral discharge, crying without consolation, and discomfort.
- Assess the child for signs and symptoms of a distended bladder or residual urine, for which bladder emptying would be required.
- Assess time of last voiding by wet diaper or by palpating bladder above symphysis. Bedside ultrasound of the bladder may be performed before the procedure to establish certainty of the presence or amount of urine in the bladder.
- Reinforce the need for catheter placement, as appropriate, to both the child and the family.
- Explain the procedure, as appropriate, to both the child and the family.

KidKare Reassure the toddler and older child that the catheter is flexible, will feel like a noodle, and will produce a feeling of pressure and a desire to urinate.

- Provide instruction on pelvic muscle relaxation whenever possible. To relax pelvic and periurethral muscles, teach the child to blow a pinwheel and to press the hips against the bed or examination table during the catheterization. Next teach the child to contract and relax the pelvic muscles and to repeat this relaxation procedure during catheter insertion.

PROCEDURE **Straight Catheter Urine Specimen Collection**

Steps	Rationale/Points of Emphasis
1a. Perform hand hygiene and gather the necessary supplies.	Reduces the transmission of microorganisms. Promotes efficient time management and provides an organized approach to the procedure. **caREminder** *Another nurse may be necessary to assist if the child is unable to cooperate for any reason.*
1b. Select catheter appropriate for child (see Table 116-1).	Selection of the catheter is based on the child's age and gender, construction material of the catheter, and the internal and external diameter of the catheter. Small catheter sizes promote comfort and are adequate for specimen collection. Use of shorter-length urinary catheters and basing length on gender and age can reduce incidence of knotting (e.g., for toddlers and younger females, insert 2 inches; for male infants, insert 3 inches; for male toddlers, insert 3 to 4 inches).
1c. Have extra catheters available to use if needed.	If a catheter becomes contaminated, is inadvertently placed in the vagina, or is the incorrect size, a new catheter will be immediately needed to maintain sterility and complete the procedure in a timely manner.
2. Close the door to the child's room or draw the curtains around the child's bed.	Provides privacy during the procedure.
3. Raise the bed to a comfortable working height or stand on a step stool at crib side.	Reduces the strain placed on your back.
4. Don gloves and protective apparel.	Standard precautions to reduce transmission of microorganisms.
5a. Place a waterproof pad under the child's buttocks while positioning the child/infant.	Prevents the bed linens from being soiled.
5b. Position females in the supine position with the heels of the feet together and the knees tilted outward (called the frog position). Use rolled blankets, pillow, or towels to support legs in this position.	This position facilitates visualization of the inner labia.

Steps	Rationale/Points of Emphasis
5c. Position males in the supine position with the legs together. Use rolled towels under knees. Raise the penis and scrotal sac to rest on top of the thighs. **KidKare** Remind the child to keep his or her buttocks on the bed or table and to keep the perineal muscles relaxed. The child will most likely need to be reminded of this several times during the procedure.	This position facilitates visualization of the urethral opening. Bending the knees slightly may be a more comfortable position for the child.
6. Place a drape over the child/infant. In females, place the drape in a diamond configuration with one corner at the child's sternum, one corner over each knee, and one corner over the perineum. In males, cover the child's chest and lower extremities with a sheet, leaving only the genital area exposed.	Allows exposure of the child's perineum while covering the rest of the body, allowing for privacy.
7. Wash the child's genital area with warm water and soap. Rinse and dry the area.	Removes secretions and feces.
8. Remove gloves and perform hand hygiene	Reduces transmission of microorganisms.
9. Establish a sterile working area, using a sterile towel spread open.	Establishes a space from which to gather sterile equipment and proceed with catheterization without contamination.
10. Using sterile technique, open the sterile catheter, sterile povidone-iodine, sterile lubricant, swabs, and sterile prefilled syringe of water and drop them on the sterile towel. Open the sterile gravity drainage and collection bag and leave it sitting in the packaging container.	Facilitates ease of access to the equipment. If lidocaine gel is to be used, assemble lidocaine applicator according to the manufacturer's instructions and follow procedure for use of lidocaine lubricant gel.
11. Aseptically place a sterile towel between the female child's legs under the perineal area or on the thighs of a male child.	The pad becomes an extension of the sterile work area.
12. Don sterile gloves.	Reduces introduction of microorganisms into the urinary tract, which is normally sterile.
13a. While laying your nondominant arm across the midsection of the lower abdomen, use the thumb and middle finger of your nondominant sterile hand to spread open the female child's labia.	Allows for exposure and visualization of the urethral opening. Swelling of the labia in neonates, due to maternal hormones, may make it difficult to visualize the urethral opening. A flashlight or examination light may be helpful in locating the urethral opening. If locating the urethra in females is difficult, have an assistant, wearing sterile gloves, grasp the labia majora and gently pull forward, forming a cave-like opening, allowing the hymen and urethra to drop open.
13b. For a male child, follow the same procedure and use your nondominant hand to position the child's penis perpendicular to the body. In an uncircumcised male, withdraw the foreskin just far enough to visualize the urethral opening. Do not pull back behind the glans.	Withdrawing the foreskin further will be painful to the child and could cause tears that could lead to potential sites of infection.
14. With your dominant sterile hand, cleanse the area around the urethral opening with the sterile povidone-iodine swabs and discard them in a nearby waste receptacle. In females, using a separate povidone-iodine swab for each stroke, cleanse both the right and left side of the inner labia with one downward stroke. Then clean midline, from the clitoris down to the rectum with one stroke. In males, cleanse the penis in an outgoing circular motion, from the urethral opening to the base of the penis, using a new povidone-iodine swab each time.	Prevents contamination of the catheter by microorganisms on the skin and prevents introduction of open organisms into the patient's urethra and bladder. **caREminder** *The labia should not be allowed to close during the entire procedure because this contaminates the sterile field. If the labia do close, stop the procedure, don new sterile gloves, and start over at this step.*

Continued

Steps	Rationale/Points of Emphasis
15. With your sterile dominant hand, place the sterile specimen container on the sterile field between the child's legs and place the open end of the sterile catheter into the sterile specimen container. (If using a prepackaged catheter kit, the catheter comes already inserted into a sterile specimen tube. Gently pull 4 to 6 inches of the length of the catheter out of the sterile collection tube.)	Placing the end of the catheter in the specimen container prevents the sterile field from becoming wet and contaminating the catheter and the sterile field.
16. With your sterile dominant hand, lubricate the tip of the sterile catheter with the water-soluble lubricant that has been squirted on the sterile field. The catheter should be lubricated about 2 inches for a female child and about 6 inches for a male child.	Lubricant decreases the friction between the catheter and the urinary tract during catheterization. In males, using lubricant on the tip of the catheter promotes opening of the sphincter mechanism.
17a. Lift the lubricated tip of the catheter with your dominant sterile hand and gently insert it into the child's urethral opening.	Allows for catheterization to obtain sterile urine specimen.
17b. Do not touch the child's perineal hair or skin as the catheter is advanced.	Hair or skin will contaminate the catheter.
17c. In males, insert the lubricated catheter tip into the urethra without allowing the intraurethral lubricant to exit the urethral meatus. Because gentle pressure may cause an erection in an adolescent male, hold the penis firmly but not tightly. If held tightly, pressure will collapse the urethra and will prevent advancement of the catheter.	If the adolescent has an erection, stop the procedure until there is a nonerectile state and then continue with the procedure.
17d. Ask the child to take a deep breath while you insert the catheter.	Taking a deep breath helps to relax the urinary tract. **KidKare** The child may state that he or she needs to urinate during catheter insertion. Tell the child to go ahead and try to do so; this opens the urethra for passage of the catheter.
18. Insert the catheter until urine begins to flow. If an obstruction is encountered, *do not* force the catheter. If the catheter is inadvertently placed in the vagina, leave it in place and put a second catheter in the other opening (urethra). Once the catheter is inserted in the urethra, remove the catheter from the vagina. In males, the prepuce is retractable; put it back in the natural position after inserting the catheter. ***Alert!*** *When the catheter reaches the striated sphincter (proximal urethra in males and midurethra in females), if the child vigorously contracts the pelvic muscles, temporarily stop insertion of the catheter. Hold the catheter in place with steady gentle pressure. Assist the child to press the hips against the bed or examination table and relax the pelvic muscles before gently advancing the catheter into the bladder. Wait for the sphincter to relax before advancing the catheter. If still unable to advance the catheter, discontinue the procedure and notify the healthcare prescriber.*	Placing the catheter too far into the bladder can cause irritation to the bladder wall and/or knotting of the catheter. Forcing the catheter can cause trauma, bleeding, and possible scar formation, which can lead to strictures and obstruction of the urethra. If lidocaine gel is used, it will increase the volume of intraurethral lubricant. Therefore urine return may not be as rapid as when minimal amounts of water-soluble lubricant are used. Urine may not appear immediately, deceiving the practitioner into inserting the catheter farther than necessary. This can cause the catheter to circle around the bladder, occasionally knotting, or to find its way out of the bladder and then to kink in the urethra. The best way to prevent these problems is to insert only the necessary length of the tubing in the bladder and then wait for urine to appear. Gently pressing the suprapubic region (Credé's maneuver) may also assist urine to drain. Avoids possible painful swelling of the glans (paraphimosis).
19. Let 10 to 20 mL of urine drain into a sterile specimen container and close container. Allow the remaining urine to drain into the urine receptacle.	Draining the urine directly into the specimen container decreases the possibility of contaminating the specimen.
20. Remove the catheter.	Once the specimen is obtained, the catheter is no longer needed.
21. Put the lid on the container, label the specimen, and place in the biohazard bag.	Standard precautions.

Steps	Rationale/Points of Emphasis
22. Wash and cleanse the child's perineal area and return the foreskin to its natural position after cleansing on the uncircumcised male.	Cleansing promotes the child's comfort and sense of well-being while removing the povidone-iodine solution from the area. Failure to return the foreskin can lead to swelling of the penis and impairment of circulation.
23. Return the child's bed to the lowest position or to a level that is age appropriate.	Reduces potential injury from falls.
24. Label specimen with child's name, medical record number, and date and time specimen was obtained and by whom; place in plastic biohazard transmittal bag following standard precautions. Send to laboratory as soon as possible.	Ensures that correct tests are performed on specimen. Prompt testing reduces changes in specimen (e.g., bacterial growth).
25. Dispose of used equipment and waste in appropriate receptacle.	Standard precautions
26. Remove gloves and perform hand hygiene.	Reduces transmission of microorganisms.

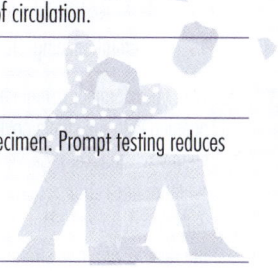

PROCEDURE Use of Lidocaine Lubricant Gel

Steps	Rationale/Points of Emphasis
1. Complete steps 1–12 above.	
2. Lidocaine gel is introduced into procedure once the perineal area has been cleansed. 2% lidocaine gel has shown effectiveness in reducing discomfort associated with insertion of the catheter. With sterile gloves on, assemble the applicator with 2% lidocaine lubricant gel. Place nickel- to quarter-size amount of lubricant on a sterile cotton ball.	Facilitates ease of access to the equipment. Standard applicators come with either 5 or 10 mL of 2% lidocaine gel.
3. For males, use forceps to place the gel-covered cotton ball on the meatus; leave in place for at least 2 minutes. For females, place a lidocaine-soaked cotton ball on the urethral meatus; leave in place for at least 2 minutes. Place the applicator with the rest of the lubricant in it on the sterile field. Set aside one cotton ball for additional lidocaine gel applications.	The lubricant is used to numb the external meatus and reduce discomfort associated with inserting the catheter. This is the first of four applications of the lubricant gel.
4. During wait period, continue to set up the catheterization kit. With your sterile dominant hand, lubricate the tip of the sterile catheter with the 2% lidocaine solution or water-soluble lubricant that has been squirted on the sterile field. The catheter should be lubricated about 2 inches for a female child and about 6 inches for a male child.	Both lubricants decrease the friction between the catheter and the urinary tract during catheterization. In males, using lubricant on the tip of the catheter promotes opening of the sphincter mechanism.
5. Attach the prefilled syringe of water to the secondary lumen balloon port of the urinary catheter and inflate the balloon with the sterile water, and then deflate the balloon retaining the sterile water in the syringe.	Ensures that the balloon of the retention catheter is working and does not have a leak.
6. After 2 minutes, use forceps to remove and discard the first cotton ball from the meatus of the male or female.	First application of lidocaine has been completed.
a. Continue with the process of sterile cleaning of the perineal area. While laying your nondominant arm across the midsection of the lower abdomen, use the thumb and middle finger of your nondominant sterile hand to spread open the female child's labia.	Allows for exposure and visualization of the urethral opening. Swelling of the labia in neonates, due to maternal hormones, may make it difficult to visualize the urethral opening. A flashlight or examination light may be helpful in locating the urethral opening. If locating the urethra in females is difficult, have an assistant, wearing sterile gloves, grasp the labia majora and gently pull forward, forming a cave-like opening allowing the hymen and urethra to drop open.

Continued

Steps	Rationale/Points of Emphasis
b. For a male child, follow the same procedure and use your nondominant hand to position the child's penis perpendicular to the body. In an uncircumcised male, withdraw the foreskin just far enough to visualize the urethral opening. Do not pull back behind the glans.	Withdrawing the foreskin further will be painful to the child and could cause tears that could lead to potential sites of infection.
7. With your dominant sterile hand, cleanse the area around the urethral opening with the sterile povidone-iodine swabs and discard them in a nearby waste receptacle. In females, using a separate povidone-iodine swab for each stroke, cleanse both the right and left side of the inner labia with one downward stroke. Then clean midline, from the clitoris down to the rectum with one stroke. In males, cleanse the penis in an outgoing circular motion, from the urethral opening to the base of the penis, using a new povidone-iodine swab each time.	Prevents contamination of the catheter by microorganisms on the skin and prevents introduction of open organisms into the patient's urethra and bladder. **caREminder** *The labia should not be allowed to close during the entire procedure because this contaminates the sterile field. If the labia do close, stop the procedure, don new sterile gloves, and start over at this step.*
8. In males, begin installation by gently touching the applicator to the meatus. Slowly instill the lidocaine gel into the meatus (see Table 116–2 for amount of lubricant to use). Place a cotton ball on the meatus. Hold the lubricant in place by gently squeezing the distal penis (behind the glans penis). Wait 2 minutes. In females, use the applicator to drip lidocaine gel downward from the clitoris onto the urethral opening. Place a second lidocaine gel–soaked cotton ball on the meatus. Wait 2 minutes.	Instilling the lidocaine too quickly causes a burning sensation and irritation of the meatus. The amount of lubricant instilled depends on length and diameter of urethra. Though the female urethra is generally shorter, the amount administered is the same for females and males.
9. For males, repeat the numbing and instillation process in step 8 two more times. For females, gently touch the meatus with the applicator and then gently instill a small amount of lubricant into the urethra. Place a cotton ball over the urethra. Wait 2 minutes. Repeat installation of lidocaine one more time and wait 2 minutes.	Repeated applications ensure efficacy of anesthetic.
10. For males, instill extra sterile water-soluble gel into urethra.	Dilates urethra and acts as additional lubricant.
11. Continue with catheterization procedure following steps 16–18 of the procedure for Insertion of an Indwelling Catheter, Chapter 116. Place end of catheter in sterile specimen container and collect urine specimen. Follow steps 10–12 of the procedure for Indwelling Catheter Urine Collection, Chapter 121. Follow steps 10–15 of the procedure for Removal of an Indwelling Catheter, Chapter 116.	Placement of catheter should proceed in atraumatic fashion as a result of lidocaine gel applications.

Child and Family Evaluation and Documentation

- Evaluate the amount, color, clarity, and odor of the urine and the presence of any sediment.
- Evaluate child for signs and symptoms of a urinary tract infection, including fever, tachycardia, foul-smelling urine or perineum, perineal discharge, cloudy or sedimented urine, or urine discoloration.
- Document the following:
  - Completion of the procedure
  - Catheter size used
  - Amount, color, clarity, and odor of the urine and the presence of any sediment
  - Child's response to the specimen collection

Community Care

- If the procedure is performed in an outpatient setting, encourage parents to offer fluids to the child on the trip to the office or clinic.
- Instruct the family to contact the healthcare provider if
  - Urine is cloudy or dark
  - Blood is present in the urine or a change in smell of the urine occurs
  - Child has nausea or vomiting
  - Child has chills or fever
  - Child has flank pain
  - Child is lethargic
  - Child has painful voiding or frequent urgency to void
  - Swelling or redness occurs around the urethral opening

Unexpected Situation

- *Catheter cannot be advanced in urethra:* Hold the catheter in place with steady and gentle pressure. Instruct child to take deep breaths. Ensure child's buttocks are resting on the table or bed and abdomen is not taut. Have the child cough or participate in diversionary tactics. Once child is more relaxed, proceed with insertion of the catheter.

Bibliography

Chen, L., Hsiao, A., Moore, C., et al. (2005). Utility of bedside bladder ultrasound before urethral catheterization in young children. *Pediatrics, 115*, 108–111.

Gray, M. (1996). Atraumatic urethral catheterization of children. *Pediatric Nursing, 22*, 306–310.

Liaw, L., Nayar, D., Pedler, S., & Coulthard, M. (2000). Home collection of urine for culture from infants by three methods: Survey of parents' preferences and bacterial contamination rates. *British Medical Journal, 320*(7245), 1312–1313.

Lifshitz, E., & Kramer, L. (2000). Outpatient urine culture: Does collection technique matter? *Archives of Internal Medicine, 160*, 2537–2540.

Milling, T., Van Amerongen, R., Melville, L., et al. (2005). Use of ultrasonography to identify infants for whom urinary catheterization will be unsuccessful because of insufficient urine volume: Validation of the Urinary Bladder Index. *Annals of Emergency Medicine, 45*, 510–513.

Witt, M., Baumann, B., & McCans, K. (2005). Bladder ultrasound increases catheterization success in pediatric patients. *Academic Emergency Medicine, 12*, 371–374.

CHAPTER

124

Urine Collection: Suprapubic Aspiration

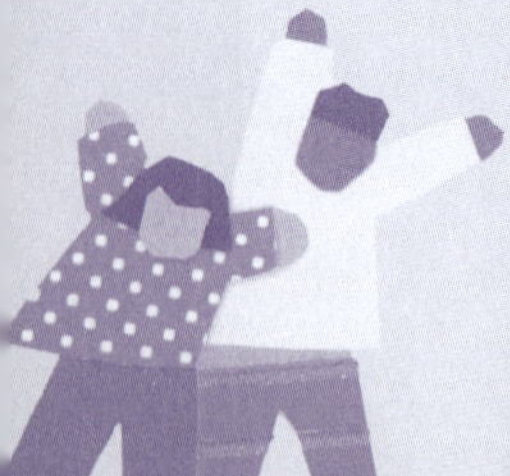

Clinical Guidelines

- A healthcare prescriber may perform suprapubic aspiration.
- A registered nurse (RN), licensed practical nurse (LPN), or unlicensed assistive personnel (UAP) may assist with the procedure to maximize efficiency and to minimize trauma and contamination of the specimen.
- To confirm the diagnosis of a urinary tract infection, suprapubic aspiration or transurethral bladder catheterization (see Chapter 123) may be obtained if a child with unexplained fever is assessed as being sufficiently ill to warrant immediate antimicrobial therapy.
- Suprapubic aspiration is typically performed on children younger than 2 years of age and on premature infants. Small bladder capacity, anterior wall infection, and bleeding disorders are considered contraindications for performing this procedure.

caREminder

The diagnosis of urinary tract infection cannot be established by a culture of urine collected in a bag.

Equipment

- Sterile gloves sized for person performing procedure
- Nonsterile gloves for assistant
- Antiseptic solution
- Sterile 20- to 23-gauge needle with syringe
- Sterile gauze pad
- Bandage or occlusive dressing
- Urine collection container with labels
- Plastic biohazard transmittal bag

Child and Family Assessment and Preparation

- Explain procedure to parents and child in appropriate developmental terms, using instructional props as necessary.
- Allow parents to stay at bedside to comfort child.
- Obtain consent as required by institution.

- Assess the child for signs and symptoms of urinary tract or bladder infection, including fever, inability to void, burning on urination, feeling of fullness, bladder spasms, foul-smelling urine, redness or irritation of urethral opening, urethral discharge, crying without consolation, and discomfort.
- Assess time of last voiding by wetness of diaper or by palpating bladder above symphysis. Bedside ultrasound of the bladder may be performed before the procedure to establish certainty of the presence or amount of urine in the bladder.
- Coordinate timing of procedure with healthcare prescriber to ensure that adequate amount of urine is present in bladder and that grouping of activities can aid in decreasing the stress and anxiety of child and family.

PROCEDURE Suprapubic Aspiration Urine Specimen Collection

Steps	Rationale/Points of Emphasis
1. Perform hand hygiene.	Reduces transmission of microorganisms.
2. Gather the necessary supplies and set up supplies for procedure, maintaining sterility. Ensure specimen collection containers are easily accessible.	Promotes efficient time management and provides organized approach to the procedure.
3. Transport infant/child to treatment area.	Child's bedside should be viewed as a safe environment where painful procedures do not occur.
4. Perform hand hygiene and don gloves.	Standard precautions to reduce transmission of microorganisms.
5. Stand at head of child. Position infant/child on back with legs extended or flexed, as practitioner prefers (Figure 124-1). Restrain as necessary.	Controls child's movement to decrease inadvertent injury.

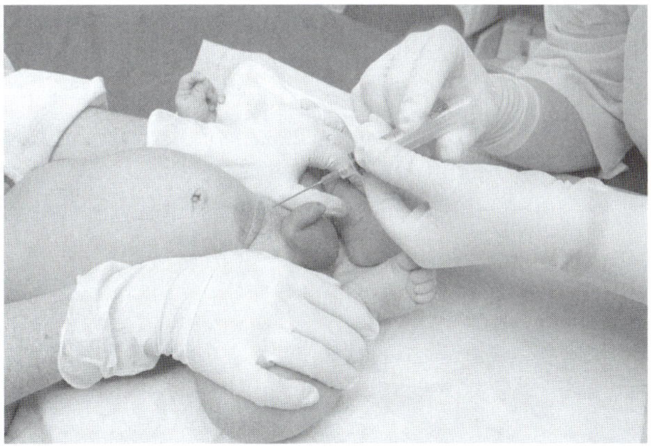

FIGURE 124-1
The nurse stands at the child's head to position the child with legs flexed. The nurse's arms help to restrain the child's trunk.

Steps	Rationale/Points of Emphasis
6. Assist practitioner performing procedure as required. Offer comfort measures such as pacifier or quiet soothing tones during procedure.	Biobehavioral measures can aid in calming infant and in minimizing movement.
7. After procedure, apply pressure to site as directed by practitioner. Ease infant/child from restrained position.	Minimizes bleeding, which is usually minimal; little pressure is needed after the procedure.
8. Apply a bandage to the site.	Protects site.
9. Allow infant/child to be held and comforted by parent.	Calms child and reduces stress.
10. Label specimen with child's name, medical record number, and date and time specimen was obtained and by whom; place in plastic biohazard transmittal bag following standard precautions. Send to laboratory as soon as possible.	Ensures that correct tests are performed on specimen. Prompt testing reduces changes in specimen (e.g., bacterial growth).
11. Perform hand hygiene.	Reduces transmission of microorganisms.

CHILD AND FAMILY EVALUATION AND DOCUMENTATION

- Address questions and concerns of child and parents regarding procedure after it is completed.
- Evaluate puncture site for bleeding.
- Document the following:
  - Time of procedure
  - Practitioner who performed the task
  - Appearance of the aspiration site
  - Amount and appearance of urine collected
  - Test the sample was sent for
  - Child's tolerance of procedure
  - Family teaching provided

COMMUNITY CARE

- Instruct family to contact the healthcare provider if
  - Oozing is present at needle insertion site
  - Child does not void

Unexpected Situation

- *One hour after assisting with a suprapubic aspiration on a 10-month-old child, you notice that the bandage over the puncture site is moist:* There may be oozing from the puncture site or the site may be wet if the child has voided. Remove the old bandage, clean the site with sterile water and gauze, and redress the site with an occlusive dressing. Reassess the site in 1 hour; if the dressing is wet again, notify the healthcare prescriber.

Bibliography

American Academy of Pediatrics. (1999). The diagnosis, treatment, and evaluation of the initial urinary tract infection in febrile infants and young children. *Pediatrics, 103*, 843–852.

Chen, L., Hsiao, A., Moore, C., et al. (2005). Utility of bedside bladder ultrasound before urethral catheterization in young children. *Pediatrics, 115*, 108–111.

Ramage, L. (1999). Accuracy of urine culture obtained by suprapubic aspiration and paired clean-catch in infancy. *Archives of Disease in Childhood, 80*(Suppl. 1), G46.

Roberts, K. (2000). The AAP practice parameter on urinary tract infections in febrile infants and young children. *American Family Physician, 62*, 1815–1822.

Thomas, J., Kurien, A., & Philipraj, S. (2006). Methods for collecting urine samples in adults and children with suspected urinary tract infection (Protocol). *The Cochrane Database of Systematic Reviews*, (2), No. CD006025.

CHAPTER

125

Ventilators: High Frequency

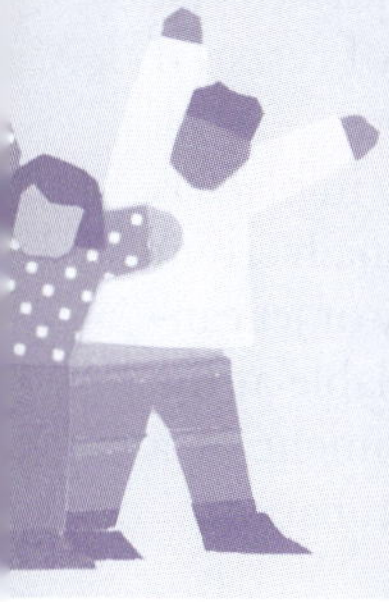

Clinical Guidelines

- High-frequency ventilation is ordered by a physician. Ventilatory parameters are set by the physician in collaboration with the respiratory therapist and RN to maintain pH, pulmonary arteriole carbon dioxide ($PaCO_2$), pulmonary arteriole oxygen (PaO_2), and arteriole saturations (SaO_2).
- It is the responsibility of the physician, respiratory therapist (RT), registered nurse (RN), and licensed practical nurse (LPN) to collaborate and manage the moment-to-moment ventilatory needs of the child.
- The RN or LPN has demonstrated knowledge and competence in basic ventilator mechanisms of action (Chart 125-1) and in the assessment, monitoring, and ongoing care of the child on a ventilator.
- High-frequency ventilation is a method of exchanging gases at a faster respiratory rate (60 to 3,000 oscillations per minute) and lower tidal volumes (equal to or less than dead-space volume). The theoretic advantages of high-frequency ventilation are that smaller applied tidal volumes result in lower peak pressures and thus reduce the incidence of barotrauma and cardiovascular depression.
- The indications for use in the child with respiratory or ventilatory failure include air leak, pneumothorax, pneumopericardium, pulmonary interstitial emphysema, bronchopleural fistulas, acute respiratory distress syndrome (ARDS), persistent pulmonary hypertension, meconium aspiration syndrome, pneumonia, pulmonary hemorrhage, hypoplastic lungs, diaphragmatic hernia, and multiorgan system failure. High-frequency ventilation is also used to reduce barotraumas when conventional ventilator settings are getting very high and when conventional ventilation is failing or as a prestep before extra corporeal membranous oxygenation (ECMO).
- The goal of high-frequency ventilation is to maintain adequate alveolar ventilation and to correct hypoxemia.
- Children receiving high-frequency ventilation may be placed on continuous drips of a sedative and/or pain medications and/or a paralytic agent to decrease the work of breathing and to allow the ventilator to work more effectively.

Equipment

- Nonsterile gloves
- Manual resuscitation bag and face mask
- Positive end-expiratory pressure (PEEP) valve (optional, for resuscitation bag)

CHART 125-1 TERMS USED WITH HIGH-FREQUENCY VENTILATION

Amplitude: the size of the pressure wave produced by the oscillator. Also can be an alternate way to describe the delivered volume.

Dead space: the amount of space from the ventilator to the lung (i.e., the length of the endotracheal tube) that is not being ventilated.

Fractional inspired oxygen concentration (FIO_2): the amount of supplemental oxygen delivered to the child through the ventilator.

Frequency (Hertz): the number of times the ventilator delivers its rate.

Oscillation: the movement of the lungs as they stay in a state of open flux.

Mean airway pressure (MAP): the distending pressure applied to the lung from the ventilator. Measured before delivery. Can be increased or decreased on the oscillation ventilator.

Minute ventilation: a mathematic formula that multiplies the rate by the tidal volume and subtracts the dead space.

Sighs: conventional breaths that may be given periodically to replenish alveoli and decrease atelectasis.

Stroke volume: the volume of gas displaced within the lung. It is produced by the vibrating device; this affects CO_2 elimination.

- Multiple sources of oxygen delivery (e.g., for high-frequency ventilator, resuscitation bag, backup ventilator)
- Functional humidification system for high-frequency ventilator
- Sterile water for humidification
- Constant electrical source (for those ventilators without battery backup)
- High-frequency positive-pressure ventilator, high-frequency oscillatory ventilator, or high-frequency jet ventilator with additional conventional ventilator (a special triple-lumen endotracheal tube or a triple-lumen endotracheal tube adapter is required with a pressure monitoring port located on the distal tip and a jet port located within the tube wall for the high-frequency jet ventilator with additional conventional ventilator method of delivery)
- Oxygen analyzer
- Suction equipment and catheters
- Stethoscope
- Sedation, pain medications, and paralytic (as ordered)

CHILD AND FAMILY ASSESSMENT AND PREPARATION

- Inform the child and the parents of the need for high-frequency ventilation. Discuss the following:
  - Purpose of high-frequency ventilation and the intended reason for use
  - Signs and symptoms that may indicate complications of high-frequency ventilation
  - The need for artificial airway change or removal
  - The need for supplemental sedation, pain control, and possibly paralyzation
  - The sensations the child may experience (i.e., noise of the ventilator, oscillations of the ventilator, alarm sounds)
- Prepare the parents for providing interaction with the child, including touch, talking, and providing other comfort measures, even while the child may be sedated. Discuss how the family can promote relaxation in the child and let the ventilator "breathe" for the child. Establish a way of nonverbal communication with the child (i.e., picture board, writing pad), so that the child can maintain communication even while intubated; have call bell within ease of reach, if appropriate.
- Observe and ensure that the artificial airway in place is secure and stable to reduce the risk for inadvertent extubation. Ensure that a replacement airway or jet cannula of the same existing size is readily available at the child's bedside to ensure quick reestablishment of a patent airway in the event of inadvertent extubation.

PROCEDURE Management of Child During System Setup

Steps	Rationale/Points of Emphasis
1. To place the child on high-frequency ventilation, begin by following Chapter 126: Managing Child During Setup procedure.	High-frequency ventilation is usually not the first ventilatory choice when ventilation is initiated for a child. Therefore, many of the steps outlined in Chapter 126 may have already been completed (e.g., the child is already intubated and on one form of ventilatory support at the time the decision is made to place the child on high-frequency ventilation).

Steps	Rationale/Points of Emphasis
2. Once the respiratory therapist or technician has set up the high-frequency ventilator at the child's bedside (and ensures settings are as prescribed), attach airway circuitry adapter from ventilator to artificial airway of child.	Provides for mechanical ventilation to be instituted in the child.
3. Confirm that ventilator setting and parameters are as prescribed and that alarms are on and functioning.	Ensures that ventilator settings have been established in the manner prescribed by the physician.
4. Ensure that the circuitry tubing is free of water and is not kinked, that all connections are secure, that the circuitry tubing has some slack so that the child can move his or her head, that manual resuscitation bag attached to 100% flowmeter oxygen is ready, and that suction equipment is at hand and ready for use.	Provides child-ready ventilation with assurance that it is working in the prescribed manner with emergency equipment at the bedside.
5. Assess ventilatory effectiveness and lung compliance: • For high-frequency oscillation ventilation, assess chest wall vibration rather than lung sounds. • For high-frequency positive-pressure ventilation, assess chest wall vibration in addition to lung sounds (secondary to high ventilatory rate). • For high-frequency jet ventilation, assess chest wall pulsation (from jet ventilator) in addition to breath sounds	Monitors efficacy of ventilator and alerts parent to potential problems. **caREminder** *The movement of the anterior chest wall on the child will appear to vibrate, rather than rise and fall as with normal respirations. This sudden decrease in chest wall movement is an indicator of lung compliance, patent airway, and effectiveness of ventilator.*
6. Dispose of used equipment in appropriate receptacles.	Standard precautions.
7. Ensure that child is placed in comfortable safe position and is free from pain.	Ensures child's safety and comfort.
8. Perform hand hygiene.	Reduces transmission of microorganisms.

PROCEDURE Ongoing Evaluation and Troubleshooting the System

Steps	Rationale/Points of Emphasis
1. To provide ongoing evaluation of the child and to troubleshoot the system, follow Chapter 126: Ongoing Evaluation and Troubleshooting of the System procedure.	The use of high-frequency ventilation at low tidal volume allows the primary goals of ventilation, oxygenation, and CO_2 removal to be achieved without some of the costs of pressure-induced lung injury. However, as with other methods of mechanical ventilation, high-frequency ventilation can also have iatrogenic complications. Potential complications may include airway obstruction from inadequate humidification of inspired gas, lung and airway damage from high-velocity streams of inspired gas, cardiac depression from the development of auto-PEEP, weaning failures, inadequate gas exchange, mechanical failure of high-frequency ventilators, and inadvertent asymmetric ventilation.
2. To troubleshoot specifically for the jet ventilator:	
a. Assess for high Servo pressures.	This may be reflected as a worsening lung condition, possible airway obstruction, tension pneumothorax, or kinked ventilator tubing.
b. Assess for low Servo pressures.	This may be reflected as improving lung compliance or as a possible leak in the patient–ventilator system. A pneumothorax being continually evacuated by a chest tube also may be a causative factor.
c. Monitor alarm tones.	If the peak inspiratory pressure (PIP) of the conventional ventilator breaths is set higher than the jet ventilator, the PIP will interrupt the jet flow. If the conventional ventilator tubing gets kinked, this could result in over-pressurization of the circuit, and alveolar rupture may occur if the expiratory gas cannot escape. If the infant's/child's head is repositioned, assessment of chest wall vibration must be made to ensure that the tracheal wall has not occluded the jet port on the endotracheal tube.

Child and Family Evaluation and Documentation

- Evaluate the child for adequacy of ventilation, oxygenation, perfusion, effect of driving pressures, and response to inspiratory time, tidal volume, or changes in PEEP or continuous positive airway pressure (CPAP). Monitor tidal volume, fractional inspired oxygen concentration (FIO_2), and mean airway pressure directly if possible. Monitor carbon dioxide levels directly with transcutaneous PCO_2 analyzer and saturations directly with pulse oximeter, if possible.
- Evaluate the child's progress toward discontinuance of high-frequency ventilation. Indicators of progress toward this goal include decreasing levels of PEEP, supplemental oxygen, and driving pressure with corresponding stability or improvement of underlying pathology for which high-frequency was instituted; stability or improvement in hemodynamic parameters; and child's ability to assume increasing proportions of minute ventilation.
- Document the following:
  - Date, time, and initial setup of ventilator
  - Ventilator settings
  - Blood gas parameters
  - Vital signs
  - Oxygen saturation
  - Response to initiation of high-frequency ventilation
  - Airway type and size (e.g., no. 4.0 endotracheal tube, no. 3.5 fenestrated trachea tube, cuffed or uncuffed tube)
  - Method used to secure airway in place
  - Tube location (e.g., oral, nasal, tracheal)
  - Change in breathing pattern (notify the physician of changes)
  - Pain and anxiety assessment and any interventions required managing the child's pain or sedation
  - Date, time, and frequency of suctioning, along with color, amount, and consistency of secretions; presence of blood; any adverse effects; and child tolerance
  - Blood gas results and interventions made to correct blood gas abnormalities

Community Care

- Children on high-frequency ventilation are not discharged home on this type of ventilation. Once progress is made to discontinuance of high-frequency ventilation, the child may be eventually discharged home on a mechanical ventilator or some other type of airway adjunct to provide ongoing respiratory support. See Chapter 126 for more information regarding community care needs of the child discharged home on a ventilator.

Unexpected Situation

- *The ventilator repeatedly alarms high pressure:* Assess child's status, and implement intervention as indicated (e.g., if unequal breath sounds, evaluate ETT placement or management of condition; if signs of tension pneumothorax, notify physician or advanced practice nurse to immediately treat this). If child appears to be stable, assess ETT and ventilator settings and system (i.e., ensure airway is patent, suction if indicated, verify that ventilator tubing is not kinked or does not have water in it).

Bibliography

Bhuta, T., Clark, R. H., & Henderson-Smart, D. J. (2001). Rescue high frequency oscillatory ventilation versus conventional ventilation for infants with severe pulmonary dysfunction born at or near term. *The Cochrane Database of Systematic Reviews*, (1), No. CD002974.

Bhuta, T., & Henderson-Smart, D. J. (1998a). Rescue high frequency oscillatory ventilation versus conventional ventilation for pulmonary dysfunction in preterm infants. *The Cochrane Database of Systematic Reviews*, (2), No. CD000438.

Bhuta, T., & Henderson-Smart, D. J. (1998b). Elective high frequency jet ventilation versus conventional ventilation for respiratory distress syndrome in preterm infants. *The Cochrane Database of Systematic Reviews*, (2), No. CD000328.

Brinker, D. (2004). Sedation and comfort issues in the ventilated infant and child. *Critical Care Nursing Clinics of North America*, *16*, 365–377.

Henderson-Smart, D. J., Bhuta, T., Cools, F., & Offringa, M. (2003). Elective high frequency oscillatory ventilation versus conventional ventilation for acute pulmonary dysfunction in preterm infants. *The Cochrane Database of Systematic Reviews*, (2), No. CD000104.

Mehta, N. M., & Arnold, J. M. (2004). Mechanical ventilation in children with acute respiratory failure. *Current Opinion in Critical Care*, *10*, 7–12.

Null, D. M., Jr., Bachman, T. E., & Ashurst, J. T. (2002). Improved pulmonary outcomes with HFOV: A meta-analysis of the 3100A trials. *Neonatal Intensive Care*, *15*(6), 10–14.

Reper, P., Van Bos, R., Van Loey, K., Van Laeke, P., & Vanderkelen, A. (2003). High frequency percussive ventilation in burn patients: Hemodynamics and gas exchange. *Burns*, *29*, 603–608.

Wratney, A. T., Gentile, M. A., Hamel, D. S., & Cheifetz, I. M. (2004). Successful treatment of acute chest syndrome with high-frequency oscillatory ventilation in pediatric patients. *Respiratory Care*, *49*, 263–269.

Wunsch, H., & Mapstone, J. (2004). High-frequency ventilation versus conventional ventilation for treatment of acute lung injury and acute respiratory distress syndrome. *The Cochrane Database of Systematic Reviews*, (3), No. CD004085.

C H A P T E R

126

Ventilators: Mechanical

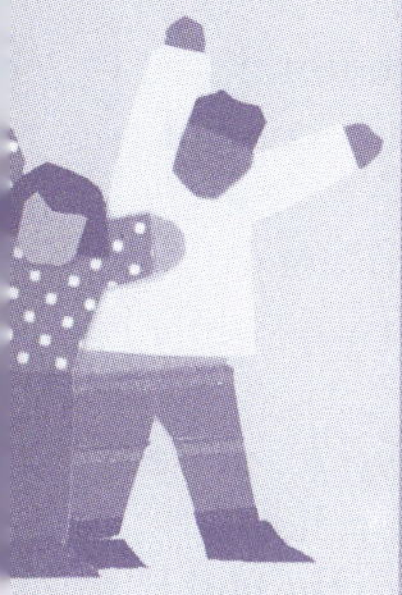

Clinical Guidelines

- Mechanical ventilation or positive-pressure ventilation is ordered by a physician. Ventilatory parameters are set by the physician in collaboration with the respiratory therapist to maintain pH, pulmonary arterial carbon dioxide ($PaCO_2$), pulmonary arterial oxygen (PaO_2), and arterial saturations (SaO_2).
- It is the responsibility of the healthcare prescriber, respiratory therapist (RT), registered nurse (RN), and licensed practical nurse (LPN) to collaborate and manage the moment-to-moment ventilatory needs of the child.
- The RN or LPN must have demonstrated knowledge and competence in basic ventilator mechanisms of action (Chart 126-1) and in the assessment, monitoring, and ongoing care of the child on a ventilator.
- The purpose of mechanical ventilation is to promote gas exchange in the lung. It does so by producing positive intrathoracic pressure and positive airway pressure. This positive pressure may be delivered to the airway through a mask, cannula, or endotracheal or tracheotomy tube. The amount of gas exchange that takes place is then dependent on the resistance and compliance of the lung itself.
- The goals of positive-pressure ventilation are to maintain adequate alveolar ventilation, to correct hypoxemia, and to decrease the work of breathing while providing adequate respirations and provide rest for the child.
- Mechanical ventilators can be categorized in three ways: those that deliver a preset amount of tidal volume, those that deliver a preset amount of peak inspiratory pressure, and those that deliver rates at high frequency (60 to 3,000 oscillations per minute) with low tidal volumes.
- Positive-pressure ventilation is indicated for the child with respiratory or ventilatory failure. Hypoxemia, metabolic acidosis, respiratory acidosis, inadequate tissue oxygenation, and respiratory muscle fatigue are all signs and symptoms of respiratory or ventilatory failure. This may be due to acute or chronic lung injury, neurologic disorders, trauma, chemical or medical respiratory depressants (i.e., sedation, anesthesia, or pain killers), multiorgan system failure, or disease entities.
- Children receiving ventilatory support may be placed on intermittent administration or continuous drips of a sedative, pain medication, or a paralytic agent to decrease the work of breathing and allow the ventilator to work more effectively.

Equipment

- Nonsterile gloves
- Manual resuscitation bag and face mask
- Suction equipment and catheters
- Positive end-expiratory pressure (PEEP) valve (optional, for resuscitation bag)

CHART 126-1 TERMS OF MECHANICAL VENTILATION

Assist-control: with each spontaneous breath the child takes, a preset tidal volume is triggered and delivered. If the child does not take spontaneous breaths, a mechanical breath is automatically given at a preset rate and tidal volume.

Continuous positive airway pressure (CPAP): a constant elevated level of airway pressure is maintained during inspiration and expiration with each spontaneous breath the child takes.

Controlled mandatory ventilation (CMV): a mechanical breath is automatically given to the child at a preset rate and tidal volume. Best used for apneic or chemically paralyzed children.

I:E ratio: the amount of inspiratory versus expiratory time taken with each breath can be adjusted to fit the individual child's needs.

Positive end-expiratory pressure (PEEP): a constant level of airway pressure is maintained during expiration, whether mechanical or spontaneous breaths are taken.

Pressure control: a mandatory amount of preset mechanical breaths at a preset peak inspiratory pressure is triggered and delivered. If the child does not take spontaneous breaths, a mechanical breath is automatically given at a preset rate and pressure.

Pressure regulated volume control (PRVC): a preset peak inspiratory pressure is maintained, along with a preset tidal volume during each spontaneous breath. Can be used as an adjunct, as with the child who has muscular dystrophy.

Pressure support: when the child takes a spontaneous breath, the ventilator delivers a preset sustained peak pressure throughout the inspiratory phase, thus resulting in increased tidal volume. The higher the pressure support, the larger the tidal volume.

Sigh: a large, hyperinflated mechanical breath that is given at a preset volume and frequency.

Synchronized intermittent mandatory ventilation (SIMV): a mandatory number of mechanical breaths are synchronized with the child's spontaneous breaths at a preset frequency and tidal volume.

Volume control: a preset tidal volume is triggered and delivered with each spontaneous respiration the child takes.

- Two sources of oxygen delivery (one with oxygen flowmeter for resuscitation bag and one to attach to mechanical ventilator)
- Air source (for ventilator connection)
- Constant electrical source (for those ventilators without battery backup)
- Sterile water
- Mechanical ventilator with heated, filtered humidifier, and in-line thermometer
- Oxygen analyzer
- Stethoscope
- Intubation equipment (if not already intubated) (see Chapter 59)
- Cardiopulmonary monitor and equipment (as needed) (see Chapter 23)
- Pulse oximetry equipment (as needed) (see Chapter 100)
- Intravascular therapy equipment (as needed) (see Chapter 55)
- Sedation, pain medication, and paralytic (as ordered)

CHILD AND FAMILY ASSESSMENT AND PREPARATION

- Inform the child and the parents of the need for mechanical ventilation or positive-pressure ventilation. Discuss the following:
  - Purpose of mechanical ventilation or positive-pressure ventilation and the reason (e.g., respiratory failure, complications of pneumonia, acid-base imbalance) for use
  - Signs and symptoms that may indicate complications of mechanical ventilation
  - The need for artificial airway change or removal
  - The need for supplemental sedation, pain control, and possible paralyzation
  - The possibility of physical restraints to keep the child from pulling out the artificial airway while being ventilated
  - The sensations the child may experience (i.e., noise of the ventilator, alarm sounds, breathing relief)
- Prepare the family to provide interaction with the child, including touch, talking with, and providing other comfort measures, even while the child may be sedated. Discuss how the family can promote relaxation in the child and let the ventilator "breathe" for the child. Establish a way of nonverbal communication with the child (e.g., picture board, writing pad), so that the child can maintain communication even while intubated. Have call bell within ease of reach, if appropriate.
- Determine the child's baseline weight. This will aid in determining how much tidal volume or pressure is required for mechanical ventilation.

PROCEDURE Managing the Child During System Setup

Steps	Rationale/Points of Emphasis
1. Notify respiratory care therapist of need for mechanical ventilator. If the child is not intubated, the respiratory therapist should be prepared to assist in intubation procedures.	In most institutions, the respiratory care therapist conducts the initiation and setup of ventilator management. Ventilator choice depends on size of the child, disease treated, severity of the disease, institutional availability of differing manufacturers' ventilators, and preference of the physician.
2a. As primary nurse completes steps 4 and following, another healthcare provider should obtain supplies and medications needed for intubation (if child not already intubated) (see Chapter 59). 2b. Place appropriately sized manual resuscitation bag, oxygen reservoir, tubing, flowmeter, and appropriately sized face mask at bedside. Place suction catheters and suction equipment at the bedside.	The child's deteriorating respiratory status will require the collaborative efforts of several healthcare professionals to work in a coordinated fashion to meet the child's emergent needs. For the child on a ventilator, emergency respiratory equipment must be maintained at the bedside at all time in case the child becomes extubated and requires manual ventilation.
3. Verify that the child has a patent IV line for administration of sedatives, paralytics, and emergency drugs. Initiate IV access if none is in place and if IV access will be needed.	IV access is needed if the child experiences cardiac arrest during intubation. Emergency medications can also be delivered by the interosseous route or by the endotracheal tube once it is verified to be in place.
4. Perform hand hygiene and don gloves.	Reduces transmission of microorganisms.
5. Initiate bag-valve mask ventilation (as required) or manual ventilation through endotracheal or tracheostomy tube until mechanical ventilator is ready to be connected to the child.	Manual ventilation may be needed if the child's respiratory status is declining rapidly. Ensure that the child is being hand ventilated with 100% oxygen from flowmeter using a manual resuscitation bag to a face mask or artificial airway (endotracheal tube or tracheotomy tube). An optional PEEP valve may be a necessary addition to the manual resuscitation bag to maintain adequate ventilation.
6. If not already completed, connect the child to cardiopulmonary monitor and pulse oximeter. Monitor for the child's heart rate, respiratory status, and oxygenation status throughout the procedure.	Provides for ongoing assessment of the infant/child for any changes in heart rate, respiratory rate or function, oxygen saturation, and level of consciousness.
7. Assess the child for signs of inadequate ventilation. Observe the child for increased work of breathing that may include shallow, irregular, or agonal respirations; apnea, tachypnea, or dyspnea; intercostal, substernal, abdominal, or tracheal retractions; nasal flaring; purse-lipped breathing; or central cyanosis.	These signs indicate respiratory distress and a need for mechanical ventilation.
8. Assess the child for signs of inadequate oxygenation. Auscultate for adventitious breath sounds that may increase respiratory distress and observe pulse oximeter for decreasing saturations. Observe for accompanying signs of respiratory distress that may include restlessness, agitation, confusion, lethargy, tachycardia, cardiac dysrhythmias, or change in blood pressure.	These signs may lead to a need for positive-pressure ventilation.
9. Obtain and assess child's blood gases (as indicated).	Determines presence of acute respiratory acidosis, hypoxemia, or hypercapnia, which would confirm the need for mechanical ventilation.
10. Suction the child's airway as needed.	Removes secretions and any potential airway blockage that may impede successful ventilation and intubation of the child.
11a. Administer pain medications, sedatives, or paralytics as ordered immediately before the intubation. 11b. Atropine may also be given pretreatment to reduce the incidence of reflex bradyarrhythmias.	The infant/child should be kept quiet and still during the procedure to prevent additional injuries. The child should be free from pain during the procedure. If paralytics are used, a physician experienced in intubation techniques should be present. Mechanical stimulation of the airway or hypoxemia may induce bradyarrhythmias in the infant and young child.

Continued

Steps	Rationale/Points of Emphasis
12. Assist in intubation procedure (see Chapter 59).	A properly placed and secure tracheal tube is the most effective and reliable method of assisted ventilation. The physician, nurse anesthetist, or nurse practitioner performs the procedure; the respiratory therapist assists in managing the airway; and the nurse monitors the child's status and suctions and tapes the endotracheal tube.
13. Once the child is intubated and the respiratory therapist has set up the ventilator, attach airway circuitry adapter from ventilator to artificial airway of child.	Provides for mechanical ventilation to be instituted to the child.
14. Confirm that ventilator settings and parameters are as prescribed and that alarms are on and functioning.	Ensures that ventilator settings have been established in the manner prescribed by the physician.
15. Ensure that the circuitry tubing is free of water and is not kinked, all connections are secure, the circuitry tubing has some slack so the child can move his or her head, a manual resuscitation bag attached to 100% flowmeter oxygen is ready, and suction equipment is at hand and ready for use.	Provides child-ready ventilation with assurance that it is working in the prescribed manner with emergency equipment at the bedside.
16. Visually assess child's chest for symmetry of movement and auscultate child's breath sounds with stethoscope to ensure that there is equal inflation in all lung fields, without adventitious sounds.	Monitors efficacy of ventilator and alerts parent to potential problems.
17. Dispose of equipment and waste in appropriate receptacles.	Standard precautions.
18. Ensure that child is placed in comfortable safe position and is free from pain.	Ensures child's safety and comfort.
19. Perform hand hygiene.	Reduces transmission of microorganisms.

PROCEDURE Ongoing Evaluation and Troubleshooting of the System

Steps	Rationale/Points of Emphasis
1. Assess for atelectasis by evaluating for decreased or bronchial breath sounds, localized dullness to percussion, increased breathing effort, tracheal deviation or localized consolidation on chest x-ray, increased peak inspiratory pressure (PIP), decreased compliance, and decreased Pa_{O_2} or oxygen saturations. If signs and symptoms of atelectasis are present: • Obtain frequent blood gases to monitor effectiveness of gas exchange in the lungs (Pa_{O_2} and Pa_{CO_2}), and report the results to the healthcare prescriber for changes in ventilator management. • Suction the child's airway to ensure there are no mucus plugs or other airway obstructions at least once per shift or more frequently as indicated. • Reposition the child at least every 2 hours, and perform percussion and postural drainage to loosen secretions and decrease atelectasis. • X-ray may be needed to confirm localized consolidation or to confirm position or malposition of the endotracheal tube.	Early detection of atelectasis is key to altering its course. Ventilatory interventions may include techniques that increase hyperinflation, hyperventilation, or supplemental oxygen. A physician is required to consult and treat atelectasis caused by tumor, pleural effusion, or other extraneous pathology. Right mainstem bronchial intubation or esophageal intubation will not provide adequate mechanical ventilation and may cause pulmonary collapse; interventions to correct tube placement will be necessary.

Steps	Rationale/Points of Emphasis
2. Assess for signs and symptoms of cardiovascular depression. Observe for • An acute or gradual fall in blood pressure • Changes in heart rate, either tachycardia or bradycardia • Increase capillary refill time • Weak peripheral pulses • Presence of dysrhythmias • Decrease in pulse pressure	Cardiovascular depression with positive-pressure ventilation is manifested by reduced venous return, shifting of the ventricular septum to the left, and increased right ventricular afterload because of increased pulmonary vascular resistance. The amount of cardiovascular depression that can occur is dependent on the level of positive pressure applied, the duration of positive pressure, the amount of positive pressure on the vasculature, the child's intravascular volume, and the adequacy of the hemodynamic compensatory mechanism. The cardiovascular effects of positive-pressure ventilation can be reduced by optimizing filling pressures to reduce the positive-pressure ventilation changes in intrathoracic pressure, by delivering minimal PIP necessary for adequate ventilation, and by optimizing the inspiratory-to-expiratory (I:E) ratio. Interventions to correct cardiovascular depression will require healthcare prescriber collaboration and changes to the ventilator settings to achieve optimum ventilation with decreased cardiovascular complications.
3. Assess for inadequate breathing patterns and inadequate ventilation.	
a. Assess for increased work of breathing; shallow, irregular, or agonal respirations; apnea, tachypnea, or dyspnea; intercostal, substernal, abdominal, or tracheal retractions; nasal flaring; purse-lipped breathing; central cyanosis; minimal chest excursion; asynchrony of respirations to ventilation; Cheyne-Stokes breathing pattern; stacking breathing pattern; abdominal breathing; asymmetric chest expansion; "see-saw" breathing pattern; or irregular breathing.	The goal in managing mechanical ventilation is to negate respiratory distress, to decrease the work of breathing, to maintain or improve ventilation, and to maintain or improve oxygenation.
b. Examine the ventilator tubing to ensure that it is properly assembled, without loose, kinked, or clamped connections that may cause obstruction, throughout the course of the shift.	The child on mechanical ventilation is dependent on the nurse to meet the multitude of his or her needs, both psychosocial and physical. Anxiety related to the inability to communicate and dependence on others may increase the resistance to ventilation.
c. Suction the child's airway at least once per shift or more frequently as indicated.	Clears airway of plugs and other obstructions.
d. Reposition the child at least once per shift or more frequently as indicated.	Prevents dependent fluid buildup.
e. X-ray or direct observation may be needed to confirm position or malposition of the endotracheal tube.	Right mainstem bronchial intubation or esophageal intubation will not provide adequate mechanical ventilation, and interventions to correct tube placement will be necessary.
f. Ensure that the child is comfortable and properly sedated with pain control, if necessary.	Pain or discomfort is likely to result in changes to the child's respiratory pattern.
4. Assess for signs and symptoms of pulmonary barotrauma. • Observe the child for acutely increased PIP, acutely decreased Pa_{O_2} or Sa_{O_2}, acutely decreased airway compliance, acute change in heart, and acute changes in vital signs. • Observe the child for acute dyspnea, restlessness, agitation, panic, acutely increased breathing effort, or new onset of subcutaneous emphysema. • Auscultate the child's lungs for acutely decreased or absent breath sounds in a specific area or lobe. • Suspect if the child complains of acute chest pain or sudden difficulty in breathing. Notify healthcare prescriber to obtain order for x-ray to confirm suspicions.	Because of increased airway resistance or decreased lung compliance, high pressures may be needed to deliver the desired tidal volume. These high pressures can put the child at risk for cardiovascular depression and pulmonary barotrauma. Pulmonary barotrauma is damage to the lung from extrapulmonary air that may result from intrapleural changes during positive-pressure ventilation. This barotrauma can manifest as pneumothorax, pneumomediastinum, pneumoperitoneum, pneumopericardium, or subcutaneous emphysema. Barotrauma in children receiving positive-pressure ventilation is increased with preexisting lung lesions (e.g., blebs, localized infections), high inflation pressures (e.g., large tidal volumes, high PEEP, right mainstem intubations, ventilatory-to-patient breath asynchrony), and invasive thoracic procedures (e.g., thoracentesis, bronchoscopy). Positive-pressure ventilation barotraumas can be reduced by decreasing or optimizing PIP, decreasing PEEP, optimizing child comfort to allow synchrony of child to ventilator breathing, ensuring proper endotracheal tube placement, and decompressing pleural or mediastinal air. Invasive surgical interventions are required to correct most of the complications from pulmonary barotraumas.

Continued

Steps	Rationale/Points of Emphasis
5. Assess for signs and symptoms of inadvertent extubation or airway malposition.	Early unplanned extubation places the child at increased risk for respiratory distress.
a. Ensure that the artificial airway in place is always secure.	Secretions and movement may loosen the tape and device holding the airway in place, requiring frequent retaping or readjustment of the tube. Tracheal tube ties may loosen, allowing the tracheostomy tube to become dislodged.
b. Be alert to vocalizations made from the child.	Endotracheal intubation requires passing a tube through the vocal chords. As such, no verbalizations should be heard. Children with large air leaks or tracheotomy tubes with fenestrations or Passey-Muir valves may be able to make some sounds; however, this usually coincides with improvement in ventilation.
c. Be alert to acute gastric distention.	Misplaced endotracheal tube position in the esophagus means that air will be forced into the stomach, causing gastric distention.
d. Be alert to low-pressure ventilator alarms and to high-pressure alarms.	Low-pressure alarms indicate hypoventilation; high-pressure alarms may indicate ventilator tubing is kinked or clamped or that there is airway obstruction.
e. Auscultate the lungs frequently for decreased, absent, or changed breath sounds.	Inadvertent extubation may be more subtle and less obvious with the endotracheal tube in the hypopharynx.
f. X-ray or direct observation may be needed to confirm position or malposition of the endotracheal tube. Observe for asymmetric chest expansion and breath sounds heard only on the right anterior side.	Right mainstem bronchial intubation or esophageal intubation will not provide adequate mechanical ventilation and may cause atelectasis, pulmonary barotrauma, or impaired gas exchange. Interventions to correct tube placement will be necessary.
6. Obtain, assess, and evaluate the child's blood gases (as frequently as needed). Notify the healthcare prescriber of any blood gas abnormality.	Indicates acidosis, alkalosis, or inadequate oxygenation. Findings may indicate need for ventilatory changes.
7. Evaluate the child for any change in secretions indicating nosocomial lung infection from artificial airway placement, invasive procedures, or mechanical ventilation. The healthcare prescriber should be notified of any signs of infection because interventions will be required.	Note presence of purulent or discolored secretions (color other than white or clear), dyspnea, decreased compliance, fever, change in vital signs, positive tracheal aspirate cultures, positive blood cultures, or positive Gram stain of secretions.
8. Evaluate the child's ongoing needs for sedation and pain management.	Provides comfort and facilitates safety for the child.

Child and Family Evaluation and Documentation

- Evaluate the child for changes in respiratory pattern or effort while being ventilated.
- Evaluate child and family responses to interventions and provide further teaching as needed.
- Document the following:
  - Airway type and size (e.g., no. 4.0 endotracheal tube, no. 3.5 fenestrated trachea tube, cuffed or uncuffed tube)
  - Method used to secure airway in place
  - Tube location (e.g., oral, nasal, tracheal)
  - Date, time, and initial setup of ventilator
  - Ventilator settings
  - Blood gas results and interventions made to correct blood gas abnormalities
  - Child's own spontaneous respirations per minute
  - Vital signs
  - Oxygen saturation
  - Response to initiation of ventilation
  - Changes in breathing pattern; notify the healthcare prescriber of changes
  - Date, time, and frequency of suctioning, along with color, amount, and consistency of secretions, presence of blood, any adverse effects, and child tolerance
  - Pain, sedation, and anxiety assessment and any interventions required to manage the child's pain, level of consciousness, and anxiety level

Community Care

- If the child is to be discharged home on a ventilator, begin discharge planning with a home health nurse and respiratory therapist as early as possible. Refer, as necessary, to occupational, physical, and speech therapists; educational or vocational teachers or counselors; respite volunteers; dietitian; Social Services; financial counseling service (including government aid); in-home medical supplier or vendor; self-help support groups; and a mental health counselor with follow-up visits and appointments.
- Communication with the home care/community providers should include
  - Child's diagnosis
  - Type of ventilator, including manufacturer and date of institution

- Practitioners responsible for follow-up care
- Tracheal tube size and type
- Ventilator protocol taught in healthcare setting
- Notification of any complications after placement on ventilator

- Provide child with the in-home ventilator before discharge; child should be stable on that ventilator for at least 48 hours before discharge.
- Collaborate with home care providers to assist the family in
  - Acquiring needed home equipment and supplies, including a spare tracheotomy tube and ties, resuscitation bag and face mask, and supplemental oxygen (home ventilators have an internal compressor that allows the ventilator to generate its own air supply), before discharge
  - Locating a vendor to provide needed equipment and supplies on an ongoing basis
  - Assessing the home environment to ensure the electrical capability of the home (e.g., that there are grounded outlets)
  - Ensuring telephone availability
  - Determining optimal locations for equipment and supplies
  - Reorganizing their daily patterns of living
  - Identifying ways of accomplishing daily tasks and household needs without jeopardizing the child
  - Training respite workers in the responsibilities of watching a ventilator-dependent child
  - Developing safe travel plans
  - Planning a clear daily schedule of child care
  - Developing an inventory list and schedule for ordering supplies
  - Maintaining a schedule and a procedure for cleaning and changing the ventilator circuitry
- Instruct family in
  - Proper hand hygiene
  - Signs and symptoms of cardiorespiratory problems and appropriate interventions
  - Measures to prevent atelectasis
  - Ventilator settings and functions
  - Appropriate response to ventilator alarms, the factors that may cause alarms and the importance of being able to hear the alarms, and the most common complications of positive-pressure ventilation (i.e., decannulation or accidental disconnect)
  - Signs and symptoms of respiratory distress and failure and appropriate interventions
  - Measures to prevent respiratory infection
  - Tracheostomy care
  - How to obtain vital signs accurately
  - Cardiopulmonary resuscitation
  - Personal hygiene, skin care
  - Emergency plans and precautions
  - Indications for calling nurse, physician, emergency medical services, vendor, and supplier
  - How to notify police, telephone and electric companies, fire department, and paramedics of presence of ventilator-dependent individual in the home
  - Importance of having electrical generator as backup power source
- Assist the child and parents in providing the opportunity to express their feelings. Allow for opportunities that facilitate the child's independent actions and decision making, if applicable. Allow the parents to verbalize acceptance of and comfort in their role. Ensure that the parents use community resources. Ensure that each member of the family participates in the child's care and expresses a feeling that the home ventilator care is manageable.
- Instruct the parents to contact the healthcare provider if
  - There is a medical emergency (e.g., child exhibits difficulty breathing, ventilator malfunctions and ceases to operate, child experiences cardiac arrest).

Unexpected Situation

- *Child is inadvertently extubated:* Assess if child is breathing and the adequacy of respiratory effort. If child's respiratory effort is insufficient, begin bag-mask ventilation and notify the physician or advanced practice nurse (APN) immediately. If respiratory effort is adequate, monitor vital signs and oxygenation and notify physician or APN.

Bibliography

Anonymous. (1995). AARC clinical practice guideline: Long-term invasive mechanical ventilation in the home. *Respiratory Care, 40*, 1313–1320.

Brinker, D. (2004). Sedation and comfort issues in the ventilated infant and child. *Critical Care Nursing Clinics of North America, 16*, 365–377.

Cheifetz, I. M. (2003). Invasive and noninvasive pediatric mechanical ventilation. *Respiratory Care, 48*, 442–453.

Deakins, K., & Chatburn, R. L. (2002). A comparison of intrapulmonary percussive ventilation and conventional chest physiotherapy for the treatment of atelectasis in the pediatric patient. *Respiratory Care, 47*, 1162–1167.

Donn, S. M., & Sinha, S. K. (2003). Invasive and noninvasive neonatal mechanical ventilation. *Respiratory Care, 48*, 426–439.

Foland, J. A., Martin, J., Novotny, T., Super, D. M., Dyer, R. A., & Mhanna, M. J. (2001). Airway pressure release ventilation with a short release time in a child with acute respiratory distress syndrome. *Respiratory Care, 46*, 1019–1023.

Gillette, M. A., & Hess, D. R. (2001). Ventilator-induced lung injury and the evolution of lung-protective strategies in acute respiratory distress syndrome. *Respiratory Care, 46*, 130–148.

Greenough, A., Milner, A. D., & Dimitriou, G. (2004). Synchronized mechanical ventilation for respiratory support in newborn infants. *The Cochrane Database of Systematic Reviews*, (3), No. CD000456.

Herrera, C. M., Gerhardt, T., Claure, N., et al. (2002). Effects of volume-guaranteed synchronized intermittent mandatory ventilation in preterm infants recovering from respiratory failure. *Pediatrics, 110*, 529–533.

Liu, Y., Zhao, W., Xie, L., et al. (2004). Aspiration of dead space in the management of chronic obstructive pulmonary disease patients with respiratory failure. *Respiratory Care, 49*, 257–262.

Pierce, L. N. B. (2000). Protocols for practice: Applying research at the bedside. Traditional and non-traditional modes of mechanical ventilation. *Critical Care Nurse, 20*, 81–84.

Woodgate, P. G., & Davies, N. W. (2001). Permissive hypercapnia for the prevention of morbidity and mortality in mechanically ventilated newborn. *The Cochrane Database of Systematic Reviews*, (2), No. CD002061.

CHAPTER

127

Ventriculostomy Drain, Assisting in Placement and Care of

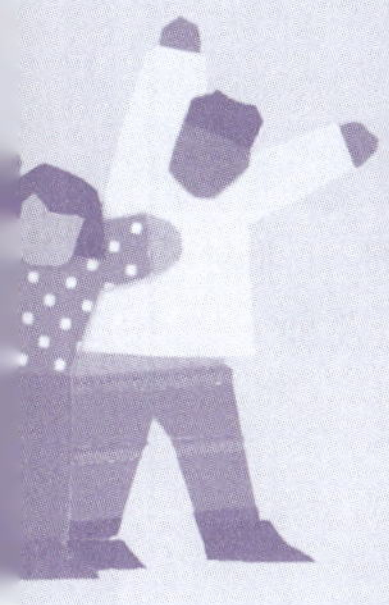

Clinical Guidelines

- Placement of an external ventriculostomy catheter (EVC) is a surgical procedure performed by a physician. EVC removal of such a device is the responsibility of the physician.
- The registered nurse (RN) is responsible for monitoring the child and system.
- Informed consent to complete the procedure must be obtained.
- Children with external ventriculostomy catheters may be maintained in either an intensive care setting or a general care unit, depending on the child's clinical presentation and acuity.

> **Alert!** *Children with ventriculostomies are at increased risk for latex allergies; therefore latex allergy precautions should be instituted and applied for the entire period in which the catheter is in place (see Chapter 60).*

- The neurosurgeon must specify the desired height of the drip chamber of the EVC in relation to the child.
- An external ventriculostomy drain (EVD) is a closed system; therefore sterility of the site and equipment must be maintained.
- Sedation and pain management of the child with ventriculostomy are implemented on an individual basis according to the child's diagnosis and unique healthcare needs.

Equipment

For setup and placement:

- External ventriculostomy drainage collection kit, which includes
  - Ventricular catheter
  - Trocar
  - Drainage bag
- Several disposable razors
- Sterile povidone-iodine prep swabs
- Sterile gowns, latex-free gloves, masks, and caps

- Sterile drapes or towels
- Lidocaine (Xylocaine) local anesthetic (0.5% or 1%)
- Sterile syringes (assortment of sizes: 3 and 5 mL and tuberculin)
- Needles (22 and 25 gauge)
- Cranial drill and bit
- Alcohol wipes
- Scalpel
- Suture material (usually, 2–0 to 3–0 nylon/silk)
- Gauze dressing (4 × 4)
- Antibacterial or chlorhexidine (Betadine) ointment
- 3-inch Kerlex dressing
- 1-inch Dermaform tape
- Preservative-free sterile normal saline for injection
- Level and tape measure to ensure height of drip chamber
- Latex allergy precaution for any supply coming in contact with child
- Sedation and pain medications (as ordered)
- Antibiotics (as ordered)
- Sterile transparent dressing (optional)
- Tincture of benzoin (optional)

For daily care:

- ICP monitor, if needed
- Level and tape measure to ensure height of drip chamber
- Latex allergy precaution for any supply coming in contact with child
- Dressing change supplies (if needed)
- Sedation and pain medications (as ordered)
- Antibiotics (as ordered)
- Surgical exam light (optional for physician)

CHILD AND FAMILY ASSESSMENT AND PREPARATION

- Assess the cognitive level, readiness, and ability to process information of the child and family.
- Reinforce the need for and identify and discuss the risks and benefits of catheter placement, as appropriate, to the child and family, reinforcing physician's explanation.
- Assess child for signs and symptoms of a change in neurologic status, including altered or decreased level of consciousness, anxiety, restlessness, irritability, agitation, lethargy, confusion, drowsiness, headaches, seizures, posturing, inappropriate motor function or dysfunction, widened pulse pressure, bradycardia, altered respiratory pattern, and pupillary dysfunction.
- Assess for allergies to latex, lidocaine, chlorhexidine, and antibacterial ointments.

KidKare Signs and symptoms of increased ICP in the infant may include all the previous ones as well as tense or bulging fontanel, separated cranial sutures, increased head circumference, projectile vomiting, a high-pitched cry indicating neurologic irritability, and paralysis of upward gaze of the eyes ("sun-setting sign").

- Ensure that informed consent has been obtained and the appropriate documents are signed and present in the child's medical record.
- Prepare the family for providing interaction with the child, including touch, talking with, and providing other comfort measures, even while the child is sedated.

PROCEDURE Preparing for Bedside Insertion of Ventriculostomy Catheter

Steps	Rationale/Points of Emphasis
1. Perform hand hygiene and gather all necessary equipment and supplies for device placement.	Hand hygiene reduces the transmission of microorganisms. Assembly of all necessary equipment facilitates quick and efficient insertion of an EVC for ICP monitoring.

caREminder

This is a sterile procedure. Reduce traffic in the patient area as much as possible during the procedure.

KidKare The neurosurgeon may request sedation or analgesia for the child before starting the invasive procedure. The neurosurgeon may also opt for IV antibiotics during preparation or after catheter insertion. Antibiotic therapy may assist in preventing infections that can occur secondary to this invasive procedure.

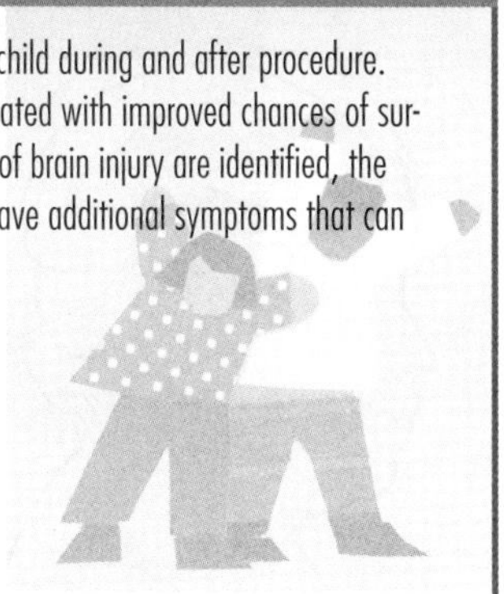

Steps	Rationale/Points of Emphasis
2. Obtain baseline data (i.e., vital signs, level of consciousness, pupil response, skeletal motor function, and sensory function) of the child.	Assists in identifying any acute changes in child during and after procedure. Prompt treatment of critical illness is associated with improved chances of survival. The earlier that signs and symptoms of brain injury are identified, the sooner treatment can begin. Infants may have additional symptoms that can aid in diagnosis.

Alert! *Two healthcare providers are needed to assist the neurosurgeon in placement of the catheter device. One nurse positions and holds the child in place, while assessing the child's condition during the procedure. The other nurse provides and gathers equipment as needed.*

Steps	Rationale/Points of Emphasis
3. Assess sedation and pain management needs of child in collaboration with the physician throughout the procedure. Administer sedation and pain management medications as indicated.	Ventriculostomy placement may be a painful procedure. The child's comfort will be enhanced by administration of medications to manage sedation and pain.
4. Prepare sterile field, and place instruments on field. Prime ventricular catheter setup with preservative-free normal saline.	Maintains aseptic technique.
5. Don sterile attire and sterile gloves.	Standard precautions for surgical sterile procedure—reduces transmission of microorganisms and maintains asepsis.
6. Position the child for access by the physician (this may include turning the child so that the head is at the side of the bed horizontally) and hold the child's head securely in midline position throughout, while maintaining sterile access for physician.	Ease of access; facilitates catheter insertion.
7. Restrain limbs as necessary to ensure sterility of procedure.	Keeps child from moving and possibly breaking sterile field required for catheter insertion.
8a. Assist physician in identifying area on scalp for catheter placement. The left frontal and temporal scalp area is the preferred access point for most physicians. 8b. Follow institution policy and procedure for ensuring preoperative verification process is completed, appropriate operative site is marked, and "time out" is completed before start of procedure.	Identifies access site (usually the right upper quadrant of the temporal cranium, because this is the least likely to cause neurologic sequelae from going through the brain to the ventricle). Implements universal protocol for preventing wrong site, wrong procedure, wrong person surgery according to the Joint Commission on Accreditation of Healthcare Organizations (JCAHO) Standards for Patient Safety.
9. Assist physician in draping head in sterile fashion for catheter system setup.	Protects insertion site from contamination.
10. Assist physician in shaving the scalp and prepping the area with sterile povidone-iodine scrub.	Visualizes insertion site, and prevents hair from falling into and thereby contaminating sterile field. Reduces risk of infection from microorganisms.

KidKare Save child's hair and place in a plastic bag; parents or child may wish to keep the hair.

Steps	Rationale/Points of Emphasis
11. The physician applies subcutaneous lidocaine (Xylocaine) to the insertion site on the scalp and makes an incision. Then, using the hand drill and scalpel, the physician bores through the skull and dura mater.	Allows for insertion of ventricular catheter.
12. The neurosurgeon threads a ventricular catheter through the brain to the ventricles, and then sutures it into place (Figure 127-1).	Allows direct access to the ventricle for monitoring of pressure, draining of cerebrospinal fluid/blood, and providing a route for medication administration.

Continued

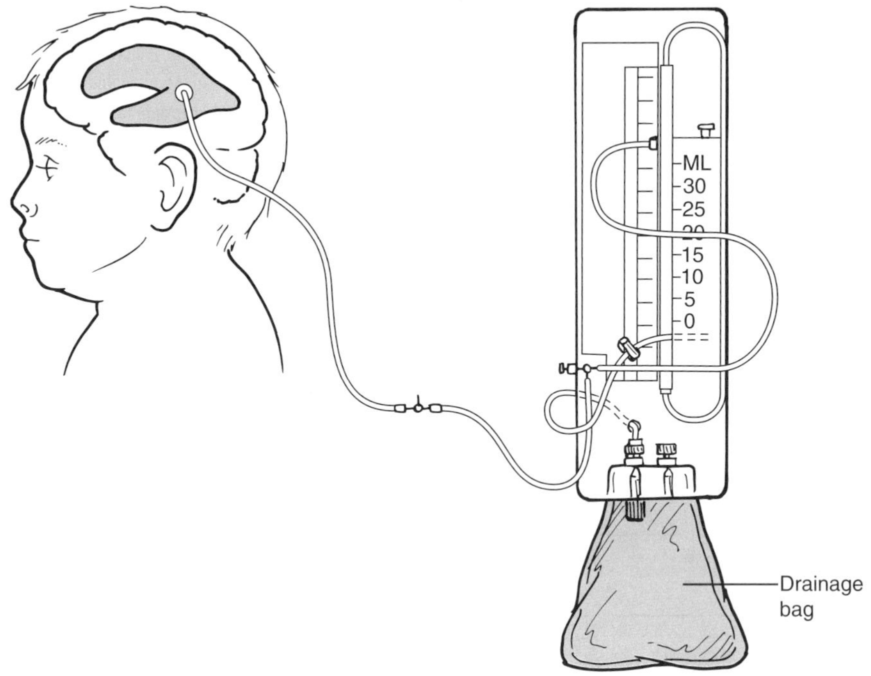

FIGURE 127-1
The ventricular catheter is threaded through the brain to the ventricles. Placement of the tube allows for monitoring of ventricular pressure, draining of cerebrospinal fluid and blood, and providing a route for medication administration.

Steps	Rationale/Points of Emphasis
13. Assist the neurosurgeon as needed throughout the procedure and continually assess the child for neurologic and vital sign changes.	Provides baseline for ongoing monitoring.
14. When the ventricular catheter is in place and sutured down, assist in placing a small amount of antibacterial or chlorhexidine ointment and semipermeable transparent dressing over the catheter insertion site on the scalp. Tincture of benzoin may be used to make the skin tackier before placement of the transparent dressing.	Protects the site from microorganisms. **Alert!** ***Use of tincture of benzoin is not advised with premature infants because it creates a stronger bond between adhesive and epidermis than the fragile cohesion of the epidermis to the dermis. Thus, epidermal stripping during adhesive removal may occur.***
15. Recheck the system for tight connections. **caREminder** *The physician may want to read and visualize ICP and waveforms from the ventriculostomy catheter. If so, the setup for ICP monitoring should be provided (see Chapter 54).*	Identifies any loose connections, which may leak cerebrospinal fluid (CSF) and be a potential site for infection, or cause an erroneous decrease in pressure readings.
16. If requested by the physician, assist in dressing the entire scalp with gauze and Kerlex dressing.	Further protects the site from contamination or from accidental disconnection by the child.
17. Reposition the child vertically in bed, with the head-of-bed (HOB) position at the prescribed angle, as ordered by the physician. Using the tape measure and level, place the drip chamber of the ventriculostomy drainage device at the prescribed height. Place a sign at head of child's bed clearly identifying the prescribed angle measurement.	The amount of ventriculostomy drainage that occurs is partially based on gravity. Therefore the position in relation to the drip chamber height is essential to this equation. Lowering the drip chamber enhances CSF drainage. Raising the drip chamber reduces CSF drainage. Positioning the child so that the head of the bed is elevated promotes venous return.

Steps	Rationale/Points of Emphasis
	caREminder *The HOB position and the level of the drip chamber must be prescribed by the physician and are not to be altered unless prescribed. An "alert" sign at the head of the child's bed should denote the prescribed angle of elevation and communicate that the level not be changed.*
18. Maintain the child's head midline at all times. The child can be turned, making sure to maintain a midline position (avoid the use of neck and shoulder rolls because these can cause skin breakdown or venous constriction).	Flexion or rotation of the head can obstruct venous return and thereby increase intracranial pressure. Positioning the child so that the head of the bed is elevated 30 degrees promotes venous return. Flexion or rotation of the neck can obstruct venous return.
19. Dispose of equipment and waste in appropriate receptacle.	Standard precautions.
20. Remove gloves and sterile attire. Perform hand hygiene.	Reduces transmission of microorganisms. Standard precautions.

PROCEDURE Daily Care of the Child With an External Ventriculostomy Device

Steps	Rationale/Points of Emphasis
1. Restrain and administer pain and sedation medications to the child when necessary and as prescribed.	Promotes safety and facilitates effective pain management of child. An agitated child may contaminate the ventriculostomy catheter insertion site increasing infection risk or may dislodge the catheter.
2. If at any time the scalp dressing appears to be contaminated, wet, or loose along the edges, change the dressing using sterile technique. **Alert!** *CSF drainage is more likely to occur if the child's ICP is elevated.*	If the dressing is wet, the nurse should be alerted to the possibility of a cerebrospinal fluid (CSF) leak at the insertion site. Report the occurrence of drainage immediately to the physician because subsequent permanent neurologic impairment may occur.
3. Observe the tubing and catheter system to ensure the system is intact, without leaks or kinks, that all clamps are open, and that all tubing and connections are secure.	A CSF leak can occur at any connection site throughout the system, thereby contaminating and introducing microorganisms into a sterile environment.
4. Note the color and characteristics of the CSF drainage. **Alert!** *Notify the physician immediately if abnormal drainage occurs.*	Normal CSF is clear and colorless; therefore yellow, bloody, or discolored drainage may be a sign of contamination or new bleeding.
5. Monitor and record the amount of CSF drainage at least every 2 hours (or per institutional policy) and allow the fluid to drain from the external ventriculostomy drip chamber into the drainage collection bag. **Alert!** *Seek to avoid prolonged elevations of ICP. Identify the need for changes in interventions, sedation, positioning, or stimulation.*	It is normal to have some CSF drainage per hour; however, a sudden increase or decrease in the amount can be a sign of increased intracranial pressure (ICP) or blockage.

Continued

Steps	Rationale/Points of Emphasis
6. Maintain the position of the child vertically in bed, with the HOB position at the prescribed angle and the drip chamber at the prescribed height.	Moving the child or altering the elevation of the head of the bed affects the relationship of the drip chamber.
7. Maintain the child's head midline at all times. The child can be turned, being sure to maintain a midline position (avoid the use of neck and shoulder rolls because these can cause skin breakdown or venous constriction).	Flexion or rotation of the head can obstruct venous return and thereby increase ICP.

Alert! *Changes in ICP require therapeutic interventions instituted immediately upon prescribed physician orders, including computed tomography and surgery.*

CHILD AND FAMILY EVALUATION AND DOCUMENTATION

- Evaluate child's response to the procedure, including level of sedation and level of pain both during insertion and on an ongoing basis.
- Observe the child with an external ventriculostomy device frequently for changes in neurologic status, such as altered or decreased level of consciousness, anxiety, restlessness, irritability, agitation, lethargy, confusion, drowsiness, headaches, seizures, posturing, inappropriate motor function or dysfunction, widened pulse pressure, bradycardia, altered respiratory pattern, or pupillary dysfunction. An infant may also display tense or bulging fontanel, separated cranial sutures, increased head circumference, projectile vomiting, high-pitched cry, or "sun-setting sign."
- Immediately report deleterious changes in status to the physician.
- Document date and time of insertion, assessments, the insertion site position and placement, catheter size used, medications, if any, and child's response to the procedure on the appropriate institutional forms.
- Document the amount, color, and consistency of drainage of CSF, if any, every 2 to 4 hours, on the appropriate institutional form.
- Document and monitor the baseline and ongoing neurologic assessments, pupil size, increased ICP, changes in level of consciousness, changes in respiratory pattern and abnormal waveforms, vital signs, and response to therapeutic interventions, at least every 2 hours, on the appropriate institutional form.
- If monitoring ICP, note trends and monitor and document the child's ICP, pressure waveform, and cerebral perfusion pressure, at least every 2 hours, on the appropriate institutional form.
- Observe the drainage tubing to ensure the system is intact, without leaks, kinks, or clots, and document at least once every shift.
- Evaluate for and document the potential of infection related to catheter placement, including temperature, white blood cell count, CSF cultures, device cultures (if obtained), inflammation at the insertion site, and signs or symptoms of meningitis, and notify the appropriate physician immediately.
- Document administration of sedation or pain medication or any other measures to provide pain management, comfort, and diversionary activities.
- Determine whether the child and family have other areas of concern to discuss.

COMMUNITY CARE

- Ensure the child and caregivers that the child's hair will regrow at the site it was shaved off for catheter placement.
- Instruct the family to contact the healthcare provider if
  - Signs of insertion site infection occur, such as redness, drainage, or swelling
  - Child develops a fever
  - Child exhibits changes in neurologic status, such as changes in level of consciousness, headache, irritability, or onset of high-pitched cry (look for bulging fontanel in infants)

Unexpected Situations

- *The catheter becomes dislodged from the insertion site:* Apply pressure to the insertion site with sterile gauze and immediately notify physician. Assess for changes in child's neurologic status. Continuously observe and assess child for signs and symptoms of increased ICP until catheter is replaced or other appropriate intervention is initiated.
- *The integrity of the catheter or drainage tubing is compromised:* A break or other compromise in the catheter or tubing should be immediately secured by occluding the damaged area with sterile gauze. Notify the physician immediately to assess for catheter repair, replacement, or other intervention.

Bibliography

Fan, J. (2004). Effect of backrest position on intracranial pressure and cerebral perfusion pressure in individuals with brain injury: A systematic review. *Journal of Neuroscience Nursing, 36,* 278–288.

Hickey, J. V. (2003). Intracranial hypertension: Theory and management of increased intracranial pressure. In J. V. Hickey (Ed.). *The clinical practice of neurological and neurosurgical nursing* (5th ed., pp. 285–318). Philadelphia: Lippincott Williams & Wilkins.

Joint Commission on Accreditation of Healthcare Organizations. (2004). *Universal Protocol for Preventing Wrong Site, Wrong Procedure, Wrong Person Surgery*™. Retrieved May 8, 2006, from http://www.jointcommission.org/PatientSafety/UniversalProtocol

Josephson, L. (2004). Management of increased intracranial pressure: a primer for the non-neuro critical care nurse. *Dimensions of Critical Care Nursing, 23,* 194–207.

Ng, I., Lim, J., & Wong, H. B. (2004). Effects of head posture on cerebral hemodynamics: Its influences on intracranial pressure, cerebral perfusion pressure, and cerebral oxygenation. *Neurosurgery, 54,* 593–597.

Pfausler, B., Spiss, H., Beer, R., et al. (2003). Treatment of staphylococcal ventriculitis associated with external cerebrospinal fluid drains: A prospective randomized trial of intravenous compared with intraventricular vancomycin therapy. *Journal of Neurosurgery, 98,* 1040–1044.

Pfisterer, W., Mühlbauer, M., Czech, T., & Reinprecht, A. (2003). Early diagnosis of external ventricular drainage infection: Results of a prospective study. *Journal of Neurology, Neurosurgery and Psychiatry, 74,* 929–932.

Yasuda, T., Tomita, T., McLone, D. G., & Donovan, M. (2002). Measurement of cerebrospinal fluid output through external ventricular drainage in one hundred infants and children: Correlation with cerebrospinal fluid production. *Pediatric Neurosurgery, 36*(1), 22–28.

CHAPTER

128

Vision Screening

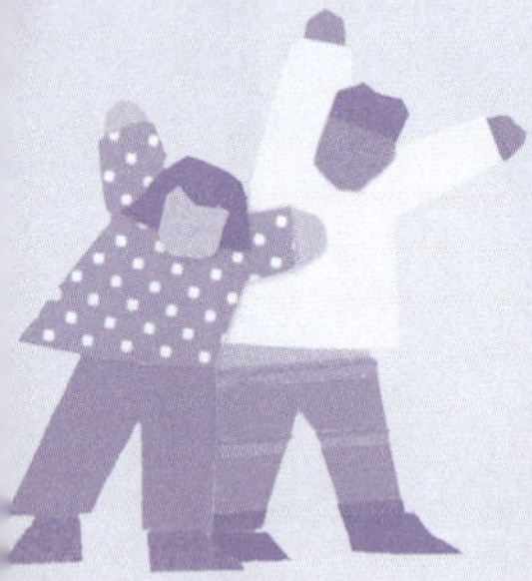

Clinical Guidelines

- Vision screening may be performed by physicians, optometrists, nurses, and other professionals certified in vision screening in accordance with state laws.
- Because early detection and treatment is vital in the prevention of long-term visual impairments, vision screening should begin from birth (Table 128-1).
  - From birth to age 3, vision screening should include ocular history, vision assessment, external inspection of the eyes and lids, ocular motility assessment, pupil examination, and red reflex.
  - From 3 years and older, screening includes all the above plus age-appropriate measurement of visual acuity and an attempt at ophthalmoscopy. Preschool-aged children, especially 3- to 4-year-olds, should be screened for amblyopia and strabismus.
  - Color deficiency screening is recommended to be performed before the child enters school. However, children aged 5 and older are better at being able to follow instructions and complete the test.
- Functional assessments that should be performed are tests of visual acuity, ocular alignment, and ocular media clarity. Based on the child's history and findings, additional tests may be performed based on cooperation by the child, such as stereoacuity testing, color vision testing, and visual fields (see Chapter 77).

Equipment

- Visual acuity chart (Snellen chart or Insta-Line, HOTV, tumbling Es or tumbling hands, Lea symbols, flash cards, or equivalent)
- Measuring tape, masking tape, or placement marker
- Occluder, small paper cup, or cardboard (3 × 5-inch card or cut-out shapes)
- Report sheet and/or documentation form
- Pen
- Plus lenses (+2.25 and +1.75 diopters) or hyperopia lens
- Timer or watch with second hand
- Ophthalmoscope or pen light
- Small, interesting or colorful objects (e.g., small stuffed animal, ceramic figure)
- Polarized glasses
- Pseudoisochromatic plates, like the Ishihara plates or equivalent
- Stereotests like the fly, circle patterns, animals, or equivalent

TABLE 128-1

Common Vision Screening Tests*

Test	Purpose
Visual acuity: distance	Tests clarity of vision; to detect myopia, amblyopia, astigmatism
Visual acuity: hyperopia	Evaluates farsightedness
Tracking and convergence	Assesses binocular vision and ability of eyes to turn inward and focus
Cover/uncover and alternate cover	Detects potential ocular misalignment such as strabismus
Hirschberg corneal light test	Detects physical misalignment of the eyes
Red reflex	Assesses ocular media clarity and detects abnormalities of the back of the eye; should be done on all newborns and infants
Pupillary reactions	Assesses retinal or optic nerve dysfunction; should be evaluated on all newborns and infants
Stereoacuity testing	Detects amblyopia and ocular misalignment by assessing depth perception
Color discrimination	Identifies inability to identify color

*Children age 3 years and older can typically follow directions and cooperate with testing; therefore, these tests are performed as indicated in children older than age 3. The red reflex and pupillary reactions can be elicited from birth because they do not require the child's cooperation.

CHILD AND FAMILY ASSESSMENT AND PREPARATION

- Obtain ocular history:
  - Have you been informed by your healthcare provider that your child has eye or vision problem?
  - Does anyone in the child's immediate family have any history of cataract, retinopathy, or any eye problem?
- Perform external assessment of the child's eyes and lids. Use the ABC checklist for vision, as appropriate:
  - A = appearance: eyes turning in or out, ptosis, swelling, differently sized pupils
  - B = behavior: head-tilting, squinting, excessive stumbling, fumbling, or awkwardness
  - C = child's statement: headaches, blurry vision, can not see the board, double vision

Alert! *Any visual complaint or manifestation of vision problems from a child warrants referral to an eye specialist, regardless of test results. Another important referral criterion is parent observation.*

- Inquire about relevant familial eye disorders such as childhood cataracts or glaucoma, strabismus, amblyopia, and parental or sibling history of wearing glasses in preschool or early childhood.
- Explain the procedure to the family and child in an age-appropriate manner (see Table 128–1 for common vision screening tests and their purpose). Assure them that the procedures are painless.

PROCEDURE **Visual Acuity: Distance**

Steps	Rationale/Points of Emphasis
1. Select a room with good lighting. If using an Insta-Line chart, ensure that it is plugged in and that all the lightbulbs work.	Good lighting prevents glare that could affect test results.
2. Measure 10 feet from the tool (e.g., Snellen chart, Insta-Line) and mark the spot with a placement marker or plain masking tape. If the tool is calibrated for 20 feet, use that distance.	Ensures accuracy of test results. The American Academy of Pediatrics Section on Ophthalmology, the American Association for Pediatric Ophthalmology and Strabismus, and the American Academy of Ophthalmology recommend a testing distance of 10 feet for all visual acuity tests.
3. Position the child so that the chart is at eye level.	Eye chart level, in reference to the eyes, influences test results.

Continued

Steps	Rationale/Points of Emphasis
4. Cover the left eye with an occluder, a small cup, a card, or the child's hand. The hand, if used as an occluder, should be cupped and not impinge on the eye. Instruct the child to keep both eyes open, even the one that is occluded. If a child has glasses, let him or her wear glasses during the testing, except when the child reports he or she only wears them for close-up reading.	Acuity is initially tested monocularly. The left eye is occluded because it is common practice to test and chart the result of the right eye first; standard routines help avoid missing elements of the examination. Both eyes are kept open to prevent vision in the occluded eye from becoming blurry for subsequent testing. Wearing glasses ensures that the child's lenses have the appropriate correction. **KidKare** Engage the child in the testing by allowing him or her to hold the occluder. It gives the child a sense of control during the testing.
5. Ask the child to read the letters on the line on which you point. An Insta-Line has a control that allows you to light up the line to be read instead of pointing to it. Make sure that the child does not peek or squint.	Initiates distance testing. Peeking or squinting may alter results. **KidKare** When testing preschoolers, children with developmental delay, or children who do not speak the language, the letter chart may be substituted with the symbol chart such as the Lea symbols, the HOTV chart, the tumbling Es, or the tumbling hands. The LEA symbols and HOTV require object naming or object matching, whereas the tumbling Es and the tumbling hands require the child to demonstrate with his or her fingers which direction the E or the hand is pointing. When using any of the symbol charts, orient the child to the objects up close and practice with the larger prints before testing the child at a distance.
6. Start testing with at least the 20/40 line and move down to the 20/20 line; typically the tool is calibrated at 10 feet but the reading is reported at 20 feet. Go down the line until the child is unable to read half of the letters or unable to name half of the objects in the line. If the child is unable to read the 20/40 line at the start, move upward until the child can read more than half of the letters.	Establishes acuity level. Failure to read half of the symbols or letters in a line constitutes a failure.
7. Chart result by recording the last line that was read correctly. Chart as "right eye 20/20" or "right eye 20/30," and so on.	This records the child's right eye acuity. To avoid transcription errors, write out right eye or left eye.
8. Occlude the right eye and repeat steps 5, 6, and 7. Chart as "left eye 20/XX."	Tests and records the left eye acuity.
9. With both eyes open, repeat steps 5, 6 and 7. Chart as "both eyes 20/XX."	Tests and records distance acuity binocularly.
10. Refer for follow-up as follows (verify your state's referral criteria): • Visual acuity of 20/50 or worse in children younger than 6 years old • Visual acuity of 20/40 or worse in children ages 6 and older • A two-line difference in visual acuity in any age group For example, a 5-year-old has a result of right eye = 20/40, left eye = 20/30 and another 5-year-old has a result of right eye = 20/40, left eye = 20/20. The first child passes, and the second child requires referral.	Facilitates child receiving needed treatment.

PROCEDURE Visual Acuity: Hyperopia

Steps	Rationale/Points of Emphasis
1. Have the child hold a plus lens, or hyperopia lens, over both eyes. **caREminder** *In individual screenings, use the age-appropriate lens, which is +2.25 for children ages 9 and younger and +1.75 for 10 years and older. In mass screenings, the +1.75 lens may be used solely because it is the most generally applicable lens to all age groups and saves time by not having to switch lenses for each child.*	Holding the equipment gives the child a sense of control during the testing.
2. Leave the lenses in place for 1 minute; use a timer or a watch with second hand.	Increases reliability of examination by preventing the eyes from falsely accommodating to the letters or objects.
3. With the lenses still over the eyes, ask the child to read the letters on the 20/30 line. Point to the line or light up the optotype. Make sure that the child does not squint.	Squinting results in false-negative results by helping the eyes falsely accommodate to the objects. **caREminder** *Memorize the letters or objects on the 20/30 line so you can watch the child during the testing.*
4. The child passes the test if he or she is unable to read the 20/30 line. Refer for follow-up care if the child is able to read the 20/30 line.	A child who is not farsighted will have blurry vision when he or she looks through the hyperopia lens.

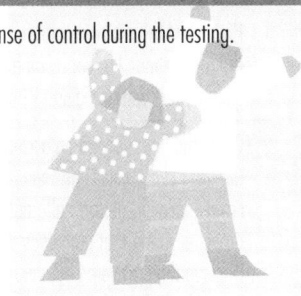

PROCEDURE Tracking and Convergence

Steps	Rationale/Points of Emphasis
1. Hold the (pen) light, ophthalmoscope, or small, interesting/colorful object about 12 inches from the child's eyes. Ask child to look at the object that you are holding in front of him or her without moving his or her head.	Establishes focus.
2. Move the object in the following direction, pausing after each angle, in the shape of the letter H: horizontally to your right, upward, downward past the midline, upward to the midline, horizontally to your left past the midline, upward, downward past the midline, upward to the midline, and horizontally to the initial starting point in front of the eyes. Note cooperativeness, head movement, and tracking with eyes. Refer for follow-up if signs of difficulty tracking are present: tracking is jerky, child cannot follow object without moving his or her head, or if it seems that child is not cooperating by not following the object.	Enables assessment of difficulty tracking. Referral allows for more specific testing and treatment.
3. Move the object closer to the child's eyes and observe for the inward turning of the eyes. Refer the child for follow-up if eyes do not turn inward as object is brought closer.	Checks for convergence. Referral allows for more specific testing and treatment.

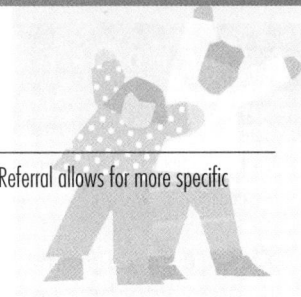

PROCEDURE Cover/Uncover and Alternate Cover Test

Steps	Rationale/Points of Emphasis
1. Have child focus on one of a few interesting objects that you have placed in the room about 10 feet away from where the child is sitting. If the child has glasses, test with the glasses on.	The eyes must be fixated when doing this test, and interesting objects to focus on increase the chance of catching a child's attention long enough to complete testing.
2. Cover the left eye with an occluder and quickly move the occluder to cover the right eye ("cover/uncover"). If no movement is elicited by cover/uncover, perform alternating cover test by occluding the eyes several times, ensuring that both eyes do not simultaneously see the object. Observe the uncovered eye and note vertical or horizontal movement. Remind the child often to fixate on the object.	Tests for ocular misalignment.
3. Refer for follow-up if vertical or horizontal movement is noted as the eye is uncovered.	This is a sign of ocular misalignment, such as strabismus, and may require treatment.

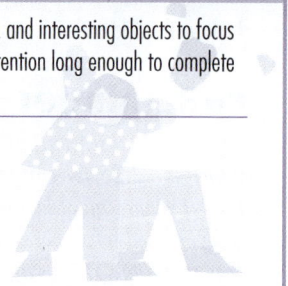

PROCEDURE Hirschberg Corneal Light Test

Steps	Rationale/Points of Emphasis
1. Dim the lights to ensure that no other light source is in front of the child. Position yourself in front of the child and ask him or her to look at a target behind you. Hold a lighted penlight or ophthalmoscope about 12 inches from the child's eye at eye level.	Dim lighting makes it easier to see the light reflex; multiple lights may result in misinterpretation of the light source. Your position enables you to see the child's eyes during testing.
2. Observe the reflection of the light in the pupils of both eyes. The reflection should fall in the same location in the cornea of each eye, even when the eyes move. Otherwise, refer for follow-up.	Any other position of the reflection indicates ocular misalignment.

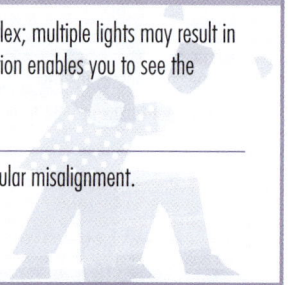

PROCEDURE Red Reflex

Steps	Rationale/Points of Emphasis
1. Dim lighting of the room, if possible. Ask an older child to focus on an object behind you. **KidKare** To prompt a young infant to voluntarily open his or her eyes, sit the awake infant upright. Hold an interesting object in front of the infant to capture his or her attention.	Dim lighting dilates the pupil; hence, it is easier to look through and behind it.
2. Hold the ophthalmoscope with your dominant hand and view the child's right eye with your right eye. (After examining the right eye, view the child's left eye with your left eye.)	Maintains a position that avoids touching the face of your patient with your face.

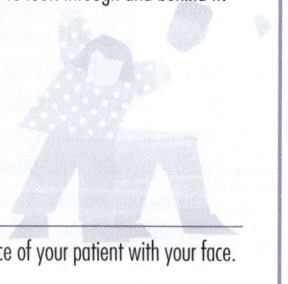

Steps	Rationale/Points of Emphasis
3. From about 12 to 18 inches away from the child's face, slowly move to his or her temporal line of sight. Focus on the retina by adjusting the focusing wheel or diopter lens.	The lens is adjusted to accommodate refraction error between your eyes and the child's.
4. Look for light reflex from the retina. A red reflex should be seen.	A retina that is clear will show a red reflex. Referral is indicated if you see any other color besides red, if you see opacity, or the two eyes are not equivalent in color, intensity, and clarity.

PROCEDURE Pupillary Reactions

caREminder

When planning the order or the flow of functional assessments, try to perform the pupillary reaction after the red reflex test. The pupillary reaction test constricts the pupil and makes performing ophthalmoscopy more difficult.

Steps	Rationale/Points of Emphasis
1. Keep the lighting of the room dim. Flash the penlight or ophthalmoscope about 12 inches away from the child on the child's right eye and observe for pupillary size, shape, and reaction. Do the same with the left eye.	Pupils should be equal, round, and reactive to light. Slow or poorly reactive pupils may indicate retinal or optic nerve dysfunction.
2. Repeat step 1. This time, watch for simultaneous constriction. When one eye is being tested, both eyes should constrict.	Unequal reaction also indicates neural dysfunction.

PROCEDURE Stereoacuity Testing

Steps	Rationale/Points of Emphasis
1. Have the child stand or be seated directly in front of the stereotest plate and don the polarized glasses. If the child has glasses, test with polarized glasses over his or her prescription glasses.	Prepares the child for testing. The object is three-dimensional when seen through the polarized glasses. The child's glasses facilitate appropriate acuity.
2. Ask the child to look at the plate and pinch the fly's wings. Note whether the child's fingers remain above or actually come in contact with the picture. Refer for follow-up care if the child pinches the surface of the test plate and pass if he or she pinches above it. When using the circle or the animal patterns instead of the fly, ask the child to identify which patterns seem to come out closer to him or her. Refer if the child does not identify more than half of the correct responses.	Passing the test indicates that the child's eyes are teaming well together (i.e., working binocularly). Those with amblyopia or with ocular misalignment have poor depth perception.

PROCEDURE Color Discrimination

Steps	Rationale/Points of Emphasis
1. Follow manufacturer's directions for equipment. For the Ishihara plates, go through the plates one at a time while the child identifies the numbers that he or she sees.	Following manufacturer's instructions ensures that the test is administered correctly. A child who has color deficiency would not be able to see the numbers or objects on some of the plates.
KidKare Use the plates toward the back of the book, which require tracing of the lines instead of number and shape identification, for children who have not yet learned numbers or shapes, who do not speak the same language, or who are developmentally delayed.	
2. Record result. Failure does not warrant referral, but notify parents of results.	Color deficiency is currently untreatable and usually not progressive.

Child and Family Evaluation and Documentation

- Document the child's level of cooperation with the testing.
- Document pertinent positives on external assessment, child report or complaint, significant family history, and results of all tests performed, be it a pass or fail, positive or negative.
- For children wearing glasses or contacts, document that they had them on during testing. Specify which: glasses or contacts. If nothing is noted it will be assumed that the child was not wearing prescriptive correction.
- Refer to an eye specialist if the child fails any of the tests. See functional assessments for specific referral criteria.

Community Care

- Inform the parent and the child, if appropriate for age, of the result of each examination.
- Color deficiency is more prevalent in males; thus in mass screenings this may be performed only on boys aged 5–6. A child needs color screening only once in his or her lifetime; therefore parents must be aware whether their child passes or fails and the results must be properly documented. Give the parent and child written information regarding color deficiency. Advise the parent to inform the child's teacher of the color deficiency so that proper classroom accommodations may be provided for the child.
- For test failures, make necessary referral to an ophthalmologist or an eye specialist. Give the parent a letter of referral to an eye specialist identifying concerns during the screening.
- If a child is in school, advise the parent to inform the child's teacher of the result of the screening so that necessary accommodations may be in place in the classroom while waiting for eye therapy.
- Instruct the family to contact the healthcare provider if
  - Child complains of blurry vision, double vision, difficulty reading, or headaches.

Unexpected Situation

- *When testing child, you notice redness of the eye structures and swelling around or discharge from the eye:* Refer child to primary care provider.

Bibliography

American Academy of Pediatrics, American Association of Certified Orthoptists, American Association for Pediatric Ophthalmology and Strabismus, & American Academy of Ophthalmology Policy Statement. (2003). Eye examination in infants, children and young adults by pediatricians. *Pediatrics, 111*, 902–907.

American Academy of Pediatrics Policy Statement. (2002). Red reflex examination in infants. *Pediatrics, 109*, 980–981.

American Optometric Association. (2003, August 7). *A school nurse's guide to vision screening and ocular emergencies.* Retrieved December 20, 2005, from http://www.eyes.org/common/attachments/articles/SNGS%2Epdf

Berry, B. E., Simons, B. D., Siatkowski, R. M., Schiffman, J. C., Flynn, J. T., & Duthie, M. J. (2001). Preschool vision screening using the MTI-Photoscreener. *Pediatric Nursing, 27*, 27–34.

Cavallini, A., Fazzi, E., Viviani, V., et al. (2002). Visual acuity in the first two years of life in healthy term newborns: An experience with the Teller acuity cards. *Functional Neurology, 17*, 87–92.

Halle, C. (2002). Achieve new vision screening objectives. *The Nurse Practitioner, 27,* 15–35.

Hered, R., & Rothstein, M. (2003). Preschool vision screening frequency after an office-based training session for primary care staff. *Pediatrics, 112,* 17–21.

Kemper, A. R., Fant, K. E., Bruckman, D., & Clark, S. J. (2004). Hearing and vision screening program for school-aged children. *American Journal of Preventive Medicine, 26,* 141–146.

Krumholtz, I. (2004). Educating the educators: Increasing grade-school teachers' ability to detect vision problems. *Optometry, 75,* 445–451.

Kvarnstrom, G., & Jakobsson, P. (2005). Is vision screening in 3-year-old children feasible? Comparison between the Lea symbol chart and the HVOT (LM) chart. *Acta Ophthalmologica Scandinavica, 83,* 76–80.

Optometric Physicians of Washington in affiliation with American Optometric Association. (n.d.). *School nurse recommendations.* Retrieved December 20, 2005, from http://www.eyes.org/educators/index.cfm?Parent=86

Powell, C., Wedner, S., & Richardson, S. (2005). Screening for correctable visual acuity deficits in school-age children and adolescents. *The Cochrane Database of Systematic Reviews,* (1), No. CD005023.

Preschoolers Study Group. (2004). Preschool visual acuity screening with HOTV and Lea symbols: Testability and between-test agreement. *Optometry & Vision Science, 81,* 678–683.

Proctor, S. (2005). *To see or not to see: Screening the vision of children in school.* Castle Rock, CO: National Association of School Nurses.

Salcido, A. A., Bradley, J., & Donahue, S. P. (2005). Predictive value of photoscreening and traditional screening of preschool children. *Journal of American Association for Pediatric Ophthalmology and Strabismus, 9,* 114–120.

United States Preventive Services Task Force. (2002). *Guide to clinical preventive services* (pp. 373–382). McLean, VA: International Medical Publishing, Inc.

CHAPTER

129

Visitor Identification and Management

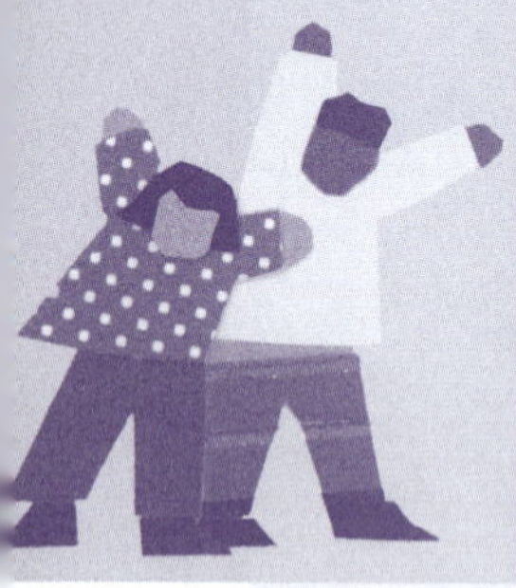

Clinical Guidelines

- All healthcare staff members are responsible for enforcement of visitor identification and management procedures.
- Institutional employees, primary care providers, and volunteers must wear official photo identification badges while on the facility premises.
- Patient visitors (including family members) must register at the security desk at the institution and wear a visitor identification badge while on the facility premises.
- Parents/guardians must present an identification band that matches the child or some other valid identification to identify them as family to the pediatric patient. Such identification will be needed to gather informed consent and to release child from the facility to parent/guardian care.
- The institution establishes visiting hours and regulations to enhance child care, comfort, and safety.
- Notify the child and family members of visiting policies on admission.
- Honor family preferences for visitation and release of information.
- Limited visitation may be enforced because of child's physical status; concerns of visitor's questionable behavior by staff, security, or other patients; or as a result of court-ordered restrictions on visitations.
- If limited visiting hours are instituted, provide the family with rationale for these limitations (e.g., change of shift report in the intensive care units to protect patient privacy). Always note whether the limitation of visiting hours significantly limits the amount of time parents can spend with their children. This is especially important if there are issues such as work or home responsibilities or transportation that limit parents' ability to visit freely.
- Encourage parents or guardians to participate in the patient rounds of their child. This facilitates communication and information sharing between staff and parents and recognizes the important role parents play in the decision making and recovery of the child.
- Encourage overnight stay by one parent or another adult family member in all patient care areas where space permits.
- Encourage sibling visitation after siblings have been screened for potential communicable diseases.
- Inform visitors, including children, before their first visitation as to what they may see and hear during their visit, such as oxygen delivery equipment, traction, and so on.
- An adult must accompany all visitors (younger than 18 years of age). The accompanying adult shall be responsible for supervising the child visitors and ensuring they do not affect the privacy or safety of other patients.

- Monitor the child's response to visit and intervene as needed to ensure that child is receiving adequate rest and quiet.
- Provide support and care to the family after the visitation.
- Contact security services immediately if the visitors become unruly or present a threat to the safety and well-being of the patient, the staff, other visitors, or other patients.

EQUIPMENT

- Hospital orientation pamphlet
- Visitor information documents
- Institutional visitor identification badge or band.
- Institutional parent identification band.

CHILD AND FAMILY ASSESSMENT AND PREPARATION

- When child is preadmitted to the hospital for a planned procedure or surgery, provide family instructions about visitation policies, unit routines, and family-centered services (e.g., chaplain, social services, parking).
- Provide child and family with written materials about family-centered care support services and visitation policies.

caREminder

Caution must be implemented to protect privacy of pediatric patients. Many hospitals give the parents/guardians a "code word" or "confidentiality code" (multidigit number) that must be supplied to nursing staff before any information can be released. The "code word" or "confidentiality code" is kept in the child's chart throughout his or her hospital stay.

CHILD AND FAMILY EVALUATION AND DOCUMENTATION

- Evaluate child's and family's understanding of visitation guidelines and support services available to visiting family members.
- Evaluate child's verbal and nonverbal response to visitations.
- Periodically evaluate with the child and the family whether the visitation practices are meeting their needs.
- After a visitation, document the following:
  - Who visited the child
  - Length of stay
  - Child's verbal and nonverbal cues during the visit (if observed)
  - Visitor's response to the visitation (if observed)
- Between visitations, document the following:
  - Telephone contacts with family members
  - Verbal and nonverbal cues of the child that address child's adjustment to absence of family members

COMMUNITY CARE

- Inform family members that they will be called at home if there is a significant change in the child's health status.
- Provide family members with unit telephone number to call when they are at home.
- Provide information to family members regarding adequate lodging, meals, laundry services, and other services they may need during child's stay.

Unexpected Situation

- *While answering a call light, you notice there are several teenagers congregated in an adolescent patient's room. The talking, laughter, and music coming from the room is loud enough to be heard from several rooms away. Other families are complaining about the noise:* There are several interventions that should be taken. First, ask them to turn the music down to a level where the music can only be heard in that room. Then ensure that all adolescent visitors have been properly identified as visitors per institutional policy. Also determine whether a supervising adult is present, per institutional policy. If no adult is present, unchaperoned adolescents may be asked to leave. If an adult is present, discuss the need to maintain a quite environment for other patients on the unit. If the number of visitors at the bedside and their response to interventions to decrease noise level are a safety concern, contact institutional security for further interventions.

Bibliography

Farrell, M., Joseph, D., & Schwartz-Barcott, D. (2005). Visiting hours in the ICU: Finding the balance among patient, visitor and staff needs. *Nursing Forum, 40*(1), 18–28.

Griffin, T. (2001). Nurses and families in the NICU. Parental visits and infant care: Understanding parent's needs. *Neonatal Network: Journal of Neonatal Nursing, 20*(1), 65.

Griffin, T. (2003). Facing challenges to family-centered care. I. Conflicts over visitation. *Pediatric Nursing, 29*(2), 135–137.

Montgomery, L., Kleiber, C., Nicholson, A., & Craft-Rosenberg, M. (1997). A research-based sibling visitation program for the neonatal ICU. *Critical Care Nurse, 17*, 29–40.

Roland, P., Russell, J., Richards, K., & Sullivan, S. (2001). Visitation in critical care: Processes and outcomes of a performance improvement initiative. *Journal of Nursing Care Quality, 15*(2), 18–26.

Schuman, A. (2005). You have a role in preventing child abduction. *Contemporary Pediatrics, 22*(3), 36, 38, 40.

C H A P T E R
130

Vital Signs: Blood Pressure

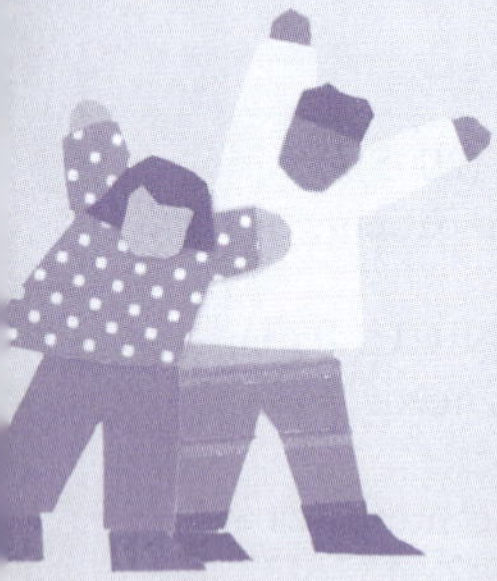

CLINICAL GUIDELINES

- A registered nurse (RN), licensed practical nurse (LPN), or unlicensed assistive personnel (UAP) may measure blood pressure. When the blood pressure is taken by the UAP, any variance from previous measures is reported to the licensed caregiver.
- Blood pressure is measured initially to obtain baseline data to assess general hemodynamic status of each child within the first hour of admission to an acute care setting.
- Blood pressure is measured to assess response to treatment regimes.

> ***Alert!*** *A decrease in blood pressure is a late sign of shock in children.*

- During acute illness, measure blood pressure every 4 to 8 hours or more frequently as clinically indicated.
- In neonates, measure blood pressure if renal disease or coarctation of the aorta is suspected or if clinical signs of hypotension are present. Universal screening of neonates is not recommended. Wide variability exists in blood pressure between limbs. Suspicion of coarctation must be followed up with echocardiography.
- Do not routinely measure blood pressure in children with osteogenesis imperfecta due to high risk of fractures; measure blood pressure only with a direct order from physician or advanced practice nurse.
- For health maintenance, blood pressure should be measured:
  - When a child older than 3 years of age is seen in a medical setting
  - In a child younger than 3 years of age with history of neonatal condition requiring intensive care; symptoms of hypertension, hypotension, elevated intracranial pressure, recurrent urinary tract infections, and renal or cardiac disease; malignancy or transplant (solid organ, bone marrow); and treatment with medications known to affect blood pressure
- Auscultation is the preferred method of measuring blood pressure in children because frequent calibration of automated devices is required and there is a lack of established reference standards for children. Automated devices are acceptable when auscultation is difficult (e.g., in young children) or when frequent measurements are required.
- Use the right arm whenever possible for consistency of measurement and comparison with standard norms.

EQUIPMENT

- Stethoscope
- Measurement device:
  - Mercury-gravity or aneroid sphygmomanometer
    Or
  - Automated device that uses oscillometric or Doppler technique
- Appropriately sized blood pressure cuff

CHILD AND FAMILY ASSESSMENT AND PREPARATION

- Assess for signs of hypotension, including weak pulse, diaphoresis, pallor, and dizziness.
- Assess for signs of hypertension, including headache, bounding pulse, and flushing.
- Explain to the child and family why monitoring is important, how it is done, and equipment used. Use language that is appropriate for developmental level (e.g., "I'm going to see how your heart is working. You will feel like your arm is getting a hug.").
- In nonemergent situations:
  - Show child equipment and let child handle equipment.
  - Demonstrate on parent, other staff, or stuffed animal how procedure is done and how equipment is used.

PROCEDURE Auscultation Method

Steps	Rationale/Points of Emphasis
1. Review child's previous blood pressure readings.	Provides baseline data for comparison, if available.
2. Analyze child's diagnosis and current medications for effect on blood pressure.	Alerts to possible problems and drugs that may affect the blood pressure.
3. Perform hand hygiene. Clean diaphragm of stethoscope.	Reduces transmission of microorganisms.
4a. Select site (Figure 130-1). Begin by checking record to see whether previous measurement was taken. If so, use same site and position. Use right arm when possible.	Extremity closest to the heart provides consistency and comparability with standard norms and child's own readings. **KidKare** Although the right arm is preferable, child's anxiety, anatomy, or condition may necessitate using another extremity.

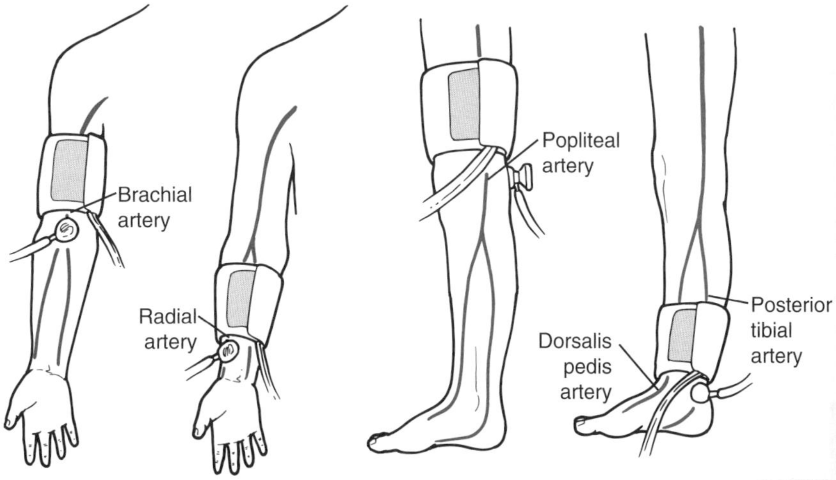

FIGURE 130-1
Arterial sites used to measure blood pressure: brachial, radial, popliteal, posterior tibial, and dorsalis pedis.

Continued

Steps	Rationale/Points of Emphasis
4b. Do not use extremity that has an injury, wound, or foreign devices (e.g., IV, arteriovenous, or renal dialysis shunt).	May cause further injury or potentiate thrombi in indwelling devices.
4c. Do not use extremity with altered circulation (e.g., Blalock-Taussig shunt, coarctation).	Measurement may be inaccurate and further compromise an already compromised extremity.
5a. Select appropriately sized cuff (Figure 130-2).	Facilitates correct cuff selection to obtain accurate measurement. The practice of labeling of BP cuffs as "infant," "pediatric," "small adult," "adult," and "large adult" is misleading, and such designation may result in the improper choice of equipment. Using upper arm circumference (UAC) as a measure for cuff size most closely reflects directly measured radial arterial pressure but significantly overestimates diastolic pressure. When two thirds or three fourths of the upper arm length are used as cuff selection criterion, they significantly underestimate systolic and diastolic blood pressure compared with directly measured radial arterial pressure.

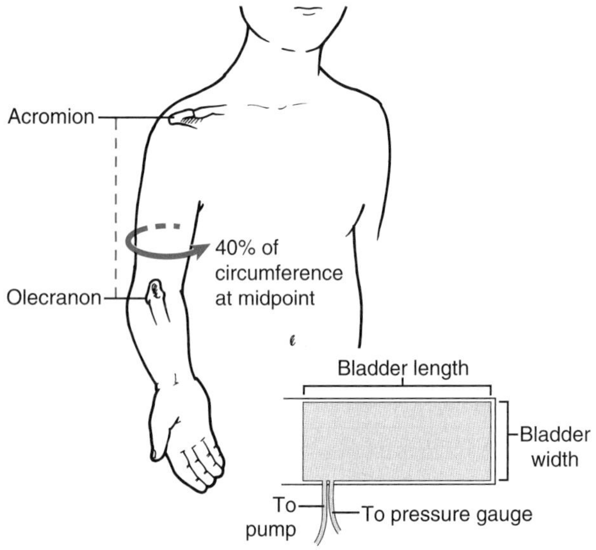

FIGURE 130-2
Determination of proper cuff size: identify midpoint between the olecranon (elbow) and the acromion (shoulder).

Steps	Rationale/Points of Emphasis
5b. Bladder width should be about 40% of the arm circumference midway between the olecranon (elbow) and the acromion (shoulder).	Increases accuracy of measurement. Using too small a cuff may falsely elevate measurement; too large a cuff may give falsely low reading.
5c. This usually corresponds to a cuff bladder that covers 80% to 100% of the arm circumference.	Use the manufacturer's lines on the cuff as a guide for cuff selection.
5d. If unable to obtain the appropriately sized cuff, choose one that is oversized rather than too small.	Too large a size tends to have less effect than too small.
6. Center the bladder of the cuff on the extremity proximal to the pulse (e.g., at the brachial site, position about 1–2 inches above the antecubital fossa) and snugly secure cuff. Do not apply cuff over clothing.	A loose cuff may give a false high reading. Clothing may interfere with correct placement of cuff.
7. Measure BP after 3 to 5 minutes of rest, when possible. Position child's arm (extremity) at heart level during the rest.	Ensures most accurate reading because agitation may falsely elevate the results. A level below the heart may cause false high readings. A level above the heart may cause false low readings.
8. Locate the pulse at the site. Place the bell of the stethoscope where the pulse is felt, below the bottom edge of the cuff.	Facilitates hearing Korotkoff sounds that are of low frequency, which the bell is best for auscultating.
9. Close sphygmomanometer valve, and inflate cuff to a pressure 30 mm Hg above the point at which artery pulsation is obliterated. Stabilize extremity during measurement.	Inflation higher than point of pulse obliteration avoids missing auscultation of first sound. Movement may cause extra sounds and interfere with ability to hear pulsations.
10. Deflate cuff at a rate of 2 to 3 mm Hg per second.	Ensures accurate measurement of blood pressure.

Steps	Rationale/Points of Emphasis
11a. Note Korotkoff sounds, beginning with the onset of tapping sound.	Correlates with phase I, which represents systolic pressure.
11b. Note muffling of the sound, if applicable	Muffling of the sound represents phase IV. This may occur several millimeters before disappearance of the sound. This occurs more commonly in preadolescents. The presence of diastolic hypertension can be excluded when Korotkoff sounds are heard to 0 mm Hg.
11c. Note disappearance of sound	Silence correlates with phase V, which corresponds with diastolic pressure.
12. Do not reinflate cuff during deflation. If necessary to repeat BP, allow a few minutes between measurements.	Ensures more accurate measurement.
13. Completely deflate cuff and remove from arm.	Measurement is complete.
14. Perform hand hygiene.	Reduces transmission of microorganisms.
15. Record findings on patient record. Also record child's position, extremity and site used, cuff size, level of activity (e.g., 90/50 mm Hg, supine, right arm, brachial, infant cuff, quiet). If BP is very high or low, note heart rate also.	Makes findings available to other health team members; indicates child's status and allows comparison of measurements. Heart rate can affect blood pressure.

PROCEDURE Automated Device Method

Steps	Rationale/Points of Emphasis
1. Follow steps 1–6 in previous procedure (Auscultation Method).	Ensures accuracy of measurement.
2. Refer to manufacturer's directions for machine use.	Increases accuracy of measurement.
3. Stabilize extremity during measurement.	Increases ability of automated device to detect pulsations and determine accurate measurement.
4. Perform hand hygiene.	Reduces transmission of microorganisms.
5. Record value on patient record. Also record the child's position, extremity and site used, cuff size, and activity level.	Makes findings available to other health team members; indicates child's status and allows comparison of measurements.

PROCEDURE Palpation Method

Steps	Rationale/Points of Emphasis
1. Follow steps 1–6 in the first procedure, Auscultation Method, and step 1 of the second procedure, Automated Device Method, for locating artery, cuff selection, and placement.	Ensures accurate measurement.
2. Palpate the artery as you inflate cuff.	Palpating pressure aids in identifying presence of ausculatory gap.
3. Inflate cuff to 30 mm Hg higher than the point at which you last felt pulse.	Pulse disappears when cuff pressure equals systolic pressure. Inflating cuff higher helps you to find exact point at which palpable pulse will be felt.
4. Slowly deflate cuff and note point at which pulse return is felt.	Correlates to systolic pressure.
5. Completely deflate cuff and remove from extremity.	Measurement is complete.
6. Perform hand hygiene.	Reduces transmission of microorganisms.
7. Record measurement on patient record as palpated systolic reading (e.g., 100/p). Also record the child's position, extremity and site used, cuff size, and activity level.	Makes findings available to other health team members; indicates child's status and how measurements can be compared. Documents assessments of care given as part of the legal record.

CHILD AND FAMILY EVALUATION AND DOCUMENTATION

- Compare child's blood pressure to previous readings and age-appropriate norms (see Appendix A) to detect change in status and potential pathology. Blood pressure is typically equal in the upper and lower extremities until about 6 to 9 months of age. At that time, blood pressure in the lower extremities is higher than in the upper extremities. Report deviations from this pattern and inequalities between upper extremities to the physician or advanced nurse practitioner.
- Note method used to obtain BP and specific method and equipment, if appropriate. Blood pressure measurements obtained from an oscillometric device (Dinamap 8100, Critikan, Tampa, FL) have been found to be higher (systolic by 10 mm Hg, diastolic by 5 mm Hg) than auscultatory measures. Measurements obtained from another oscillometric device (BpTRU) were closer to auscultated measures. Thus use the same method for measurements each time because measures obtained by the two different methods may not be interchangeable.
- Blood pressure measured in the arm is not equivalent to measurement obtained from the calf and should not be compared as such.
- Note child's response to interventions.
- Document on patient record the blood pressure value obtained, extremity and site used, cuff size, child's position, and activity level.

COMMUNITY CARE

- If measurement of blood pressure in a child is required in the home setting:
  - Assess equipment needs (appropriate cuff size, method of measurement: automated or auscultation).
  - Contact vendor to supply equipment and appropriately sized cuffs.
  - Instruct parent on how to obtain the measurements; evaluate return demonstration.
  - Give written instructions on how to obtain measurement and frequency of measurement.
- Instruct the family to contact the healthcare provider if
  - Change from baseline value is noted (give specific parameters based on age, diagnosis, health status)

Unexpected Situation

- *Measurements from a newborn show BP is significantly higher in the arms than in the legs:* Wait a few minutes and then obtain repeat BP measurements. If difference persists, it may indicate coarctation of the aorta. Document and notify physician or advanced practice nurse.

Bibliography

AAP Committee on Fetus and Newborn, 1992 to 1993. (1993). Routine evaluation of blood pressure, hematocrit, and glucose in newborns. *Pediatrics, 92*, 474–476.

Arafat, M., & Mattoo, T. (1999). Measurement of blood pressure in children: Recommendations and perceptions on cuff selection. *Pediatrics, 104*, e30.

Clark, J. A., Lieh-Lai, M. W., Sarnaik, A. & Mattoo, T. K. (2002). Discrepancies between direct and indirect blood pressure measurements using various recommendations for arm cuff selection. *Pediatrics, 110*, 920–923.

Crapanzano, M. S., Strong, W. B., Newman, I. R., Hixon, R. L., Casal, D., & Linder, C. W. (1996). Calf blood pressure: Clinical implications and correlations with arm blood pressure in infants and young children. *Pediatrics, 97*, 220–224.

Crossland, D. S., Furness, J. C., Abu-Harb, M., Sadagopan, S. N., & Wren C. (2004). Variability of four limb blood pressure in normal neonates. *Archives of Disease in Childhood: Fetal and Neonatal Edition, 89*, 325–327.

Hegyi, T., Anwar, M., Carbone, M. T., et al. (1996). Blood pressure ranges in premature infants. II. The first weeks of life. *Pediatrics, 97*, 336–342.

Mattu, G. S., Heran, B. S., & Wright, J. M. (2004). Comparison of the automated non-invasive oscillometric blood pressure monitor (BpTRU) with the auscultatory mercury sphygmomanometer in a paediatric population. *Blood Pressure Monitoring, 9*, 39–45.

National High Blood Pressure Education Program Working Group on Hypertension Control in Children and Adolescents. (2004). The fourth report on the diagnosis evaluation and treatment of high blood pressure in children and adolescents. *Pediatrics, 114*, 555–576.

Nwankwo, M. U., Lorenz, J. M., & Gardiner, J. C. (1997). A standard protocol for blood pressure measurement in the newborn. *Pediatrics, 99*, e10.

Park, M. K., Menard, S. W., & Yuan, C. (2001). Comparison of auscultatory and oscillometric blood pressures. *Archives of Pediatrics & Adolescent Medicine, 155*, 50–53.

CHAPTER
131

Vital Signs: Heart Rate

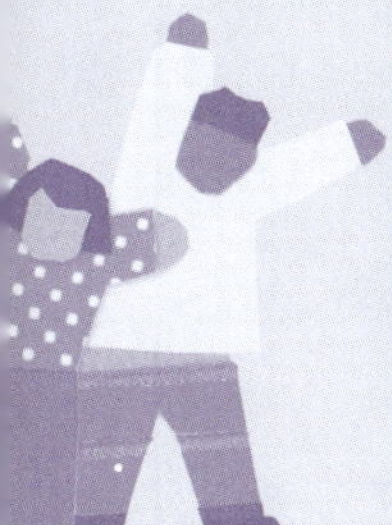

Clinical Guidelines

- A registered nurse (RN), licensed practical nurse (LPN), or unlicensed assistive personnel (UAP) may measure heart rate. When the heart rate is measured by the UAP, any variance from previous measurements is reported to the licensed caregiver.
- Heart rate is measured to assess the general status of each child within the first hour of admission to an acute care setting.
- Monitor heart rate every 4 to 8 hours during acute illness while child is a patient on a general care unit and every 1 to 2 hours in the intensive care unit.
- Heart rate is reassessed to monitor response to treatment regimens and as indicated by nursing or medical judgment.

Equipment

- Watch or clock with a second hand or digital readout
- Stethoscope
- Alcohol wipes

Child and Family Assessment and Preparation

- Assess for associated factors that affect heart rate and quality, including hypoxia, hyperthermia, hypothermia, hypovolemia, hemorrhage, pain, anxiety, crying, and level of activity. Children may normally have a sinus arrhythmia in which heart rate increases with inspiration and decreases with expiration.
- Review patient record for medical diagnosis, current medications, or past history of arrhythmias.
- Explain to the child and family what you are going to be doing and why. Use terms appropriate for developmental level. For example, instead of saying, "I am going to take your pulse," say, "I am going to see how fast your heart is beating." Demonstrate on parent, self, or stuffed animal first. Offer the child a chance to manipulate the stethoscope if appropriate.

PROCEDURE Preprocedural Care

Steps	Rationale/Points of Emphasis
1. Review child's record for baseline data on pulse rate; know range for age (see Appendix A).	Provides data base for comparison. Cardiac output is dependent on heart rate in infants; therefore heart rate is normally much faster in infants than in older children.
2. Determine site: • In child younger than 2 years of age, apical auscultation is easier to obtain. • In older children, apical auscultation may be performed or a peripheral pulse may be palpated.	Yields most accurate values.
3. Calm child, if required. Obtain measurement when child is quiet whenever possible.	Factors such as agitation, crying, pain, and anxiety alter (usually increase) heart rate.
4. Perform hand hygiene.	Reduces transmission of microorganisms.

PROCEDURE Measuring Heart Rate by Auscultation of Apical Pulse

Steps	Rationale/Points of Emphasis
1. Cleanse stethoscope chest piece and ear pieces with alcohol wipe before and after examination.	Reduces the spread of microorganisms.
2. Insert ear pieces into your ears with tips bent forward toward face.	Earpiece placement should conform to the normal anatomy of ear canal.
3. Identify site. Palpate the chest wall to determine the point of maximal impulse (PMI): • In children younger than 7 years of age—just left of the midclavicular line and fourth intercostal space • In children older than 7 years of age—left midclavicular line and fifth intercostal space (Figure 131-1).	These positions approximate where heart sounds are best heard at these ages.

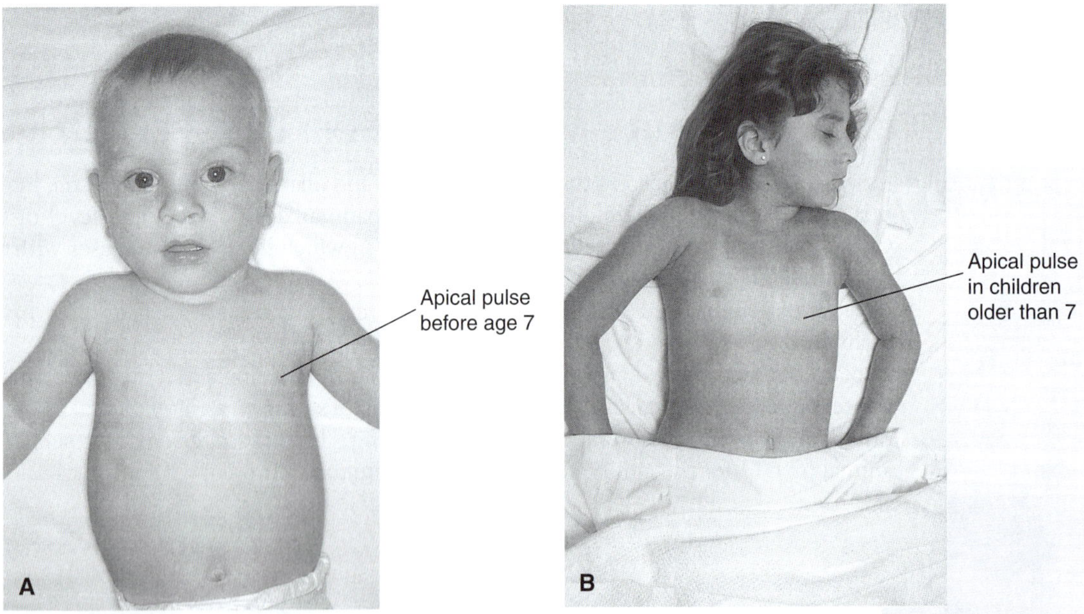

FIGURE 131-1
(**A**) Location of point of maximal impulse in child younger than 7 years. (**B**) Location of point of maximal impulse in child older than 7 years.

Steps	Rationale/Points of Emphasis
	caREminder *Optimally, a quiet room and a quiet, cooperative, or sleeping child will contribute to more success when auscultating the heart. Noisy respirations, crying infants, and environmental noises detract from the ability to detect heart sounds and possible murmurs.*
4a. Place diaphragm of stethoscope over the PMI and count HR: • If child's pulse is regular, count for 30 seconds and multiply by 2. • If pulse is irregular, count for 1 full minute. 4b. Note rhythm and quality of sound.	Counting for a full minute gives you a more accurate rate, particularly when a sinus arrhythmia or other irregularity is present. **caREminder** *Warm chest piece of the stethoscope by rubbing it in the palm of your hand. A cold stethoscope can cause discomfort or startle the child.*
4c. Report murmur to the physician or advanced practice nurse.	Murmurs are not uncommon in infants but must be evaluated for potential pathology.
5. Perform hand hygiene.	Reduces transmission of microorganisms.
6. Record heart rate, site used to obtain, and child's activity level (e.g., asleep, quiet, crying, fussing) in patient record.	Communicates findings to other healthcare team members and provides basis for comparison; activity impacts heart rate. Documents assessments and care given to child as part of the legal record.

PROCEDURE **Measuring Heart Rate by Palpation of Peripheral Sites**

Steps	Rationale/Points of Emphasis
1. Identify site; radial and brachial pulses are most frequently used (Figure 131-2).	Provides easiest accessibility.
2. Locate the child's pulse and palpate with your first two or three fingers; do not use excessive pressure. Note rhythm.	Do not use thumb to check pulse because the thumb has a pulse and may be confused with the child's. Excessive pressure may occlude the pulsation.
3. If child's pulse is regular, count for 30 seconds and multiply by 2. If irregular, count for 1 full minute.	Pulse rate is recorded in beats per minute. Irregular rhythms should be counted for 1 full minute to ensure accuracy.
4. Perform hand hygiene.	Reduces transmission of microorganisms.
5. Record heart rate, site used to obtain, and child's activity level (e.g., asleep, quiet, crying, fussing) in patient record.	Communicates findings to other healthcare team members and provides basis for comparison; activity impacts heart rate. Documents assessments and care given to child as part of the legal medical record.

CHILD AND FAMILY EVALUATION AND DOCUMENTATION

- Compare child's heart rate to previous readings and age-appropriate norms (see Appendix A) to detect change in status and potential pathology.
- Document time and site where measurement is obtained, rate, rhythm, strength of pulse (if obtained by palpating pulse), and child's activity level. If appropriate, note interventions and child's response to interventions.
- Notify physician or advanced practice nurse if any abnormal sounds are detected.

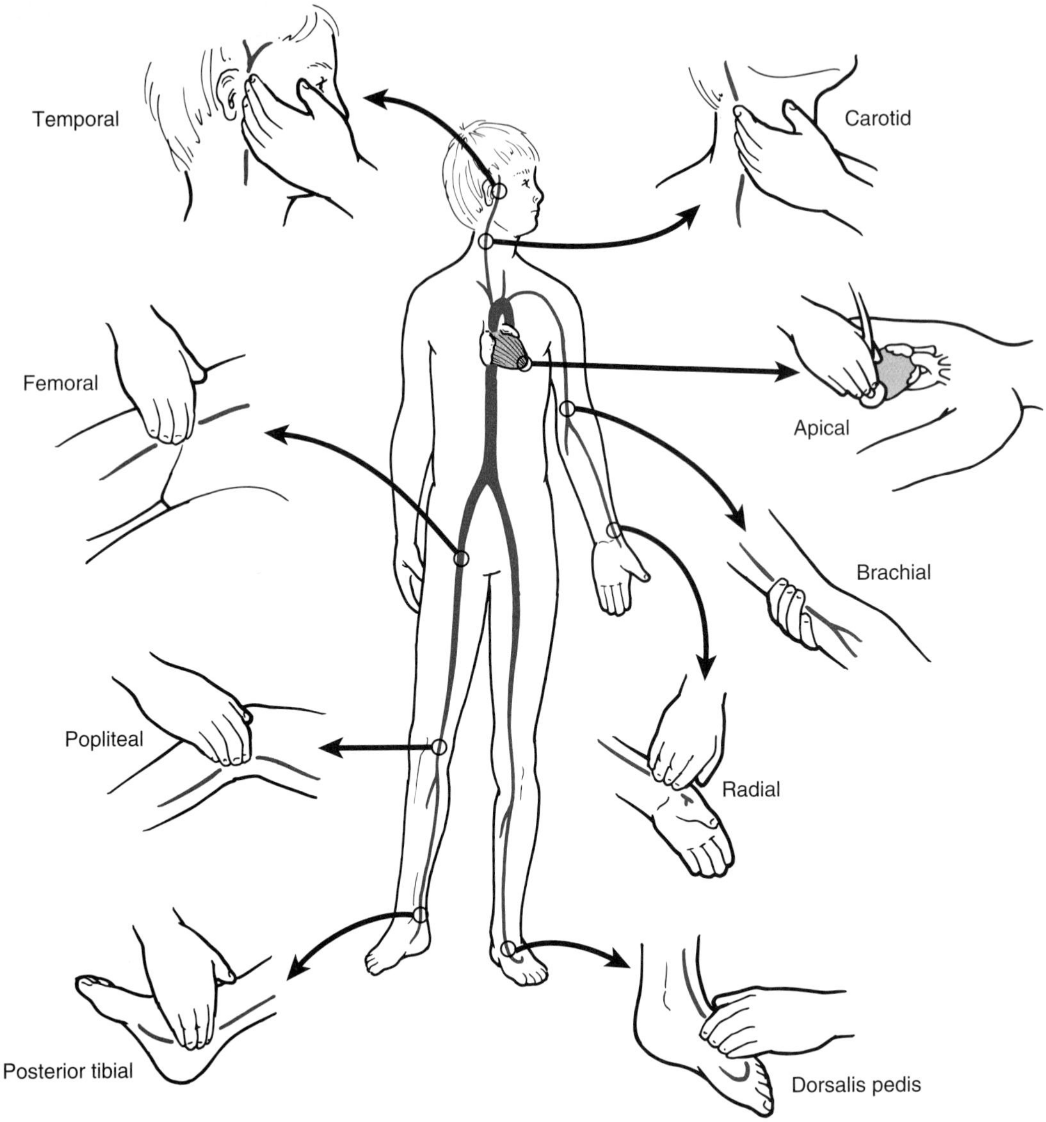

FIGURE 131-2
Pulse sites.

COMMUNITY CARE

- Instruct the child (as appropriate) and parent on proper technique to assess heart rate. In a child younger than 2 years of age, apical sites are used; in older children, radial or carotid sites are used because these are easily accessible. The apical site can be used in older children per their preference.
- Provide written instructions on technique with drawings to demonstrate sites.
- Evaluate child's or parents' return demonstration of technique.
- Children with identified heart murmurs require follow-up and further evaluation by a cardiac specialist.
- Instruct the family to contact the healthcare provider if
  - Child experiences decreased exercise tolerance; chest pain, especially with exercise; dizziness; dyspnea; syncope; signs of congestive heart failure; or abnormal vital signs
  - Infant experiences poor feeding with failure to thrive, respiratory distress, cyanosis, signs of congestive heart failure, or abnormal vital signs

Unexpected Situation

- *Child's heart rate accelerates and decelerates:* Take the pulse for 1 full minute and note if the rhythm varies with respiration. Have an older child hold his or her breath and note if rhythm is still irregular. Assess for signs of disruption in cardiac output (i.e., weak, thready pulse; increased heart rate; cyanosis; tachypnea; fussiness; decreased activity; poor feeding); if present, notify physician or advanced practice nurse. Sinus arrhythmia, where the heart rate varies with respiration, is common in infants and young children and not associated with cardiac problems.

Bibliography

Smith, K. M. (1997). The innocent heart murmur in children. *Journal of Pediatric Health Care, 11*, 207–214.

White, J., Shepperd, S., Yudkin, P., Harnden, A., & Mant, D. (2004). Parents measuring pulses: An observational study. *Archives of Disease in Childhood, 89*, 274–275.

Yakowich Moody, L. (1997). Pediatric cardiovascular assessment and referral in the primary care setting. *Nurse Practitioner, 22*(1), 120–134.

C H A P T E R

132

Vital Signs: Pain Assessment

Clinical Guidelines

- The physician, registered nurse (RN), licensed practical nurse (LPN), or unlicensed assistive personnel (UAP) is responsible for assessment of pain and may obtain subjective reports of pain. When measurement is obtained by the UAP, any variance from baseline is reported to the licensed caregiver.
- Each facility should identify two or three pain assessment tools appropriate for use in each age group or patient group (e.g., use an appropriate tool for cognitively impaired children). Select from these tools when choosing a method of pain assessment for an individual child; if the first tool does not work, try one of the others. After identifying a tool that works for the child, use this consistently unless the situation changes (e.g., the child is comatose and can no longer use a self-report tool) (see Chapter 7).
- Assess pain level within the first hour of admission to an acute care setting or during an outpatient contact to obtain baseline data regarding the comfort status of the child.
- For a child who has chronic pain, frequency of pain assessments are based on child's condition but are performed at least monthly.
- Assess pain level every 8 to 12 hours in an acutely ill child and more frequently as clinically indicated. Pain assessment is an ongoing process; each caregiver performs a comprehensive pain assessment when initially assuming care of the child. After the initial assessment, if the child's status changes, if the child demonstrates signs of pain or is subjected to a presumably painful event, or if there is change in infusion rates of sedation, analgesic medication, or anesthetic medication, perform another comprehensive pain assessment.

Alert! *If the child is comfortable, it is not necessary to perform a comprehensive pain assessment with each set of vital signs. However, be aware of each state's law, because some require that pain assessment be recorded each time vital signs are recorded.*

- Assess pain level before and after pain interventions within 1 hour of any intervention for an acutely ill child (time interval is dependent on the specific intervention) to assess response to treatment regimes.

EQUIPMENT

- Pain assessment tool, developmentally appropriate for child; use a self-report tool when possible. If self-report is not an option, use a reliable and valid multidimensional tool (see Chapter 7)

CHILD AND FAMILY ASSESSMENT AND PREPARATION

- Obtain an initial history from the child and/or family members of the current pain, including
  - What words the child uses to communicate pain (use these words when talking with the child)
  - Presence of pain: "Are you having any pain?" If yes, then obtain the following:
    - Character and quality: "Tell me what the pain feels like" (e.g., burning, stabbing, aching, pinching)
    - Onset: "When did the pain start? Did anything happen to set off the pain?"
    - Location and radiation: "Where is the pain? Does it go to other places?" For younger children: "Point to where the pain is." Coloring pain location on a body outline tool may help a child identify the site.
    - Duration: "How long have you been feeling this pain?"
    - Frequency: "How often does the pain occur? Is it all the time or just at certain times?"
    - Exacerbation: "Does anything make the pain worse?"
    - Relief and present pain regimen: "Does anything help make the pain better?" "What are you doing to try to make the pain go away?" Ask about medications—prescription and over-the-counter medications, herbs, nonpharmacologic interventions, effectiveness of regime, side effects of regime
    - Association: "Have daily routines and habits changed because of the pain?" "What is the effect on eating, sleeping, elimination, activity, or other behavior patterns?"
- For a child who is preverbal or has special needs, ask parents and record in child's plan of care how the child usually behaves when he or she is in pain and what interventions may help.
- Assess what coping techniques the child and family have previously used successfully.
- Reinforce to the child that pain is not a punishment for misdeeds, particularly for preschool-aged and young school-aged children.
- Teach child and family how to use a developmentally appropriate pain assessment tool, before a painful event, when possible. Select tool based on developmental age of the child and type of pain or medical condition (e.g., procedural or postoperative pain). Assess the child's ability to understand tool (e.g., understands the concept of seriating, greater than, less than). Introduce a different tool if the child does not understand how to use the first tool to express his or her pain level.
- Use the same assessment method over time to determine adequacy of pain management (see Chapter 7).

PROCEDURE **Pain Assessment**

Steps	Rationale/Points of Emphasis
1. Review the child's initial pain history and previous pain level, when available.	Provides basis from which to make comparison.
2. Note the child's medical diagnosis and history of events that are assumed to be painful or cause tissue trauma.	Alerts to potential pain. **caREminder** *Be alert for causes of pain other than the primary diagnosis or complaint.*
3. Determine whether child is taking any medications that may affect perception of pain or ability to communicate pain.	Some medications sedate or reduce anxiety (e.g., benzodiazepines, phenothiazines, barbiturates) but do not provide analgesia.
4. Perform hand hygiene.	Reduces transmission of microorganisms.
5. Assess for presence of pain indicators, considering the child's age and sleep state: • **Acute pain** ▪ *Subjective:* statement of pain; if unable to report, ask parent for input ▪ *Physiologic:* increased respiratory or heart rate, shallow respirations, decreased oxygen saturation, diaphoresis, pupil dilation	A multidimensional assessment provides the most accurate assessment and provides guidance for pain management. Preterm infants may not respond with behavioral or physiologic changes because they do not have the reserves available to mount a response. Infants in deeper sleep states are less likely to demonstrate as robust a response to pain as active awake infants. Acute and chronic pain have different manifestations because the body adapts to pain that is ongoing.

Continued

Steps	Rationale/Points of Emphasis
▪ *Behavioral:* crying, moaning, fussiness, anxiety, anger, decreased activity level, alteration in sleep, the position that child assumes (e.g., laying very still, fetal position, flexed or rigid extremity), facial grimace, guarding of painful area, touching painful area • **Chronic pain** ▪ Vital signs stable ▪ Disrupted sleep ▪ Developmental regression ▪ Change in eating patterns ▪ Behavior or school problems ▪ Withdrawal from peer group activities ▪ Depression ▪ Aggression • **For a child receiving neuromuscular blockade:** ▪ Assess physiologic parameters ▪ Assess pupillary size ▪ Stop paralytic agents for a short period to assess pain behaviors.	***Alert!*** *The presence of severe pain is a medical emergency and requires immediate intervention; report it to the appropriate healthcare professional.*
6. Assess pain level using a validated developmentally appropriate pain assessment tool; use the same tool over time to compare adequacy of pain management (e.g., the same tool as taught previously to child and family).	A valid and reliable tool increases confidence that the tool is accurately measuring pain. Multidimensional assessments are more accurate than are single parameters. Tools for infants usually use physiologic and behavioral indicators; those for older children typically include self-report in addition to physiologic or behavioral indicators.
7. Perform a physical examination of the painful area.	Provides additional assessment data.
8. Determine child's pain level and appropriate interventions; consider the specific situation (age, coping style, environment) and type and intensity of pain. Implement pain management interventions (see Chapter 7).	Appropriate assessment of pain and adequate management avoid prolonging the child's suffering.
9. Perform comprehensive reassessment of pain level: • If clinical indicators of pain are present • After implementation of pain interventions, with change in infusion rates of sedation, analgesic, or anesthetic medication; assessment must be performed within 1 hour after intervention; may be performed sooner depending on intervention (e.g., 5 to 20 minutes after IV bolus).	Evaluates adequacy of pain management intervention and helps in detection of unmanaged pain.
10. Perform hand hygiene.	Reduces transmission of microorganisms.

CHILD AND FAMILY EVALUATION AND DOCUMENTATION

- Consider age-related norms when evaluating vital signs (see Appendix A).
- Document date and time of assessment, signature of person assessing child, and presence of pain and comfort indicators.
- Describe behavior (e.g., "shallow, rapid breathing; lying rigid in bed" or "sleeping comfortably"), position of comfort, and activity level.
- Evaluate changes from previous measurements; indicate intervention if applicable (e.g., "repositioned," "cold pack applied to right knee for 15 minutes," "massaged area," "acetaminophen administered") and response to interventions.
- Document outcomes of interventions (e.g., "settled to sleep," "pain decreased to 3/10," "no change in pain level").
- Reassess pain as indicated.

COMMUNITY CARE

- Instruct the parents regarding developmentally appropriate techniques for pain assessment, nonpharmacologic techniques for pain management, and pain medications, including dosing, side effects and methods to reduce side effects, and reassessment after interventions.

- Instruct the family to notify the healthcare provider if
  - Pain is not maintained below the goal determined desirable by child and family

Unexpected Situation

- *Four hours after abdominal surgery, you ask a 7-year-old to rate his current pain level using the 0 to 10 numeric rating scale that he was taught preoperatively. The child rates it a 0:* He has had no medication postoperatively and is lying immobile in bed, intermittently crying and moaning. You are concerned that he is in pain because of his behaviors, and review the use of the numeric rating scale with him. He then tells you that his pain is really an 11, but his mommy said he would get a shot if he said his tummy hurt and he doesn't want a shot. Quickly explain use of intravenous analgesic and administer as ordered.

Bibliography

Beyer, J. E., Turner, S. B., Jones, L., Young, L., Onikul, R., & Bohaty, B. (2005). The alternate forms reliability of the Oucher pain scale. *Pain Management Nursing, 6*(1), 10–17.

Boldingh, E. J., Jacobs-van der Bruggen, M. A., Lankhorst, G. J., & Bouter, L. M. (2004). Assessing pain in patients with severe cerebral palsy: Development, reliability, and validity of a pain assessment instrument for cerebral palsy. *Archives of Physical Medicine and Rehabilitation, 85*, 758–766.

Chambers, C. T., Hardial, J., Craig, K. D., Court, C., & Montgomery, C. (2005). Faces scales for the measurement of postoperative pain intensity in children following minor surgery. *Clinical Journal of Pain, 21*, 277–285.

Crandall, M., & Savedra, M. (2005). Multidimensional assessment using the adolescent pediatric pain tool: A case report. *Journal for Specialists in Pediatric Nursing, 10*, 115–123.

Franck, L. S., Greenberg, C. S., & Stevens, B. (2000). Pain assessment in infants and children. *Pediatric Clinics of North America, 47*, 487–512.

Ramelet, A. S., Abu-Saad, H. H., Rees, N., & McDonald, S. (2004). The challenges of pain measurement in critically ill young children: A comprehensive review. *Australian Critical Care: Official Journal of the Confederation of Australian Critical Care Nurses, 17*, 33–45.

Rutledge, D. N., Donaldson, N. E., & Pravikoff, D. S. (2002). Update. Pain assessment and documentation. Pediatrics. *Online Journal of Clinical Innovations, 5*(3), 1–45. Retrieved October 5, 2006, from http://www.cinahl.com/cexpress/ojcionline

Solodiuk, J., & Curley, M. Q. (2003). Pain assessment in nonverbal children with severe cognitive impairments: The individualized numeric rating scale (INRS). *Journal of Pediatric Nursing, 18*, 295–299.

Willis, M. H. W., Merkel, S. I., Voepel-Lewis, T., & Malviya, S. (2003). FLACC Behavioral Pain Assessment Scale: A comparison with the child's self-report. *Pediatric Nursing, 29*, 195–198.

CHAPTER

133

Vital Signs: Respiratory Rate

Clinical Guidelines

- A registered nurse (RN), licensed practical nurse (LPN), or unlicensed assistive personnel (UAP) may measure respiratory rate. When measurement is obtained by the UAP, any variance from previous measures is reported to the licensed caregiver.
- Respirations are measured initially to obtain baseline data to assess the general status of each child within the first hour of admission to an acute care setting.
- Respirations are measured before and immediately after respiratory interventions to assess response to treatment regimens.
- Measurement of respirations is done every 4 to 8 hours in an acutely ill child and more frequently as clinically indicated.

Equipment

- Clock or watch with a second hand or digital readout

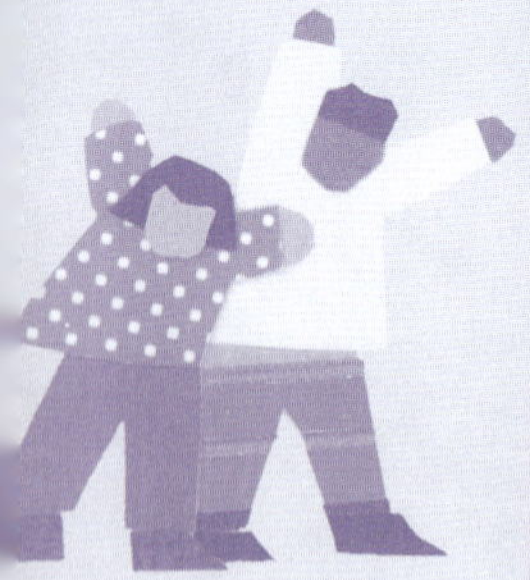

Child and Family Assessment and Preparation

- Assess the child's color, depth of respirations, presence of nasal flaring, grunting, retractions and type, use of accessory muscles and rhythm of respirations, the position that child assumes to breathe (e.g., sitting up or leaning forward), fussiness, and anxiety.

Alert! *The presence of respiratory distress or apnea is a medical emergency and requires immediate intervention.*

- Explain to the child and family, using developmentally appropriate language, what you are assessing and why it is important. It is best to make a general statement about measuring how the heart and lungs are working rather than specifying that the respiratory rate is counted to avoid the child consciously controlling his or her respirations.
- Measure the child's respiratory rate first, before disturbing the child for other procedures that may affect the rate.

PROCEDURE Respiratory Rate

Steps	Rationale/Points of Emphasis
1. Review the child's previous respiratory rate, when available.	Provides basis from which to make comparison.
2. Note the child's medical diagnosis and history of respiratory problems or difficulties.	Alerts to potential respiratory problems.
3. Determine whether child is taking any medications that may affect respiratory rate or depth.	Medications can alter respiratory pattern (e.g., morphine can decrease rate and depth of respirations, salicylates can increase rate and depth).
4. Perform hand hygiene.	Reduces transmission of microorganisms.
5. Count respirations: • Observe the abdomen for movement in infants and young children. • Observe thoracic movement in older children. • If respirations are regular, count number of respirations for 30 seconds and multiply by 2. • If respirations are irregular, count the number of respirations for 1 full minute.	Ensures accurate measurement. Young children are primarily diaphragmatic breathers; older children depend more on their intercostal muscles. **Alert!** *Count respirations in infants for 1 minute. Infants are episodic breathers; it is normal for them to vary their respiratory rate and pattern. Counting for a full minute obtains a more accurate measure.*
6. Note depth and pattern of respirations, presence of anxiety, restlessness, irritability, and position of comfort. Observe child's color, including extremities, noting cyanosis or pallor.	Alerts to respiratory distress and signs of hypoxia. Child may need immediate medical attention to prevent respiratory failure. Helps evaluate possible causes of respiratory distress. **Alert!** *If respiratory distress is noted, immediately auscultate breath sounds and immediately report this information to appropriate healthcare professional.*
7. Perform hand hygiene.	Reduces transmission of microorganisms.
8. Record results; respiratory rate is recorded in breaths per minute.	Communicates the findings to other healthcare team members. Documents assessments and care given to patient as part of the legal record.

CHILD AND FAMILY EVALUATION AND DOCUMENTATION

- Consider age-related norms when evaluating respiratory rates (see Appendix A).
- Evaluate and document color, respiratory rate, rhythm, depth of respirations, presence of respiratory distress, position of comfort, level of activity, changes from previous measurements, and response to interventions.

COMMUNITY CARE

- Instruct the parent on the above technique for counting respirations when indicated, signs of respiratory distress, and when to administer medications or aerosol treatment (e.g., for asthma).
- Instruct the family to contact the healthcare provider if
  - Child has signs of respiratory distress
  - Child has a respiratory rate outside of normal parameters for age

Unexpected Situation

- *Infant has slow respiratory rate:* Count respirations for 1 full minute; infants may have an irregular respiratory rate, and counting for less than a minute may underestimate the rate. Assess for signs of respiratory distress (cyanosis, head bobbing, nasal flaring, grunting, wheezing, coughing, labored respirations, tachypnea). The diaphragm is the primary muscle of respiration in an infant. Abdominal distention may cause significant respiratory distress. Notify physician or advanced practice nurse if signs of respiratory distress are present.

Bibliography

Armitage, G. (1999). Nursing assessment and diagnosis of respiratory distress in infants by children's nurses. *Journal of Clinical Nursing, 8*, 22–30.

CHAPTER

134

Vital Signs: Temperature

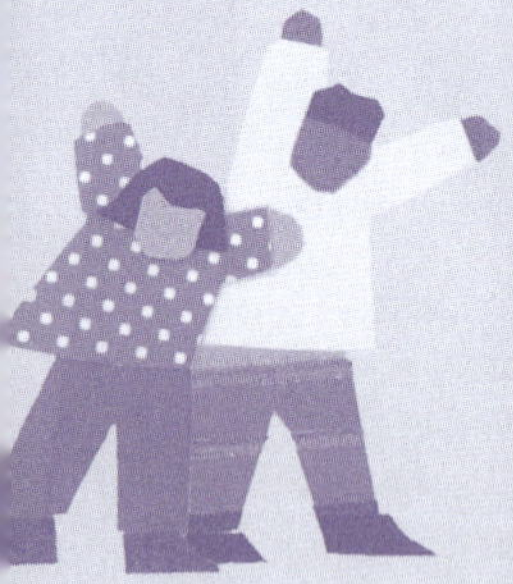

Clinical Guidelines

- A registered nurse (RN), licensed practical nurse (LPN), unlicensed assistive personnel (UAP), or healthcare prescriber may take temperatures. When the temperature is taken by the UAP, any variance from baseline or deviance from previous measurement is reported to the licensed caregiver.
- Temperature is measured to assess the baseline status of each child within the first hour of admission and to detect change in child's status (e.g., hypothermia, presence of infection, or other changes in the child's condition).
- Reassess temperature 30 minutes to 1 hour after an intervention to measure response to treatment regime.
- Measure temperature every 4 to 8 hours or more frequently when child is unstable, acutely ill, or has problems with thermoregulation.
- When using a temperature-regulating device (e.g., isolette, hypothermia blanket, overhead radiant warmer), assess the child's temperature every 1 to 3 hours.
- Do not use mercury-containing thermometers.
- The oral route is contraindicated if the child has developmental delay, oral surgery, seizures, altered level of consciousness, or will not cooperate (e.g., children under 5 years of age).
- Use the axillary route in the immediate postdelivery infant; use the rectal route only when the axillary is out of range.
- The rectal route is contraindicated if the child has neutropenia, thrombocytopenia, a bleeding disorder, is preterm birth, or has had rectal or bowel surgery.
- Tympanic (infrared) measurement is not recommended for use in children younger than 3 months of age. Studies demonstrate children and parents prefer tympanic thermometers over electronic and chemical dot thermometers.
- Temporal artery measurements can be used for infants, children, and adolescents.
- Disposable thermometers (e.g., Tempa-DOT) are accurate for children younger than 5 years of age.

***Alert!** Studies demonstrate conflicting findings regarding the accuracy and reliability of different measurement methods. Users must be knowledgeable as to how to accurately employ the method and operate the device being used. Use the same method and route of measurement whenever possible.*

Equipment

- Thermometer: electronic, tympanic, temporal artery, or disposable (e.g., chemical dot thermometers such as Tempa-DOT)
- Disposable probe cover: necessary for electronic or tympanic thermometer
- Gloves

- Water-soluble jelly
- Tissues or dry cloth

CHILD AND FAMILY ASSESSMENT AND PREPARATION

- Assess for history or risk factors for latex allergy (see Chapter 60); if present, do not use Tempa-DOT thermometers, which contain latex.
- Explain to child and family, in developmentally appropriate language (e.g., "I'm going to see how warm your body is."), the reason for measuring temperature, equipment being used, and how temperature will be assessed.
- Show child and family equipment you will use.
- Demonstrate on parent (or self) how equipment is used.

PROCEDURE Preprocedural Care

Steps	Rationale/Points of Emphasis
1a. Review child's medical record for • Vital signs over the past 24 hours • Evaluation of current medical problems	Provides baseline data for comparison. Indicates problems that may cause hypothermia or hyperthermia.
1b. Check record for desired temperature parameters (see Appendix A: Vital Signs).	Identifies goals of treatment and when to notify healthcare prescriber.

PROCEDURE Measuring Oral Temperature in a Child Older Than 5 Years of Age Using an Electronic Thermometer

Steps	Rationale/Points of Emphasis
1. Perform hand hygiene.	Reduces transmission of microorganisms.
2. Remove probe from holder and note display that thermometer is charged.	Display indicates charged and ready for use.
3. Select appropriate probe: blue—oral.	Eliminates oral–fecal cross-contamination.
4. Place probe cover on probe.	Protects from cross-contamination from child to child.
5. Gently insert probe with probe cover into the child's posterior sublingual pocket (see Figure 134-1) until the unit emits signal.	Tone indicates that temperature measurement is complete. **KidKare** Letting child hold the thermometer helps promote cooperation and involvement in self-care; remind child to keep lips closed. Sealing lips ensures an accurate reading not altered by ambient (room) air temperature.

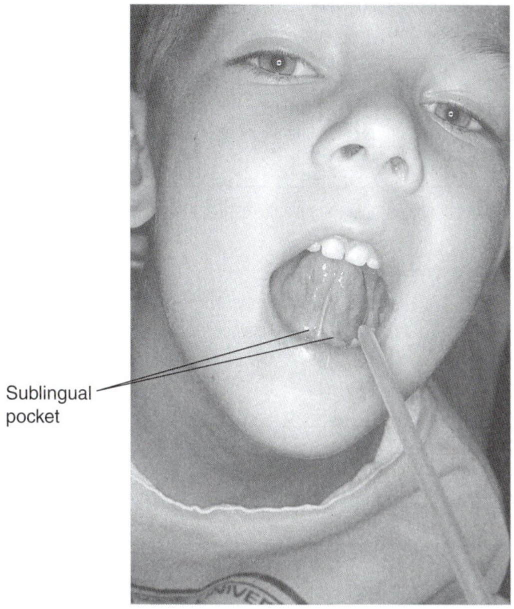

FIGURE 134-1
Oral thermometer placement.

Continued

Steps	Rationale/Points of Emphasis
6. Remove probe from mouth and note temperature on display. Be sure to note if in Celsius or Fahrenheit.	Measurement is complete.
7. Discard probe cover. **Alert!** *Do not leave probe cover in crib or bed; dispose of in a location where a young child may not retrieve from trash as covers present a choking hazard.*	Covers are disposable to prevent cross-contamination from child to child.
8. Return unit to charger base.	Ensures that unit will be charged for the next use.
9. Perform hand hygiene.	Reduces spread of microorganisms.

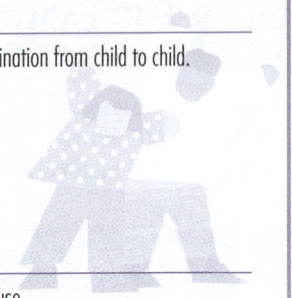

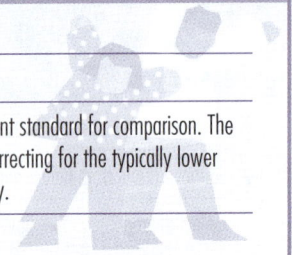

PROCEDURE Measuring Tympanic Temperature in a Child Older Than 3 Months of Age

Steps	Rationale/Points of Emphasis
1. Perform hand hygiene.	Reduces transmission of microorganisms.
2. Remove probe from base unit and note display that unit is charged.	Ensures that unit is ready for use.
3. Ensure that display indicates tympanic mode (some units assess surface, rectal, core, and tympanic temperature).	Ensures accurate measurement and a consistent standard for comparison. The thermometer may calculate several values, correcting for the typically lower value obtained through tympanic thermometry.
4. Place disposable cover on the probe tip.	Prevents cross-contamination.
5. Perform ear tug—retract the pinna posteriorly (upward and backward pull).	Straightens ear canal to more completely expose the tympanic membrane so that the scanner obtains a more accurate reading.
6. Insert probe into ear canal while pressing scan button; check to ensure that patient's ear canal is sealed.	The probe measures heat generated from the tympanic membrane. Sealing the canal increases accuracy of measurement by preventing ambient air from altering the temperature sensed from the tympanic membrane.
7. Release scan button.	Activates the machine.
8. Remove probe when thermometer emits signal. Note display reading and whether reading is Celsius or Fahrenheit	Indicates measurement is complete.
9. Discard probe cover by pressing release button.	Probe covers are disposable to prevent cross-contamination from child to child. **Alert!** *Do not leave discarded probe in crib or bed; dispose of in a location where child cannot retrieve from trash as the small covers present a choking hazard.*
10. Return unit to charger base.	Ensures that unit will be charged for the next use.
11. Perform hand hygiene.	Reduces transmission of microorganisms.

PROCEDURE Measuring Rectal Temperature Using an Electronic Thermometer

Steps	Rationale/Points of Emphasis
1. Perform hand hygiene. Don examination gloves.	Reduces transmission of microorganisms.
2. Remove probe from holder and note display that thermometer is charged.	Indicates thermometer is ready for use.
3. Select appropriate probe: red—rectal.	Use of appropriate probe prevents cross-contamination and spread of microorganisms.
4. Place probe cover on probe.	Protects from cross-contamination from child to child.
5. Lubricate tip with water-soluble jelly.	Makes insertion easier and prevents irritation to rectal mucosa.
6. Gently spread the child's buttocks and insert probe ½ inch (1.3 cm) for infant and 1 inch (2.5 cm) for child.	Deep insertion may cause trauma or perforation to rectal mucosa. **Alert!** *If unable to insert thermometer, STOP. In an infant, this may indicate imperforate anus.*
7. Hold the child's buttock closed with one hand and keep probe in place with other (Figure 134-2). 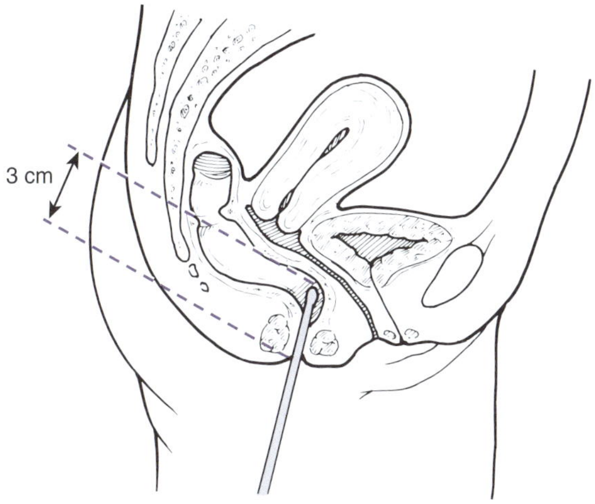 **FIGURE 134-2** Rectal thermometer placement. Note curve of rectum at approximately 1¼ inches (3 cm) from anus, where risk for perforation is greatest.	Prevents expulsion of probe.
8. Monitor changing temperature display until unit emits a tone. Note temperature on display and if measured in Celsius or Fahrenheit.	Indicates that temperature measurement is complete.
9. Discard probe cover by pressing release button.	Probe covers are disposable to prevent cross-contamination from child to child. **Alert!** *Do not leave discarded probe cover in crib or bed; dispose of in a location where child cannot retrieve from trash as the small covers present a choking hazard.*
10. Return unit to charger base.	Ensures that unit will be charged for the next use.
11. Perform hand hygiene.	Reduces transmission of microorganisms.

PROCEDURE Measuring Axillary Temperature Using an Electronic Thermometer

Steps	Rationale/Points of Emphasis
1. Perform hand hygiene.	Reduces transmission of microorganisms.
2. Remove probe from holder and note display that thermometer is charged.	Indicates that unit is ready for use.
3. Select appropriate probe: blue—oral.	Reduces potential for fecal contamination.
4. Place probe cover on probe.	Prevents spread of microorganisms from child to child.
5. Place covered probe in child's axilla and hold child's arm firmly to child's side.	Positions probe correctly for accurate measurement of body temperature.
6. Note temperature when digital display has stabilized and unit emits tone; note whether measured in Celsius or Fahrenheit.	Indicates temperature measurement is complete.
7. Return unit to charger base.	Ensures that unit will be charged for the next use.
8. Perform hand hygiene.	Reduces transmission of microorganisms.

PROCEDURE Measuring Temperature Using Temporal Artery Thermometer

Steps	Rationale/Points of Emphasis
1. Perform hand hygiene.	Reduces transmission of microorganisms.
2. Follow manufacturer's instructions for use.	Ensures correct use of equipment and most accurate results.
3. Apply disposable cover to probe, if using covers.	Prevents spread of microorganisms between patients. Institutions may choose to use probe covers or cleanse unit between uses.
4. Position the probe in the middle of the child's forehead.	Puts probe in position to scan path of temporal artery.
5. Depress and hold the "ON" button.	Prepares instrument for measurement.
6. While holding the "ON" button, move the probe laterally to the hairline and stop.	The sensor within the instrument scans the naturally emitted infrared heat from the arterial blood supply and records the highest temperature.
7. Release the "ON" button.	Indicates measurement is complete and displays recorded temperature. **caREminder** *If the child is diaphoretic, keep the "ON" button depressed and touch the concave depression behind the earlobe before releasing the "ON" button. Touching behind the earlobe compensates for any cooling that might result from perspiration on the forehead.*
8. Read thermometer output according to manufacturer's instructions.	Ensures most accurate reading.
9. If temperature registers over 98.6°F (37°C), retake temperature using a different method appropriate for child's age and condition.	Verifies accuracy of measurement, although it may not be directly comparable.
10. If not using disposable probe covers, cleanse with institution approved disinfectant.	Reduces spread of microorganisms between patients.
11. Perform hand hygiene.	Reduces transmission of microorganisms.

PROCEDURE **Measuring Temperature Using a Disposable Thermometer**

Steps	Rationale/Points of Emphasis
1. Perform hand hygiene.	Reduces transmission of microorganisms.
2. Remove single unit from package.	Individual packaging ensures cleanliness.
3. Peel off disposable thermometer's protective tape.	Exposes the adhesive.
4. Place temperature strip per manufacturer's directions for use: • Press strip firmly to child's forehead or axilla. • Place in sublingual pocket.	Ensures thermometer will be appropriately used. Must be secure to register accurately.
5. Use the strip to monitor temperature after color stops changing.	Indicates measurement is complete.
6. Read temperature according to manufacturer's directions, for example: • Read block indicated by color change; green indicates registered temperature. If green does not appear, the temperature is midway between that indicated by tan and blue. • Last dot on temperature grid that has changed color	Obtains temperature reading. Studies indicate that fevers can easily be missed using liquid crystal forehead strips, especially in children younger than 2 years of age.
7. If temperature registers over 98.6°F (37°C), retake temperature using a different method appropriate for child's age and condition.	Verifies accuracy of measurement, although it may not be directly comparable.
8. Perform hand hygiene.	Reduces transmission of microorganisms.

CHILD AND FAMILY EVALUATION AND DOCUMENTATION

- If temperature is outside of normal range (see Appendix A), note environmental factors: ambient temperature, layers of clothing, and activity level. Note child's hydration level, level of consciousness, and response to environment.
- Remeasure temperature if reading is widely out of range or inconsistent with previous measurements.
- Document the following:
  - Temperature, route, and time obtained
  - Interventions implemented to alter temperature and child's response to these

COMMUNITY CARE

- Digital or disposable thermometers are recommended for home use because they are easier to read and safer than a mercury thermometer; advise parents to dispose of mercury-containing thermometers properly.
- Instruct child and family in proper techniques for use of equipment; give written instructions.
- Observe return demonstration.
- Instruct child and family to contact healthcare provider if
  - Temperature is outside designated parameters for age and condition; for example, greater than 105°F (40.6°C)
  - In a neonate, temperature greater than 100.4°F (38°C) or less than 97.5°F (36.5°C) may indicate sepsis and is an emergent situation

Unexpected Situation

- *Temperature is higher or lower than expected based on how child's skin feels:* Reassess temperature, ensuring that correct technique for the method is used. If it still seems inconsistent, use a different thermometer.

Bibliography

Barton, S. J., Gaffney, R., Chase, T., Rayens, M. K., & Piyabanditkul, L. (2003). Pediatric temperature measurement and child/parent/nurse preference using three temperature measurement instruments. *Journal of Pediatric Nursing, 18*, 314–320.

Chaturvedi, D., Vilhekar, K. Y., Chaturvedi, P., & Bharambe, M. S. (2004). Comparison of axillary temperature with rectal or oral temperature and determination of optimum placement time in children. *Indian Pediatrics, 41*, 600–603.

Craig, J. V., Lancaster, G. A., Williamson, P. R., & Smyth, R. L. (2000). Temperature measured at the axilla compared with rectum in children and young people: Systematic review. *British Medical Journal, 320*, 1174–1178.

Falzon, A., Grech, V., Caruana, B., Magro, A., & Attard-Montalto, S. (2003). How reliable is axillary temperature measurement? *Acta Paediatrica, 92*, 309–313.

Goldman, L. R., Shannon, M. W., and the Committee on Environmental Health. (2001). Technical report. Mercury in the environment: Implications for pediatricians (RE109907). *Pediatrics, 108*, 197–205.

Houlder, L. C. (2000). The accuracy and reliability of tympanic thermometry compared to rectal and axillary sites in young children. *Pediatric Nursing, 26*, 311–314.

Lanham, D. M., Walker, B., Klocke, E., & Jennings, M. (1999). Accuracy of tympanic temperature readings in children under 6 years of age. *Pediatric Nursing, 25*, 39–42.

Leichk-Rude, M. K., & Bloom, L. F. (1998). A comparison of temperature taking in neonates. *Neonatal Network, 17*(5), 21–37.

Martin, S. A., & Kline, A. M. (2004). Can there be a standard for temperature measurement in the pediatric intensive care unit? *AACN Clinical Issues, 15*, 254–266.

Maxton, F. J., Justin, L., & Gillies, D. (2004). Estimating core temperature in infants and children after cardiac surgery: A comparison of six methods. *Journal of Advanced Nursing, 45*, 214–222.

McKenzie, N. E. (2003). Evaluation of a new, wearable, precision phase-change thermometer in neonates. *Pediatric Nursing, 29*, 117–125.

Pontious, S., Kennedy, A. H., Shelley, S., & Mittrucker, C. (1994). Accuracy and reliability of temperature measurement by instrument and site on children. *Journal of Pediatric Nursing, 20*, 114–123.

Potter, P., Schallom, M., Davis, S., Sona, C., & McSweeney, M. (2003). Evaluation of chemical dot thermometers for measuring body temperature of orally intubated patients. *American Journal of Critical Care, 12*, 403–407.

Roy, S., Powell, K., & Gerson, L. (2003). Temporal artery temperature measurements in healthy infants, children and adolescents. *Clinical Pediatrics, 42*, 433–437.

Rush, M., & Wetherall, A. (2003). Temperature measurement: practice guidelines. *Pediatric Nursing, 15*(9), 25–28.

Silberry, G. K., Diener-West, M., Schappell, E., & Karron, R. A. (2002). Comparison of temple temperatures with rectal temperatures in children under two years of age. *Clinical Pediatrics, 41*, 405–414.

CHAPTER 135

Warming Devices, Use of

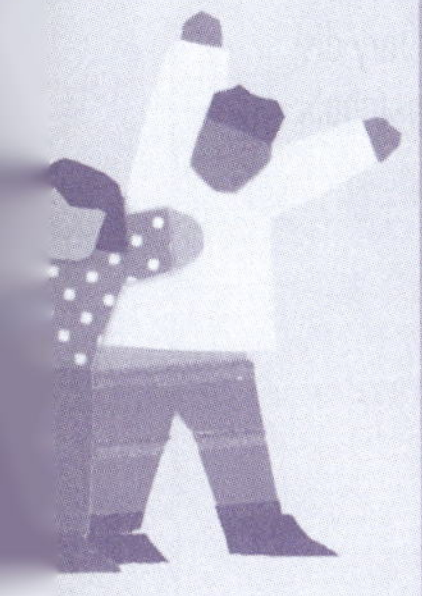

Clinical Guidelines

- Use of selected warming devices to maintain the child's temperature may be implemented by the registered nurse (RN) or licensed practical nurse (LPN). Follow institutional protocols.
- Use of hypothermia blanket may only be implemented by the RN or LPN by order of a physician or nurse practitioner.
- The child's temperature is maintained between 97.7 and 99.5°F (36.5 and 37.5°C). For more information on the environmental temperature range needed for infants, see Chapter 79.
- The preterm infant's temperature is maintained between 97.3 and 98.9°F (36.3 and 36.9°C).
- Hypothermia is considered to be a body temperature under 97.2°F (36.2°C) and may occur in premature infants and in children with intracranial birth injury, shock, or critical illness or in those under heavy sedation.
- All preterm infants are maintained under a radiant warmer or in an isolette until they are able to maintain their body temperature within normal ranges without adjunct therapy.
- Warming measures are initiated when a child's axillary temperature is less than or equal to 97.2°F (36.2°C).
- The child's temperature is closely monitored during warming measures and until it has returned to within normal parameters.
- Profoundly hypothermic children are placed on a cardiorespiratory monitor.

Equipment

- Temperature measurement device (see Chapter 134 for types of temperature measurement devices)
- Blankets
- Head covers
- Booties

For radiant warmer:

- Radiant warmer
- Servo temperature probe

For isolette:

- Double-walled isolette (use of porthole sleeves, when available, decreases the amount of ambient heat loss)
- Servo temperature probe

For chemically heated mattress:

- Chemically heated mattress
- Linen to cover mattress

For hypothermia blanket:

- Electronic warming blanket
- Hypothermia machine with thermometer probe
- Protective sheets

For heat lamp:

- Heat lamp
- Yardstick or tape measure

CHILD AND FAMILY ASSESSMENT AND PREPARATION

- Assess child's clinical history and related symptoms to determine reasons for hypothermia:
  - Injury to or disease of the hypothalamus or pituitary gland, which can produce changes in the child's ability to thermoregulate
  - Lack of clothing or covers
  - Cold environment (e.g., crib placed near a window or air-conditioning vent)
  - Diagnosis related
  - Dehydration
  - Hypoglycemia
  - Sepsis
  - Wet linen and covers
  - Pooling of secretions under the body
  - Ventilation with cold, dry oxygen
  - Starvation

Alert! *Cold-stressed children may have electrolyte and cardiac disturbances that require close observation.*

- Explain to the child and parents what you will be doing to moderate or alter the child's temperature and make the child more comfortable. Include in discussion
  - Measures used to provide warmth to the child
  - Manner in which the parents can assist with the child's care while maintaining the child's temperature
  - Explanation of all equipment to be used to assist in warming the child
  - Measures to be used to monitor the child's temperature
  - Providing skin-to-skin contact ("kangaroo care") to the infant
- Encourage parents to be present in the room and to participate in measures to warm the child.
- Use diversionary techniques with the child if needed for cooperation.

PROCEDURE Preintervention Measures

Steps	Rationale/Points of Emphasis
1. Perform hand hygiene and gather the necessary supplies to assess child's temperature.	Reduces the transmission of microorganisms. Promotes efficient time management and provides an organized approach to the procedure.
2. Determine child's temperature (see Chapter 134), compare with normal temperature, and observe the child for clinical manifestations of hypothermia.	Evaluates degree of hypothermia. Signs of hypothermia include pallor, acrocyanosis or central cyanosis, mottling of the skin, and signs of respiratory distress. Consistently cold-stressed neonates exhibit poor weight gain, metabolic acidosis, apnea, and bradycardia. **caREminder** *Avoid rectal temperatures because they can cause tissue damage and are stressful to the child.*
3. Notify physician/nurse practitioner of child's temperature and if there is evidence of dehydration, hypoglycemia, or diagnosis-related condition that would impact thermoregulation.	Alerts physician/nurse practitioner to order laboratory tests to determine causative agent. Orders for implementing warming measures can also be acquired at this time. Heat transfer between the child and the environment is altered by thickness of the body (amount of subcutaneous fat) and degree of dilation and blood flow through the skin blood vessels. Hypoglycemia and hypothermia are early signs of sepsis in neonates and infants.
4. Select intervention method to warm the child. Gather needed equipment to proceed with intervention measures. Follow manufacturer's instructions for prewarming selected equipment (e.g., radiant warmer, isolette). (See Chapter 79 for additional information on selected warming devices for the newborn.)	Prevents hypothermia, which can increase oxygen consumption and cause respiratory distress. Warming measures are selected based on child's temperature, age, diagnosis, healthcare setting (emergency department, intensive care unit, general care unit), and resources available.
5. Perform hand hygiene before initiating interventions with the child.	Reduces transmission of microorganisms when initiating contact with the child.

PROCEDURE Basic Warming Measures

Steps	Rationale/Points of Emphasis
1. Provide adequate or extra clothing and blankets to the child. Store blankets and clothing in a warm place before use.	Decreases heat loss.
2. Cover the infant's head with a head covering and feet with socks or booties. Cover the child's feet with socks or slippers.	The infant's head represents a large percentage of the body surface area. Heat can be lost rapidly when the head remains uncovered.
3. Ensure that the crib or bed is placed away from windows or ventilation systems.	Prevents loss of heat by convection and radiation.
4. Encourage parent to provide kangaroo care to the infant and, if desired, assist them with this.	Skin-to-skin contact has demonstrated effectiveness in stabilizing and often raising the temperature of infants.

PROCEDURE Radiant Warmer and Isolette

Steps	Rationale/Points of Emphasis
1. Place infant under a prewarmed radiant warmer or in a double-walled isolette with porthole covers (may require physician's order).	Radiant warmers provide heat by an infrared energy source. Isolettes circulate warm air around the infant. Prewarming decreases the heat loss from conduction from the mattress. Double walls and porthole covers help decrease heat loss from radiant and convection loss. Preterm infants require placement in these environments because they are unable to initiate thermogenesis because of their limited stores of fat and insufficient amounts of other chemicals, such as glucose, liver enzymes, and hormones.
2a. Place Servo temperature probe on the infant, ensuring that the infant is not lying on the probe/probe wires.	Servo temperature probes allow monitoring temperature without disturbing the infant and monitoring the trend of temperature. Probes provide more accurate measures of body temperature. **caREminder** *Place temperature probe over a solid meaty area, not over a hollow organ such as lung or stomach; a probe placed over the stomach fluctuates with the temperature of the feeding.*
2b. Verify probe temperatures with electronic thermometer every 2–4 hours and as needed.	Correlates temperatures to ensure accuracy because probe temperatures will also control the environmental temperatures.
2c. Change temperature probe site every 12–24 hours or whenever the infant is repositioned in a manner that results in the infant lying on the probe.	Probe electrodes can dry out and thus not adhere to the skin well. Poor skin adherence may alter probe readings. Accidental dislodgment can lead to overheating.
3. Minimize the number of entries into the isolette.	Entering the isolette changes the ambient temperature of the environment.

PROCEDURE Chemically Heated Mattress

Steps	Rationale/Points of Emphasis
1. Follow manufacturer's instructions for activating the mattress.	These mattresses are portable and can maintain heat for several hours. When the pack is activated, it will heat automatically.
2. Place the mattress on the child's bed and cover it with a sheet.	Because of the possibility of contact burns, covering the mattress with light linen (e.g., pillowcase) will allow the heat to penetrate while preventing skin injury.
3. Place child on mattress that has been covered with a sheet.	Increases transmission of heat to child.
4. Discard the mattress after use.	Chemical mattresses are not reusable.

PROCEDURE Hypothermia Blanket

Steps	Rationale/Points of Emphasis
1. Obtain equipment and place in open air; do not cover machine base with linen.	Unit needs to be ventilated.
2. Ensure that equipment is in good working condition.	Ensures child safety during use of device.
3. Follow manufacturer's instructions for setting up equipment.	Ensures child safety during use of device.
4. Place the hypothermia blanket on the child's bed, cover it with a sheet, and connect the blanket to the machine.	Readies unit for use.

Alert! *Do not use safety pins because these will damage the thermal blanket and may injure the child.*

Steps	Rationale/Points of Emphasis
5. If available, insert the rectal temperature probe at least 2 inches (5 cm) and tape to the child's buttocks.	Allows for constant and accurate monitoring of the child's temperature. This is also less stressful than repeatedly disturbing the child to obtain temperature measurements; rectal probe sizes are much smaller than a rectal thermometer, reducing the risk of tissue injury.
6. Set the machine to the desired temperature.	Allows the blanket to begin warming.
7. Assess the child's temperature every 15 to 30 minutes. Turn off the machine when the child's temperature is within 1 or 2 degrees of the desired temperature.	Prevents child from becoming hyperthermic.
8. Periodically assess the child's temperature using axillary or oral devices.	Helps to determine accuracy of rectal thermometer reading.
9. Observe for sign of skin redness or irritation.	External warming may lead to skin breakdown or burns.
10. Position the child for comfort and turn every 1 to 2 hours.	Prevents tissue damage and promotes circulation.

PROCEDURE Heat Lamp

Steps	Rationale/Points of Emphasis
1. Obtain equipment and make sure it is in good working order.	Ensures child's safety while using device.

> ***Alert!*** *Monitor the child closely during heat lamp use because of the risk for burns. Heat lamps are not recommended for home use with children because of this risk.*

Steps	Rationale/Points of Emphasis
2. Position the heat lamp using a yardstick or tape measure to ensure the lamp is 18 inches (0.5 meter) from the child's body (Figure 135-1). Follow manufacturer's instructions.	Prevents skin injury from lamp being too close and also prevents hypothermia if lamp is too far to provide adequate heat.

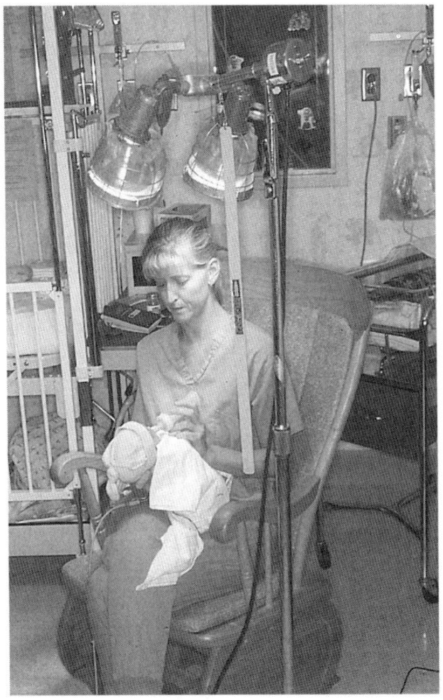

FIGURE 135-1
Position the heat lamp 18 inches from the infant's body.

Steps	Rationale/Points of Emphasis
3. Monitor child's skin for redness. Monitor for skin injury to child. Discontinue after 30 minutes.	Prevents overheating.

CHILD AND FAMILY EVALUATION AND DOCUMENTATION

- Compare child's temperature with previous readings.
- Evaluate child's response to warming measures.
- Evaluate parents' understanding of methods used to monitor and maintain infant's temperature.
- Notify healthcare prescriber if the infant's temperature does not maintain stability in response to the measures used.
- Document the following:
  - Temperature, route obtained, and device used. Include manual readings and readings from warming devices (e.g., Servo control on radiant warmer).

- Interventions implemented to maintain temperature
- Child's response to interventions
- The set point of radiant warmer temperature, incubator, isolette temperature
- Education provided to the family
- Family's participation in child's care

- Document that physician was notified of child's condition and chart specific orders given and completed at that time.

COMMUNITY CARE

- Assess family's ability to take the child's temperature and to read the device accurately.
- Educate the parents about normal temperature and signs and symptoms of decreased temperature.
- Provide teaching instructions for warming measures to include
  - Dressing child warmly with head and foot coverings
  - Bundling the child in more than one blanket as needed
  - Encouraging fluid intake
  - Keeping the temperature in the room at about 70.8°F (21.5°C)
  - Positioning child with arms drawn close to the body and the thighs drawn up toward the abdomen
- Instruct the family to contact the healthcare provider if
  - Child's extremities are cold to touch and blue in color
  - Child complains of being very cold, despite warming measures
  - Child experiences difficulty breathing
  - Child's temperature remains outside normal parameters despite appropriate environmental management (e.g., adding or removing layers of clothing, altering room temperature)

Unexpected Situations

- *Child's temperature continues to decrease despite use of warming device:* Evaluate the warming device for proper settings and functioning; correct malfunction as indicated. When using an isolette, check for sources of heat loss—the infant may require transfer to a radiant warmer to increase his or her temperature.
- *Child's skin is reddened:* Evaluate the warming device for proper functioning and proper distance from child. Adjust settings, switch to alternate warming device, or discontinue as indicated.

Bibliography

Blake, W. W., & Murray, J. A. (2006). Heat balance. In G. B. Merenstein & S. L. Gardner (Eds.), *Handbook of neonatal intensive care* (6th ed., pp. 122–138). St. Louis: Mosby.

Flenady, V. J., & Woodgate, P. G. (2005). Radiant warmers versus incubators for regulating body temperature in newborn infants. *The Cochrane Database of Systematic Reviews*, (1), No. CD000435.

Hackman, P. S. (2001). Recognizing and understanding the cold-stressed term infant. *Neonatal Network, 20*(8), 35–41.

Horns, K. M. (2002). Comparison of two microenvironments and nurse caregiving on thermal stability of ELBW infants. *Advances in Neonatal Care, 2*, 149–160.

Laroia, N., & Phelps, D. (2003). Double wall vs. single wall incubator for reducing heat loss in very low birth weight infants in incubators. *The Cochrane Database of Systematic Reviews*, (2), Art. No. CD004215.

New, K., Flenady, V., & Davies, M. W. (2004). Transfer of preterm infants from incubator to open cot at lower versus higher body weight. *The Cochrane Database of Systematic Reviews*, (2), No. CD004214.

Noerr, B. (2004). Thermoregulation. In M. T. Verklan & M. Walden (Eds.), *Core curriculum for neonatal intensive care nursing* (3rd ed., pp. 125–134). St. Louis: Elsevier Saunders.

Sinclair, J. C. (2002). Servo-control for maintaining abdominal skin temperature at 36°C in low birth weight infants. *The Cochrane Database of Systematic Reviews*, (1), No. CD001074.

C H A P T E R

136

Wound Care

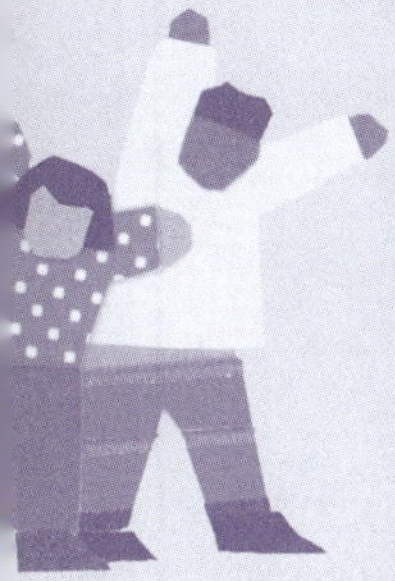

Clinical Guidelines

- A healthcare prescriber orders wound care. Optimally, specific written directions are given for the type of cleansing solution, topical antimicrobial or antiseptic agent, and dressing material.
- Wound care is performed by a registered nurse (RN), licensed practical nurse (LPN), healthcare prescriber, or family member who has been taught techniques of wound management and dressing change for the child.
- The child's skin and bony prominences are assessed at least daily for pressure sores.
- The child receives topical wound therapy that supports a healing environment and minimizes the risk for complications. This includes dressing materials, wound-cleansing solutions, wound-cleansing technique, topical medications, methods to secure the dressing, and support surfaces, such as specialty beds, mattress overlays, and seating surfaces.
- The child receives or maintains adequate systemic care to promote wound healing and to minimize the risk for complications. This includes nutrition, fluids, gas exchange, circulation, and systemic medications.
- The child receives interventions to reduce or eliminate causative factors in wound formation, such as moisture, pressure, shear, and friction, as well as interventions to minimize the deleterious effects of immobility, neuropathy, paralysis, impaired circulation, and impaired oxygenation. If the wound is a result of pressure, keep pressure off this area even if a support surface is used.
- Aseptic technique is used to perform wound care. Care and management techniques may vary based on the type of wound and the setting of the child (acute care versus home care).
- Sterile technique (sterile dressings and sterile gloves) or a modified clean technique (nonsterile gloves and sterile dressings) is used in the acute care and outpatient settings per institutional policies.
- Clean technique (nonsterile dressings and nonsterile disposable gloves or freshly washed clean hands) is used in the home, school, and other community settings.
- Any wound that appears suspicious for infection should be cultured.
- Pharmacologic and nonpharmacologic measures are used before and during wound care procedures to minimize child's discomfort during the procedure (see Chapter 7).

Equipment

- Nonsterile gloves
- Sterile gloves (if needed for sterile dressing change)
- Cotton balls
- Sterile water

- Mineral oil or petrolatum (as needed)
- Wound-cleansing solution
- Cotton-tipped applicators
- Wound-cleansing delivery method
- Topical antimicrobial or antiseptic (if ordered)
- Dressing materials (primary dressing; secondary dressing if necessary)
- Material to secure dressing
- Biohazard bag (as needed)
- Trash can

CHILD AND FAMILY ASSESSMENT AND PREPARATION

- Assess pertinent history, focusing on primary reason child has a wound (e.g., surgical incision, intravascular access site, pressure ulcer, accidental injury).
- Assess chart to determine presence of any allergies, including those to latex, alcohol, and any skin preparation products (e.g., povidone-iodine).
- Inform child and family of frequency and type of wound care.
- Assess the child's developmental level and readiness to learn.
- Assess the child's and family's ability and desire to participate in the dressing change process.
- Assess the child's pain level with each dressing change and deliver appropriate pain relief interventions before initiating wound care.
- Prepare child and family by describing the procedure and, if appropriate, demonstrating on a doll.
- Determine whether dressing change should be performed in the treatment room to ensure the child's room remains a "safe location" free from painful experiences.

PROCEDURE Providing Wound Care

Steps	Rationale/Points of Emphasis
1. Gather the necessary supplies.	Promotes efficient time management and provides an organized approach to the procedure.
2. Raise the bed and place the child in a position of comfort so that the wound site can be easily reached during wound care. Protect the child's privacy by keeping other body parts well covered.	Promotes good body mechanics.
3. Perform hand hygiene. Don nonsterile gloves.	Standard precautions to reduce transmission of microorganisms.

caREminder

There are many arguments supporting and rejecting clean versus sterile technique for dressing changes. It is important to consider the strength of the host system when deciding on the dressing change technique. Children who are immunocompromised, have multiorgan system failure, severe nutritional deficits, or impaired ventilation and circulation are better served by a sterile technique because the threats of cross-contamination or new contamination are likely to overwhelm the system. Every wound is contaminated, but not every wound is infected!

Steps	Rationale/Points of Emphasis
4a. Carefully remove old dressing. It may be necessary to use sterile water to loosen dressing. For the neonate, remove adhesives slowly and carefully using water-soaked cotton balls. Pull tape on a horizontal plane, folding tape back onto itself while continuously wetting the adhesive–skin interface. Alternatively, use mineral oil or petrolatum to loosen tape unless retaping is necessary at that site.	Applying sterile water helps loosen the dressing and therefore decreases pain of removal as well as trauma to the skin and the wound. Ensure sterile water does not run onto another wound and thus spread bacteria to that wound site.

Alert! *Adhesive removal from the skin of the premature infant has been documented to cause epidermal detachment. Measures must be used to minimize the trauma from adhesive removal (Chart 136-1).*

CHART 136-1 STRATEGIES TO REDUCE TRAUMA FROM ADHESIVE REMOVAL FOR NEONATES

- Use skin barriers such as Karaya rings and pectin products under adhesives.
- Do not use solvents to assist in adhesive removal because they present a danger of toxicity to the neonate.
- Mineral oil may be helpful in removing adhesive, but not if the site must be used again for reapplying adhesives.
- Skin bonding agents (tincture of benzoin and Mastisol) are not recommended because they may result in epidermal stripping during adhesive removal.
- Minimize use of tape when possible by using smaller pieces.
- Back adhesive tape with cotton or pieces of tape.
- Delay tape removal until at least 24 hours after application.
- Delay removal of tape and pectin barriers for more than 24 hours after application.
- Use soft gauze wraps to secure probes rather than adhesive.
- Use hydrogel adhesives for electrocardiogram electrodes.
- Remove adhesive slowly, using only warm water and cotton balls.

Steps	Rationale/Points of Emphasis
4b. Inspect dressing with attention to type and current environment. Dispose of old dressing in trash receptacle. Use a biohazard bag if needed to designate medical waste that contains significant amounts of blood or other body fluids.	The dressing tells a story of the wound's progress and amount of drainage and odor. Biohazard bags are an essential item to control the spread of diseases from human waste, discarded medical supplies, and biologic contaminates. The red bags are marked with the international symbol to alert others of the hazardous waste contained within to ensure proper handling.
4c. Change gloves.	Reduces transmission of microorganisms.
5. Cleanse wound bed with appropriate solution. Clean using moist cotton-tipped applicators or gauze pads, moving from clean area to dirty area. **caREminder** *If the wound has been noted to have suspicious drainage, the site should be cultured. Cleanse the wound surface well with sterile water or normal saline before culture is obtained.*	Normal saline, tap water, and commercially prepared wound-cleansing solutions are recommended for cleansing. Although more research is needed, clinical evidence has suggested that the use of tap water to cleanse acute wounds reduces the infection rate, whereas other trials conclude there is no difference in the infection and healing rates between wounds that were not cleansed and those cleansed with tap water and other solutions. The quality of the tap water should be considered before its use, and in the absence of potable tap water, boiled and cooled water as well as distilled water can be used as wound-cleansing agents. Use antiseptic solutions with caution, with low frequency, and at weak dilutions because they are nonselective and cytotoxic to healing tissue as well as bacteria. Piston irrigation and rinsing under a running faucet are acceptable methods of cleansing the wound surface. **Alert!** ***Isopropyl alcohol should not be used on preterm or term infants for any skin care because of the risk for toxicity. Because of the high risk for percutaneous absorption, povidone-iodine should not be used in premature infants or with term infants with an open wound or a wound under an occlusive dressing. It should be used with caution in pregnant women.***
6. Inspect the wound bed and document findings with attention to size, type of tissue in base, color, borders, exudates, odor, condition of surrounding tissue, and pain.	Measure length, width, depth, and for the presence or absence of undermining tracts. Viable granulation tissue is red, glistens, and bleeds easily due to its vascular makeup. Tough yellow tissue is nonviable slough and must be débrided. Dark-brown, black, necrotic, or leathery tissue is nonviable and must be débrided. All nonviable tissue is a foreign body that impedes wound healing. Serous and serosanguinous drainage are normal. Purulent drainage is abnormal. Wounds heal from edges to center and from base to top. New skin is first evident on wound borders.

Continued

Steps	Rationale/Points of Emphasis
7. Apply topical medication if ordered.	Topical medication requires contact with wound surface to be effective.
8. Apply primary dressing to wound surface only.	Maintain moist wound surface to promote healing but keep moist dressing off surrounding skin to prevent maceration. There is overwhelming support of maintaining a moist wound surface to promote wound healing. A moist surface permits faster and more efficient migration of tissue cells (vascular, collagen, and epithelial), enhances nutrient delivery, and facilitates waste removal (dead cells and secretions). Most wound care products support moist healing when used correctly. It is important to match wound characteristics with dressing features to obtain the desired outcome. For example, if a wound has slough or necrotic tissue, choose a dressing that facilitates débridement; similarly, if a wound is exudating heavily, choose an absorptive dressing. Dressing change frequency is determined by wound condition and dressing choice. Several methods are available to débride wounds, including sharp (surgical), mechanical (dressings), autolytic (dressings), and enzymatic (enzymes). Necrotic tissue impedes wound-healing progress, increases the risk for infection, and must be removed.
9. Apply secondary dressing if necessary.	Secondary dressings are absorptive and provide cover to the primary dressing.
10. Secure the dressing with tape, a semipermeable dressing, or Montgomery straps. A soft gauze bandage can be used for extremities. For neonates, minimize contact between adhesive tape and skin by "backing" tape or applying cotton to adhesive.	Choose a method for securing the dressing that maintains integrity of the dressing, minimizes trauma to surrounding tissue, and is compatible with the dressing change frequency. Avoid adhesive methods when the dressing change frequency is greater than once a day. **KidKare** Montgomery straps can be made for younger children by using a small piece of pectin wafer, cloth tape, and tracheostomy ties.
11. Dispose of waste in appropriate receptacle. Return reusable supplies to secure location.	Reusable supplies, such as cleansing solutions, should be placed in a location out of the child's reach to prevent potential injury.
12. Remove gloves and perform hand hygiene.	Reduces transmission of organisms.

CHILD AND FAMILY EVALUATION AND DOCUMENTATION

- Evaluate child's and family's understanding of the wound care and their ability to complete such care independently (if needed).
- Evaluate need for referral to wound or ostomy care specialist (if not previously consulted)
- Document the following:
  - General appearance of child's skin and bony prominences
  - Location and appearance of wound site
  - Presence of drains or tubes
  - Drainage present on old dressing
  - Date, time, and type of dressing applied
  - Child's tolerance of dressing change, including use of pain medications and their effectiveness
  - Involvement of child and family members in the procedure
  - Teaching implemented and response of the family members

COMMUNITY CARE

- Arrange home care visits for complex wounds or draining fistulas.
- Make appointment for follow-up visit with the healthcare prescriber or wound care nurse. Follow-up visit should include
  - Visualizing and documenting the status and progress of the wound and healing
  - Addressing any concerns the family may have about school and activity restrictions
  - Monitoring compliance with dressing change procedures

- Ensure that family has the following before discharge:
  - Written instructions on how to complete wound care and administer any medications
  - Supplies to complete wound care
  - Community locations to acquire more supplies if needed
- Teach family the following:
  - Hand hygiene techniques
  - Correct disposal of contaminated dressings
  - Signs of skin breakdown
  - Signs of infection
  - Methods to manage pain during dressing change
- Instruct the family to contact the healthcare provider if
  - Child has redness, warmth, pain, or other signs of infection at the wound site
  - Child develops a fever
  - Child demonstrates a change in behavior (e.g., more agitated)

Unexpected Situation

- *As you perform the dressing change, you note that the incision edges are not approximated at the distal end and the surrounding tissue is red and swollen. The suture line has separated. Purulent drainage is on the old dressing:* Documentation about a child's abdominal incision from the previous day states that the wound was clean and dry and the wound edges were approximated. The sutures were intact. There was no inflammation, edema, or erythema of the surrounding tissue. Determine whether the child has other signs and symptoms such as pain, malaise, fever, and paresthesias. Cleanse the wound site with sterile water. Obtain a culture of the drainage. Redress the wound with a dry sterile dressing. Notify the healthcare prescriber of your findings.

Bibliography

Beitz, J. (2005). Wound debridement: Therapeutic options and care considerations. *Nursing Clinics of North America, 40*(2), 233–249.

Fernandez, R., Griffiths, R., & Ussia, C. (2002). Water for wound cleansing. *The Cochrane Database of Systematic Reviews*, (4), No. CD003861.

Garcia-Gonzalez, E., & Rivera-Rueda, M. (1998). Neonatal dermatology: Skin care guidelines. *Dermatology Nursing, 10*(4), 274–279.

Howard, R. (2001). The appropriate use of topical antimicrobials and antiseptics in children. *Pediatric Annals, 30*(4), 219–224.

Lund, C., Kuller, J., Lane, A., Lott, J., & Raines, D. (1999). Neonatal skin care: The scientific basis for practice. *Journal of Obstetric, Gynecologic, and Neonatal Nursing, 28*(3), 241–254.

Lund, C. H., Kuller, J., Lane, A., et al. (2001). Neonatal skin care: Evaluation of the AWHONN/NANN research-based practice project on knowledge and skin care practices (clinical studies). *Journal of Obstetric, Gynecologic, and Neonatal Nursing, 30*(1), 30–40.

Lund, C. H., Osborne, J. W., Kuller, J., et al. (2001). Neonatal skin care: Clinical outcomes of the AWHONN/NANN evidence-based clinical practice guideline (clinical studies). *Journal of Obstetric, Gynecologic, and Neonatal Nursing, 30*(3), 41–51.

Suddaby, E., Barnett, S., & Facteau, L. (2005). Skin breakdown in acute care pediatrics. *Paediatric Nursing, 31*(2), 132–138, 148.

Taquino, L. (2000). Promoting wound healing in the neonatal setting: Process versus protocol. *The Journal of Perinatal & Neonatal Nursing, 14*(1), 104–118.

Valencia, I., Falabella, A., & Schachner, L. (2001). New developments in wound care for infants and children. *Pediatric Annals, 30*(4), 211–218.

Walker, L., Downe, S., & Gomez, L. (2005). Skin care in the well term newborn: Two systemic reviews. *Birth, 32*(3), 224–228.

Wound, Ostomy, and Continence Nurses Society (WOCN). (2003). *Guidelines for prevention and management of pressure ulcers.* Glenview. IL: WOCN.

APPENDIX

A

Ranges for Vital Sign Measurements

TABLE 1

Normal Heart Rate and Respiratory Rate Ranges

Age	Heart Rate Normal Range (beats per minute)	Respiratory Rate Normal Range (breaths per minute)
Neonate	70–190	30–50
1–11 months	80–160	30–45
1–2 years	80–130	20–30
3–4 years	80–120	20–30
5–7 years	75–115	20–25
8–11 years	70–110	14–22
12–15 years	Female 70–110 Male 70–100	12–20
>15 years	Female 60–100 Male 55–95	12–20

TABLE 2

Normal Temperature Ranges*

Age	Fahrenheit (degrees)	Celsius (degrees)
Preterm infant	97.7–98.6	36.5–37
Term infant	97.2–99.9	36.2–37.7
0–6 months	97.2–99.4	36.2–37.4
6–12 months	96–99.7	35.6–37.6
1–13 years	95.9–99	35.5–37.2
>13 years	96.4–99.6	35.8–37.6

*Measurement method and circadian rhythm must be considered in evaluating normal temperatures.

TABLE 3

Blood Pressure*

BP Levels for Boys by Age and Height Percentile

		SBP, mm Hg							DBP, mm Hg						
		Percentile of Height							Percentile of Height						
Age, y	BP Percentile	5th	10th	25th	50th	75th	90th	95th	5th	10th	25th	50th	75th	90th	95th
1	50th	80	81	83	85	87	88	89	34	35	36	37	38	39	39
	90th	94	95	97	99	100	102	103	49	50	51	52	53	53	54
	95th	98	99	101	103	104	106	106	54	54	55	56	57	58	58
	99th	105	106	108	110	112	113	114	61	62	63	64	65	66	66
2	50th	84	85	87	88	90	92	92	39	40	41	42	43	44	44
	90th	97	99	100	102	104	105	106	54	55	56	57	58	58	59
	95th	101	102	104	106	108	109	110	59	59	60	61	62	63	63
	99th	109	110	111	113	115	117	117	66	67	68	69	70	71	71
3	50th	86	87	89	91	93	94	95	44	44	45	46	47	48	48
	90th	100	101	103	105	107	108	109	59	59	60	61	62	63	63
	95th	104	105	107	109	110	112	113	63	63	64	65	66	67	67
	99th	111	112	114	116	118	119	120	71	71	72	73	74	75	75
4	50th	88	89	91	93	95	96	97	47	48	49	50	51	51	52
	90th	102	103	105	107	109	110	111	62	63	64	65	66	66	67
	95th	106	107	109	111	112	114	115	66	67	68	69	70	71	71
	99th	113	114	116	118	120	121	122	74	75	76	77	78	78	79
5	50th	90	91	93	95	96	98	98	50	51	52	53	54	55	55
	90th	104	105	106	108	110	111	112	65	66	67	68	69	69	70
	95th	108	109	110	112	114	115	116	69	70	71	72	73	74	74
	99th	115	116	118	120	121	123	123	77	78	79	80	81	81	82
6	50th	91	92	94	96	98	99	100	53	53	54	55	56	57	57
	90th	105	106	108	110	111	113	113	68	68	69	70	71	72	72
	95th	109	110	112	114	115	117	117	72	72	73	74	75	76	76
	99th	116	117	119	121	123	124	125	80	80	81	82	83	84	84
7	50th	92	94	95	97	99	100	101	55	55	56	57	58	59	59
	90th	106	107	109	111	113	114	115	70	70	71	72	73	74	74
	95th	110	111	113	115	117	118	119	74	74	75	76	77	78	78
	99th	117	118	120	122	124	125	126	82	82	83	84	85	86	86
8	50th	94	95	97	99	100	102	102	56	57	58	59	60	60	61
	90th	107	109	110	112	114	115	116	71	72	72	73	74	75	76
	95th	111	112	114	116	118	119	120	75	76	77	78	79	79	80
	99th	119	120	122	123	125	127	127	83	84	85	86	87	87	88
9	50th	95	96	98	100	102	103	104	57	58	59	60	61	61	62
	90th	109	110	112	114	115	117	118	72	73	74	75	76	76	77
	95th	113	114	116	118	119	121	121	76	77	78	79	80	81	81
	99th	120	121	123	125	127	128	129	84	85	86	87	88	88	89
10	50th	97	98	100	102	103	105	106	58	59	60	61	61	62	63
	90th	111	112	114	115	117	119	119	73	73	74	75	76	77	78
	95th	115	116	117	119	121	122	123	77	78	79	80	81	81	82
	99th	122	123	125	127	128	130	130	85	86	86	88	88	89	90
11	50th	99	100	102	104	105	107	107	59	59	60	61	62	63	63
	90th	113	114	115	117	119	120	121	74	74	75	76	77	78	78
	95th	117	118	119	121	123	124	125	78	78	79	80	81	82	82
	99th	124	125	127	129	130	132	132	86	86	87	88	89	90	90
12	50th	101	102	104	106	108	109	110	59	60	61	62	63	63	64
	90th	115	116	118	120	121	123	123	74	75	75	76	77	78	79
	95th	119	120	122	123	125	127	127	78	79	80	81	82	82	83
	99th	126	127	129	131	133	134	135	86	87	88	89	90	90	91
13	50th	104	105	106	108	110	111	112	60	60	61	62	63	64	64
	90th	117	118	120	122	124	125	126	75	75	76	77	78	79	79
	95th	121	122	124	126	128	129	130	79	79	80	81	82	83	83
	99th	128	130	131	133	135	136	137	87	87	88	89	90	91	91
14	50th	106	107	109	111	113	114	115	60	61	62	63	64	65	65
	90th	120	121	123	125	126	128	128	75	76	77	78	79	79	80
	95th	124	125	127	128	130	132	132	80	80	81	82	83	84	84
	99th	131	132	134	136	138	139	140	87	88	89	90	91	92	92
15	50th	109	110	112	113	115	117	117	61	62	63	64	65	66	66
	90th	122	124	125	127	129	130	131	76	77	78	79	80	80	81
	95th	126	127	129	131	133	134	135	81	81	82	83	84	85	85
	99th	134	135	136	138	140	142	142	88	89	90	91	92	93	93
16	50th	111	112	114	116	118	119	120	63	63	64	65	66	67	67
	90th	125	126	128	130	131	133	134	78	78	79	80	81	82	82
	95th	129	130	132	134	135	137	137	82	83	83	84	85	86	87
	99th	136	137	139	141	143	144	145	90	90	91	92	93	94	94
17	50th	114	115	116	118	120	121	122	65	66	66	67	68	69	70
	90th	127	128	130	132	134	135	136	80	80	81	82	83	84	84
	95th	131	132	134	136	138	139	140	84	85	86	87	87	88	89
	99th	139	140	141	143	145	146	147	92	93	93	94	95	96	97

The 90th percentile is 1.28 SD, the 95th percentile is 1.645 SD, and the 99th percentile is 2.326 SD over the mean.

BP Levels for Girls by Age and Height Percentile

		SBP, mm Hg							DBP, mm Hg						
		Percentile of Height							Percentile of Height						
Age, y	BP Percentile	5th	10th	25th	50th	75th	90th	95th	5th	10th	25th	50th	75th	90th	95th
1	50th	83	84	85	86	88	89	90	38	39	39	40	41	41	42
	90th	97	97	98	100	101	102	103	52	53	53	54	55	55	56
	95th	100	101	102	104	105	106	107	56	57	57	58	59	59	60
	99th	108	108	109	111	112	113	114	64	64	65	65	66	67	67
2	50th	85	85	87	88	89	91	91	43	44	44	45	46	46	47
	90th	98	99	100	101	103	104	105	57	58	58	59	60	61	61
	95th	102	103	104	105	107	108	109	61	62	62	63	64	65	65
	99th	109	110	111	112	114	115	116	69	69	70	70	71	72	72
3	50th	86	87	88	89	91	92	93	47	48	48	49	50	50	51
	90th	100	100	102	103	104	106	106	61	62	62	63	64	64	65
	95th	104	104	105	107	108	109	110	65	66	66	67	68	68	69
	99th	111	111	113	114	115	116	117	73	73	74	74	75	76	76
4	50th	88	88	90	91	92	94	94	50	50	51	52	52	53	54
	90th	101	102	103	104	106	107	108	64	64	65	66	67	67	68
	95th	105	106	107	108	110	111	112	68	68	69	70	71	71	72
	99th	112	113	114	115	117	118	119	76	76	76	77	78	79	79
5	50th	89	90	91	93	94	95	96	52	53	53	54	55	55	56
	90th	103	103	105	106	107	109	109	66	67	67	68	69	69	70
	95th	107	107	108	110	111	112	113	70	71	71	72	73	73	74
	99th	114	114	116	117	118	120	120	78	78	79	79	80	81	81
6	50th	91	92	93	94	96	97	98	54	54	55	56	56	57	58
	90th	104	105	106	108	109	110	111	68	68	69	70	70	71	72
	95th	108	109	110	111	113	114	115	72	72	73	74	74	75	76
	99th	115	116	117	119	120	121	122	80	80	80	81	82	83	83
7	50th	93	93	95	96	97	99	99	55	56	56	57	58	58	59
	90th	106	107	108	109	111	112	113	69	70	70	71	72	72	73
	95th	110	111	112	113	115	116	116	73	74	74	75	76	76	77
	99th	117	118	119	120	122	123	124	81	81	82	82	83	84	84
8	50th	95	95	96	98	99	100	101	57	57	57	58	59	60	60
	90th	108	109	110	111	113	114	114	71	71	71	72	73	74	74
	95th	112	112	114	115	116	118	118	75	75	75	76	77	78	78
	99th	119	120	121	122	123	125	125	82	82	83	83	84	85	86
9	50th	96	97	98	100	101	102	103	58	58	58	59	60	61	61
	90th	110	110	112	113	114	116	116	72	72	72	73	74	75	75
	95th	114	114	115	117	118	119	120	76	76	76	77	78	79	79
	99th	121	121	123	124	125	127	127	83	83	84	84	85	86	87
10	50th	98	99	100	102	103	104	105	59	59	59	60	61	62	62
	90th	112	112	114	115	116	118	118	73	73	73	74	75	76	76
	95th	116	116	117	119	120	121	122	77	77	77	78	79	80	80
	99th	123	123	125	126	127	129	129	84	84	85	86	86	87	88
11	50th	100	101	102	103	105	106	107	60	60	60	61	62	63	63
	90th	114	114	116	117	118	119	120	74	74	74	75	76	77	77
	95th	118	118	119	121	122	123	124	78	78	78	79	80	81	81
	99th	125	125	126	128	129	130	131	85	85	86	87	87	88	89
12	50th	102	103	104	105	107	108	109	61	61	61	62	63	64	64
	90th	116	116	117	119	120	121	122	75	75	75	76	77	78	78
	95th	119	120	121	123	124	125	126	79	79	79	80	81	82	82
	99th	127	127	128	130	131	132	133	86	86	87	88	88	89	90
13	50th	104	105	106	107	109	110	110	62	62	62	63	64	65	65
	90th	117	118	119	121	122	123	124	76	76	76	77	78	79	79
	95th	121	122	123	124	126	127	128	80	80	80	81	82	83	83
	99th	128	129	130	132	133	134	135	87	87	88	89	89	90	91
14	50th	106	106	107	109	110	111	112	63	63	63	64	65	66	66
	90th	119	120	121	122	124	125	125	77	77	77	78	79	80	80
	95th	123	123	125	126	127	129	129	81	81	81	82	83	84	84
	99th	130	131	132	133	135	136	136	88	88	89	90	90	91	92
15	50th	107	108	109	110	111	113	113	64	64	64	65	66	67	67
	90th	120	121	122	123	125	126	127	78	78	78	79	80	81	81
	95th	124	125	126	127	129	130	131	82	82	82	83	84	85	85
	99th	131	132	133	134	136	137	138	89	89	90	91	91	92	93
16	50th	108	108	110	111	112	114	114	64	64	65	66	66	67	68
	90th	121	122	123	124	126	127	128	78	78	79	80	81	81	82
	95th	125	126	127	128	130	131	132	82	82	83	84	85	85	86
	99th	132	133	134	135	137	138	139	90	90	90	91	92	93	93
17	50th	108	109	110	111	113	114	115	64	65	65	66	67	67	68
	90th	122	122	123	125	126	127	128	78	79	79	80	81	81	82
	95th	125	126	127	129	130	131	132	82	83	83	84	85	85	86
	99th	133	133	134	136	137	138	139	90	90	91	91	92	93	93

The 90th percentile is 1.28 SD, the 95th percentile is 1.645 SD, and the 99th percentile is 2.326 SD over the mean.

*Determine the child's height percentile on the CDC growth charts; then, compare the child's systolic and diastolic blood pressures with the numbers provided in the table (boys or girls) according to the child's age and height percentile.

Reproduced with permission from American Academy of Pediatrics. (2004). The fourth report on the diagnosis, evaluation, and treatment of high blood pressure in children and adolescents. *Pediatrics, 114*, 555–576. Copyright© 2004, AAP.

APPENDIX B

Internet References

Measurement Conversion
http://www.onlineconversion.com

Pediatric Developmental Milestones and Health Promotion
Bright Futures Guidelines for Health Supervision
Bright Futures in Practice Series:
Mental Health
Nutrition
Oral Health
Physical Activity
http://www.brightfutures.org/

Pediatric Growth Charts
Centers for Disease Control Growth Charts: United States
http://www.cdc.gov/growthcharts/

Pediatric Immunization Schedule
Centers for Disease Control: Vaccines and Immunizations
http://www.cdc.gov

Preventing Accidental Injury
Safe Kids USA
http://www.usa.safekids.org/

N

Q

R

Z